a LANGE medical book

CURRENT
Diagnosis & Treatment
Psychiatry

FOURTH EDITION

T0293627

Edited by

Michael H. Ebert, MD
Emeritus Professor of Psychiatry
Yale University School of Medicine
New Haven, Connecticut

Peter R. Martin, MD
Professor of Psychiatry and Behavioral Sciences
Professor of Pharmacology
Vanderbilt University School of Medicine
Nashville, Tennessee

Molly McVoy, MD
Associate Professor of Child and Adolescent Psychiatry
Case Western Reserve University School of Medicine
Cleveland, Ohio

Robert J. Ronis, MD, MPH
Professor and Chair Emeritus of Psychiatry
Case Western Reserve University School of Medicine
Cleveland, Ohio

Sidney H. Weissman, MD
Clinical Professor of Psychiatry and Behavioral Sciences
Northwestern University Feinberg School of Medicine
Chicago, Illinois

McGraw Hill

1 2 3 4 5 LBC 28 27 26 25 24

ISBN 978-1-265-41109-1
MHID 1-265-41109-3
ISSN 1528-1124

Notice

Medicine is an ever-changing science. As new research and clinical experience broaden our knowledge, changes in treatment and drug therapy are required. The authors and the publisher of this work have checked with sources believed to be reliable in their efforts to provide information that is complete and generally in accord with the standards accepted at the time of publication. However, in view of the possibility of human error or changes in medical sciences, neither the authors nor the publisher nor any other party who has been involved in the preparation or publication of this work warrants that the information contained herein is in every respect accurate or complete, and they disclaim all responsibility for any errors or omissions or for the results obtained from use of the information contained in this work. Readers are encouraged to confirm the information contained herein with other sources. For example and in particular, readers are advised to check the product information sheet included in the package of each drug they plan to administer to be certain that the information contained in this work is accurate and that changes have not been made in the recommended dose or in the contraindications for administration. This recommendation is of particular importance in connection with new or infrequently used drugs.

This book was set in Minion Pro by KnowledgeWorks Global Ltd.
The editors were Timothy Y. Hiscock, Sydney Keen, and Peter J. Boyle.
The production supervisor was Richard Ruzycka.
Project management was provided by Tasneem Kauser, KnowledgeWorks Global Ltd.

This book is printed on acid-free paper.

McGraw Hill books are available at special quantity discounts to use as premiums and sales promotions or for use in corporate training programs. To contact a representative, please visit the Contact Us pages at www.mhprofessional.com.

Dedicated to the memory of Barry Nurcombe, MD,
one of the founding editors of this textbook
and an esteemed leader in academic psychiatry
in Australia and the United States

Contents

Contributors

Sarah B. Abdallah, MD
Post-doctoral Fellow in Psychiatry
Yale University School of Medicine
New Haven, Connecticut
Chapter 30

Peter H. Addy, PhD
Associate Research Scientist
Yale University School of Medicine
New Haven, Connecticut
Chapter 22

Akhil Anand, MD
Assistant Clinical Professor of Psychiatry
Cleveland Clinic Lerner College of Medicine
Case Western Reserve University
Cleveland, Ohio
Chapter 27

Alan Apter, MD
Professor of Psychiatry
Baruch Ivcher School of Psychology
Herzliya, Israel
Chapter 49

Christopher W. Austelle, MD
Postdoctoral Research Fellow in Psychiatry and
    Behavioral Sciences
Stanford University School of Medicine
Palo Alto, California
Chapter 10

Kara S. Bagot, MD
Assistant Professor of Psychiatry
Icahn School of Medicine at Mount Sinai Medical
New York, New York
Chapter 46

Richard Balon, MD
Professor of Psychiatry and Behavioral Neurosciences
Professor of Anesthesiology
Wayne State University School of Medicine
Detroit, Michigan
Chapter 34

Anahita Bassir Nia, MD
Assistant Professor of Psychiatry
Yale University School of Medicine
New Haven, Connecticut
Chapter 22

Pablo Vidal-Ribas Belil, MSc
Investigator
Institut de Recerca Sant Joan de Déu
Barcelona, Spain
Chapter 57

William Bernet, MD
Emeritus Professor of Psychiatry and Behavioral Sciences
Vanderbilt University School of Medicine
Nashville, Tennessee
Chapters 51 & 60

Wade Berrettini, MD, PhD
Professor of Psychiatry
Perelman School of Medine, University of Pennsylvania
Philadelphia, Pennsylvania
Chapter 3

Boris Birmaher, MD
Distinguished Professor of Psychiatry
Western Psychiatric Institute and Clinic
Pittsburgh, Pennsylvania
Chapter 48

Daniel G. Blazer, MD, PhD
JP Gibbons Distinguished Professor Emeritus of Psychiatry
    and Behavioral Sciences
Duke University School of Medicine
Durham, North Carolina
Chapter 2

Michael H. Bloch, MD, MS
Associate Professor of Psychiatry
Yale University School of Medicine
New Haven, Connecticut
Chapter 53

William V. Bobo, MD
Professor and Chair of Psychiatry and Psychology
Mayo Clinic
Jacksonville, Florida
Chapter 24

Douglas L. Boggs, PharmD, MS
Associate Research Scientist in Psychiatry
Yale University School of Medicine
New Haven, Connecticut
Chapter 21

David A. Brent, MD
Professor of Psychiatry, Pediatrics, and Epidemiology
University of Pittsburgh School of Medicine
Pittsburgh, Pennsylvania
Chapter 47

Simona Bujoreanu, PhD
Assistant Professor of Psychology
Harvard Medical School
Boston, Massachusetts
Chapter 56

Muhammet Celik, MD
Resident in Psychiatry
New York Medical College at Saint Joseph's Medical Center
Yonkers, New York
Chapter 33

Catherine Chiles, MD
Associate Clinical Professor of Psychiatry
Yale University School of Medicine
New Haven, Connecticut
Chapter 59

Camellia P. Clark, MD
Private practice, former Associate Professor of Psychiatry
University of California San Diego
La Jolla, California
Chapter 36

Judith Cooney, PhD
Associate Professor of Psychiatry
University of Connecticut School of Medicine
Farmington, Connecticut
Chapter 20

David R. DeMaso, MD
George P. Gardner & Olga E. Monks Professor of
   Child Psychiatry & Professor of Pediatrics
Harvard Medical School, Boston, Massachusetts
Chapter 56

Rasim Diler, MD
Professor of Psychiatry
Western Psychiatric Institute and Clinic of the
   University of Pittsburgh Medical Center
Pittsburgh, Pennsylvania
Chapter 48

Kenneth A. Dodge, PhD
William McDougall Distinguished Professor at
   Sanford School of Public Policy
Duke University
Durham, North Carolina
Chapter 4

Deepak Cyril D'Souza, MD
Albert E. Kent Professor of Psychiatry
Yale University School of Medicine
New Haven, Connecticut
Chapters 21, 22, & 24

Daniel H. Ebert, MD, PhD
Assistant Professor of Psychiatry and Behavioral Science
The Johns Hopkins University School of Medicine
Baltimore, Maryland
Chapter 58

Michael H. Ebert, MD
Emeritus Professor of Psychiatry
Yale University School of Medicine
New Haven, Connecticut
Chapters 5 & 35

Ellen L. Edens, MD, MPE
Associate Professor of Psychiatry
Yale University School of Medicine
New Haven, Connecticut
Chapter 18

James W. B. Elsey, BSc
Senior Behavioral Scientist
Rethink Priorities
San Francisco, California
Chapter 23

S. Hossein Fatemi, MD, PhD
Bernstein Professor Emeritus of Psychiatry and
   Behavioral Sciences
University of Minnesota Medical School
Minneapolis, Minnesota
Chapter 24

Thomas V. Fernandez, MD
Associate Professor of Psychiatry
Yale University School of Medicine
New Haven, Connecticut
Chapter 30

Charles V. Ford, MD
Professor of Psychiatry and Neurobiology
Heersink School of Medicine
University of Alabama at Birmingham
Birmingham, Alabama
Chapters 31 & 32

Sandra L. Friedman, MD, MPH
Professor, Pediatrics-Developmental Pediatrics
University of Colorado School of Medicine
Aurora, Colorado
Chapter 40

Brian Fuehrlein, MD, PhD
Associate Professor of Psychiatry
Yale University School of Medicine
New Haven, Connecticut
Chapter 33

Suhas Ganesh, MD
Assistant Professor
National Institute of Mental Health and Neurosciences
Bengaluru, India
Chapter 24

Keming Gao, MD, PhD
Joseph R. Calabrese Professor of Psychiatry
Case Western Reserve University School of Medicine
Cleveland, Ohio
Chapter 26

Mark S. George, MD
Distinguished University Professor of Psychiatry,
   Radiology and Neuroscience
Medical University of South Carolina
Charleston, South Carolina
Chapter 10

J. Christian Gillin, MD†
Formerly Professor of Psychiatry
University of California, San Diego School of Medicine
San Diego, California
Chapter 36

Matthew N. Goldenberg, MD, MSc
Associate Professor of Psychiatry
Yale University School of Medicine
New Haven, Connecticut
Chapter 58

Benjamin I. Goldstein, MD, PhD, FRCPC
Professor of Psychiatry, Pharmacology, and
   Psychological Clinical Science
University of Toronto
Toronto, Ontario, Canada
Chapter 48

Christoffer Grant, PhD
Assistant Professor of Psychiatry
University of Connecticut School of Medicine
Farmington, Connecticut
Chapter 20

Stephan H. Heckers, MD,
William P and Henry B Test Professor of Psychiatry and
   Behavioral Sciences
Vanderbilt University School of Medicine
Nashville, Tennessee
Chapter 24

Edmund S. Higgins, MD
Affiliate Associate Professor of Psychiatry and Family
   Medicine
Medical University of South Carolina
Charleston, South Carolina
Chapter 10

Lauren Hoffman, PharmD
Assistant Professor of Psychiatry
Case Western Reserve University School of Medicine
Cleveland, Ohio
Chapter 8

Steven D. Hollon, PhD
Gertrude Conaway Vanderbilt Professor of Psychology
Vanderbilt University
Nashville, Tennessee
Chapter 9

Jolomi Ikomi, MD
Medical Director, Project Recovery ChristianaCare
ChristianaCare Behavioral Health Services
Wilmington, Delaware
Chapter 17

Mihaela Cristina Ivan, MD
Clinical Assistant Professor of Psychiatry
Menninger Department of Psychiatry & Behavioral Sciences
Baylor College of Medicine
Houston, Texas
Chapter 7

†Deceased.

Douglas C. Johnson, PhD
Staff Neuropsychologist, Neurology Service
John J. Pershing VA Medical Center
Poplar Bluff, Missouri
Chapter 28

Yifrah Kaminer, MD, MBA
Professor of Psychiatry
University of Connecticut School of Medicine
Farmington, Connecticut
Chapter 46

Kristopher A. Kast, MD
Assistant Professor of Psychiatry and Behavioral Sciences
Vanderbilt University School of Medicine
Nashville, Tennessee
Chapters 17 & 20

Robert A. King, MD
Professor of Child Psychiatry
Yale University School of Medicine
New Haven, Connecticut
Chapters 49 & 50

Howard S. Kirshner, MD
Professor Emeritus of Neurology
Vanderbilt University School of Medicine
Nashville, Tennessee
Chapter 15

John H. Krystal, MD
Professor Psychiatry
Yale University School of Medicine
New Haven, Connecticut
Chapter 28

Mary M. LaLonde, MD, PhD
Assistant Clinical Professor of Psychiatry
Mount Sinai School of Medicine
New York, New York
Chapter 45

Eli R. Lebowitz, PhD
Associate Professor
Yale University School of Medicine
New Haven, Connecticut
Chapter 50

James F. Leckman, MD, PhD
Neison Harris Professor of Child Psychiatry, Pediatrics, and Psychology
Yale University School of Medicine
New Haven, Connecticut
Chapter 53

Robert F. Leeman, PhD
Professor of Health Sciences
Bouvé College of Health Sciences
Northeastern University
Boston, Massachusetts
Chapter 19

Elizabeth L. Leonard, PhD
Assistant Professor of Psychiatry
Creighton University School of Medicine
Omaha, Nebraska
Chapter 40

James W. Lomax, MD
Distinguished Emeritus Professor of Psychiatry
Menninger Department of Psychiatry & Behavioral Sciences
Baylor College of Medicine
Houston, Texas
Chapter 7

Peter T. Loosen, MD, PhD
Professor Emeritus of Psychiatry and Behavioral Sciences
Vanderbilt University School of Medicine
Nashville, Tennessee
Chapter 26

Fadi Maalouf, MD
Professor of Psychiatry
American University of Beirut
Beirut, Lebanon
Chapter 47

Andrés Martin, MD, MPH
Riva Ariella Ritvo Professor in the Child Study Center and Professor of Psychiatry
Yale University School of Medicine
New Haven, Connecticut
Chapter 13

Ashley M. Schnakenberg Martin, PhD
Assistant Professor of Psychiatry
Yale University School of Medicine
New Haven, Connecticut
Chapter 21

Peter R. Martin, MD
Professor of Psychiatry and Behavioral Sciences
Professor of Pharmacology
Vanderbilt University School of Medicine
Nashville, Tennessee
Chapter 16

Brett McDermott, MD, FRANZCP
Associate Professor of Child and Adolescent Psychiatry
The University of Queensland
South Brisbane
Queensland, Australia
Chapter 52

Molly McVoy, MD
Associate Professor of Psychiatry
Case Western Reserve University School of Medicine
Cleveland, Ohio
Chapters 11, 43, & 57

Herbert Y. Meltzer, MD
Professor of Psychiatry and Behavioral Sciences,
    Pharmacology and Neuroscience
Feinberg School of Medicine
Northwestern University Feinberg School of Medicine
Chicago, Illinois
Chapter 24

Andrew E. Molnar, Jr., PhD
Assistant Professor of Psychiatry and Behavioral Sciences
Vanderbilt University School of Medicine
Nashville, Tennessee
Chapter 6

Stephen Montgomery, MD
Assistant Professor of Psychiatry and Behavioral Sciences
Vanderbilt University School of Medicine
Nashville, Tennessee
Chapter 60

Polly J. Moore, PhD
Director of Sleep Research
California Clinical Trials
Chapter 36

Kerim M. Munir, MD, MPH, DSc, MD
Associate Professor of Psychiatry and Pediatrics
Harvard Medical School
Boston, Massachusetts
Chapter 40

Myo Thwin Myint, MD
Associate Professor of Psychiatry
Tulane University School of Medicine
New Orleans, Louisiana
Chapter 54

Jeffrey H. Newcorn, MD
Professor of Psychiatry and Pediatrics
Icahn School of Medicine at Mount Sinai
New York, New York
Chapter 45

Barry Nurcombe, MD[†]
Formerly Emeritus Professor of Psychiatry
The University of Queensland, Australia, and Vanderbilt
    University School of Medicine
Nashville, Tennessee
Chapters 5, 11, 12, 13, 42, & 54

John I. Nurnberger, Jr., MD, PhD
Distinguished Professor Emeritus of Psychiatry and
    Medical and Molecular Genetics
Indiana University School of Medicine
Indianapolis, Indiana
Chapter 3

Stephanie S. O'Malley, PhD
Elizabeth Mears and House Jameson Professor of Psychiatry
Yale University School of Medicine
New Haven, Connecticut
Chapter 17

Ismene L. Petrakis, MD
Professor of Psychiatry
Yale University School of Medicine
New Haven, Connecticut
Chapter 18

William M. Petrie, MD
Professor Emeritus of Psychiatry and Behavioral Sciences
Vanderbilt University School of Medicine
Nashville, Tennessee
Chapter 15

Marc N. Potenza, PhD, MD
Steven M. Southwick Professor of Psychiatry
Yale University School of Medicine
New Haven, Connecticut
Chapter 23

Rajiv Radhakrishnan, MD
Assistant Professor of Psychiatry, Radiology, and
    Biomedical Engineering
Yale University School of Medicine
New Haven, Connecticut
Chapter 24

Sean D. Regnier, PhD
Postdoctoral Fellow in Psychiatry
Yale University School of Medicine
New Haven, Connecticut
Chapter 19

Howard B. Roback, PhD
Emeritus Professor of Psychiatry and Psychology
Vanderbilt University School of Medicine
Nashville, Tennessee
Chapter 6

Robert J. Ronis, MD, MPH
Professor Emeritus of Psychiatry
Case Western Reserve University School of Medicine
Cleveland, Ohio
Chapter 2

Rebecca E. Salomon, PhD
Assistant Professor of Nursing
School of Nursing, University of North Carolina
Chapel Hill, North Carolina
Chapter 38

Ronald M. Salomon, MD
Private practice of Psychiatry, recently Professor of
    Psychiatry
University of Arkansas for Medical Sciences
Little Rock, Arkansas
Chapter 38

George E. Sayde, MD, MPH
Postdoctoral Clinical & Research Fellow in Psychiatry
Columbia University Irving Medical Center
New York, New York
Chapter 37

Elizabeth K.C. Schwartz, MD, PhD
Resident in Psychiatry
Yale University School of Medicine
New Haven, Connecticut
Chapter 19

R. Taylor Segraves, MD, PhD
Professor Emeritus of Psychiatry
Case Western Reserve University School of Medicine
Cleveland, Ohio
Chapter 34

Richard C. Shelton, MD
Charles B Ireland Professor of Psychiatry and Behavioral
    Neurobiology
University of Alabama Heersink School of Medicine
Birmingham, Alabama
Chapters 8, 25, & 27

Wendy K. Silverman, PhD
Alfred A. Messer Professor in the Child Study Center and
    Professor of Psychology
Yale University School of Medicine
New Haven, Connecticut
Chapter 50

Deborah R. Simkin, MD
Adjunct Associate Professor of Psychiatry
University of South Alabama College of Medicine,
    Mobile, Alabama
Clinical Assistant Professor
Florida State University College of Medicine
Tallahassee, Florida
Chapter 46

Mehmet Sofuoglu, MD, PhD
Professor of Psychiatry
Yale University School of Medicine
New Haven, Connecticut
Chapter 19

Steven M. Southwick, MD[†]
Formerly Professor Emeritus of Psychiatry
Yale University School of Medicine
New Haven, Connecticut
Chapter 28

Thomas J. Spencer, MD
Associate Professor of Psychiatry
Harvard University Medical School
Boston, Massachusetts
Chapter 44

William W. Stoops, PhD
Dr. William R. Willard Professor in Behavioral Science
University of Kentucky Departments of Behavioral Science,
    Psychiatry and Psychology
Lexington, Kentucky
Chapter 19

Griffin A. Stout, MD
Assistant Professor in Psychiatry
Nationwide Children's Hospital
Columbus, Ohio
Chapter 35

[†]Deceased.

Argyris Stringaris, MD, PhD, MRCPsych
Chair of Child and Adolescent Psychiatry
University College London
London, England
Chapter 57

John W. Thompson, Jr., MD
Professor of Psychiatry and Behavioral Sciences
Tulane University School of Medicine
New Orleans, Louisiana
Chapter 37

Travis Thompson, PhD†
Formerly Professor of Pediatrics
University of Minnesota Medical School
Minneapolis, Minnesota
Chapter 9

Halle Thurnauer, MA
Clinical Psychologist
Icahn School of Medicine at Mt. Sinai
New York, New York
Chapter 21

Michael G. Tramontana, PhD
Clinical Associate Professor of Psychiatry and
    Behavioral Sciences
Vanderbilt University School of Medicine
Nashville, Tennessee
Chapters 12, 41, & 42

Louis Trevisan, MD
Associate Professor of Psychiatry, Adjunct
Yale University School of Medicine
New Haven, Connecticut
Chapters 31 & 32

Fred R. Volkmar, MD
Irving B. Harris Professor of Child Psychiatry,
    Professor of Pediatrics and Psychology
Yale University School of Medicine
New Haven, Connecticut
Chapter 43

James S. Walker, PhD†
Formerly Assistant Professor of Psychiatry,
    Neurology, and Psychology
Vanderbilt University School of Medicine
Nashville, Tennessee
Chapter 6

Sidney H. Weissman, MD
Clinical Professor of Psychiatry and Behavioral Sciences
Northwestern University Feinberg School of Medicine
Chicago, Illinois
Chapters 1, 5, 14, 29, & 39

Larry Welch, EdD
Consulting Psychologist
Social Security Administration
Chapter 6

Thomas N. Wise, MD
Professor of Psychiatry
George Washington University School of Medicine
Washington, DC
Chapter 59

Yvonne H.C. Yau, MSc
Post-doctoral Student
McGill University
Montreal, Canada
Chapter 23

Charles Zeanah, MD
Professor of Psychiatry and Pediatrics
Tulane University School of Medicine
New Orleans, Louisiana
Chapter 54

Kenneth J. Zucker, PhD
Professor Emeritus of Psychiatry
University of Toronto
Toronto, Canada
Chapter 55

†Deceased.

Preface

Current Diagnosis & Treatment: Psychiatry, Fourth Edition, reflects the current evolving knowledge base of psychiatry which informs clinical practice. Woven into the text are advances in our knowledge of all areas which impact human behavior and inform our clinical work. They include neurobiology, genetics, psychology, and the impact of society. This volume translates this enhanced understanding in a practical and succinct form that is useful for all healthcare professionals who provide care for individuals dealing with mental health and behavioral disturbance.

Today's mental health professional must be knowledgeable in understanding factors that affect behavior not thought of a few years ago. Previous theories of the biological and psychological forces impacting on human development today appear simplistic and arbitrary. Developments in neurobiology, genetics, cognitive, developmental psychology, and our understanding of the impact of society have made and are continuing to make inroads into our understanding of psychiatric syndromes. This volume further integrates these advances into our current appreciation and clinical work, which impact on our application of pharmacotherapy, somatic therapy and psychotherapy. Concurrently the reader is prepared to comprehend the next generation of new "understandings." For example, 10 years ago it was felt that certain psychoses were the result of one gene. Today, we know they are the result of the interaction of possibly hundreds of genes with other genetic material and an individual's life experiences. This has altered both our understanding of the biology of psychosis and potential therapies.

Section I identifies some of the major tributaries of scientific knowledge that inform the current theory and practice of psychiatry and also presents techniques for the evaluation of psychiatric patients. Section II presents the diagnosis, phenomenology, and psychopathology of the major adult psychiatric syndromes and their evidence-based treatments. Section III presents the same material for the major syndromes seen in child and adolescent psychiatry. Section IV presents specialized settings for diagnosis and treatment in psychiatry.

Current Diagnosis & Treatment: Psychiatry, Fourth Edition, is written from an empirical viewpoint, with recognition that the boundaries of psychopathological syndromes may change unexpectedly with the emergence of new knowledge. Eventually, the accumulation of new knowledge will sharpen our diagnostic techniques and improve the treatment of these illnesses that have such a high impact on normal development, health, and society.

Acknowledgments

The editors would like to thank our McGraw Hill editors and their colleagues, especially Timothy Y. Hiscock, Peter Boyle, Sydney Keen, and Tasneem Kauser, for their thoughtful guidance and help.

We thank Ellen Levine Ebert for her editorial assistance in the preparation of the text.

Clinical Decision-Making in Psychiatry

1

Sidney H. Weissman, MD

FIRST: BECOMING A PSYCHIATRIST

To become a physician, one must first study to obtain and sustain fundamental knowledge of the workings of the human body. When accomplished, the student physician must then learn how to examine, evaluate, and diagnose an individual who is ill. After accomplishing these tasks, the student physician learns therapeutics. After graduating medical school and a residency a student can become an independent practicing physician. There remains one other crucial requirement. One must live by the oath of Hippocrates, "first, do no harm." Our ability to heal as physicians has evolved over centuries in sync with our expanded knowledge.

The requirements for becoming a psychiatrist follow an additional more complex course than for other physicians. Other physicians assess patients initially by an examination, which includes history taking, listening, looking, feeling, and using instruments. They may also then interview family members, examine tissue, or obtain other laboratory or radiologic exams. The results of the information they obtain are then compared to external standards to determine a diagnosis. The diagnosis can directly be communicated to colleagues.

An example of this process is seen in the work of the pathologist. The pathologist uses a microscope to examine a slide of tissue. The characteristics of the slide are compared either by the pathologist from memory or with other physical slides of similar tissue. The pathologist uses shared standard observable criteria to determine if tissue is cancerous or benign. Other pathologists can physically examine the slide to concur on the diagnosis of the tissue.

The psychiatrist, in initially evaluating a patient, also assesses their patients by listening and observing and gathering data. The psychiatrist, like the pathologist, has a peer-developed diagnostic standard (DSM-5-TR) as to what to call or label certain behaviors. However, in the psychiatric diagnostic system unlike in pathology, the data noted for one diagnosis may not be identical between two patients with the same diagnosis. For example, in the DSM-5-TR in describing Antisocial Personality Disorder it states, "A pervasive pattern of disregard for and violation of rights of others … as indicated by three (or more) of the following": The DSM then lists seven behaviors. This complicates the psychiatrist's diagnostic decision-making. Some of the characteristics of Antisocial Personality Disorder are seen in other diagnoses.

To assess patients every psychiatrist must develop their own internal guide in order or obtain and order information obtained from observing and listening to their patients. This guide is formed both by knowledge of psychiatry and also by the psychiatrist's unique life experiences.

After making an initial DSM-5-TR diagnosis on the basis of the patient's behavior, the psychiatrist has an additional task. They must develop a hypothesis derived from the unique factors that shaped the patient's life to account for why they developed the disorder they did. To accomplish this, the psychiatrist examines four areas of the patient's life, which impact and shape their behavior. First are biological factors, for example a head injury, medical disorder, or the presence of a major psychiatric disorder in the family. Next are psychological factors. These address specific actions that may have disrupted the patient's psychological well-being, for example experiencing a major loss or death. Then social factors are evaluated. In a psychiatric diagnosis, this is usually but not restricted to immediate or childhood family interactions, which may have affected their behavior. Finally, it is critical to undertake a broad examination of the external societal pressures that may have impacted on the individual and/or their family, for example the experience of prejudice.

The psychiatrist now weighs and measures all of the factors in their life that may have impacted on a patient's behavior to develop the hypothesis that explains their behavior. Then a treatment plan can be developed.

The psychiatrist's interpretation and application of diagnostic standards are impacted by the psychiatrist's life experiences and beliefs. These may play critical roles in the psychiatrist's formulation and treatment approach. In pathology, we are not concerned about the pathologists' private beliefs since the standards are public and agreed upon. They will not affect their assessment of a patient's tissues, but for the psychiatrist, they might. A patient with life experiences similar to their own might assume a patient is "psychiatrically ill" because they do not address these experiences as they have. The psychiatrist, because of how psychological data are gathered and assessed, must constantly focus on themselves and their responses to situations a patient describes. They must be able to distinguish their unique responses and values from those of their patient's.

This process is not easy. Physicians do not routinely assess the rationale for their actions. The psychiatrist must. Knowing oneself for psychiatrists is also a strength. Self-experience may enable us to develop empathy to appreciate the experience and feelings of others. But we must be clear that we maintain a focus on understanding our patients and their needs and that they are not the same as ours.

Psychiatrists in their clinical work have an additional task. They must develop and maintain relationships with patients such that they do not look for or create a personal nonclinical engagement. Friendships and business relationships create special expectations and feelings. When they occur between the psychiatrist and the patient, they can stimulate feelings in both the psychiatrist and patient that interfere with both a diagnostic assessment and further psychiatric therapy. This may prevent ongoing therapeutic work with a patient.

In this chapter, we now address psychiatric clinical reasoning. This process is an art utilizing the unique skills of every practitioner in their application of scientific principles. This volume provides an in-depth presentation of the current knowledge of psychiatric disorders that is essential to perform psychiatric diagnoses and treatment. The integration of this knowledge with the essential knowledge of oneself is the responsibility of every psychiatric practitioner.

THE PURPOSE OF CLINICAL REASONING

It is through clinical reasoning that clinicians collect, weigh, and combine the information required to reach diagnosis; decide which treatment is required; monitor treatment effectiveness; and change plans and at times a diagnosis if a treatment does not work. The study of clinical reasoning, therefore, concerns the cognitive processes of the clinician that underlie diagnosis and the planning and implementation of treatment and an awareness of factors in the physician which might interfere in the process.

In our first encounters with a patient, we develop a diagnosis. For clinicians, the chief purpose of diagnosis is to summarize information in such a way as to guide treatment. In one approach to organizing and summarizing data, the clinician matches a pattern of clinical phenomena elicited from the patient against his learned patterns of disease entities. In psychiatry, the names of these patterns are stated and described in DSM-5-TR. The psychiatrist selects the disorder that best matches his data. In the absence of a good or clear match, the clinician uses an auxiliary approach. The clinician attempts to understand each element of the particular environmental, biological, psychological, and existential factors that may have led to or perpetuated the patient's current problem. The clinician then attempts to find the best "match" for the disorder, again using DSM-5-TR. The first approach lends itself to developing commonly accepted treatment approaches that may apply to many patients. The second stresses the adaptation of the clinical data to a diagnosis unique to a given patient but more clearly derived from the psychiatrist's clinical practice.

▶ The Start of the Diagnostic Process

Even before the patient is seen, the clinician may have gathered cues, for example, from the referral source. As the patient enters the office, before the interview begins, the clinician scans the patient's eyes, face, skin, clothes, gait, coordination, posture, and voice in order to perceive salient cues (e.g., "pale, elderly, frail, shabbily dressed, worried looking, using a cane, favoring one leg). Initially, the net is cast widely to maximize the chance of correctly recognizing salient cues, perhaps at the expense of perceiving data that turn out to be irrelevant. As the diagnostic process proceeds, however, the gathering of evidence becomes more and more focused. During the patient interview the clinician's demeanor, receptiveness, and empathic communication encourage the patient to tell their story. More cues are elicited from the patient's spontaneous comments.

▶ Evaluating Cues & Making Inferences

Out of the enormous amount of data obtained, the experienced clinician knows what to look for and evaluate. Freckles, for example, are less likely to be pertinent than are blue lips (although, in certain circumstances, freckles could be relevant). Blue lips, however, must be evaluated before they are regarded as significant, e.g., abnormal). For example, has the patient been eating berries, or is the blueness circulatory in origin? If the blueness is circulatory in origin, is it due to central or peripheral dysfunction?

If a patient says that people are talking about them, the clinician must decide whether this complaint is based on reality, whether it is an exaggeration of reality, or whether it is based on a false conviction (i.e., a delusion). As the interview progresses the experienced clinician makes tentative inferences.

Assembling Cues & Inferences as a Clinical Pattern

The clinician begins to form cues and inferences into tentative patterns that form the foundation set of clinical reasoning; for example, (1) potentially lethal suicide attempt; (2) angry and depressed; (3) uncooperative and dismissive toward the examiner; (4) said to have made one previous suicide attempt (the time and lethality of which are uncertain at this point). The efficiency, thoroughness, and accuracy of information distinguish the expert from the novice. It is from this data that the clinician first attempts a diagnosis from pattern recognition. If unable, the clinician undertakes a more exhaustive assessment of the patient and determines the need for obtaining clinical data from other sources to make a DSM-5-TR diagnosis.

Generating a Formulation (Dynamic Hypothesis)

In addition to developing DSM-5-TR pattern or categorical diagnosis the clinician develops a dynamic assessment of the factors which may have led to the observed symptomatic behavior. This is known as the bio-psycho-social and societal assessment of these factors or the formulation. It is the most difficult element in the diagnostic process. Its purpose is to understand the forces that shape a patient's behavior. The formulation is used subsequently to guide the patient's treatment, But the formulation is governed by the rules of general system theory. We may learn the forces that may have impacted upon a patient but do not know the specific impact of each individually or collectively as causal agents for their symptomatic behavior.

A clinical example will highlight the problem. A 60-year-old business executive presented for treatment because of depression. At the time of his first visit, the country was in the midst of a major recession. The patient's stated major concern was that he could not save his company from bankruptcy. The psychiatrist's DSM-5-TR diagnosis was depression. In his formulation, the psychiatrist viewed the patient's concerns as related to the patient's feeling of powerlessness and shame. For these reasons he began intensive psychotherapy. After 6 weeks he had not improved. In reassessing the forces which may have triggered the depression he considered the possibility they were biologic. Further that his depression and self-doubts exaggerated his business fears. Antidepressants were then started. Four weeks later, the patient had improved and reported his company was not going bankrupt after all. Two months later, the patient was not interested in psychotherapy but wished to continue on medication. The reported and observed behaviors all met criteria for depression. The biopsychosocial factors and society issues integrated into a formulation which could support a psychotherapeutic treatment. The psychiatrist's first treatment approach was based on his knowledge and experience

in assessing all of the data he had about the patient but was incorrect. DSM-5-TR diagnosis and the formulation are both simply initial hypothesis used to understand a patient in order to develop a therapeutic plan. They must be altered as new data become available. In this case when the treatment was not effective.

In following interviews after the initial assessment and commencement of treatment, the clinician develops an inquiry process (e.g., further history and assessment of cognitive functioning, need for a physical examination by a primary care doctor, laboratory testing, special investigations, and information from collateral sources, past records, and consultations). Clinicians organize their data collected (e.g., past medical history, mental status examination) to gather important cues and evidence. The depth and thoroughness of enhanced data gathering will depend on the ambiguities and complexity behavior of the patient in understanding a patient's behavior. It is designed to elicit information either to make or confirm the categorical diagnosis, to enrich knowledge of the factors leading to the formulation and to enable the development and if needed alteration of a treatment plan.

Revising, Deleting, or Accepting Hypotheses

Modification of the initial diagnosis and subsequent treatment plan is a continuous process. As new information is learned the clinician reassesses the initial categorical diagnosis.

At times, the initial DSM-5-TR diagnosis does not change, but with further knowledge obtained working with the patient the formulation and understanding of the factor impacting on a patient do. When this occurs, changes in therapeutic strategy are essential.

CONCLUSION

Developing a psychiatric diagnosis begins with an initial clinical interview with the patient. The initial interview utilizes the unique talents and knowledge of the psychiatrist to assess the patient. In this interview, the psychiatrists learn about the patient's current problem, their premorbid functioning, relevant past history, family history, and medical history. The information that the psychiatrist obtains from the initial interview and any other sources is then uniquely synthesized by the psychiatrist into a plan of further action. Sometimes a diagnosis is initially clear, but frequently further interviews and information may be needed. They may include interviews with family members or assessments by a psychologist or a neurologist to determine possible brain malfunction. In some situations, medical examination may be required. When satisfied with enough clinical information a tentative DSM-5-TR diagnosis is made. It is tentative and should be considered a working hypothesis that must be repeatedly tested, and may need to be altered with further information.

At this point, the psychiatrist integrates the data used to make the descriptive DSM-5-TR diagnosis with their bio-psycho-social and societal assessment of the patient. This is possibly the most difficult element in the diagnostic and decision-making process. The experienced psychiatrist knows that although symptoms or behaviors may be common, they are unique expressions for each patient. Knowing this the psychiatrist develops an initial treatment plan for their patient. Initial treatment plans must also be understood as working hypotheses, which may need to be altered as more data are obtained about a patient. With more data, the psychiatrist over time develops a more detailed and complex therapeutic plan. This may require individual, family, or group psychotherapy, medications, a combination of the therapies, or a somatic therapy in conjunction with medications or psychotherapy. If the psychiatrist believes they have the requisite skills to treat the patient, they may progress to treat the patient. If they do not, they must refer the patient to a clinician who does.

Cox K: Perceiving clinical evidence. *Med Educ* 2002;36:1189.

Diagnostic and Statistical Manual of Mental Disorders, 5th edn. text revision, DSM-5-TR, American Psychiatric Association, Washington DC, 2022.

Dowe J, Elstein A: *Professional Judgment*. Cambridge, UK: Cambridge University Press, 1988.

Edelstein, L: *The Hippocratic Oath*, text translation p. 56. ISBN 970-081-00184-6, 1943.

Elstein AS, Shulman LS, Sprafka SA: *Medical Problem Solving*. Cambridge, MA: Harvard University Press, 1978.

Engel G: The clinical application of the biopsychosocial model. *AM J Psychiatry* 1980;137: 535–544.

Eva LW: What every teacher needs to know about clinical reasoning. *Med Educ* 2004;39:98.

Groves M, O'Rourke P, Alexander H: Clinical reasoning: the relative contribution of identification, interpretation, and hypothesis errors to misdiagnosis. *Med Teach* 2003;25:621.

Kushniruk AW, Patel VL, Marley AA: Small worlds and medical expertise. *Int J Med Inform* 1998;49:255.

Lighthall G, Vazquez-Guillamet C: Understanding decision making in critical care. *Clin Med Res* 2015;133(3–4):156–168.

Psychiatric Epidemiology

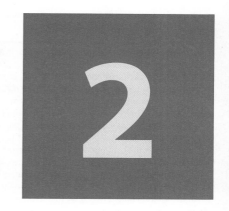

Daniel G. Blazer, MD, PhD
Robert J. Ronis, MD, MPH

THE BIOPSYCHOSOCIAL MODEL & THE WEB OF CAUSATION

George Engel promulgated a theoretical model, based on general systems theory, of the etiology of mental disease that remains central to epidemiologic investigations into the twenty-first century. Research demonstrates that unitary explanations are not adequate to explain disease etiology or thus inform appropriate prevention and treatment strategies. Engel suggested an interrelatedness among biological, psychological, and social factors. Biological factors include hereditary, anatomic, and molecular factors and those factors related to gender, age, and ethnicity. Psychological factors include temperament, personality, motivation, emotion, attention, and cognition. According to Engel's theory, social factors included family, society, culture, and environment; other authors would include religious and spiritual as well as economic factors in this group. This model pervades epidemiology, yet recent efforts focus not on simply integrating the different elements but rather moving toward a transdisciplinary approach that breaks down traditional disciplinary barriers. From this perspective, psychiatric epidemiologists explore the frequency, distribution, outcome, and causation of psychiatric disorders.

Identifying a case becomes the first task of the epidemiologist. An essential component of all these uses is the determination of valid **denominators** to compare the characteristics of populations with and without disease. For example, to determine the **prevalence** of a case (i.e., the frequency of the case in a given population at a given point in time), one must know the number of persons both with and without the disorder in the population. To determine the **incidence** of a case (the number of new cases that emerge in the population over a given interval—usually 1 year), one must know the number of people in the population at the beginning of an interval who do not experience the disorder. A list of key terms in epidemiology can be found in Table 2–1.

In recent years, psychiatric epidemiologists have recognized that cases often occur simultaneously in the same person (the cases are **comorbid**). Recent studies have emphasized not only the prevalence and incidence of individual cases but also comorbid cases.

Engel GL: The clinical application of the biopsychosocial model. *Am J Psychiatr* 1980;137:537–544.

Hernandez L, Blazer D: *Genes, Behavior, and the Social Environment: Moving Beyond the Nature/Nurture Debate.* Washington, DC: The National Academies Press, 2006.

Lilienfeld DE: Definitions of epidemiology. *Am J Epidemiol* 1978; 107:87.

CONCEPT OF THE "CASE"

The *Diagnostic and Statistical Manual of Mental Disorders,* 5th edition (DSM-5), and other psychiatric diagnostic systems disaggregate psychiatric disorders into discrete cases. For example, either an individual meets criteria for a diagnosis of major depressive disorder or he or she does not. To identify a case, one must have criteria for identifying cases, but these criteria may vary from one nomenclature to another. For example, the criteria for a case in DSM-5-TR differ from those in DSM-5 or DSM-4-TR in some circumstances.

The use of the concept of a case in epidemiology makes it easier for practicing clinicians to interpret the types of studies performed by epidemiologists, although by arbitrarily assigning an individual to a category of either "case" or "noncase," one loses considerable data. Several early epidemiologic studies were cognizant of this dilemma and attempted to assign patients to groups based on how well they met the predetermined criteria for each group: these researchers recognized that the ability of clinicians to assign individuals as either cases or noncases was not perfect and was more applicable to a probability function than to a simple yes–no decision. Similarly, the use of symptom rating scales does not require that an individual be assigned to a case or noncase category but rather permits the assessment of depressive psychopathology

Table 2–1 Key Terms in Epidemiology

Prevalence: The frequency of a given disorder in a population at a particular point of time (i.e., it is the ratio of the number of cases of a disorder in the population divided by the number of persons in the population). Although community surveys take time to complete (usually 3 months to 1 year), it is assumed that the results of such studies estimate the frequency of a disorder within a population (usually given as a percentage) on a given day. In some cases, prevalence is measured not as the frequency on a given day but as the frequency of all cases of the disorder that are present during some interval of time, such as 1 month or 1 year.

Denominator: In the prevalence ratio, the denominator is the number of persons in the population. This number becomes important because the prevalence may vary depending on the population from which cases are selected. For example, the denominator may be all persons in a community, all females in a community, all persons attending a clinic, all persons 65 years of age or older attending a clinic, or all African Americans in the community. For each denominator, prevalence may vary.

Incidence: The likelihood, over a period of time (usually 1 year), that an individual who is free from a given disorder will develop it. For example, if 1000 persons are free of a disorder on January 1 and 100 develop the disorder during the next 12 months, then the incidence of that disorder is 10%. In most cases, incidence is much lower than prevalence, and, naturally, because incidence reflects a rate, the collection of data at two or more points in time is necessary to determine incidence.

Risk: The likelihood that an individual will experience a psychiatric disorder. In this sense, risk is basically a measure of incidence.

Risk factor: Any factor that may increase the likelihood that a person will develop a psychiatric disorder. For example, it is known that female gender, younger age, lower socioeconomic status, and being divorced are risk factors for developing major depression. A risk factor may not necessarily be causal.

Risk profile: The array of risk factors associated with a specific disorder.

Relative risk: The increased (or decreased) risk for developing a disorder among persons with a risk factor, compared to persons without a risk factor.

Comorbidity: The presence of at least two distinct disorders in the same individual, each with its own etiology, presentation, and course.

as a continuum. (Examples of "case finding" in psychiatric epidemiology are provided later in the description of individual studies.)

American Psychiatric Association: *Diagnostic and Statistical Manual of Mental Disorders*, 4th edn. Text revised. Washington, DC: American Psychiatric Publishing, 1994.

American Psychiatric Association: *Diagnostic and Statistical Manual of Mental Disorders*, 5th edn. Text revised. Washington, DC: American Psychiatric Publishing, 2022.

American Psychiatric Association: *Diagnostic and Statistical Manual of Mental Disorders*, 5th edn. Washington, DC: American Psychiatric Publishers, 2013.

OTHER EPIDEMIOLOGIC CONCEPTS

To discern the relationship(s) between factors that contribute to the emergence of a case, epidemiologists explore what has been described as the **web of causation**. The concept of a web of causation is that specific relationships, such as the relationship between social stressors and a mental disorder, may be connected through a variety of intervening variables that interrelate in a way best illustrated by a web consisting of nodes (etiologic factors) and strings (interrelationships of these etiologic factors). For example, genetic factors may lead to endophenotypes (such as dysfunction of a neurotransmitter system), which lead to intermediate phenotypes (such as a depressed mood), which in turn are shaped by the social environment of the individual. Social factors, in turn, may alter genetic expression, even directly through the process of epigenesis. Epidemiologic studies assist investigators in sorting out the different nodes and interactions within this web of causation.

According to Morris, epidemiology has several vital uses: (1) study of the historical health of communities and the estimation of morbidity for different disorders, (2) assessment of the efficiency of health programs and services, (3) determination of individuals **at risk** of acquiring a disease or disability in all their various presentations, (4) identification of syndromes as the unified collection of related signs and symptoms, and (5) assisting in "the search for the causes of health and disease." Proper epidemiologic studies can promote sound health policy, enable more rational health care planning, and facilitate cost-effective prevention and treatment.

MacMahon B, Pugh TF, Ipsen J: *Epidemiological Methods*. Boston: Little, Brown, 1960.

Morris JN: *Uses of Epidemiology*. Philadelphia: Williams & Wilkins, 1964.

HISTORICAL PERSPECTIVE

▶ First-Generation Studies

The earliest formal psychiatric epidemiologic studies were undertaken during the first part of the twentieth century. They were generally of limited scale, relied on institutional records, and used small groups of informants for their data. These were "convenience" studies in which, instead of initiating the surveys themselves, epidemiologists assembled health data from those persons who had already received treatment for a medical problem or had committed suicide. Faris and Dunham's relatively large pre–World War II study examined the geographic distribution of patients with mental disorders in mental hospitals in the Chicago area. They found that manic–depressive illness was distributed equally throughout the geographic area, whereas schizophrenia clustered in the lower socioeconomic areas.

Second-Generation Studies: The Stirling County & Midtown Manhattan Studies

In comparison to pre–World War II investigations, the studies that followed World War II took advantage of the considerable health information gathered on the military forces during the war. This was the beginning of the "community survey" era of epidemiology. Postwar studies—such as the Stirling County (Nova Scotia) Study, the Midtown Manhattan Study, and the Baltimore Study of mental illness in an urban population—were second-generation studies that attempted to determine the prevalence rates of mental illness (not specific psychiatric disorders) in community residents with the help of nonpsychiatrist clinical interviewers. The postwar studies examined general health as well as psychiatric disorders and tended to gather and interpret rates of symptom presentation in groups rather than assess the presence of discrete cases. The gathering of often-isolated symptoms, or the finding of psychopathology or emotional illness by using the data collection system of the World War II era, was not helpful to health planners or policymakers.

Contributing to the ascension of psychiatric epidemiologic research during the early postwar period was the realization that the increase in mortality and morbidity associated with chronic disease (including that of mental disorders) was more important than was the mortality and morbidity associated with acute, generally infectious, disorders. Difficulty with case identification in the community continued to preclude the determination of prevalence rates for specific clinical disorders.

The initial paradigms for these newer studies were often quite different. The Stirling County Study attempted to determine rates for qualitatively different disorders as well as for overall impairment. The Midtown Manhattan Study assumed that mental disorders were on a continuum and—reflecting the thinking at that time (that mental illness differed in degree and not kind)—that all clinical manifestations of illness could be evaluated in terms of functional impairment. The overall prevalence of psychiatric impairment from both of these studies was approximately 20%. Leighton and colleagues demonstrated in Stirling County that the mental illness of the individual could be influenced, for benefit or detriment, by the attributes of the community, thus ushering in an emphasis, during the late 1950s and early 1960s, on social psychiatry.

Third-Generation Studies

Third-generation epidemiologic studies were based on more advanced epidemiologic and statistical techniques and on a move toward scientific or evidence-based medicine.

These studies began with the important development of operational criteria for mental disorders (specifically DSM-3). Newer methodological techniques helped address the increasing need for more exact rates of specific disorders for specific persons in specific settings. Indeed, effective treatment has been shown to be related directly to accurate and thus specific assessment and diagnosis. Similarly, appropriate mental health policy planning for the unique health needs of persons with various psychiatric disorders depends greatly on an accurate and precise definition of boundaries between disorders. Further, research into the etiology and thus effective treatment and, it is hoped, eventual prevention of psychiatric disorders must derive from the specificity of operational criteria. Otherwise, the blurring that has occurred between symptom patterns can lead only to similar blurring in the assessment of treatment and prevention effectiveness.

The American Psychiatric Association's DSM-3 was a clear departure from its predecessors in that the specificity and boundaries that demarcated a foundation of this evolving instrument led to specific case and noncase determinations. Many etiologic assumptions in DSM-2 that were not demonstrated by empirical research were abandoned in DSM-3. Although interview instruments have been derived from each of these criteria sets, the Diagnostic Interview Schedule (DIS), associated with the development of DSM-3, was the first instrument designed for use by (trained) lay interviewers in community-based epidemiologic studies, a decision based on cost–benefit considerations. The DIS became the preferred instrument for use in most large epidemiologic studies during the 1980s, such as the Epidemiologic Catchment Area (ECA) study (see next section).

The National Institute of Mental Health's Epidemiologic Catchment Area Study

The National Institute of Mental Health's ECA study was the most comprehensive and sophisticated epidemiologic study accomplished in its time in the United States. When it was undertaken between 1980 and 1984, its purpose was to provide the best estimates, for the United States, of the prevalence of alcohol and drug abuse and other mental disorders, based on a formalized criteria set (DSM-3) rather than global impairment. Unlike previous studies, this investigation included not only data from institutional and community samples but also longitudinal data and information on disease severity. The ECA investigators explored the specific demographic, biological, psychosocial, and environmental factors that might influence the presence and the severity of a mental disorder (i.e., the biopsychosocial model). The study not only allowed investigators to follow up on possible clinical change but also assessed the service utilization of both mental health and general health services. The ECA study has assisted greatly in the planning for future health care service needs including physical resources, financing, personnel, and educational requirements. The ECA study also confirmed the capability of DSM-3 criteria to discriminate among mental disorders and generally helped sharpen the nosology of mental illness. Although the methodology of the ECA study was a great improvement on previous work, the use of DSM-3 as the basis for case identification tended to emphasize reliability rather than validity. DSM-3 diagnostic criteria, in contrast to DSM-2 criteria, were intended to enhance diagnostic reliability, which, although necessary, is insufficient to establish diagnostic validity. Further, because lay interviewers were employed in the ECA study, in-depth, qualitative, and intuitive clinical data were not collected.

Compared to previous surveys, the ECA study found lower rates of virtually all disorders than many had assumed, except for phobic disorders (as shown in Table 2–2). Women exhibited higher rates of mental disorders than did men, although there were important differences in the rates for specific disorders. Men had higher rates of substance abuse and antisocial personality disorder, and women had significantly higher rates for anxiety-based, affective, and somatization disorders. Men and women exhibited similar rates for schizophrenia and manic episodes. The ECA study showed that individuals with comorbid conditions were more likely to receive treatment than were those with a single disorder; yet, fewer than one third of persons with mental illness, a substance abuse disorder, or both received any treatment. An important methodological finding was that, in comparison to international studies (after adjusting for differences in diagnostic categories and time frames), disease rates based on the DIS were found to be essentially compatible with previous epidemiologic studies based on the Present State Examination. Yet similar to the second-generation studies, around 20% of the population experienced at least one mental disorder.

▶ The National Comorbidity Study and Its Replicate

The National Comorbidity Study (NCS) was the first attempt in the United States to estimate the prevalence of specific psychiatric disorders, with and without comorbid substance abuse, in a national population sample. The NCS was designed to further the findings of the ECA study, but in contrast to the ECA study (which was drawn from local and institutional groups), the NCS had a national focus. The NCS sought risk factors as well as prevalence and incidence rates, in contrast to the ECA study, which focused only on the latter (see Table 2–2). With its national focus, the NCS made possible regional comparisons, including rural and urban differences, and it was possible to establish, on a national basis, more precise investigations into unmet mental illness treatment needs. Furthermore, the NCS was referenced to the DSM-3-R rather than DSM-3 and also contained some questions that would allow comparison to the future DSM-4 and the *International Classification of Diseases,* 10th edition (ICD-10). The Composite International Diagnostic Interview (CIDI) was the instrument used in the NCS. The NCS found a higher prevalence of mental disorders in the U.S. population, and this prevalence was aggregated in approximately one-sixth of the population (i.e., in individuals who had three or more comorbid disorders).

In the NCS, risk profiles were constructed for depression alone and when found in association with other psychiatric disorders: 4.9% of persons studied were found to have current major depression (i.e., within the past 30 days) and 10.3% to have major depression within the past 12 months (see Table 2–2). The lifetime prevalence of depression was 17.1%. Risk factors for both current and lifetime depression were as follows: being female; having a lower level of education; and being separated, widowed, or divorced. The NCS investigators fielded a new survey between 2001 and 2003 (the NCS Replicate) and found even higher 1-year prevalence of specific psychiatric disorders:

Table 2–2 Comparison Data from the NCS and ECA Study[1]

Disorder	Prevalence Rates (12 months)	
	NCS (12 months)	ECA Study
Any disorder	27.7	20
Substance abuse disorders	16.1	N/A
Alcohol abuse and dependence	10.7 dependence only	6.8
Drug abuse and dependence	3.8 dependence only	2.41
Schizophrenia/schizophreniform disorders	0.5 (0.1)	1.0
Affective (mood) disorders	8.5	5.1
Manic episode	1.4	
Major depressive episode	7.7	2.7
Dysthymia	2.1	2.3
Anxiety disorders	11.8	N/A
Social phobia	6.4	6.2
Panic	1.3	0.9
Obsessive-compulsive disorder	N/A	1.65
Antisocial personality disorder (life time)	4.8	1.2
Cognitive impairment	N/A	1.3

[1]ECA study data are from Robins LN, Regier DA (eds). *Psychiatric Disorder in America.* New York: The Free Press. NCS data are from Kessler RC, McGonagle KA, Zhao S, et al: Lifetime and 12-month prevalence of DSM-3 psychiatric disorders in the United States. Results from the National Comorbidity Survey. *Arch Gen Psychiatry* 1994;51:8–19. N/A, not available.

major depression (6.7), bipolar disorder I and II (2.6), dysthymic disorder (1.5), generalized anxiety disorder (3.1), panic disorder (2.7), obsessive compulsive disorder (1.0), alcohol abuse (3.1), alcohol dependence (1.3), posttraumatic stress disorder (3.5), and a diagnosis of any disorder (26.2). The rates for all time frames and the demographic distributions in the NCS and NCS-R were higher than those found in the ECA study. The fact that a different method of case identification was used probably explains most of the difference in prevalence between the NCS and the ECA study. The sample from the NCS was younger, and younger persons are known to have a higher prevalence of many disorders, such as substance use disorders and major depression. The NCS data also suggested that although "pure" depression may have a strong biogenetic contribution, comorbid depression may be more environmentally determined. Furthermore, as in the ECA study and other international investigations, more recent birth cohorts were found to be at increased risk for major depression.

Many explanations have been offered for the striking finding of high estimates of childhood depression and the unexpectedly low estimates of depression in the elderly: methodological limitations including the bias found in diagnostic instruments for the assessment of psychopathology in both children and the elderly, differential morbidity, faulty sampling, response-biased memory, institutionalization, and selective migration. Some or all of these explanations may play a role.

Continued investigation of the NCS data, building on the findings of the Medical Outcome Study (which showed that depressive symptoms themselves were a significant risk factor for other diseases) found that major and minor depression were not distinct entities but were actually on a continuum. Further, and also using the NCS data, the lifetime prevalence of major and minor depression associated with seasonal affective disorder (SAD) was found to be much lower (1%) than that found in previous studies. This was probably because the instrument used more accurately reflected DSM-3-R criteria for SAD. Another study, using the NCS data, found a significant lifetime association between panic disorder and depression in patients who first present with panic disorder and a less powerful but statistically valid association for those who first present with depression. An investigation from Germany, using the revised version of the CIDI on a community sample of adolescents and young adults, found that agoraphobia and panic disorder had "marked differences in symptomatology, course, and associated impairments" and were not necessarily linked, a finding at odds with some earlier studies. If confirmed, this study, which used a more sophisticated epidemiologic design than was available in much earlier studies, will demonstrate a more precise separation between several disorders previously considered to be closely related. This finding may lead to a more definitive basis for both prevention and treatment strategies.

▶ The National Epidemiologic Survey on Alcohol and Related Conditions (NESARC)

The NESARC is a representative sample ($N = 43,093$) of the adult population of the United States, with the target population, the civilian population of 18+ years of age. NESARC oversampled Black and Hispanic subjects and young adults (aged 18–24). The Alcohol Use Disorder and Associated Disabilities Interview Schedule-DSM-4 was used, a structured in-person interview. Though focused on alcohol use and comorbid conditions, the NESARC provides yet another estimate of the prevalence of psychiatric disorders in the United States. Prevalence varies somewhat from the NCS-R and the ECA but not dramatically. (See Table 2–2 for a comparison of NESARC estimates of 1-year prevalence compared to the ECA and NCS.)

More narrowly focused epidemiologic studies have contributed to increased understanding of psychiatric disorders associated with social conditions. For example, through a population survey, Breslau and colleagues demonstrated that posttraumatic stress disorder occurred in 9.2% of the population following exposure to trauma. Not only was this prevalence lower than that reported previously, but the most common trauma experienced was the unexpected death of a loved one, not the usually reported combat, rape, or other serious physical assault. Bassuk and colleagues investigated the prevalence of mental illness and substance abuse disorders among homeless and low-income housed mothers, compared to the prevalence of these disorders among all women in the NCS, and found the prevalence of trauma-related disorders among poor women to be significantly higher than that found among women in the general population.

American Psychiatric Association: *Diagnostic and Statistical Manual of Mental Disorders*, 3rd edn. Washington, DC: American Psychiatric Publishers, 1980.

Bassuk EL et al: Prevalence of mental health and substance use disorders among homeless and low-income housed mothers. *Am J Psychiatry* 1998;155:1561.

Blazer DG, Kessler RC, Swartz M: Epidemiology of recurrent major and minor depression with a seasonal pattern. The National Comorbidity Survey. *Br J Psychiatry* 1998;172:164.

Breslau N et al: Trauma and post traumatic stress disorder in the community: the 1996 Detroit Area Survey of Trauma. *Arch Gen Psychiatry* 1998;55:626.

Faris REI, Dunham HW: *Mental Disorders in Urban Areas: An Ecological Study of Schizophrenia and Other Psychoses*. Chicago: University of Chicago Press, 1939.

Kessler RC et al: Lifetime and 12-month prevalence of DSM-3-R psychiatric disorders in the United States. Results from the National Comorbidity Study. *Arch Gen Psychiatry* 1994;51:8.

Kessler RC et al: Lifetime panic-depression comorbidity in the National Comorbidity Survey. *Arch Gen Psychiatry* 1998;55:801.

Kessler RC et al: Prevalence, correlates, and course of minor depression and major depression in the National Comorbidity Survey. *J Affect Disord* 1997;45:19.

Kessler RC et al: Prevalence, severity, and comorbidity of 12-month DSM-4 disorders in the National Comorbidity Survey replication. *Arch Gen Psychiatry* 2005;62:617.

Leighton DC et al: *The Character of Danger: Psychiatric Symptoms in Selected Communities*. New York: Basic Books, 1963.

Narrow WE, Rubio-Stipec M: Epidemiology. In: Sadock BJ, Sadock VA, Ruiz P (eds). *Kaplan and Sadock's Comprehensive Textbook of Psychiatry*, 9th edn. Philadelphia: Lippincott Williams & Wilkins, 2009, pp. 754–770.

Pasamanick B et al: A survey of mental disease in an urban population. *Am J Public Health* 1956;47:923.

Robins L, Helzer J, Croughan J: Diagnostic Interview Schedule: Its history, characteristics and validity. *Arch Gen Psychiatry*, 1981;38:381–389.

Robins L, Regier D: *Psychiatric Disorders in America: The Epidemiologic Catchment Area Study*. New York: Free Press, 1991.

Strole L, Fisher AK: *Mental Health in the Metropolis: The Midtown Manhattan Study*. New York: McGraw-Hill, 1982.

Wittchen HU, Reed V, Kessler RC: The relationship of agoraphobia and panic in a community sample of adolescents and young adults. *Arch Gen Psychiatry* 1998;55:1017.

RURAL–URBAN DIFFERENCES & THE SOCIAL DRIFT HYPOTHESIS

Another important finding of most epidemiologic studies is that the prevalence of some mental disorders, particularly schizophrenia, has been found to be higher in urban and industrialized areas than in rural areas. A number of explanations for this finding have been suggested: social migration (the downward drift of persons and families experiencing schizophrenia to lower socioeconomic levels), inbreeding among the mentally ill, and the greater availability in urban areas of services for the chronically mentally ill. These differences may also reflect the comparative integration and stability of rural areas. Leighton and colleagues, in their study of rural Nova Scotia, found that depression and other psychiatric disorders were more common for all ages in "disintegrated" communities. Given the recent emphasis on the genetic basis of many psychiatric disorders, more research must be done on the degree of possible inheritance of these disorders in populations, and on the social drift hypothesis, before firm conclusions can be reached.

Leighton AH: *My Name Is Legion*. New York: Basic Books, 1959.

Mental Disorder, Physical Health, & Social Functioning

A survey of the point prevalence of schizophrenia within three regions of Scotland was undertaken in 1996, replicating a similar survey conducted in 1981. In comparison to the 1981 study, the patients studied in 1996 had both more positive and negative symptoms and more nonschizophrenic symptoms. Some of the symptoms encountered involved physical health.

An increasing number of epidemiologic studies have demonstrated that depression is a serious illness in its own right and that depressive disorder, and depressive symptoms without a formal depressive disorder being present, can have a serious impact on the general physical health of an individual. The Medical Outcome Study looked carefully at this association by evaluating processes and outcomes of care for patients with the chronic conditions of hypertension, diabetes, coronary heart disease, and depression. Patients with either a current depressive disorder or depressive symptoms in the absence of a disorder tended to have worse physical health, poorer social role functioning, worse perceived current health, and (perceived) greater bodily pain than did patients without a chronic depressive condition. Further, the poor functioning associated with depression or depressive symptoms was equal or worse than that associated with eight major medical conditions, and the effects of depressive symptoms and chronic medical conditions were addictive. For example, the combination of advanced coronary artery disease and depressive symptoms was associated with roughly twice the reduction in social functioning found with either condition alone. These authors and subsequent studies concluded that it was important to correctly assess and treat depression in all health care settings in order to improve overall patient outcome, reduce patient and family suffering, and reduce societal costs. The Medical Outcome Study was one of the first to directly compare the social and occupational costs of physical and psychiatric disorders, emphasizing that psychiatric disorders are a major public health concern. More recent research has extended these findings.

Spitzer and colleagues found that depression, anxiety, somatoform disorders, and eating disorders were associated with considerable impairment in health-related quality-of-life scales. As in the Medical Outcome Study, impairment was found in patients with subclinical symptoms and in those with clinically diagnosable disorders. Mental disorders appeared to contribute to overall impairment to a greater degree than did medical conditions.

From 1982 to 1996, the comorbidity of physical and psychiatric disorders was studied in an unselected 1966 northern Finland birth cohort. In comparison to individuals without a psychiatric diagnosis, psychiatric patients were found to have been hospitalized more frequently for injuries, poisonings, or indefinite symptoms. Men were more commonly hospitalized with a variety of gastrointestinal and circulatory disturbances; women with a comorbid psychiatric disorder were more commonly hospitalized with respiratory disorders, vertebral column disorders, gynecologic disorders, or induced abortions. Epilepsy, nervous and sensory organ disorders in general, and inflammatory disorders of the bowels were more common in patients with schizophrenia as compared to those without the disease.

The National Treatment Outcome Research Study, the first large-scale prospective, multisite treatment outcome study of drug users in the United Kingdom, found an extensive range of psychological and physical health problems among this population. Studies looking at the comorbid features of physical and psychological health have consistently demonstrated a high correlation, and these findings have given leaders in the health, social service, and criminal justice systems impetus to plan integrated approaches to this vulnerable, and at least dually afflicted, population.

Gossop M et al: Substance use, health, and social problems of service users at 54 drug treatment agencies. Intake data from the National Treatment Outcome Research Study. *Br J Psychiatry* 1998;173:166.

Kelly C et al: Nithsdale Schizophrenia Surveys. 17. Fifteen year review. *Br J Psychiatry* 1998;172:513.

Makikyro T et al: Comorbidity of hospital-treated psychiatric and physical disorders with special reference to schizophrenia: a 28 year follow-up of the 1966 Northern Finland General Population. *Public Health* 1998;112(4):221–228.

Spitzer RL et al: Health related quality of life in primary care patients with mental disorders. *JAMA* 1995;274:1511–1517.

Wells KB et al: The functioning and well-being of depressed patients. *JAMA* 1989;262:914.

▶ Social Determinants of Health: Efforts to Address Care Inequities

Efforts to address health inequities and consequent poor health outcomes are broadly categorized under the rubric of Social Determinants of Health (SDOH).

Studies suggest that the quality of clinical care impacts only about 20% of county-to-county variation in health outcomes, while SDOH account for as much as 50%. SDOH are fundamental social and structural factors that touch people's lives and impact their wellness and longevity.

Within SDOH factors such as poverty, education, and employment have been shown to have the most significant impact. Other factors such as housing, food and nutrition, transportation, social and economic mobility, and environmental conditions also contribute to SDOH.

Health-related social needs (HRSN) refer to an individual's needs, such as affordable housing, nutritious food, or accessible transportation. An unequal distribution of SDOH results in HRSN at the individual level. Interventions such as providing supportive housing for individuals with serious health including behavioral health conditions have been shown to improve health outcomes and, in some cases, reduce health care costs. Addressing health risks in the home such as exposure to lead paint or second-hand smoke, improving access to healthy foods and applying evidence-based nutrition standards, increasing access to preventive care through use of nonemergency medical transportation, and other such interventions may show similar benefits.

Distinguishing between SDOH and HRSNs is key to developing measures, assessing evidence and formulating policy responses. The Centers for Disease Control and Prevention (CDC)'s public health programs address SDOH and HRSNs in a number of ways. Within the National Center for Chronic Disease Prevention and Health Promotion for example, CDC's *Racial and Ethnic Approaches to Community Health* (REACH) grants have funded locally based solutions to addressing health inequities for more than 20 years. Between 2014 and 2018, REACH provided better access to healthy foods to nearly 3 million people and opportunities for physical activity and access to local chronic disease programs for countless others. In 2021, CDC launched the *Closing the Gap with Social Determinants of Health Accelerator Plans* project, developing action plans to reduce chronic diseases among people experiencing health disparities. Another project, the *Good Health and Wellness in Indian Country* program, focuses on improving HRSNs and strengthening links between community programs and clinical services in order to promote health and help prevent chronic diseases.

In August 2021, CDC launched the *Community Health Workers for COVID Response and Resilient Communities* initiative to put additional trained community health workers (CHWs) in communities with high rates of COVID-19 and long-standing health disparities related to race, income, geographic location, or other sociodemographic characteristics. The *Health Impact in 5 Years* (HI-5) initiative highlights nonclinical, community-wide approaches that have evidence for reporting positive health impacts within 5 years.

CDC has also established cross-departmental relationships aimed at addressing SDOH. For example, CDC and the Department of Housing and Urban Development established an agreement to build a sustainable, collaborative partnership to advance shared priorities related to health and housing. In addition, the Federal Transit Administration in the Department of Transportation has partnered with CDC on the Interagency Coordinating Council on Access and Mobility (CCAM), which is charged with increasing transportation access for low-income populations, older adults, and people with disabilities. CCAM is jointly working across 11 federal departments to develop a 2023–2026 Strategic Plan for Human Services Transportation.

These are only a few examples of the ways the CDC and Department of Health and Human Services (HHS) have incorporated a better understanding of SDOH and HRSNs in the development of agendas and prioritization of programs and policies promoting public health and preventing chronic disease. Much of the research to date has focused on shorter-term outcomes and medically complex populations or those with high health care utilization. Further research can help us better understand how interventions to address risks related to SDOH and HRSNs in less medically complex individuals impact health and well-being over the life course, as well as the longer-term impacts of interventions; the impact on a wider range of populations and individuals without chronic illnesses; and the most appropriate "dose" of various interventions. Additional research is needed that focuses on health outcomes, in addition to health utilization, health costs, and healthy behaviors.

Hood CM, Gennuso KP, Swain GR, et al: County health rankings: relationships between determinant factors and health outcomes. *Am J Prevent Med* 2016;50(2):129–135.

Muenning P, Fiscella K, Tancredi, et al: The relative health burden of selected social and behavioral risk factors in the United States: implications of policy. *Am J Public Health* 2010; 100(9):1758–1764.

U.S. Department of Health and Human Services: Healthy People 2030, Social Determinants of Health. https://health.gov/healthypeople/objectives-and-data/social-determinants-health

U.S. Department of Health and Human Services, Office of the Assistant Secretary for Planning and Evaluation, April 1, 2022: Addressing social determinants of health: examples of successful evidence-based strategies and current federal efforts. https://aspe.hhs.gov/sites/default/files/documents/e2b650cd64cf84aae8ff0fae7474af82/SDOH-Evidence-Review.p

▶ Conclusion: Epidemiology, Etiology, & Public Health

Epidemiology places psychiatric disorders in a broad context, which is not always apparent with individual patients. This comprehensiveness is the basis of the biopsychosocial model. Three kinds of factors may be operative: those that promote vulnerability (or indeed resilience), those that "release" symptoms at a particular time, and those that determine how long a particular disorder will last. Koopman (1996) adds that there is now a shift to studying complex systems that create patterns of disease. Such studies are conducted by the comprehensive monitoring of individuals as individuals and when they interact with others and their environment.

Research by Kendler and colleagues (1993), investigating the risk factors for depression among twins, is among the first in an increasing number of epidemiologic studies based on an integrated biopsychosocial approach. Henderson (1996) extends this approach along the causal continuum in a slightly different way, noting that "the concept of populations having different frequency distributions of morbidity, not just different prevalence rates for clinical cases, carries with it the implication that some factor or factors are pushing up the over-all distribution in some groups, but not in others." He suggests that there may be some instrumental "force" in the environment that promotes disease. According to Susser and Susser (1996), epidemiology historically offered the paradigm of the "black box," in which exposure was related directly to outcome, without much interest in (and thus investigation into) contributing factors or pathogenesis. Moving toward a more fundamental, comprehensive, and integrative

goal, these authors would suggest the alternative paradigm of "ecoepidemiology" or the study of "causal pathways at the societal level and with pathogenesis and causality at the molecular level." Among the lessons that may be drawn then are (1) that intervention by those in health policy and practice must involve a population-based strategy rather than a singular focus on afflicted or vulnerable individuals, (2) that the web of causation is multidimensional, and (3) that theory and practice are interdependent.

Korkeila and colleagues (1998) investigated factors predicting readmission to a psychiatric hospital during the early 1990s in Finland. Frequently admitted patients were found to be an identifiable group with three defining characteristics: previous admissions, long length of stays, and a diagnosis of psychosis or personality disorder. This study was particularly important because it reconfirmed earlier work that showed that, in this era of an emphasis on community care, there may be a small group of patients who, with the current treatment strategies available, may always need frequent or longer hospital treatment.

Public health prevention and treatment strategies drawn from any research must be carefully and critically constructed. This will not be easy. Intervention with individuals and even populations of individuals may be both more difficult and less effective when the real "target is a social entity with its own laws and dynamics." To begin to address these issues of profound complexity and increasing topical relevance, many authors have strongly supported the reintegration of population-driven epidemiology into public health. Adding support and some urgency to this drive has been the advent of managed care, which has created information needs that only more sophisticated epidemiologic investigations can address. Questions on specific treatments for specific patient populations in specific settings; the effectiveness of various forms of health care, including management and finance strategies; and the relentless quest for ways to improve quality while simultaneously attending to related costs will all require methodologically sound investigations.

Henderson AS: The present state of psychiatric epidemiology. *Aust N Z J Psychiatry* 1996;30:9.

Kendler KS et al: The prediction of major depression in women: towards an integrated etiologic model. *Am J Psychiatry* 1993; 150:1139.

Koopman J: Comment: emerging objectives and methods in epidemiology. *Am J Public Health* 1996;86:630.

Korkeila JA et al: Frequently hospitalized psychiatric patients: a study of predictive factors. *Soc Psychiatry Psychiatr Epidemiol* 1998;33:528.

Susser M, Susser F: Choosing a future for epidemiology. I. Eras and paradigms. *Am J Public Health* 1996;86:668.

Psychiatric Genetics

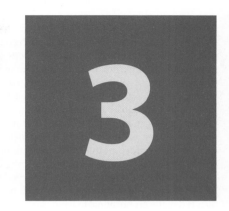

John I. Nurnberger, Jr, MD, PhD
Wade Berrettini, MD, PhD

METHODS IN PSYCHIATRIC GENETICS

A scientific revolution has occurred in the field of genetics with the advent of genome-wide studies of sequence, allelic association, copy number variation (CNV), and transcription. New analytic and bioinformatic tools have permitted the analysis of ever larger and more complex multiomic datasets. At the same time, a broader knowledge base of regulatory loci in the genome has increased our understanding of the function of intronic and intergenic regions of the genome.

Using these advances, gene variants influencing risk for most neuropsychiatric diseases have been identified. Solid evidence now supports specific common and rare risk-increasing variants for most neuropsychiatric diseases.

CLINICAL EPIDEMIOLOGY: TWIN, FAMILY, AND ADOPTION STUDIES

Three types of population genetic studies—twin, family, and adoption studies—are conducted to ascertain whether a particular human phenomenon is substantially genetically influenced.

Twin studies are based on the fact that monozygotic (MZ) or identical twins represent a natural experiment in which two individuals have exactly the same DNA sequence for each of their genes. This is in contrast to dizygotic (DZ) or fraternal twins, who share 50% of their DNA sequences and are no more genetically similar than any pair of siblings. A phenomenon that is influenced by genetic factors should be more "concordant" (similar) in MZ twins compared to DZ twins.

Family studies can answer three critical questions concerning the inheritance of a disorder:

1. Are relatives of an affected subject at **increased risk** for the disorder compared to relatives of control subjects?
2. What other disorders are found at increased rates among the relatives of an individual with a given illness, compared to relatives of control subjects? Is there a **spectrum**?

3. Can a specific mode of inheritance be discerned? All major psychiatric disorders now appear to be **polygenic** and **multifactorial**.

A family study typically begins with a **proband** or initially ascertained patient, whose relatives are then studied.

> Nurnberger JI Jr, Wiegand R, Bucholz K, et al: A family study of alcohol dependence: coaggregation of multiple disorders in relatives of alcohol-dependent probands. *Arch Gen Psychiatry* 2004;61:1246–1256.

In **adoption studies**, the risk for the disorder may be evaluated in four groups of relatives: the adoptive and biological relatives of affected adoptees and the adoptive and biological relatives of control adoptees. If the disorder is heritable, one should find an increased risk among the biological relatives of affected subjects, compared to the other three groups of relatives. One can also compare risk for illness in adopted-away children of ill parents versus adopted-away children of well parents.

Segregation analysis may be used to determine whether the pattern of illness in families is consistent with a specific mode of transmission (most useful for conditions in which a single gene accounts for a substantial portion of the variance). Some of the complexities of major psychiatric disorders are as follows:

Variable penetrance (some individuals with strong genetic predisposition will not manifest the disease)

Phenocopies (individuals with very limited genetic predisposition who manifest the symptoms of the disease)

Genetic heterogeneity (multiple combinations of risk-increasing alleles can produce the same syndrome)

The diagnostic boundaries of a syndrome may be uncertain

Pleiotropy (the same allele may increase risk for various phenotypes in a population)

Linkage Analysis

At any genetic locus, each individual carries two copies of the DNA sequence that defines that locus (alleles). One of these alleles is inherited from the mother and the other from the father. These alleles will be transmitted with equal probability (i.e., ½), one of the two alleles to each offspring. If two genetic loci are "close" to each other on a chromosome, their alleles tend to be inherited together (not independently) and they are known as "linked" loci. During meiosis, crossing over (also known as **recombination**) can occur between homologous chromosomes, thus accounting for the observation that alleles at linked loci are not *always* inherited together.

The rate at which crossing over occurs between two linked loci is directly proportional to the distance on the chromosome between them. In fact, the genetic distance between two linked loci is defined in terms of the percentage of recombination between the two loci (this value is known as **theta**). Loci that are "far" apart on a chromosome will have a 1 in 2 chance of being inherited together and they are not linked. Thus, the maximum value for theta is 0.5, whereas the minimum value is 0. Linkage analysis is a method for estimating theta for two or more loci.

Although linkage analysis has been tremendously valuable in the study of Mendelian disordrers in medicine, it has not generally been useful in studies of major psychiatric disorders, as these disorders appear to be complex in their inheritance patterns. With advances in molecular genetic techniques, genome-wide association studies and sequencing studies have supplanted linkage studies in most cases. However, linkage studies have identified rare loci of substantial effect. Examples include three subtypes of early onset Alzheimer disease (AD) caused by amyloid precursor protein, or presenilin 1 or presenilin 2.

Libiger O, Schork NJ: A basic overview of contemporary human genetic analysis strategies. In: Nurnberger JI Jr, Berrettini W (eds). *Principles of Psychiatric Genetics*. Cambridge: Cambridge University Press, 2012.

Association Studies and Candidate Gene Studies

In association studies one compares allele frequencies for a given locus in two populations, one of which is composed of unrelated individuals who have a disease, while the "control" population is usually composed of ethnically similar unrelated persons who do not have the disease. If a particular allele commonly predisposes individuals to the disease in question, then that allele should occur more frequently in the diseased population, compared to the control population.

There are potential pitfalls to the case-control association approach. False-positive results can occur if the two populations are not carefully matched for ethnic background. One alternative control group is the parents of affected individuals (the alleles *not* transmitted to the affected child compose the "control group"—this is known as the Transmission Disequilibrium Test or TDT).

Association studies using a preselected "candidate gene" were often conducted several decades ago, but are less common since the advent of genomewide association studies in about 2006. Reviews have demonstrated that most candidate gene hypotheses of psychiatric disorders have not been supported by genome-wide association studies (GWAS) studies and nearly all earlier positive reports of common alleles being associated with a psychiatric disorder are now generally regarded as false positives. Notable exceptions include the association of APOE4 alleles in late-onset Alzheimer's disease (rs7412 and rs429358) and the association of an OPRM1 allele in opioid use disorder (rs1799971).

Seifuddin F, Mahon PB, Judy J, et al: Meta-analysis of genetic association studies on bipolar disorder. *Am J Med Genet B Neuropsychiatr Genet* 2012 Jul;159B(5):508–518. doi: 10.1002/ajmg.b.32057. Epub 2012 May 9. PMID: 22573399.

MOLECULAR GENETIC METHODS

A class of common DNA markers, known as **single nucleotide polymorphisms (SNPs)**, are now usually used to detect association. An SNP is a variation at one base in a DNA sequence (e.g., compare GATACA with GATGCA, in which the fourth nucleotide can be either the "A" allele or the "G" allele). It is estimated that there are at least several million common (allele frequency > 1% in at least one ethnicity) SNPs in the human genome, evenly distributed across the 3 billion bases of the human genome.

Genome-wide Association Studies

GWAS were introduced in 2006. They were made possible by chip technology in which as many as ~5 million common SNPs may be genotyped by incubating a person's fragmented genomic DNA with one such chip. This methodology enables examination of virtually every gene in the genome with multiple SNPs and, because of linkage disequilibrium (the fact that nearby variants tend to be transmitted together not only within families but also across a population), even detection of association with alleles some distance from the actual SNP tested is possible. The major limitation of GWAS studies is data interpretation, since the number of simultaneous tests is massive, requiring complex statistical corrections because not all events are independent. The presently accepted standard is a p value of 5×10^{-8} or smaller for an SNP association with a phenotype in a GWAS study, based on empirical probability of a type I error. Because the effect size of variants associated with psychiatric disorders is generally quite small (odds ratios of 1.01–1.2 are the norm), achieving p values that meet this threshold requires very large sample sizes. Thousands of complex traits such as height, weight, blood pressure, cognitive ability and disease risk have now been analyzed extensively with GWAS methods, including sample sizes approaching or exceeding 1,000,000 individuals. These samples are achievable now only by extensive collaborations involving multiple sites, across at

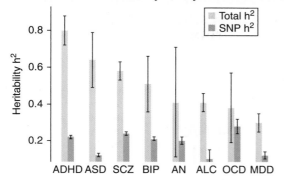

Total & SNP Heritability for Psychiatric Disorders

▲ **Figure 3-1** Comparison of total heritability (based on twin studies) and SNP heritability (based on the single nucleotide polymorphisms (SNPs) assessed in a genome-wide association study). The difference between the two for each disorder may be due to interactions between loci, epigenetic effects, and rare variants, among other factors. ADHD, Attention-deficit hyperactivity disorder, ASD, Autism spectrum disorder, SCZ, Schizophrenia, BIP, Bipolar diorder, AN, Anorexia nervosa, ALC, Alcohol use disorder, OCD, Obsessivecompulsive disorder, MDD, Major depressive disorder. (From Pettersson et al, Psychological Medicine, 2019, PMID: 30221610.)

least several continents. Each set of cases should be matched with controls from a similar ethnic background because of the extensive variation in allele frequencies on the basis of ancestry. This ethnic variability is generally assessed formally using multidimensional scaling (MDS) or a similar method.

GWAS methods have now proven to be useful in psychiatric disorders, with hundreds of common risk alleles identified for schizophrenia, bipolar disorder and unipolar depression, and studies in many other disorders underway. Recent statistical analyses show that common variants indexed by GWAS likely account for 25–30% of the heritability for major psychiatric disorders (Figure 3-1).

It will be very valuable to assemble the large samples of cases necessary to identify those variants specifically and to understand the biologic pathways that they perturb. Additional variance will be explained by gene–gene interaction (known as epistasis) and rare variants.

Output from a GWAS study is usually displayed in a plot of individual SNP association *p* value versus genomic location (indexing each chromosome). This is often referred to as a **"Manhattan plot,"** because of its resemblance to a city skyline (Figure 3-2).

In recent years, it has become increasingly recognized that GWAS studies in psychiatric disorders are substantially biased toward inclusion of subjects of European ancestry. This is a problem in terms of scientific and clinical equity since findings from subjects from one ancestry do not always

apply to those of other ancestries. It has also been noted that transancestral studies, with good representation of subjects of other ancestries, may be more successful at identifying functional risk loci. For these reasons massive efforts are now underway to broaden the scope of GWAS studies to include subjects from African, Asian, and Latino ancestries and increasing attention is being paid to indigenous populations who may have distinctive ancestral genetic histories.

Approximately a decade ago, a technique of polygenic risk score (PRS) was developed to assess the extent to which GWAS results explained the total heritability (estimated from twin and family studies) for a trait. A PRS is a single value estimate of an individual's common allele genetic liability to a phenotype, calculated as a sum of their genome-wide genotypes, each risk allele weighted by a corresponding effect size estimate (or Z-scores) derived from GWAS data. In practice PRS is calculated by summing all GWAS risk alleles surpassing an assumed level of statistical significance (e.g., $p < 0.05$, 0.01, or 0.001), weighted by the effect size of the allele on risk, using GWAS data. There may be as many as 100,000 such "risk" alleles in a GWAS, each contributing a very small amount to the PRS. In more recent methods, all SNPs are included in the PRS calculation. The PRS (also designated as PGS for polygenic score) has been useful to assess the degree to which common alleles for one disorder (or trait) overlap with those of another disorder or trait, as shown in the analysis by below Lee et al. (2013).

Genetic overlap, or coheritability, may also be observed by correlation of genetic effects using all common SNPs examined in genomewide association studies. One observation using these methods was that most of the genetic variation explaining schizophrenia and bipolar disorder is in fact shared between the two conditions (Figure 3-3).

▶ Sequencing Studies

Large-scale sequencing studies have been completed for many major psychiatric disorders, including autism, schizophrenia, unipolar and bipolar disorder. The two strategies generally employed are whole genome sequencing and exome sequencing, the former involving determination of every base pair in a subject's genome and the latter involving just the ~2% of the genome that is directly transcribed or lies in adjacent regulatory regions. An important variable in sequencing endeavors is the "read frequency," or the number of times that an area is analyzed for sequence information. Up to 30× coverage may be necessary to identify some rare mutations precisely, but 8× may be sufficient to identify most variants. The major advantage of sequencing over GWAS is that sequencing allows for identification of rare variants (e.g., <1% frequency in cases), some of which have large effects on illness vulnerability.

Analysis of whole genomic sequence data presents challenging computational problems, because there are 3×10^9 datapoints per person, including several hundred thousand rare variants and 250–300 loss-of-function variants in annotated genes in each person's genome. How does one identify

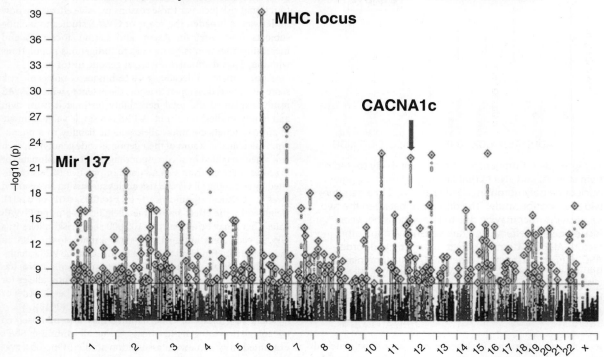

SZ Working Group of the Psychiatric Genetics Consortium GWAS of 76,755 persons with SZ and 243,649 control individuals.

▲ **Figure 3–2** Example of a Manhattan plot for a genomewide association study. The x-axis shows loci across the genome, organized by chromosome. The y-axis shows the *p*-value for association between locus and disease at each locus. The generally accepted threshold for genomewide significance is 5 × 10-8, if only one phenotype is analyzed. More extreme *p*-values may be required for analysis of multiple phenotypes in the same population. (Reproduced with permission from Trubetskoy V, Panagiotaropoulou G, Awasthi S, Braun A, Kraft J, Skarabis N et al: Mapping genomic loci implicates genes and synaptic biology in schizophrenia. *Nature.* 2022 Apr;604(7906):502–508.)

the pathogenic variants within these huge datasets? Current studies have relied on lists of genes previously reported to be associated with the disorder in question, as well as strategies of collapsing different variants within single genes or even single regions. We expect that statistical methods will evolve quickly in this area to help answer this question and strengthen the value of sequencing methods for defining the genetics of psychiatric disorders. Already, studies in autism have identified dozens of loss-of-function variants considered pathogenic.

▶ **Copy Number Variation**

Studies of CNVs have been reported over the past two decades in neuropsychiatric disorders. CNVs may be insertions, deletions, duplications, or inversions of hundreds to millions of base pairs. They are not rare and are found across the genome in healthy individuals, but in disease populations, certain CNVs are found at significantly high frequencies for

autism, intellectual disability (ID), schizophrenia, and other disorders. They may either be *inherited* or *de novo,* and the *de novo* events have appeared to be of more importance, at least for the childhood onset disorders. *De novo* status is demonstrated by examination of the parents' genomes and confirmation of the absence of the CNV in them.

Cross-Disorder Group of the Psychiatric Genomics Consortium: identification of risk loci with shared effects on five major psychiatric disorders: a genome-wide analysis. *Lancet* 2013;381: 1371–1379; erratum *Lancet* 2013;381:1360.

Malhotra D, Sebat J: CNVs: harbingers of a rare variant revolution in psychiatric genetics. *Cell* 2012;148(6):1223–1241. (Review)

Peterson RE, Kuchenbaecker K, Walters RK, et al: Genome-wide association studies in ancestrally diverse populations: opportunities, methods, pitfalls, and recommendations. *Cell* 2019 Oct 17;179(3):589–603. doi: 10.1016/j.cell.2019.08.051. Epub 2019 Oct 10. PMID: 31607513.

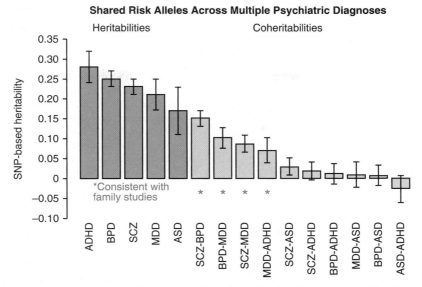

Shared Risk Alleles Across Multiple Psychiatric Diagnoses

▲ **Figure 3–3** Heritability and coheritability for common disorders. The first five columns of the figure presents SNP heritability estimates for Attention-Deficit Hyperactivity Disorder, Bipolar Disorder, Schizophrenia, Major Depressive Disorder, and Autism Spectrum Disorder. Columns 6–15 shows the genetic covariance (coheritability) between allele frequencies for SNPs assessed in each pair of disorders. The relationship between coheritability and SNP heritability for each pair of disorders gives an estimate of shared genetic influences (e.g., 0.68 + 0.04 for schizophrenia and bipolar disorder). (Reproduced with permission from Lee SH, Ripke S, Neale BM, et al: Genetic relationship between five psychiatric disorders estimated from genome-wide SNPs. *Nat Genet* 2013; 45:984–994.)

▶ High-Risk Studies

Studies of individuals with psychiatric diseases are always confounded by the issue of disease effects: are differences between affected individuals and controls related to the cause of the disorder, or are they related to the effects of the disorder (or its treatment)? When investigating possible differences for a genetic disease, this difficult issue can be addressed by studying a group of individuals (usually adolescents or young adults) who are at high risk to develop the disorder under study (usually because they have parents and/or other relatives with the disorder). The high-risk group may then be followed over time to assess whether the abnormalities observed are truly predictive of the disease.

Nurnberger JI Jr, McInnis M, Reich W, et al: A high-risk study of bipolar disorder: childhood clinical phenotypes as precursors of major mood disorders. *Arch Gen Psychiatry* 2011;68(10): 1003–1011.

Schuckit MA, Smith TL, Chacko Y: Evaluation of a depression-related model of alcohol problems in 430 probands from the San Diego prospective study. *Drug Alcohol Depend* 2006;82(3): 194–203.

▶ Epigenetics of Psychiatric Disorders

Epigenetics is the study of heritable biological modifiers of DNA transcription. The most common mechanisms discussed are (1) DNA methylation at cytosine residues in the promoter region of a gene and (2) chromatin remodeling. Methylation of DNA effectively prevents transcription of a particular gene. Chromatin (the protein framework supporting DNA in the nucleus) may exist in an active state (allowing transcription) or an inactive state (preventing transcription). Various stimuli, including environmental events, may be responsible for epigenetic changes that turn genes on or off. Substantial additional gene regulation occurs at the level of RNA transcription, including by regulatory micro RNAs (miRNA).

Differential methylation does appear to be important in Prader-Willi syndrome, which includes intellectual disabiltity, disordered eating and sometimes mood disorders as part of the clinical picture. This condition is related to imprinting on 15q; the DNA segment for this chromosomal region that is transcribed is generally the segment from the father. The mother's DNA from that region tends to be methylated and not transcribed. In Prader-Willi, there is deletion of the father's DNA in that region as well, so neither segment is functional. In Angelman syndrome, there is usually duplication of the father's chromosome, or uniparental disomy.

ALCOHOL USE DISORDERS

1. Epidemiologic Genetic Studies

A. Twin Studies

Twin studies tend to show heritability of drinking behavior (about 40%) and heritability of alcoholism (about 40–60%). More recently, genome-wide association studies demonstrate that about 10–20% of the variance in prevalence of alcohol use disorder (AUD) appears to be related to detectable common genetic variation.

B. Adoption Studies

Adoption studies of AUD have generally been consistent with genetic hypotheses. Starting with adoption data, Cloninger, Bohman, and Sigvardsson postulated a familial distinction of AUD: a milieu-limited (type I) and a male-limited (type II) group. Persons with type I usually have onset after age 25, manifest problems with loss of control, and have a great deal of guilt and fear about alcohol use. Persons with type II have onset before age 25, are unable to abstain from alcohol, and have fights and arrests when drinking, but less frequently show loss of control and guilt and fear about alcohol use.

C. Family Studies

A report from the Collaborative Study of the Genetics of Alcoholism (Nurnberger et al, 2004, referenced in Methods section) shows significant coaggregation of drug dependence, mood disorders, and anxiety disorders as well as alcohol dependence in the relatives of persons with AUD.

2. Disorders Genetically Related to AUD

Winokur reported an increased prevalence of depression in the female relatives of patients with AUD, roughly comparable to the increased prevalence of AUD in male relatives. Some forms of illness may result from shared vulnerability factors. Recent studies suggest that comorbid disorders (including AUD and affective illness) themselves run in families.

Bohman and Cloninger observed that adopted-away daughters of type II (male-limited) alcoholics manifest no increase in alcoholism but do show an increase in somatization disorder.

Persons with AUD and antisocial personality disorder may transmit both AUD and sociopathy as part of the same syndrome.

Offspring of persons with AUD appear to have a greater risk for conduct disorder and related conditions.

4. Association Studies

ADH—Alcohol dehydrogenase (ADH) is the major metabolic enzyme for alcohol, catalyzing its breakdown into acetaldehyde, which is then further metabolized by aldehyde dehydrogenase (ALDH). Both the *ADH* and *ALDH* genes have variants that have been associated with the "flushing" reaction to alcohol (a feeling of warmth that is accompanied by reddening of the skin and sometimes nausea and tachycardia). These variants are most common in East Asian populations, and they tend to protect against the development of AUD. In recent studies, single nucleotide polymorphisms in some of the ADH enzymes (genes for several isoenzymes of ADH are located on chromosome 4q) have been associated with AUD in European-origin populations and in Native Americans. The strongest single finding is in the *ADH1B* gene, and a variant at this locus appears to be associated with early onset of regular drinking.

DRD2—Originally reported about a decade ago, a meta-analysis of 21 studies shows an increased risk of 50–100% for persons carrying a variant in this gene. Recent GWAS studies confirm this association.

▶ Genome-wide Association Studies

GWAS studies have been reported using phenotypes related to AUD and alcohol consumption. To the surprise of many investigators, the genetic correlation between consumption and AUD is modest (~50%).

A recent GWAS featured >1 million subjects of multiple ethnicities (see below). *ADH1B* variation is strongly associated with AUD and variants at other *ADH* genes are associated as well. *DRD2* variation is also prominently associated, as is *FTO*, a gene related to fat mass and obesity.

Zhou H et al: Multi-ancestry study of the genetics of problematic alcohol use in over 1 million individuals. *Nat Med* 2023 Dec; 29(12), 3184–3192. doi: 10.1038/s41591-023-02653-5. PMID: 38062264.

▶ Endophenotypes

A poorly synchronized resting EEG (lower alpha) has been thought to be related to AUD predisposition. Changes in beta and theta rhythms have also been demonstrated. Measurements of event-related potentials have shown smaller P300 waves following visual stimuli in 7- to 13-year-old sons of persons with AUD compared to controls. Low P300 appears to be a familial marker of the predisposition to AUD. Schuckit has studied behavioral and neuroendocrine responses to alcohol administration in a series of high-risk populations. Offspring of fathers with AUD displayed less subjective intoxication than controls. A follow-up identified decreased subjective intoxication as a risk factor for later development of an AUD. Intravenous infusion studies of alcohol have suggested a more complex dissection of subjective effects but continue to show differences in response based on familial risk.

King AC, Cao D, deWit H, et al: The role of alcohol response phenotypes in the risk for alcohol use disorder. *BJPsych Open.* 2019 Apr 22;5(3):e38. doi: 10.1192/bjo.2019.18. PMID: 31685074.

Kranzler HR, Zhou H, Kember RL, et al: Genome-wide association study of alcohol consumption and use disorder in 274,424 individuals from multiple populations. *Nat Commun* 2019 Apr 2; 10(1):1499. doi: 10.1038/s41467-019-09480-8. PMID: 30940813.

Salvatore JE, Han S, Farris SP, et al: Beyond genome-wide significance: integrative approaches to the interpretation and extension of GWAS findings for alcohol use disorder. *Addict Biol* 2019 Mar;24(2):275–289. doi: 10.1111/adb.12591. Epub 2018 Jan 9. PMID: 29316088.

Saunders GRB, Wang X, Chen F, et al: Genetic diversity fuels gene discovery for tobacco and alcohol use. *Nature* 2022 Dec;612 (7941):720–724. doi: 10.1038/s41586-022-05477-4. Epub 2022 Dec 7. PMID: 36477530.

ALZHEIMER DISEASE

Genetic etiologies are clear for some forms of AD. Early-onset cases are more likely to be hereditary and may be determined by single genes. Later-onset cases are more likely to be multifactorial.

Family Studies

Most of the relatives of later-onset AD probands will have died of other causes before passing the age of risk. However, the risk to siblings of probands whose age of onset was less than 70 years is close to 50% if they have an affected parent. The morbid risk may be 40% for first-degree relatives of a proband with AD when the relative reaches age 90. Heun reported a 30% incidence of dementia in first-degree relatives of Alzheimer probands compared to 22% in controls.

A subset of early-onset AD cases is highly familial. At least some AD cases (primarily those with later onset) are sporadic (no close relatives affected).

Molecular Genetic Studies

In 1987, St. George-Hyslop et al reported linkage of familial AD to restriction fragment length polymorphism (RFLP) markers on chromosome 21. Subsequently, certain isolated, rare AD families have been found to have a point mutation in the gene for amyloid precursor protein. These studies suggest that abnormalities in this gene (encoding the amyloid protein, which accumulates in the form of "plaques" in the extracellular space in brains of persons with AD) can cause the disease by itself. Another cause of early-onset familial Alzheimer is a gene on chromosome 14 (*presenilin 1*), while other families are linked to a gene on chromosome 1 (*presenilin 2*). These two genes are highly homologous.

Many late-onset families show linkage to a region of chromosome 19 coding for lipoprotein E (usually abbreviated as ApoE), which is also implicated in cardiovascular illness. One copy of the E4 allele will increase AD risk fourfold compared to that with E2. Two copies of E4 increase risk by a factor of ~12. The influence of APoE4 is detectable in most ethnic groups. The molecular mechanisms for the Alzheimer vulnerability genes are now the subject of intense investigation. There is reason to suspect that they all affect the accumulation of amyloid and the phosphoprotein tau, which is found in neurofibrillary tangles.

Apart from the large effect size of ApoE alleles, the remaining common risk alleles for AD have comparatively small influences on risk. A recent GWAS publication of more than 111,000 AD cases and 677,000 controls revealed 75 risk loci, including 42 new to this publication. All the alleles except ApoE4 were of small effect. Tau, amyloid, microglia and tumor necrosis factor alpha pathways were implicated in the analyses. The roles of these genes in the pathogenesis of AD are poorly understood (Figure 3–4).

ANTISOCIAL PERSONALITY DISORDER

Twin Studies

Recent twin studies show stability of antisocial personality characteristics over time and some overlap between antisocial traits and borderline personality disorder traits.

Adoption Studies

Adoption studies (primarily in Scandinavian countries with central records for both adoption and criminality) have tended to show both genetic and environmental influences on antisocial personality disorder (AP). In an adoption study by Cloninger, when environmental factors predisposed to criminality, 6.7% of male adoptees were criminal compared to 2.9% of male adoptees with nonpredisposing postnatal and genetic backgrounds. When the genetic background, but not the postnatal environment, was predisposing, 12.1% of male adoptees were criminal compared to 2.9% of control male adoptees. When both genetic and postnatal backgrounds were judged to predispose to criminal behavior, 40% of male adoptees were criminal. These results are consistent with the additive effects of genes and postnatal influences. The environmental influences implicated were multiple foster homes (for men) and extensive institutional care (for women).

Epidemiologic Studies: Family Studies

Of 223 male criminals, 80% were found to have a diagnosis of AP in a study by Guze. Sixteen percent of interviewed male first-degree relatives also had this diagnosis, whereas only 2% of female relatives had AP, compared to 3% and 1% in the relatives of controls. Increased rates of alcoholism and drug abuse were also found among the first-degree relatives of these criminals.

A family study of 66 female felons and 228 of their first-degree relatives revealed increased rates for AP (18%), alcoholism (29%), drug abuse (3%), and hysteria (similar to DSM-5 somatic symptom disorder) (31%) in the relatives, all the hysteria occurring in the female relatives. Predictably,

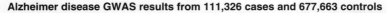

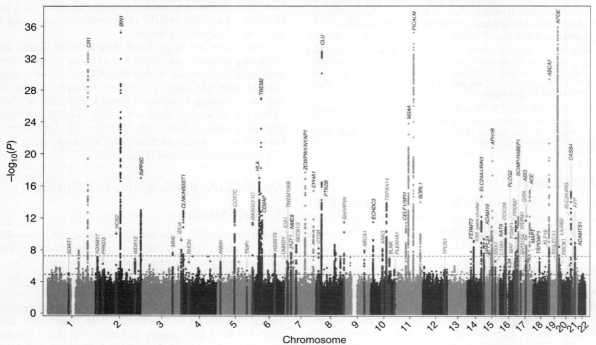

▲ **Figure 3–4** Manhattan plot for genomewide association study of Alzheimer disease. (Reproduced from Bellenguez C, Küçükali F, Jansen IE, Kleineidam L, Moreno-Grau S, Amin N, Naj AC, et al. New insights into the genetic etiology of Alzheimer's disease and related dementias. *Nat Genet.* 2022;54(4):412–436.)

male relatives had a threefold increase in AP (31%) compared to the female relatives (11%). The increased risk for AP among first-degree relatives of female felons (31%) compared to the risk for relatives of male felons (16%) may suggest greater genetic (or environmental) risk factors in female felons as compared to male felons.

▶ Cytogenetic Studies

Several reports have suggested that the prevalence of XYY males in prisons and penal/mental institutions is higher than the prevalence in the general population. The XYY karyotype is associated with slightly lower than normal intelligence, tall stature, and cystic acne. This karyotype is found in approximately 1 in 1000 male newborns. Hook found XYY in 1 in 53 of 3813 males in 20 penal/mental institutions. Witkin surveyed all tall Danish men from a birth cohort, finding 12 of 4139 (0.29%) who had the XYY anomaly. Five of these 12 XYY men had a criminal record, primarily petty criminality. Witkin suggests that lower than average intelligence may account for the excess of criminal activity among XYY males. This karyotype does not seem to be associated with a predisposition to impulsive violence, as once thought.

▶ Biological Markers

Nielsen identified a variant of the *tryptophan hydroxylase* gene (which codes for the synthetic enzyme for serotonin) associated with low 5-hydroxyindoleacetic acid (5-HIAA) in cerebrospinal fluid and suicide attempts in violent criminal offenders. Low 5-HIAA has been associated with impulsivity and violence in experimental colonies of rhesus monkeys. A Dutch family was reported with lowered monoamine oxidase A activity caused by a point mutation on the eighth exon of the *MAOA* gene. Males with this mutation (both *MAO* genes are on the X chromosome) show impulsive aggression, arson, attempted rape, and exhibitionism. It is likely that other familial monoamine defects will be found to be associated with aggressive behavior.

For various reasons, including modern interpretations of ethical limitations on research among prisoners, it has been difficult to study large samples of persons with antisocial behavior in relation to genetically predisposing factors, and genomewide studies have yet to be undertaken in these conditions.

▶ GWAS studies

A recent meta-analysis of multiple GWAS studies of related traits found that variation in *FOXP2* and its target gene

CNTNAP2 were associated with antisocial phenotypes in an animal model and in man. The authors were also able to establish substantial genetic covariation between antisocial behavior and Conduct Disorder and Depression, with negative relationships between antisocial behavior and intelligence and educational attainment.

A large GWAS of externalizing behavioral traits was able to derive PRSs (see methods) for antisocial phenotypes and a number of related phenotypes.

Barr PB, Dick DM. The genetics of externalizing problems. *Curr Top Behav Neurosci* 2020;47:93–112. doi: 10.1007/7854_2019_120. PMID: 31845132.

Karlsson Linnér R, Mallard TT, Barr PB, et al: Multivariate analysis of 1.5 million people identifies genetic associations with traits related to self-regulation and addiction. *Nat Neurosci* 2021 Oct;24(10):1367–1376. doi: 10.1038/s41593-021-00908-3. Epub 2021 Aug 26. PMID: 34446935.

Tielbeek JJ, Uffelmann E, Williams BS, et al: Uncovering the genetic architecture of broad antisocial behavior through a genome-wide association study meta-analysis. *Mol Psychiatry* 2022 Nov;27(11):4453-4463. doi: 10.1038/s41380-022-01793-3. Epub 2022 Oct 25. PMID: 36284158.

ANXIETY DISORDERS

The increased familial risk for anxiety disorders has been known for more than 100 years. Disorder types are often mixed within families, which may include subjects with panic disorder, phobic disorders, and generalized anxiety disorder. One family study of pure panic disorder probands found a significantly higher risk of panic episodes among first-degree relatives compared to relatives of controls. There was a fivefold increase in risk for any anxiety disorder. Similarly, an increased (11.6%) risk for agoraphobia has been reported for the relatives of agoraphobic probands, compared to 1.9% for relatives of panic probands and 1.5% for control probands. A study of simple phobia found an increased risk (31%) for simple phobia among relatives of probands with that diagnosis (but no other anxiety disorder) compared to relatives of well probands (11%). A family history study of social phobia demonstrated that relatives of phobic probands are at increased risk for this disorder (6.6%) compared to relatives of panic disorder probands (0.4%) or relatives of controls (2.2%).

A separate genetic transmission for generalized anxiety disorder has not been established. Thus, although there is some evidence for familial transmission of generalized anxiety, the transmission may not be specific.

▷ Twin Studies

In a Norwegian sample, the concordance of all anxiety disorders for MZ twins (34.4%) was significantly greater than that for DZ twins (17.0%).

▷ Association Studies

A GWAS report of scores (ranging from 0 to 6) on a generalized anxiety disorder screening questionnaire, the GAD-2, has implicated diverse common alleles as conveying very small amounts of risk (Levey et al, 2020). These alleles were in the *SATB1* gene, a regulator of gene expression, the *MAD1L1* gene (implicated in bipolar disorder and schizophrenia genetics) and the estrogen receptor alpha gene (*ESR1*).

Levey DF, Gelernter J, Polimanti R, et al: Reproducible genetic risk loci for anxiety: results from ~200,000 participants in the million veteran program. *Am J Psychiatry* 2020;177:223–232.

ATTENTION-DEFICIT HYPERACTIVITY DISORDER

Twin studies suggest that attention-deficit hyperactivity disorder (ADHD) has a substantial heritability, estimated at ~80% (Faraone and Larsson, 2019). As is true in most complex psychiatric disorders, the SNP-based heritability is much smaller, estimated at 28% (Lee et al, 2013). The remaining heritability may be explained partially by CNVs, which have been detected in ADHD kindreds (Martin et al, 2020).

▷ Genome-wide Association Studies

A meta-analysis of ADHD, including 38,691 persons with ADHD and 186,843 controls identified 27 genome-wide significant loci (Demontis et al, 2023). These loci were found among genes active in early brain development. ADHD genetic risk was enriched in genes associated with midbrain dopaminergic neurons, a fact consistent with the efficacy of genes activating brain presynaptic dopamine release.

Demontis D, Walters GB, Athanasiadis G, et al: *Nature Genetics* 2023 Feb;55(2):198–208.

Faraone SV, Larsson H: Genetics of attention deficit hyperactivity disorder. *Mol Psychiatry* 2019;24:562–575.

Martin J, Hosking G, Wadon M, et al: A brief report: de novo copy number variants in children with attention deficit hyperactivity disorder. *Transl Psychiatry* 2020;10:1–6.

AUTISM SPECTRUM DISORDER (PERVASIVE DEVELOPMENTAL DISORDER)

The frequency of autism spectrum disorder (ASD) in siblings of ASD probands has consistently remained elevated at several times the population rate, even with increased diagnosis in recent years. The overall heritability of autism is estimated at 60–70%.

What is striking about the genetics of autism is its association with multiple single-gene disorders. The most clearly documented of these disorders is the fragile X syndrome.

Perhaps 8% of autistic subjects have the cytogenetic fragile X; 40–50% of fragile X males may have autism spectrum disorder. There are also probable associations between autism and tuberous sclerosis, neurofibromatosis, and phenylketonuria (Table 3-1).

The recent literature on autism genetics has been dominated by three types of reports: (1) CNVs, (2) sequence variants, and (3) common variant influences based on GWAS.

▶ Copy Number Variant Studies of Autism

Sebat et al reported *de novo* (found in the subject but not in parents) CNVs in 7% of subjects with autism compared to 1% of controls. When he divided subjects into simplex (one affected per family) or multiplex (multiple affected subjects per family), the simplex subjects had a 10% rate of CNVs. Pinto et al found that the difference between cases and controls was

Table 3–1 List of the More Common Copy Number Variants Found in Persons With Autism Spectrum Disorder

	ASD Penetrance (rate of ASD in carriers)	Neuropsychiatric Pleiotropy (associated neuropsychiatric phenotypes)	Somatic Pleiotropy (associated somatic phenotypes)
Del1q21.1	8%	ID, ADHD, schizophrenia	Microcephaly, heart defect, eye abnormalities, short stature, epilepsy
Dup1q21.1	36%	ID, ADHD, schizophrenia, speech delay	Epilepsy, macrocephaly, heart defect
Del2q23.1	100%	ID, ADHD, language disorder, motor delay	Epilepsy, obesity, brachycephaly, microcephaly, short stature
Del2q37	25%–42%	ID, ADHD	Epilepsy, short stature, obesity, heart defect
Del3q29	27%	ID, speech delay, language disorder, anxiety disorder, schizophrenia, bipolar disorder	Gastrointestinal problems, heart defect, feeding problems, recurrent ear infections, abnormal dentition
Del5q14.3	43%	ID, absent speech	Epilepsy, capillary malformation
Dup7q11.23	41%	ID, ADHD, anxiety disorder, oppositional defiant disorders, speech delay	Epilepsy, macrocephaly, brachycephaly dilatation of ascending aorta, patent ductus arteriosus, chronic obstipation, kidney abnormalities
Del8p23		ID, ADHD	Heart defect, congenital diaphragmatic hernia
Dup15q11-q13	69%	ID, ADHD	Epilepsy, defect, muscle hypotonia, short stature
Del15q11.2	32%	ID, ADHD, schizophrenia, OCD, speech delay	Epilepsy, ataxia, defect
Dup15q11.2	43%	ID, ADHD, speech delay	Epilepsy, ataxia, hypotonia
Dup15q13.2–q13.3	80%	ID, speech delay	Epilepsy, urogenital anomalies, recurrent infections
Del15q13.2–q13.3	60%	ID, ADHD	
Del16p11.2	15%	ID	Epilepsy, hypotonia, sacral dimples, speech articulation problems
Dup16p11.2		Schizophrenia, bipolar disorder	Epilepsy, hypotonia, tremor, ataxia, sacral dimples, speech articulation problems
Dup16p13.11	25%	ADHD, speech delay	Epilepsy
Del17p11.2	Unknown		Epilepsy
Del17q12		Schizophrenia	Macrocephaly, renal anomalies
Del22q11.2	30%	Schizophrenia, ADHD, speech delay, anxiety disorders	(amongst others:) Heart defect, palate abnormalities, hypocalcaemia, feeding difficulties, recurrent infections
Dup22q11.2	18%	ID, ADHD	Heart defect, hearing loss, urogenital anomalies, palate abnormalities
Del22q13.3	>50%	ID, language disorder	Epilepsy, heart defect, renal anomalies, strabismus

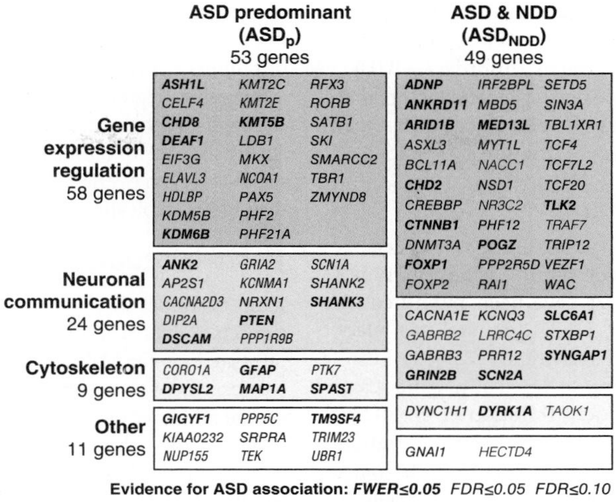

	ASD predominant (ASD$_p$) 53 genes			ASD & NDD (ASD$_{NDD}$) 49 genes		
Gene expression regulation 58 genes	ASH1L	KMT2C	RFX3	ADNP	IRF2BPL	SETD5
	CELF4	KMT2E	RORB	ANKRD11	MBD5	SIN3A
	CHD8	KMT5B	SATB1	ARID1B	MED13L	TBL1XR1
	DEAF1	LDB1	SKI	ASXL3	MYT1L	TCF4
	EIF3G	MKX	SMARCC2	BCL11A	NACC1	TCF7L2
	ELAVL3	NCOA1	TBR1	CHD2	NSD1	TCF20
	HDLBP	PAX5	ZMYND8	CREBBP	NR3C2	TLK2
	KDM5B	PHF2		CTNNB1	PHF12	TRAF7
	KDM6B	PHF21A		DNMT3A	POGZ	TRIP12
				FOXP1	PPP2R5D	VEZF1
				FOXP2	RAI1	WAC
Neuronal communication 24 genes	ANK2	GRIA2	SCN1A	CACNA1E	KCNQ3	SLC6A1
	AP2S1	KCNMA1	SHANK2	GABRB2	LRRC4C	STXBP1
	CACNA2D3	NRXN1	SHANK3	GABRB3	PRR12	SYNGAP1
	DIP2A	PTEN		GRIN2B	SCN2A	
	DSCAM	PPP1R9B				
Cytoskeleton 9 genes	CORO1A	GFAP	PTK7	DYNC1H1	DYRK1A	TAOK1
	DPYSL2	MAP1A	SPAST			
Other 11 genes	GIGYF1	PPP5C	TM9SF4	GNAI1	HECTD4	
	KIAA0232	SRPRA	TRIM23			
	NUP155	TEK	UBR1			

Evidence for ASD association: *FWER≤0.05* *FDR≤0.05* *FDR≤0.10*

▲ **Figure 3–5** Genes containing rare variants associated with autism spectrum disorder (ASD). On the left are genes with variants associated with ASD and not with other neurodevelopmental disorders (NDD). On the right are genes associated with NDD in general (including ASD). The divisions on the y-axis show predominant gene functions for each group. The shading for each gene shows the strength of evidence corrected for multiple testing. (Reproduced with permission from Satterstrom FK, Kosmicki JA, Wang J, et al. Large-Scale Exome Sequencing Study Implicates Both Developmental and Functional Changes in the Neurobiology of Autism. *Cell.* 2020;180(3):568–584.)

particularly striking when considering CNVs that disrupted genes implicated in autism and intellectual disability on the basis of cytogenetic reports. Current studies implicate more than 20 chromosomal regions that are associated with autism spectrum conditions. CNVs are commonly detected by chromosomal microarray or whole exome sequencing.

Sequencing Studies of Autism

Extensive sequencing in subjects with ASDs has identified >100 sequence variants associated with the condition; these are primarily *de novo* and are generally associated with loss of function of the gene product. Prominent gene functions include gene expression regulation and neuronal communication. The studies have included both whole exome and whole genome sequencing efforts. Exome sequencing is now commonly recommended for clinical screening of patients with ASD. The clinical yield of genetic screening is generally estimated at 10–15% (Figure 3–5).

Genome-wide Association Studies of Autism

A recent study in >18,000 cases and 27,000 controls identified five significant gene variants associated with ASD plus seven additional variants shared with related phenotypes (schizophrenia, depression, educational attainment). Although individual common variants have very small effects, their combined effects account for most of the heritability of ASD. In contrast, rare variants, including CNV and SNV (single nucleotide variation), account for substantial liability within individuals but much less of the heritability of ASD within the population.

Gaugler T, Klei L, Sanders SJ, et al: Most genetic risk for autism resides with common variation. *Nat Genet* 2014 Aug;46(8): 881–885. doi: 10.1038/ng.3039. Epub 2014 Jul 20. PMID: 25038753.

Grove J, Ripke S, Als TD, et al: Identification of common genetic risk variants for autism spectrum disorder. *Nat Genet* 2019 Mar;51(3):431–444. doi: 10.1038/s41588-019-0344-8. Epub 2019 Feb 25. PMID: 30804558.

Satterstrom FK, Kosmicki JA, Wang J, et al: Large-scale exome sequencing study implicates both developmental and functional changes in the neurobiology of autism. *Cell* 2020 Feb 6;180(3):568–584.e23. doi: 10.1016/j.cell.2019.12.036. Epub 2020 Jan 23. PMID: 31981491.

Vorstman JAS, Parr JR, Moreno-De-Luca D, et al: Autism genetics: opportunities and challenges for clinical translation. *Nat Rev Genet* 2017 Jun;18(6):362–376. doi: 10.1038/nrg.2017.4. Epub 2017 Mar 6. PMID: 28260791.

DRUG USE DISORDERS

Genetic Epidemiology: Twin, Adoption, and Family Studies

A study of the Vietnam Era Twin Registry revealed evidence for a common genetic factor operating across pharmacologic classes. These authors also found evidence for class-specific genetic factors, especially in opioid use disorder, similar to results of a family study. The relatively clear conclusion from twin, family, and adoption studies is that there are general genetic factors increasing risk for drug use disorders (DUDs), and there are pharmacologic class-specific genetic factors that appear to increase risk predominantly for a use disorder limited to a single pharmacologic class of drugs (e.g., opioids).

Association Studies

Multiple large GWAS reports of association between variants in the cluster of nicotinic receptor subunit genes on 15q25 and nicotine use disorder (NUD) have been published. A multiancestral meta-analysis of NUD (derived via electronic health records) in 898,680 individuals (739,895 European, 114,420 African American, 44,365 Latin American) identified 72 independent risk loci (Toikumo et al, 2023). One implicated SNP (rs16969968) is a missense variation (N398D) in the alpha-5 subunit gene (*CHRNA5*). The high-risk (N) allele is deficient in fluxing calcium in cellular models. The high-risk allele also remains desensitized to a greater extent after agonist exposure. These results implicate the risk allele as a hypofunctional variant. Several other variants have been identified in nicotinic receptor subunit genes, clearly implicating multiple nicotinic receptor complexes in NUDs.

A multiancestry GWAS report of opioid use disorder (Kember et al, 2022) identified 14 loci, including alleles in the mu opioid receptor gene. Larger sample sizes are needed to identify additional alleles, perhaps because the SNP heritability is only 11%.

Smaller-scale stimulant use disorder (Cox et al, 2021) and cannabis use disorder (Johnson et al, 2020) GWAS reports have identified a small number of loci, but larger sample sizes are needed.

Cox J, Sherva R, Wetherill L, et al: Genome-wide association study of stimulant dependence. *Transl Psychiatry* 2021 Jun 29;11(1):363.

Johnson EC, Demontis D, Thorgeirsson TE, et al: A large-scale genome-wide association study meta-analysis of cannabis use disorder. *Lancet Psychiatry* 2020 Dec;7(12):1032–1045.

Kember RL, Vickers-Smith R, Xu H, et al: Cross-ancestry meta-analysis of opioid use disorder uncovers novel loci with predominant effects in brain regions associated with addiction. *Nature Neuroscience* 2022 25:1279–1287.

Toikumo S, Jennings MV, Pham B, et al: Multi-ancestry meta-analysis of tobacco use disorders based on electronic health record data prioritizes novel candidate risk genes and reveals associations with numerous health outcomes. medRxiv 2023 29:2023.03.27.23287713. doi: 10.1101/2023.03.27.23287713.

EATING DISORDERS

Family Studies

Controlled family studies have been conducted over the past two decades. These studies suggest that there is considerable familial aggregation. The overall pattern suggests substantial risk in family members, with an odds ratio almost certainly greater than 10 and perhaps much larger. There are increased rates of anorexia nervosa (AN) among first-degree relatives of bulimia nervosa (BN) probands, and increased rates of BN among first-degree relatives of AN probands. This clustering of eating disorders in families of AN and BN individuals provides strong support for familial transmission of both disorders and is consistent with overlap in risk alleles. There is diagnostic crossover to BN, typically, in the course of AN over years of illness.

Twin Studies

If one examines the AN twin studies with the largest number of subjects and most appropriate methodology, mean concordance rates are 64% for MZ twins and 14% for DZ twins. Differences between these rates suggest a modest additive heritability with a large influence of nonadditive genetic and/or shared environmental factors. More recent studies have used structural models to estimate the fraction of risk attributable to additive genetic factors. The estimates of heritability range from 0.48 to 0.76.

One of the first twin studies of eating disorders described pairwise concordance of 56% in MZ and 5% in DZ pairs (71% and 10% with probandwise figures). Family history assessment (including additional informant data from parents) showed that 4.9% of the female first-degree relatives and 1.16% of the female second-degree relatives had had anorexia at some point in their lives, a risk considerably higher than the reported population prevalence. The MZ cotwins were much more similar in "body dissatisfaction," "drive to thinness," weight loss, length of amenorrhea, and minimum body mass index (BMI). Estimates indicate that roughly 58–76% of the variance in the liability to AN, and 54–83% of the variance in the liability to BN, can be accounted for by genetic factors. For both AN and BN, the remaining variance in liability appears to be due to unique environmental factors (i.e., factors that are unique to siblings in the same family) rather than shared or common environmental factors (i.e., factors that are shared by siblings in the same family).

Twin studies of the specific symptoms of binge eating, self-induced vomiting, and dietary restraint suggest that these behaviors are roughly 46–72% heritable. Likewise, pathological attitudes such as body dissatisfaction, eating and weight concerns, and weight preoccupation show heritabilities of roughly 32–72%. Taken together, findings suggest a significant genetic component to AN and BN as well as the attitudes and behaviors that contribute to, and correlate with, clinical eating pathology.

Molecular Studies

The first AN GWAS included ~1000 cases, but there were no genome-wide significant findings (Wang et al, 2011). However, a larger study of 16,992 AN cases and 55,525 controls revealed eight genome-wide significant loci, including alleles implicating CADM1, MGMT, FOXP1, and PTBP2. Analysis of genetic correlations with other behavioral traits revealed substantial overlap with OCD, anxiety and major depressive disorder (MDD), but less-than expected overlap with obesity-related traits, such as body fat percentage and BMI. This suggests that the alleles for AN and alleles for obesity may be two extremes of a body weight distribution. Despite searches for rare variants of large effect on AN, none have been identified.

Abdulkadir M, Hübel C, Herle M, Loos RJF, Breen G, Bulik CM, Micali N. The impact of anorexia nervosa and BMI polygenic risk on childhood growth: a 20-year longitudinal population-based study. *Am J Hum Genet* 2022;109:1242–1254.

Wang K, Zhang H, Bloss CT, et al; The Price Foundation Collaborative Group: a genome-wide association study on common SNPs and rare CNVs in anorexia nervosa. *Mol Psychiatry* 2011;16:949–959.

Watson, H Yilmaz Z, Thornton LM, et al: Genome-wide association study identifies eight risk loci and implicates metabo-psychiatric origins for anorexia nervosa. *Nat Genet* 2019;51:1207–1214.

INTELLECTUAL DISABILITY

Epidemiologic Studies

Classical twin studies tend to support moderate heritability for ID. Recurrence risk for siblings of a child with ID has been estimated to range from 9.5% to 23% depending on severity of the disorder and the mother's reproductive history. For mothers who have already had more than one child with ID, the risk is 25–50% for sibs.

Specific Etiologic Causes

Many medical syndromes are manifest as ID, such as specific errors of metabolism and chromosomal anomalies. Polani estimated that of the 4% of human conceptions that are chromosomally abnormal, 85–90% are selectively eliminated as spontaneous abortions. Of live births, 6% may have a genetic or developmental abnormality of some type; 0.5% survive with chromosomal abnormality; 4% with another developmental anomaly; and 1.5% with a single gene disorder. Among single-gene causes of ID, Koranyi listed five dominant diseases (tuberous sclerosis, neurofibromatosis, Sturge-Weber disease, von Hippel–Lindau, and craniosynostosis), and four recessive diseases (Hurler–Hunter disease, galactosemia, G-6 phosphodehydrogenase deficiency, and familial hypoglycemia), as well as three recessive aminoaciduria and three lipid-related disorders. Many more are listed in McKusick's compendium *Mendelian Inheritance in Man.*

Down syndrome accounts for ID in 1.5 persons per 1000 and is the most common single cause of the condition. The prevalence of Down varies greatly and is primarily determined by maternal age. Familial microcephaly is present in about 1/40,000 births but may account for a significant proportion of ID because of its effects in heterozygotes (see later discussion). Fragile X syndrome accounts for about 0.5/1000, and other X chromosome syndromes for another 1/1000. All metabolic causes together are responsible for 1/1000 and chromosomal abnormalities for 3/1000.

Down Syndrome

This condition, well studied, is accounted for by a triplication of genetic material on chromosome 21. The area is being localized more and more precisely using molecular techniques combined with cytogenetics. It is probable that sections of 21q22.2 and 21q22.3 are involved, though 21q21 may also be implicated. The areas involved include genes for amyloid and superoxide dismutase. The *ETS-2* proto oncogene is near this area as well, and its presence may be related to the well-described increased incidence of leukemia in persons with Down syndrome and their relatives. Human 21q21–22.3 is homologous to portions of mouse chromosome 16. A mouse model of Down has been described based on a laboratory-generated reciprocal translocation involving this area.

The reasons for triplication or nondisjunction in Down are not entirely clear. The likely etiologic factors are environmental rather than genetic. Vulnerability for the condition does not seem to be inherited. A small proportion of Down patients have a translocation rather than a triplication.

As noted earlier, the clearest correlate is maternal age. Yet it has been known for some years that the origin of the nondisjunction might be paternal as well as maternal. Serum markers contribute to prenatal determination (decreased alpha-fetoprotein and estriol and increased human chorionic gonadotropin) and aid in the selection of women for referral to amniocentesis.

It has been reported that a familial association exists between Alzheimer and Down syndrome, but this is unlikely to suggest a common pathology for all cases of Downs syndrome. Recent studies suggest that triplication of a critical region on chromosome 21 is not likely to be the sole cause of clinical variation in Down syndrome and that other genomic areas are probably important as well. Patients with Down syndrome do seem to be at increased risk for Alzheimer pathology as they age.

Fragile X Syndrome

Fragile X syndrome is named after a cytogenetic observation; cultured cells from some patients show chromosomal breakage under appropriate conditions. There are actually multiple "fragile sites" on human chromosomes. The fragile X (breakage at Xq27.3) is merely the best known. The syndrome itself was originally described by Martin and Bell, who described a large pedigree with ID segregating in an X-linked recessive pattern.

Fragile X is the most common form of X-linked ID and is, in general, the most common heritable form of ID (Down being genetic but not inherited). It is estimated that 1/850 persons carry the defect. Of those, four in five males will express the clinical phenotype as compared with one in three females (some homozygotes are nonpenetrant, and some heterozygotes are penetrant). Genetic tests are now available to determine carrier status in nonpenetrant individuals. The precise genetic error in the Xq27.3 region is now known to be a triplet repeat of variable length. Increased numbers of repeats (associated with greater severity of illness) occur as the gene is passed to succeeding generations. When the number of repeats exceeds a threshold, clinical manifestations are seen. The gene involved is *FMR1*, and it codes for the protein FMRP. This is an RNA-binding protein. Recent functional studies have centered on its role in metabotropic glutamate receptor activity.

Most female fragile X heterozygotes do not have ID. However, schizotypal features are seen in about one-third of a sample of carriers, and there is an association with affective disorders as well. Some subjects with fragile X develop an autistic syndrome.

▶ Molecular Genetic Studies of Intellectual Disability

CNVs have been found to be associated with ID, just as they are with autism. These studies are producing a number of promising candidate genes and neurobiological pathways.

Other developmental disorders with well-defined genetic influences include Rett disorder, Prader-Willi syndrome, Angelman syndrome, and Smith-Magenis syndrome. For discussion, see Erickson et al (2012).

Genetic screening is generally recommended for children with neurodevelopmental disorders that include ID. The diagnostic yield averages about 25% in various clinical cohorts. An optimal testing strategy would include fragile X testing plus chromosomal microarray or exome sequencing (and increasingly exome sequencing appears to be the most cost-effective).

Jansen S, Vissers LELM, de Vries BBA. The genetics of intellectual disability. *Brain Sci* 2023 Jan 30;13(2):231. Doi: 10.3390/brainsci13020231. PMID: 36831774.

Mollon J, Almasy L, Jacquemont S, et al: The contribution of copy number variants to psychiatric symptoms and cognitive ability. *Mol Psychiatry* 2023 Feb 3. Doi: 10.1038/s41380-023-01978-4. Online ahead of print. PMID: 36737482.

MOOD DISORDERS

1. Genetic Epidemiologic Studies

A. Family Studies

Family studies in affective disorder have continually demonstrated an aggregation of illness in relatives (Tables 3–2 and 3–3). In a study at the National Institute of Mental Health (NIMH), 25% of the relatives of bipolar (BP) probands were found to have bipolar or unipolar (UP) illness, compared to 20% of relatives of UP probands and 7% of relatives of controls. In the same study, 40% of the relatives of schizoaffective probands demonstrated affective illness at some point in their lives. These data demonstrate increased risk in relatives of patients. They also show that the various forms of affective illness appear to be related in a hierarchical way: relatives

Table 3–2 Lifetime Risk for Major Mood Disorder in Different Groups

General population	2%
Relatives of UP	20%
Relatives of BP	25%
Relatives of SA (BP)	40%
Children of two ill parents	50%+
Identical twin ill	60%

of schizoaffective probands may have schizoaffective illness themselves, but are more likely to have BP or UP illness. Relatives of BP probands have either BP or (more likely) UP illness.

Age of onset may be useful in dividing affective illness into more genetically homogeneous subgroups. Early-onset probands have an increased morbid risk of illness in relatives in some datasets. A birth cohort effect was observed in several family studies, with an increasing incidence of affective illness among persons born more recently. The cohort effect was observed among relatives at risk to a greater degree than in the general population. The reasons for this increase in incidence are not yet clear.

B. Twin Studies

Twin studies show consistent evidence for heritability. On the average, MZ twin pairs show concordance 65% of the time and DZ twin pairs 14% of the time.

C. Adoption Studies

Several adoption studies have been performed in the area of affective illness. The results have been generally consistent with genetic hypotheses.

2. The Affective Spectrum

Following are the types of affective disorders and other disorders that are genetically related:

BPI—Bipolar I. Classic "manic–depressive illness" with severe mania, generally including episodes of major depression as well.

Table 3–3 Lifetime Risk for Bipolar Disorder in Different Groups

Controls	0.5–1%
Relatives of UP	3%
Relatives of BP	8%
Relatives of SA	17%
MZ twin	80%

BPII—Bipolar II. Periods of hypomania and major depression. This disorder is genetically related to BPI and UP. There is some evidence in recent family studies for an excess of BPII illness in relatives of BPII probands. It has been demonstrated that BPII tends to be a stable lifetime diagnosis, that is, patients do not frequently convert to BPI.

Rapid cycling—Rapid-cycling BP illness has been the subject of great theoretical and clinical interest. A link with thyroid pathology has been proposed. Rapid cycling may be familial.

UP mania—This entity includes BPI patients with no history of major depression. This group is not distinguishable from other BPI patients on the basis of family pattern of illness.

Cyclothymia/Other specified bipolar and related disorder—This condition includes persons with repetitive high and low mood swings, generally not requiring clinical attention; it is probably genetically related to BP disorder.

Schizoaffective disorder—A group of patients with intermittent psychosis during euthymia have an increase in affective illness and schizophrenia in relatives. This group may have the highest genetic load (total risk for affective or schizophrenic illness in relatives) of any diagnostic category among mood and psychotic disorders. They may carry gene variants related to both BP illness and schizophrenia. Patients with chronic psychosis and superimposed episodes of mood disorder confer risk for both chronic psychosis and mood disorder to relatives but have less overall genetic load.

Schizophrenia—An overlap in linkage areas and vulnerability genes has been identified in recent years, including in genome-wide association studies. This is especially true for BPI disorder and not so much for BPII (which is more closely related to major depression).

Eating disorders—Family studies of anorexia and bulimia have generally found excess affective illness in relatives. Relatives of persons with anorexia may have similar risk for affective disorders to that of relatives of BP probands.

Attention-deficit hyperactivity disorder (ADHD)—Children with this disorder appear to have increased depression in their relatives. The opposite has not been demonstrated (BP/UP probands have not been reported to have increased risk of attention-deficit disorder in their offspring).

Alcohol use disorder—There may be overlapping vulnerability traits. Alcohol use disorder appears to be comorbid with UP and BP disorders (each appears to confer an increased risk for the other within individuals). There is some evidence that alcohol use disorder with affective disorder may itself aggregate within families.

3. Linkage Studies

Linkage studies in mood disorders are less pertinent in the era of genome-wide association studies. They still may be useful in identifying risk alleles of large effect in extended kindreds by using data from sequencing studies.

4. Endophenotypes

A number of endophenotypic markers have been suggested:

- Amygdala activation on functional MRI (fMRI)
- Hippocampal size
- Response to sleep deprivation
  - Cognitive deficits in bipolar disorder
  - Emotion-related processing tasks
  - Polygenic risk scores

5. Gene Expression Studies

Studies have begun on brain samples from autopsy studies of patients with mood disorders, and in peripheral tissues such as blood. These studies should be helpful in identifying candidate genes for mood disorders and for related phenotypes such as suicidal behavior.

6. High-Risk Studies

More offspring of patients with BP than controls have a diagnosed Axis I disorder. Offspring of BP parents may be more prone to respond to dysphoric feeling states with "disinhibitory" behavior. Offspring with a childhood-onset anxiety or externalizing disorder appear to be at greater risk for later development of major mood disorder. Early symptoms of hypomania or mood instability may be predictive of later onset of BP.

7. GWAS Studies of Bipolar Disorder

Fifteen high confidence genes were identified in the most recent bipolar GWAS study by Mullins et al (see below), using gene expression data to validate genetic association findings. These include the serotonergic receptor gene *HTR6*, the melanin-concentrating hormone receptor gene *MCHR1*, and the neurodevelopmental gene *FURIN* (Figure 3–6).

8. Specific Genes Related to Bipolar Disorder

Several genes have now been identified in multiple GWAS studies, including combined samples:

Ankyrin 3 (ANK3) was the first gene identified in a major psychiatric disorder using GWAS methods. This gene codes for a structural membrane protein related to sodium channels. Sodium transport has been reported to be abnormal in studies of bipolar disorder and major depression since the 1960s.

The calcium channel gene **CACNA1C** reached genome-wide significance in the report of Ferreira et al, which has been replicated several times. **Recent data show that calcium**

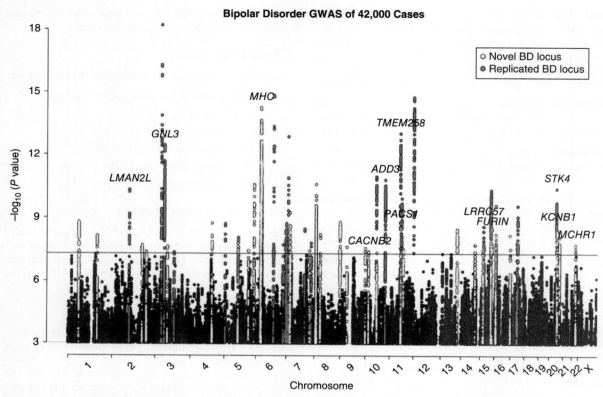

▲ **Figure 3–6** Manhattan plot for genomewide association study of bipolar disorder (BP). The gray horizontal line at 5×10^{-8} shows the threshold for genomewide significance. Loci designated with open circles are novel (not identified in previous genomewide association studies of BP). Loci designated with closed circles were identified in previous studies and replicated in this study. Labeled genes are those with corroborative evidence from gene expression analyses in postmortem brain studies or notable genes in novel loci (*MHC, CACNB2, KCNB1*). (Reproduced with permission from Mullins N, Forstner AJ, O'Connell KS, et al. Genome-wide association study of more than 40,000 bipolar disorder cases provides new insights into the underlying biology. *Nat Genet*. 2021 Jun;53(6):817–829.)

channel genes as a set appear to be associated with major psychiatric disorders in general and bipolar disorder in particular.

Neurocan (NCAN) was identified by a large international consortium studying bipolar illness and using GWAS methods. It codes for an extracellular matrix glycoprotein. In the mouse, this is localized in cortical and hippocampal brain areas.

The Major Histocompatibility Locus: A signal in the Human Leukocyte Antigen (HLA) region was identified in the most recent GWAS study of bipolar disorder. This may be distinct from the HLA signal already identified for schizophrenia.

Sequencing studies have produced evidence for other high-confidence candidates, including *NCKAP5, SYNE1/CPG2, AKAP11*, and the class of GABAergic genes.

A general increase in ultra-rare protein-truncating variants was observed in the largest sequencing study of bipolar disorder to date, continuing the evidence for genetic heterogeneity in bipolar disorder.

9. GWAS Studies of Major Depression

The largest sample to date in mood disorders was studied by Howard et al (including >200,000 cases and >500,000 controls, with a replication sample of >1 million participants). One hundred and two variants, 269 genes, and 15 genesets were associated with depression, including prominently genesets related to synaptic structure and neurotransmission (see below). Enrichment studies emphasized the importance of prefrontal brain regions. A strong genetic relationship was identified between depression and the trait of neuroticism. Gene-drug relationships with the dopaminergic gene *DRD2* and several of the calcium-channel genes were featured (Figure 3–7).

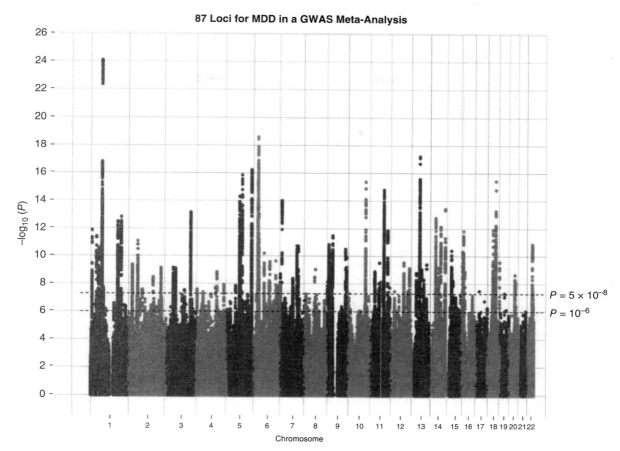

▲ Figure 3–7 Manhattan plot for genomewide association study of major depressive disorder. (Reproduced with permission from Howard DM, Adams MJ, Clarke TK, et al. Genome-wide meta-analysis of depression identifies 102 independent variants and highlights the importance of the prefrontal brain regions. *Nat Neurosci*. 2019 Mar;22(3): 343–352.)

Joint analyses of bipolar disorder and major depression have shown that BP2 shares substantial genetic variance with major depression (~70%) and much less with schizophrenia (~40%). On the other hand BPI shares substantial variance with schizophrenia (~70%) and much less with major depression (~40%). Genetic correlation between educational attainment and mood disorders was positive for bipolar disorder but negative for major depression. The two disorders (BP and UP) are related but clearly distinct genetically.

10. CNV Studies in Bipolar Disorder

Rare CNVs were reported to be elevated in a study by Zhang et al in subjects with bipolar disorder from the NIMH Genetics Initiative Database. A subsequent study showed increased CNVs in patients with bipolar disorder

who had early onset (before age 21), but not patients with later onset.

Coleman JRI, Gaspar HA, Bryois J, et al: The genetics of the mood disorder spectrum: genome-wide association analyses of more than 185,000 cases and 439,000 controls. *Biol Psychiatry* 2020 Jul 15;88(2):169–184. Doi: 10.1016/j.biopsych.2019.10.015. Epub 2019 Nov 1. PMID: 31926635.

Howard DM, Adams MJ, Clarke TK, et al: Genome-wide meta-analysis of depression identifies 102 independent variants and highlights the importance of the prefrontal brain regions. *Nat Neurosci* 2019 Mar;22(3):343–352. Doi: 10.1038/s41593-018-0326-7. Epub 2019 Feb 4. PMID: 30718901.

Mullins N, Forstner AJ, O'Connell KS, et al: Genome-wide association study of more than 40,000 bipolar disorder cases provides new insights into the underlying biology. *Nat Genet* 2021 Jun;53(6):817–829. Doi: 10.1038/s41588-021-00857-4. Epub 2021 May 17. PMID: 34002096.

Palmer DS, Howrigan DP, Chapman SB, et al: Exome sequencing in bipolar disorder identifies AKAP11 as a risk gene shared with schizophrenia. *Nat Genet* 2022 May;54(5):541–547. doi: 10.1038/s41588-022-01034-x. Epub 2022 Apr 11. PMID: 35410376.

OBSESSIVE–COMPULSIVE DISORDER

1. Epidemiologic Research

A. Twin Studies

There are no large twin studies of obsessive–compulsive disorder (OCD). Rasmussen and Tsuang reviewed reported series and noted that 32 of 51 (63%) MZ pairs were concordant. Lenane studied 145 first-degree relatives of 46 children with OCD. Of the 90 parents personally evaluated, 15 (17%) received a diagnosis of OCD, compared to 1.5% of the parents of 34 conduct-disordered children who served as a control group. The 17% prevalence rate is significantly higher than the population prevalence rate of about 2%. Fathers were three times as likely as mothers to receive a diagnosis of OCD. Of the 56 siblings personally evaluated, three (5%) met criteria for OCD. When age correction was applied, the rate rose to 35%. This figure should be viewed with caution because of the magnitude of the age correction for siblings. It should be noted that all probands had severe childhood-onset OCD and were referred to the authors for treatment. It is possible that childhood-onset OCD represents a more severe form of the OCD spectrum. Nevertheless, this carefully conducted family study reveals an increased risk of OCD among the first-degree relatives of OCD probands.

When OCD occurs in the familial context of Tourette syndrome, it may be part of the spectrum of Tourette syndrome. However, most OCD occurs in individuals who have no first-degree relatives affected by Tourette. Occasionally, an individual destined to develop Tourette will present with symptoms of OCD, and the motor tics appear subsequently. These patients are often diagnosed as having OCD until motor tics develop.

An OCD GWAS report described ~2090 cases and 4567 matched controls, but no allele reached genome-wide significance, suggesting that larger sample sizes are needed and that no common allele conveys more than a small amount of risk (Mahjani et al, 2022). A GWAS report on Tourette syndrome, with a sample size of 6133 individuals with TS and 13,565 ancestry-matched control participants, identified a locus on chromosome 5q15 locus, which includes the *NR2F1* gene (Tsetsos et al, 2023).

Mahjani B, Klei L, Mattheisen M, et al: The genetic architecture of obsessive-compulsive disorder: contribution of liability to OCD from alleles across the frequency spectrum. *Am J Psychiatry* 2022 Mar;179(3):216–225.

Tsetsos F, Topaloudi A, Jain P, et al: Genome-wide association study points to novel locus for Gilles de la Tourette syndrome. *Biol Psychiatry* 2023 Feb 2:S0006-3223(23)00051-3. doi: 10.1016/j.biopsych.2023.01.023.

SCHIZOPHRENIA

A. Twin Studies

MZ twin concordance is greater than DZ twin concordance in each study of schizophrenia, consistent with genetic hypotheses. Second, the heritability of broadly defined schizophrenia is greater than the heritability of strictly defined schizophrenia. This is consistent with a spectrum concept: some individuals with the genetic loading for schizophrenia manifest a different condition. Third, the amount of discordance is considerable; even in MZ twins the discordance is 51% when a broad definition of illness is used.

Twin study paradigm to generate data regarding environmental effects in schizophrenia—Examining age of onset in the Maudsley Hospital twin series, it was found that there was a high incidence of illness in the second of a pair of twins within 2 years of onset in the first twin. Further categorizing the group on the basis of whether the twins lived together or apart, the 2-year incidence was elevated only in those living together. That is, twins living together are concordant in age of onset, whereas twins living apart are not. This intriguing finding suggests an environmental factor.

B. Family Studies

Pooled European family study data show an age-corrected morbid risk of 5.6% in parents, 10.1% in siblings, and 12.8% in children. The lower rate in parents is thought to be related to a relative decrease in fertility among persons with schizophrenia. The estimate of risk for schizophrenia in the general population is about 1%; thus, all classes of first-degree relatives of persons with schizophrenia have a clear increase in prevalence. The risk for offspring of two parents with schizophrenia is difficult to estimate because of the small number of cases. It is probably between 35% and 45% (in pooled data it is 46.3%). Among second-degree relatives (uncles, aunts, nephews, nieces, grandchildren), half-siblings, and cousins, the risk is 2–4%.

Thus, close relatives of persons with schizophrenia have about a 5- to 10-fold excess risk for the illness. The risk diminishes in more distant relatives. A further group of first-degree relatives appear to develop "schizophrenic spectrum" disorders (see later). Nevertheless, the majority of close relatives of persons with schizophrenia have no psychiatric diagnosis.

There is no strong evidence for genetic determination of the conventional subtypes of schizophrenia (hebephrenic, catatonic, and paranoid forms). Though there is significant concordance in MZ twins for subtype, this does not hold true in family studies.

The question of the distinctness of schizophrenia and affective disorders is not settled. In a large family study using lifetime diagnoses and separately examining relatives of probands with schizophrenia, chronic schizoaffective disorder, acute schizoaffective disorder, BP affective disorder, UP affective disorder, and controls, it was concluded that there was evidence for overlap in genetic liability (Lichtenstein et al, 2009). Specifically, an increase in UP disorder was seen in all groups of relatives of patients. Relatives of probands with schizoaffective disorder (both chronic and acute) showed both an excess of affective disorders and an excess of chronic psychoses. However, probands with BP showed an excess of relatives with schizophrenia, and probands with schizophrenia showed an excess of relatives with BP. The overlap from family study data has been confirmed by comparison of BP, MD and schizophrenia GWAS data, showing greater than expected overlap among susceptibility alleles (Lee et al, 2013).

With regard to mode of transmission, the available data have been analyzed extensively. The results have generally been interpreted as favoring a multifactorial rather than a single-locus model.

C. Adoption Studies

The adoption study methodology was first applied to schizophrenia ~40 years ago. It was reported that there is an excess of schizophrenia in the adopted-away offspring of women with schizophrenia compared to control adoptees. A series of large, systematic studies were carried out by Kety and Rosenthal, who analyzed adoption and psychiatric hospitalization registries in Denmark. In the later studies, subjects were directly interviewed. In all studies, adoptees were separated from their biologic parents at an early age and adopted by nonrelatives. It was found that there were more schizophrenia and schizophrenia spectrum disorders diagnosed in the biologic relatives of schizophrenic adoptees than in the biologic relatives of psychiatrically normal adoptees. The prevalence of psychiatric illnesses in the adoptive relatives of the two groups was comparable but small.

The frequency of schizophrenia spectrum disorders is higher in adopted-away offspring of parents with schizophrenia than in the adopted-away offspring of control parents. All of these studies have been criticized on the grounds of selection bias and the validity of diagnosis, and comparisons. However, further independent analysis of the data has confirmed the results: that is, biologic relatives of schizophrenics who have not shared the same environment have a significantly higher prevalence of schizophrenia and schizophrenic spectrum disorders than do biologic relatives of comparable control groups.

D. Spectrum Studies

Thirty percent of first-degree relatives of persons with schizophrenia have associated disorders. The particular diagnostic categories that seem to be implicated are paranoid personality disorder and schizotypal personality disorder. Schizotypal personality disorder is most likely part of the schizophrenia spectrum, with suggestive evidence for paranoid and schizoid personality disorders as well.

A separate entity characterized by paranoid delusions only (simple delusional disorder) may also exist, for which the inheritance is independent of that for schizophrenia and affective disorder.

E. Molecular Studies

The most recent schizophrenia GWAS study included more than 76,000 cases, identifying more than 200 loci (Trubetskoy et al, 2022; see Figure 3-2 in the Methods section). Risk alleles were concentrated among genes involved in neuronal function including genes related to CNS development, brain cell differentiation, and synaptic transmission. Also, risk alleles were clustered in genes encoding ion channels, synapses, axonal structures and dendritic compartments. Lastly, sequencing thousands of exomes from individuals with schizophrenia demonstrated that genes harboring common risk alleles also contained rare schizophrenia risk alleles of potentially large effect (Singh et al, 2022).

The locus of largest effect in SZ (see Figure 3-2 in Methods) is on chromosome 6, at the major histocompatibility (MHC) region. Within this region, complement C4 exists in two isoforms, C4A and C4B. Sekar et al (2016) showed that a human endogenous retrovirus (HERV) insertion into C4A is largely responsible for this locus, with an odds ratio of 1.3 for those who are homozygous for the HERV insertion. Furthermore, Sekar et al (2016) demonstrated that the effect of this allele was to increase expression of C4A in the CNS. This is important because C4 directs pruning of synapses in the CNS, suggesting that excessive synaptic pruning may occur in SZ, thereby offering an explanation for the fact that people with SZ have a thinner frontal cortex that matched controls (Cannon et al, 2015).

CNVs are collectively an uncommon source of genetic risk for schizophrenia, occurring perhaps in no more than 4–5% of cases. Marshall et al (2017) found eight CNVs to be significantly enriched among the genomes of indiviuals with schizophrenia. These eight include CNVs at 1q21.1, 2p16.3 (NRXN1), 3q29, 7q11.2, 15q13.3, distal 16p11.2, proximal 16p11.2 and 22q11.2.

▶ Endophenotypes in Schizophrenia

The concept of endophenotypes in psychiatric disorders has been developed over the past several decades. The term defines an illness-related characteristic, observable through biochemical testing or microscopic examination. A valid endophenotype should be more closely related to pathophysiologic gene variants than are symptoms for that disorder.

The utility of endophenotypes in psychiatric research is now more appreciated, because we have a more accurate understanding of the genetic complexity of operationally defined disorders in the current psychiatric nosology. Endophenotypes should create more homogeneous subtypes, which may cut across current nosologic boundaries.

Valid endophenotypes would enable more rapid advances in understanding these disorders at the molecular level.

Criteria for an Endophenotype

Criteria for an endophenotype have been derived.

- It must be associated with illness in the general population.
- It should be stable and state-independent. In other words, it must be observable despite the fact that the patient is in partial or complete remission.
- It should be heritable.
- It should segregate with illness within families.
- Among kindreds in which the proband has the endophenotype, it should also be observable at a higher rate among unaffected family members compared to the general population.

Several useful schemes have now been developed for the quantitative assessment of endophenotypes, including those by Glahn and by Gershon.

Possible endophenotypes in schizophrenia include deficits in working memory and a reduced P50 evoked potential following repeated auditory stimulation. A number of endophenotypes have been investigated by the ongoing BSNIP consortium.

In summary, genetic studies of schizophrenia have identified numerous promising candidate genes through GWAS and sequencing. GWAS studies have now identified calcium channel–related genes as implicated in both schizophrenia and bipolar disorder. Research has revealed several promising endophenotypes, particularly auditory evoked potential abnormalities and neurocognitive deficits.

Cannon TD, Chung Y, He G, et al: Progressive reduction in cortical thickness as psychosis develops: a multisite longitudinal neuroimaging study of youth at elevated clinical risk. *Biol Psychiatry* 2015;77:147–157.

Lee SH, Ripke S, Neale BM, et al: Genetic relationship between five psychiatric disorders estimated from genome-wide SNPs. *Nat Genet* 2013;45:984–994.

Lichtenstein P, Yip BH, Björk C, et al: Common genetic determinants of schizophrenia and bipolar disorder in Swedish families: a population-based study. *Lancet* 2009;373(9659):234–239.

Marshall CR, Howrigan DP, Merico D, et al: Contribution of copy number variants to schizophrenia from a genome-wide study of 41,321 subjects. *Nat Genet* 2017 Jan;49(1):27–35.

Sekar A, Bialas AR, de Rivera H, et al: Schizophrenia risk from complex variation of complement component 4. *Nature* 2016;530:177–183.

Singh T, Poterba T, Curtis D, et al: Rare coding variants in ten genes confer substantial risk for schizophrenia. *Nature* 2022 Apr;604(7906):509–516.

Trubetskoy V, Panagiotaropoulou G, Awasthi S, et al: Mapping genomic loci implicates genes and synaptic biology in schizophrenia. *Nature* 2022 Apr; 604(7906):502–508.

SOMATIZATION DISORDER (SOMATIC SYMPTOM DISORDER)

In a family history study, Coryell evaluated first-degree relatives of 49 probands with Briquet syndrome, now called somatic symptom disorder (SSD) in DSM-5. First-degree relatives of nonsyndromic subjects with similar complaints and mood disorder probands formed the control groups. The risk for a complicated medical history was 8% in the first-degree relatives of SSD probands compared to control values of 2.3% and 2.5%, respectively.

In a family study of severe SSD, Guze and colleagues reported a significantly increased risk for similar disorders among the first-degree female relatives of probands (7/105), compared to female relatives of control probands (13/532). In addition, they reported an increased risk for antisocial personality disorder among the male (18/96) and female (9/105) relatives of the SSD probands, compared to the risk for male (44/420) and female (14/532) relatives of controls.

Torgersen studied 14 MZ twin pairs and 21 DZ twin pairs in which one member had a somatoform disorder (somatization disorder, conversion disorder, psychogenic pain disorder, or hypochondriasis). Of MZ twin pairs, 29% were concordant for somatoform disorder, compared to 10% of DZ twin pairs. This difference was not significant.

Adoption Studies

In an analysis of a large Swedish adoption cohort, Sigvardsson identified a set of discriminant function variables that distinguished female adoptees with repeated brief somatic complaints and psychiatric disability ("somatizers") from other female adoptees. In a subsequent analysis, Bohman divided somatizers into two groups, "high-frequency somatizers" (those who have high prevalence of psychiatric, abdominal, or back complaints) and "diversiform somatizers" (those who have a lower frequency of complaints, but multiple, highly variable symptoms). Thirty percent of the high-frequency somatizers had histories of alcohol abuse and/or criminality (based on the national registries for these behaviors). Their male biological relatives were at increased risk for violent criminal behavior and alcohol abuse. For both types of somatizers, a cross-fostering analysis provided evidence for both congenital and postnatal influences on the development of somatoform disorder. These studies suggest a familial connection between some types of somatoform disorder, alcoholism, and criminality. Additional work is needed in this area.

Molecular Genetic Studies

To our knowledge no GWAS or sequencing studies have been performed in persons with these disorders.

Torgersen S: Genetics and somatoform disorders. *Tidsskr Nor Laegeforen* 2002;122(14):1385–1388.

TOURETTE SYNDROME

▶ Epidemiologic Research

A. Twin Studies

Price studied 30 MZ and 13 DZ same-sex pairs defined by one twin having Tourette syndrome. MZ twin concordance was 77% for any tics, compared to 23% concordance for DZ twins. For Tourette disorder proper, the MZ concordance rate was 53%, compared to the DZ rate of 8%. These are all significant differences.

Pauls studied 338 biological relatives of 38 Tourette disorder probands, 21 adoptive relatives, and 22 relatives of normal controls. Among the biological relatives, 8.3% had Tourette disorder, whereas 16.3% had chronic tics and 9.5% had OCD. These risks are all significantly greater than the risks for the 43 relatives of controls.

B. Linkage Studies

A collaborative effort to use systematic genomic screening to find gene variants implicated in Tourette has been underway for several years. Recent results suggest that variants on chromosome 2p may be involved. Rare mutations in the gene coding for dendritic growth protein SLITRK1 (chromosome 13q) have been associated with this condition.

C. Genome-Wide Association Studies

Tsetsos et al (2023) identified a genome-wide significant locus on chromosome 5q15, implicating the *NR2F1* gene. Larger sample sizes are needed to identify additional risk alleles.

Karagiannidis I, Dehning S, Sandor P, et al: Support of the histaminergic hypothesis in Tourette syndrome: association of the histamine decarboxylase gene in a large sample of families. *J Med Genet* 2013;50(11):760–764.

Paschou P. The genetic basis of Gilles de la Tourette syndrome. *Neurosci Biobehav Rev* 2013;37(6):1026–1039.

Tsetsos F, Topaloudi A, Jain P, et al: Genome-wide association study points to novel Locus for Gilles de la Tourette syndrome. *Biol Psychiatry* 2023 Feb 2:S0006-3223(23)00051-3. doi: 10.1016/j.biopsych.2023.01.023.

GENETIC COUNSELING

Empirical data for genetic counseling is summarized in Table 3–4. These data assume that the other parent is unaffected. The percentages in parentheses after the family history provide the unselected general population risk. For example, the general population lifetime risk for UP illness (defined narrowly) is 8%. If a subject has a parent with UP depression, the lifetime risk is double that of the general population (16%). Such individuals are also at fourfold increased risk for BP illness.

Table 3–4 Family Study Data for Genetic Counseling*

Family History*	Unselected General Population Risk	Increased Risk for Offspring
Unipolar disorder (UP)	8%	2-fold (16%) for UP
		4-fold (4%) for BP
Bipolar disorder (BP)	1%	9-fold (9%) for BP
		2-fold (16%) for UP
Schizophrenia (SZ)	1%	10-fold (10%) for SZ
		2-fold (15%) for UP
Alcoholism	18% males, 10% females	~2-fold
Panic disorder	0.5%	12-fold (6%)
Tourette syndrome	0.25%	100-fold (25%)
Alzheimer disease	3%	5-fold (15%) at age 75
Attention-deficit/ hyperactivity disorder	3%	5-fold (15%)
Anorexia nervosa	0.5%	10-fold (5%)

*These data assume that only one parent is affected.

Some illnesses have narrow age-at-onset distributions in the general population. For example, first episodes of BP illness almost always occur before age 60. Fully 50% of BP individuals have their initial episode (depressive or manic) before age 20. This should be considered in a general way when assessing risk. For example, an unaffected 40-year-old son of a parent with BP illness has already passed through most of the age at risk, and thus, his risk for BP is substantially less than 9%. An estimate of 2% would be more accurate in this case.

It is anticipated that genotypic methods will be adapted for use in genetic counseling in the coming years. Such methods are not yet widely applicable aside from use in certain unusual families with a rare CNV or other rare allele of large effect. PRSs for psychiatric disorders are being studied for eventual clinical application but require large controlled trials in diverse populations prior to use. Genetic testing using HLA typing or metabolic enzymes *CYP2D6* or *CYP2C19* may be useful in treatment planning for mood stabilization or antidepressant therapy.

Gershon ES, Alliey-Rodriguez N: New ethical issues for genetic counseling in common mental disorders. *Am J Psychiatry* 2013 Sep;170(9):968–976. doi: 10.1176/appi.ajp.2 013.12121558. PMID: 23897273.

Nurnberger JI Jr, Austin J, Berrettini WH, et al: What should a psychiatrist know about genetics? Review and recommendations from the Residency Education Committee of the International Society of Psychiatric Genetics. *J Clin Psychiatry* 2018 Nov 27; 80(1):17nr12046. doi: 10.4088/JCP.17nr12046. PMID: 30549495.

https://ispg.net/genetic-testing-statement. Accessed 5/8/23.

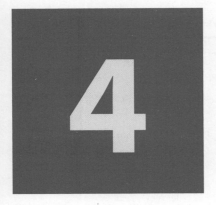

4

Developmental Psychology

Kenneth A. Dodge, PhD

DEVELOPMENTAL CONCEPTS

The concept of development is the backbone of modern behavioral science. Psychiatric practitioners and behavioral scientists are concerned primarily with change, its origins, and its control. **Developmental psychology** is the scientific study of the structure, function, and processes of systematic growth and change across the life span. Systems of classification of behavior (including psychiatric nosology) take into account not only contemporaneous features and formal similarities among current symptoms and syndromes but also past qualities, immediate consequences, long-term outcome, and likelihood of change (naturally or through treatment).

Whereas developmental psychology is concerned with species-typical patterns of systematic change (and central tendencies of the species), the discipline of **developmental psychopathology** is concerned with individual differences and contributes greatly to the understanding of childhood disorders.

The organizing framework of developmental psychopathology is a movement toward understanding the predictors, causes, processes, courses, sequelae, and environmental symbiosis of psychiatric illnesses in order to discover effective treatment and prevention. This movement is guided by a developmental framework that integrates knowledge from multiple disciplines (e.g., psychobiology, neuroscience, cognitive psychology, social psychology) and levels of analysis (e.g., neuronal synapse, psychophysiologic response, mental representation, motor behavior, personality pattern). The relation between developmental psychology and developmental psychopathology is reciprocal: The study of normal development gives context to the analysis of aberrations, and the study of psychopathology informs our understanding of normative development.

A developmental orientation forces a scholar to ask questions that move beyond the prevalence and incidence of disorders. Table 4–1 lists some of these questions.

THE ORTHOGENETIC PRINCIPLE

The **orthogenetic principle** proposes that development moves from undifferentiated and diffuse toward greater complexity, achieved through both differentiation and consolidation within and across subsystems. The newborn infant is relatively undifferentiated in response patterns, but through development achieves greater differentiation (and less stereotypy) of functioning. Each period of development is characterized by adaptational challenges resulting from environmental demands (e.g., a mother who has become unwilling to breastfeed) and from emerging internal influences across subsystems (e.g., growing recognition of the self as able to exert control). The challenges are best conceptualized not as mere threats to homeostasis; rather, change and the demand for adaptation define the human species, and challenges push the individual toward development. The inherent adaptational response of the species is toward mastery of new demands. The mastery motive is as yet unexplained by science, although it is characteristic of the human species (see "Adaptation & Competence" section later in this chapter).

Thus, development is characterized by periods of disruption in the homeostasis of the organism brought on by new challenges, followed by adaptation and consolidation until the next challenge is presented. The adaptive child uses both internal and external resources to meet a challenge. **Successful adaptation** is defined as the optimal organization of behavioral and biological systems within the context of current challenges. Adaptation requires the assimilation of past organizational structures to current demands as well as the generation of new structures equipped to meet the demands.

Piaget described two types of change: **assimilation**, which involves incorporation of the challenge into existing organizational structures (e.g., an infant might treat all adults as the same kind of stimulus); and **accommodation**, which involves

Table 4–1 Questions Related to a Developmental Orientation

How and why do some at-risk individuals become psychologically ill, whereas others do not?

How do the capacities and limitations of the human species at various life stages predispose individuals to disorder? (For example, why are females at relatively high risk for depression during adolescence?)

How do genes and the environment interact to produce psychopathology?

How are various disorders related developmentally? (For example, how does oppositional defiant disorder lead to conduct disorder, which leads to antisocial personality disorder?)

Where are the natural boundaries between normal and abnormal?

Are there critical periods, and if so, why? (For example, why is a high lead level in the blood more detrimental early in life?)

What does the concept of multifactorial causation imply for the likely success of intervention?

Lerner RM (ed): Theoretical models of human development. In: Damon W (series ed), Lerner RM (vol ed), *Handbook of Child Psychology, Vol. 1. Theoretical Models of Human Development*, 6th edn. New York: Wiley, 2006.

MAJOR PRINCIPLES OF ONTOGENY & PHYLOGENY

Cairns and Cairns outlined seven principles that characterize the human organism in interaction with the environment over time: conservation, coherence, bidirectionality, reciprocal influence, novelty, within-individual variation, and dynamic systems. The first principle is that of **conservation**, or connectivity in functioning across time. Even with all the pressure to change, social and cognitive organization tends to be continuous and conservative. The constraints on the organism and the multiple determinants of behavior lead to gradual transition rather than abrupt mutation. Observers can recognize the continuity in persons across even long periods of time; that is, we know that a person remains the same "person." For Piaget, who began his career by writing scientific papers on the evolution of mollusks, this within-person continuity principle is consistent with his view that species-wide evolution is gradual. Piaget believed that development within individuals reflects development of the species (i.e., ontogeny recapitulates phylogeny).

The second principle is **coherence**. Individuals function as holistic and integrated units, in spite of the multiple systems that contribute to any set of behaviors. One cannot divorce one system from another, because the two systems function as a whole that is greater than its component parts. This fact is another conservative force, because an adverse effect on one part of a system tends to be offset by compensatory responses from other parts of the system. This phenomenon applies to all human biological systems and can be applied to psychological functioning.

The third principle is a corollary of the second: Influence between the organism and the environment is **bidirectional**. The person is an active agent in continuous interaction with others. Reciprocal influences are not identical; rather, at each stage of development, the person organizes the outer world through a mental representational system that mediates all experience with the world. Nevertheless, reciprocity and synchrony constrain the person, and the relative weight of these constraints varies at different points in development. At one extreme, it is possible to speak of symbiosis and total dependency of the infant on the mother; at the other extreme, behavior geneticists refer to genetic effects on environmental variables (such as the proposition that genes produce behavior that leads to the reactions that one receives from others in social exchanges).

Another corollary of the second principle is the principle of **reciprocal influence** between subsystems within the individual. Behavioral, cognitive, emotional, neurochemical,

reorganization of the organism's structures to meet the demands of the environment (e.g., a developing infant learns to discriminate among adults and to respond differently to different adults) (see "Organismic Theory" section later in this chapter). Accommodation is more complex than assimilation, but successful adaptation requires a balance of both.

Maladaptation, or incompetence in responding to challenge, is characterized by the inadequate resolution of developmental challenges (as in the psychoanalytic concept of fixation). Maladaptation may be evidenced by developmental delays or lags, such as the continuing temper tantrums of an emotionally dysregulated child beyond the period when such behavior is normative. At any phase, the organism will manifest some form of regulation and functioning, even if it is not advantageous for future development. Thus, the child's tantrums might serve to regulate both a complex external environment of marital turmoil and an internal environment of stress. However, suboptimal regulation will prevent or hamper the individual from coping with the next developmental challenge.

Sometimes, apparently effective responses to a particular challenge lead to maladaptation at a more general level. Consider a toddler who responds to the withdrawal of a mother's undivided attention by ignoring her. Although this pattern of response may mean calmer evenings temporarily, the toddler will be ill equipped to respond to other challenges later in development. Consistent social withdrawal may cause the child to fail to acquire skills of assertion; however, continued ignoring of the mother may lead to a phenotypically distinct response in the future (e.g., depression in adolescence). Thus, the orthogenetic principle calls to mind the functioning of the entire organism (not merely distinct and unrelated subsystems) and the readiness of that organism to respond to future challenges.

hormonal, and morphologic factors affect each other recip-rocally. Mental events have biological implications and vice versa. Among the most exciting research directions in devel-opmental psychopathology has been afforded by the technol-ogy of functional magnetic resonance imaging (fMRI), which enables the understanding of how environmental stimuli and behavioral displays are mediated through brain activity.

The fifth principle of ontogeny is that **novelty** arises in development. Change is not haphazard. The forces of recip-rocal interaction within the individual and the environment lead not only to quantitative changes in the individual but also to the emergence of qualitatively distinct forms, such as locomotion, language, and thought. These changes represent growth rather than random events, in that previous forms typically remain and are supplemented by novel forms.

The sixth principle of phylogeny is that of **within-individual variation** in developmental rates across subsys-tems. Change within a subsystem occurs nonlinearly, as in language development or even physical growth. Some of this nonlinearity can be explained by species-wide phenomena, such as puberty, but much of it varies across individuals. In addition, rates of change vary within an individual across subsystems. Consider two young children, identical in age. Child A may learn to crawl before child B, but child B might catch up and learn to walk before child A. Likewise, child B might utter a recognizable word before child A, but child A might be talking in sentences before child B. This unevenness within and across individuals characterizes development and makes predictions probabilistic rather than certain. Some of the variation is attributable to environmental factors that have enduring personal effects (such as the lasting effects on cognitive achievement of early entry into formal schooling) or biological factors that have enduring psychological effects (such as the effect of early puberty on social outcomes), whereas other factors may have only temporary effect (such as efforts to accelerate locomotion onset) or no effect at all.

Finally, according to the seventh principle, development is extremely sensitive to unique configurations of influence, such as in **dynamic systems**. Growth and change cannot be reduced to a quantitative cumulation of biological and envi-ronmental units. Also, development is not simply hierarchi-cal, with gradual building of functions on previous ones. Rather, development often follows a sequence of organiza-tion, disorganization, and then reorganization in a different (possibly more advanced) form. In physical sciences, this principle is called **catastrophe theory**, reflecting the hypoth-esis that during the disorganization, events are literally ran-dom. But reorganization occurs eventually, in lawful and predictable ways.

Dynamic systems theory incorporates several postulates about growth and change. First, change occurs nonlinearly. Second, minor quantitative changes can lead to dramatic qualitative changes in state. Consider how flow of water from a spigot changes from a succession of droplets to a stream or how water itself turns to ice. These major qualitative shifts occur in a regulated way with only minor quantitative changes in a parameter. Third, microlevel events that occur repeatedly often precipitate macrolevel changes in an organism's state.

Granic and Patterson (2006) have described how dynamic systems theory contributes to our understanding of the development of serious conduct disorder. Early difficult temperament and minor conduct problems sometimes shift dramatically to serious violence and antisocial personality disorder through a series of subtle changes in the micro-level characteristics of a parent–child relationship. Coercive exchanges, positive reinforcement, and capitulation by one party at a microlevel can lead a child to emerge from the interaction with macrolevel changes in the propensity for antisocial behavior in other relationships.

Cairns RB, Cairns BD: *Lifelines and Risks: Pathways of Youth in Our Time.* New York: Cambridge University Press, 1994.

Granic I, Patterson GR: Toward a comprehensive model of antisocial development: a dynamic systems approach. *Psychol Rev* 2006;113(1):101.

AGE NORMS

A simple but powerful developmental concept that has affected psychiatric nosology is that of **age norms**. Rather than evaluating a set of behaviors or symptoms according to a theoretical, absolute, or population-wide distribution, diag-nosticians increasingly use age norms to evaluate psychiat-ric problems. Consider the evaluation of temper tantrums. In a 2-year-old child, tantrums are normative, whereas in an adult, angry outbursts could indicate an intermittent explo-sive disorder or antisocial personality. More subtle examples affect the diagnosis of many disorders in the *Diagnostic and Statistical Manual of Mental Disorders, Fifth Edition* (DSM-5-TR), such as attention-deficit/hyperactivity disorder, mental retardation, and conduct disorder. With regard to major depressive episodes and dysthymic disorder, age-norming has resulted in consideration of different symp-toms at different ages in order to diagnose the same disorder (e.g., irritability and somatization are common in prepubes-cent depression, whereas delusions are more common in adulthood). DSM-5-TR explicitly requires consideration of age, gender, and culture features in all disorders, suggesting the importance of evaluating symptoms within the context of their expression.

The importance of age-norming suggests the need for empirical studies of symptoms in large epidemiologic sam-ples and the linking of research on normative development to psychopathology. In this way, developmental psychopathol-ogy is similar to psychiatric epidemiology (see Chapter 2). Despite the increased emphasis on age-norming, ambiguity pervades current practice. DSM-5-TR defines disorders in terms of symptoms that are quantified as "often," "recurrent," and "persistent" without operational definition. Some clini-cians intuitively contextualize their use of the term "often" relative to a child's age-mates (so that "often displays temper tantrums" might mean hourly for a 2-year-old child and weekly for a teenager), whereas other clinicians do not (so that "often" has the same literal meaning across all ages). The specific meaning of these terms is not clear in the context of some DSM-5-TR disorders. Complete age-norming might imply the removal of all age differences in prevalence rates (reducing disorder merely to the statistical extremes of a distribution at an age level), whereas complete neglect of age norms implies that at certain ages a disorder is ubiquitous. To resolve these problems, developmental researchers need to learn which patterns of symptoms ought to be examined epidemiologically, and psychopathologists need to compare their observations to empirical norms.

American Psychiatric Association: *Diagnostic and Statistical Manual of Mental Disorders*, 5th edn. Washington DC: American Psychiatric Association, 2022.

DEVELOPMENTAL TRAJECTORIES

Diagnosticians must consider not only the age-normed profile of symptoms but also the developmental trajectories of those symptoms (both age-normed and individual). For example, consider three 10-year-old children who exhibit aggressive behavior. As depicted in Figure 4–1, child A has displayed a relatively high rate of aggression historically, but the trajectory is downward. Child B has displayed a constant rate of aggressive displays, and child C's aggressive displays have accelerated geometrically. Which child has a problematic profile? The diagnostician will undoubtedly want to consider not only current symptom counts (in relation to age norms) but also the developmental trajectory of these counts (and the age norm for the trajectory). Child C might be most problematic because of the age trend, unless this trend were also age normative (e.g., some increase in delinquent behavior in adolescence is certainly normative). In contrast, child

B's constant pattern might be problematic if the age-normed trend were a declining slope.

Some DSM-5 disorders explicitly take into account the trajectory of an individual's symptoms. For example, Rett disorder, childhood disintegrative disorder, and dementia of the Alzheimer type involve deviant trajectories. The diagnosis of other disorders may require trajectory information that is not yet available. This information must be based on longitudinal study of individuals and not cross-sectional data, because only longitudinal inquiry allows for the charting of growth curves within individuals over time. Population means at various ages indicate little about within-individual changes. Population-wide symptom counts might grow systematically across age even when individual trajectories are highly variable.

Recent advances in quantitative methodology have enabled researchers to identify trajectories of development that mark different risk. Growth curve analyses are being used to identify predictors of trajectories so that dimensions can forecast future change in behavior based on normative profiles.

A related concept to trajectories is a **dynamic cascade.** Once a trajectory is set in motion, it may set off a series of events that account for an accelerating trajectory or a particular pathway. For example, early childhood harsh physical discipline of a child may lead that child to become anxious and to engage in disruptive behavior in the school classroom, which, in turn, leads peers and teachers to reject the child. This induced social isolation may prevent the child from learning essential social skills of cooperation, which further isolates the child and gets the child into trouble at school, which gets reported back to the parents as a disciplinary problem, leading the parents to increase their harsh discipline. The events "cascade" into an enlarging circle of problems, which accelerate the child's trajectory of disruptive behavior. Diagnostically, the problems grow from early oppositional defiant disorder to conduct disorder to intermittent explosive disorder to antisocial personality disorder.

Costello EJ: Developments in child psychiatric epidemiology. *J Am Acad Child Adolesc Psychiatry* 1989;28:836.

Masten A, Cicchetti D: Developmental cascades. *Dev & Psychopath* 2010;22(3): 491–495. doi:10.1017/S0954579410000222.

Nagin DS: Analyzing developmental trajectories: A semi-parametric, group-based approach. *Psychol Methods* 1999;4:139.

THE BOUNDARY BETWEEN NORMAL & ABNORMAL

One of the tenets of developmental psychology is that a knowledge of normal development informs psychopathology partly because the boundaries between normal and abnormal are sometimes vague, diffuse, or continuous. Many disorders (e.g., conduct disorder, dysthymic disorder) are defined on the basis of cutoffs in dimensional criteria rather than on

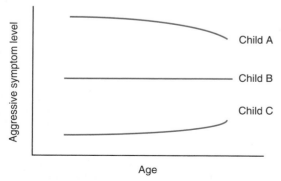

▲ **Figure 4–1** Three hypothetical developmental trajectories for aggressive behavior.

qualitative distinctions that are more easily recognizable. Criteria such as "low energy" and "low self-esteem" (for dysthymic disorder) and "marked or persistent fear" (for social phobia) are matters of degree. One of the central questions is where to locate the boundary between normal and abnormal when the criteria of psychopathology are dimensional.

In some cases, the boundary is arbitrary. In other cases the "true" boundary might be identified on the basis of three considerations: (1) a noncontinuous pattern of the distribution of scores, (2) a qualitatively distinct change in functioning that accompanies a quantitative difference in a score, or (3) unique etiology at the extreme of a distribution.

The first consideration is whether the population of scores is distributed normally with a single mode or bimodally with an unusually large number of cases at one extreme. A large number of cases at one extreme would suggest that a second causal agent is operating, beyond whatever agent caused the normal distribution. A second causal agent might suggest a deviant (i.e., psychopathologic) process. Consider the relation between the intelligence quotient (IQ) score (a continuous measure) and mental retardation. The distribution of IQ scores in the U.S. population is not normal. Far more cases of IQs below 70 occur than would be expected by a normal distribution. Thus, the distinction between normal and abnormal IQ scores is not merely one of degree.

The second consideration is whether qualitative differences in functioning occur with quantitative shifts in a criterion. For example, if a decrement of 10 IQ points from 75 to 65 makes it significantly more difficult for a child to function in a classroom than a decrement from 100 to 90, then a case can be made for locating the cutoff point near an IQ of 70.

The third consideration is the possible distinct etiology of scores at an extreme end of the distribution. A single set of causes will ordinarily lead to a normal distribution of scores. A disproportionate number of scores at an extreme often suggests a separate etiology for those scores. In the case of IQ scores, one set of forces (e.g., genes, socialization) leads to a normal distribution, whereas a second set of forces (e.g., Down syndrome, anoxia, lead toxicity) leads to a large number of cases at the low extreme.

Cicchetti D, Toth SL: Developmental psychopathology and preventive intervention. In: Damon W (series ed), Renninger KA, Sigel IE (vol eds). *Handbook of Child Psychology, Vol 4. Child Psychology in Practice*, 6th edn. New York: Wiley, 2006, p. 497.

MULTIPLE PATHWAYS

A vexing problem highlighted by research in developmental psychology is that some disorders involve multiple etiologic pathways. The principles of equifinality and multifinality, derived from general systems theory, hold for many disorders. **Equifinality** is the concept that the same phenomenon may result from several different pathogens. For example, infantile autism results from congenital rubella, inherited metabolic disorder, or other factors. **Multifinality** is the concept that one etiologic factor can lead to any of several psychopathologic outcomes, depending on the person and context. Early physical abuse might lead to conduct disorder or to dysthymic disorder, depending on the person's predilections and the environmental supports for various symptoms; poverty predisposes one toward conduct disorder but also substance abuse disorder.

The diversity in processes and outcomes for disorders makes the systematic study of a single disorder difficult. Unless scholars consider multiple disorders and multiple factors simultaneously, they cannot be sure whether an apparent etiologic factor is specific to that disorder. Inquiry into one disorder benefits from a conceptualization within a larger body of development of normal adjustment versus problem outcomes. The broad coverage of developmental psychology provides the grounding for inquiry into various disorders.

Rutter M: Psychosocial resilience and protective mechanisms. In: Rolf J, Masten AS, Cicchetti D, et al. (eds). *Risk and Protective Factors in the Development of Psychopathology*. New York: Cambridge University Press, 1990.

BIOSOCIAL INTERACTIONS

The discovery of biosocial interactions in psychiatric disorders has been called one of the most important discoveries in all of science in the past several decades. Not only are multiple distinct factors implicated in the genesis of a disorder, the profile of factors often conspires to lead to psychopathologic outcomes. Empirically, this profile is the statistical interaction between factors (in contrast with the main effects of factors). Thus, a causal factor might operate only when it occurs in concert with another factor. For example, the experience of parental rejection early in life is a contributing factor in the development of conduct disorder, but only among that subgroup of children who also display a biologically based problem such as health difficulties at the time of birth. Likewise, health problems at birth do not inevitably lead to conduct disorder; the interaction of a biologically based predisposition with a psychosocial stressor is often required for a psychopathologic outcome.

Caspi et al. (2002) hypothesized that risk for conduct disorder grows out of the early experience of physical maltreatment, but only among a subpopulation characterized by polymorphism in the gene encoding the neurotransmitter-metabolizing enzyme monoamine oxidase A (MAOA). They found that physically maltreated children with a genotype conferring high levels of MAOA expression were less likely to develop antisocial problems than children without this genotype. These findings help us understand why not all victims of maltreatment grow up to victimize others, and they also indicate that environmental experiences may be necessary to potentiate the action of a genotype.

The same group of researchers has discovered a biosocial interaction in the development of depressive disorder. Life stressors precipitate the onset of depressive episodes, but only among a subpopulation characterized by a functional polymorphism in the promoter region of the serotonin transporter (5-HT T) gene. Individuals with one or two copies of the short allele of the 5-HT T promoter polymorphism exhibit more depressive symptoms, diagnosable depression, and suicidality in response to stressful life events than individuals homozygous for the long allele. The importance of biosocial interactions suggests the importance of examining multiple diverse factors simultaneously, in both empirical research and clinical practice.

Caspi A, McClay J, Moffitt TE, et al: Role of genotype in the cycle of violence in maltreated children. *Science* 2002;297:851.

Caspi A, Sugden K, Moffitt TE, et al: Influence of life stress on depression: moderation by a polymorphism in the 5-HTT gene. *Science* 2003;301:386.

CRITICAL PERIODS & TRANSITION POINTS

A **critical period** is a point in the life span at which an individual is acutely sensitive to the effects of an external stimulus, including a pathogen. Freud argued that the first 3 years of life represent a critical period for the development of psychopathology, through concepts such as regression, fixation, and irreversibility. The concept of critical stages gained credence with studies of social behavior in animals by the ethologist Lorenz and the zoologist Scott. This concept is part of several central theories of social development, such as Bowlby's attachment theory (discussed later in this chapter). The rapid development of the nervous system in the first several years, coupled with relatively less neural plasticity in subsequent years, renders this period critical. The effects of exposure to lead and alcohol, for example, are far more dramatic when the exposure occurs in utero or in early life.

A variation of the concept of a critical period is the hypothesis of gradually decreasing plasticity in functioning across the life span. As neural pathways become canalized, mental representations become more automatic and habits form. However, the notion of the primacy of early childhood has been thrown into question by empirical data that indicate greater malleability in functioning than was previously thought. Rutter, for example, suggests that a positive relationship with a parental figure is crucial to the prevention of conduct disorder and that this relationship can develop or occur at any point up to adolescence, not just during the first year of life.

Some developmental psychologists have argued for other critical periods in life, such as puberty and giving birth, as critical periods for the development of major depressive disorder in women, although this assertion has been contested. Critical periods might be defined not only by biological events but also by psychosocial transitions. Developmental psychologists have increasingly recognized the crucial role of major life transitions in altering developmental course, accelerating or decelerating psychopathologic development, and representing high-risk periods for psychopathology. These **transition points** include but are not limited to entry to formal schooling, puberty and the transition to junior high school, high school graduation and entry into the world of employment, marriage, birth of children, and death of loved ones (particularly parents or spouse). These transitions have been associated with elevated risk for some forms of psychopathology. One task of developmental psychologists is to discover which life transitions are most crucial and how these transitions alter the course of development of some but not other forms of psychopathology.

Kandel ER, Hawkins RD: Neuronal plasticity and learning. In: Broadwell RD (vol ed). *Decade of the Brain. Vol 1: Neuroscience, Memory, and Language.* Washington DC: Library of Congress, 1995.

BRAIN DEVELOPMENT AND THE PRIMACY OF EARLY LIFE EXPERIENCES

Over the past two decades, advances in the measurement of brain activity through fMRI and related technologies, coupled with emerging findings from long-term prospective panel studies following children from birth through adulthood, have led developmental scientists to recognize the primacy of early life experiences in shaping a child's life course.

Beginning at birth, the human brain responds to environmental input by forming over a million new neural connections (not neurons—that number is stable—but connections) every second, a far more rapid rate of growth than at any other time in the life span. Basic sensory pathways for vision and hearing develop first, followed by higher cognitive functions and language. By age 3, brain volume reaches about 80% of its adult brain size, even though overall body volume is much less. By this age, however, some of the weaker connections begin to whittle away through a process called **pruning**, in order for stronger brain circuits to become more efficient. With the growth of neural connections, the capacity for change (called **plasticity**) is high; with pruning, the capacity for change declines.

Complementing brain development studies are epidemiological panel studies that demonstrate the strong predictive power that comes from early life experiences, particularly trauma. Children who experience child maltreatment in the first 5 years of life are at several times higher risk for poor health, mental health, and behavioral outcomes in adulthood, even controlling for possible confounding factors. The process is that early adverse childhood events (called ACEs) lead children to develop a defensive mindset that is encoded in neural connections that, in turn, leads children to respond adaptively to future threat but maladaptively to common life circumstances. Once set in neural connections, these associations are difficult to disconnect and maladaptive life outcome are likely to cascade. This work, and a long line of accompanying research, suggest the importance of prevention and early intervention.

Center on the Developing Child. (2023). *The science of early childhood development (InBrief)*. Retrieved from www.developingchild.harvard.edu.
Dodge KA: Toward population impact from early childhood psychological interventions. *Am Psychol* 2018;73(9):1117–1129. PMCID: PMC6416783. https://doi.org/10.1037/amp0000393.

THE ONSET AND ORIGIN OF DISPARITIES

One of the most pervasive yet vexing phenomena in developmental psychology and psychiatry is the disparities in maladaptive outcomes that develop across race and income groups. These disparities are evident in employment, education, the justice system, and the mental health system. Although race and income are highly correlated, over the past 30 years, the gap in education outcomes has shifted from one of primarily race disparities to primarily income disparities. One of the most robust findings in developmental psychology is the discovery that the gaps in outcomes are highly attributable to gaps in early-life opportunities. Persons of color experience poorer adult outcomes because they experience fewer opportunities in the first years of life. Furthermore, early intervention that is successful in reducing gaps in opportunities is also likely to be successful in reducing gaps in outcomes.

Bailey ZD, Feldman JM, Bassett MT: How structural racism works—racist policies as a root cause of US racial health inequities. *N Engl J Med* 2021;384:768–773. https://doi.org/10.1056/NEJMms2025396.
Dodge KA, Goodman WB, Bai Y, et al: Impact of universal perinatal home-visiting program on reduction in race disparities in maternal and child health: two randomized controlled trials and a field quasi-experiment. *Lancet Reg Health Am* 2022;5:1–11. https://doi.org/10.1016/j.lana.2022.100356.

THE CHAOS OF ADOLESCENCE

Just as the years following birth are a sensitive period of rapid brain development, so, too, is the adolescent period beginning with puberty and lasting through age 25 or so. Parents, school teachers, and physicians are well aware of the heightened risk-taking and sensation seeking that adolescents crave, and the seemingly long delay before more rational decision-making takes hold. Recent studies of neurodevelopment have identified two important dramatic changes in brain function during this period that have been integrated by B.J. Casey and Laurence Steinberg into a theory of the adolescent brain.

The first development that occurs during puberty is growth in the reward system. To adolescents, sensationalized activities hold huge rewards, take on larger meaning, and attract more attention. The second development does not occur until years later, that is, the control system that identifies punishments and realistic appraisals of the actual consequences of engaging in sensationalized behaviors. The period in between is the "chaos" that adults observe in their teenagers. One might construe these dual systems as the gas pedal and brake pedal of an automobile. The "gas" pedal develops sooner than the brake. Optimal functioning balances the reward and control functions but does not take full shape until the mid-20s. Steinberg has applied this model to an understanding of the culpability of teenagers in their misbehavior and the responsible decision-making that we can, or cannot, expect of teenagers, with important implications for U.S. Supreme Court decisions to abolish capital punishment for juveniles based on their neuro-immaturity.

Casey BJ, Heller A, Gee D: Development of the emotional brain. *Neurosci Lett* 2019;693:29–34. PMCID:PMC5984129, DOI: 10.1016/j.neulet.2017.11.055.
Steinberg L, Icenogle G: Using developmental science to distinguish adolescents and adults under the law. *Annu Rev Dev Psychol* 2019;1:21–40.

IMPORTANCE OF CONTEXT

One of the most important contributions of developmental psychology has been the discovery that patterns of behavior, and of process–behavior linkage, vary across contexts. In the context of U.S. society, a child who is teased by peers might find support for retaliating aggressively, whereas the same teasing experience in Japanese society might cause shame, embarrassment, and withdrawal. Thus, reactive aggressive behavior might be stigmatized as psychopathology in one culture but not another. Context shapes single behaviors and may also shape patterns of psychopathology.

Context also provides the frame or ground through which individual behaviors are given meaning. For example, a child interprets a parent's discipline in relation to norms that are observed culture-wide. In cultures that endorse the use of corporal punishment as appropriate, a child who is punished in this manner (at mild, nonabusive levels) is not at particularly high risk for anxiety problems or conduct problems. However, in cultures that do not endorse this type of parenting, a child who is corporally punished is likely to interpret it as a signal that the parent rejects the child as aberrant or is an aberrant parent, and either interpretation is likely to lead to anxiety and conduct problems.

Context can be defined at many levels, from discrete situational features to broad cultural features and from internal states such as mood to external factors such as geography or time of day. Bronfenbrenner's continuum of environmental contexts forms the basis of his ecological theory (discussed later in this chapter).

Bronfenbrenner U: *The Ecology of Human Development: Experiments by Nature and Design*. Cambridge, MA: Harvard University Press, 1979.

Dodge KA, Coie JD, Lynam D: Aggression and antisocial behavior in youth. In: Damon W (series ed), Eisenberg N (vol ed), *Handbook of Child Psychology, Vol. 3. Social, Emotional, and Personality Development*, 6th edn. New York: Wiley, 2006, pp. 719–788.

Lansford JE, Chang L, Dodge KA, et al: Physical discipline and children's adjustment: cultural normativeness as a moderator. *Child Dev* 2005;76(6):1234–1246.

ADAPTATION & COMPETENCE

Research in developmental psychology has sometimes enabled sharper distinctions between normal and abnormal (such as when a genetic marker of a disorder is identified), but more often it has articulated the continuity between normal and abnormal. Research has suggested that disorders might be defined less by noncontextualized behavioral criteria (e.g., a score on an IQ test) and more by an assessment of the individual's level of adaptation and functioning. This concept has been embraced by the term **competence**, or adaptive functioning, which is the level of performance by an individual in meeting the demands of his or her environment to the degree that would be expected given the environment and the individual's age, background, and biological potentials.

Empirical research has shown that measures of childhood social competence are important predictors of adolescent psychiatric disorders, including conduct disorder and mood disorders. Impaired social competence is a premorbid marker for the onset of schizophrenia and is a predictor of relapse.

The concurrent importance of adaptive functioning is so obvious that this concept has become part of the diagnostic criteria for some disorders. For example, a diagnosis of mental retardation requires impairment in adaptive functioning above and beyond the score on an IQ test. A diagnosis of generalized anxiety disorder requires impairment in social functioning in addition to the absolute pattern of anxiety. A diagnosis of obsessive–compulsive disorder requires marked personal distress or significant impairment in functioning. Some broad definitions of mental disorder are based on a general assessment of an impairment in adaptive functioning due to cognitive or emotional disturbance.

Kazdin AE: *Conduct Disorders in Childhood and Adolescence*. Thousand Oaks, CA: Sage, 1995.

Kupersmidt JB, Dodge KA (eds): *Children's Peer Relations: From Development to Intervention*. Washington, DC: American Psychological Association, 2004.

RISK FACTORS & VULNERABILITY

Epidemiologic and developmental researchers have introduced the notion of **risk factors** to identify variables known to predict later disorder. A risk factor is defined by its probabilistic relation to an outcome variable, without implying determinism, early onset of disorder, or inevitability of outcome. Risk factors are either markers of some other causal process or causal factors themselves. One goal of developmental research is to determine the causal status of risk markers. As noted earlier in this chapter, social competence, or level of adaptive functioning, is a broad risk factor for many disorders, but empirical research must determine whether this factor merely indicates risk that is caused by some other factor (e.g., genes) or constitutes a contributing factor in itself.

Risk factors often accumulate in enhancing the likelihood of eventual disorder. For example, the probability of conduct disorder is enhanced by low socioeconomic status, harsh parenting, parental criminality, marital conflict, family size, and academic failure. The number of factors present seems to be a stronger predictor of later disorder than is the presence of any single factor, suggesting that causal processes are heterogeneous and that risk factors cumulatively increase vulnerability to a causal process.

The concept of **vulnerability** has been applied to individuals who are characterized by a risk factor. Many empirical studies of the development of disorder use samples that are defined by a risk factor (such as offspring of alcoholics and first-time juvenile offenders); however, it is not clear that the causal and developmental factors are similar in disordered individuals who come from high-risk and low-risk populations.

Biederman J, Milberger S, Faraone SV, et al: Family-environment risk factors for attention-deficit hyperactivity disorder. *Arch Gen Psychiatry* 1995;52:464.

Cicchetti D, Cohen DJ (eds): *Developmental Psychopathology*, Vols. 1–3. New York: Wiley, 2006.

MEDIATORS & PROCESS

Developmental psychologists study the causal process through which disorder develops. The identification of a risk factor does not necessarily imply a causal process for these reasons: (1) a risk factor might be a proxy for a causal factor and empirically related to a disorder only because of its correlation with this causal factor (the so-called third-variable problem), (2) a risk factor might occur as an outcome of a process that is related to a disorder rather than as the antecedent of the disorder, or (3) a risk factor might play a causal role in a more complex, multivariate process. Indeed, individuals who are predisposed to a disorder often select environments that are congruent with the disorder. The environment might appear to "cause" the disorder but instead merely be a marker of risk. Therefore, developmental psychologists often attempt

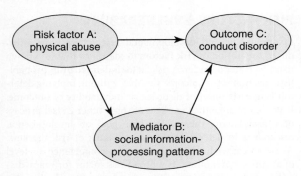

▲ **Figure 4–2** Mediation of the effect of physical abuse on the development of conduct disorder.

to understand the process through which risk factors are related to eventual disorder. The factors that are identified as intervening variables in this process are called **mediators**, or variables that account for (or partially account for) the statistical relation between a risk factor and a disorder.

Four empirical steps are required to demonstrate at least partial mediation (Figure 4–2). First, risk factor A must be empirically related to outcome C (i.e., there must be a phenomenon to be mediated, called the **total effect**). Second, A must be related to mediator B. Third, B must be related to C. Finally, in a stepwise regression or structural equation model analysis, when B has been added to the prediction of C, the resulting relation between A and C (called the **direct effect**) must be reduced significantly from the original bivariate relation. The difference between the total effect and the direct effect is called the **indirect effect**, that is, the magnitude of the mediation of the effect of A on C by B.

An example (depicted in Figure 4–2) is the biased pattern of social information-processing that often results from an early history of physical abuse. Early abuse (A) is a known risk factor for the development of conduct disorder (C) (i.e., it is statistically correlated with later conduct disorder, but many abused children do not develop this disorder nor do all persons who have conduct disorder show a history of abuse). Early abuse is also correlated with the development of a social information-processing pattern (B) of hypervigilance to threatening cues, perceiving the social world as a hostile and threatening place, and poor social problem-solving skills. These mental factors (B) are associated statistically with later conduct disorder (C) and account for about half of the effect of early abuse (A) on later conduct disorder (C).

Baron RM, Kenny DA: The moderator-mediator variable distinction in social psychological research: conceptual, strategic, and statistical considerations. *J Pers Soc Psychol* 1986;51:1173.

Dodge KA, Pettit GS: A biopsychosocial model of the development of chronic conduct problems in adolescence. *Dev Psychol* 2003; 39(2):349.

MODERATORS & PROTECTIVE FACTORS

Rutter found that the effect of a risk factor on a disorder can vary across contexts, populations, or circumstances. That is, the magnitude of an effect might be reduced (or enhanced) under different conditions. For example, the effect of early harsh discipline on the development of conduct disorder is reduced under circumstances of a warm parent–child relationship. This phenomenon is called a **moderator effect** and is defined by a significant interaction effect between a risk factor and a moderating factor in the prediction of a disorder.

Moderator variables have also been called **protective**, or **buffering**, factors. A protective factor protects, or buffers, the individual from the pathogenic effects of a risk factor. Intelligence and a positive relationship with a caring adult have been the most commonly studied protective factors for a variety of disorders. One remaining question is whether protective factors operate more strongly in high-risk than in low-risk groups; that is, if a variable buffers both low-risk and high-risk groups from risk, it is not clear whether that variable would be defined as a protective factor (or simply another predictor variable).

Rutter M, Sroufe LA: Developmental psychopathology: concepts and challenges. *Dev Psychopathol* 2000;12:265–296.

INTERVENTION & PREVENTION AS EXPERIMENTS

There is a reciprocal relation between the scientific study of behavior in developmental psychology and the application of scientific principles to psychiatry. Concepts from developmental psychology have been applied in psychiatric practice, but psychiatric intervention can also be viewed as a field experiment to test hypotheses about behavioral development. Systematic intervention and prevention can be viewed as experiments to test basic principles. In fact, given the complexity of human behavioral development and the ethical restraints against known iatrogenic manipulations, clinical practice may be the most powerful scientific tool available to test hypotheses from developmental psychology. Thus, the relation between these disciplines is reciprocal, and communication between the disciplines must be preserved.

Renninger KA, Sigel IE (vol eds). *Handbook of Child Psychology.* New York: Wiley, 2006, p. 497.

▼ GENERAL DEVELOPMENTAL THEORIES

Seven major theories of development are listed in Table 4–2, along with key concepts and criticisms of each theory. These theories, along with their applications, are described in detail in the sections that follow.

Table 4–2 General Developmental Theories

Theory	Key Concepts	Criticisms
Temperament theory	Traits, genetic origins of behavior	Imprecise measurement, static view of human beings
Organismic theory	Stages of development, transformational role	Empirical refutation
Attachment theory	Patterns of relationships, working models	Too much emphasis on destiny from infancy
Social learning theory	Observational learning, imitation, reinforcement	Exclusive emphasis on environmental influences and cognitive mediation
Attribution theory	Mental heuristics, causal influences	Lack of emphasis on development, too narrow
Social information processing theory	Mental processes during social interaction	Nonbiological
Ecological theory	Levels of systems	Vague and not falsifiable

TEMPERAMENT THEORY

Since the "human bile" theories of ancient Greeks, scholars have speculated that persons are born into the world with varying predispositions to behave in particular ways, called **traits**. Trait theorists have postulated a variety of dispositional tendencies, from Eysenck's neuroticism and extraversion to the "Big Five" traits of agreeableness, openness, extraversion, neuroticism, and conscientiousness. In developmental inquiry, temperament theory has received the greatest attention. It has been hypothesized that infants are born with biologically based temperaments that vary on a continuum from difficult to easy. This trait is evidenced in ease of early care, including feeding, soothing, and cuddling. As children grow older, these differences are evidenced in ease of manageability (e.g., the temper tantrums of 18-month-old children and the behavior difficulties of the preschool period). The trait of difficultness has been hypothesized as a risk factor for conduct disorder. Empirical studies have found significant but modest support for this hypothesis. Prospective studies indicate that infants characterized as difficult are indeed at risk for conduct problems in the early school years, but the relation is somewhat weaker (although still present) for predictions from infancy to adolescence.

A different temperament theory, proposed by Kagan, has focused on the continuum of biological inhibition as the marker variable. Some infants regularly withdraw from novel social stimuli (**inhibited pattern**) whereas others seek out social stimulation (**uninhibited pattern**). Optimal levels of inhibition may fall between these extremes. Highly inhibited infants exhibit separation anxiety from parents and are likely to grow into shy, fearful, and withdrawn children. They are thought to be at risk for panic disorder in adulthood. Inhibited individuals demonstrate an increase in heart rate and stabilization of heart rate variability in response to a stress challenge. Individuals vary systematically in the degree to which the hypothalamus, pituitary gland, and adrenal gland (called the HPA axis)

respond with glucocorticoid secretion during stress. Inhibited children have a lower threshold of sympathetic nervous system response and display a greater rise and stabilization of heart rate than uninhibited children exhibit. This pattern acts as a traitlike temperamental characteristic throughout life that may be associated with symptoms of anxiety.

Another postulate of temperament theories is that temperament elicits environmental treatment that perpetuates behavior consistent with that temperament. For example, it is hypothesized that "difficult" children elicit harsh discipline, which exacerbates difficult behavior, whereas inhibited children seek secure environments that pose minimal challenge and risk. In the last decade, it has been demonstrated through twin and adoption studies that environmental experiences have a heritable component; that is, inherited genes lead either to behavior patterns that elicit environmental reactions or to behaviors that seek particular environments, a phenomenon known as niche-picking.

▶ Applications of the Theory

Most temperament theorists recognize the importance of both inherited and environmental sources of development, so this theory has spawned empirical research directed toward understanding how these forces interact. It may be that infants with a particular temperament will develop more favorably under certain environmental conditions than others, and the task of inquiry is to identify optimal temperament–environment matches. Researchers are examining whether temperamentally difficult (or highly inhibited) infants develop more favorably under conditions of environmental restraint and structure or flexibility and freedom.

Another application has been to encourage research on the process through which genetic effects may operate on human development, thus informing the age-old debate between the influence of nature and nurture on human behavior (see Chapter 3).

Criticisms of the Theory

One problem with research on temperament theory has been the reliance on parents for assessments of temperament. Parents may be biased or inaccurate, or they may lack a broad base of knowledge of other infants. A parent's perceptions about his or her child may be legitimate factors in the child's development, but these perceptions confound information about the child's actual behavior with the parent's construal of the behavior. Direct observational measures of behavior have been developed to assess temperament, as have measures of biological functions, including heart rate reactivity, cortisol secretions, and skin conductivity. These measures also show some stability across time and some predictive power, but the number of studies is small and the statistical effects weak.

Another problem is the difficulty of distinguishing genetic–biological features from reactions to environmental treatment. A 6-month-old infant brings both a genetic heritage and a history of environmental experiences to current interactions. Even biological measures (e.g., resting heart rate, cortisol levels) have a partial basis in past social exchanges, so that the task of sorting genetic from environmental sources in biobehavioral measures is difficult.

Rothbart MK, Bates JE: Temperament. In: Damon W (series ed), Eisenberg N (vol ed), *Handbook of Child Psychology, Vol. 3. Social, Emotional, and Personality Development*, 6th edn. New York: Wiley, 2006, p. 99.

ORGANISMIC THEORY

No one has had more influence in developmental psychology than Piaget. The coherence of behavior across diverse domains and the tendency for changes in abilities to occur simultaneously across domains form the basis of the organismic theory of Piaget and others such as Gesell, Werner, and Baldwin. This theory attempts to describe general features of human cognition and the systematic changes in thought across development. The organizing principle in organismic theory is **structure**, which is a closed system of transformational rules that govern thought at a particular point in development. Consider the 5-year-old girl who observes one row of nine beads placed near each other and a second row of six beads stretched across a greater distance than the first row. Even though the girl has counted the beads in each row and knows that nine is greater than six, in response to the question, "Which row has more beads?" she will answer, "The row with six beads." Moreover, the girl will see no contradiction in her answer. According to Piaget, this nonobvious phenomenon occurs because the girl's structural transformation law is to consider the whole of a stimulus, not each part separately. The child's rule structure is closed; that is, it is internally consistent and not easily altered by external contradictions.

Piaget hypothesized that infants are born with a general wiring for a crude set of transformational rules common to all sensorimotor coordination. These rules are part of the evolutionary inheritance of the human organism. Development occurs over a 12- to 15-year period in nonlinear chunks, called **stages**. Within each stage, functioning is internally consistent and stable (called an **equilibrium**). Change from one stage to the next occurs as a result of interaction between the child and the realities of the environment. When contradictory realities accumulate sufficiently, change occurs rapidly and globally. As discussed earlier in this chapter, processes of change involve assimilation and accommodation. Assimilation is the act of interpreting environmental experiences in terms that are consistent with existing rule structure (a form of generalization), whereas accommodation is the act of altering rule structures to account for environmental experience (a form of exception noting). Children engage in both assimilation and accommodation in order to maintain coherence (and the perception of consistency), until their overgeneralizations and exceptions become so contradictory that they must create higher-level, more flexible, novel structures that account for the contradictions of earlier stages. When a novel structure (i.e., a new set of rules) is achieved, **equilibration** consolidates the rules until contradictions accumulate to set the scene for the next stage change. Piaget's four broad stages of cognitive development are (1) the sensorimotor period, (2) the preoperational stage, (3) the concrete-operational stage, and (4) the period of formal operations.

Applications of the Theory

Many of Piaget's concepts continue to have heuristic value even today and to provide hypotheses relevant to psychopathology. The notions of egocentrism, the invariant sequences of skill acquisition, and increasing differentiation (i.e., development rather than mere change) provide hypotheses regarding the behavior of children who have conduct problems and of adolescents who are lagging developmentally. Furthermore, Piaget's discoveries of the limits of young children's abilities have inspired cognitive educational strategies.

Criticisms of the Theory

Even though Piaget's influence has been tremendous, crucial features of organismic theory have been refuted. Children have repeatedly been shown to be more competent than Piaget suggested they could be at a particular age. Piaget's proposed cross-domain universality in type of thought has been shown to be false, suggesting to some scholars that the stage concept is faulty. It has been replaced by concepts of learning strategies, information-processing patterns, and the parsing of multiple components in complex task completion.

Piaget J: Piaget's theory. In: Kesson W (ed). *Handbook of Child Psychology. Vol 1: History, Theory, and Methods*, 4th edn. New York: Wiley, 1983.

ATTACHMENT THEORY

Bowlby generated a theory of attachment that has had enormous influence in contemporary developmental psychology. According to Bowlby, infants are born with innate tendencies to seek direct contact with an adult (usually the mother). In contrast to Freud's perspective that early attachment-seeking is a function of a desire for the mother's breast (and food), Bowlby argued that attachment seeking is directed toward social contact with the mother (the desire for a love relationship) and driven by fear of unknown others. By about 6–8 months of age, separation from the mother arouses distress, analogous to free-floating anxiety. The distress of a short-term separation is replaced quickly by the warmth of the reunion with the mother, but longer separations (such as those that occur in hospitalization or abandonment) can induce clinging, suspicion, and anxiety upon reunion. Similar effects are seen in older children until individuation occurs, at which point the child is cognitively able to hold a mental representation of the mother while she is gone, enabling the child to explore novelty.

Bowlby hypothesized that individual differences exist in patterns of parent–infant relationship quality and that the infant acquires a mental representation (or working model) of this relationship that is stored in memory and carried forward to act as a guiding filter for all future relationships. This working model of relationships generalizes to other contexts and allows future interactions to conform to the working model, thereby reinforcing the initial representation of how relationships operate. Thus, the quality of the initial parent–infant relationship has primary and enduring effects on later adjustment, relationships, and parenting.

Individual differences in attachment patterns have been assessed through a laboratory procedure called the Strange Situation, devised by Ainsworth. The parent and 12-month-old child are brought to an unfamiliar room containing toys, after which a stranger enters. The parent then leaves the room for a short period, followed by a reunion. The child's behavior, especially toward the parent upon reunion, is indicative of the quality of the overall parent–child attachment. Attachment classifications are summarized in Table 4–3.

About two-thirds of children fit the "secure" response pattern (type B), in which they demonstrate distress when the parent leaves and enthusiasm (or confident pleasure) upon her return. An "avoidant" response pattern (type A) involves little distress and little relief or pleasure upon reunion with the parent. A "resistant or ambivalent" response pattern (type C) involves panicky distress upon the parent's departure and emotional ambivalence upon reunion (perhaps running toward the parent to be picked up but then immediately, angrily struggling to get down). Recently, scholars have identified a fourth class of response, "disorganized" (type D, empirically linked to early physical or sexual maltreatment), in which the child's behavior involves great distress and little systematic exploration or seeking of adults.

▶ Applications of the Theory

Follow-up studies have shown that these patterns of attachment are somewhat stable over time (although not strongly correlated across relationships with different adults) and predictive of behavioral adjustment in middle childhood. Infants of types A, C, and D are all at risk for later maladjustment, although more specific patterns of outcome for each type have not been detected reliably. Developmental scholars have created methods for assessing relationship quality and working models at older ages and have related these assessments to current behavioral functioning.

▶ Criticisms of the Theory

Critics of attachment theory suggest that the initial relationship does not determine destiny as strongly as Bowlby argued, and that long-term predictive power is due partly to consistency in the environment that led to the child's initial response pattern. Attachment theory has been used to condemn the practice of early out-of-home daycare (because it interferes with the development of a secure attachment with the mother), even though most studies find little long-term effect of such care after other confounding factors (e.g., economics, family stability, stress, later caregiving) are controlled. More broadly, the reversibility of the effects of early social deprivation and trauma remain controversial. The current general conclusion is that even though early experiences shape later experiences through the filter of mental representations, the plasticity of the human organism is greater than previously hypothesized, but only up to a point.

Ainsworth MDS et al: *Patterns of Attachment.* Hillsdale, NJ: Erlbaum, 1978.

Bowlby J: *Attachment and Loss. Vol 3: Loss, Sadness, and Depression.* New York: Basic Books, 1980.

SOCIAL LEARNING THEORY

Bandura's social learning theory, though acknowledging the constraints of biological origins and the role of neural mediating mechanisms, emphasizes the role of the individual's

Table 4–3 Attachment Types and Associated Working Models and Outcomes

Attachment Type	Working Model	Outcome
A: Avoidant	Fearful	Risk
B: Secure	Exploration with confidence	Healthy
C: Ambivalent	Panicky distress and anger	Risk
D: Disorganized	Great distress	Risk

experience of the environment in development. Other learning theories are based on the organism's direct performance of behaviors, whereas social learning theory posits that most learning occurs vicariously by observing and imitating models. For survival and growth, humans are designed to acquire patterns of behavior through **observational learning**. Social behavior in particular is a function of one's social learning history, instigation mechanisms, and maintaining mechanisms.

Four processes govern social learning: (1) attention, which regulates exploration and perception; (2) memory, through which observed events are symbolically stored to guide future behavior; (3) motor production, through which novel behaviors are formed from the integration of constituent acts with observed actions; and (4) incentives and motivation, which regulate the performance of learned responses. Development involves biological maturation in these processes as well as the increasingly complex storage of contingencies and response repertoires in memory.

Instigation mechanisms include both biological and cognitive motivators. Internal aversive stimulation might activate behavior through its painful effect (on hunger, sex, or aggression). Cognitively based motivators are based on the organism's capacity to represent mentally future material, sensory, and social consequences. Mentally represented consequences provide the motivation for action.

Maintaining mechanisms include external reinforcement (e.g., tangible rewards, social and status rewards, reduction of aversive treatment), punishment, vicarious reinforcement by observation, and self-regulatory mechanisms (e.g., self-observation, self-judgment through attribution and valuation, self-applied consequences). Development in social learning theory is decidedly not stagelike and has few constraints. For example, Bandura argued that even relatively sophisticated moral thought and action are possible in young children, given relevant models and experiences.

▶ Applications of the Theory

Social learning theory has been applied most effectively to aggressive behavior, where it has provided powerful explanations for the effects of coercive parenting, violent media presentations, and rejecting peer interactions on the development of chronic aggressive behavior. Furthermore, it provides the basis for most current behavior-modification interventions in clinical practice.

▶ Criticisms of the Theory

Critics dispute the primacy of cognitive mediation in understanding learning effects and the relative emphasis on environment over genetic and biological influences.

Bandura A: *Social Foundations of Thought and Action: A Social Cognitive Theory.* Englewood Cliffs, NJ: Prentice-Hall, 1986.

ATTRIBUTION THEORY

The emphasis on cognition in social learning theory is largely consequence oriented (i.e., based on individuals' cognitions about the likely outcomes of their behavior). Attribution theory is more concerned with how people understand the causes of behavior. Its origins are in the naïve or common-sense psychology of Heider, who suggested that an individual's beliefs about events play a more important role in behavior than does the objective truth of events. For social interactions, an individual's beliefs about the causes of another person's behavior are more crucial than are the true causes. For example, in deciding whether to retaliate aggressively against a peer following a provocation (such as being bumped from behind), a person often uses an attribution about the peer's intention. If the peer acted accidentally, then no retaliation occurs, but if the peer acted maliciously, then retaliation may be likely. The perceiver's task in social exchanges is to decide which effects of an observed action are intentional (reflecting dispositions) and which are situational.

When judging whether another person's behavior (such as aggression) should be attributed to a dispositional rather than a situational cause, perceivers use mental heuristics, such as correspondent inference and covariation. Perceivers examine whether the person's actions are normative or unique (if unique, they may indicate a dispositional rather than situational cause). They examine the other person's behavioral consistency over time and distinctiveness across situations (if the behavior is consistent, it more likely reflects a disposition). Finally, they examine whether the action has personal hedonic relevance to the perceiver (if the action is relevant to the perceiver, perceivers tend to attribute dispositional causes).

These principles predict the kinds of causal attributions that people make about the events around them, the circumstances under which people will make errors in inference, and people's behavioral responses to events. Extensions of attribution theory have addressed differences in the causal attributions made by people about themselves versus others (actor–observer effects), the kinds of explanations that people give for their own behavior and outcomes (internal versus external attributions), and the circumstances under which people spontaneously make attributions.

▶ Applications of the Theory

Attribution theory has been applied to problems in several domains of psychiatry and health. Studies have shown that attributions predict behavioral responses to critical events such as interpersonal losses and failure. People who attribute their failure to a lack of ability on their part are likely to give up and to continue to fail, whereas people who attribute their failure to a lack of effort are likely to intensify future efforts to succeed. People who regularly attribute their failures to global, stable, and internal causes (i.e., they blame themselves) are at risk for a mood disorder and somatization disorder. People who attribute their own negative outcomes to the fault of others are likely to direct aggression toward the perceived cause of the outcome (and to develop a conduct disorder). Interventions have been developed to help people redirect attributions more accurately or more adaptively, most notably in cognitive therapies for depression.

▶ Criticisms of the Theory

Until recently, the problem of development was relatively ignored in attribution theory. Studies only recently have begun to address topics such as the age at which attributions come to be made spontaneously, the relevance of spontaneous attribution tendencies for age differences in depression, and the experiential origins of chronic attributional tendencies.

Dodge KA. Translational science in action: hostile attributional style and the development of aggressive behavior problems. *Dev Psychopathol* 2006;18:791.

SOCIAL INFORMATION-PROCESSING THEORY

The comprehensive extension of social learning theory and attribution theory is to consider all of the mental processes that people use in relating to the social world. Simon's work in cognitive science forms the basis for social information-processing theory. This theory recognizes that people come to social situations with a set of biologically determined capabilities and a database of past experiences (Figure 4–3).

They receive as input a set of social cues (such as a push in the back by a peer or a failing grade in a school subject). The person's behavioral response to the cues occurs as a function

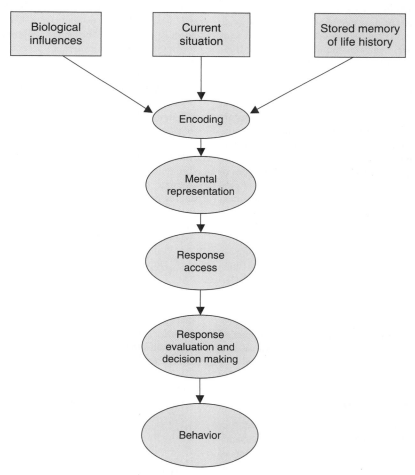

▲ **Figure 4–3** Social information-processing theory.

of a sequence of mental processes, beginning with encoding of cues through sensation and perception. The vastness of available cues requires selective attention to cues (such as attention to peers' laughter versus one's own physical pain). Selective encoding is partially predictive of ultimate behavior. The storage of cues in memory is not veridical with objective experience. The mental representation and interpretation of the cues (possibly involving attributions about cause) is the next step of processing. A person's interpretation of a stimulus is predictive of that person's behavioral response (e.g., a hostile attribution made about another's ambiguously provocative push in the back will predict a retaliatory aggressive response). Once the stimulus cues are represented, the person accesses one or more possible behavioral responses from memory. Rules of association in memory, as well as the person's response repertoire, guide this retrieval. For example, one person might follow the rule "when intentionally provoked, fight back," whereas another person might follow the rule "when provoked, run away." Accessing a response is not the same as responding behaviorally, however, as in the case of a withheld impulse. The next step of processing is response evaluation and decision making, wherein the person (not necessarily consciously) evaluates the interpersonal, intrapersonal, instrumental, and moral consequences of accessed behavioral responses and decides on an optimal response. Clearly, evaluations that a behavior is relatively likely to lead to positive consequences are predictive of that behavioral tendency. The final step of processing involves the transformation of a mental decision into motor and verbal behavior.

Social information-processing theory posits that people engage in these mental processes over and over in real time during social interactions and that within particular types of situations, individuals develop characteristic patterns of processing cues at each step in the model. These patterns form the basis of psychopathologic tendencies. For example, in response to provocations, one person might regularly selectively attend to certain kinds of cues (such as threats), attribute hostile intentions to others, access aggressive responses, evaluate aggressing as favorable, and enact aggression skillfully. This person is highly likely to develop conduct disorder. Likewise, in response to academic failure, another person might selectively attend to his or her own contributing mistakes, attribute the outcome to personal failure, access self-destructive responses, evaluate all other responses as leading to further failure, and enact self-destructive responses effortlessly. This person is likely to develop dysthymic disorder or major depressive disorder.

Applications of the Theory

Social information-processing theory has been used successfully to predict the development of conduct problems in children and depressive symptoms in adolescents. Not all individuals with conduct problems display the same deviant processing patterns at all steps of the model; however, most people with conduct problems display at least one type of processing problem. Some children with conduct problems show hostile attributional tendencies, whereas others evaluate the likely outcomes of aggressing as positive. These processing differences accurately predict subtypes of conduct problems: children with hostile attributional tendencies display problems of reactive anger control, whereas children who make positive evaluations of the outcome of aggressing display instrumental aggression and bullying.

The development of processing styles has shed light on the development of psychopathology. For example, children with early histories of physical abuse are likely to become hypervigilant to hostile cues and to display hostile attributional tendencies. These tendencies predict later aggressive-behavior problems and account for the empirical link between early physical abuse and the development of aggressive-behavior problems.

Social information-processing theory has the potential to distinguish among types of psychopathology. In one investigation, groups of children with depressive, aggressive, comorbid, or no symptoms were found to display unique profiles of processing patterns. The aggressive group tended to attribute hostile intentions to others, to access aggressive responses, and to evaluate the outcomes of aggressing as favorable. The depressive group, in contrast, tended to attribute hostile intentions to others as well, but they also attributed the cause of others' hostile intentions to self-blame, and they accessed self-destructive responses and evaluated aggressive responses negatively.

Social information-processing theory has suggested interventions designed to help people construe situations differently and to act on the social world more effectively. For example, one intervention has been directed toward helping aggressive adolescents attribute interpersonal provocations in a less personalized and hostile way. This intervention has been successful in reducing the rate of aggressive behavior in these adolescents, relative to untreated control subjects.

Criticisms of the Theory

By focusing on in situ mental actions, processing theory relatively neglects enduring structural components of personality that are emphasized in psychoanalytic and Piagetian theories. Another criticism is that social information-processing theory locates the sources of deviant behavior in the individual, in contrast to the broader social ecology.

Dodge KA, Coie JD, Lynam D: Aggression and antisocial behavior in youth. In: Damon W (series ed), Eisenberg N (vol ed), *Handbook of Child Psychology, Vol. 3. Social, Emotional, and Personality Development*, 6th edn. New York: Wiley, 2006, p. 719.

Dodge KA, Bai Y, Godwin J, et al: A defensive mindset: a pattern of social information processing that develops early and predicts life course outcomes. *Child Development.* 2022;93(4):e357–e378. http://doi.org/10.1111/cdev.13751.

ECOLOGICAL THEORY

Ecological theory evolved from the recognition that even though the environment has a major effect on development, many models of development have limited generalizability across contexts. Consider, for example, classic studies by Tulkin and his colleagues on the effect of mother–infant interaction patterns on the infant's development of language and mental abilities. This effect is stronger among socioeconomic middle-class families than among lower-class families. Likewise, Scarr has found that the magnitude of genetic influences on intellectual development varies according to the cultural group being studied. Greater genetic effects are observed in middle-class White groups than in lower-class African American groups. Among lower-class families, different influences on development are operating. Findings such as these led ecological theorists such as Lewin, Bronfenbrenner, and Barker to conclude that models of development are bounded by the context in which they are framed.

Ecological theory suggests that process models of development have no universality; rather, they must be framed within the limits of a cultural and historical context. This theory must be distinguished from the radical postmodernist perspective that scientific principles have no objective basis. Ecological theorists conceptualize the environment systematically and attempt to understand how it affects development.

Bronfenbrenner has articulated an ecological model that includes developmental influences at the individual (person), person-by-environment (process), and context levels. He categorizes contextual settings into three types: microsystems, mesosystems, and exosystems. As discussed earlier in this chapter, the most proximal type is the microsystem, which includes the immediate physical and social environment. Examples of microsystems are homes, schools, playgrounds, and work places. Each microsystem has a structure and a set of rules and norms for behavior that are fairly consistent across time. Developmental scientists study processes within each of these settings, and ecologists warn them not to overgeneralize process phenomena from one microsystem to another.

The next type is the mesosystem, which is defined as a combination of microsystems that leads to a new level of developmental influence. For example, in understanding the effects of parental versus peer influences on adolescent development, one must consider not only each of the family and peer microsystems but also the effect of the combined mesosystem, that is, the effect of the conflict between the family's values and the peer group's values on the child's development.

The final type is the exosystem, a combination of multiple mesosystems. Research on the effects of maternal employment on child development has been enhanced by an understanding of this exosystem. That is, in order to understand how maternal employment affects a child's social development, one must understand not only the family and work context but also the cultural and historical contexts of women's employment.

▶ Applications of the Theory

Ecological theory has led clinicians to question the generalizability of their practices across cultural, gender, and ethnic groups. Group-specific interventions are being developed. Ecological theory has also led to policy changes in the funding of research at the federal level, in that large research studies are now required to address questions of generalizability across groups. Finally, ecological theorists have pressed clinicians to consider the possibility that interventions at a broader level might exert a powerful effect at the microsystem level.

▶ Criticisms of the Theory

Ecological theory is not a theory in the formal sense. Rather, it is a structured framework for identifying influences at numerous levels. Thus, it is not falsifiable. Its value is in alerting clinicians to factors that otherwise might be neglected.

Bronfenbrenner U, Morris PA: The bioecological model of human development: In: Damon W (series ed), Lerner RM (vol ed), *Handbook of Child Psychology, Vol. 1. Theoretical Models of Human Development*, 6th edn. New York: Wiley; 2006, p. 793.

SYNTHESIS: DIATHESIS–STRESS MODELS & OTHER INTERACTIONIST THEORIES

It has been increasingly recognized that interactionist models of development apply to most forms of psychopathology. These models focus on the confluence of forces that must coalesce in order for a disorder to develop. The most basic of these models is the diathesis–stress model. A **diathesis** is a dispositional characteristic that predisposes an individual to a disorder. The disposition may be biological (as in a genetic predisposition for schizophrenia), environmental (as in poverty), or cognitive (as in low IQ). A disorder is probabilistically related to the presence of a diathesis, but the process of development of psychopathology requires that the individual with the diathesis also be exposed to a stressor, which, again, might be biological or environmental. Only those individuals with both diathesis and stressor are likely to develop the disorder.

Consider the diathesis–stress model of major depressive disorder. According to this model, individuals who display the cognitive diathesis of self-blame for failure are at risk for the development of depression, but only if they subsequently experience a stressor that is linked to the diathesis (such as failure). Statistically, this model hypothesizes an interaction effect, and it has been supported for a variety of problems, from depression to physical illness.

Theorists have noted that individual and environmental factors interact not only in static models such as the case of major depressive disorder but also over time in transactional models. These models articulate the reciprocal influences between person and environment and the unfolding of disorder across experience. Finally, theorists have come to recognize that the unfolding occurs in nonlinear, nonuniform ways that lead to qualitative changes in the individual, as in dynamic systems (see "Major Principles of Ontogeny & Phylogeny" earlier in this chapter). Dynamic systems models are borrowed from phenomena in physics to describe the development of novel behavior in infancy (such as the onset of locomotion and language) and have the potential to be applied to the development of novel deviant behavior in psychopathology.

Magnussen D, Stattin H: The person in context: a holistic-interactionist approach: In: Damon W (series ed), Lerner RM (vol ed), *Handbook of Child Psychology, Vol. 1. Theoretical Models of Human Development*, 6th edn. New York: Wiley; 2006, p. 400.

LIFE-COURSE PROSPECTIVE INQUIRY

One of the most powerful methods in developmental clinical research is that of life-course prospective inquiry, closely linked to developmental epidemiology. By identifying an important sample (either a high-risk sample or a representative sample) and then following that sample with repeated assessments across time using hypothesis-driven measures, researchers have been able to identify risk factors in the development of a disorder, moderators of that risk, and mediating processes in the etiology of the disorder. Two such longitudinal studies are described in this section as examples of ongoing research in this field.

THE DEVELOPMENT OF DEPRESSION PROJECT

The Development of Depression Project has tested the diathesis–stress model of the development of major depressive disorder in adolescents. According to Garber, some children develop cognitive styles for attributing their failures and losses to internal, global, and stable characteristics of themselves, and they begin to have negative automatic thoughts in response to life events. Later, when confronted with failures and losses, these children are at elevated risk for developing major depressive disorder. It is the interaction of the cognitive diathesis and the life stressor, not either factor in isolation, that leads to depression. In order to rule out competing hypotheses that cognitive styles or problem life events result from, rather than lead to, depression, a research design is needed that follows children across time.

The research strategy in this study was to identify a sample of children prior to adolescence; to assess cognitive diatheses, life events, family processes, and psychopathology in this sample at that time; and then to follow the children with repeated assessments throughout adolescence in order to determine which ones develop depression following common stressors of adolescent life.

At the first wave of assessment in sixth grade, 188 children and their parents were assessed for psychopathology, life events stressors, family processes, and most pertinent, the cognitive diathesis for depression. Analyses of the initial wave revealed that children of depressive parents demonstrated more subthreshold symptoms of depression and more negative attributional styles than did the children of nondepressed parents. Even though these findings are consistent with the hypothesized model, the critical test would come over time if initial depressive symptom levels could be controlled statistically to see whether attributional styles and life stressors interact to predict onset of depressive disorder. Annual follow-ups through young adulthood indicate that among those children who displayed at least some depressive symptoms, controlling for initial depressive symptom levels, the interaction of early cognitive diathesis and subsequent stressful life events significantly predicted later depressive symptom levels as determined by psychiatric interviews. That is, only those children with a combination of initial negative automatic thoughts and subsequent stressful life events showed elevated depressive symptoms later; all other groups showed lower levels of symptoms. This is a moderator effect: The cognitive diathesis moderates (or alters) the effect of stressful life events on depressive symptoms.

This prospective study has provided empirical support for a model in which early family interactions involving psychological control and lack of acceptance lead a child to develop cognitive styles of negative self-worth, negative automatic thoughts, and negative attributions for failure. Later, in adolescence, those children who show the unique combination of experiencing stressful life events and having negative automatic thoughts about those events are most likely to develop depression. This model integrates biological (genetic risk), family process, cognitive, and ecological (stressful life events) factors in the onset and course of depression. It also suggests three points for intervention with children who are at risk for depression. First, early family interactions involving acceptance and control might be targeted through parent training. Second, the child's cognitive styles might be addressed in brief preventive cognitive therapy. Third, the child's ecology might be modified by altering the child's exposure to stressful life events (or at least the child's experience of inevitable stressful events).

The findings of this seminal study have been used as the empirical basis for innovative intervention programs to prevent depressive disorder in early adolescents. Prevention scientists, including Gregory Clarke, Martin Seligman, Timothy Strauman, and Judy Garber, have developed individual- and group-based multisession programs designed to help adolescents alter their cognitive responses to failure, loss, and other stressors. Evaluation of these programs through randomized trials has revealed proximal success in altering targeted cognitive styles and distal success in preventing depressive symptoms in response to future stressors.

Hilsman R, Garber J: A test of the cognitive diathesis–stress model in children: academic stressors, attributional style, perceived competence and control. *J Pers Soc Psychol* 1995;69:370.

Horowitz JL, Garber J: The prevention of depressive symptoms in children and adolescents: a meta-analytic review. *J Consult Clin Psychol* 2006;74:421.

THE CHILD DEVELOPMENT PROJECT

The Child Development Project was initiated to understand the role of family experiences and patterns of social information processing in the development and growth of aggressive conduct problems and conduct disorder. The design is a developmental epidemiologic one: 585 preschool children at three geographic sites were selected randomly at kindergarten matriculation to participate in a 20-year longitudinal study. The hypotheses guiding the study were based on the social learning theory in developmental psychology and the social information-processing theory in cognitive science, namely, that early family experiences of physical abuse and harsh discipline would predict later serious conduct problems; and that this relation would be mediated by the child's intervening development of problematic patterns of processing social information.

In-home family interviews and direct observations of family interactions provided information about the child's experience of physical abuse and harsh discipline in the first 5 years of life. About 12% of this random sample was identified as having experienced physical abuse at some time in their lives, a high rate that is consistent with national surveys of community samples. At subsequent annual assessments, video-guided interviews with each child provided measures of the child's patterns of social information processing. Finally, teacher ratings, peer nominations, direct observations, and school records provided evidence of externalizing conduct problems. The study followed this sample from preschool into high school.

Analyses indicated that the physically abused group of children had a fourfold increase in risk for clinically significant externalizing problems by middle school. This risk could not be statistically accounted for by confounding factors, such as socioeconomic status, child temperament, or exposure to other violent models. Thus, it seems that the experience of harsh parenting, especially if extreme, is partially responsible for conduct problems in some children.

Consistent with the original hypotheses, the physically abused children were also at risk for problems with social information processing. Specifically, physically abused children were relatively likely to become hypervigilant to hostile cues, to develop hostile attributional biases, to access aggressive responses to social problems, and to believe that aggressive behaviors lead to desired outcomes. Also consistent with hypotheses, children who demonstrated these processing patterns were likely to develop clinically significant externalizing problems in middle school and high school. Finally, the mediation hypothesis was supported, in that the child's social information-processing patterns accounted for about half of the statistical relation between early physical abuse and later conduct problems.

Lansford JE, Dodge KA, Pettit GS, et al: A 12-year prospective study of the long-term effects of early child physical maltreatment on psychological, behavioral, and academic problems in adolescence. *Arch Pediatr Adolesc Med* 2002;156:824–830.

CONCLUSION

Developmental psychology plays an important role in psychiatric science and practice. Concepts such as the orthogenetic principle, ontogeny, phylogeny, age-norming, and developmental trajectories can help the practicing psychiatrist to place a patient's current symptoms into developmental and ecological context. Common patterns in the development of psychopathology (e.g., biosocial interactions, multiple pathway models, mediational models, and bidirectional effects) enrich the psychiatrist's understanding of the etiology of psychiatric disorders.

Even though major developmental theories (e.g., temperament, attachment, social learning) have historical significance, most contemporary thinking is not directed at contrasting these theories at a macrolevel. Rather, it is understood that psychiatric phenomena usually involve complex interactions of factors at multiple levels. Current research is aimed at understanding how variables implicated by various theories interact to produce psychiatric disorder, rather than proving one general theory to be more meritorious than another.

The relation between developmental psychology and psychiatry is reciprocal. That is, knowledge gained from developmental theory and empirical findings has been useful to psychiatrists in both scientific understanding and practice, and the findings and concerns of psychiatrists have modified developmental theory and guided developmental empirical inquiry. These disciplines have been fused even more tightly in the emerging discipline of developmental psychopathology, which seeks to understand the etiology, process, and life course of psychiatric phenomena.

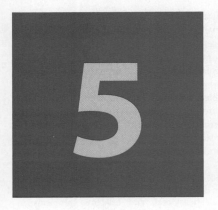

The Psychiatric Interview[1]

Sidney H. Weissman, MD
Barry Nurcombe, MD[†]
Michael H. Ebert, MD

Human behavior is complex. When it becomes dysfunctional because of environmental stress or brain disease, it can mystify the inexperienced clinician. This is especially true of neurobehavioral disorders, which involve neuropsychiatric changes in cognition and emotion that overlap the boundary of psychiatry and neurology. The clinician must appreciate and assess the signs and symptoms of a neurobehavioral disorder with the same discernment as in physical syndromes such as myocardial infarction or infectious disease.

This chapter describes the psychiatric history and mental status examination (MSE), in the conduct of an effective psychiatric interview. The patient interview process actually begins prior to the clinician meeting the patient. It begins when the clinician first learns that they are to see a particular patient and obtain initial diagnostic data and what their role will be in the care of a patient. Additionally, they will learn if they are to see the patient alone or with others. Further will they be able to interview the patient at a later date to obtain any additional information. With this background the clinician formulates an initial interview strategy. It will vary determined by the circumstances surrounding the initial interview and how it unfolds. A guideline to the steps of the interview process is described along with the techniques the clinician must master in order to elicit information relevant to developing a diagnostic hypothesis in an orderly, reliable, and comprehensive manner. The components of psychiatric history and the MSE are described in accordance with the stages of the interview during which they would usually be obtained.

What can be achieved at the initial psychiatric interview depends on the situation in which it is conducted and what the physician and the patient are seeking. For example, a brisk, focused interview in an emergency room contrasts with the more extensive survey appropriate to an outpatient clinic. Both of these interviews would differ from what is possible at the bedside of a patient who is severely ill in a medical or surgical ward. Despite these distinctions, fundamental issues can be addressed to varying degrees in any clinical situation, as illustrated in Table 5–1. We will return to these issues in our discussion of the elements of psychiatric history.

THE STAGES OF THE PSYCHIATRIC INTERVIEW

▶ Note Taking

Prior to commencing an interview, the interviewer must have established how they will record the information they obtain from a patient during the interview. In obtaining a complex detailed history and patient assessment notes will be essential. The interviewer must develop a technique whether using handwritten notes or a computer to maintain contact with the patient.

▶ Inception

If the interviewer works in a clinic, at the opening of the psychiatric interview he or she goes to the waiting room, introduces himself or herself to the patient, accompanies the patient to the interview room, and shows them to a seat. After taking identifying data from the patient, the interviewer can tell the patient what he or she already knows. This approach avoids unnecessary mysteries and clears the way for action. Consider the following example:

Psychiatrist: Your parents came to see me yesterday. They told me they're worried because your schoolwork has fallen off, although you've always been a good student; you've dropped most of your friends; and you seem to have become depressed. Last week they found one of your assignments in which you spoke about suicide. They think you may need help with an emotional problem.

[1]Some of this material also appears in Nurcombe B, Gallagher RM: *The Clinical Process in Psychiatry: Diagnosis and Management Planning.* Cambridge University Press, 1986. Reprinted with the permission of Cambridge University Press.
[†]Deceased

Table 5–1 Issues to be Addressed in the Psychiatric Interview

Chronology of events and development of symptoms; subjective concerns of the patient; and concerns of patient's family, friends, neighbors, or employers
Insight, judgment, and motivation for treatment
Precipitation of illness and relevant stressors
Predisposition and family history of psychiatric illness
Presentation
Previous psychiatric illness and behavioral problems
Previous psychiatric treatment and/or mental health intervention

Table 5–2 Content of the Psychiatric History

Identifying data
Presenting problem
History of present illness
History of past psychiatric illnesses
Medical history
History of drug or alcohol intake or of antisocial behavior
Early development and childhood environment
Educational history
Vocational history
Family history
Sexual history
Marital history
Characteristic coping mechanisms, values, ideals, aspirations

Patient (a 16-year-old boy): So?

Psychiatrist: So, they asked you to see a psychiatrist. I get the impression you're not too happy about that.

Patient: No.

Psychiatrist: Maybe we can start by you telling me how you feel about it.

Interviews are not always conducted in an office; they may be transacted beside a patient's bed, or between pieces of equipment in the examination room of an emergency clinic, or even while driving a car. Wherever they occur, the beginning has a pattern, a certain formality. The interviewer introduces himself or herself, says why he or she is there, and invites the patient to respond by telling his or her story. If the patient does not want to do so, the interviewer helps the patient to explain why.

Reconnaissance (Obtaining Initial Data on the Present Illness)

The interviewer helps the patient tell their story as spontaneously as possible. He or she listens and does not interrupt any more than is necessary to keep the story flowing. The interviewer does not rush the data gathering or try to direct it prematurely. If the interviewer only asks direct questions, all he or she will get are brief marginally helpful answers. Open-ended probes should be used as much as possible. The more leading the probe, the less useful the response, unless the issue in question is a simple, unequivocal one. The facilitating techniques we describe later in this chapter are particularly appropriate for the reconnaissance stage.

Detailed Inquiry

After the patient has finished his or her story, the interviewer seeks further information about the present illness, past illness, medical history, early environment, education, and other relevant matters from the psychiatric history. A full detailed inquiry may take several interviews, but a scanning of the features most important for a provisional diagnosis can be accomplished within an hour.

Table 5–2 lists the content of the psychiatric history. The order suggested in the table should not be followed blindly. The interviewer should be prepared to deal with topics in whatever manner they unfold. In accordance with the case, some areas will be emphasized, and others pursued in less detail.

Detailed inquiry involves questioning, but the questions are kept as open ended as possible at the outset, moving from general to specific as more detail is required. Compare the following questions:

- How are things in your marriage?
- How are things between you and your wife?
- How do you and your wife get on?
- Is your marriage a happy one?
- Do you love your wife?

This approach is similar to the way a surgeon approaches a guarded section of a painful abdomen: from the outside in. Direct questions may provoke circumscribed responses and are most appropriate to issues of fact (e.g., What year were you married?).

Some issues are left to a later time after a joint decision regarding working with the patient has been made. Unless the patient presents his or her sexual life as a problem at the outset, exploration of this area is usually postponed.

Transitions

The interview setting and time constraints can interfere with transitions. Ideally the interviewer never moves abruptly from one topic to another. Change should be signaled. For example, the psychiatrist could say, "Okay. I'd like to go on from there to something else. Could you tell me about the jobs you've had? What did you do after you left school?"

CHAPTER 5

▶ Standard Versus Discretionary Inquiry

Part of the detailed inquiry is standardized, including essential questions to assess patients of a given age, in a specific clinical situation, or as part of a minimum database. The components of an ideal standard inquiry should be defined for each clinical setting. The rest of the detailed inquiry is largely determined by the interviewer and is discretionary and involves the eliciting of evidence supporting or refuting the initial diagnostic hypotheses.

ELEMENTS OF THE PSYCHIATRIC HISTORY

We will now address the components of psychiatric history, which are shown in Table 5–1. Each issue addressed in Table 5–1 should be addressed, and the information related to one of the categories shown in Table 5–2.

▶ The Present Illness

An accurate psychiatric history serves as the guide to diagnosis, intervention, and treatment. To accomplish this, it is essential to define the present episode. This enables the determination of its potential precipitants and whether the present episode constitutes a discrete psychiatric illness or is an episode in a chronic psychiatric disorder.

Some patients present a variety of not well-defined concerns. Others have a more focused complaint and can identify particular issues as problematic. Whatever the problem(s) for which the patient, their family or associates seek help, the clinician attempts to delineate them; to understand how the patient experiences them; and to ascertain their duration, onset, development, and persistence.

▶ Precipitation of Illness & Relevant Stressors

From the onset of the patient's problem's the interviewer attempts to determine whether the patient experienced physical or psychosocial stress at that time. The mere coincidence of stress at the onset does not substantiate a causal association; indeed, causation remains speculative in some cases. Causation is supported, however, if the patient previously had a breakdown when exposed to a similar stress or if the patient's account of the stress indicates its personal significance.

Some stressors have universal impact. Others are highly idiosyncratic, and painstaking work may be required before they can be unraveled in psychotherapy. In some cases, it is an open question whether an event was a true precipitant, or secondary to a disorder in its early stages, or mere coincidence.

▶ Previous Psychiatric Illness & Behavioral Problems

The interviewer considers the following questions in evaluating the patient for previous psychiatric illness and behavioral problems: Has the patient had any problems of a similar nature in the past? What precipitated them if anything? Has the patient had any other emotional disorders or physical symptoms related to their experience of stress? Has the patient had, or do they have, physical or neurologic disease that could contribute to the present problem? Does the patient have, or had, personal habits (e.g., substance use) that could cause, precipitate, or complicate the present problem?

▶ Previous Psychiatric Treatment & Mental Health Intervention

The interviewer should be aware of any therapeutic interventions prior to the current evaluation, including formal psychiatric treatment (or treatment by another mental health professional), emergency evaluations, hospitalizations, or mental health treatment rendered by a primary care physician. The clinician who carried out the treatment and the treating facility should be identified, as should the approximate date(s) and duration of treatment. The patient's response to each pharmacologic agent and associated side effects should be documented. The type, duration, frequency of sessions and results of psychotherapy should be identified. The interviewer will usually verify and amplify this information by requesting records from previous treating professionals and facilities, with appropriate written consent from the patient.

▶ Predisposition & Potentials

The interviewer considers the following questions in evaluating the patient for predisposition to and family history of psychiatric illness: What was the patient like before they became ill? What biopsychosocial strengths and weaknesses may have predisposed the patient prior to their symptomatic behavior? These questions require a comprehensive evaluation, and it is unrealistic to expect all of this information to be elaborated in a single interview. However, important pieces of the jigsaw puzzle are usually available. The interviewer can also seek information about the following additional concerns: What personal and environmental strengths, resources, and liabilities are apparent at the present time? What hurdles do they face? The information obtained can be summarized as an inventory of the patient's physical, intellectual, emotional, and social assets and deficiencies. This inventory is crucial to the design of an individualized plan of management.

▶ Presentation

The interviewer considers the following questions in evaluating the patient's current presentation for treatment: Why is the patient presenting now for help? Is the patient being seen at the onset of a disorder. If later, do they have a relatively defined pattern of symptoms or are their symptoms left after the patient has recovered partially but remains troubled by residual difficulties? Did the patient come of his or her own accord, or were they required or persuaded to do so? Did others bring the patient for treatment? If so, Why?

Insight, Judgment, & Motivation for Treatment

The interviewer considers the following questions in evaluating the patient's insight, judgment, and motivation for treatment: Does the patient think they have a mental health problem? Does the patient think they have been referred inappropriately? The patient may be correct. If the patient recognizes and acknowledges their mental health problem, do they have any ideas of its nature or cause? How realistic are these notions?

If the patient appreciates, they have a problem what kind of help does the patient seek, if any? Is this in line with what is advisable, appropriate, or feasible? Is the patient troubled by either doubts concerning their problem or the kind of treatment they will receive? Fears of craziness or unknown to the patient psychiatric treatments are likely to be inflamed by deep-seated anxieties about helplessness and victimization. These fears are often aggravated by images derived from family or cultural values, including those depicted in the media. It is better that such concerns be addressed as soon as possible and addressed when they are the result of misinformation.

Family History

The family history is an important component of the initial interview. Understanding the patient's family structure and the varied family influences on the patient's growth and development are essential to "knowing" the patient. They may document a genetic predisposition to psychiatric illness. This initial inquiry is the beginning of a genogram that can be developed in more detail in subsequent interviews. The initial interview, if time permits should identify each family member for one or two generations and needs to also identify individuals with psychiatric illness and if possible fort two generations. This line of questioning is subtle because of social stigma and the natural reluctance of individuals to disclose family problems. It is desirable to inquire about the presence of psychiatric illness in several ways. The interviewer may begin with an open-ended question such as inquiring whether any family member has had emotional or behavioral problems. Follow-up questions can include whether any family member has been treated by a behavioral health provider and whether anyone in the family has been hospitalized for psychiatric illness.

Social History

An initial even if limited social history should be elicited in the first diagnostic interview. This part of the initial interview informs the examiner of the social, cultural, and family structural influences that contribute to the patient's personality, values, and social integration. Open-ended questions that invite the patient to describe the structure and membership of the nuclear and extended family are a good start. Often the description will be colored by feelings and attitudes toward each person. They can be explored in depth in a subsequent interview. Marriages, children, divorces, major illnesses, and deaths within the immediate family should be documented as part of the social history. This part of the interview can be interwoven with the family history of illness, particularly psychiatric illness. The social history is often ignored in initial psychiatric interviews, but the absence of this information limits the diagnostic formulation.

Educational & Occupational History

The initial diagnostic interview should include a brief educational and occupational history. During this part of the interview, the diagnostician is forming a timeline to register major events in the patient's life and evaluating developmental milestones. The educational history helps to give a developmental history extending through the second decade of life, as well as an indirect indication of intellectual capacity and social adjustment. Interruptions in education are often a sign of emerging psychopathology or a discrete behavioral setback or crisis. The occupational history is valuable life history information but can also indicate periods in a person's life when an acute psychiatric illness occurred or when the gradual development of psychopathology altered a person's life, including his ability to attend schoolwork. Choices of educational and occupational paths may provide a window into understanding a patient's personality, motivation, identification with people who are important to the patient, and family values and influences.

A military history is important when it is relevant to the patient's presenting difficulties. Major psychiatric illnesses often present for the first time under the stress of military service when the individual is in their late teens and early twenties away from home. Military health care may provide substantial documentation of symptoms in an acute psychiatric illness, diagnosis, and response to treatment. If an individual has a medical discharge from the military, the documentation of the illness is very useful data for diagnostic impression, treatment response, and prognosis.

Legal History

A legal history addresses two points. Is the patient having any immediate difficulty with the law or are lawsuits, divorce and custody disputes, bankruptcy, arrests, convictions, and imprisonment elements of their immediate life? To omit this inquiry because it is a difficult subject is an error. It may be a critical point in developing a diagnosis.

Forming Hypotheses

Throughout the initial interview, the diagnostician is working to form hypotheses about the etiology of the current problem under evaluation. This involves an acquired skill set that includes memory, a questioning technique that draws the patient out in a nonintimidating manner, a capacity to convey empathy, and an ability to make each part of the interview productive in terms of information gathering, while also building an alliance with the patient. It is reasonable to take occasional notes, but it is a not helpful technique to focus on note taking instead of the patient. Likewise, following a rigid interview outline and not following leads that the patient offers when they occur. It is precisely this mixture of structure and completeness in acquiring clinical data which serves to enrich our knowledge of the patient. Knowledge allows us to form hypotheses about the patient's defining life events and diagnosis. Using this model over time allow us to develop skills which will lead to our becoming skilled the experienced clinicians.

MSE: CONTENT, PURPOSE, & FORMAT

The MSE is a set of systematic observations and assessments undertaken by a diagnostician during the clinical interview. Properly conducted, the MSE provides a detailed and systematic description of the patient's cognitive and affective functioning. This information is essential to the consolidation of those patterns of clues, and inferences that are required for the generation of diagnostic hypotheses. The MSE, guided by the hypothetico-deductive approach to diagnosis, is an essential part of the subsequent inquiry plan. In this section we offer a comprehensive description of the components of the MSE. In regard to a particular patient and in accordance with the clinical context, background information, and psychiatric history—the interviewer will apply the MSE tactically and empathically, pursuing brief, comprehensive, or discretionary lines of inquiry, as warranted.

The Need for Standardization

The MSE, like the psychiatric history, involves routine and questions necessitated by the behavior of a unique patient. The information obtained guides the development of diagnostic hypotheses. The examiner must develop in assessing specific answer to MSE questions clear standardized for themselves answers. The interpretation of these responses is essential in developing diagnostic hypotheses. The techniques of eliciting MSE data should be formalized, the phenomena in question clearly defined, and the weight to be placed on each phenomenon clarified.

Reliability

The **reliability** of a test (question) refers to the likelihood (usually expressed as a correlation) that similar results will be obtained on retesting (**test–retest reliability**) or that similar results will be obtained by different observers (**interrater reliability**). Test–retest reliability applies to relatively stable characteristics such as the use of language or cognitive function; it is not to be expected in characteristics (e.g., mood) that are changeable and often linked to a current situation.

When psychiatrists test a patient's abstracting ability, for example, by asking the patient to explain proverbs in his or her own words, how certain can the psychiatrist be that the clinical test is a true measure of the ability in question? In other words, what is the **validity** of the test? The interpretation of proverbs is culturally impacted. A clinician from a different cultural background than the patient may have a differing interpretation. In examining various tests used in the MSE we will address their validity along with the mental faculties required of the patient for its adequate performance.

Types of MSEs

A. Brief Screening MSE

When a patient has been referred to an outpatient clinic for a situational or personality problem, and none of the indications for a comprehensive screening examination pertain (see next section), a brief, informal screen may be sufficient. The brief screening MSE is completed during the inception, reconnaissance, and detailed inquiry stages of the psychiatric interview. In particular, the interviewer notes the patient's general appearance, motor behavior, quality of speech, relationship to the interviewer, and mood. From the patient's demeanor, conversation, and history, the interviewer makes inferences about consciousness, orientation, attention, grasp, memory, fund of information, general intellectual level, language competence, and thought process. Abnormal thought content is not investigated unless clinical clues indicate the need for inquiry (e.g., into hallucinations, obsessions, depersonalization). Physiologic functions (e.g., sleep, appetite, libido, menstrual cycle, energy level) and insight should always be assessed.

B. Comprehensive Screening MSE

The interviewer should be alerted to the need for a comprehensive screening MSE whenever there is a reasonable possibility that the patient has psychosis or primary or secondary brain dysfunction. Table 5–3 summarizes the settings and clues that mandate a comprehensive MSE. If the clinician has any doubts, the comprehensive screen should be completed.

Components of the MSE

Table 5–4 summarizes the areas to be covered in the MSE. The following sections describe these areas in more detail.

A. Appearance & Behavior

From the moment the interviewer first greets the patient, he or she will be aware of the patient's appearance. The interviewer

Table 5–3 Indications for a Comprehensive Screening Mental Status Examination

The patient is seen in a hospital emergency room or crisis clinic; is being managed on a nonpsychiatric ward and has been referred for consultation; or is being admitted to a psychiatric unit.
The patient is older than 60 years.
The patient has a history of psychiatric disorder, substance abuse, organic brain disorder, or physical disorder that could affect brain function.
The patient's personal habits, memory, concentration, or grasp have deteriorated recently.
The patient or other informant presents clinical clues that suggest current mood disorder, psychosis, or organic brain dysfunction (e.g., persistent or intermittent depression, withdrawal, elation, overactivity, bizarre ideation, hallucinations, delusions, ideas of influence and reference, headaches, loss of memory and grasp, disorientation, disordered language, headaches, seizures, motor weakness, tremor, or sensory loss).
Physical examination indicates or suggests brain dysfunction.
In forensic referrals, when mental competence or legal insanity are in question.

needs to be able to describe it in detail before making any inferences. The clinician stores in their memory an image of the patient's physique and habits. Is there evidence of weight loss or gain? Does the patient have any conspicuous marks or disfigurement? The interviewer should describe the patient's face and hair. Does the patient look ill? What is the expression of their eyes and mouth? Does the patient appear to be in touch with the surroundings? Is the patient clean and neat, or do they exhibit deficiencies in personal hygiene revealed by poor grooming of the skin, hair, or nails? How is the patient dressed? Is the patient's clothing neat? Is it appropriate or peculiar? After the interviewer considers these characteristics, they determine whether an inference may be made about the patient that relates to their reason for being seen.

The interviewer notes general overactivity or underactivity, abnormalities of posture, gross incoordination, or impairment of large muscle function. What is the patient's gait like, and how they sit? The interviewer notes any abnormalities of finer movement and posture, such as tremor, tics, or fidgeting.

Table 5–4 Sections of the Mental Status Examination

A. Appearance and behavior
B. Relationship to the interviewer
C. Affect and mood
D. Cognition and memory
E. Language
F. Disorders of thought
G. Physiologic function
H. Insight and judgment

Stereotypies are organized, repetitive movements or speech or perseverative postures. They may be associated with schizophrenia. A striking variant of postural stereotypy is called **waxy flexibility**, in which the patient with a severe psychiatric disorder will remain for extended periods in a position into which the interviewer or examiner places them (e.g., standing on one leg). Other disorders of movement associated include a stiff expressionless face; facial grimacing or contortions; stiff, awkward, or stilted body movement; and unusual mannerisms of expressive movement or speech. The last should not be confused with the awkward movements of someone who is anxious in interpersonal situations. The interviewer also notes whether the patient exhibits any rituals such as a need to touch objects repetitively, as in obsessive–compulsive disorder, or any habits such as nail biting, thumb sucking, lip licking, yawning, or scratching.

The interviewer attends to the accent if different from theirs, pitch, tone, and tempo of the patient's speech, paying particular attention to unusually high or low pitch and abnormal tone.

If the patient is mute, or unwilling or unable to utter anything which may occur in advanced brain disorder, severe melancholia, catatonia, conversion disorder or in the elective mutism of children.

B. Relationship to the Interviewer

The interviewer infers how the patient is engaged in the interview process by how they behave and by what they say. The relationship may be consistent or vary in response to the topic being discussed, or it may be influenced by other factors. (e.g., when the patient is distracted by an auditory hallucination).

Affective states are difficult to assess, aside from noting whether they are inconsistent or are apparently influenced by obscure factors not apparent to the interviewer. The interviewer draws on a number of behavioral clues to assess the quality of the patient's relationship and mood. As a rule, the more inferential the judgment, the more unreliable the conclusion. Interviewers may differ in the inferences they make concerning a patient's affect, especially when it is unstable, ambiguous, complex, or shielded by interpersonal caution.

The interviewer's behavior will inevitably affect the ebb and flow of the patient's feelings. The patient may be responding appropriately to the interviewer's friendly approach (or rudeness, for that matter). They will also be responding to highly idiosyncratic internal predispositions. For example, a patient may harbor mingled anxiety and deference for somebody they perceive as a threatening authority figure who must be placated.

Given the fallibility of inference, the interviewer is well advised to stick closely to observations and be able to cite them. This skill requires training. The beginner may be overly impressed by their seemingly correct intuitive leaps; while the expert heeds intuition but realizes how unreliable it is.

The beginner may grasp for, and hold firmly to, an inference, sometimes in spite of contrary evidence. The expert makes the inference, cites the clues on which it is based, can offer alternative explanations, and discards the inference for a better one if contrary evidence emerges.

The quality of the patient's eye contact is of significant importance in gauging affective states. Negativistic patients may avert their gaze from the interviewer. A delirious patient whose sensorium is impaired may stare into space, as may a depressed patient or patient with schizophrenia whose thoughts are dominated by gloomy ruminations or delusional preoccupations. Intermittent staring may be a feature of different forms of epilepsy. The interviewer notes whether they can engage the patient's attention even if briefly. If not, the interviewer might suspect an organic brain disorder.

Some patients may simply stare at the interviewer. He or she should distinguish the wide eyes of awe or fear from the narrowed slits which might signify hypervigilant suspiciousness. Other patients may make hesitant eye contact, particularly when they are embarrassed about what they are saying. Not all patients with shifty gaze are liars, and some prevaricators have learned to deliver their lines without batting an eyelash.

The impact of the eyes on interpersonal relations cannot be overestimated. The configuration of supraorbital, circumorbital, and facial musculature; eyelids; palpebral fissure; gaze; depth of ocular focus; pupil size; and conjunctival moisture combine to produce a range of social signals of great significance. They may be interpreted as quests for interpersonal dominance, or competitiveness, attraction, hostility or avoidance, the initiation and punctuation of conversation. They also provide the feedback a person requires to know how the other person has responded to what one has said.

The expression of the eyes and face are with our appreciation of combined posture and movement offer a global sense of the patient. The facial expression may provide clues to remoteness, bewilderment, and perplexity and sadness in the patient's responses to questions. Whole body movement and posture may reveal potential tenseness (e.g., clenched fists, sweaty palms, stiff back, leaning forward), restlessness, preoccupation, and boredom.

Patients convey varied attitudes toward interviewers. The interviewer notes and describes the following attitudes in the patient: shyness, fear, suspiciousness, cautiousness, assertiveness, indifference, passivity, clowning, interest in the interviewer, clinging, coyness, seductiveness, or invasiveness. This is all data used in the diagnostic hypothesis.

C. Affect & Mood

Affect refers to a feeling or emotion, experienced typically in response to an external event or to a thought. In the patient's relationship to the interviewer the clinician can observe and experience particular manifestations of affect. Affects are usually associated with feelings about the self or about others who have a personal significance to the individual. Less often, an affect is experienced without a clear reference point. Affect may be the conscious and observable component of a system that signals a positive or negative response to the success or failure of attaining one's goals.

In contrast to an affect, which may be momentary, **mood** refers to an inner state that persists for some time and can inhibit the experience of a particular emotion or affect. For example, a mood of depression may inhibit an individual from deriving momentary diversion and pleasure from a joke; however, the expression of gloom, sadness, or desolation returns and prevails moments after hearing the joke. Affects and mood are inferred from the patient's demeanor and spontaneous conversation. A general query such as "How are you feeling, now?" or "How have your spirits been?" can be helpful. The interviewer should try to avoid leading questions such as "Do you feel depressed?"

Demeanor and affect usually coincide, but sometimes they do not. For example, a stiff smile can mask anxiety or depression. If the interviewer suspects this to be the case, he or she can offer an indicating or clarifying interpretation to help the patient acknowledge suppressed emotion, such as "I notice that even though you speak of sad things, you are smiling" or "It's hard to smile when you feel bad inside."

The interviewer describes in the mental status report the general qualities of the patient's emotional expression. Particular morbid affects or moods are noted. For example, is the patient **affectively flat**, that is, emotionally dull, monotonous, and lacking in resonance? Is the patient **emotionally constricted**, with a narrow range of affect, as in obsessional or schizoid personality? Does the patient exhibit **inappropriate or incongruous affect**, in that it is not in keeping with the topic of conversation?

Does the patient show evidence of **lability**, suddenly changing from neutral to excited or from one emotional pole to the other? Lability is often associated with emotional intemperateness, an abrupt unreflective expression of heightened emotion (e.g., excited anticipation, affection, irritation).

The interviewer notes the presence of **histrionic affect**, the blatant but rather shallow expression of emotion often observed in those who exaggerate their feelings in order to avoid being ignored and who need to capture, or who fear losing, the center of the interpersonal stage. Histrionic affect is often encountered in people with histrionic, narcissistic, or borderline personality disorder.

Euphoria, a sense of well-being expressed in inexorable good spirits, is encountered in a number of disorders. These include hypomania or mania, less commonly in schizophrenia and organic brain disorders including frontal lobe dysfunction, neurosyphilis, disseminated sclerosis, and after traumatic brain injury. Silliness is sometimes encountered in histrionic or immature people overwhelmed by the enormity of a difficult situation. Excessive silliness is also characteristic of some disorganized schizophrenic patients.

As euphoria becomes heightened it merges into elation and excitement. Patients in heightened states may also exhibit irritation if obstructed or thwarted.

Apathy, a pervasive lack of interest and drive (also known as **anergia**), may be observed in patients suffering from schizophrenic, depression, or have an organic brain disorder. The apathetic patient has little or no enthusiasm for work, social interaction, or recreation. Anergia is usually associated with a decrease in sexual activity. **Anhedonia**, a subjective sense that nothing is pleasurable, is commonly associated with anergia and nay be observed in schizophrenic and depressive patients. **Excessive fatigue**, which may be manifest as hypersomnia, is associated with many diverse disorders such as organic brain disorder, schizophrenia, anxiety disorders, depressive disorders, and somatization disorder.

When applied to an affect or mood, **depression** refers to a pervasive sense of sadness. It is often used to describe a feeling state triggered or related to a life event involving loss, rejection, defeat, or disappointment. It may be associated with tearfulness and anger about the event. In severe depression the patient feels emotionally deadened or empty, their world is stale, the future hopeless. The patient is preoccupied with dark foreboding thoughts, and they may be agitated by persistent self-recrimination about past misdeeds. Diminished concentration and a slowing of thinking and movement characteristically accompany depressed affect and gloomy ruminations. In some patients agitated depression is associated with psychomotor restlessness. Severe depression has important somatic features, including characteristic posture and facies, headache, irritability, precordial heaviness, gastrointestinal slowing, anorexia, weight loss, loss of sexual interest, and insomnia. Depression typically has a diurnal variation: Dysphoria, hopelessness, and agitation are worse in the morning, and the patient brightens up by evening.

The interviewer will readily recognize **openly expressed anger** and **irritability**. These feelings may be quite understandable in the context of the patient's circumstances. Morbid or pathological anger, however, is defined by its pervasiveness, frequency, disproportionate quality, impulsiveness, and uncontrollability. Morbid anger may be associated with organic brain disorder, usually in the form of catastrophic reactions to frustration, especially when the patient can no longer complete a familiar or easy task. Abnormal anger is also associated with some forms of epilepsy; personality disorders of the aggressive, antisocial, borderline, or paranoid type; attention-deficit and disruptive behavior disorders of childhood; drunkenness; paranoid disorders; hypomania or mania; and intermittent or isolated explosive disorders.

Controlled hostility may be expressed as sullenness, uncooperativeness, superiority, or mockery. It can be helpful to invite the patient to express anger or resentment directly and to determine when it began or what triggered it. This is particularly the case with adolescents. When working with adolescents, the interviewer might consider saying, "Whenever I ask you a question, you close up. Something about being here is making you pretty uptight. Can you help me to understand what you are feeling?

Anxiety and **fear** refer to the subjective apprehension of impending danger, together with widespread manifestations of an autonomic nervous system discharge (e.g., dilated pupils; cold, sweaty palms; tachycardia; tachypnea; nausea; bowel hurry; urinary urgency). Fear has an identifiable object: the need to defend, respond and protect oneself against danger. Anxiety may be associated with the threat of a loss of what is perceived as an essential element in one's life. Loss of a love relationship. It may also be a response to a concern of not being able to perform or address a situation as well as you feel you "should." Direct action (i.e., fight or flight) can address or respond to a fear, whereas the adaptive solution may be more complex. Fear is biologically advantageous because they signal the need for constructive responses.

In some anxiety states, the patient may report an intense anxiety in certain situations (e.g., "a fear" of heights). In these situations, the anxiety appears disproportionate or eccentric to an observer and may be recognized as pathologic by the patient. Many of the disorders of thought content (described later in this chapter) can be regarded as unconsciously determined.

D. Cognition & Memory

Table 5–5 lists the cognitive functions that can be assessed in an MSE. We describe them in more detail in the following sections:

1. Level of consciousness & awareness—The psychiatrist may be asked to consult on a comatose or stuporous patient if a nonorganic cause is hypothesized. A **coma** is a state of non-awareness from which the patient cannot be aroused. Diminished awareness is called semi coma or **stupor**, in which case the subject is temporarily rousable (e.g., by pain or noise) but reverts to stupor when the stimulus ceases. In stupor, eye movements become purposeful when a painful stimulus is applied, and wincing or pupillary constriction may occur, but the patient remains akinetic and mute. Stupor occurs in a number of quite varied disorders including metabolic states, encephalopathy, brain tumors, and injury including infections and in some psychiatric disorder (e.g., dissociative disorder, depression, and schizophrenia).

Table 5–5 Cognitive Functions

Level of consciousness and awareness
Orientation, attention, and concentration
Memory
Information
Comprehension
Conceptualization and abstraction

Coma related to psychological causes, psychogenic coma, is suggested by normal vital and neurologic signs, resistance to opening the eyes, normal pupillary reactions, and staring (rather than wandering) eyes. Swallowing, corneal, and gag reflexes are usually intact, and electroencephalography and oculovestibular reflexes are normal. Intravenous barbiturate may increase verbalization in psychogenic stupor while it will depress awareness further in organic conditions.

Torpor denotes a lowering of consciousness short of stupor. Awareness is narrowed and restricted, and apathy, perseveration, and psychomotor retardation are observed, but the more dramatic phenomena of delirium (i.e., illusions, hallucinations, and agitation) are lacking. Torpor is associated with severe infection and multi-infarct dementia.

In **twilight or dreamy states**, restricted awareness is manifested as disorientation for time and place, with reduced attention and impaired short-term memory. In addition, the patient may report that they have the feeling of being in a dream.

Delirium is a common not infrequently seen in medical and surgical inpatients. It is caused by diffuse cerebral dysfunction of acute or subacute onset and depending on its cause may be reversible. After an initial prodromal restlessness and insomnia, delirium typically presents with obtundation, emotional lability, visual illusions, and cognitive impairment. The clinical features tend to worsen at night ("sundowning"). So-called quiet deliria are common, with the patient demonstrating little more to note than clouding of consciousness, mild disorientation for time and place, and reduced concentration. Restlessness, tremor, asterixis (irregular, asymmetrical jerking of the extremities), myoclonus, and disturbance of autonomic function are also common. Patients vary in their psychological reactions to delirium: depressive, paranoid, schizophreniform, anxious, and somatoform responses may be encountered. Delirious patients may be fearfully or combatively hypervigilant, or torpid and apathetic.

Visual illusions, which are characteristic of delirium, involve the patient misinterpreting moving shadows, curtains, and surrounding furniture. Physical sensations may also be misperceived. For example, the patient may mistake abdominal pain for the knives of malefactors and tinnitus for radio waves. If delusional beliefs arise, the patient may act on them, seeking escape or defense. Visual hallucinations are more common than auditory hallucinations in delirium. Visual hallucinations may be playful (e.g., animals romping), sometimes personal (e.g., the face of a dead relative), or sometimes horrible or threatening (e.g., dismembered bodies, accidents). They are most evident at night and can be provoked when the eyes are closed, especially when the orbits are pressed. Affect is usually labile in delirium, but persistent blunting, anxiety, suspiciousness, hostility, depression, or euphoria may be encountered and is usually congruent with the prevailing illusions or hallucinations.

Delirious patients may exhibit wandering attention and concentration; their thinking may become disconnected or incoherent and their memory impaired. These patients sometimes confabulate or link memories out of correct sequence. Subtle restriction of consciousness often occurs during acute anxiety and results in vagueness or amnesia for traumatic experiences. Rarely, the amnesia is accentuated. The patient may wander off in a daze, turning up in an emergency room unaware of his or her name or address. This is known as **dissociative fugue state** and should be differentiated from epilepsy or postictal conditions.

2. Orientation, attention, & concentration—Disorders of orientation are most often involved when the sensorium is clouded, as in torpor, obtundation, dreamy states, delirium, or fugue. Orientation is usually lost in the following order: time, place, and person. Disorientation for time (day and date) and place usually indicates organic brain disorder. Disorientation for personal identity is rare and is associated with psychogenic or postictal fugue states, other dissociative disorders, and agnosia (loss of the ability to recognize sensory inputs). The interviewer assesses the patient's orientation by asking him or her for the information listed in Table 5–6. The reliability of the clinical assessment of orientation is high, but its predictive validity is uncertain.

Attention is involved when a patient is alerted by a significant stimulus and sustains interest in it. Concentration refers to the capacity to maintain mental effort despite distraction. An inattentive patient ignores the interviewer's questions, for example, or soon loses interest in them. The distractible patient is diverted from mental work by incidental sights, sounds, and ideas.

Table 5–7 describes simple clinical tests for attention and concentration. These tests have high reliability in assessing attention but have limited predictability regarding causation. Primarily they test the ability to concentrate. A patient's ability to answer arithmetic questions requires not only concentration but also knowledge. Errors are common and may

Table 5–6 Clinical Tests of Orientation

Time
Hour
Day
Date
Month
Year

Place
Building
City
State

Person
Name
Address and telephone number
Age
Occupation
Marital status

Table 5–7 Clinical Tests of Attention and Concentration

Subtract sevens or threes, serially, from 100.
Reverse the days of the week or months of the year.
Spell simple words backwards (e.g., *world*).
Repeat digits (two, three, four, or more) forward and backward.
Perform mental arithmetic (Number of nickels in $1.35? Interest on
   $200 at 4% for 18 months?).

be related to psychiatric disturbance, socioeconomic status, intelligence, or the patient's ability to cope with an interview situation. The procedures help to identify organic brain disorders but have little diagnostic specificity.

3. Memory—Memory has several stages. Information must first be registered and comprehended. It is then held in short-term storage. If the material is to be retained beyond immediate recall, a more durable memory trace is formed. Memory traces in long-term storage will decay, consolidate, or become simplified and schematized, partly as a result of subsequent experience. Long-term memories are retrieved or recalled from storage by tagging a pattern of sensory phenomena and matching it with long-term memory schemata.

In clinical practice, abnormal memory is manifest as **amnesia** (memory loss) or **dysmnesia** (distortion of memory). Psychogenic amnesia occurs in several forms. During and after an experience of severe anxiety, memory is likely to be defective. Some people have the ability to repress unwelcome anxiety-laden ideas rendering their memory as patchy or selective. In dissociative disorders, such as psychogenic amnesia and fugue, the patient usually loses memory for a circumscribed period of time during which profoundly disturbing events for them were experienced. Less commonly the amnesia is generalized (i.e., total) or subsequent (i.e., amnesia for everything after a particular time).

In addition to displaying generalized amnesia, patients in a psychogenic fugue state may travel a distance from home and assume a new identity. Often it is unclear in such cases whether unconscious self-deception or conscious imposture is involved.

Organic amnesia occurs in acute, subacute, and chronic forms. After acute head trauma, **retrograde amnesia** (loss of memory of past events) is likely to occur resulting in a disruption of short-term memory. The extent of **anterograde amnesia** (inability to form new memories) after head trauma is an index of the severity of brain injury. Amnesia also occurs in association with alcoholic blackouts and after acute intoxication, delirium, or epileptic seizures.

Subacute amnesia is the amnestic syndrome that occurs in Wernicke encephalopathy, a disease caused by thiamine deficiency and encountered most commonly in individuals with inadequate diet after extended severe alcohol abuse. Wernicke encephalopathy is characterized by conjugate gaze ophthalmoplegia, nystagmus, ataxia, and delirium. After the

delirium clears, most patients experience a residual syndrome with disorganized memory in an otherwise clear sensorium referred to Korsakoff syndrome. Patients with Korsakoff syndrome have difficulty recalling events from before the onset of encephalopathy. They also experience severe impairment of the ability to lay down new memories after the encephalopathy. The retrograde amnesia affects the patient's ability to remember the precise order in which events occurred. The anterograde amnesia, however, tends to be even more marked; the most severely affected patients, for example, are unable to store new information. As a consequence, these patients are often disoriented for place and time and may make up answers (confabulation) to fill the memory gap in their memories. Thus, the characteristic pattern of Korsakoff syndrome is amnesia, disorientation, confabulation, a facile lack of concern, and a tendency to get stuck in one groove of thought (**perseveration**). Chronic amnesia, as seen in dementing illnesses, extends back for years. In these cases, recent memory is lost before remote memory.

Disorders of recognition involve the sudden uncanny feeling that one has experienced the present situation, or heard precisely the same current conversation, on a previous occasion. This is referred to as déjà vu. These phenomena are associated with anxiety and less commonly with temporal lobe epilepsy. **Psychotic misidentification** may occur in some patients with schizophrenia who either describe familiar people as strangers or claim to recognize people they never met. Patients who regard familiar individuals (such as family members) as doubles or impersonators of themselves have a behavior referred to as Capgras syndrome.

Disorders of recall include retrospective falsification and confabulation. All people indulge at times in forms of **retrospective falsification**, embellishing the past to present a more appealing, tragic, or amusing impression of themselves. Histrionic and narcissistic individuals sometimes invent such an extensive and impressive past history of themselves that they appear to believe it and convince others to believe it. Depressed individuals in addressing their past may focus on sin, failure, and self-recrimination in their perceived unexceptional lives. After recovery from psychosis, patients often repress their memories of illness and retain only bland or vague recollections of the acute disorder. It is usually inadvisable to ask them to recall their experiences in detail.

A **confabulation** is a false memory that the patient believes is true. Confabulations may be quite detailed, but they are often inconsistent and fanciful. Confabulations commonly fill memory gaps, especially in the amnestic syndrome. Some schizophrenic patients spin complicated fantasies about telekinesis, extrasensory perception, nuclear radiation, and the like. These are part of their delusional thinking. It is frequently difficult to draw the line between confabulation, delusion and deception. This is the case in understanding the hysterical impostor or the dramatic abnormal illness behavior of the individual without any medical disorder referred to as Munchausen syndrome.

Table 5–8 Clinical Tests of Memory

Testing immediate recall

Repeat digits forward and backward. (Present digits at 1-second intervals. The average adult performance is up to six forward and four backward.)

Repeat three unrelated words (e.g., *apple, table, grass*) immediately.

Repeat three three-part words (e.g., 33 *Park Avenue, brown mahogany table, 12 red roses*).

Testing recent memory

Repeat the three one-part phrases after 1, 3, and 5 minutes.

Repeat the three three-part phrases after 1, 3, and 5 minutes.

Recall events in the recent past (e.g., a chronological account of the present illness, the last meal, an account of how the patient got to the office, the names of the physicians and nurses who are caring for the patient in the hospital).

Repeat this sentence: *One thing a country must have to become rich and great is a large, secure supply of wood.*

Recount the following story with as many details as possible: *William Stern/ a 63-year-old/ state representative/ from Walton County,/ Utah,/ was planning his reelection campaign/ when he began experiencing chest pain./ He entered Logan Memorial Hospital/ for 3 days of medical tests./ A harmless virus was diagnosed/ and he, his wife,/ Sandra,/ and their two sons,/ Rick and Tommy,/ hit the campaign trail again.* (The average patient should be able to reproduce 8 of the 15 separate ideas in this paragraph. Less adequate performance suggests defective recall of information that requires hierarchical analysis, short-term memory storage, and sequential recall.)

Testing remote memory

Recall parents' names, date and place of birth, graduation dates, age and year of marriage, and occupational history.

Table 5–8 lists the clinical tests for immediate, recent, and remote memory. These tests have good test–retest and inter-rater reliability. Patient performance may be affected by intelligence and age and by emotional states such as depression and to a lesser extent anxiety. The most useful tests for detecting organic lesions appear to be orientation, delayed recall, sentence repetition, and general information.

4. Information—The patient's fund of general knowledge depends on education and current interest in contemporary affairs. Table 5–9 provides a clinical test of information. Organicity is suggested if the patient makes 12 or more

Table 5–9 Clinical Test of Information

Name the last four presidents, starting with the current president

Name the mayor, state governor, and state senators

Name four large United States cities

Discuss four important current events

For what are these people famous: George Washington, Christopher Columbus, William Shakespeare, Albert Einstein?

mistakes ($\varepsilon = 60\%$) on this test if performed in a standardized fashion. The test is quite useful as an estimate of organicity.

5. Comprehension—A patient's comprehension is evaluated by his or her grasp of the importance of the immediate situation. For example, does the patient know why they are where they are? Does the patient appreciate that they are ill or in need of treatment? Does the patient understand the purpose of the examination?

There are no tests for comprehension. It is evaluated as the interview proceeds. Although comprehension is often disturbed in delirium and dementia, for example, there is no evidence that this disturbance contributes anything to the diagnosis of organicity beyond what is provided by other tests of the sensorium (i.e., orientation, concentration, memory).

6. Conceptualization & abstraction—Simple levels of conceptualization are assessed by testing the patient's capacity to discern the similarities and differences between sets of individual words. The patient's capacity to abstract is tested by asking the patient to discern the meaning of well-known metaphors (Table 5–10). The tests listed in Table 5–10 have limited reliability and validity. They are affected by intelligence, educational level, culture, and age. Responses give the interviewer limited diagnostic power. Research has demonstrated that clinicians using these tests could not distinguish among manic patients, schizophrenic patients, and creative writers. They are of most use when they tap unmistakable formal psychotic thought disorder. Consider the following examples:

A young man with disorganized and accelerated thinking responds to the proverb "People in glass houses should not throw stones": "Oh yeah. My California uncle passed the shotgun out the windows and started firing!"

To the proverb "A rolling stone gathers no moss," he answers, "Put a few pebbles in your mouth when you're hiking. You'll go a few more miles."

Table 5–10 Clinical Tests of Conceptualization and Abstraction

1. How are the following pairs similar or alike?
   a child and a dwarf
   a tree and a bush
   a river and a canal
   a dishwasher and a stove
2. How are the following pairs different?
   a lie and a mistake
   idleness and laziness
   poverty and misery
   character and reputation
3. What is the meaning of the following proverbs? (Ask the patient if he or she has heard them before.)
   "A rolling stone gathers no moss."
   "People who live in glass houses should not throw stones."
   "Strike while the iron is hot."

Another young patient, who has the delusion that he is Christ, responds to the glass houses proverb as follows: "Those who know that it has been seen what they have done—and believe me it has all been seen—let him who is without sin cast the first stone. Okay? That's what I believe it means."

The same patient responds to the rolling stone proverb in this way: "If you can continue to move and always move and always follow yourself and no one else, you'll never have the evil one within yourself."

Unfortunately, the sample of thinking provoked by these tests is usually so small, and its pathology so equivocal, that these tests are of dubious virtue.

E. Language

Language is a system of communication that facilitates thinking by the way semantics hierarchically organizes ideas and concepts. Syntax indicates the way words are used to connect the relationship between ideas and concepts.

Language competence is assessed from the patient's speech during the psychiatric interview. Any history of spoken or written language difficulty, or any observation of clumsy articulation, disordered rhythm, and difficulty in the understanding or choice of words, should be noted and investigated further. **Language comprehension** is tested by asking the patient to point to single objects, and then to point to a number of objects in a particular sequence. The interviewer may also ask the patient to perform a series of actions in an arbitrary sequence (e.g., "Touch your nose with your right index finger, then point that finger at me, then put it behind your back."). **Language expression** is evaluated by asking the patient to repeat words, phrases, and sentences and to name correctly a number of objects. Expression and comprehension are evaluated by asking the patient to read a passage aloud and to answer questions about it. Asking the patient to take dictation tests graphic language. Any errors and slowness in performance should be noted. The following sections describe some common disorders of language.

1. Aphasia—Aphasia is a dysfunction in the patient's ability to express himself or herself. The three most common forms of aphasia are all manifest as difficulty in repeating words or phrases. In **Broca aphasia**, comprehension is relatively intact but expression dysfluent, sparse, telegraphic, and full of circumlocution. In **Wernicke aphasia**, comprehension is impaired. Expression, though fluent, rambles, lacks meaning, and is full of errors to which the patient seems oblivious. In **conduction aphasia**, comprehension is intact, expression is fluent but full of errors and pauses, and repetition is difficult; however, reading is relatively intact.

2. Muteness—Muteness is seldom found in neurologic disease, except in the acute phase, in seizure disorder, or in advanced cerebral degeneration. The aphasic patient is never mute. Muteness is much more commonly a sign of major depression, stupor, catatonia, somatoform disorder, dissociation, or an anxiety disorder in children (i.e., elective mutism).

3. Schizophrenic language—The psychiatrist must distinguish the language of the schizophrenic from the "jargon" of Wernicke aphasia. Untreated or acutely symptomatic schizophrenic patients tend to be heedlessly bizarre in thought content; aphasic patients are more aware of their errors and are more likely to use substitutions to overcome their language defects. The confused speech of schizophrenic patients is frequently referred to as **word salad**. It may be so chaotic as to be barely comprehensible.

4. Paralogia—Paralogia, or talking past the point, occurs when the patient gives answers that are erroneous but reveal knowledge of what should be the correct answer. For example, the interviewer may ask, "How many legs has a cow?" and the patient responds, "Five." Talking past the point occurs in Ganser syndrome (also called the syndrome of approximate answers). It is most likely to be observed in individuals who regard hospitalization for insanity as preferable to incarceration for crime.

5. Neologisms—Neologisms are new words coined by the patient. They are often condensations of ideas that attempt to capture an idea or concept difficult to describe. Neologisms are most commonly observed in schizophrenia; they must be distinguished from aphasic paraphasia, and circumlocution, where the patient attempts to overcome expressive difficulty. Sometimes a neologism reveals that the patient has been "derailed" by the sound or sense of an associated word or idea. At other times, neologisms are a response to hallucinations or a defense (in the patient's private code) against the intrusion by the interviewer upon the patient's private thoughts.

F. Disorders of Thought

Pathological thought may be found in the process, in the form, or in the content of thinking. The process and form of thinking may be disordered in terms of tempo, fluency (including continuity and control), logical organization, and intent. In normal thinking an individual responds to the setting. In a nonstressful setting it is characterized by appropriate, reasonable but not excessive speed, and a smooth and continuous flow from one idea to the next between two conversant. It has a clear goal-directed organization, and consensual logic in the links between, and the sequence of, its constituent ideas.

In psychological illness, particularly the turmoil associated with psychoses such as schizophrenia and mania, any or all of the foregoing characteristics may be disorganized. Pathologic thinking can be observed as sluggish, abrupt, disconnected, meandering or halting, and prone to wander off at tangents in illogical directions.

Abnormal thinking can be experienced by the thinker as invasive, inserted, or controlled by alien forces (**thought insertion**). It can also be sensed as leaking, stolen, lost, or broadcast from the mind into the outside world (**thought withdrawal** or **broadcasting**). Finally, the psychotic thinker may become oblivious to or unconcerned about the need to make sense, and lose contact with their audience or use language to mask their confused thinking.

1. Abnormalities of thought process & form

i. Tempo—**Accelerated thinking** is referred to as flight **of ideas. It may** reach such a pitch that goal direction is lost and the connection between ideas is governed not by logical sense but by sound or idiosyncratic verbal or conceptual associations. Alliteration, assonance, rhyme referred to as **clang associations**, and punning are examples of speech where ideas in a conversation are distracted readily by internal or environmental stimuli. Flight of ideas is usually associated with **pressured speech** and may be experienced by the patient as racing thoughts. Flight of ideas is characteristic of mania, but it may occur also in excited schizophrenic patients or individuals who are frightened. In hypomania the flight of ideas is less marked, the tempo being accelerated but the associations less disorganized than in mania.

The tempo of thinking may also be slowed as in **retardation of thought**, seen especially in major depression. The patient often complains of fuzziness, woolliness, and poor concentration. Response time in speech to questions is increased. There are long silences during which the patient may lose the thread of the conversation. In the extreme, retardation of thought becomes mutism or even stupor.

ii. Fluency—In **circumstantiality**, although the goal direction of thinking is retained, associations meander into fruitless, overly detailed, or barely relevant byways. The listener may feel impelled to hurry the speaker along. Circumstantiality is frequently seen in some epileptic patients whose peculiar combination of pedantry, perseveration, religiosity, and cliché lend their thinking to a so-called "viscous" quality.

Perseveration refers to a tendency to persist with a point or theme, even after it has been dealt with exhaustively or the listener has tried to change the subject.

iii. Continuity—In **thought blocking**, the patient's speech is interrupted abruptly by silences that last less than a second or much longer, even a minute or more. During the pause the patient's eyes often flicker, particularly if they are experiencing an auditory hallucination. Sometimes the patient manifests a blank expression. Blocking is often precipitated by questions or ideas that have personal significance, particularly if they are experienced as dangerous. Blocking is an uncommon but striking sign. It is often misidentified. The observer mistaking the retarded thinking of a depressed or preoccupied patient for the abrupt roadblock of the true phenomenon. It is almost pathognomonic of schizophrenia but must be differentiated from the absences of petit mal epilepsy, the hesitation caused by anxiety, and the peculiar mental fixity associated with amphetamine intoxication.

During the period of blocking, intermediate associations may be lost, and the patient recommences on an apparently different track (**tangential thinking**). This can give rise to a phenomenon known as the **knight's move in thought**: The listener can sometimes intuit how the patient got from A to E and realizes that the unspoken intermediate associations (B, C, and D) were quite indirect. On other occasions, the patient's thinking appears subject to **derailing** (jumping the track to proceed on a different subject), particularly when a painful to the patient point has been touched on. Patients are often aware of disturbances in the continuity of their thinking and will describe how their thoughts become paralyzed, interrupted, or jumbled.

iv. Control—Akin to the subjective phenomena described in the previous section is the patient's sense that speed, direction, form, or content of their thought are out of control. Complaints such as "confused," "racing thoughts," "unable to concentrate," "scatterbrained," "jumbled," and "going crazy" often reflect the subjective perception of pathologically accelerated, dysfluent, or discontinuous thinking.

Sometimes schizophrenic patients report that their thinking is controlled by external forces or people, for example, by means of radio waves or other transmissions. Thinking may be perceived as directed by the external agency, or particular thoughts experienced as having been implanted by it. This is known as **thought insertion** or **thought alienation**.

In **thought deprivation** or **thought broadcasting**, the patient senses that ideas are escaping their mind, being stolen by others, or being broadcast via radio, television, or the internet. The perception that the television picks up and repeats one's thoughts may provoke a grandiose or persecutory delusional misinterpretation.

v. Logical organization—Psychotic thinking may reflect a deterioration in the capacity to think formally or logically. Commonly, the schizophrenic patient when experiencing a psychotic episode uses a private logic, with over personalized concrete symbols. Within this logical framework, conceptual boundaries are blurred, and the thinking patterns are metaphorical and idiosyncratic, almost as if they emerged directly from a dream state. Thus, to the observer, when thoughts are expressed in this manner, they may appear on the surface to be diffuse, bizarre, and lacking in clarity. However, it is at times possible to interpret their meaning in the context of the patient's personal situation and the issues that he or she is struggling with.

vi. Intent of communication—The conventional purpose of discourse allows individuals to share ideas. Patients may use an interaction to consciously or unconsciously obscure the communication of their inner thoughts and ideas. A schizophrenic patient may attempt to retain the privacy of their thoughts by conversing in an obscure, remote, supercilious, attacking, mocking, or farcical manner.

2. Abnormalities of thought content—Several disorders are defined by the presence of abnormalities of thought content. In many instances the patient will complain of a unique fear for them (e.g., a phobia of heights); in other cases, the patient appears to have accepted an eccentric idea (e.g., the delusion of being a reincarnation of Christ) and to be acting accordingly. Abnormal thought may be divided into the following categories: abnormal perceptions, abnormal convictions, abnormal preoccupations and impulses, and abnormalities in the sense of self. **Abnormal perceptions**—Perception is the ability to integrate sensory stimuli to form an image or impression and give it a personal meaning. The uniqueness of the personal meaning is influenced by past experience. Perception may be increased or decreased in intensity. **Heightened perception** refers to increased intensity of personal meaning which to an observer alters the physical reality of the perception. This occurs in delirium, mania, after use of hallucinogens, and in the rare ecstatic states that occur as part of acute schizophrenia or exhilarated hysterical trances. **Dulled perception** is the converse and occurs in depression and organic delirium.

In **derealization**, the external world seems different, changed, vague, unreal, or distant. This symptom when seen during adolescence is associated with **depersonalization**, the sense that one is distanced from the environment or a spectator of one's own actions. It is also associated with anxiety or dissociative disorders, depression, schizophrenia, organic brain disorder, and after hallucinogen use. In **synesthesia**, the subject perceives color in response to music, for example. It is a common psychedelic experience.

Time may be experienced as accelerated under the influence of hallucinogens, in mania, or during an epileptic aura. Time may seem slowed or stopped in depression or epilepsy. In some conditions, time seems to lack continuity and the subject feels uninvolved in the temporal stream. This is particularly likely to be encountered in depersonalization, amnestic syndromes, depression, schizophrenia, or toxic-confusional states.

An **illusion** is sensory stimulation, perception which is given a false, personalized interpretation. Illusions are common in delirium and may be visual (e.g., fluttering curtains seen as intruders), auditory (e.g., a slamming door interpreted as the report of a pistol), tactile (e.g., skin sensations thought to be caused by vermin), gustatory (e.g., poison detected in the taste of food), kinesthetic (e.g., flying), or visceral (e.g., abdominal pain thought to be caused by ground glass). Illusions may also occur in hysteria, depression, and schizophrenia, particularly when perception is subordinated to a delusional idea (e.g., of guilt or persecution) or an intense emotion (e.g., abandonment or erotic yearning).

A hallucination occurs when an individual reports a perception in their waking state in the absence of any sensory stimulus. It is not merely a sensory distortion or misinterpretation. The individual is convinced the stimulus occurred. A true hallucination appears to the individual to be substantial and to occur in external objective space. In contrast, a normal mental image is insubstantial and experienced within internal subjective space. Deafness, tinnitus, or blindness, usually in association with dementia or delirium, may determine the modality of hallucinations.

Sensory deprivation experiments have produced visual and auditory hallucinosis in many subjects. Cortical disease may be associated with hallucinations (usually visual). Tumors of the olfactory or basal temporal regions may cause olfactory hallucinosis, for example, as an aura. Hallucinations, especially visual in modality (though sometimes vestibular and kinesthetic), are common in the delirium caused by toxins (e.g., drugs, hallucinogens, alcohol), fever, cerebrovascular disease, and central degenerative disorders. Aside from these medical circumstances, hallucinatory experiences are common and normal, in some people, when falling asleep (hypnagogic) or waking (hypnopompic). Severe sleep deprivation can cause hypnagogic hallucinosis.

Hallucinations can be auditory, visual, olfactory or gustatory, tactile, or somatic. In form, they may be amorphous, elementary, or complex. They may be experienced as emanating from inner or outer space and, if from outside, from near or far. Hallucinations may be unsystematized, appearing to have no link to life circumstances, or systematized and part of a causally interconnected delusional world.

Auditory hallucinations may be inchoate (e.g., humming, rushing water, inaudible murmurs), fragmentary (e.g., words or phrases such as "fag," "get him," or "beastly") or complex. Typically, the schizophrenic patient locates complex hallucinations as a voice or voices speaking to or about him or her. The voice may be soothing, mocking, disparaging, or noncommittal. Sometimes the voice echoes the patient's thoughts or comments neutrally on his or her actions. Sometimes the voice orders the patient to perform actions, or the patient feels the voice puts thoughts into their head, a perception referred to as thought insertion. A hallucinatory voice may be perceived as coming from the radio, television, computer or cell phone, from outside a window, or even from a distant place. In alcoholic hallucinosis, typically, a conspiracy of threatening whisperers plan to injure the patient, provoking the patient to self-defense or flight.

Visual hallucinations vary from elemental flashes of light or color, as in disorders of the visual pathways and cortex, to well-formed scenes of people, animals, insects, and things. In delirium, insects or other small objects may be seen moving on the bed or in the surroundings. Lilliputian hallucinations, of little people on the bed, for example, occur in delirium and other organic brain syndromes. Complex audiovisual hallucinations may occur in temporal lobe epilepsy. In general, visual hallucinosis suggests acute brain disorder rather than functional psychosis and tends to occur in a setting of confusion or obtundation. Sometimes, however, a schizophrenic patient will report visual hallucinations (e.g., trips in flying saucers) aligned with his or her prevailing delusions. The visual hallucinations of hysteria or dissociative disorder have a pseudo-hallucinatory (i.e., "unreal,") quality. In post-traumatic stress disorder they may represent the intrusive memory of the traumatic event, as when a war veteran reexperiences a battle incident.

Olfactory and gustatory hallucinations (e.g., burning rubber, steak, and onions) may occur in epilepsy. Schizophrenic patients may perceive gas being pumped into their bedrooms by persecutors or may think they taste poisonous substances in their food. Severely depressed patients may be conscious of the stench of corruption rising from their unworthy bodies or may complain of the changed, metallic, tasteless quality of their meals.

Tactile hallucinations are characteristic of cocaine and amphetamine intoxication; the patient being distracted by the sensation of insects crawling on the skin. Schizophrenic patients may report the effect on the skin of radioactivity beamed at them from a hostile source.

Somatic hallucinations occur in schizophrenia, whereby genital, visceral, intracerebral, or kinesthetic sensations are often referred to the influence of persecutors or machines. The melancholic patient may have the sense of having no stomach, with food dropping from the throat into a void.

In schizophrenia, or under the influence of hallucinogens, the patient may have the belief that somebody, a presence, is behind them. This can occur in states of extreme fear, but it may become a central feature of schizophrenia, in the guise of a hallucinatory double of the self (Doppelganger) who always lurks just behind the periphery of vision.

ii. Abnormal convictions—A **delusion** is a false belief not susceptible to argument and inconsistent with the subject's sociocultural background. Bordering on delusion is an **overvalued idea.** This may be an idea not supported by fact but may become a governing force in the patient's life.

It is not always easy to draw the line between an individual, who holds unfamiliar views that are nevertheless consistent with a different sociocultural system, someone who holds a belief not supported by the majority of individuals in their society and a deluded person. In political discussions individuals may express as fact situations that do not exist. Indeed, some people drift across unclear boundaries between these categories. An active delusion or belief in a false political reality may dominate an individual's life, subordinating all other matters. It is private, idiosyncratic, ego-centered, and inconsistent with the common experience of people from the same background. Either a true delusion or false belief may isolate the subject from others.

Severe sensory deprivation, or exhaustion and physical privation, may lead to delusional misinterpretation, often associated with wish-fulfilling hallucinations. A delusion can act as a transcendental escape from the self-experience of an existential wasteland. This is the ground from which cosmic, messianic, and redemptive delusions grow.

As for the content of delusions, the most common are persecution, jealousy, love, grandeur, disease, poverty, and guilt. **Delusions of persecution** are most frequently encountered in schizophreniform disorders or schizophrenia, organic mental disorder (especially alcoholic hallucinosis, amphetamine delirium or delusional disorder, other hallucinogenic syndromes, epilepsy, and all forms of delirium) and, less commonly, in major depression or during transitory psychotic episodes. Patients may perceive others as talking conspiratorially about them (delusions of reference) or spying. External organizations or the government (e.g., communists, FBI) may be experienced as disrupting, interfering or attempting to harm a patient by acting alone or with other groups. They are believed by the patient to accomplish this by diverse means. They may include radiation, poisonous gases, radio and television waves, intruders, assassins, and so on. The patient may allude to the use of cell phones to spy on them.

Delusions of jealousy occur in the same syndromes as delusions of persecution. They may be woven into family strife between spouse or siblings.

Delusions of grandeur occur in mania, schizophrenia, paranoid disorders, and organic delusional syndromes (e.g., neurosyphilis). In mania and organic grandiosity, the patient's megalomania (e.g., of being God, the governor, the Virgin Mary, Napoleon) are in line with their general high spirits. In schizophrenia and paranoid disorders, an inflated sense of importance may be reinforced by auditory hallucinations and the grandiosity of a delusional explanation for ideas of persecution: Why else would important agencies (e.g., the FBI, the Vatican) be looking for them?

Erotic delusions is a belief that a person of higher status is in love with them (erotomania). A lonely person may develop a crush on a celebrity or prominent citizen or an acquaintance. Fantasies of mutual involvement evolve into delusions, and the subject bombards the other person with telephone calls and text messages. The failure of the perceived loved one to reciprocate is put down to conspiratorial forces that stand in the way of destiny. The schizophrenic patient believes that they are receiving erotic messages (hallucinations) from their beloved.

Somatic delusions, usually of disease or ill health, occur in many psychiatric disorders. Schizophrenic patients may have bizarre complaints, possibly in an attempt to explain somatic hallucinatory experiences, for example, of blood running backward in the head, of radiation being trained on the genitals by an outside agency, or of objects placed inside the body by malevolent forces. In melancholia, the patient may have delusions of being dead (no blood in the body), of their internal organs rotting away, or of their brain being destroyed by syphilis, in retribution for an unpardonable sin. The boundary between hypochondriasis, disease phobia, and disease conviction, physical disease, and somatic delusions may be difficult to determine.

The wide breadth of hallucinatory experiences that may be reported by our patient are affected and altered by prescribed antipsychotic medications. Patients on less-than-optimal therapeutic dosages nay alternately report hallucinations which they at one moment firmly believe and then report the next that they know they are not real. A few minutes later they again believe the reality of their hallucination.

Seriously depressed patients are prone to **delusions of poverty** and **delusions of nihilism**. The future is hopeless, the present desolate, the patient destitute and abandoned to a bleak fate. Depressive patients may also complain of inordinate guilt, with the most extreme punishments being meted out to them for unremarkable, long ago ancient transgressions.

iii. Abnormal preoccupations & impulses—A **phobia** is an irrationally exaggerated dread with an intense anxiety that focuses on a particular object, situation, or act. The anxiety generated by phobias differs from generalized anxiety in their being elicited by specific triggers, Diffuse anxiety unfocused anxiety sometimes precedes the development a phobic disorder. Phobic patients are aware of the exaggerated, irrational nature of their phobia and regard it as symptomatic. The patient often tries to avoid the phobic situation. If unable they may feel compelled to perform actions (such as hand washing) in order to eradicate the object of the fear or atone for tabooed action.

An **obsession** is a persistent idea, desire, image, phrase, or fragment of music that cuts into the stream of conscious thinking. The patient recognizes the alien nature of the obsession and attempts to resist it, without success. The obsession often presses the subject to perform compulsive acts, to relieve anxiety. The key characteristics of obsessions are their persistent, irresistible, imperative nature; their ego-alien quality; and their repetitiousness. Obsessional symptoms have been reported after encephalitis. They may occur in the premonitory phase of schizophrenia or as part of a major depression (e.g., the patient may experience persistent ruminations that old tax returns were in error and that ruin will result). Obsessive–compulsive symptoms are most characteristic of the anxiety disorder that bears the same name (see Chapter 30).

An impulsive act—an **Impulsion**—differs from compulsions in that they may occur with little warning and may create dangerous situations for the patient and others. The negative effect of impulsive acts frequently harms individuals and causes legal entanglements for the impulsive actor. Impulsive acts spring from a diverse number of affects including anger, anxiety, frustration, rejection, sadness, or humiliation. Alcohol intoxication which disinhibits behavior may lead to impulsive acts. Common impulsions include violent assault, fast driving, sexual assault, sexual exhibitionism, shoplifting, stealing, and fire-setting. Sudden, episodic, if not explosive, onset is the hallmark of these phenomena. The perpetrator of impulsive actions is unable to exercise control over their actions.

iv. Abnormalities of the sense of self—The normal person has a sense of selfhood composed of the following elements: a sense of existing and being involved in one's own body and activity; a sense of personal continuity in time between past, present, and future; a sense of personal integrity; and a sense of distinction between self and outside world. In psychiatric disorders, any or several of these phenomena may be disturbed. An individual may feel uninvolved in his or her own body or actions and experience themselves like a spectator looking at another person (as in depersonalization). An individual's sense of temporal continuity may be dislocated, and present is confused with past. The future may seem remote and the present but a series of disconnected scenes. The individual may feel as though they are falling apart, fragmented, or split in two; or the difference between themselves and other persons or objects may have become blurred.

The sense of depersonalization, often associated with derealization, can occur in adolescence, epilepsy, dissociative disorders, schizophrenia, and depression. Adolescents experiencing severe emotional turmoil sometimes develop a sense of discontinuity, disintegration, and dedifferentiation. These symptoms are very common after ingestion of hallucinogens (and may be reexperienced as flashbacks) and in reactive psychosis, schizophreniform disorder, or schizophrenic disorders.

G. Physiologic Function

Sleep disturbances are often encountered in psychiatric practice. Sleep deprivation may precipitate or accentuate psychiatric disorder. Sleep disturbance may be a prodrome, a symptom, or a sequel of psychiatric disorder. Many psychopharmacologic agents also affect sleep. See Chapter 36 for more on sleep disorders.

Appetite may be increased in dysthymic personality and after psychotropic drug medication. Eating binges (not necessarily determined by increased appetite) may occur in bulimia nervosa as a condition separate from, in alternation with, or following, anorexia nervosa (see Chapter 35).

Anorexia and weight loss can occur in almost any stress condition but are particularly likely in major depression, paranoid schizophrenia, somatoform disorders, alcoholism or drug addiction, and, anorexia nervosa. A comprehensive physical screening investigation is always required when anorexia and weight loss are present.

Sexual desire may be increased in mania, in some forms of acute schizophrenia, and in narcissistic or borderline personality under stress. Sexual behavior may be disinhibited after alcohol or drug ingestion, in delirium, or in organic dementia. Sexual desire is decreased by any debilitating disorder, by anxiety, worry, tiredness, age, poor nutrition, and lack of affection for the partner. It is usually reduced by depression, schizophrenia, alcoholism, or substance abuse and by antipsychotic, antihypertensive, and antidepressant medication.

Absent, irregular, infrequent, and scanty menstrual periods may occur in psychiatric disorder, particularly in depression, anorexia nervosa, anxiety disorders, schizophrenia, and substance abuse. Any condition that reduces total body fat to below 14%, in the female, produces anovulation and amenorrhea. Dysmenorrhea, dyspareunia, vaginismus, and other pelvic complaints are common in somatoform disorders, and in abnormal illness behavior generally, but a discretionary physical screen is required before a stress-related condition is diagnosed. See Chapter 34 for a more complete discussion of sexual dysfunctions.

Any or all body systems may be accelerated in the hyperdynamic states of anxiety, delirium, mania, and schizophrenic catatonic excitement or slowed in the general hypomotility of depression, organic dementia, and hypothyroidism. The patient's level of energy, or fatigue, may also be affected by disorders with accelerated or sluggish mental processes. Anergia, weakness, or obscure bodily discomfort are encountered frequently in somatoform disorders.

H. Insight & Judgment

1. Insight—The patient's attitude or insight into their presenting for a mental health evaluation has several aspects. For example, does the patient recognize that he or she has a problem? Do they identify their problems as personal and psychological in nature? Do they understand the nature and cause of the illness? Do they want help and, if so, what kind of help? Did they make the appointment?

The hypomanic patient has no problem. They feel very well (e.g., high-spirited, amusing, energetic, expansive, and optimistic). The manic or schizophrenic patient may view the reason for the appointment as an external problem (i.e., other people or agencies are stupidly obstructive or malevolent). Many patients with externalizing personality disorders (e.g., borderline, antisocial, narcissistic) blame others for their predicament.

Sophisticated patients, particularly those who have undergone previous psychotherapeutic treatment, may have considerable knowledge of their formal diagnosis and the theoretical or potential causes of their disorder. Indeed, sometimes this causes problems in treatment:

The patient may be aware of having a problem but want no help, or they may want help of a particular sort or from a particular kind of clinician. Whenever this is reasonable and feasible, it should be arranged. The patient's desires should be respected as much as possible in the negotiation phase of the clinical process.

2. Judgment—The interviewer can ask the patient one of the following questions to test judgment: What would you

do if you found a stamped, addressed envelope in the street? Why are there laws? Why should promises be kept? Good judgment requires intact orientation, concentration, and memory. There is no evidence that a finding of poor judgment adds anything to diagnosis beyond that provided by the detection of deficits in the lower-order functions, such as accomplishing household chores, maintaining personal hygiene, or selecting appropriate attire.

▶ Termination

A psychiatric interview may last 15 minutes or go on for much longer. The usual time is about 45 minutes: long enough for a rapid survey but not so long as to exhaust the patient. The interviewer can signal the approach of the conclusion by saying, for example, "Our time is almost finished, and there are a few additional things we need to discuss."

A concluding summary of the material points of the interview can be very helpful. It allows the patient to correct or modify misinterpretations and leads naturally into the interviewer's plan for what happens next—another interview, for example, or special investigations.

PRACTICAL MATTERS

▶ Facilitating the Interview

If an interview is to achieve its purpose (i.e., to gather information), the interviewer must develop an atmosphere favoring the expression of ideas, feelings, and attitudes. The patient must develop a sense of trust and confidence in the interviewer, in order to be as spontaneous as possible. They need to see the interviewer as encouraging participation and collaboration toward a therapeutic end, through free expression and self-exploration.

The interviewer must accept the patient, without moral judgment. If he or she cannot do so, it is better to be honest about it and refer the patient to another physician. Anybody can help somebody, but nobody can help everybody. If a patient angers, repels, or frightens the interviewer, and the feeling persists, the interviewer in assessing the cause of these feelings should seek help in a consultation with a colleague.

The interview is facilitated if the interviewer understands the patient and conveys this understanding by facial expression, intonation, and well-timed reflections of the content and emotion behind the patient's story. The deepest affective understanding of a patient is empathy. The clinician communicates to their patient an appreciation of their life situation and the difficulties they are experiencing. This contrasts with sympathy, which may not communicate an appreciation of a patient's life situation but expresses feeling **for** a specific painful event.

The open-ended style of questioning described earlier in this chapter for most initial psychiatric interviews helps to convey the spirit of collaboration, free expression, and self-exploration. An atmosphere of trust is fostered if the interviewer is relaxed and receptive, not preoccupied, rushed, abrupt, or irritable. Over time interviewers may modify the techniques and the interview format they have learned to fit in their own style and format. Nonetheless that must obtain the critical information needed in an assessment.

▶ Interview Setting

A skilled interviewer can be effective walking along a corridor, playing catch, or sitting by the side of a bed. Nevertheless, offices are preferable to closets, and chairs are an improvement over a packing box. If the interviewer has the opportunity, he or she should arrange the interview room to take advantage of its size, proportions, furnishings, and design.

The fundamental principles are simple. The room should be large enough to fit the patient, a desk, chairs, and other equipment, without crowding the interviewer. The arrangement of the desk and chairs should allow entry and egress, but if possible, the interviewer should not sit between the patient and the door. He or she should try not to interview people from across a desk. Harsh lighting should be avoided. The patient should not be blinded by glare shining directly from a window or a lamp. The chairs should be comfortable, and the interviewer should not tower over the patient. The interviewer should not leave the patient stranded in the middle of the room; people feel less exposed with something solid behind them. The interviewer should not sit too close (i.e., knee to knee) or too far away. He or she should be near enough to make arm contact by leaning forward.

▶ Interview Techniques

The interviewer should encourage free expression during the opening and detailed inquiry stages of the psychiatric interview. He or she does so by the setting they have created, the atmosphere created, and the interview techniques used. The interviewer should be at ease with these techniques, and they should be used naturally, without flamboyance or stiltedness. If a particular technique does not suit the interviewer, he or she should not use it; an alternative should be found that conveys the same spirit and has a similar purpose.

The following are examples of useful techniques: Attentive listening, subtle vocal and nonvocal encouragement, support and reassurance, the reflection of feeling, gentle indication, and judicious paraphrasing.

Having invited the patient to tell his or her story, the interviewer waits and listens. The interviewer. meets the patient's gaze from time to time to indicate they are following. The interviewer's intent but relaxed posture indicates involvement. If the interviewer takes notes, they should be as brief as possible and unobtrusive.

While the flow of associations proceeds, the interviewer needs to do little but maintain relaxed concentration, signaled by posture, eye contact, and subtle nonvocal or vocal encouragement A nod or an "uh-huh" or "mmmm" at strategic points may be all that is needed. Sometimes, when the flow seems to waver or slow, it is very effective to pick up and repeat a significant phrase or the last word the patient has said. But the interviewer should not be mechanical and should not do something unless it feels natural.

The interviewer needs to be alert to the patient's reactions, particularly to changes in voice intonation and speech tempo, tensing of facial muscles, alterations of skin color, and moistening of conjunctivae, which may herald a flush of anxiety or anger or a sudden feeling of sadness.

Silences are a unique difficulty in patient interviews. If the patient is thinking and engaged with the interviewer, all the interviewer need do is wait. Similarly, if the patient has broken down in tears, it may be better to wait calmly until the patient can continue. If the silence occurs when the patient has lost track of or has confused feelings about the topic, the interviewer can facilitate associations with a subtle oral reflection, picking up a key word, phrase, or idea from the recent conversation and repeating it gently, sometimes with a questioning intonation. Reflecting on the comments of a patient speaking circumstantially is frequently useful to helping patients to refocus on the interview.

Reflecting on the feelings is a variant of this technique. The interviewer picks up and echoes feelings explicit or implicit in what the patient has spoken. But the interviewer beliefs they can be expressed more clearly and completely.

▶ Transference & Countertransference

Transference refers to the unreasonable displacement of attitudes and feelings that originated in earlier life experiences or in childhood to people in the here and now. This phenomenon is particularly likely to affect the doctor–patient relationship when patients feel vulnerable in needing to rely on a health care provider or in telling their story they experience fear, anxiety, guilt, despair, or hope.

The patient who is upset by the overt rudeness of the interviewer is not displaying transference. However, if the patient is angered because the interviewer has a moustache or dresses differently than they do; it is apparent that they are adding something that is unique to them in an objectively neutral situation.

The patient may unconsciously regard the physician as a parent or a sibling. experiencing them in a caring or antagonistic role. Some examples of the commonest roles are of nurturing mother, demanding mother, protective father, punitive father, and rivalrous sibling. Sometimes older patients will relate to the physician as though they are parents in the clinical encounter.

The interviewer can suspect a potential transference patient response when the patient's affective state does not match the feeling tone of the doctor–patient interaction. When the patient is exceptionally deferential, hanging onto the interviewer's opinions, the interviewer may suspect a positive transference. When the patient is unexpectedly hostile, suspicious, or competitive, and there is no reasonable explanation for such antagonism, a negative transference is likely.

A positive transference can become eroticized, for example with the patient falling in love with an idealized parental figure. Most of these infatuations are transitory, like the crushes of adolescence. If the interviewer recognizes them and responds in a professional manner, they will go no further. Occasionally, however, after an initial visit the patient makes unscheduled visits, writes notes, telephone calls, or send unasked-for gifts. The interviewer should not respond impulsively, out of fear or affront, lest a vulnerable patient be hurt. The interviewer may need to consult a psychiatric colleague to decide how to proceed.

Transference has its counterpart in a physician's reactions to a patient, **countertransference**, which occurs when a physician irrationally transfers to a patient his or her attitudes and feelings derived from their earlier or childhood experiences. Psychiatric interviewers must be alert for countertransference. They should suspect it whenever they have powerful feelings of affection, protectiveness, fear, frustration, irritation, hatred, or erotic excitement toward a patient; when they very much look forward to the next appointment; or when they cannot tolerate a particular patient. If the interviewer recognizes these feelings, he or she will be much less likely to respond impulsively with rejection, flight, or self-indulgence. Once again, the interviewer should seek the help of a colleague or group of colleagues if he or she is unsure how to proceed in the patient's best interests.

Experienced clinicians know that these emotional displacements are ubiquitous and inescapable. They are most likely to be problematic when the interviewer is overworked, preoccupied, or rendered emotionally vulnerable by the vicissitudes of his or her personal life. The interviewer must look after himself or herself physically and emotionally. If transference reactions become disruptive forces in clinical work the psychiatrist needs to consider a consultation regarding their life situation.

STRUCTURED INTERVIEWS AND RATING SCALES

There is a role for standardized rating scales and structured interviews in developing a psychiatric history and evaluating changes in psychopathology while a patient is under treatment. However, these instruments are rarely appropriate to substitute for a traditional psychiatric interview in clinical practice. Screening questionnaires are used in primary care practice or in identifying psychopathology in large populations. Examples are depressive screening instruments in primary care and posttraumatic stress disorder screening instruments in military populations.

Symptom-based scales are designed to measure change in a particular symptom or a syndrome-based group of symptoms, rather than establish a diagnosis in the framework of a particular diagnostic system. These scales can be useful in clinical practice to document, objectively and quantitatively, the change in response to a therapeutic intervention or simply change over time. They can be self-rating scales completed by the patient or rater-administered scales completed by the clinician. Obviously, the disadvantage of self-rated scales is the reliability of the measurement.

The Brief Psychiatric Rating Scale measures major psychotic and nonpsychotic symptoms in patients with a major psychiatric disorder. It is a widely used rater-administered scale for evaluating baseline psychopathology and treatment response, particularly in inpatient populations. The Hamilton Rating Scale for Depression is one of the most widely used rater-administered scales for assessing symptoms of depression and measuring their change over time. It is frequently used in clinical trials. The Beck Depression Inventory and the Zung Depression Scale are both self-rating scales that are frequently used to evaluate severity of depression in patients engaged in treatment. The Zung scale is also used as a screening instrument for depression. The Hamilton Rating Scale for Anxiety is a frequently used rater-administered scale for evaluating the severity of anxiety symptoms. There are a variety of symptom-based scales designed to be used in child psychiatric disorders, substance-abuse disorders, and geriatric psychiatric syndromes. The reader is directed to the bibliography for further details in these areas.

CONCLUSION

The purpose of the psychiatric interview is to obtain information from the patient about their presenting problem and its potential precipitants. Additionally, we learn about any previous disorders, predisposition, strengths and limitations, reason for the current presentation, insight, and desire for help. The psychiatric history covers topics that range from identifying data to coping mechanisms. The four stages of the interview—inception, obtaining initial data, detailed inquiry, and termination—are adapted to different topics.

In the inception stage, the interviewer makes introductions, gets the patient or family seated, takes identifying information, and may summarize what they understand or know about the patient. The quality of the interview is enhanced if the interviewer creates an atmosphere of trust, spontaneity, and expressiveness by their acceptance, empathic understanding, open-ended interview style, and natural manner. The decor, lighting, furnishings, and arrangement of the room can also promote (or subvert) the desired atmosphere.

During the initial data gathering of the present illness, the interviewer helps the patient describe the presenting problem and its precipitation and development.

During the detailed inquiry, stage, the interviewer in varying degrees of depth explores past illness; early development and environment; later educational, occupational, social, and marital history; interests, values, and aspirations; habitual coping style; family history; and mental status.

LAST STEPS

During the interview, the clinician has fostered the patient's free expression of why they are there. This was accomplished by being attentive and demonstrating an empathic appreciation of the patient's difficulties. The clinician will seldom, if ever, need to or be able to pursue every detail in the initial interview regarding the patient's presenting symptoms and behavior. They will however need enough data to develop a working clinical formulation (hypothesis), a diagnosis, decide whether a comprehensive or brief MSE is indicated and develop a tentative future plan of action.

At this point if the initial interview was requested by the patient the interviewer will summarize and present their recommendations to the patient. Time must be available for the patient to ask questions. The conclusion of the interview occurs after the interviewer and patient agree on the development of the next step on the patient's clinical experience or treatment.

Basch MF: *Doing Psychotherapy*. New York: Basic Books, 1980.

Carlat DJ: *The Psychiatric Interview*. Philadelphia: Lippincott Williams & Wilkins, 1999.

Colby KM: *A Primer for Psychotherapists*. New York: Ronald Press, 1951.

Guze BH, James M: Medical assessment and laboratory testing in psychiatry. In: Sadock BJ, Sadock VA, Ruiz P (eds). *Kaplan and Sadock's Comprehensive Textbook of Psychiatry*, 9th edn. Philadelphia: Lippincott Williams & Wilkins, 2009, pp. 995–1012.

Leckman JF, Taylor E: Clinical assessment and diagnostic formulation. In: Thapar A, Pine DS, Leckman JF, et al. (eds). *Rutter's Child and Adolescent Psychiatry*, 6th edn. Oxford: Blackwell, 2015.

Maj M, Gaebel W, López-Ibor JJ, Sartorius N: *Psychiatric Diagnosis and Classification*. New York: Wiley, 2002.

McIntyre KM, Norton JR, McIntyre JS: Psychiatric interview, history and mental status examination. In: Sadock BJ, Sadock VA, Ruiz P (eds). *Kaplan and Sadock's Comprehensive Textbook of Psychiatry*, 9th edn. Philadelphia: Lippincott Williams & Wilkins, 2009, pp. 886–907.

Sadock BJ: Signs and symptoms in psychiatry. In: Sadock BJ, Sadock VA, Ruiz P (eds). *Kaplan and Sadock's Comprehensive Textbook of Psychiatry*, 9th edn. Philadelphia: Lippincott Williams & Wilkins, 2009, pp. 918–928.

Sajatovic M, Ramirez LF: *Rating Scales in Mental Health*. Hudson, OH: Lexi-Comp Inc., 2001.

Scheiber SC: The psychiatric interview, psychiatric history, and mental status examination. In: Hales RA, Yudofsky SC, Talbott JA (eds). *The American Psychiatric Press Textbook of Psychiatry*, 2nd edn. Washington, DC: American Psychiatric Press, 1994, pp. 187–220.

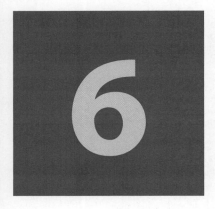

Psychological Assessment

Andrew E. Molnar, Jr., PhD
James S. Walker, PhD[†]
Howard B. Roback, PhD
Larry Welch, EdD

WHAT IS PSYCHOLOGICAL ASSESSMENT?

Psychological assessment is the systematic process by which psychologists evaluate characteristics of people (Weiner, 2010). Characteristics may include personality traits, intelligence, neuropsychological functions, psychiatric symptoms or disorders, behaviors and their contingencies, attitudes and beliefs, learning disabilities, academic achievement, school readiness, adaptation to medical illness and disabilities, appropriateness for surgery or organ donation, adaptive and social functioning, coping skills, quality of life, fitness for duty, criminality, and competency to stand trial, among others. It may extend beyond individual characteristics to the assessment of parent–child or couple interactions, family functioning, or group and organizational factors. The outcome of the assessment involves a report that can be instrumental in securing services for patients, whether through educational or other social service systems.

Psychological assessment usually involves the integration of multiple sources of data for characterizing people, including interviews, behavioral observations, administration of standardized assessments, collateral reports, and historical documents. A key component of most psychological assessment is the use of reliable, standardized, norm-referenced and valid psychological tests or measures to gather data. These tests often have norms by which psychologists can compare an individual's performance with those of others (e.g., age groups, psychiatric populations). Depending on the nature of the assessment, psychologists rely on one or more methods or tests to make their determinations. The use of multiple tests within a single assessment is called a "battery." A "common battery" refers to the use of the same core set of tests across individuals based on contemporary research and practice findings within an area of psychological assessment. Common batteries help standardize the assessment and measure change in testing performance over time. Psychologists often supplement common batteries with other measures to further refine and individualize the assessment process. There are many different cognitive and psychological assessments, and specific instruments that are suitable to evaluate infants/toddler, preschoolers, school-age children and adolescents, adults, and geriatric populations.

Weiner IB: Psychological assessment. In: IB Weiner, WE Craighead (eds). *The Corsini Encyclopedia of Psychology*, 4th edn., Vol 3. Hoboken, NJ: Wiley, 2010, pp. 1319–1321.

PSYCHOLOGICAL ASSESSMENT IN PSYCHIATRIC SETTINGS

Psychological assessment in psychiatric settings generally focuses on the determination of patients' psychiatric diagnoses, symptom expression and severity, personality functioning, and cognitive and neuropsychological functioning. Referral questions often center on differential diagnosis, the contribution of personality factors to psychiatric symptomatology, central nervous system dysfunctions, neurodevelopmental disorders, potential risk for suicide or homicide, primary defense mechanisms and coping styles, malingering, and identification of major therapeutic issues. The results of the assessment are used to directly answer referral questions and inform treatment recommendations. When repeated at follow-up time points, psychological assessment can play an important role in determining treatment effectiveness for a given patient.

The psychiatrist's ability to call upon and use psychological assessment on complex clinical cases in the course of practice has many diagnostic advantages, particularly in today's health care environment that emphasizes documentation, the use of psychometrically validated measures, and the demonstration of treatment effectiveness. In particular, psychological assessment can improve the reliability and validity of conclusions drawn solely from standard clinical interviews or observations. Further, psychological assessments may help psychiatrists make well-considered judgments about the appropriateness of psychosocial treatments, pharmacological treatments, or their combination. For example, a physician who had been minimally successful in treating a chronically depressed patient with several antidepressant medications referred the patient for a psychological assessment to determine the nature of the patient's depression and what might be targeted using a psychotherapeutic approach. The assessment revealed a consistent set of negative assumptions the patient held about himself, best summarized in a core belief, "I am never good enough," which then drove the patient's longstanding pattern of procrastination, incomplete projects, and perfectionism. A course of psychotherapy was strongly recommended to help the patient recognize his negative beliefs, establish reasonable expectations for performance and self-worth, and engage in and complete tasks.

TYPES OF ASSESSMENT MEASURES

Psychologists may use a variety of measures in psychiatric settings to assess patients. These may include structured diagnostic measures, general and disorder- or symptom-specific measures, personality disorder or trait measures, and clinical neuropsychological measures to evaluate cognitive functions. These measures may include self-report inventories that ask patients directly about issues related to the purpose of the psychological assessment. They also include performance-based measures in which patients perform specific tasks as a means of assessing their functioning in a certain area. In general, diagnostic, disorder, symptom-specific, and personality measures involve self-report. Cognitive and other neuropsychological measures are performance-based and administered by a qualified examiner or psychologist. As tests are formally reviewed in this chapter, be aware that although examples and descriptions are provided, it is not legally permissible or wise to publish exact test items in an effort to preserve the integrity of the instruments.

RELIABILITY AND VALIDITY OF MEASURES

Psychologists select tests or measures that are relevant to the referral questions and are reliable and valid (Blacker & Endicott, 2008). Reliability is the consistency of the measure in discriminating targeted characteristics. Three standard forms of reliability often are reported: internal consistency, interrater reliability, and test–retest reliability. Internal consistency is a measure of agreement among the items of a measure. Said differently, each of the items within a measure (e.g., cognitive, physiologic, and behavioral) should be tapping the same underlying construct or dimension (i.e., depression). Because some characteristics of patients are multidimensional (e.g., psychosis includes positive and negative symptoms) and not necessarily similarly present across patients or periods of illness, the internal consistency of each subscale of a measure often is reported separately.

Interrater reliability is the demonstrated agreement between two or more test administrators evaluating the same patients using the same psychological measures. For example, two psychologists who separately test the same patient to determine the patient's cognitive functioning using the same testing materials should reach the same conclusions, assuming similar assessment conditions. Interrater reliability is dependent on the careful training of psychologists to understand the measures and administer them in a standardized way, namely with uniform testing, scoring, and interpretation procedures. This requires extensive training and skill, integrating both the standardized administration as well as efforts to establish rapport and cooperation from patients across the lifespan.

Test–retest reliability is the extent of agreement between assessments at two different time points. The interval between assessment time points may vary for different measures but should be long enough for patients not to recall their original responses and short enough for the characteristic being measured to remain stable. All forms of reliability are important in psychological assessment to ensure that the tests have items of direct relevance to the targeted area of assessment (internal consistency), different examiners make similar determinations using the same tests (interrater), and changes in test performance represent actual shifts in functioning rather than fluctuations largely produced simply by test re-administration (test–retest).

Validity refers to the degree to which the test actually measures what it claims to be measuring. The validity of a test is determined in several ways: content validity, construct validity, and criterion-related validity. Content validity means that a test's items measure all the critical facets of the area being assessed. For instance, an anxiety symptom survey would likely cover somatic (e.g., sweating, palpitations, shaking), cognitive (e.g., concern about having an attack), and behavioral components of anxiety (avoidance of situations in which escape would be difficult) for it to gather information sufficient for making a valid anxiety disorder diagnosis (e.g., Panic Disorder with Agoraphobia). Content validity also means that the patient will feel comfortable with the test's items, wording, and perceived intent. Content validity increases the chance that the patient will engage in the testing process.

Construct validity refers to the degree to which a test actually measures what it claims to measure. For example, the Wechsler Adult Intelligence Scale—Fourth Edition (Wechsler, 2008) purports to measure four areas of intelligence including verbal comprehension, perceptual reasoning, working memory, and processing speed, all of which determine a person's overall or full-scale intelligence level (i.e., their "IQ"). For the WAIS-IV to have construct validity, the items in the subtests should coalesce to capture these different constructs. A statistical procedure called factor analysis is often used to explore or test a priori theorized constructs presumed to underpin a particular measure, thus deriving indices that represent an individual's cognitive abilities.

Criterion-related validity is the extent to which a measure predictably relates to other measures or outcomes. Many forms of criterion-related validity exist. The results of tests designed to assess similar characteristics or related concepts should show agreement or positive association. Similarly, tests designed to measure different characteristics should have little relationship with each other. When a gold standard of comparison exists (e.g., established structured diagnostic interview), this often serves as the criterion to which a measure is compared (Blacker & Endicott, 2008). Using the gold standard criterion, a test should be able to accurately identify true cases of the characteristic being assessed (referred to as sensitivity) as well as noncases (referred to as specificity). For example, the structured clinical interview called the Scale for Impact on Suicidality—Management Assessment and Planning of Care (Nelson et al., 2010) was developed to classify incoming psychiatric patients with suicidal ideation to the appropriate level of psychiatric care (inpatient hospitalization vs. outpatient care). The scale correctly identified 66.7% of those who required hospitalization admission (sensitivity) and 78.1% of the patients who did not require admission (specificity), indicating that it may be a reasonably valid tool for assessing suicide risk and guiding the planning of care for these patients.

Blacker D, Endicott J: Psychometric properties. In: AJ Rush, MB First, D Blacker (eds). *Handbook of Psychiatric Measures*, 2nd edn. Washington, DC: American Psychiatric Publishing, 2008, pp. 7–13.

Nelson C, Johnston M, Shrivastava A: Improving risk assessment with suicidal patients: a preliminary evaluation of the clinical utility of The Scale for Impact of Suicidality—Management, Assessment and Planning of Care (SIS-MAP). *Crisis* 2010;31: 231–237.

Wechsler D: *Wechsler Adult Intelligence Scale—Fourth Edition*. Bloomington, MN: Pearson, 2008.

ASSESSMENT PROCEDURES TO ENSURE ACCURACY

Beyond measurement reliability and validity, psychologists employ additional procedures to ensure the accuracy of conclusions derived from psychological assessments. Use of normative data, multiple measures, validity testing, and optimal assessment circumstances are important procedural matters. First, psychologists ensure that the measures used in the assessment have normative data that are sufficient and culturally appropriate for the patient. Use of proper normative data allows the examiner to determine the extent to which a person's age, education, gender, or race may potentially moderate assessment results. If a measure has not been psychometrically developed with specific groups, the measure's norms may not accurately convey the patient's true level of functioning; the examiner must consider this type of testing bias when interpreting patient performance. There have been extensive efforts recently to include socio-cultural factors as part of the assessment process, being an extension to just age-based norms.

Second, psychologists often select multiple measures that broadly tap the same domain in order to acquire a convergence of information that increases confidence in conclusions made about a patient's relative performance strengths and weaknesses. The use of multiple measures to characterize an individual's traits or characteristics is a hallmark of psychological assessment (Campbell & Fiske, 1959).

Third, psychologists often include symptom or performance validity measures. These measures are constructed to determine if the patient has put forth his or her best effort during the assessment process (Iverson, 2003). They may be stand-alone instruments or consist of critical items embedded within other tests (e.g., the F or "infrequency" scale in the Minnesota Multiphasic Personality Inventory [MMPI]-2 measures the extent to which a person answers in an atypical and deviant manner). When performance on these measures falls below normative expectations, it is possible that the patient's performance is less than credible. In more significant and pervasive deviations from expectancies, the patient may be seen as malingering as opposed to displaying symptom exaggeration. In clinical and legal contexts, there are formal criteria of how symptom/performance validity measures should be used (Heilbronner et al., 2009; Bush et al., 2005).

Fourth, psychologists conduct psychological assessments under circumstances that optimize patient performance. This means that the patient is well rested, is motivated to participate, and has minimal acute confounds (e.g., recent substance use or change in medications may undermine true baseline abilities), and that the assessment setting is private, quiet, adequately lighted, and comfortable. Furthermore, psychologists provide patients with breaks as needed (e.g., due to fatigue) or reschedule the assessment if necessary. Psychologists also properly manage requests by third parties (e.g., family member, attorney) to observe the evaluation. Several professional organizations (American Academy of Clinical Neuropsychology, 2001; National Academy of Neuropsychology, 2000) recommend that psychologists minimize third-party observation because it can unduly influence both test standardization and interpretation, unless the purpose of the assessment is to evaluate specific interpersonal relationships (e.g., parent–child interaction). Finally, psychologists use an informed consent process, consistent with the American Psychological Association's professional ethics codes (APA, 2002) with all patients to fully engage them in the assessment process. Prior to formal assessment, psychologists cover the reason for the assessment, costs associated with the assessment, how privacy is maintained, where the report findings will go, and the qualifications of those administering and interpreting the assessment measures. This has become particularly important with the establishment of electronic medical record systems, where professionals, providers, and others have ready access to patient information.

American Academy of Clinical Neuropsychology: Policy Statement on the Presence of Third Party Observers in Neuropsychological Assessments. *Clin Neuropsychol* 2001;15(4):433–439.

American Psychological Association: Ethical principles of psychologists and code of conduct. *Am Psychol* 2002;57: 1060–1073.

Bush SS, Ruff RM, Tröster AI, et al: Symptom validity assessment: Practice issues and medical necessity: NAN Policy & Planning Committee. *Arch Clin Neuropsychol* 2005;20(4):419–426.

Campbell DT, Fiske DW: Convergent and discriminant validation by the multitrait-multimethod matrix. *Psychol Bull* 1959;56: 81–105.

Heilbronner RL, Sweet JJ, Morgan JE, et al: American Academy of Clinical Neuropsychology Consensus Conference Statement on the neuropsychological assessment of effort, response bias, and malingering. *Clin Neuropsychol* 2009;23(7):1093–1129.

Iverson G: Detecting malingering in civil forensic evaluations. In: A MacNeill, LC Hartlage (eds). *Handbook of Forensic Neuropsychology*. New York: Springer, 2003.

National Academy of Neuropsychology: Presence of third party observers during neuropsychological testing: Official statement of the National Academy of Neuropsychology. *Arch Clin Neuropsychol* 2000;15(5):379–380.

ASSESSMENT PREPARATIONS

Obtaining as much information about the patient as possible is essential in preparation for the assessment. This will often include discussions with referring providers, obtaining medical records to review, speaking with collaterals (e.g., family, teachers), and, most importantly, speaking with the patient by means of a clinical interview. A good interview includes questions that clarify a patient's developmental, familial, educational, medical, psychiatric, social, vocational, and legal histories (unless a more structured process is used, as will be described later). Skilled examiners make initial judgments about the patient's awareness, as well as his or her ability to process information, track conversations, access memory, produce coherent thoughts, and describe expectations. This process helps the examiner understand the patient's readiness for testing and provides information that can guide the design and construction of the psychological assessment and inform interpretation of testing data.

STRUCTURED DIAGNOSTIC ASSESSMENTS

Structured diagnostic assessments are used to determine psychiatric diagnoses based on the definitions and criteria of the *Diagnostic and Statistical Manual of Mental Disorders* (DSM) or the World Health Organization *International Classification of Diseases* (ICD). With the revision of the DSM, the most commonly used semistructured interview is The Structured Clinical Interview for DSM-5. This is commonly used within psychiatric research protocols to determine, verify, or characterize a patient's psychiatric condition. They are also useful clinically to diagnostically decipher patients who present in complex ways and when clinical interviewing alone is deemed inadequate. It is also now more common for clinicians to utilize semistructured interviews, helping to target the reason for consultation and strengthen rapport with patients and families.

GENERAL PSYCHIATRIC SYMPTOM MEASURES

General psychiatric symptom measures provide comprehensive assessment of psychopathology but not specific to formal psychiatric disorder categories. Most of these measures are relatively brief (e.g., Symptom Checklist-90 Revised). A few are lengthier (e.g., Minnesota Multiphasic Personality Inventory), though commonly used for the purposes of psychological assessment. General psychiatric symptom measures may be used for multiple assessment purposes, including (1) baseline assessment of distress or dysfunction; (2) intervention outcome determination; and (3) screening tools to identify people likely to have psychiatric difficulties. Two quite popular general psychiatric symptom measures, Symptom Checklist-90 Revised and Minnesota Multiphasic Personality Inventory, are presented next.

▶ Symptom Checklist-90 Revised

The Symptom Checklist-90 Revised (Derogatis, 1994) is a 90-item self-administered questionnaire. Items fall into nine subscales: Somatization, Obsessive-Compulsive, Interpersonal Sensitivity, Depression, Anxiety, Hostility, Phobic Anxiety, Paranoid Ideation, and Psychoticism. The number of items varies across subscales. Patients are asked to indicate how much distress each item causes them during the past week using a Likert-type scale of 0 = not at all, to 4 = extremely. It usually takes 15–20 minutes to complete the SCL-90-R. A briefer version (53 items) derived from the SCL-90, called the Brief Symptom Inventory (Derogatis, 1993), takes only 8–10 minutes to finish.

Patients are given a short introduction to the measure. After completion, scores are obtained for each of the nine subscales. Gender-keyed norms are available for a variety of adult samples (e.g., psychiatric inpatients, psychiatric outpatients, community samples of psychiatrically healthy adults [>17 years of age] and adolescents [13–17 years old]). Three levels of interpretation are possible. First, the SCL-90 has three global indices including the Global Severity Index (mean of all items), Positive Symptom Total (number of items rated >0), and Positive Symptom Distress Index (mean distress rating for items comprising the Positive Symptom Total). These indices convey overall psychiatry symptom severity. Second, subscale scores indicate possible syndromal presentations. Third, attention to individual item responses may be useful (e.g., thoughts of death or dying). The SCL-90-R has been translated into multiple languages and norms are available across a range of patient (psychiatric and medical) and nonpatient groups, making the instrument widely applicable as a broad general screening instrument of global psychiatric distress and some symptom profiles.

▶ Minnesota Multiphasic Personality Inventory—2nd Edition for Adults and Adolescents

The Minnesota Multiphasic Personality Inventory—2nd Edition for Adults (Butcher et al., 1989) and Adolescents (MMPI-A) are very comprehensive self-report/administered inventories designed to assess general psychopathology in adults and adolescents, respectively. The MMPI-2 has 567 items, and the MMPI-A has 478 items. The items, presented in a largely random fashion, coalesce into eight basic syndrome scales: Hypochondriasis, Depression, Hysteria, Psychopathic Deviance, Paranoia, Psychasthenia, Schizophrenia, and Hypomania. Subscales for each syndromal scale capture symptom characteristics contributing to the full-scale score. Additional scales include two basic clinical scales involving Masculinity-Femininity and Social Introversion and three validity scales to assess how the patient approached the testing: Lie, Infrequency, and Correction. Moreover, several other scales have been developed and routinely scored to assist with interpretation (e.g., Bizarre Mentation and MacAndrew Alcoholism Scale—Revised). The MMPI-2 and MMPI-A have extensive research bases to support their use for multiple clinical applications and are among the most extensively used psychological assessment measures in the field. The MMPI-2 and MMPI-A take about 1–1.5 hours to complete. It is expected that a revision to the MMPI-2 will be released in 2024.

The MMPI-2 and MMPI-A scores are obtained for all scales. Fractions of the Correction scale are added to some of the syndrome scales to "correct" for symptom over- or under-reporting. Scale scores are reported on a form that displays them in a graphical profile. Interpretation of the MMPI-2 is based primarily on a profile analysis consisting of the two or three highest scale elevations. Scales with T scores of 65 or above are considered clinically significant. Abnormally low scores also are interpretable. For example, an individual who has elevated scores for Depression and Psychasthenia is likely to be extremely sensitive and feel victimized. If scale 8 is also elevated, then concerns about paranoid trends within a depressed, victimized stance are present. Numerous books are available to help interpret specific code types.

Butcher JN, Dahlstrom WG, Graham JR, et al: *Minnesota Multiphasic Personality Inventory-2 (MMPI-2): Manual for administration and scoring.* Minneapolis: University of Minnesota Press, 1989.

Derogatis LR: *Brief Symptom Inventory (BSI): Administration, Scoring, and Procedures Manual*, 3rd edn. Minneapolis: National Computer Systems, 1993.

Derogatis LR: *The SCL-90-R: Administration, Scoring, and Procedures Manual*, 3rd edn. Minneapolis: National Computer Systems, 1994.

DISORDER- OR SYMPTOM-SPECIFIC MEASURES

Numerous measures exist to assess the range of clinically important symptoms that commonly occur in particular psychiatric disorders (e.g., psychotic, mood, and anxiety disorders). These measures are useful for obtaining a fine-grained assessment of the type and nature of the disorder when the condition is suggested by the findings from a clinical interview, structured diagnostic assessment, or general psychiatric symptom measure. As with most measures, disorder- or symptom-specific measures vary in length and format. When relatively brief and self-administered, these measures can be used as screening tools. Examples of psychotic (Positive and Negative Syndrome Scale), mood (Beck Depression Inventory—II), anxiety (Yale-Brown Obsessive Compulsive Scale; Beck Anxiety Inventory), and substance use disorder specific measures (Addiction Severity Index) are described next.

▶ Positive and Negative Syndrome Scale

The Positive and Negative Syndrome Scale (Kay et al., 1987) is a semistructured interview that measures the severity of psychosis in adult patients with schizophrenia, schizoaffective disorder, and other psychotic disorders. The scale has 30 items, with three subscales including the Positive Scale covering positive psychotic symptoms such as delusions or hallucinations, Negative Scale covering negative psychotic symptoms such as social withdrawal and blunted affect, and General Psychopathology Scale detailing a range of other symptoms commonly associated with psychosis (e.g., disorientation, somatic concerns). A 30-item version called the Kiddie-PANSS (Fields et al., 1994) also has been developed to measure positive and negative symptoms in severely disturbed children and adolescents. The PANSS takes 30–45 minutes to administer and score.

The PANSS is designed for use only by mental health professionals who have clinical experience working with patients who have psychotic spectrum disorders. The interview begins by asking the patient to generally discuss his or her condition and life circumstances. The interviewer then explores any symptoms that the patient may have volunteered. This portion of the interview allows for behavioral observation of the patient and data gathering to substantiate ratings (e.g., guarded presentation). Next, the interviewer asks specific questions to determine the presence and severity of other symptoms not already evident in the interview. Individual items are scored on 7-point Likert scales, with 1 indicating the presence of a symptom and subsequent numbers representing ascending levels of symptom severity. Ratings across items per scale are summed to obtain scores on the Positive, Negative, and General Psychopathology Scale. A Composite Scale score (i.e., the difference between the Positive and Negative Scale score) is used to indicate which symptom typology predominates. Normative data are available to further interpret the scores.

Beck Depression Inventory—II

The Beck Depression Inventory—II (Beck et al., 1996) measures the severity of depression in adolescent and adult patients with previously diagnosed depressive illness. It consists of 21 multiple-choice items in which patients report the severity of affective (e.g., irritability), cognitive (e.g., suicidal thoughts), and physical symptoms (e.g., fatigue) of depression in the past 2 weeks along an ordinal continuum to characterize the symptom severity. The BDI-II may be used to characterize major components of a patient's depressive experience; however, it does not provide complete coverage of DSM-5 criteria and, hence, should not be solely used for diagnostic purposes. Given its easy self-administration format, it can also be used to screen patients for depression, with low scores being used as a cutoff to reduce rates of false negatives, followed by a clinical interview or structured diagnostic assessment. In addition, when repeated, the BDI-II can be used to monitor a patient's response to treatment over time.

The BDI total score (sum of all individual item scores) indicates the overall severity of depression. Beck and colleagues suggest the following interpretation guidelines: 0–13 = minimal; 14–19 = mild; 20–28 = moderate; and 29–63 = severe. Subscale scores involving somatic-affective and cognitive factors may be calculated. The BDI-II takes 5–10 minutes to complete. It should be interpreted within the full context of the clinical interview and psychological assessment encounter.

Yale-Brown Obsessive Compulsive Scale

The Yale-Brown Obsessive Compulsive Scale (Goodman et al., 1989a, 1989b) is a clinician-administered, semistructured interview developed to measure the severity of obsessive–compulsive symptoms in patients diagnosed with Obsessive Compulsive Disorder (OCD). The Y-BOCS examines patients' obsessions and compulsions, and both are rated on the time spent on them, interference with functioning, distress, resistance, and control. The scale may be used to screen patients and monitor change with treatment. It is not a diagnostic instrument in that it does not specifically assess criteria according to the DSM-5 standards for OCD. A version for children called the CY-BOCS (Riddle et al., 1992) is available. The Y-BOCS takes about 30 minutes to administer.

The interviewer first asks the patient to complete a 64-item checklist used to identify the content of any obsessive–compulsive symptoms. Subsequently, the interviewer asks the patient to identify the three most distressing ones and then focuses on them for the rest of the interview. The interviewer assesses five areas to determine how much time they occupy, the degree to which they interfere with normal functioning, how much subjective distress they cause, how much the patient actively resists them, and the extent to which the patient feels he or she can control them. Each area is rated from 0 = no symptoms to 4 = extreme symptoms. Scores are summed to yield one total score and two subscale scores (Obsessions, Compulsions). The Y-BOCs has become the gold standard for assessing obsessive–compulsive symptom severity.

Addiction Severity Index

The Addiction Severity Index (McLellan et al., 1992) is a 200-item clinician- or technician-administered semistructured interview designed to assess information on seven functional areas often negatively affected by substance abuse: medical status, employment and support, drug use, alcohol use, legal status, family or social status, and psychiatric status. It is one of the most commonly used instruments in the substance abuse treatment field in the United States and worldwide. Information generated from the ASI is used to guide initial assessment and treatment planning for patients seeking inpatient or outpatient alcohol or drug abuse treatment. Abbreviated 30-day follow-up versions can be used over the course of treatment to track patient progress and adjust the treatment plan accordingly. The ASI is available in multiple languages and has normative data available for numerous populations (e.g., males and females treated for alcohol, opiate, and cocaine abuse; patients treated within different levels of care; or special populations such as pregnant women or people incarcerated). The initial ASI takes 45–50 minutes to complete. The follow-up versions take approximately 15–20 minutes to finish.

The ASI begins with a demographic information gathering section and then covers each of the seven functional areas separately, using a common format. Questions in each section target frequency, duration, and severity of problems over the patient's lifetime and in the past 30 days. Both objective indicators of problems and the patient's subjective experience of the problems are considered. For example, a patient may be asked how many times he or she has been treated for any psychological or emotional problems, followed by another question that asks the patient how troubled or bothered he or she had been by these psychological or emotional problems in the past 30 days. Based on the patient's report and the interviewer's interpretation of the information for each functional area, the interviewer renders severity ratings (0–9) that reflect the degree to which the interviewer believes the patient needs additional treatment or assistance. Finally, composite scores are calculated to have an overall severity index for each functional area. These are particularly useful for monitoring patient treatment progress over time.

Beck AT, Steer RA, Brown GK: *Beck Depression Inventory—II Manual*. San Antonio, TX: Psychological Corporation, 1996.

Fields JF, Kay SR, Grosz D, et al: Assessing positive and negative symptoms in children and adolescents. *Am J Psychiatry* 1994; 151:249–253.

Goodman WK, Price LH, Rasmussen SA, et al: The Yale-Brown Obsessive-Compulsive Scale, I: development, use and reliability. *Arch Gen Psychiatry* 1989a;46:1006–1011.

Goodman WK, Price LH, Rasmussen SA, et al: The Yale-Brown Obsessive-Compulsive Scale, II: validity. *Arch Gen Psychiatry* 1989b;46:1012–1016.

Kay SR, Fiszbein A, Opler LA: The positive and negative syndrome scale (PANSS) for schizophrenia. *Schizophr Bull* 1987;13: 261–276.

McLellan AT, Kushner H, Metzger D, et al: The fifth edition of the Addiction Severity Index. *J Subst Abuse Treat* 1992;9:199–213.

Riddle MA, Scahill L, King RA, et al: Double-blind, crossover trial of fluoxetine and placebo in children and adolescents with obsessive-compulsive disorder. *J Am Acad Adolesc Psychiatry* 1992;31:1062–1069.

PERSONALITY DISORDER OR TRAIT MEASURES

Numerous personality disorder or trait measures may be used for the purposes of psychological assessment. Some measures assess for personality disorders (e.g., Personality Assessment Inventory). Others assess for specific personality traits (e.g., NEO Personality Inventory). Personality measures are useful for determining intrapersonal (e.g., emotions, self-perceptions) and interpersonal factors that inform psychiatric symptom expression and vulnerability. Conventionally, personality measures administered in a structured manner using a standardized self-report format, scored in a quantitative manner, and using normative samples for comparison and interpretative purposes are referred to as objective measures. Personality measures that use unstructured or ambiguous images (e.g., inkblots, human figures) to reveal hidden or unconscious aspects of a patient's mental life are referred to as projective measures. Two of the most well-known measures are the Rorschach Inkblot Test and the Thematic Apperception Test. A few objective and projective personality disorder or trait measures are described next.

▶ Personality Assessment Inventory

The Personality Assessment Inventory (Morey, 1991) contains 344 items to assess major clinical DSM-5 Axis I and II syndromes. As a personality assessment instrument, the PAI focuses on four areas: (1) a Borderline Features Scale with four subscales that assess affective instability, identity problems, negative relationships with others, and impulsive self-harm; (2) an Antisocial Scale with three subscales to capture antisocial behaviors, egocentricity/poor empathy, and stimulus seeking; (3) an interpersonal scale assessing

a dominating/controlling versus meek/submissive dimension; and (4) an interpersonal scale assessing a warm/affiliation versus cold/rejecting dimension. In addition, the PAI has treatment scales (Suicidal Ideation, Treatment Rejection, Nonsupport, Stress, and Aggression) to provide clinicians with pertinent information for treatment planning, an especially useful feature of this measure.

Patients answer all items on a 4-point Likert-type scale (0 = false, not at all true, to 3 = very true). Scores for each scale are obtained by summing all the item scores that make up each scale. Only trained mental health professionals should interpret these scores. Normative community and patient sample data are provided to guide interpretation. The PAI takes 40–50 minutes to complete.

▶ NEO Personality Inventory—Revised

The NEO Personality Inventory—Revised (Costa & McCrae, 1992) is a 240-item self-administered questionnaire for patients that assesses five major domains or dimensions of the five-factor model of personality, namely, Neuroticism (sensitive/nervous vs. secure/confident); Extraversion (outgoing/energetic vs. solitary/reserved); Openness (inventive/curious vs. consistent/cautious); Agreeableness (friendly/compassionate vs. cold/unkind); and Conscientiousness (efficient/organized vs. easy-going/careless). Each domain contains facets of the dimension being assessed. For example, the Agreeable domain contains the facets of trust, straightforwardness, altruism, compliance, modesty, and tender-mindedness. In addition, the NEO-PI-R has validity scales that are used to determine the extent to which the respondent answered the items accurately and honestly. Given that the NEO-PI-R is a measure of common traits rather than one that ascertains disorder, it is most useful for determining the nature and degree of these traits within a patient and in what ways they may affect the patient's functioning.

Each item is scored on a 5-point Likert-type scale, with 0 = strongly disagree, to 4 = strongly agree. Items are summed to obtain scores for overall domains and the facets that compose them. Normative group data are available to aid interpretation. It takes 35–40 minutes to complete the NEO-PI-R.

▶ Rorschach Inkblot Test

The Rorschach Inkblot Test was developed by a Swiss psychiatrist, Hermann Rorschach, who first published the test in 1921; it was subsequently translated into English in 1942. It contains 10 bilaterally symmetrical inkblot configurations. Five of the inkblots are achromatic, two have additional spots of red, and three combine several colors. During the test administration, the examiner asks the patient what each card looks like (i.e., "What might this be?"). The examiner then records the patient's responses verbatim, the time it takes to generate responses, and any nonverbal reactions. After the responses are compiled, the examiner asks the patient to go through the cards again. This is referred to as the inquiry phase. In the latter phase, the examiner is attempting to identify the factors influencing the response—what parts of the blot are used and what features made the blot look a certain way (e.g., color, movement, texture, shading, and form). All of these factors are interpretable. For example, perception of movement (e.g., the percept of a bird in flight) is considered to relate to the richness of an individual's fantasy life. The form determinant (e.g., how closely the response corresponds with the selected area of the inkblot) is believed to indicate an individual's reasoning powers and reality testing. Color responses are believed to reflect the emotional life of the respondent. For example, pure color responses (i.e., the blot color itself stimulates the respondent's associative process) are considered to reflect an individual with poorly integrated emotional reactions. Moreover, idiosyncratic responses such as contaminated ones (seeing two different things at the same blot area and then fusing them together, as in, "This is a dog. It's a bug. No, it's a dog-bug") may suggest confusion, thought disorder, or psychosis proneness.

Responses are analyzed in terms of the number that fall into various categories (e.g., movement, form, location), the normative frequency of these categories for different clinical groups, and the relationships among determinants (i.e., ratios such as percentage of conventional form). Psychodynamically oriented examiners also interpret the content of responses in terms of symbolic meaning (e.g., perception of an island may reflect a sense of isolation). When interpreted within the respondent's specific experiences, the latter analyses are believed to reveal a great deal about a patient's unique personality style (Allison et al., 1988). There are objective scoring systems for some projective tests, such as the Exner Comprehensive Scoring System (Exner, 2002), one of the most widely used for the Rorschach. However, some clinicians prefer to make psychodynamic interpretations from the thematic content of the patient's Rorschach responses, arguing that they are achieving a much richer understanding of the patient than that provided through more sterile numerical analysis of the person. Time needed for administration and interpretation of the Rorschach using the Exner scoring system will vary with the length and complexity of the patient's responses, but the test usually takes an hour or more to complete.

▶ Thematic Apperception Test

The Thematic Apperception Test (TAT), developed in 1938 by Henry Murray, consists of 29 pictures and one blank card. The cards have recognizable human figures, and the patient is asked to generate a story of what is happening in the scene. Each card is intended to elicit information about a specific type of relationship (e.g., child–mother, child–father) or an important psychological area (e.g., sexuality). The examiner asks the patient to tell what led up to the situation, what the people are thinking and feeling, and how the situation will end. The patient's responses are recorded verbatim for later

analysis. As needed, the examiner may encourage the patient to elaborate on something said during the inquiry. The TAT is used primarily to generate hypotheses about an individual's family and social relationships, areas of conflict, and related personality issues. Examiners often use a subset of the cards instead of all of them to capture a range of situations likely to generate important clinical information. For example, one card shows a human figure looking out a large opened window. Patients who tell a story of someone struggling with loneliness, isolation, and despair or who indicate the person might be contemplating suicide may themselves be struggling with depression and suicidality.

There is significant variability in the scoring of TAT responses. Some examiners prefer a more intuitive approach to understanding the psychodynamic implications of a story (Allison et al., 1988), whereas others favor a more complex scoring system such as Murray's drive system analysis (Murray, 1938). In the former case, the psychologist attempts to identify significant emotions and attitudes projected onto the cards. Themes that recur with unusual frequency are judged to reflect prominent psychological needs. Time to administer and analyze the TAT will vary with the number of cards used and length of patient responses. The interpretation of these instruments requires specific training and competences.

Allison J, Blatt SJ, Zimet CN: *The Interpretation of Psychological Tests*. New York: Hemisphere, 1988.

Costa PT, McCrae RR: *NEO-PI-R Professional Manual*. Odessa, FL: Psychological Assessment Resources, 1992.

Exner JE: *The Rorschach, Basic Foundations and Principles of Interpretation*, 4th edn. New York: Wiley, 2002.

Morey LC: *Personality Assessment Inventory: Professional Manual*. Odessa, FL: Psychological Assessment Resources, 1991.

Murray HA: *Explorations in Personality*. New York: Oxford University Press, 1938.

Rorschach H: *Psychodiagnostics*. Trans. P Lemkau, B Dronenberg. Bern: Huber, 1942; New York: Harper & Row, 1942.

CLINICAL NEUROPSYCHOLOGICAL ASSESSMENT

Clinical neuropsychology, broadly defined, examines the cognitive and behavioral manifestation of brain function and dysfunction. Clinical neuropsychologists address assessment questions relevant to early in life (e.g., Does a child have an intellectual disability? Does the child need academic accommodations? Are intentional difficulties influencing their ability to learn? What are the changes in their cognitive abilities following a concussion?), throughout life (e.g., Is a profile consistent with schizophrenia? Is a person suffering from depression or dementia?), and at the end of life (e.g., Can the patient live independently? From what type of dementia are they suffering?). In addition, clinical neuropsychologists are involved in many settings, ranging from medical and legal to forensic and academic environments. Clinical neuropsychologists are broadly expected to have obtained specific training experiences and competencies before entering practice (Rey-Casserly et al., 2012). This now includes a 2-year fellowship specifically in clinical neuropsychology beyond receiving a doctorate, whether in child, adult, or geriatric settings.

Although an extensive discussion of the full range of neuropsychological practice is beyond the scope of this chapter, there is a fairly common set of activities that make up the typical neuropsychological assessment. In neuropsychology, referrals can come from patients, parents, lawyers, physicians, psychologists, and insurance companies in addition to other entities. In some settings, the referral question may be for a simple screening of cognitive abilities to provide a baseline against which changes in abilities can be tracked and measured. In other settings, the referral questions can be quite complex and may require the neuropsychologist to engage in many hours of testing, scoring, conceptualizing, writing, and disseminating the results. Most evaluations start with gathering background information to understand the question being asked and determine whether the referral is appropriate. After a decision to test is made, the process typically begins with an interview and test selection/administration. Measurement selection is based on the specific referral question and can range from a simple screening to an extended battery. In general, most neuropsychological assessments include measures that assess the domains of intellectual abilities, attention, motor skill, visuo-spatial abilities, language, memory, and executive functioning.

Instead of attempting to present all possible neuropsychological measures to the reader, categories and representative examples of them are described here in order to convey a sense of the range and utility of neuropsychological testing. An example of an inclusive neuropsychological assessment battery also is provided. It is important to keep in mind that these are just examples and that the approach is extensive and involves many different instruments that are appropriate to patient age, developmental level, and sensory impairments.

Rey-Casserly C, Roper BL, Bauer RM: Application of a competency model to clinical neuropsychology. *Prof Psychol Res Pract* 2012;43(5):422–431.

SCREENING MEASURES

Before practitioners make a referral for a neuropsychological evaluation, quite often they will use a screening measure to help identify salient cognitive issues as part of their mental status exam. An initial gauge of cognitive status is important because it may allow clinicians to determine if someone is broadly cognitively intact, mildly impaired, or exhibiting significant declines. In some cases, the screening may suggest that a referral is not needed. Although many measures for screening cognitive disorders are available, the Mini Mental State Exam (MMSE), the Montreal Cognitive Assessment (MoCA), and Clock Drawing Tests are common examples.

Mini Mental State Exam

For many decades the gold standard for a cognitive screening has been the Mini Mental State Exam (Folstein et al., 1975). A key strength of this MMSE is that it has been used by countless numbers of practitioners, across many disciplines, and has decades of research behind its use. Alternative forms for repeated testing, updated normative data, and translation into multiple languages are new additional strengths of the measure. The MMSE takes about 5 minutes to complete and has items that tap attention, learning, language, and working and immediate memory. It is scored on a 30-point scale, and studies have proposed cutoff scores for identifying population members (e.g., 23 or below may be consistent with a dementia group). Limitations of the MMSE are: (1) it is less sensitive in detecting mild forms of cognitive impairment when compared to other instruments; (2) its normative data often are not used by clinicians when interpreting the findings; and (3) the MMSE is copyrighted and, thus, can be costly to use.

Montreal Cognitive Assessment

Because of the limitations of the MMSE, practitioners are starting to use other measures, such as the Montreal Cognitive Assessment test (MoCA), for screening purposes. The MoCA is another 30-point scale that takes about 10 minutes to complete (Nasreddine et al., 2005). The authors' initial validation study suggests that their instrument has improved sensitivity and specificity over the MMSE for certain diagnoses (e.g., mild cognitive impairment). Although the amount of research on the MoCA pales in comparison to the MMSE, several professional groups support its use, and multiple versions are available, including those translated into many languages. The MoCA website also has an extensive listing of references for specific populations. In comparison to the MMSE, the MoCA is a more demanding task for patients to complete. Given the increased research on and proliferation of more publicly available screening measures such as the MoCA, these kinds of measures may become more commonly accepted alternatives to the MMSE.

Clock Drawing Test

A common screening tool among clinicians, especially geriatricians, is the Clock Drawing Test. It became standardized in the 1980s as part of the Parietal Lobe Battery Boston Diagnostic Aphasia Examination (Borod et al., 1980). The task is deceptively complex in that it asks the patient to produce a contour, sequence numbers into their correct location, recode the time into numbers on a dial, and produce the appropriate "hands." Hence, the task requires a medley of visual, motoric, attentional, memory and executive abilities. The test can be administered under different conditions (e.g., copy vs. command) in order to determine if a patient has the executive skill to complete all of the task demands on their own or if the patient needs the assistance of a predrawn clock face to correctly set the hands. Clock drawing is useful for providing initial insight into important cognitive issues that range from a possible neglect syndrome to the demonstration of significant executive reductions, and it can cue the clinician to refer for more detailed follow-up testing. Most clinicians use qualitative methods to evaluate patient performance. Methodological advances in scoring Clock Drawing have been proposed by several authors (Royall et al., 1998).

Borod JC, Goodglass H, Kaplan E: Normative data on the Boston diagnostic aphasia examination, parietal lobe battery, and the Boston naming test. *J Clin Exp Neuropsychol* 1980;2(3):209–215.

Folstein MF, Folstein SE, McHugh PR: Mini-mental state. A practical method for grading the cognitive state of patients for the clinician. *J Psychiatric Res* 1975;12(3):189–198.

Nasreddine ZS, Phillips NA, Bédirian V, et al: The Montreal Cognitive Assessment (MoCA): a brief screening tool for mild cognitive impairment. *J Am Geriatr Soc* 2005;53:695–699.

Royall D, Cordes J, Polk M: CLOX: an executive clock drawing task. *J Neurol Neurosurg Psychiatry* 1998;64(5):588–594.

ATTENTION MEASURES

Attention is one of the most widely used, yet difficult to define, concepts within the field of neuropsychology. Attention is not a solitary function. It demands the involvement of multiple brain systems to focus on the full range of sensory input available to process, to sustain these attentional resources in the face of distraction, and to disengage from one stimulus to pay attention to the next. Measures in this domain focus on specific senses (e.g., tests of visual discrimination) or on processes that relate to attention (e.g., shifting attention efficiently and effectively from one stimulus to another). Furthermore, many factors can influence a patient's performance on attention tasks (e.g., sleep difficulties, fatigue, pain, psychiatric disorders, and acute substance use).

One way to initially assess attentional abilities is through the clinical interview. Neuropsychologists consider if a patient understands what has been said, as well as the extent to which the patient loses track after a sentence or two, or monitors and corrects his or her mistakes in the conversation. In addition, neuropsychologists observe the patient's level of distractibility and thought organization (e.g., tangentiality, perseveration). If significant difficulties are present (e.g., a patient is in a state of delirium), further testing may not be appropriate until acute symptoms resolve. In less confounding cases, attentional reductions or fluctuations may partially account for variable or poor performance in other domains (e.g., memory).

Many attention measures are available. Overall, they tap comprehension of information, span of apprehension, visual scanning and attention to detail, discrimination, processing speed, and working memory. Two common measures

of attention are the Digit Span subtest from the WAIS-IV and Continuous Performance Tests. Each is described here. Parenthetically, attention measures are not in themselves useful for determining the diagnosis of Attention-Deficit/ Hyperactivity Disorder. Attention-Deficit/Hyperactivity Disorder is largely a behavioral diagnosis that requires observations in real-world settings and the use of measures such as the Conners' Rating Scales—Revised (Conners, 1997) or the Wender Utah Rating Scale (Ward et al., 1993) that are specifically designed to assess this condition. There are now multiple revisions to these instruments that have been tailored to children and adolescents, with forms available for parents/ caregivers, teachers, or even self-report.

▶ Digit Span

The digit span subtest from the WAIS-IV (Wechsler, 2008) is broadly a measure of a person's ability to process aural information. The psychologist starts the test by reciting numbers at approximately one per second. If the patient is able to correctly repeat each number in the sequence, the test will continue with longer strings of numbers until either failure or a maximum is reached in this "digits forward" task. In the second stage of the test the patient repeats the sequence of numbers in reverse order (i.e., digits backward), whereas in the third stage, the patient repeats the numbers back in numerical sequence. The latter two tasks are more difficult, as they have greater working memory demands than digits forward. In addition to comparing overall performance to peers, examiners will frequently look at the type of performance patterns to get a sense of whether the person was inattentive or if they had variable effort (e.g., if they performed better on digits backward than on digits forward). Further, some psychologists compare performance on digit span to the first trial of learning on the CVLT (a word list test discussed later) to see how the patient handles different methods of processing incoming information. The child version of the Wechsler system also has working memory tasks.

▶ Continuous Performance Tests

Continuous Performance Tests (CPT), such as the Conners CPT (Conners & Staff, 2000), are computer-administered vigilance measures that require a patient to process visual information over a sustained period of time and selectively respond to targets on the screen. In the most common setup, letters of the alphabet will flash on the computer screen at varying speeds. Every time one is presented, the patient is required to hit the spacebar, and reaction time is measured. However, when a specific letter is presented (e.g., "X"), the subject is required to inhibit their response. CPT tests are considered measures of sustained attention in that patients are asked to maintain their vigilance in what can be considered a relatively boring test. By varying rates of stimulus presentation and task demands, data are generated that identify how the patient performed overall and as a function of time (e.g., evaluating errors of omission and commission). Ultimately, performances across indices are tabulated and compared to known groups of test responders.

Conners CK: *Conners' Rating Scales—Revised: Technical Manual.* New York: Multi-Health Systems, 1997.

Conners CK, Staff MHS: *Conners' Continuous Performance Test II (CPT II V. 5).* North Tonawanda, NY: Multi-Health Systems, 2000.

Ward MF, Wender PH, Reimherr FW: The Wender Utah Rating Scale: an aid in the retrospective diagnosis of childhood attention deficit hyperactivity disorder. *Am J Psychiatry* 1993; 150(8):885–890.

MOTOR MEASURES

Prior to the widespread clinical use of computed tomography (CT) and magnetic resonance imaging (MRI) scans, neuropsychological testing, and more specifically motor and language testing, was quite useful in helping physicians localize potential brain lesions. For example, by combing neuropsychological data, behavioral observations, and an understanding of human neuroanatomy (e.g., a person is able to walk but has difficulty with language production following a stroke), psychologists could make predictions about lesion location (e.g., what specific artery is implicated). Many conditions, including Parkinson disease, multiple sclerosis, and neurotoxin exposure, produce significant changes in motor functioning. Repeated testing over time can help track motor changes as indicators of the progression of these kinds of conditions. Commonly used motor measures include finger tapping task, grip strength task, and the grooved pegboard task, and all have been co-normed (Heaton et al., 2004).

▶ Finger Tapping, Grip Strength, and Grooved Pegboard

Finger tapping (Reitan & Wolfson, 1993), or finger oscillation, is a measure of motor performance in which a person taps his or her index finger as quickly as possible over a 10-second interval on a standardized apparatus. This is repeated over multiple trials, with rest periods, for both the dominant and nondominant hand. In general, a dominant-hand advantage is expected. On measures of grip strength (Reitan & Wolfson, 1993), where a dominant-hand advantage is expected, patients squeeze a hand dynamometer to measure this ability over several trials. The grooved pegboard test (Klove, 1963) requires a patient to use one hand to pick up and rotate small, grooved metal pegs to fit simple keylike openings on a board. Clinicians will record the speed with which the task is completed, whether any pegs were dropped, and if other problems are noted secondary to possible conditions such as visual reductions or peripheral neuropathy. By examining the performances both within and across these measures, the neuropsychologist will have a better idea about the intactness of the motor systems or if a weakness might be related to a specific etiology. These tests can also help clinicians discriminate one etiology from another. For example, patients with early Alzheimer disease tend to have reasonably preserved performance on motor tests when compared to other forms of dementia.

Heaton RK, Miller SW, Taylor MJ, Grant I: *Revised Comprehensive Norms for an Expanded Halstead-Reitan Battery: Demographically Adjusted Neuropsychological Norms for African American and Caucasian Adults (HRB).* Psychological Assessment Resources, 2004.

Klove H: Clinical neuropsychology. *Med Clin North Am* 1963;47: 1647–1658.

Reitan RM, Wolfson D: *The Halstead-Reitan Neuropsychological Test Battery: Theory and Clinical Interpretation*, 2nd ed. Tucson, AZ: Neuropsychology Press, 1993.

LEARNING AND MEMORY MEASURES

Across the age spectrum, learning problems and memory dysfunction are two of the most common referral concerns posed to neuropsychologists. A wide range of factors may contribute to this multifaceted skill area, including reductions in attention, language, vision, and motor skills (and motivation). In the verbal domain, neuropsychologists often look at how patients process incoming information that is presented in a structured format (e.g., a story) or an unstructured one (e.g., a list of words). Visually, they might look at how patients encode a complex design, a small series of designs, or even a repeated set of designs. A main goal is to determine how and the extent to which the patient encodes different types of information. More specifically, after a delay, neuropsychologists consider the degree to which the patient can freely recall the information, retrieve more with cues, or recognize it over time. The answers to these considerations assist with differential diagnosis. For example, broadly speaking, many etiologies that are more "subcortical" in nature may have intact recognition abilities, whereas someone with a primary progressive process such as Alzheimer disease does not. Commonly used measures of learning and memory include word lists, stories, or the recall of visually based information. The Wechsler Memory Scale, Fourth Edition (PsychCorp, 2009) is a well-normed battery of memory measures for people aged 16–90 that includes the types of measures described next. However, because of the significant time to complete the full battery, clinicians often choose a selected sample of WMS-IV subtests (e.g., logical memory, a measure of story learning, or the visual reproduction subtest). Two frequently used learning and memory measures are the California Verbal Learning Test—II and the Rey-Osterrieth Complex Figure Test. While the CVLT-II is still used, there is now a revision to the instrument, referred to as the CVLT-III with similar testing parameters.

California Verbal Learning Test—II

The California Verbal Learning Test—II (Delis et al., 2000) is a word list task where patients listen to 16 simple items (called list A) presented by the neuropsychologist, one at a time, and are asked to repeat back all the words they can remember in any order. This pattern of learning is repeated five times. Then, a second 16-item list is similarly processed (list B). Next, the patient is asked to recall as many items as possible from only list A, both on their own and when prompted with cues. After a 20-minute delay, the patient is asked to recall what they can from list A on their own and under cued conditions. Finally, the patient is asked to discriminate list A items from foils in a larger word list. From all this information, neuropsychologists determine the patient's ability to learn information and recall it over time, and the degree to which the information can be "pulled out" through either cuing or discrimination formats. Also, the CVLT-II shows the extent to which intrusions occur (i.e., "recalled" words that were never presented as part of the original list A). The number of intrusions is a valuable predictor in differentiating patients with Alzheimer from healthy controls (Zakzanis et al., 1999). There is now a 3rd revision to the instrument which includes similar approaches to administration.

Rey-Osterrieth Complex Figure Test

The Rey-Osterrieth Complex Figure Test (Rey, 1941; Osterrieth, 1944) is exactly what the name implies; patients are first asked to copy a complex figure that is presented to them. While the patient is copying, neuropsychologists note how he or she accomplishes the task (e.g., in an organized or haphazard manner). After both brief and longer delays, wherein verbal tasks are administered so that interference is minimized, the patient is asked to reproduce whatever he or she can recall. This procedure is often followed by a discrimination test of segments contained in the figure among distracters. If reductions in recall are noted, beyond primary deficits in memory, it may be that the patient's approach to the task (e.g., a haphazard one) led to poor initial learning of the figure.

Delis DC, Kramer JH, Kaplan E, Ober BA: *California Verbal Learning Test, Second Edition (CVLT-II)*. San Antonio, TX: Psychological Corporation, 2000.

Osterrieth PA: Le test de copie d'une figure complex: contribution a l'etude de la perception et de la memoire. *Arch Psychol* 1944;30:286–356.

PsychCorp: *Wechsler Memory Scale, Fourth Edition (WMS-IV): Technical and Interpretive Manual*. San Antonio, TX: Pearson, 2009.

Rey A: L'examen psychologique dans les cas d'encephalopathie traumatique. *Arch Psychol* 1941;28:286–340.

Zakzanis KK, Leach L, Kaplan E: *Neuropsychological Differential Diagnosis*. Swets & Zeitlinger, 1999.

LANGUAGE MEASURES

Concerns about the development or changes in language abilities often prompt requests for neuropsychological assessment. Evaluations of academic performance are a common focus of referral (e.g., spelling, reading comprehension), as are cases of language loss following a tragic event such as stroke. The range of language measures are vast and cross both clinical and academic environments. In addition, batteries of tests have been developed to more extensively evaluate all aspects of language comprehension and production in multiple modalities (e.g., spoken and written).

One of the most effective "tests" of language is the clinical interview. By speaking with a patient, neuropsychologists begin to assess the patient's ability to comprehend questions, respond, engage in turn taking, and remain on topic. Language difficulties noted during the clinical interview can be more thoroughly evaluated later in the formal examination. Moreover, if a person has significant limitations with basic language functions, other cognitive and personality testing may be very difficult to accomplish.

Some of the most commonly used language measures include the Boston Naming Test, the Controlled Oral Word Association Test, and the Boston Diagnostic Aphasia Exam.

Boston Naming Test

The Boston Naming Test (Goodglass et al., 2000) is a 60-item measure of simple line drawings that patients are asked to name. After a brief interval, if they cannot surmise the correct word because of stimulus misperception, they are given a semantic cue. If the drawing is still incorrectly identified, they are given initial phonemic information to determine if that cue can assist in recall. There is also a follow-up recognition/discrimination procedure. These ancillary tasks are included to help determine if the information being requested is potentially available yet difficult to retrieve. The test takes about 10–15 minutes to administer. This brief task helps determine if the patient is having difficulty with naming common objects and the degree to which the results correspond with the patient's self-observations or performance declines noted by significant others that might be consistent with a specific etiology (e.g., a dementia). There are now norms available for children and adolescents, as well as gender-specific comparisons.

Controlled Oral Word Association Test

Neuropsychologists often use measures of fluency in to examine language production. In the Controlled Oral Word Association Test (Benton & Hamsher, 1976), patients are asked to provide in 1 minute as many words as they can that begin with a specific letter of the alphabet. This procedure is repeated with two different letters of the alphabet. Normative data for specific letter combinations are referenced. Often, the information generated from this test is compared to a measure of semantic fluency (i.e., when someone asks them to name all the items they can within a certain category). The relative performance on these measures is important: Most people are able to do better with a semantic/categorical cue to structure the search of their lexicon; however, some etiologies, such as patients with Alzheimer disease, are less likely to take advantage of this aid (Monsch et al., 1994).

Benton AL, Hamsher K: *Multilingual Aphasia Examination*, 2nd edn. Iowa City, IA: AJA Associates, 1976.

Goodglass H, Kaplan E, Barresi B: *BDAE: The Boston Diagnostic Aphasia Examination (BDAE-3)*. San Antonio, TX: Pearson, 2000.

Monsch A, Bondi M, Butters N, et al: A comparison of category and letter fluency in Alzheimer's and Huntington's disease. *Neuropsychology* 1994;8:25–30.

EXECUTIVE FUNCTIONING MEASURES

The domain of executive functioning is arguably one of the most intriguing and complicated domains to accurately measure. Simply stated, executive functions refer to tasks or behaviors that require volition, planning and decision making, purposeful action, self-regulation, and monitoring of effective performance (Lezak et al., 2012). There are many measures in each of these areas that can be used. As examples, the Wisconsin Card Sorting Test and Trail Making Test are described next.

Wisconsin Card Sorting Test

The Wisconsin Card Sorting Test (WCST) (Berg, 1948; Grant & Berg, 1948) is a complex measure that requires many facets of cognitive ability to successfully complete the task demands. The test itself is anomalous in that the patient is not given much instruction on how the task is to be completed, other than being presented with four stimulus cards that differ on multiple dimensions and asked to logically match them. The patient is only provided with yes/no feedback on each attempt. The sorting principles change without notice, and the patient's task is to recognize when this happens and shift set appropriately. Patients are evaluated on their effectiveness in figuring out the task demands and on their use of strategies. An extensive error analysis is performed (e.g., variables such as perseverations and loss of set). Some of the robust findings over the years include a relationship between dorsolateral, frontal cortex lesions and an elevated number of perseverations (Lezak et al., 2012). There are now modified and electronic variations of the task available, including programs intended to assess executive functions in youth.

Trail Making Tests

The Trail Making Test (Army Individual Test Battery, 1944) is one of the oldest paper-and-pencil measures still in use and remains one of the most sensitive tests of executive

functioning available to both clinicians and researchers. The test is divided into A and B sections. Trails A asks patients to connect 25 numbers in sequence. They are timed on their efficiency, and the number of mistakes is noted. Trails B follows and asks patients to complete the test with a similar sequencing methodology, but in this case, alternate between numbers and letters in order to create a significant executive demand. Neuropsychologists look at the relationship between Trails A and B scores to help determine if scores are more consistent with global motor slowing (i.e., slowed Trails A performance) or if there are more specific reductions when an executive component is added (i.e., Trails B performance in relationship to Trails A performance). The Delis-Kaplan Executive Function Systems (DKEFS) is now available, as well as portions of The Developmental Neuropsychological Assessment to measure executive skills.

Army Individual Test Battery: Manual of Directions and Scoring. Washington, DC: War Department, Adjutant General's Office, 1944.

Berg EA: A simple objective technique for measuring flexibility in thinking. *J Gen Psychol* 1948;39:15–22.

Grant DA, Berg EA: A behavioral analysis of degree of impairment and ease of shifting to new responses in a Weigl-type card sorting problem. *J Exp Psychol* 1948;39:404–411.

Lezak MD, Howieson DB, Bigler ED, Tranel D: *Neuropsychological Assessment*, 5th edn. New York: Oxford University Press, 2012.

GENERAL INTELLECTUAL AND ACHIEVEMENT MEASURES

Testing instruments that measure IQ have a long history of development and acceptance within both neuropsychology and school psychology. Although there are many measures in the areas of general intellectual and achievement testing, the Wechsler series of tests represent the gold standard and are continually revised and updated to be in step with current demands and to provide updated meaningful cohort group comparisons. To fully complete an assessment in this domain alone, several hours of testing may be required, and specific standards on achievement evaluations are often defined state by state.

The Wechsler Tests

The more recent versions of Wechsler tests (e.g., the WPPSI-IV for preschoolers [Wechsler, 2012]; the WISC-IV for ages 6 years through 16 years and 11 months [Wechsler, 2003; WISC-V revision in 2014]; and WAIS-IV for age 16–90 [Wechsler, 2008]) provide index scores based on a series of smaller tests that aim to provide data in how general abilities are understood, processed, and accessed by a person. These and other intelligence tests generally provide a composite standard score, known as the intelligence quotient (IQ), that represents the patient's overall performance on the test as compared to others of the same age group. IQ scores are typically expressed as a standard score in which 100 is the mean, with a standard deviation of 15. Thus, a Wechsler Full-Scale IQ (FSIQ) score of 115 would correspond to a percentile of 84. In the WAIS-IV, an FSIQ can be derived from a series of subtests that make up the four primary index scales: verbal comprehension (subtests: information, vocabulary, and similarities), perceptual reasoning (subtests: block design, matrix reasoning and visual puzzles), working memory (subtests: digit span and arithmetic), and processing speed (subtests: symbol search and coding). There are also one or more supplemental subtests within each of the index scales that can be administered separately or substituted for a core subtest.

The WAIS-IV is conormed with the WMS-IV (memory) and the publisher has developed specific scoring programs that can compare the results of these tests with achievement measures such as the Wechsler Individual Achievement Test—Third Edition (Wechsler, 2009). The WIAT-III, which provides a number of tests that measure achievement levels in areas such as reading comprehension, is frequently used to help educators determine strengths and weaknesses of a student and can help them in making recommendations for accommodation, in evaluating responses to intervention, or in diagnosing learning disabilities.

Wechsler D: *Wechsler Intelligence Scale for Children—Fourth Edition*. San Antonio, TX: Pearson, 2003. Revision in 2014.

Wechsler D: *Wechsler Adult Intelligence Scale—Fourth Edition*. Bloomington, MN: Pearson, 2008.

Wechsler D: *Wechsler Individual Achievement Test—Third Edition*. Bloomington, MN: Pearson, 2009.

Wechsler D: *Wechsler Preschool and Primary Scale of Intelligence—Fourth Edition*. Bloomington, MN: Pearson, 2012.

GERIATRIC EMPHASIS AND TESTS DESIGNED FOR REPEATED USE

Some of the measures described previously may be too complex or time-consuming for geriatric patients. Instead, shorter neuropsychological screening instruments are frequently used with this population. In addition, given that geriatric patient performance is often tracked over time, these instruments may have alternate forms to minimize practice effects with repeated testing, as well as data predicting expected rates of change. Both instruments mentioned here (Dementia Rating Scale—II; Repeatable Battery for Adult Neuropsychological Assessment) have these capacities. In addition, they have data methodologies that highlight patterns of performance that are more consistent with either cortical or subcortical based etiologies common in geriatric patient populations. More recently, efforts have moved forward to develop measures to determine specific capacities or make predictions about someone's ability to live independently. The Independent Living Scale (Loeb, 1996) is one such measure and looks at multiple face-valid constructs such as money management and health reasoning abilities.

▶ Dementia Rating Scale—II

The Dementia Rating Scale—II (Mattis, 1988; Jurica et al., 2004) is a popular, global screening tool for dementia that takes about 30–45 minutes to complete. The test is broken down into five subscales that are named attention (with items that include a simplified digit span), immediate memory (with items that include the recognition of a word list), conceptualization (with items that ask how are two things are similar), initiation and perseveration (with items that include a fluency test and the request to perform simple motor commands), and construction (with items that include the reproduction of simple line drawings). Individual subtest scores are calculated and an overall score is generated that is compared to an age-matched sample with education corrections. Suggested cutoff scores can assist with differentiating healthy controls from a dementia group (van Gorp et al., 1999).

▶ Repeatable Battery for Adult Neuropsychological Assessment (RBANS)

The Repeatable Battery for Adult Neuropsychological Assessment (Randolph et al., 1998) is an adult screening measure that takes about 45 minutes to complete and has measures that tap the domains of immediate memory, visuo-spatial/constructional, language, attention, and delayed memory. Tests in the battery include familiar tests such as a word list, story, and visual design that need to be learned and remembered after a delay. Supplementing these tasks are measures that include a simple naming test, digit span task, and semantic fluency. The RBANS has an alternative form, with normative data, that allows a clinician to calculate scores representing a reliable change over time. Clinically, pre–post evaluations with the RBANS might be requested to help evaluate the effect of a medication or to track suspected progressive declines in degenerative conditions.

Jurica PJ, Leitten CL, Mattis S: *DRS-2 Dementia Rating Scale-2: Professional Manual*. Psychological Assessment Resources, 2004.

Loeb PA: *Independent Living Scales (ILS) Manual*. Psychological Corporation, 1996.

Mattis S: *Dementia Rating Scale*. Odessa, FL: Psychological Assessment Resources, 1988.

Randolph C, Tierney MC, Mohr E, Chase TN: The Repeatable Battery for the Assessment of Neuropsychological Status (RBANS): preliminary clinical validity. *J Clin Exp Neuropsychol* 1998;20(3):310–319.

van Gorp WG, Marcotte TD, Sultzer D, et al: Screening for dementia: comparison of three commonly used instruments. *J Clin Exp Neuropsychol* 1999;21(1):29–38.

INCLUSIVE BATTERIES

Another option available to neuropsychologists is to use prepackaged inclusive batteries. A major advantage of these batteries is their provision of normative data across all the inclusive tests. This feature allows neuropsychologists to take full advantage of scoring methodologies that may help them better predict if someone is truly impaired. Because these batteries can take many hours to complete, neuropsychologists sometimes select a subset of tests to administer to patients rather than administering the entire battery.

▶ Halstead-Reitan Neuropsychological Test Battery

The Halstead-Reitan Neuropsychological Test Battery (Reitan & Wolfson, 1993) contains many commonly used neuropsychological tests and is likely the most common fixed battery compendium. It originated from the work of Ward Halstead, who in 1947 at the University of Chicago published his observations of several hundred case studies of patients who had frontal lobe damage. By using 10 scores, Halstead blindly distinguished patients with confirmed brain lesions from control subjects. Ralph Reitan, a student of Halstead's, modified the battery in 1955 to identify lateralizing features of patient performances such as motor deficits expected in subtle stroke, the effect of temporal lobe epilepsy on memory, and the loss of abstraction ability associated with frontal damage. The battery had utility in being reasonably reliable in differentiating the presence of organicity before other techniques (e.g., neuroimaging) were available to do so (Lezak et al., 2012). A well-known measure from this battery, not already described, is the Category Test, an abstract reasoning task consisting of 180 items. The patient is required to use mental flexibility and problem solving to form concepts, using feedback from the examiner about the accuracy of attempts.

Reitan RM, Wolfson D: *The Halstead-Reitan Neuropsychological Test Battery: Theory and Clinical Interpretation*, 2nd edn. Tucson, AZ: Neuropsychology Press, 1993.

Lezak MD, Howieson DB, Bigler ED, et al: *Neuropsychological Assessment*, 5th edn. New York: Oxford University Press, 2012.

SUMMARY

This chapter described the wide range of psychological assessments used in psychiatric settings for the purposes of diagnostic formulation, specification of specific Axis I disorders or psychiatric symptoms, personality disorders and traits, and areas of neuropsychological functioning. The nature and extent of the psychological assessment and the measures used within it will depend on the referral questions being asked about the patient and the judgment of the psychologists conducting the evaluation. Although psychiatrists and other practitioners may not have the specific competencies to properly administer and interpret all of the measures described in this chapter, it is important they be aware of the domains of functioning in which psychological assessment may be helpful to their overall understanding and care of their patients. The measures described in this chapter provide some examples of how assessments yield useful clinical information. However, the measures described in this chapter are not exhaustive. For more detailed information about the plethora of measures available for the purposes of psychological assessment, readers are referred to comprehensive textbooks such as the Handbook of Psychiatric Measures (Rush et al., 2008) and Neuropsychological Assessment (Lezak et al., 2012).

Lezak MD, Howieson DB, Bigler ED, Tranel D: *Neuropsychological Assessment*, 5th edn. New York: Oxford University Press, 2012.

Rush AJ, First MB, Blacker D: *Handbook of Psychiatric Measures*, 2nd edn. Washington, DC: American Psychiatric Publishing, 2008.

Hannay HJ, Bieliauskas L, Crosson BA, et al: Special issue: Proceedings of the Houston Conference on Specialty Education and Training in Clinical Neuropsychology. *Arch Clin Neuropsychol* 1998;13:2.

Psychodynamic Psychotherapy and the Therapeutic Relationship

James W. Lomax, MD
Mihaela Cristina Ivan, MD

Human beings are subject to a multitude of adverse influences arriving from both external and internal sources. These adverse influences include internal conflicts (between one's aims and goals or urges and prohibitions), interpersonal disputes, certain cognitive and/or behavioral "errors" (e.g., catastrophizing and avoidance of exaggerated anticipated danger), personal and relational loss (both loss of significant attachment figures and loss of physical or cognitive abilities through illness, injury, or aging), and sociocultural or spiritual struggles. Through psychotherapy, physicians provide assistance in the managing of suffering resulting from these adverse influences. Structured professional relationships have been developed to address each of these adversities as the different forms of psychotherapy. Psychotherapy may also be focused on modifying the patient's overall pattern of adaptation to life (or personality). As Cloninger and others (1993) have demonstrated, personality is best considered an interactive combination of factors that are gene and environment based. The gene-based elements are relatively immutable, while behaviors stemming from environmental experience can potentially be altered. Some of the expressive psychotherapies make modifications in "character" as defined by Cloninger. The challenge to psychotherapists is to develop interventions not always knowing which ones relate to temperament and are genetically determined, and those related to environmental experience. To address behavioral problems related to temperament, the psychotherapist helps the patient to *accommodate* or learn new means of expression of the gene-based determinants of behavior. This enables their expression in ways that create less chaos or conflict in the person's relational world.

Psychotherapeutic treatment is an important tool in the professional skill set of the physician. It is a necessary component for the successful management of many forms of human illness and suffering. Illness and suffering are eased by a relationship with another caring human being that helps the suffering individual feel less isolated and more connected with a social community. In psychotherapy, this easing of suffering is conceptualized to be an enhanced product of a unique therapeutic relationship between patient and therapist. The terms of that relationship are defined implicitly or explicitly in a therapeutic alliance with its terms developed between patient and therapist.

The psychodynamic therapist needs to learn the evidence-based and technical principles of the psychotherapeutic management of the various adverse influences on human development and functioning. However, it is not proven that a particular psychiatric disorder (e.g., depression) should always be treated with a particular type of psychotherapy (e.g., cognitive, interpersonal, or psychodynamic). In fact, Wampold (2001) has documented that the theoretical orientation of the therapist is only modestly predictive of patient outcome. Because an individual's suffering is unique, and life circumstances in any individual are so varied, psychotherapy must be custom designed for every patient. Even though learning a manualized therapy is often helpful in the early phases of a therapist's professional development, the therapist must also learn when to deviate from the manual or any systematized therapeutic approach. In any therapy conducting a coherent and useful psychotherapeutic experience for a patient is more important than following any particular therapeutic approach. Allen (2012) conveys a superb approach of melding new conceptual models while retaining basic principles of dynamic therapy in a recent book on restoring the ability to mentalize in traumatized patients. Overreliance on a particular therapeutic approach often leads therapists to an overly rigid and inadequately empathic therapeutic relationship.

This chapter also comments on the management of the therapist's career and life. There is a significant downside to the many blessings and pleasures that derive from the privilege of knowing other humans so intimately. Physicians are subject to the same suffering that afflicts all people and also must be mindful of the exquisite and potentially devastating suffering that can follow when their neediness or emotional distress distorts the physician–patient relationship.

To increase the likelihood of a long, happy, and productive professional life, the psychiatrist must manage not only their patient's "medical" care, but also the human relationship with the patient. The term "secondary traumatic stress" refers to a specific therapeutic suffering related to patients with posttraumatic stress disorder. However, suffering is a part of many physician–patient relationships when treating the spectrum of other diagnostic categories because of our empathic engagement with suffering. Awareness of this "adverse effect" of professional caring plus the acquisition of principles of good self-care helps to avoid a chronic state of excessive fear of the clinical relationship. Fear in the patient–therapist relationship may arise from several sources: (1) fear that the patient will cross some boundary between a therapeutic alliance and a personal relationship, provoking insecurity and uncertainty about the appropriate therapeutic response—fear of this sort (especially with patients suffering from borderline, narcissistic, and histrionic personality disorders) may lead the therapist to be or to behave in an excessively, distant, and artificial manner; (2) fear that the patient will commit some form of aggression against the therapist (physical, lawsuit, etc.) because of some dissatisfaction; (3) the fact that an empathic connection to any suffering patient is inherently a painful experience and sometimes has been considered a diagnostic of certain types of psychopathology (the "praecox feeling" associated with treating individuals with schizophrenia). Fear of patients is especially intense in the early phases of professional development, when the learner is appropriately insecure about his or her professional abilities. Fear-based detachment from patients often must be unlearned in order to have a gratifying and steadily developing professional life. Fearful professionals cannot be creative, convey hope, or model joy in living. By doing four things, the physician can come to enjoy life and the art of medicine. The physician must (1) understand the nature of human vulnerability, both of the patient and of the physician; (2) understand the mechanisms whereby patients construct their experience of the physician and other attachment figures in their environment (and our own analogous constructions); (3) learn to apply the concepts of empathy, transference, and boundaries; and (4) develop a lifelong habit of meaningful continuing education, which includes the discussion of our clinical experiences in settings that are both very professional and very personal.

Allen JG: *Restoring Mentalizing in Attachment Relationships: Treating Trauma with Plain Old Therapy.* Washington, DC: American Psychiatric Press, 2012.

Cloninger CR, Surakic DM, Przyeck TR: A psychobiological model of temperament and character. *Arch Gen Psychiatry* 1993;50:975–990.

Wampold BE: *The Great Psychotherapy Debate: Models, Methods, and Findings.* Hillsdale, NJ: Erlbaum, 2001.

DEFINITION OF PSYCHOTHERAPY

Psychotherapy can be defined in general terms as the use of verbal means in a professional relationship to diminish effects of adverse influences and to increase positive, health-promoting capacities of another person. Such a definition does not concern itself with the academic training of the therapist and does not completely distinguish the activities of a well-intentioned friend from those of a paid professional. Psychotherapy is a process wherein an individual (the patient) participates in a structured encounter or a series of encounters with another person who—by dint of training, licensure, certification, and ethical proscription—is qualified to influence the mental state of another in a way that decreases the suffering and/or increases the healthy psychological, interpersonal, and behavioral options of the patient. There is no fundamental difference between the patient and the therapist other than the training of the therapist for the role. This point is made to emphasize that a psychotherapist is not superior to the patient, even though the therapist is always the party responsible for the management of the therapeutic relationship. The patient may be inclined to think of the therapist as superior, but the therapist must judiciously temper the patient's expectations and avoid being unprofessionally distracted by them. Nevertheless, understanding the difference inherent in the training and preparation for the therapeutic role between therapist and patient is crucial.

QUALIFICATIONS OF A PSYCHOTHERAPIST

Personal Traits

Although professional education is the chief distinguishing feature of a psychotherapist, educational programs cannot make a good psychotherapist out of every individual. Predictors of psychotherapeutic competency include fascination by the human condition, compassion, a vision of self that includes service to others, and persistence. Intelligence is certainly important, but more important are reflective capacity, empathy, patience, and sensitivity. Somewhat counterintuitively, the right amount of self-doubt is also a positive predictor of eventual psychotherapeutic and professional competency. In fact, some individuals who have no diagnosable psychiatric disorder have strongly developed personality traits (pessimism, narcissism) or cognitive styles (suspiciousness, catastrophizing, or overgeneralization) that undermine patient care. Some individuals actually represent a potential danger, both to themselves and to their patients, if allowed to manage a psychotherapeutic relationship. These individuals include the charismatic leader overly gratified by idealization and deference, and emotionally needy or love-starved individuals. These individuals have powerful personal agendas or needs that may exploit the patient's inherent vulnerability in the therapeutic relationship.

Training

Psychoanalytic training institutes evolved a tripartite structure for training to become a psychoanalyst that has served as a prototypical model for many models of psychotherapy education. Candidates for psychotherapy education must first pass through a screening process to assess their personal attributes outlined in the preceding section. Other qualifications are generally specified, such as a particular terminal degree. The student therapist then enters a course of psychoanalytic education and training, a number of supervised psychoanalytic treatments and a personal psychoanalysis. Psychotherapy education programs involve didactic classes and cases supervised by a faculty member or a designated mentor with competency in a specific form of psychotherapy. Unlike in psychoanalytic training, a personal psychotherapeutic experience is not required but is frequently "recommended." The length and content of such training programs vary considerably in practice. Some are embedded in discipline-specific educational programs such as psychiatry residency, psychology graduate school, internship and postdoctoral programs, clinical social work, and nurse practitioner programs. The length of psychotherapy education programs varies from months to many years, reflecting the ideals and scope of the practitioners of the particular therapeutic modality. In each of the programs, however, mechanisms are in place to identify educational milestones and to ensure the competence of their graduates. For most psychotherapeutic modalities, graduates are eligible to present their work to specific national oversight organizations that qualify training programs, set standards for the profession, credential new graduates into the national professional community, and require members of the professional organization to remain accountable to the established standards.

There are many psychotherapy education programs in the United States. Many are dedicated to teaching a specific psychotherapeutic discipline. The learner is expected to master a particular body of theoretical knowledge, which, in conjunction with the supervised cases, is structured to provide a framework for understanding the patient's experience and for structuring therapeutic interventions while avoiding either neglect or exploitation of the patient. A great deal of what is marketed as psychotherapy is practiced by individuals who have had less education than the version just outlined.

Psychiatry Residency Programs, for example, are obligated to help residents develop competence in applying supportive, psychodynamic, and cognitive–behavioral psychotherapies to both brief and long-term individual practice, as well as providing exposure to family, couples, group, and other individual evidence-based psychotherapies. However, the actual administrative oversight and supervision of cases is frequently uneven and psychiatry residencies do not require a personal psychotherapy experience. Some therapists practice various forms of psychotherapy with little training and in an unregulated way.

ACGME Program Requirements for Graduate Medical Education in Psychiatry, Effective: July 1, 2007 (http://acgme.org/400_psychiatry_07012007_u04122008.pdf).

Robertson MH: *Psychotherapy Education and Training: An Integrative Perspective*. Madison, CT: International Universities Press, 1995.

Rogers CR, Dymond R: *Psychotherapy and Personality Change*. Chicago, IL: University of Chicago Press, 1954.

MAJOR FORMS OF PSYCHOTHERAPY

There may be hundreds of forms of psychotherapy; considerable overlap exists in their theories and practices because of the many general principles that they share. The different forms of psychotherapy place special emphasis on one or another of these general principles.

Four major forms of psychotherapy result from the different ways workers conceptualize the nature and development of psychic distress: dynamic, experiential–humanistic, cognitive–behavioral, and integrated. There is also a strong evidence base for dialectical behavioral therapy, mentalization-based psychotherapy, motivational interviewing, and other psychotherapies. These will also be considered "integrative psychotherapies" for the purposes of this short chapter, which focuses on psychodynamic psychotherapy.

Dynamic Psychotherapies

The dynamic psychotherapies are based on the belief that much of human behavior, especially that which is troublesome to the individual, is determined by life experiences that produced psychological factors outside of the individual's awareness, including mental blind spots for both the therapist and the patient. One is compelled, therefore, to maintain self-defeating perspectives and repeat unsuccessful and maladaptive behaviors, for unrecognized, unconscious reasons (Gabbard, 2005). Defense mechanisms operate to avoid anticipated dangers or to stabilize the individual's emotional state, but often at a loss of other emotional or relational opportunities. The development of these problematic behaviors, personality traits, affective states, and other symptoms is generally understood to have occurred because of some unfortunate mix between the individual's inherent traits (intelligence, temperament) and the caregiving surround (developmental interferences) in which he or she has developed. In the dynamic therapies, improvement is measured by improved function in various realms of the person's life and by integrating the new understandings gained in the context of a therapeutic relationship with the therapist into the relational and vocational world of the patient. Traditionally, the dynamic therapies have been seen to exist along a continuum with "supportive psychotherapy" at one end and insight-oriented therapy and psychoanalysis at the other. Recent developments have placed increased emphasis on the quality of the therapist–patient relationship as a central factor in a beneficial therapy experience.

Experiential–Humanistic Psychotherapies

The experiential–humanistic models of psychotherapy attempt to eliminate the theoretical or excessively detached perspectives seen as inherent in older (especially the ego psychological psychoanalytic psychodynamic) models of engaging patients. They replace them with "perspectivalist" attitudes. The individual's lived experience is viewed as the most, or only, important consideration. No attempt is made to decode any of the patient's potentially distorted vision of the therapist (transference) in order to "revisit and repair" an early childhood experience, inferred by the therapist based on knowledge of human development as the cause of their distortions. These therapy approaches take the patient's experience, including the patient's experience of the therapist, at face value. Psychopathology is viewed as resulting from the failure of caregivers and other attachment figures to provide the empathic responsiveness necessary for the development of a self-structure that organizes experiences in the most adaptive way. The therapist will play a wider array of roles than in the more classically dynamic approaches, determined by the patient's needs and characteristics. Therapeutic effects derive from the patient developing a new personal narrative. A therapeutic framework of safe, gratifying, and development-enhancing relationship allows for a healthier reordering of the processing of personal experience.

Cognitive–Behavioral Psychotherapies

Cognitive–behavioral models of psychotherapy view psychopathology as the result of distorted thoughts (catastrophizing and overly generalizing cognitions) that result in maladaptive behaviors (such as avoidance of anticipated catastrophic events). Various forms of mental illness (anxiety, inhibitions, and depression) result from the powerful influence of these cognitions. The therapist does not attempt to explain the etiology of these beliefs. The concept from psychoanalytic theory of a dynamic unconscious is seen as unnecessary to explain behavior. The patient's unsubstantiated beliefs ("others would be better off if I were dead") are challenged, with more adaptive beliefs implicitly or explicitly suggested and supported. The patient is encouraged to test irrational perspectives ("no one will want you if you are not perfect") and replace them with more realistic beliefs that can be validated. Although other psychotherapies frequently include cognitive elements, the behavioral components of cognitive–behavioral therapy (flooding, blocking, and prolonged exposure) involve interventions that carry these methods into specific actions of a therapist with patients (such as "prolonged exposure" to environmental situations that become associated with subsequent trauma).

Eclectic or Integrated Psychotherapies

In the practice of psychotherapy, most patients and clients receive a therapy that is an amalgam of the dynamic, experiential–humanistic, and cognitive–behavioral perspectives. This reality is created by an inherent difficulty of every therapy to stay within the confines of a particular method because each of the methods alone fails to account for the multifaceted presentation of human psychopathology. Most patients present clinical material best handled by first one and then another perspective.

The following case is presented to illustrate the typical complexity of the clinical picture that confronts the psychotherapist, and the usefulness of being familiar with a range of theoretical perspectives and techniques:

> The patient was an early-middle-aged mother of two healthy children. She was an intelligent, sensitive, and kind woman who had been married for 15 years to a hard-working man who she felt did not understand her. Indeed, he was frustrated by her manifest pessimism, her guilt, and her inability to enjoy the many fruits of their hard work. She was chronically depressed, anxious, phobic, and compulsive. She was also hypochondriacal, sexually unresponsive, and indecisive. Her father died when she was 12 years old. Her older brother had sexually abused her, and her sister had committed suicide. As the eldest girl in the family, she had been assigned domestic responsibilities inappropriate to her age following her father's death. Her older brother's idealization by both parents made it hard for her ever to feel special. She grew up embittered and thinking that she was not, and never would be, "good enough." Her sense of self was defined by her failures. Her successes were discounted as aberrations.

Although the patient might have benefited from pharmacotherapy, she said that she did not wish to take medication. She wanted a psychotherapy experience that would help her learn to enjoy her life more and unlock what she experienced as untapped potential. She feared that she might be contaminating her children's worldview. She felt that she was being unfair to her husband and restricting their life together. She saw her problem as chronic and severe and worried that she might one day follow her sister's suicidal path, an act that, for her family's sake, she desperately wanted to avoid.

In planning a psychotherapy for this patient, the therapist was struck by the myriad of symptoms she exhibited. She did not abuse substances and had no psychotic thought content. She endorsed both irrational thoughts and personal isolation. Her low self-esteem was related to chronic abusive experiences, and her guilty fears and inhibitions suggested unconscious themes of an oedipal nature. The pervasiveness of the patient's suffering and the history of her personal losses suggested that short-term work would not be effective and might even be damaging. A purely cognitive approach seemed inappropriate given the patient's overwhelming symptomatology: It would not address her many interpersonal needs. An open-ended and integrative therapy seemed indicated.

Gabbard GO: *Psychodynamic Psychiatry in Clinical Practice*, 4th edn. Washington, DC: American Psychiatric Publishing, 2005.

Gill MM: *Psychoanalysis in Transition: A Personal View*. New York: Analytic Press, 1994.

Stolorow RD, Atwood GE, Brandchaft B: *The Inter-Subjective Perspective*. Northvale, NJ: Jason Aronson, 1994.

EXPECTATIONS OF PSYCHODYNAMIC PSYCHOTHERAPY

Patients approach psychotherapy with a mixture of hopes, fears, and expectations, many of which are conscious and some of which are unconscious. Some of the patient's goals are perceived by the therapist as reasonable, but some are not. Patients do not intend to be unreasonable; their demands are a function of their perception of their needs and may be affected by their lack of information or personal experiences about life and experiences that are vastly different from their own. Therapists acquire knowledge through training and experience of what is and what is not attainable from psychotherapy. The therapist's ambitions and goals for the therapy may not, however, coincide with the patient's. With sustained clinical practice, therapists become increasingly confident in the usefulness of their work as psychotherapists while simultaneously becoming impressed with the unpredictable and nonspecific nature of its benefit. They have learned to understand the importance of allowing the patient to use therapy in a uniquely personal and creative way.

Therapists are not immune from influences that generate unreasonable expectations for therapy. These influences include pressures to move more quickly, more efficiently, and more definitively from their patients or themselves. They may unwittingly accept the plea or demand to become a magician whose aims would be accomplished by special power, not hard work. Some therapists feel apologetic for their limitations, ashamed of their imperfections, and guilty about their fees. These vulnerabilities may signal a need for supervision or personal treatment. They may combine with a patient's unreasonable demands to create a "misalliance" in which goals are implied but never stated, boundaries are fluid, and roles are not defined.

Patients and therapists should agree explicitly on the goals of the work they are mutually performing. If goals are not made explicit, they will likely become immeasurable, unreasonable, and unattainable. Goals can be changed; indeed, it is good practice to review goals from time to time, especially in a longer treatment, to ensure that patients and therapists are still on the same track. One goal should always be to provide the patient with a positive, useful experience. The therapist may be the first significant person in the patient's life who does not wish to exploit the patient, or who genuinely wishes to hear and understand the patient's problems. Such quite general influences may be profoundly salutary. Setting idealized changes as goals runs the risk of predetermining treatment failure and adding another negative event in the patient's life and sense of self-efficacy. Humans are frequently ambivalent about changes. Some patients will continue to suffer and be unable to completely let go of an unrealistic wish. A positive experience with the therapist will likely have a continuing effect on the patient even long after the treatment is ended, and positive changes may occur after "termination" of the "in-person" relationship.

THE PSYCHOTHERAPEUTIC PROCESS

PATIENT SELECTION & THERAPY PLANNING

What principles should guide the therapist in deciding whom and how to treat? Many individuals may be recognized as needing therapy, in the sense that their loved ones or personal acquaintances recognize them as suffering or causing others to suffer. Needing therapy in this sense is not the same as having the potential to use a psychotherapy experience. The process of assessing the likelihood that a prospective patient can benefit from a psychiatric treatment including psychotherapy begins with the first encounter (often via the telephone) and should continue until the mental health practitioner and patient are ready to close the evaluation phase and begin the treatment.

The first level of decision includes the question of the need for hospitalization or the likelihood that hospitalization will be necessary in the near future. Psychotherapy other than crisis intervention therapy is not feasible in the face of active psychosis or immediate suicide threat. Similarly, a patient who is in the throes of active deleterious substance use or who is currently involved in a legal proceeding probably should be referred to for specialized help.

A telephone assessment may be used to screen out patients whose difficulties are beyond the therapist's reach of expertise in counseling, or if the patient needs a higher level of care than outpatient psychotherapy. The patient should be asked how he or she came to call the particular mental health practitioner as well as about his/her understanding of psychotherapy and should be made aware of fees to be charged. The therapist should consider the following questions: What is the nature of complaint? Is the problem within their competence? Does the prospective patient indicate a degree of reflectiveness, or is there excessive demandingness or unrealistic expectation? Does the patient "reflect upon" the therapist's questions during the phone call? In a fee-for-service setting, the patient should be informed that a professional fee will be charged for the evaluation session.

An initial phone call need not be lengthy, but it can be useful, and the patient should not be scheduled for a first visit unless the therapist feels a sense of curiosity or interest about working with the patient. The patient may have some questions about the therapist or mentioned having looked up the professional on the Internet. This should neither threaten nor offend the therapist.

Occasionally, the telephone exchange will indicate that referral to a different resource is the best strategy. It is better not to evaluate a patient than to have to refer the patient to another therapist unless that possibility is mutually understood beforehand.

FIRST SESSION: EVALUATING THE PATIENT

The prospective patient is told that one session will be scheduled for evaluating the problem. At the end of that hour, the therapist and patient will compare notes and discuss options. Treatment at this point has not been offered and no long-term contract has been established. A first psychiatric session will generally be a mixture of medical interviewing, with a focus on the symptom picture and the patient's mental status, and open-ended interviewing, wherein the patient is given an opportunity not only to be heard but also to demonstrate capacity for utilizing a psychotherapeutic modality at the current point in time. Given a reasonably cooperative patient, the first session should yield three things: (1) a DSM-5-TR diagnosis (if any); (2) a sense of goodness-of-fit between patients and therapists; and (3) a sense that the patient's story is beginning to make sense according to the therapist's understanding of the nature and development of psychopathology (often conceptualized in reference to one or more clinical "models of the mind" for the dynamic psychotherapies) or therapeutic approach (of the therapy under consideration).

If the therapist is to plan a psychotherapy experience for the patient, an understanding of what is "wrong" with the patient must be developed. This extends beyond a clinical diagnosis and addresses the question of how a psychotherapy is structured to enable the patient to do a useful piece of psychological work. A succinct statement of the patient's problem should be communicated to the patient as a foundation for the therapeutic alliance. If the therapist is unable to explain to an observer (or to the patient) what he or she proposes to do and what the therapist and patient will do together and why, it is unlikely that a useful psychotherapy will be undertaken.

It bodes well for psychotherapy when the prospective patient engages the therapist in a personal way. Psychotherapeutic work in the realm of what has traditionally been referred to as transference adds depth to a psychodynamic treatment and is likely to be important if the history includes significant developmental interferences. Psychotherapy can be done without using the patient's experience of the therapist and therapeutic alliance, but such treatments tend to be intellectual and less integrated into the rest of the

patient's life. Patients with narcissistic personality disorder, especially, need a considerable period of time before they feel comfortable revealing what to them represents humiliating notions about actually needing therapy or the help of a therapist. The therapist cannot force the development of a transference relationship into the foreground, rather it is a powerful tool when the patient will allow it to develop. It is a useful tool when the "repair" of attachment relationships is necessary.

As the allotted time for the first evaluation session draws to a close, a number of complex and interlocking issues must be answered. If the evaluator is a psychiatrist, then four decisions must be made: (1) Is hospitalization indicated? If so, the administrative and practical details of getting the patient hospitalized become the focus of attention. (2) Is a different immediate intervention demanded by the patient's condition? If the therapist is required immediately to assume the role of prescribing a psychotropic medication, certain other roles may be less easily established in the future. (3) Does the therapist feel comfortable that they have appreciated the patient's situation? The patient will also want to feel that the time has been well spent and that the therapist is forming a clear understanding of their situation. (4) Does the therapist feel that they and the patient are a good therapeutic fit? Is it likely to strengthen and is it worth pursuing, or should this session be the last? Referral for whatever reason is best done at the time of the first visit.

A recommendation of no treatment is always a possibility. If the therapist is beginning to develop an understanding of the patient near the end of the session and believes that they can work together, it is appropriate that near the end of the first hour, the therapist shares with the patient their reflections on the interview. It is often useful to begin this portion with some version of, "I think I have a picture of your situation and problems, but I want to clarify your hopes and expectations for our meeting today." Asking the patient if they have any preformed ideas about what the therapist might do to be helpful is often a useful strategy at this time. These exchanges will set the stage for an agreed-upon second evaluative session that explores areas that both parties feel are important. In most cases, the therapist can reassure the patient that things should be clearer, both for the therapist and the patient, by the end of a second or third interview, and that a recommendation for treatment will be discussed at that time. The second interview should be scheduled as near as possible to the first., preferably a week or less. Patients who have made the decision to seek help generally have delayed for some time, but having begun the process, hope that it will move swiftly.

Dilts SL: *Models of the Mind: A Framework for Biopsychosocial Psychiatry*. Philadelphia, PA: Brunner-Routledge, 2001.

Gedo JE: A psychology of personal aims. In: *Beyond Interpretation*. New York: International Universities Press, 1979, pp. 1–25.

SECOND SESSION: PROCESS & CONTRACT

A second evaluation session is potentially helpful for several reasons. The therapist may not be ready to present the patient with a specific therapy recommendation because their formulation is incomplete, or they may not want to rush the patient or may want to assess the patient's reaction to the first session. For example, will the patient be able to share thoughts and reactions to the first hour? Does the patient feel more hopeful of an improved future? Was there any evidence of self-reflection that generated fresh associations?

The therapist may begin the second session with a statement that it will be useful to further explore a number of areas, but first, what were the patient's thoughts and reactions to the first meeting? An important clue to the patient's psychological mindedness may be gleaned from an invitation by the therapist for the patient to ask about "where the session went," including any dreams and memories after the initial appointment had ended. These interventions create alliance building. They further demonstrate that some of the responsibilities for the treatment rest with the patient and that both patient and therapist will be working on an important "project" that requires intimate collaboration. The patient will often report that new information or details have been recalled. An exploration of this material generally will enable the therapist to call attention to areas noted after the first session that need exploration, with the upcoming therapy recommendation clearly in mind. If left unexplored, these areas (substance use, legal trouble, and experience with other therapists) may erupt later and disrupt the treatment.

The therapist is also further considering the nature of the problem and the type of treatment to be recommended. The therapist needs to know the patient's capacity to fund therapy, ability to fit with the therapist's work schedule and office hours. In this process, the therapist experiences how the patient handles negotiations. The therapist is also assessing how easily the patient talks, and about what. Patients who wish to discuss situational issues may need more time between sessions to allow events to occur. Patients who have strong reactions to the therapy encounters may have difficulty waiting for the next session. Patients who live a bit far from the therapist's office, or who must exert considerable effort to get back and forth, may have trouble sustaining their initial enthusiasm. How motivated does the patient seem to address changes after the therapy has begun? How stable and supportive is the patient's social support network? Does the patient have the resources to effect changes? At least a rudimentary developmental history of the patient (if not taken in the first session) is usually essential for the development of the therapeutic contract.

By the midway point of the second session, an experienced therapist may have assessed and decided upon three key issues: (1) whether or not to prescribe medication; (2) whether tests (psychological, chemical and neuropsychological) are needed; and (3) what type of psychotherapy to recommend and at what frequency.

If third-party payment will be used, the therapist must determine if the patient understands that confidentiality cannot be complete and that the future may bring difficult questions regarding the history of treatment. Can the patient defer making significant life decisions that could interfere with the course and outcome of psychotherapy? What are the dynamic forces at work between the patient and their most significant ones over the need for and possible result of therapy?

The therapist will then tell the patient what is being recommended and why. Three areas must be covered: (1) the rationale for the proposed therapy and its techniques, its frequency, its anticipated length, and its cost; (2) the "hoped-for outcome" of the treatment, couched in terms that express optimism for realistic and attainable goals, and the likelihood of that outcome; and (3) alternative treatments, their anticipated lengths and costs, and their risks and likely outcome.

A schedule for visits will be negotiated, and a clear description will be provided of procedures regarding the payment of the bill, appointment cancellations, and lateness on the part of the patient or the therapist. A written policy statement may be helpful. If third-party payment, an electronic medical record, or certification procedures for managed care organizations will be a part of the picture, these factors, including the provision of a diagnosis, should be outlined clearly. The therapist should explain to the patient the diagnosis and should tell the patient what is expected of him or her during the treatment and what can be expected of the therapist. Some issues may be addressed only when they arise and become integrated into the context of the treatment. These issues include details such as chance meetings outside the office and what names will be used.

By the end of the second session, the therapist and the patient should be looking forward with optimism and anticipation to the beginning of a psychotherapeutic endeavor or "project." Their work together will be an exploratory and shared experience built upon a jointly owned respective foundation.

BEGINNING OF PSYCHOTHERAPY

It can be said that the patient experienced the onset of therapy with the first encounter with the therapist. Nevertheless, the therapist must make a point of separating evaluation from treatment, because of the wish to not enter into a formal medico-legal contractual responsibility for the patient's ongoing welfare (beyond handling any immediate needs the patient may have) until they are confident that the psychotherapy is appropriate.

Whatever goals for the treatment enterprise the patient and therapist have agreed upon, the therapist knows that there is one overarching goal: to provide the patient with an experience that will enable some measure of healing to occur. The therapist cannot will the patient into mental health, and the patient may find that for some issues, their inability to change is too great to overcome. The therapist is confident, however, that through the use of considered strategies and tactics, informed by an in-depth understanding of the patient's psychopathology and unique developmental experiences, they will, over time, create a healthy therapeutic atmosphere that will enable the patient to facilitate change.

Whatever the nature of the therapy be, the opening phase is understood to involve two parts. First, the patient passes through the stages of engagement into the therapy process. The signs of the patient experiencing to be "in therapy" will vary according to the structure of the particular therapy being used. In psychodynamic therapy, for instance, patients might be said to be "in therapy" when they begin to experience the feeling of states in life experiences that are painful and bring them into their therapy. Understanding them leads to a change in their subjective feelings. In therapy designed along more educational or supportive lines, the patient may report having been reflecting on the last session and provide additional thoughts about it. In some cases, the engagement will be revealed in a dream or in an unconscious, displaced action (symptomatic anger or fondness about someone in their environment who had been previously emotionally "neutral").

After engagement has occurred, the second part of the opening phase plays out, with the unfolding and illumination before the eyes of the patient and the therapist of the nature of the problem. The way the problem is conceptualized is intensely personal. It is worked out between the patient and the therapist in language that they will refer to by mutual agreement. This language is a derivative of the blending of the therapist's methods of organizing the experience of the therapy with the patient's organization of the experience. The words used to describe the nature of the problem will reveal the predominant theoretical orientation of the therapist merging with the narrative that the patient is constructing in the rest of their life. Once the problem has been defined in this mutual and co-created manner, the opening phase is established.

MIDDLE PHASE OF PSYCHOTHERAPY

Before the middle phase of psychotherapy can begin, the alliance between a patient and a therapist must be established firmly and the core conflict of the issue is identified and agreed upon. The process of "working through" begins. The patient is confronted repeatedly with manifestations of problematic ways of organizing experiences and relating to others. In some therapies, this process occurs in the therapeutic relationship, including transference and countertransference reactions. In other therapies, "working through" takes place once removed, by examining relationships outside the therapy, both current and past. This confrontation has variable effects on the patient. There may be moments of new understanding and growth. There may be periods of flight away from explicitly discussing the process via resistance,

avoidance, and sometimes regression, including substance misuse. The therapist's role is to follow the theme of the patient's unconscious and automatic attitudes and behaviors and—through a mixture of empathic responsiveness, probing, clarifying, confronting, and interpreting—to help the patient adhere to the work of the treatment and pursuit of healthy and agreed-upon goals.

Many difficulties are encountered during the middle phase; some are inevitable and some are incidental to therapist errors, including inevitable "empathic failures." Desirable personal attributes and therapeutic competence will not ensure a smooth middle phase. Empathic failures by the therapist will include failures to intervene and mismatches between patient's needs and therapist's interventions. The therapist will lose the sight of the patient's experience, and the patient's feelings will be hurt. What is done by both members of the therapeutic dyad at such times determines whether the error eventually deepens the therapy and increases the tolerance of the patient for imperfections in important attachment figures or ruptures the therapeutic alliance and bond beyond repair. A number of "middle-phase" problems are typical and are mentioned individually in the sections that follow.

A. Acting Out

The term "acting out" is used in different ways, but it is generally understood to refer to behavior that expresses issues and emotions generated by the therapy process, but expressed in some other relationship. A variety of behaviors are seen, involving both conscious and unconscious motivations. Individuals who are prone to impulsiveness or destructive behavior make relatively problematic psychotherapy subjects. The most flagrant behavior, such as substance use, suicide attempts, and middle-of-the-night phone calls, may be so difficult to manage as to make therapy impossible. If the therapist lacks the ability to generate shared collaborative discussions in order to preserve the treatment, he or she can be placed in the untenable position of being responsible for generating the patient's unhealthy actions.

Less dramatic forms of "acting out" must be recognized by the therapist, who should then confront the patient and bring the effects and associated thoughts into the therapy. The patient may quote the therapist to another person and arouse ire, especially if the other person is paying the bill. The patient may fail to pay the bill, miss sessions, cancel appointments, or be late; or the patient may make serious life decisions abruptly, especially regarding love relationships.

A single female mental health professional in her midthirties sought treatment with a male therapist for recurrent major depression. She also described a disturbing behavioral propensity to make particularly poor choices for her romantic involvements. Her treatment involved pharmacotherapy for the depression and expressive psychodynamic psychotherapy. The latter was far more in-depth than her previous treatments, which were predominantly pharmacologically based. As the therapy unfolded, she began to recall experiences from her childhood, which involved sexually overstimulating "play" with a reclusive uncle who had been repeatedly entrusted with childcare and babysitting responsibilities. As this "play" was recognized as sexual exploitation, the patient increased the frequency of sessions in her therapy and became engaged in the therapy in a lively fashion. However, she soon found herself preoccupied with a female patient of hers who had characteristics of a borderline personality disorder. In a highly uncharacteristic manner, her preoccupation included urges to be involved in her patient's personal life in a way that would have clearly been both professionally damaging for the professional and disastrous for her patient.

The therapist suggested (interpreted) to his patient that she was displacing feelings of an erotic, loving transference relationship into the relationship with her female patient. This "displacement" was a compromise that transiently allowed her to feel less vulnerable, but also would result in the "punishment" she felt she deserved for her childhood sexual behavior with her uncle. Because their relationship was still rather early in its development, the therapist elected to communicate in a more direct and "educational" manner. The potential danger to his patient's professional well-being required proactive and more educational intervention than might be the case in a situation that did not involve such danger for the primary and secondary patients involved in this case.

Shared understanding of such behaviors nearly always leads to an improved alliance and forward motion. Failure to confront the behavior retards or disrupts therapy.

The patient may demonstrate ego-syntonic "acting out," in which he or she enacts unconscious themes through behavior that causes no harm. For example, the patient may come early for the appointment (hoping to see the therapist's other patients or given their time), or the patient may watch the clock so as not to overstay (the unconscious fear is of feeling dismissed).

B. Acting In

Novice therapists are frequently troubled when patients do things in their presence that throw them off balance, disorient, or even frighten them. Many of these behaviors merely need to be experienced once in order to know how to handle them next time. Some behaviors may prompt the therapist to seek personal treatment in order to understand their responses.

A patient may put the therapist off balance by exhibiting overly familiar behavior. For example, a patient calls the therapist by his/her first name or asks to be called by the first name; a patient brings the therapist a small gift; or a patient asks personal questions about the therapist's life. The smooth and empathic management of these personal moments requires self-awareness, compassion, flexibility and objectivity. It also requires knowledge of the nature of therapeutic

boundaries, boundary violations, and medical ethics, as well as theoretical knowledge of the nature of psychopathology and of the science of psychotherapy. Beginning therapists need regular forums in which they can process such events. Even very experienced therapists need access to consultation anytime they are inclined to engage in atypical therapeutic behavior or recognize that they are anticipating a "boundary crossing." In general, it is best to err on the side of an awkward deferral or refusal than on the side of boundaryless permissiveness. One's technique becomes smoother with time, but there is a lifelong need for consultation and professional discussions about our work.

Some behaviors by the patient are more provocative and troublesome. For example, a patient asks for hugs or other personal contact or asks for a gift from the therapist; a patient wears revealing clothing or directly propositions the therapist; or a patient requests out-of-the-office contact. In such situations, the therapist should begin with gentle limit setting accompanied by sensible explanations. One does not say "I'd like to, but the ethics of my profession won't let me." One might say, "I wonder if this is a case testing whether our project will be another exploitation?" (In psychoanalysis as opposed to psychotherapy, the therapist often will "interpret" the patient's behavior without much further elaboration, somewhat like a sports announcer's "calling the play by play." This use of words where there would more naturally be behavior is what led Freud to describe psychoanalysis as an endeavor for which there is "no model in other human relationships.") Occasionally a patient will persist, despite firm but gentle limit setting. The therapist then confronts the patient with his or her seeming inability to reflect and dangerous testing of the safety and viability of the therapeutic relationship.

A common behavior on the border between "acting out" and "acting in" involves encounters between the patient and the therapist's office personnel. The patient may ask a secretary for personal information about the therapist. The patient may attempt to befriend or even romance the office staff. These situations are easily dealt with when the staff is knowledgeable and well trained. Considerable trouble can result, however, when the office person has no understanding of the nature of a patient–therapist relationship or, even worse, harbors resentment toward the therapist–boss. Beginning therapists must take nothing for granted in the hiring and training of office personnel. Such individuals represent the therapist to the public, for better or for worse.

Gutheil TG, Gabbard GO: Misuses and misunderstandings of boundary theory in clinical and regulatory settings. *Am J Psychiatry* 1998;155(3):409–414.

C. Stalemate

The term "stalemate" covers a variety of conditions, the essence of which is that the patient becomes dissatisfied with the therapy, makes no progress, and considers quitting. This phenomenon has traditionally been seen from an objectivist perspective and understood as a manifestation of resistance (negative therapeutic reaction). More contemporary views of the therapy process interpret these states as commentaries on the nature of the relationship between the two parties. Active interpretation is usually required to restore the alliance and the therapy, and generally some degree of therapist self-disclosure involving the immediate interaction calls to the patient's attention or the failure to get something from the therapist that the patient very much wants. It is not, of course, the gratification of these wishes that is the purpose of the therapy but rather their identification. Using first person plural language ("We are having a problem.") when describing transferential problems and difficulties of the treatment is useful in communicating the therapist's awareness of his or her role in the creation of their therapeutic relationship. When the patient's history includes physical or sexual exploitation by an attachment figure, it generally taints all subsequent intimate relationships in significant ways.

D. Third-Party Interferences

Threatened spouses and parents are joined by third-party players of all varieties in placing pressures on the very existence of psychotherapy. For example, an angry wife may request equal time to "set the record straight"; a jealous husband may knock on the door during a therapy hour; or a managed care organization may need more information before a claim for benefits can be processed or take the position that "insurance" is not to be used for reconstructive psychotherapy. Sensitivity, flexibility, and strength are required of the therapist in order to protect the patient's confidentiality and preserve the life of the therapy.

E. Other Negative Effects

Many complications are possible in psychotherapy. Constant pressure against the frame of a therapy is created by necessary restrictions. It is not easy to avoid boundary crossings, but the task is made easier if the therapist has knowledge of behaviors that are considered to be indicators of the "slippery slope" toward boundary violations. It is inappropriate to expect the patient to understand and control these matters. This is the therapist's responsibility.

The vulnerabilities of the psychotherapist are all too real, and patients can present many attractions to a therapist. The therapist is of course in danger of participating in boundary violations but is also vulnerable to painful and affective states tied to the rigors and restrictions of the work. Commonly experienced signs of untoward therapist stress include excessive fatigue at the end of the day; depression, depletion, and having nothing left for life outside the office; inability to take time off; or loss of objectivity and overidentification with the patient.

The therapist sometimes realizes that a serious mistake has been made in the original conceptualization of the therapy and that the therapy should not be allowed to continue. It is better to interrupt treatment than to persist in the face of an untenable situation. The therapist may, for example, realize that the patient has been misdiagnosed and that significant antisocial or borderline personality disorder elements are present. The patient may become engaged in behavior that runs counter to the contract or that the therapist finds intolerable (an HIV-positive patient who continues to expose unknowing partners). Consultation with a colleague may show the therapist the way out of the dilemma. If not, the only path may be to make alternative arrangements with careful consideration of the therapist's legal and ethical responsibilities.

In a gratifyingly high percentage of cases, when the patient–therapist fit has been a good one and the alliance has held together, the patient achieves most of the shared goals. The patient is easier to be with, both for the therapist and significant others. The patient reports that life is better. Symptoms attenuate, and characteristic ways of organizing experiences become less rigid and stereotyped. Relationships with other people improve. The patient begins to talk about life without the therapy, and the therapist begins to think that a successful ending for the therapy is in view. The middle phase is finished.

TERMINATION OF PSYCHOTHERAPY

The ending of a psychotherapy can occur under a variety of circumstances, some very satisfying for both parties, and some painful or traumatic, especially for the patient.

▶ Termination by Mutual Agreement: Satisfied

In this situation, circumstances are optimal. The therapist and the patient are in agreement that the therapy should end because the work has gone well and the desired effect has occurred. If the therapy has been open ended, the classic phases of termination will be seen, colored by the patient's individual circumstances. The therapist will have begun to muse that termination has become a consideration, seeing that the patient is functioning well, both within and outside the therapy hour: There is no "acting out," the original symptoms are no longer problematic, and the patient is being affirmed by the environment. When the patient raises the issue, it feels congruent to the therapist. It is discussed, and a mutually agreeable ending date is set. During the ensuing phase (brief or extended, according to agreement), a resurgence of symptomatology may occur, and the pain of loss of a relationship is experienced by both parties. The therapist knows the pain must be worked through by the patient and does not collude in any defensive maneuvers of the patient. The therapy ends on a bittersweet note, with recognition that good work was done and each party has devoted appreciated effort; but the work is over, and the patient is ready to move on. The therapeutic relationship is left intact. The therapist does not cross previously respected boundaries. The patient may well never return, but if the need arises, there would be no barriers. Even when a patient and a therapist work in the same institution, the therapist remains "responsible" for therapeutically managing the personal dimensions of the relationship.

▶ Termination by Mutual Agreement: Elements of Dissatisfaction

A common situation is the one in which the patient and the therapist agree to the ending of the therapy, but one or both feel a degree of dissatisfaction with what has been accomplished and would prefer to continue. In psychotherapy training programs, all therapeutic experiences are time limited. In others, the therapy may also have been time limited from the beginning, either because the therapist conceptualized a time-limited treatment as optimal or because the patient had limited resources. Artificial limits may have been set by a managed care organization. Nevertheless, one or both parties may wish that either the therapeutic relationship or a new, personal relationship could continue when a useful change on the part of the patient seems highly unlikely. The patient and the therapist may agree that a hoped-for goal for the treatment will not be realized. These endings are painful to a degree, but they are not traumatic. The limitations of the experience are acknowledged, but there is a sharing in appreciation of the good work. The pain of separation is experienced, but there is little recrimination or bitterness.

▶ Interruption of Psychotherapy: Disagreement

When one or both parties disagree with the ending of psychotherapy, the word "interruption" is a more descriptive designation than is "termination." In some instances, the treatment is ending because of a factor being beyond the control of the patient. For example, the therapist is leaving (relocating for a career move, rotating off residency service), or the financial support for the treatment is withdrawn unexpectedly. In these situations, psychological trauma may be experienced, generally more acutely, by the patient, although losing a therapy case can be a staggering blow to a therapist's self-esteem. In any case, the nature of the felt trauma will be a function of the reason for the interruption and the psychological structure of the injured party.

When the patient initiates a disruption in a treatment, it is important that the therapist remains in his/her role and focused. Despite being shocked, insulted, or frightened, the therapist must help the patient deal with the emotions surrounding the decision. Any impulse to counter with threats or excessively dire predictions must be stifled, perhaps to be worked through in an ad hoc personal therapy encounter for the therapist. Because of the chronic nature of psychopathology, there is a good chance that the patient who interrupts therapy will seek therapy elsewhere, sooner or later. Therapists should always endeavor to make any encounter with a patient as therapeutic as possible.

When the therapist leaves the patient, the scene is ripe for damage to be inflicted on the patient, although the degree of damage can be controlled by sensitive and thoughtful management of the situation. To do so, the therapist must transcend the narcissistic investment in the reason for the interruption. The excitement that one is feeling over an upcoming relocation or graduation or a new baby will not be shared by the patient. The patient will feel variously bereft, abandoned, devalued, jealous, envious, or a plethora of other feelings determined by circumstances and character structure. The patient must be allowed to explore these states and express the attached affects. The therapist must remain in role, acknowledging nondefensively as many of the facts as is consistent with his or her established way of working. The patient's pain is not underestimated, and the patient's individuality is respected within reason as a schedule for the interruption is worked out.

In announcing the interruption, the therapist has two decisions to make: (1) when to announce it and (2) whether transfer to another therapist is indicated. Patients need adequate time to process an interruption, but announcing the interruption too soon may cause the remaining time to be a "lame duck" period in which little is accomplished. Likewise, the patient may be soothed to know that therapy will continue, but the new therapist will immediately assume great importance in the patient's mind even if never met, which will distract the patient from dealing with feelings about the interruption.

In assessing when and how to optimally inform a patient that their treatment will be terminated by changes in the therapist's life, it is essential to review in-depth your work with the patient and how they deal with separations. In some cases, it will be obvious that further treatment will be needed, and the therapist will offer help in locating a replacement therapist. In these cases, the therapist can leave the interruption announcement until relatively late in the sequence. Other patients may not need a replacement therapist. The patient may be near enough to a termination that the work can be truncated. The patient may feel that transfer to a new therapist is not worth the trouble involved. The patient may wish to find further therapy in the future but wants to take a break from the process after the interruption. The therapy will profit from avoiding a premature and unilateral decision to recommend continued treatment. Such a recommendation may be more defensive against the therapist's guilt over leaving than it is sensitive to the patient's individuality. In such situations, where there is a good chance that the patient's therapy experience will end with the interruption, the therapist must give the patient more time. The therapist must assess the patient's record of dealing with separations. Some patients may need several months, and various tapering schedules and other modifications of the usual ways of working may be useful.

The management of an interruption or a termination requires sensitivity and skill. Having had the experience of being in therapy oneself adds immeasurably to the therapist's ability to be sensitive to the importance one attains in the eyes of the patient.

Gutheil TG, Gabbard GO: The concept of boundaries in clinical practice: theoretical and risk-management dimensions. *Am J Psychiatry* 1993;150:188.

Ogden TH: *Subjects of Analysis*. Northvale, NJ: Jason Aronson, 1994.

Strupp H, Binder J: *Psychotherapy in a New Key: A Guide to Time-Limited Psychotherapy*. New York: Basic Books, 1984.

CONCURRENT TREATMENTS

Individual psychotherapy as the sole therapeutic agent is the best treatment for some patients who present themselves to mental health professionals. Individuals with common personality disorders such as narcissistic personality and borderline personality, and those troubled by what may be called disorders of the spirit, are frequently best managed in the containing acceptance of an individual psychotherapy. Such patients may seek psychotherapy from psychologists, social workers, and pastoral counselors, reasoning not only that such professionals are uniquely qualified to help. Some may believe that psychiatrists are not interested in psychotherapy and are only interested in prescribing medication. Although this limited view of psychiatry is true for some psychiatrists, many continue to engage in the practice of psychotherapy.

Many patients, especially those encountered by psychiatrists, need more than individual therapy to manage their conditions. Combined psychotherapy and pharmacotherapy for mood and anxiety disorders has become commonplace. Frequently, the psychiatrist refers some of these patients to a nonpsychiatrist for psychotherapy and continues in a collaborative fashion to prescribe medications. Amidst this sea of change in the perception of the clinical work performed by psychiatrists, it is easy to trivialize truths about the importance of the doctor–patient relationship when the doctor only prescribes medications or provides both medication and psychotherapy. Fortunately, the concept of dynamic pharmacotherapy has provided a framework within which to consider the positive and negative effects of combining psychotherapy and medication.

It is now well established that problems with medication compliance in patients who have chronic illnesses such as bipolar disorder and schizophrenia are common and costly realities in psychopharmacology. The sensitive application of psychotherapeutic principles by psychopharmacologists makes for more successful pharmacotherapy. In some psychotherapies, the psychotherapist's zeal could bias them against potentially helpful pharmacologic agents. Paradoxically, in apparent "therapeutic stalemates," they may prescribe unneeded medications. In many clinical situations, the determination of the need for a psychopharmacologic agent is far from clear-cut. In these situations, many patients do not want to take medication; they only want the physician's time, person, and perceptual, conceptual, and executive skills. Many patients do not like the way medication affects them and fear that the therapist will lose interest in talking to them. Psychotherapists, including psychiatrists, commonly see patients who have been dissatisfied with their experience with a physician who seemed too quick to prescribe medication in lieu of engaging them in even a brief psychotherapy. Psychiatric treatment is clearly more satisfying to all concerned when the physician makes time and has the freedom to prepare a truly patient-oriented treatment plan.

Levey M: *A Clinical Method for Selecting Psychotherapy or Pharmacotherapy in Psychiatry in the New Millennium*, ed by Weissman S, Sabshin M, Eist H. Washington, DC: American Psychiatric Press, 1999.

CONCLUSION

In undertaking to learn the basic principles of psychotherapeutic management, contemporary beginning psychiatric residents and medical students considering psychiatry as a career are inclined to question whether the effort is worthwhile. The ideas and the history of the field intrigue them, but they are overwhelmed by what seems a mysterious skill set, vast in scope and only slowly acquired. They question whether they will be "allowed" (by managed care organizations) to perform psychotherapy. They question whether they or their patients will be able to afford to spend an hour (or any significant portion thereof) together when they can see a nonpsychiatrist or a psychotherapist at less expense. Medical trainees at this level may be reminded that psychiatry as practiced in the emergency room of a city hospital at 3:00 AM, although necessary, represents only a small portion of both the influence they can bring to bear on the toll taken by mental illness and of their future clinical activities.

Advanced psychiatric residents and other advanced mental health students discover in their clinical work and individual growth of the central role of relatedness in the definition of emotional well-being, and they learn to appreciate the pernicious impact of its loss in the manifestations of emotional despair. The road to the recovery of lost human relatedness is through the process of relatedness, and many times this requires a therapist. The quality and meaning of human life, both the professional's and the patient's, derive from relatedness.

Nemiah JC: The idea of a psychiatric education. *J Psychiatr Educ* 1981;5(3):183–194.

Weissman S, Thurnblad R: *The Role of Psychoanalysis in Psychiatric Education: Past, Present and Future*. Madison, WI: International Universities Press, 1987.

Psychopharmacologic Interventions

Lauren Hoffman, PharmD
Richard C. Shelton, MD

Many psychiatric disorders remain without well-established biological substrates; however, standardized diagnostic nosology has gained acceptance, primarily in the form of the *Diagnostic and Statistical Manual of Mental Disorders, Fifth Edition, Text Revision* (DSM-5-TR). As with other areas of medicine, there is no substitute for a careful diagnostic evaluation using externally validated diagnostic criteria. Whenever possible, the diagnostic evaluation should draw on a comprehensive database that includes family members, previous or concurrent providers, and other sources of information, and the evaluation should focus more on longitudinal data than just acute presentation.

PHARMACOKINETICS & PHARMACODYNAMICS

An understanding of the basic pharmacokinetics and pharmacodynamics of psychotropic drugs is required for their safe and effective utilization. These drugs interact with neurotransmitter-binding sites, which confer their psychotropic effects. For example, most antidepressants act by allosteric binding to catecholamine- or indolamine-uptake binding sites (or with the monoaminergic catalytic enzyme monoamine oxidase), which enhances the synaptic availability of monoamines such as norepinephrine and serotonin. These effects can produce direct antidepressant actions but also may produce side effects such as nausea or anxiety. Some drugs can also interact with muscarinic cholinergic-binding sites, producing significant side effects such as dry mouth, blurred vision, and constipation, and with histamine-binding sites, producing drowsiness and weight gain. The relative profile of receptor-binding affinities will allow the clinician to predict both the beneficial effects and side effects of specific drugs.

Many psychotropic drugs are fairly rapidly and completely absorbed from oral and intramuscular sites and, because of their relatively high lipid solubility, readily cross the blood–brain barrier. Intramuscular administration of short-acting injectable medications yields rapid absorption and distribution and bypasses first-pass hepatic metabolism. Therefore, therapeutic plasma levels can be achieved more rapidly. Intramuscular delivery of antipsychotic drugs (e.g., haloperidol, olanzapine, ziprasidone) or antianxiety agents (e.g., lorazepam) is reserved primarily for the acute management of agitated patients or for those without enteral access. An exception to this is the use of long-acting injectable (LAI) antipsychotics such as aripiprazole lauroxil, paliperidone palmitate, haloperidol decanoate, or fluphenazine decanoate. Each LAI has a specific injection frequency which can range from every 2 weeks to every 6 months depending on the formulation. LAIs may help with medication adherence depending on patient-specific factors. For example, they tend to be most helpful for patients who have difficulty remembering to take oral medication on a daily basis or for those who would rather not have oral medication with them whether out of convenience or fear of the stigma associated with taking an antipsychotic. It is important to be mindful of the fact that LAIs cannot be used as a panacea to improve adherence for patients who lack insight into the need for medication or those with other barriers to treatment such as lack of transportation to their appointments.

Many psychotropic drugs can have high levels of protein (e.g., α_1 glycoproteins) binding. Notable exceptions include lithium and venlafaxine. Therefore, drug interactions could occur at the level of protein binding, in which case these drugs will displace (and be displaced by) other drugs with significant binding. This can result in unexpected toxicities; therefore, clinicians should take a careful drug history whenever they plan to prescribe a new drug to a patient.

With the exception of lithium, all psychotropic drugs are metabolized, at least in part, via cytochrome enzymes. After one or more metabolic steps, water-soluble products (e.g., glucuronides) are formed and eliminated via the kidneys. Certain psychopharmacologic agents may induce or inhibit metabolism by cytochrome P-450 (CYP) enzymes.

For example, carbamazepine can induce CYP 3A4, 2B6, 1A2, and 2C9 enzymes, whereas certain selective serotonin reuptake inhibitor (SSRI) antidepressants, such as fluoxetine and paroxetine, may inhibit metabolism via CYP 2D6. These metabolic interactions must be considered when drugs are co-administered.

Psychotropic drugs can produce widely varying plasma levels, and monitoring may be helpful. However, plasma level ranges are established only with certain tricyclic antidepressants (e.g., imipramine, desipramine, nortriptyline), with antipsychotics such as haloperidol and clozapine, with anticonvulsants such as valproic acid and carbamazepine, and with lithium. Because of the narrow therapeutic index, plasma level monitoring of lithium is part of accepted practice. With other drugs, where there are no established plasma level–response relationships, plasma level monitoring can be used to check for adherence or when severe side effects suggest abnormally increased levels. In addition, plasma levels may clarify a situation in which one drug may be increasing or decreasing the level of another. For example, an SSRI such as paroxetine may elevate plasma levels of other drugs that are metabolized by CYP 2D6 (e.g., haloperidol). Unexpected side effects could occur that would be clarified by a plasma level measurement. Laboratory turnaround times for specific tests should be considered prior to ordering, as situations that warrant an immediate clinical decision from the provider may not benefit from results that will only be available days later. In those scenarios, it may be more prudent to be judicious with health care resources and avoid undue burden to the patient, as opposed to obtaining a plasma level that will not actually impact the treatment plan.

Nemeroff CB, DeVane CL, Pollock BG: Newer antidepressants and the cytochrome P450 system. *Am J Psychiatry* 1996;153:311.

Preskorn SH: Clinically relevant pharmacology of selective serotonin reuptake inhibitors: an overview with emphasis on pharmacokinetics and effects on oxidative drug metabolism. *Clin Pharmacokinet* 1997;32(Suppl 1):1.

Preskorn SH, Dorey RC, Jerkovich GS: Therapeutic drug monitoring of tricyclic antidepressants. *Clin Chem* 1988;34:822.

PHARMACOKINETICS IN SPECIAL POPULATIONS

Pharmacokinetics can differ by population. For example, children have a higher relative percentage of hepatic mass and a greater-than-expected elimination of drugs by first-pass metabolism. Older patients often have relatively reduced hepatic clearance and protein binding, which increases the relative plasma levels of most psychotropic drugs. Dosage adjustments must be made for differences in kinetics, and these adjustments should be based on research data, when available.

Pregnancy poses its own set of considerations for treatment as high-quality, controlled trials in this patient population are often lacking. Exposure of women of reproductive potential to psychotropic drugs may raise the possibility of birth defects or spontaneous abortion should pregnancy occur; however, untreated or under-treated mental illnesses can also come with repercussions for mothers and babies. All women of reproductive potential should be counseled about pregnancy and drug exposure. Lithium, anticonvulsant mood-stabilizing agents (e.g., carbamazepine or divalproex), and benzodiazepines have been associated with increased rates of specific birth defects and, generally, should be avoided, especially in the first trimester. The effects of antidepressants and antipsychotics are less clear, except for the case of paroxetine. If the patient is able to safely stop the medication during pregnancy with a low risk for exacerbation of symptoms, that may be the preferred option. Often this may not be possible depending on a variety of factors such as diagnosis, the severity of symptoms, and previously failed medication trials. In fact, some studies demonstrated a relapse rate of up to 70% for women with a history of major depressive disorder who discontinued their antidepressants during pregnancy. A risk–benefit analysis should be undertaken in which the potential risks of drug exposure are weighed against the hazards of strictly using nonpharmacologic therapy. Because the first trimester is the most important period of organogenesis, this may be considered the period of highest risk for many medications. Another consideration is that drugs may be withdrawn prior to delivery and reinstated afterward. This will help prevent untoward reactions such as excessive sedation, withdrawal, or discontinuation reactions in the newborn.

Psychotropic medications can largely be used safely by lactating mothers after the birth of their babies. Most drugs are excreted into breast milk. Drug levels in breast milk tend to be low and often lead to undetectable levels in the infant. The absolute short-term and long-term risks for infants exposed to psychotropic medication via breast milk are unknown. An appropriate risk–benefit discussion should be undertaken with the patient. Providers may refer to the LactMed database via the National Library of Medicine website for more detailed information regarding specific medications.

Altshuler LL, Cohen L, Szuba MP, et al: Pharmacologic management of psychiatric illness during pregnancy: Dilemmas and guidelines. *Am J Psychiatry* 1996;153:592.

Ambrosini PJ: Pharmacotherapy in child and adolescent major depressive disorder. In: Meltzer HY (ed). *Psychopharmacology: The Third Generation of Progress.* New York: Raven Press, 1987, pp. 1247–1254.

Catterson ML, Preskorn SH, Martin RL: Pharmacodynamic and pharmacokinetic considerations in geriatric psychopharmacology. *Psychiatr Clin North Am* 1997;20:205.

Drugs and Lactation Database (LactMed®) [Internet]. Bethesda (MD): National Institute of Child Health and Human Development; 2006. Fact Sheet. Drugs and Lactation Database (LactMed®) Available from: https://www.ncbi.nlm.nih.gov/books/NBK547437/

Payne JL. Psychiatric medication use in pregnancy and breastfeeding. *Obstet Gynecol Clin North Am* 2021 Mar;48(1): 131–149.

Simeon JG: Pediatric psychopharmacology. *Can J Psychiatry* 1989; 34:122.

Stowe ZN, Owens MJ, Landry JC, Kilts CD, Ely T, Llewellyn A, Nemeroff CB: Sertraline and desmethylsertraline in human breast milk and nursing infants. *Am J Psychiatry* 1997;154:1255.

Vitiello B: Treatment algorithms in child psychopharmacology research. *J Child Adolesc Psychopharmacol* 1997;7:3.

PRINCIPLES OF PSYCHOPHARMACOLOGIC MANAGEMENT

Clinical practice involves establishing and maintaining an effective working relationship with a patient—the therapeutic alliance. This process requires the therapist and the patient to establish mutually acceptable goals and to agree on a plan to achieve these objectives. This is especially important in psychiatry because the beneficial effect of a drug may be delayed and because some patients may lack insight into the illness being treated. The challenge of psychopharmacologic management is to maintain an effective working relationship with patients in the face of such obstacles.

The effective pharmacotherapist will maintain a broad biopsychosocial view of the patient and will plan accordingly. Medications will help to address identified symptoms but will not be able to alter psychosocial stressors (e.g., family and work issues) and more purely psychological factors that put the patient at risk for further problems. Pharmacotherapy, therefore, shares significant elements with psychotherapy. The pharmacotherapist must establish rapport and a working relationship with the patient, based on the expertise of the therapist and on mutual trust. It is important to actively engage the patient in shared decision making regarding potential medication trials. This therapeutic alliance can then be leveraged to continue to make any needed adjustments to the medication regimen and provide ongoing education.

▶ Analyzing Risks & Benefits

The risk–benefit analysis considers many factors. The most basic of these factors is the presence of any medical or psychiatric contraindications to the use of a particular drug, including the potential for drug interactions. For example, although bupropion is an effective antidepressant, it generally is not given to patients with an active seizure disorder or a current psychotic condition because the drug has the potential to aggravate these diagnoses. However, bupropion may be a preferred option for patients with concerns regarding sexual dysfunction. Other factors to consider when selecting a medication regimen include affordability and ease of administration. Even the most effective medication will not have any therapeutic benefit for the patient if they are

unable to afford it. Similarly, if multiple daily administrations or food requirements are needed, this also can serve to be a barrier for optimal treatment efficacy. Alternatively, in milder forms of some diagnoses, the pharmacotherapist may determine that medications are not required at all, instead recommending a course of individual or family therapy. The risk–benefit analysis involves the process of maximizing the potential benefits while minimizing the possible harms of pharmacotherapy.

▶ Managing Nonresponse

Lack of complete response to a given treatment is common. The management of nonresponse should begin before treatment is initiated. The clinician should inform the patient of the possibility of nonresponse and the steps that might be taken in such a circumstance. Patients must be warned of the possible delay in response and of the importance of continuing adherence in the face of incomplete improvement. If the response to treatment is inadequate, the clinician should review the treatment plan with the patient and explain to him or her the rationale for each next step. This review should always include setting expectations for both the timeline and the degree of symptom improvement. The risk of the patient to self and others should also be evaluated, especially while making medication adjustments.

▶ Managing Side Effects

The review, documentation, and management of side effects is an important part of pharmacologic treatment. The clinician should inform patients of the possibility of side effects and should review with them those that are common. A general rule of thumb is that any side effect that occurs in 10% or more of patients in clinical trials should be discussed. However, the clinician should address any serious adverse experience, even those that might be rare. For example, although hypothyroidism is an uncommon outcome of lithium treatment, patients should be advised of this possibility. The clinician should review and document the side effects with each patient and undertake a plan to manage unacceptable effects. Most side effects will improve with time, but nonadherence may be the price of ongoing adverse reactions. Due to the wide range in the severity of side effects that the patient may experience, it can be difficult to predict if they will be at a tolerable or intolerable level. The provider may have a patient present to the outpatient clinic who has been experiencing involuntary movements for months, but who only mentions it when directly prompted. Conversely, there may be a patient who experiences such severe gastrointestinal symptoms upon starting an antidepressant, that it takes many failed trials and potentially ancillary medications to make it through the initial titration.

Laboratory evaluations may be required to determine if certain serious reactions have occurred (e.g., hepatotoxicity or nephrotoxicity). Certain drugs may benefit from regular plasma-level monitoring to provide the patient with a margin of safety. Regular absolute neutrophil counts are a requirement for clozapine therapy in order to monitor for agranulocytosis, and annual thyroid-stimulating hormone and serum creatinine tests may be performed for patients on lithium to ensure adequate thyroid and kidney function. Proper medication management can require regularly scheduled laboratory evaluations for many patients.

Addressing Concurrent Alcohol or Drug Use

Another safety issue is the concurrent use of alcohol or drugs of abuse. The clinician must take a careful drug and alcohol history; however, ongoing evaluation of the patient's use also is required. In most cases, alcohol use is not strictly contraindicated while a patient is taking psychotropic drugs; however, patients must be warned of potential drug interactions. Often, this may be the potentiation of the sedative effects of both the alcohol and the prescribed medication such as a benzodiazepine. Other times, the interaction may involve the potential for altered drug metabolism secondary to liver dysfunction, depending on the frequency and the severity of alcohol use. An additional consideration when evaluating substance use is the drug interaction caused by cigarette smoke. The polycyclic aromatic hydrocarbons (PAHs) found in the smoke of burning organic matter, in this case tobacco, cause cytochrome P450 1A2 (CYP1A2) induction. There are numerous medications that are substrates of CYP1A2, but perhaps the most significant are olanzapine and clozapine. The serum levels of both medications will see a significant decrease in situations where a patient begins smoking or resumes use after a period of abstinence. While the data are less robust, there is evidence to suggest that this metabolism induction occurs with the smoke from marijuana as well. This is an important consideration as an increasing number of states are allowing medical and recreational use of this substance. If the patient meets the criteria for a substance use disorder, engaging the patient in motivational interviewing in order to determine readiness for treatment is of paramount importance. In addition to nonpharmacologic approaches, opioid and alcohol use disorders specifically have medication options available to aid in maintaining sobriety.

Evaluating Response

The clinician should target specific symptoms as indicators of response to treatment. In the case of psychosis, the presence and severity of hallucinations or agitation can be effective indicators of early response; however, a more comprehensive view of the patient's condition is required for longer term management. This involves an ongoing evaluation of a variety of symptomatic domains, including cognitive and mood symptoms and social impairments. As a result, symptoms such as occupational impairment may be important indicators of the effectiveness of pharmacotherapy. Whatever the condition, the goal of pharmacotherapy is to minimize or eliminate the symptoms and to return the patient to his or her maximal level of functioning. To this end, the clinician should review and document in each patient the change in a broad range of symptoms.

CONCLUSION

Psychopharmacotherapy ultimately represents a human endeavor in which the challenge to the clinician is the competent synthesis of the scientific basis of pharmacology with the psychosocial skills of the psychiatrist. The most successful pharmacotherapists have a thorough knowledge about the nature of psychiatric disorders, the mechanisms of drug action, and the applications of drug therapies, but they also have remarkable interpersonal skills in the management of patients. This integrative skill set in many ways defines competent contemporary psychiatry.

Anderson GD, Chan LN: Pharmacokinetic drug interactions with tobacco, cannabinoids and smoking cessation products. *Clin Pharmacokinet* 2016;55:1353–1368.

Faber MS, Jetter A, Fuhr U: Assessment of CYP1A2 activity in clinical practice: Why, how, and when? *Basic Clin Pharmacol Toxicol* 2005;97(3):125–134.

Marder SR: Facilitating compliance with antipsychotic medication. *J Clin Psychiatry* 1998;59(Suppl 3):21.

Behavioral and Cognitive–Behavioral Interventions

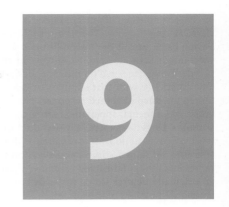

9

Travis Thompson, PhD[†]
Steven D. Hollon, PhD

ROOTS OF BEHAVIORAL & COGNITIVE–BEHAVIORAL INTERVENTIONS

Although their roots can be found at the beginning of the twentieth century, modern behavioral and cognitive–behavioral therapies arose during the 1950s and early 1960s when the scientific study of behavior emerged as a subject with validity in its own right. Disordered behavior was no longer taken to be purely a symptom or indicator of something else going on in the mind. Of inherent concern was its relation to the past and current environmental events thought to be causally related to that behavior. Methods developed in animal laboratories began to be tested—in laboratories, institutional, clinical, and school settings—with people who had chronic mental illnesses or intellectual disabilities and with pre-delinquent adolescents. Improvements in patient behavior and functioning were often striking. These changes took place against a backdrop of growing dissatisfaction with the prevailing notion that psychopathology typically arose from unobservable psychic causes that were assessed and treated using techniques that seemed to be based more on art than science. In addition, an accumulating literature of outcome studies revealed that much of psychotherapy as it had been practiced until the early 1960s, engendered very modest and largely unpredictable results. Thus, contemporary behavior therapies emerged from three distinct psychological traditions: classical or Pavlovian conditioning, instrumental or operant conditioning, and cognitive–behavioral and rational–emotive therapies.

CLASSICAL CONDITIONING

The first major perspective within learning theory approaches is typically referred to as **classical conditioning**. This perspective dates to the first decade of the twentieth century and is largely attributed to the Russian neurophysiologist Ivan

Pavlov. Pavlov was interested in studying the structure of the nervous system, in particular, simple reflex arcs between external events (**stimuli**) and an organism's behavior (**response**). He chose to study salivation in dogs in response to food and developed an apparatus that held the dogs suspended in a harness while a small amount of meat powder was deposited on their tongues. He would vary the amount and the timing of the delivery of the meat powder and recorded the subsequent variation in the nature and the amount of salivation.

What happened next confounded his simple neurologic experiments but opened the way to revolutionary new insights regarding how organisms learn to adapt their behaviors in response to novel environments. Pavlov found that, after a few trials, his dogs began to salivate when strapped into the harness, well in advance of any exposure to the meat powder on a particular trial. Naïve dogs placed in the harness for the first time did not salivate; experienced dogs that had been through the procedure earlier began to salivate well in advance of the delivery of the food. In effect, the dogs' response came to precede the food stimulus, something that could not be explained in terms of a simple reflex arc.

Pavlov's genius lay in recognizing the importance of this observation. He shifted his attention from the study of simple reflex arcs to those conditions necessary to support changes in behavior as a consequence of prior experience, that is, **learning**. He sounded a bell to signal the start of a trial that was followed by the delivery of meat powder and found that he could reliably train the dogs to salivate to the sound of a bell and not to respond to other aspects of the experimental situation. In effect, he introduced a particularly salient stimulus that carried all the predictive information contained in the situation (ringing the bell predicted subsequent delivery of meat powder, whereas nothing happened until the bell was sounded), and the dogs came to salivate reliably only after the bell was rung. Once the bell was established as a particularly informative stimulus, he could occasionally omit the meat powder on subsequent trials, and the dogs continued to salivate to the sound of the bell.

[†]Deceased

This simple paradigm contained the key elements of classical conditioning. The meat powder represented what Pavlov came to call the **unconditioned stimulus**. All dogs with intact nervous systems salivate in response to meat powder being deposited on their tongues, whether they have any experience with that stimulus or not. Salivation represented the **unconditioned response**. The bell (or earlier, the entire experimental apparatus) represented the **conditioned stimulus**. Dogs do not naturally salivate to the sound of a bell, but they come to do so if it is paired with the meat powder (the unconditioned stimulus). Salivation to the bell alone represented the **conditioned response**, a learned response to an originally neutral stimulus that is not found universally among all members of the species.

▶ Early Demonstrations in Humans

J. B. Watson, one of the leading figures in American psychology, recognized the potential relevance of classical conditioning as an explanation for the development of symptoms of psychopathology. Watson and a graduate student conducted a demonstration of how the principles of classical conditioning explicated by Pavlov could be extended to humans. In this study, Watson first showed that a 3-year-old boy called Little Albert had no particular aversion to a small white laboratory rat: He would reach for it and try to pet it, as young children are inclined to do. Watson and his assistant then placed a large gong out of sight behind Little Albert and sounded it loudly every time they brought the rat into the room. Although Little Albert had shown no initial aversion to the rat, he showed a typical startled response to the sounding of the gong (again, as most young children would). Before long, he became upset and burst into tears at the sight of the rat alone and would try to withdraw whenever it was brought into the room.

According to Watson, this study demonstrated that phobic reactions could be acquired purely on the basis of traumatic conditioning. Although Little Albert had previously been intrigued by the presence of the rat and showed no evidence of any fear in its presence, pairing of the rat (the conditioned stimulus) with the loud, and unpredictable noise produced by the gong (the unconditioned stimulus) led him to become anxious and upset in the rat's presence (the conditioned response), just as he had naturally become upset by the sound of the gong (unconditioned response). He had not only acquired a fear response to the rat but also tried to escape from it or avoid exposure to it. According to Watson, Little Albert had acquired the two hallmarks of a phobia (unreasonable fear, and escape or avoidance behaviors) purely as a consequence of simple classical conditioning.

The next major study in the sequence was conducted by Mary Cover Jones in 1924. She reasoned that, if classical conditioning could engender a phobic reaction in an otherwise healthy child, the same laws of learning could be used to eliminate that reaction. She trained a young child to have a conditioned fear response to a small animal (a rabbit) and then proceeded to feed the child in the presence of the rabbit. She found that pairing of the conditioned stimulus (the rabbit) with a second, the unconditioned stimulus (food)—which produced a different unconditioned response (contentment) that was incompatible with the first (anxiety)—came to override the original learning. The child began to relax in the presence of the rabbit and no longer showed the fear response that he had acquired earlier. Thus, Jones argued, she was able to provide relief via **counter-conditioning**.

Despite these early demonstrations, it was several decades before behavioral principles were applied systematically to the treatment of psychiatric disorders. This delay resulted partly from the sense that these procedures were just too simplistic to be of practical use in the treatment of complex human problems. Required were methods based on these learning principles that could be adapted to deal with more complex problems of living. Andrew Salter provided the first such method. In a text that was ahead of its time, Salter described a series of procedures based on the principles of conditioning that were suitable for addressing emotional and behavioral problems in human patients. Although that text attracted little attention when it was published in 1949, it described (in vestigial form) many of the strategies and procedures that would later be used in the clinical practices of behavior therapy.

▶ Applications to Clinical Treatment

Joseph Wolpe provided the first coherent set of clinical procedures, based on the principles of classical conditioning that had a major impact on the field. Wolpe had studied experimental neuroses in cats. In the course of his studies, which involved shocking animals when they tried to feed and observing the results of the conflict this produced, Wolpe replicated the essential features of Jones's earlier attempt to reduce a learned fear via the process of counter-conditioning. He soon extended his work to people with phobic disorders and was able to reduce his patients' distress by pairing the object of their fear with an activity that reliably produced an incompatible response. Like Salter, he experimented with the induction of anger and sexual arousal before finally settling on a set of isometric exercises developed to help reduce stress in patients with heart conditions. This procedure, called **progressive relaxation**, consists of having patients to alternately tense and relax different muscle groups in a systematic fashion and can lead to a state of profound relaxation. The isometric exercises could be paired with the presumably conditioned stimulus (whatever the patients feared) in order to have the new conditioned response (relaxation) override the existing arousal and distress that the patients experienced in the presence of the phobic stimulus.

Wolpe called his approach **systematic desensitization**. In progressive relaxation training, a hierarchy is developed that represents successive degrees of exposure to the feared object or stimulus. For example, a patient with fear of flying might be asked to visualize a variety of scenes that induce differing amounts of anxiety. Simply watching someone else board an airplane might induce only a minimal amount of anxiety, whereas boarding a plane oneself and flying through a thunderstorm would be expected to elicit more anxiety. Wolpe worked with the patient to develop a hierarchy of such imagined experiences and grade them on a scale from 0 to 100 in terms of how much distress they produced. He would then expose the patient to these stimuli (typically in imagination). He proceeded on to the next item in the hierarchy only when the client could tolerate a particular image without experiencing distress. If the patient started to become upset while visualizing an image, Wolpe would instruct the patient to stop the image and reinitiate the relaxation exercises until the feelings of arousal had passed. In this fashion, he systematically worked the patient through the hierarchy of representations of the feared object, proceeding as rapidly as the patient could without experiencing distress until the stimulus no longer elicited any anxiety.

Hundreds of studies have suggested that systematic desensitization (or its variants) is effective in the treatment of phobia and related anxiety-based disorders. Systematic desensitization has been applied widely to a host of problems and represents a safe and effective way of reducing anxious arousal in both adults and children. Major variations include substituting meditation or biofeedback for progressive relaxation as a means of producing the relaxation response (some people do not respond well to muscular isometrics) or arranging experiences in a graduated fashion. The basic approach appears to be robust to these minor modifications and is one of the few examples of a treatment intervention that is truly more effective than other interventions.

▶ Extinction & Exposure Therapy

Despite its evident clinical utility, systematic desensitization is based on a misperception of the laws of classical conditioning. Classical conditioning is essentially ephemeral. Organisms stop responding to the conditioned stimulus when it is no longer paired with the unconditioned stimulus. Pavlov's dogs may have learned to salivate to the ringing of the bell, but if Pavlov kept ringing the bell after it was no longer paired with the meat powder, the dogs soon stopped salivating to its rings. This is referred to as the process of **extinction**, in which conditioned stimuli lose their capacity to elicit a response when they are presented too many times in the absence of the unconditioned stimulus.

This basic feature was considered so troublesome by early behaviorally oriented psychopathologists that they felt compelled to explain how such an ephemeral process could account for a long-lasting disorder such as a phobia (most phobias do not remit spontaneously over time). O. Hobart Mowrer solved the riddle when he postulated that phobic reactions essentially involve two learning processes:

classical conditioning, to instill the anxiety response to a previously neutral stimulus; and operant conditioning, to reinforce the voluntary escape or avoidance behaviors that remove the patient from the presence of the conditioned stimulus before the anxious arousal can be extinguished. In essence, people who acquire a phobic reaction to a basically benign stimulus do not extinguish (as the laws of classical conditioning predict they should), because they do not stay in the situation long enough for classical extinction to take place.

This conclusion led some behavior theorists to suggest that although systematic desensitization was undoubtedly effective, it was unnecessarily complex and time consuming. The essential mechanism of change, they suggested, was extinction, not counterconditioning, and the only procedure needed was to expose the patient repeatedly to the feared object or situation. Of course, the therapist would also have to do something to prevent the patient from running away or otherwise terminating contact with the feared situation. Thus, according to exposure theorists, it was not necessary to ensure that the patients experienced no fear in the presence of the phobic stimulus (as Wolpe claimed). Rather, all that was required was to get them into the situation and to prevent them from leaving until the anxiety had diminished on its own.

Several decades of controlled research have suggested that the extinction theorists were correct and that exposure (plus response prevention) is at least as effective as systematic desensitization and is more rapid in its effects. That does not necessarily mean that it is more useful than systematic desensitization in practice; many patients find exposure therapy very distressing and prefer the gentler alternative provided by systematic desensitization. Although exposure typically works more rapidly than does systematic desensitization (and both work more rapidly than do nonbehavioral alternatives), it often takes as long to persuade a patient to try exposure techniques as it does to complete a full course of systematic desensitization. Nonetheless, it is now clear that exposure (with response prevention) is a sufficient condition for symptomatic change and that Wolpe was in error when he suggested that allowing a patient to experience anxiety in the presence of the phobic situation delayed the process of change. Although patients who already have acquired a conditioned fear response will undoubtedly experience distress when exposed to the object of their fears, and the fact that they become anxious during the course of that exposure neither facilitates nor retards the extinction process. (This is why most behavior therapists no longer use the term "flooding" to refer to exposure therapy; although it may be descriptive of the level of anxiety induced, it is misleading in that it seems to imply that the induction of anxiety is itself curative in some way.)

Exposure plus response prevention have a clear advantage over systematic desensitization (and virtually every other type of nonbehavioral intervention) in the treatment of more complex disorders related to anxiety. It appears to be particularly helpful in the treatment of obsessive–compulsive disorder (OCD) and severe agoraphobia. For example, treatment for a patient who has a fear of contamination and repetitive hand-washing rituals might involve having a therapy team spend a weekend locked in the patient's home, having the patient intentionally contaminate their hands and food with dirt (by shutting off the water to prevent hand washing). Similarly, a patient with severe agoraphobia would be encouraged to visit settings that they typically avoid (e.g., shopping malls or grocery stores) during the busiest times of the day and would be prevented (again by a therapy team or group) from leaving until their anxiety had subsided. Although systematic desensitization has had limited success with such severe disorders, the process of constructing and working through the literally dozens of hierarchies required typically makes the approach wildly impractical.

Summary

Strategies based on classical conditioning have been used in the treatment of depression, somatoform disorders, dissociative disorders, substance abuse, sexual difficulties, medical problems, and a variety of other disorders. In general, these approaches represent some of the most effective of the therapeutic interventions. As is the case with other types of behavioral strategies, they rest on a solid foundation of empirical work, much of it with non-human animals, and on the creative adaptation of those basic principles to human populations.

Kazdin AE, Weisz JR: *Evidence-Based Psychotherapies for Children and Adolescents.* New York: Guilford Press, 2003.

Marks IM: *Fears, Phobias and Rituals.* Oxford, UK: Oxford University Press, 1987.

Rachman S, Hodgson RJ: *Obsession and Compulsions.* New York: Prentice-Hall, 1980.

Wilson GT: Behavior therapy. In: Corsini RJ, Wedding D (eds). *Current Psychotherapies*, 5th edn. Itasca, IL: FE Peacock Publishing, 1995, pp. 197–228.

Wolpe J: *Psychotherapy by Reciprocal Inhibition.* Palo Alto, CA: Stanford University Press, 1958.

EMERGENCE OF INSTRUMENTAL & OPERANT LEARNING THEORY

As a graduate student at Columbia University, Edward Thorndike began a series of experiments that set a new course in the study of processes underlying behavior change and learning. He placed a cat in an enclosed chamber and attached a vertical pole in the center of the compartment to a rope that passed over several pulleys. When the cat bumped against the pole, the pole would tilt, causing the rope to open the door. The cat could then leave the compartment and drink milk from a nearby bowl outside the cage. At first, the cat seemed to move about unpredictably each time it was returned to the compartment. The time required for the cat to tilt the pole

grew shorter on successive repetitions of the task, and the cat's method for opening the door on each trial became progressively similar to the method used on the preceding trial. The trial-by-trial record of time to escape from what Thorndike called his "puzzle box" was the first instrumental learning curve published in a scientific journal. Eventually, each cat quickly approached the pole—seemingly purposively—and tilted it to one side, opening the door. Thorndike described this as an **instrumental conditioning** process because the pole tilting was instrumental in releasing the cat from the chamber and permitting access to a reward. Thorndike's method differed from Pavlov's classical conditioning because no specific response was elicited by a conditioned stimulus. The form of each cat's behavior that tilted the pole was idiosyncratic and variable. There was nothing fixed about the behavior, as was typical of classically conditioned behavior. Thorndike's Law of Effect described the necessary and sufficient conditions for instrumental learning to occur.

Skinner & Operant Behavior

Whereas Thorndike studied the process of behavior change, three decades later, B. F. Skinner, a graduate student at Harvard University, was interested in discovering a method for identifying the functional components of sequences of behavior. Skinner was drawn to the writings of the physiologists Charles Sherrington and Ernst Magnus. Skinner was particularly taken with Sherrington's notion of the reflex arc. He believed that psychologists had gotten seriously off on the wrong track by focusing on unobservable phenomenological events, which no amount of experimentation could verify, rather than following the example of physiology in studying observable events. Skinner wondered whether Thorndike's Law of Effect might explain how a single component could be isolated from the continuously free-flowing activities of an organism, so that the component could be studied scientifically, much as Sherrington had done. Using a method very similar to Thorndike's, Skinner placed a rat in an enclosed chamber, and each time the rat depressed a telegraph key protruding through the wall of the chamber, a pellet of food dropped into a receptacle near the rat. The lever-pressing methods each rat used varied: most pressed with their paws, some pushed with their muzzles, and others held the telegraph key between their teeth and pulled down. All methods produced the same result—the delivery of a pellet of food that the hungry rats seized and ate. Skinner said that the rat "operated" on its environment to produce reinforcing consequences, and the type of behavior was correspondingly called **operant behavior**.

In operant behavior, typically no stimulus was presented before an operant response that "caused" the behavior to occur (i.e., there was no conditioned stimulus). When Skinner analyzed the sequence of the rats' activities in an operant chamber, he found that after many repetitions when a rat approached the lever, depressed it, and heard the device click, which had been followed by food pellet presentation, the click sound produced by the lever press began to be rewarding without food pellet presentation. If a light were illuminated above the lever (indicating periods when food would be available), alternating with periods when the light was off (indicating lever presses would not produce food), soon the rat pressed nearly exclusively when the light was illuminated. The rat's behavior continued to be variable, changing from moment to moment even when the light was illuminated, unlike a classically conditioned reflex. Skinner called the food pellet a **reinforcer** and the light that signaled that operant responding would lead to reinforcer presentation a **discriminative stimulus**. Skinner spelled out in surprisingly accurate detail, the laws of operant conditioning that have stood the test of time. Immediacy, magnitude, and the intermittency of reinforcement affected the pattern of behavior maintained and also determined the persistence of behavior in the absence of reinforcement.

Skinner also observed that a stimulus repeatedly paired with food presentation (e.g., the "click" sound of the food pellet dispenser) came to serve as a reinforcer in its own right and would maintain considerable amounts of behavior over extended periods of time in the absence of a primary reinforcement. Such previously neutral stimuli that took on reinforcing properties because of their pairing with primary reinforcers were called **conditioned reinforcers** or **secondary reinforcers**. Skinner recognized that, in most developed parts of the world, relatively limited aspects of human conduct seem to be directed toward seeking food or shelter. Instead, most human conduct seems to be governed by parent or teacher approval, threat of loss of affection, or symbols of recognition from employers or peers (e.g., paychecks, awards). Skinner reasoned that these reinforcers had developed their reinforcing properties (usually very early in an individual's life) from their repeated pairing with primary reinforcers. In short, they were powerful conditioned reinforcers. This observation led later educators, drug abuse counselors, psychologists, and psychiatrists working in applied settings to develop treatment methods based on conditioned reinforcers such as social approval or concrete objects paired with other reinforcers (e.g., check marks, stars, tokens, money).

▶ Applications to Clinical Treatment

The practical utility of the operant apparatus and measurement approach was adopted quickly in experimental psychology, physiology, neurochemistry, pharmacology, and toxicology laboratories throughout the world. The methodology provided the springboard for the field of behavioral pharmacology, the study of sub-cortical self-stimulation, animal models of addictive behavior, and the study of psychophysics and complex human social behavior in enclosed experimental spaces. Skinner's pragmatic theory struck a popular chord with many young psychologists, special educators, and practitioners in training. In 1948, Sidney Bijou began an applied research program and experimental

nursery school for children with intellectual disability at the Rainier School in Washington, applying operant principles. Bijou was joined by Donald Baer, a recent graduate of the University of Chicago, and they conducted seminal research on early child operant behavior. In 1953, Ogden Lindsley and Skinner began applying operant methods to study the behavior of patients with schizophrenia at the Metropolitan State Hospital in Waltham, Massachusetts.

Several major events brought the emerging field of behavior modification to the attention of psychiatry. First, Teodoro Ayllon and Nathan Azrin were granted limited funds in 1961 for an experimental program to motivate and improve the functioning of a group of severely mentally ill, mostly schizophrenic, women who were institutionalized in Illinois. The program used a token reinforcement system originally developed by Roger Kelleher, who had studied the behavior of chimpanzees in laboratory settings. Tokens resembling poker chips were given to patients immediately after they completed agreed-upon therapeutic activities. Later the tokens could be exchanged for supplementary preferred activities or commodities. The changes in patient behavior were often dramatic and included markedly increased participation in therapeutic programs such as those aimed at employment, bathing, self-care, and related daily living skills.

Leonard Ullman headed a similar treatment unit in Palo Alto, California. Both programs operated on the principle that chronically and mentally ill patients, primarily those with schizophrenia, had been largely unresponsive to conventional psychological therapeutic methods. Although older neuroleptic medications managed many of the florid symptoms of schizophrenia, they did little to increase the patients' general adjustment and often produced problematic side effects. These programs demonstrated that it was possible to use laboratory-based management methods to motivate patients with chronic schizophrenia, increasing their participation in hospital therapeutic programs and decreasing the amount of disturbed behavior. Although no one claimed these methods changed the underlying disorder, they were very effective tools for improving patient compliance and management.

A less frequently cited but still important study conducted during this era was Gordon Paul and coworkers' comparison of the effectiveness of a social learning theory approach to that of a more traditional milieu therapy approach to managing the behavior of patients with chronic mental illnesses in an institutional setting. It is the single best study of its kind, demonstrating persuasively the effectiveness of a behavior therapy strategy for activating socially resistant patients who have schizophrenia. It also carefully documented reductions in schizophrenic disorganization and cognitive distortion; improvements in normal speech and social interactions; reductions in social isolation; and greatly reduced aggressive, assaultive, and other intolerable behavior.

The second major event was the demonstration in 1963 by Ivar Lovaas, a clinical psychologist working at UCLA, that positive reinforcement methods could be used to teach children with autism a variety of skills. Until that time, there were no known effective treatments for autism. Lovaas worked with children who were mute and with echolalic children who had autism (labeled "schizophrenic children" at that time). These children were severely intellectually disabled, were self-injurious, displayed severe tantrums, and were extremely noncompliant. Lovaas used a combination of hugs and praise, edible reinforcers, and highly controversial aversive stimulation techniques to reduce self-destructive behavior. In 1987, Lovaas published a report in which he used an intensive behavioral treatment regimen (40 hours per week of one-to-one contact), targeting language and social skills. He reported that 47% of the experimental group (9 of 19 children) functioned similar to typical peers after 2–3 years of treatment, compared with 2% of the control group. In 1993, he published a follow-up on those children at age 12 and found that of the 9 children with the best outcomes, 8 continued to function in the normal range. Lovaas was the first researcher to document such marked improvement in such a large proportion of treated children with autism; however, other interventions using similar methods of behavior analysis appear to produce similar results.

The third major event that paved the way for modern behavior therapy methods was the work of Gerald Patterson and colleagues in developing a coercion model of the relationships between families and their children with conduct disorder. In the early and mid-1960s, Patterson began working with children of normal intelligence who displayed a wide array of predelinquent behavior. Some of the children displayed characteristics of attention-deficit/hyperactivity disorder (ADHD), others seemed to have learning disabilities, and others were aggressive and noncompliant at home and school but exhibited no indications of other psychiatric or cognitive disability. On the basis of a series of laboratory and clinical studies, Patterson and his colleagues proposed that children who had conduct disorder and their families gradually learn a set of mutually coercive relationships based on interpersonal aversive stimulation and avoidance. On the basis of this model, he developed a behavioral treatment method drawing on basic operant methods (i.e., positive, social and tangible reinforcement and loss of reinforcement resulting from behavior problems, both of which were based on unambiguous and consistent contingencies). He combined these techniques with what would later be called cognitive–behavioral therapy methods (i.e., the use of verbal self-instruction to mediate behavior change).

Finally, in the late 1960s and early 1970s several large-scale programs were developed that applied operant behavioral principles in residential services for people with intellectual disability. These early institution-based programs paved the way for subsequent community-based services and treatment programs for people with intellectual disability, especially those with significant behavior problems.

Cooper JO, Heron TE, Heward WL: *Applied Behavior Analysis*, 2nd edn. New York: Prentice Hall, 2006.

Lord C, McGee J(eds): *Educating Children with Autism*. Washington DC: Commission on Behavioral and Social Sciences and Education of the National Academy of Sciences, 2001.

Patterson GR, Gullion ME: *Living with Children: New Methods for Parents and Teachers*. Champaign, IL: Research Press, 1968.

Skinner BF: *Science and Human Behavior*. New York: Macmillan, 1953.

COGNITIVE & COGNITIVE–BEHAVIORAL INTERVENTIONS

One of the major changes in behavioral approaches in the past several decades has been the emergence of the cognitive and cognitive–behavioral intervention. Based largely on social learning theory, these approaches posit that organisms are not just the passive recipients of stimuli that impinge on them but instead interpret and try to make sense out of their worlds. These approaches do not reject traditional classical and operant perspectives on learning; rather, they suggest that cognitive mediation plays a role in coloring the way those processes work in humans and other higher vertebrates.

▶ Roots of Cognitive Therapy

The roots of cognitive therapy can be found in the early writings of the Stoic philosophers Epictetus and Marcus Aurelius, and in the later works by Benjamin Rush and Henry Maudsley, among others. It was Epictetus who wrote, in the first century AD, "People are disturbed not by things, but the view which they take of them." Benjamin Rush, the father of American psychiatry, wrote in 1786 that by exercising the rational mind through practice, one gained control over the otherwise unmanageable passions that he believed led to some forms of madness. A century later, Henry Maudsley reiterated the notion that it was the loss of power over the coordination of ideas and feelings that led to madness and that the wise development of control over thoughts and feelings could have a powerful effect. In modern times, Alfred Adler's approach to dynamic psychotherapy was cognitive in nature, stressing the role of perceptions of the self and the world in determining how people went about the process of pursuing their goals in life. George Kelly is often accorded a central role in laying out the basic tenets of the approach, and Albert Bandura's influential treatise on learning theory provided a theoretical basis for incorporating observational learning in the learning process.

▶ Modern Approaches

Modern cognitive and cognitive–behavioral approaches to psychotherapy got their impetus from two converging lines of development. One branch was developed by theorists originally trained in dynamic psychotherapy. Theorists such as Albert Ellis, the founder of rational–emotive therapy, and Aaron Beck, the founder of cognitive therapy, began their careers adhering to dynamic principles in theory and therapy. They became disillusioned with that approach and came, over time, to focus on their patients' conscious beliefs. Both subscribe to an ABC model, which states that it is not just what happens to someone at point A (the antecedent events) that determine how the person feels and what they do at point C (the affective and behavioral consequences), but that it also matters how the person interprets those events at point B (the person's beliefs). For example, a man who loses a relationship and is convinced that he was left because he is unlovable is more likely to feel depressed and fail to pursue further relationships than one who considers his loss a consequence of bad luck or the product of mistakes that he will not repeat the next time around. Both theorists work with patients to actively examine their beliefs to be sure that they are not making situations worse than they necessarily are. Ellis typically adopts a more philosophical approach based on reason and persuasion, whereas Beck operates more like a scientist, treating his patients' beliefs as hypotheses that can be tested and encouraging his patients to use their own behavior to test the accuracy of their beliefs.

The other major branch of cognitive behaviorism involves theorists originally trained as behavior therapists who became increasingly interested in the role of thinking in the learning process. Bandura and Michael Mahoney represent two exemplars of this tradition, as do other theorists such as Donald Meichenbaum and G. Terence Wilson. These theorists tend to stay closer to the language and the tenets of traditional behavior analysis and are somewhat less likely to talk about the role of meaning in their patients' responses to events. They are also as likely to focus on the absence of cognitive mediators (i.e., covert self-statements) as on the presence of distortions. For example, Meichenbaum developed an influential approach to treatment, called self-instructional training, in which patients with impulse-control problems are trained to modulate their own behavior via the process of verbal self-regulation.

These approaches focus on the role of information processing in determining subsequent effect and behavior. Beck, for example, has argued that distinctive errors in thinking can be found in each of the major types of psychopathologies. For example, depression typically involves negative views of the self and the future; anxiety, an over-determined sense of physical or psychological danger; eating disorders, an undue concern with shape and weight; and obsessions, an overbearing sense of responsibility for ensuring the safety of oneself and others. Efforts to produce change involve having the patient first monitor fluctuations in mood and relate those changes to the ongoing flow of automatic thoughts, subsequently using one's own behavior to test the accuracy of these beliefs. For example, a depressed patient who believes that they are incompetent will be asked to provide

an example of something they should be able to do but cannot. The patient is then invited to list the steps that anyone else would have to do to carry out the task. The patient is then encouraged to carry out those steps just to determine whether they are as incompetent as they believe (typically, the patient is not).

Similarly, patients with panic disorders often misinterpret innocuous bodily sensations as signs of impending physical or psychological catastrophe, such as having a heart attack or "going crazy." The therapist provides a rationale that stresses the role of thinking in symptom formation and encourages the patient to test their beliefs in the imminence of the impending catastrophe by inducing a panic attack right in the office. As the patient experiences extreme states of arousal and panic with no subsequent consequences (i.e., neither dying nor "going crazy"), they come to recognize that the initial arousal is not a harbinger of impending doom (as first believed), and the patient no longer begins to panic at the occurrence of arousal. In essence, like the behavioral approaches based on classical conditioning, modern cognitive and cognitive–behavioral interventions emphasize the curative process of exposing oneself to the things one most fears as a way of dealing with irrational or unrealistic concerns.

These approaches are well established in the treatment of unipolar depression, panic disorders, social phobias, generalized anxiety disorders, and bulimia. For these disorders, cognitive and cognitive–behavioral interventions appear to be at least as effective as other competing alternatives (including medication) and quite possibly more enduring. There are consistent indications that cognitive–behavioral therapy produces long-lasting change that reduces the likelihood that symptoms will return after treatment ends. The evidence is mixed with respect to substance abuse, marital distress, and childhood conduct disorder, although at least some indications are promising. Cognitive and cognitive–behavioral interventions are typically not thought to be particularly effective in patients who have formal thought disorder, although recent studies suggest that such interventions may reduce delusional thinking in psychotic patients who receive neuroleptic drugs.

Beck AT: *Cognitive Therapy and the Emotional Disorders*. Madison, CT: International Universities Press, 1976.

Ellis A: *Reason and Emotion in Psychotherapy*. New York: Lyle Stuart, 1962.

Hollon SD, Beck AT: Cognitive and cognitive behavioral therapies. In: Lambert MJ (ed). *Garfield and Bergin's Handbook of Psychotherapy and Behavior Change: An Empirical Analysis*, 5th edn. New York: Wiley, 2004, pp. 447–492.

Meichenbaum D: *Cognitive-Behavior Modification: An Integrative Approach*. New York: Plenum, 1977.

O'Donohue WO, Fisher JE, Hayes SC: *Cognitive Behavior Therapy: Applying Empirically Supported Techniques in Your Practice*. New York: Wiley, 2003.

FUNDAMENTAL ASSUMPTIONS OF THERAPIES BASED ON LEARNING THEORY

Several basic assumptions are common to most learning-based interventions. Perhaps most fundamental is that the behavior of the individual who has been referred for psychiatric treatment is of concern in its own right. Behavior is not necessarily an indication of pathology at some other level of analysis (e.g., brain chemical or psychic). Pathologic behavior is often seen as the result of the demands of the environment in which the person is living, working, or going to school (or, in the case of the cognitive approaches, the person's perception of the environment). What appears to be pathologic may be a person's best adaptation to an impossible situation given the person's cognitive or personality limitations (e.g., living with alcoholic parents, residing in an abusive institutional or community residential setting, interacting with people who do not use the same communication system).

Although major mental illnesses have neurochemical substrates, much of the pathologic behavior observed by psychiatrists has been learned in much the same way that normal behavior is learned. Pathologic behavior generally follows the same scientific laws as normal behavior. Vulnerability to learning pathologic behavior is shaped by the biological substrate of inherited traits and neurochemical predispositions upon which the collective history of experiences is imposed. Individual differences in normal and pathologic behavior are attributable to dispositions created by variations in genetic makeup or differences in histories that predispose an individual to differences in motivation. Some people, by virtue of their genetic and associated neurochemical makeup, are prone to respond to mild, negative comments by other people as though such comments were aversive and to be avoided at all costs. Others, with different genetic makeup and correspondingly different neurochemical predisposition, may be largely impervious to similar negative reinforcers and cues. The former individuals are prone to develop avoidant behavior and extreme anxiety, whereas the latter individuals tend to be insensitive to aversive social situations.

In the early days of behavior modification and behavior therapy treatments, targets of treatment were often circumscribed responses (e.g., nail-biting, failing in school, encopresis). Since then, researchers have recognized that narrowly defined instances of pathologic behavior (i.e., presenting symptoms) are usually members of larger classes of problematic responses. The treatment task is not to treat the isolated behavior (e.g., arguing with parents or making self-deprecating remarks) but rather to identify the factors that determine the likelihood that any one of an entire class of responses may occur. Such factors could include, for example, the child having no legitimate mechanism for determining what is going on in their lives, combined with parental submission to unpleasant, coercive responses. Failure to assess properly the full breadth of the members composing a functional response class could lead to symptom substitution. For example, the successful reduction of arguing by a defiant teenager by implementing a behavioral contract limited to arguing will, in most instances, lead to the emergence of other defiant behaviors (e.g., staying out beyond a curfew, experimenting with alcohol). The task is to identify a broader class of problem behavior, develop hypotheses concerning the purposes served by that class of behavior, and then develop an intervention plan that makes the entire class of behavior ineffective and unnecessary.

Most of the causes of pathologic behavior are found in the relation between the individual, the environmental antecedents, and the consequences of their actions. An individual's history creates the context within which current environmental circumstances serve as either discriminative stimuli (e.g., a spouse coming home late from work) or conditioned negative reinforcers (e.g., threatened disapproval). An individual's history could also establish the motivational framework that governs most of the individual's actions. As a result, assessment usually requires obtaining information from the individual or other informants about events taking place in the individual's natural environment in order to obtain valid data concerning the circumstances surrounding the pathologic behavior. The meaning of an environmental cue or a putative motivating consequence is determined contextually. Whether a social stimulus is alarming, neutral, or positive will depend on the person's history and the circumstances in which the stimulus is being experienced. Similarly, a consequence can be positive, neutral, or negative depending on the individual's history and the circumstances in which the consequence is encountered. Thus, Thorndike's original Law of Effect has been contextualized. Whether this contextualization is conceptualized as residing in the cognitive domain or in the observable environment is a matter of some theoretical dispute, but the learning-based approaches emphasize idiosyncratic experiences as the shaper of behavioral proclivities.

Bandura A: *Principles of Behavior Modification.* Austin, TX: Holt, Rinehart & Winston, 1969.

Craighead WE, Craighead LW, Ilardi SS: Behavior therapies in historical perspective. In: Bonger BM, Buetler LE (eds). *Comprehensive Textbook of Psychotherapy: Theory and Practice.* Oxford, UK: Oxford University Press, 1995.

Kazdin AE: *History of Behavior Modification: Experimental Foundations of Contemporary Research.* Baltimore, MD: University Park Press, 1978.

Krasner L: History of behavior modification. In: Bellack AS, Hersen M, Kazdin AE (eds). *International Handbook of Behavior Modification and Therapy*, 2nd edn. Springer, 1990, pp. 3–25.

COMBINATIONS WITH MEDICATION

Many of the disorders treated with behavioral or cognitive–behavioral therapy can also be treated pharmacologically, although some cannot. In some disorders, a combination of drugs and behavioral (or cognitive–behavioral) therapy is more effective than either alone. For example, stimulant medication and cognitive–behavioral therapy produces greater behavioral improvements than either treatment alone among many children with ADHD. Combined treatment for depression retains the rapidity and the robustness of the medication response and the enduring effects of cognitive or behavioral treatment. Despite the theoretically based concerns of advocates for each approach, one modality rarely interferes with the other, although such interference sometimes occurs. For many disorders, there simply are not adequate data to guide clinical practices; we often know that both modalities are effective in their own right but do not know whether their combination enhances treatment response.

Drugs and other somatic interventions appear to be essential to the treatment of the more severe disorders, particularly those that involve psychotic symptoms. Nonetheless, behavioral and cognitive–behavioral interventions can often play an important adjunctive role. Recent studies indicate that D-cycloserine administered during exposure therapy for phobias facilitates extinction of the exaggerated fear response to the phobic stimulus. Antipsychotic medications remain the most effective means of reducing the more florid symptoms of psychosis, and the newer, atypical antipsychotics show promise in relieving the negative symptoms of schizophrenia. Rehabilitation programs based on behavioral skills training appear to help redress impairments in psychosocial functioning in such patients and may allow the use of newer low-dose neuroleptic medications (see Chapter 15). Lithium and anticonvulsants provide the most effective means of treatment of the bipolar disorders, but cognitive–behavioral therapy can enhance compliance with drug therapy (see Chapter 17).

The relative importance of pharmacotherapy is less pronounced among even the more severe, nonpsychotic disorders and quite possibly is nonexistent among the less severe disorders. Cognitive therapy appears to be about as effective as pharmacotherapy for all but the most severe nonbipolar depressions and may be more enduring in its effect (see Chapter 17). Exposure-based therapies are quite helpful in reducing compulsive rituals in OCD (see Chapter 20) and behavioral avoidance in severe agoraphobia (see Chapter 18). Such therapies are often combined with medication to treat these disorders. Cognitive–behavioral therapy appears to be at least as effective and possibly longer-lasting than pharmacotherapy in the treatment of panic disorders and social phobia (see Chapter 18), and the same can be said with respect to the treatment of bulimia (see Chapter 25). Exposure-based treatment is clearly superior to pharmacotherapy (or any other form of psychotherapy) in the treatment of social phobia. There is little evidence that drugs are particularly helpful in the treatment of the personality disorders (see Chapter 29); however, a dialectic-type behavior therapy appears to reduce the frequency of self-destructive behavior in patients with borderline personality disorder.

In general, the more severe the psychopathologic disorder, the greater the relative efficacy of pharmacotherapy and the more purely behavioral the psychosocial intervention should be. Medication is often useful to control disruptive symptoms, but behavioral interventions (especially operant ones) are uniquely suited to promoting new skills or restoring those that have been lost to illness or institutionalization. Behavioral interventions based on classical conditioning are particularly helpful in reducing undesirable states of arousal and affective distress; cognitive interventions reduce the likelihood of a subsequent relapse by correcting the erroneous beliefs and attitudes that contribute to recurrence. These strategies rarely interfere with one another. It is often useful to combine them in practice to achieve multiple ends.

Klerman GL, Weissman MM, Makkowitz JC, et al.: Medication and psychotherapy. In: Bergin AE, Garfield SL (eds). *Handbook of Psychotherapy and Behavior Change*, 4th edn. Hoboken, NJ: Wiley, 1994, pp. 734–782.

Panksepp J: *Textbook of Biological Psychiatry*. New York: Wiley-Liss, 2003.

Reiff MI, Tippin S: *ADHD: A Complete and Authoritative Guide*. Elk Grove Village, IL: American Academy of Pediatrics, 2004.

COMBINED INTERVENTIONS IN DEVELOPMENTAL DISABILITIES

Behavioral interventions can be highly effective in improving the quality of life for people who have developmental disabilities and display serious behavior problems. Sometimes behavioral methods are insufficient by themselves. Psychopharmacologic treatments can control psychopathologic symptoms and behavior in some people with intellectual and related disabilities (e.g., ADHD, major depression, bipolar disorder, anxiety disorder, schizophrenia) in nondevelopmentally delayed individuals.

In elucidating how psychotropic drugs reduce problem behavior, it is helpful to examine the behavioral as well as the neurochemical mechanisms of drug action. Behavioral mechanisms refer to psychological or behavioral processes altered by a drug. Neurochemical mechanisms refer to the receptor-level events that are causally related to those changed behavioral processes. Some psychopathologic problems are associated so frequently with specific developmental disabilities that pharmacotherapy is among the first treatments to be explored. Anxiety disorder, especially OCD, is commonly associated with autism and Prader-Willi syndrome. Anxiety disorder manifests itself as ritualistic, repetitive stereotypic motor responses (e.g., rocking or hand-flapping) and rigidly routinized activities (e.g., repeatedly lining up blocks, insisting that shoelaces be precisely the same length) that, if interrupted, provoke behavioral outbursts or tantrums. Selective serotonin reuptake inhibitors alleviate agitation, anxiety, and ritualistic behavior, such as skin-picking and self-injurious behavior. At times, aggression results from an anxiety disorder. For example, a patient with autism who has severe anxiety may strike out against others who are crowding too closely, in order to keep them at a distance. Fluvoxamine reduces anxiety and the need for increased social distance, thereby diminishing the need to strike out against others to keep them at a distance. Aggression, in this example, serves as a social avoidance response that fluvoxamine renders unnecessary. The behavioral mechanism of action is the reduction of anxiety and associated avoidance. The neurochemical mechanism is thought to be mediated by the inhibition of serotonin reuptake with increased binding to the serotonin-2 receptors.

An individual with autism or intellectual disability who strikes his or her head in intermittent bouts throughout the day may do so because head blows cause the release of β-endorphin, which binds to the μ-opiate receptor, thereby reinforcing self-injury. In this way, a self-addictive, vicious cycle is established and maintained and through years of repetition becomes a firmly entrenched behavioral pattern. An opiate antagonist, such as naltrexone, blocks the reinforcing effects consequent to the binding of β-endorphin to the opiate receptor. Naltrexone reduces self-injurious behavior in approximately 40% of patients, primarily in those engaging in high-frequency, intense self-injury directed at the head and hands. Evidence indicates that elevated baseline levels of plasma β-endorphin after bouts of self-injury are predictive of a therapeutic response to naltrexone.

Repetitive self-injurious behavior, such as head banging and self-biting, can be treated effectively with complementary behavioral and pharmacologic strategies, as described in the following case example.

A 13-year-old boy with autism and severe intellectual disability had no communication system at baseline. An observational functional assessment of the boy's self-injurious behavior in his natural environment (a special education classroom) indicated that approximately two thirds of this behavior was motivated by the desire to obtain attention or to escape from situations he did not like or found disturbing. Self-injury dropped 50% from baseline during the first naltrexone treatment phase. Next the patient was taught to use pictorial icons to make requests and indicate basic needs to others around him (Figure 9–1). His self-injury dropped subsequently by another 50% (i.e., a reduction of a total of 75% from baseline) when communication treatment was initiated. On follow-up 1 year later, during which time naltrexone treatment had continued, the boy's self-injurious behavior had dropped to nearly zero. In this case, naltrexone blocked the neurochemical reinforcing consequences of self-injury, and communication training provided an appropriate behavioral alternative to indicate basic needs and wants. In short, combined treatment produced complementary, additive salutary effects.

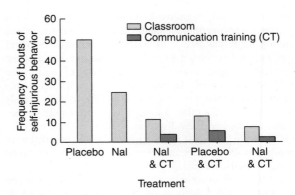

▲ **Figure 9–1** Efficacy of treatment for self-injurious behavior. Nal, naltrexone.

Emerson E, Hatton C, Parmeter T, Thompson T(eds): *International Handbook of Applied Research in Intellectual Disabilities.* Chichester, UK: Wiley, 2004.

Kelley ME, Fisher WW, Lomas JE, et al.: Some effects of stimulant medication on response allocation: A double-blind analysis. *J Appl Behav Anal* 2006;39:243–247.

Thompson T, Moore T, Symons F: Psychotherapeutic medications and positive behavior support. In: Odom S, Horner R, Snell M, Blacher J (eds). *Handbook on Developmental Disabilities.* New York: Guilford Press, 2007.

CONCLUSION

Modern behavioral and cognitive–behavioral interventions emphasize the role of learning and adaptation to the environment in shaping and maintaining normal life functions and in the emergence of maladaptive symptomatology. These interventions treat behavior as important in its own right and often seek to change instances of disordered behavior by the application of clearly articulated, basic principles of learning. There are three fundamental, interrelated perspectives: classical conditioning, which emphasizes the learning of associations between classes of stimuli; operant conditioning, which emphasizes the learning of relations between behaviors and their consequences; and the cognitive perspective, which emphasizes the role of idiosyncratic beliefs and misconceptions in coloring each of the two earlier perspectives. Learning-based approaches have sparked a major revolution in the treatment of psychiatric disorders. Each perspective can point to notable gains. Behavioral approaches can often be combined beneficially with medication and should be part of the armamentarium of any well-trained clinician.

Brain Stimulation Therapies

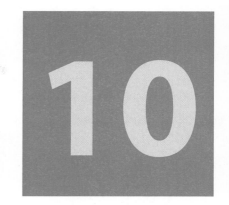

Christopher W. Austelle, MD
Edmund S. Higgins, MD
Mark S. George, MD

INTRODUCTION

Overview

The field of brain stimulation has emerged as an essential part of psychiatric practice based on research activity across basic and clinical domains. Stimulation techniques are a unique and complementary form of treatment distinctly different from pharmacology, psychotherapy or physical therapy. This chapter will give readers an overview of the current state of brain stimulation therapies, including clinical applications and emerging research directions.

The Brain as an Electrical Organ

Electricity is the currency of the brain. The ability of the brain to coordinate complex behaviors relies on inherent electrical-chemical functions of individual neurons. Psychiatrists tend to focus almost exclusively on the chemical part of the process, but the electrical aspect deserves equal attention. The neuron is the basic unit of *decision* in the brain. It all boils down to the ability of each neuron to generate an action potential—or not. The neuron can receive thousands of inputs from surrounding nerve cells. Some neurons are excitatory, meaning they raise the electrical polarity of (depolarize) the neurons they stimulate. Others are inhibitory, meaning they reduce the polarity of (hyperpolarize) the neuron, so the neuron is less likely to fire. Whether the neuron responds is based on the sum of all those inputs and how that alters the electrical charge within its membrane moment to moment. If a neuron receives sufficient depolarizing inputs, it will fire an action potential and transmit the electrical signal distally to its synaptic terminals (see Figure 10–1).

With nearly 100 billion neurons and trillions of signals being processed every second, the brain is literally buzzing with electricity. Brain stimulation interventions tap into this basic function in order to affect the electrical excitation or the inhibition and treat neuropsychiatric disorders.

Overview of Parameters and Approaches to Brain Stimulation

The goal of treatment with brain stimulation is to apply enough electricity to the brain, but no more than is needed. All treatment modalities have a specific range of voltage (intensity of the electrical charge), frequency (number of pulses delivered per second), or duty cycle (on/off time) used to treat psychiatric disorders. Duration of the electrical stimulation as well as the intertrain interval, or the time between "jolts," also impacts the effectiveness of treatment. Clinicians can manipulate the parameters (although not all in every modality), effectively adjusting the dose of electricity that the brain receives during treatment (see Figure 10–2). Over time, brain stimulation treatments have become more efficient in their delivery of electricity to the brain, utilizing less electrical charge and in a more focal manner.

Similarly, each brain stimulation method has specific characteristics that influence the way it is used and the effect it has on the patient. Some methods are more invasive and require surgical placement of electrodes, like deep brain stimulation (DBS) or invasive vagus nerve stimulation (VNS). Others are noninvasive and can stimulate the brain from outside of the body, like transcranial magnetic stimulation (TMS). The invasive modalities tend to deliver electricity to the brain intermittently all day long (turned "off" only when the battery dies or the device is removed) and the noninvasive techniques are usually administered episodically (daily or several times per day), although there are exceptions. Investigations into each device have shown that some methods work better when paired with a certain behavior (often a behavior related to the disorder being treated). Recently, there has been an interest emerging in closed-loop brain stimulation systems where electricity is delivered in response to specific inputs related to the illness being treated. However, this is only being utilized in neurological interventions and has not yet transitioned to psychiatry.

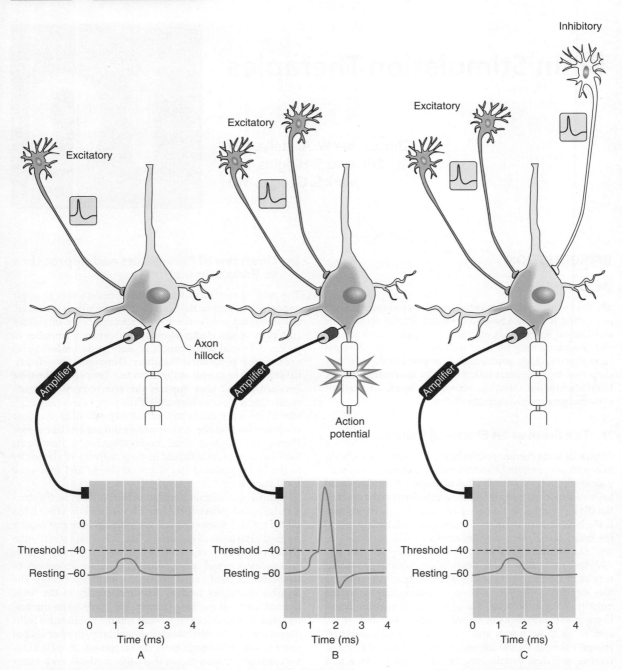

▲ **Figure 10–1** Excitatory and inhibitory neurotransmission. (A) Excitatory neuronal input isn't enough to depolarize the cell to reach the threshold and fire an action potential. (B) Two excitatory neurons (it is likely thousands) are sufficient to depolarize the neuron over the threshold and send an electrical signal down the axon. (C) The presence of an inhibitory neuron hyperpolarizes the neuron which mitigates the electrical summation. (Adapted with permission from Higgins and George. *The Neuroscience of Clinical Psychiatry*. 3ed. Wolters Kluwer Health; 2019.)

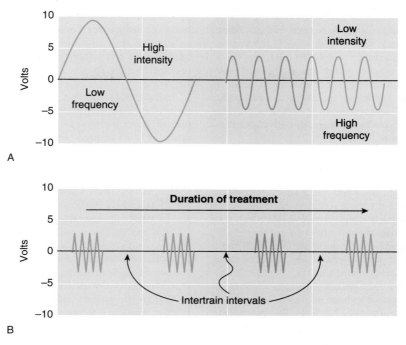

▲ **Figure 10–2** Dosing electricity. (A) Electrical parameters are adjusted by clinicians to change the dose of electricity delivered to the brain. These include current (Volts) (the intensity of the electrical wave), and frequency (Hz) (number of waves per second). (B) The various brain stimulation interventions may have varying durations of treatment or intertrain intervals (or the time between "jolts").

Raghavan M, Fee D, Barkhaus PE: Generation and propagation of the action potential. *Handb Clin Neurol* 2019;160:3–22.

von Bartheld CS, Bahney J, Herculano-Houzel S: The search for true numbers of neurons and glial cells in the human brain: A review of 150 years of cell counting. *J Comp Neurol* 2016;524(18):3865–3895.

ELECTROCONVULSIVE THERAPY

▶ Overview and History

Electroconvulsive therapy (ECT) remains the most effective treatment for depression and continues to have a range of other psychiatric indications. The idea that seizures may promote mental health and wellness has existed since the sixteenth century. In fact, the misguided theory that epilepsy and schizophrenia were inversely related inspired scientists to investigate the clinical benefits of induced convulsions. In 1934, Ladislaw Meduna, a Hungarian psychiatrist, began treating schizophrenic patients with camphor oil, inducing seizures to cure their psychotic symptoms. It actually helped, but was difficult to control as the volatile gases would affect everyone in the room. This success with seizures however led to the development of ECT by Cerletti and Bini in 1938, who successfully delivered electricity causing a seizure. With the introduction of chlorpromazine in 1954 and other medication, and the film adaptation of One Flew Over the Cuckoo's Nest in 1975, ECT use declined over the latter half of the twentieth century. However, with the improved efficiency and safety of modern treatments, ECT is experiencing a revival.

▶ Procedure

The most important part of the ECT procedure is the induction of a seizure, proven to be necessary but not sufficient for therapeutic benefit. The general parameters of electricity (intensity, frequency, duration) are applicable to ECT. Finding the sufficient (but not excessive) dose of electrical stimulation to produce a seizure is key to limiting the side effects from treatment. For clinicians administering ECT, published algorithms are available to assist with finding the dose needed to produce a seizure. Remarkably, the seizure threshold tends to rise over a course of ECT as the brain adapts to the stimulus and attempts to prevent future seizures. Patients commonly require an increased dose as the course progresses.

Reducing the side effects of ECT is an ongoing area of interest among brain stimulation researchers and clinicians. The shape of the electrical wave is a key topic in this regard. The original waveform used by the earliest clinicians was a sine wave (see Figure 10–3A); bulky and inefficient (pulse width of around 7 millisecond!), this waveform increases the risk of side effects. Shortening the electrical wave's pulse width reduces the total electrical dose and correlates with less side effects. Most machines in use currently deliver an ultra-brief (0.25–0.3 millisecond) waveform.

Electrode placement is also essential to optimizing outcomes and limiting unwanted effects. Figure 10–3B demonstrates two of the three potential options for electrode placement in ECT (right unilateral and bilateral positions). Bilateral ECT was once the most common electrode placement, but a greater association with cognitive side effects was one of several factors that shifted the field toward greater utilization of right unilateral placement. A seminal study from Sackeim and colleagues placed right unilateral and bilateral positions in a head-to-head competition (Figure 10–3C). The study demonstrated that right unilateral stimulation was just as efficacious for depression as bilateral treatment, but with less severe and persistent memory deficits. Early investigations of inducing focal seizures (limited to mood regulating network and avoiding the areas involved in memory) has been promising.

Potential Mechanisms

The therapeutic mechanism or mechanisms of action of ECT remain unsolved. Theories are based on the neurophysiological changes induced by ECT and what we already know about other mood enhancing treatments. The anticonvulsant effects of ECT are likely related to increases in inhibitory neurotransmitters (GABA) and inhibitory receptor antagonism. Functional suppression (associated with an increase in the seizure threshold) in response to a course of ECT is associated with positive clinical outcomes – some might say the brain is relearning how to regulate itself. ECT is also associated with increases in monoamines, the main targets of antidepressant medication. Additionally, ECT increases levels of neurotrophic factors, like brain derived neurotrophic factor (BDNF). These molecules are linked to neurogenesis in the hippocampus, a region essential to mood regulation. Lastly, response to ECT acutely increases the levels of various hormones (e.g. prolactin, thyrotropin, oxytocin); engagement with the neuroendocrine system is also thought to play a role in ECT's antidepressant mechanism of action.

Psychiatric Indications

Although ECT remains a viable and effective treatment for patients with schizophrenia who have not responded to antipsychotic medication, major depression is now the most common indication for its use. Clinical trials since the 1940s have demonstrated ECT's efficacy in the treatment of depression, with reported response rates of up to 90%. ECT is also an effective option for patients with bipolar depression. In head-to-head trials, there has never been an antidepressant to outperform ECT in terms of depression response or remission rates.

In the 1940s and 1950s, ECT was the first-line treatment for mania. However, with the dawn of psychotropic medication, ECT is now reserved for manic cases refractory to medication or those in need of emergent stabilization. Similarly, antipsychotic medications have replaced ECT as the first line treatment for patients with schizophrenia. However, ECT should be considered for patients who fail to respond to medication, as trials have shown its efficacy in this population. Additionally, ECT is efficacious for patients who are catatonic and have not fully responded to trials of benzodiazepines.

ECT is rarely used outside of the scope of psychiatric indications. As discussed earlier in this section, ECT can act as an anticonvulsant that raises the seizure threshold over the course of treatment. Given this information, it makes sense that ECT has been used successfully in patients in status epilepticus. In patients with Parkinson disease, ECT has a positive transient effect on motor function, although it is not officially approved to treat these symptoms. Finally, ECT has had success in the treatment of refractory neuroleptic malignant syndrome (NMS).

Adverse Effects

Representations of ECT like that shown in the popular film One Flew Over the Cuckoo's Nest have stigmatized ECT and adversely affected patient expectations of the risks and benefits of this procedure.

ECT is a relatively safe intervention, with an overall mortality rate of 1 per 10,000–80,000 treatments. Most of the risk of ECT stems from the need to have brief general anesthesia during the actual seizure. Nausea and headache may follow the ECT procedure and are usually mild and self-limiting. Other musculoskeletal side effects are less common and can be prevented with proper dosing of the anesthetic and muscle relaxant. Risk of arrhythmia is also present in the post-ECT period, but this tends to be self-limiting as well. Prior cardiovascular history increases the likelihood of this adverse effect.

Cognitive side effects from ECT can be difficult for patients to understand, considering media portrayals discussed above. Acute deficits in attention, memory, and orientation occur in most patients immediately following ECT. These are often self-limiting, and patients now largely recover within an hour. Subacute memory deficits, including anterograde and retrograde amnesia, are less common and occur in the weeks to months surrounding the acute ECT course. Chronic cognitive adverse effects are rare but may persist for months after ECT. Most of these problems are related to the type of ECT used (see Figure 10–3).

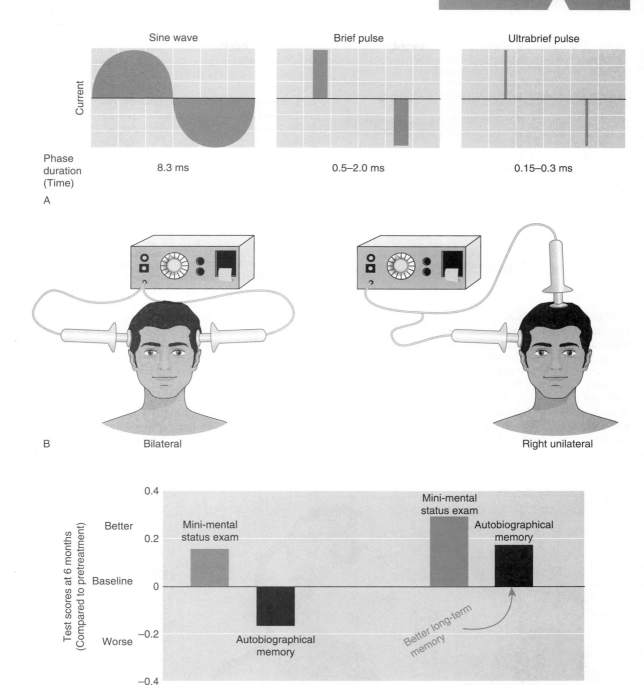

▲ **Figure 10–3** Delivering electrical stimulation. Ultrashort electrical wave pulse (A), administered unilaterally on the right (B), diminished ECT-induced decrements in cognitive functioning and long-term memory recall (C), when compared to bilateral ECT. (Adapted with permission from Higgins and George. *The Neuroscience of Clinical Psychiatry*. 3ed. Wolters Kluwer Health; 2019.)

Sackeim HA: The anticonvulsant hypothesis of the mechanisms of action of ECT: current status. *J ECT* 1999;15(1):5–26.

Sackeim HA, et al: A prospective, randomized, double-blind comparison of bilateral and right unilateral electroconvulsive therapy at different stimulus intensities. *Arch Gen Psychiatry* 2000;57(5):425–434.

Prudic J, Sackeim HA, Devanand DP: Medication resistance and clinical response to electroconvulsive therapy. *Psychiatry Res* 1990;31(3):287–296.

Weiner RD, Reti IM: Key updates in the clinical application of electroconvulsive therapy. *Int Rev Psychiatry* 2017;29(2): 54–62.

Andrade C, Arumugham SS, Thirthalli J: Adverse effects of electroconvulsive therapy. *Psychiatr Clin North Am* 2016;39(3): 513–530.

TRANSCRANIAL MAGNETIC STIMULATION

▶ Overview

TMS is based on the concept of electromagnetic induction, first described by Faraday in 1832. Faraday showed that passing a magnet through a coil generates an electrical current. Doing this repetitively creates a series of electromagnetic pulses. In turn, focally targeted electromagnetic pulses can influence underlying brain activity (ex. when a pulsating TMS coil is placed over the scalp). The first device resembling modern TMS was developed by Anthony Barker in 1985. In the early 1990s, George and colleagues started a long series of clinical trials to use repetitive TMS (rTMS) with depressed patients.

▶ Procedure

Over time, evidence from clinical trials refined the way TMS is administered in the clinic. The device itself has evolved over time and there are a growing number of devices with FDA clearance for treating depression. Figure 10–4 shows the typical TMS setup consisting of a comfortable chair that can recline and the TMS coil, which is attached to a bank of large capacitors that is charged through the wall's electrical outlet. Once the patient is comfortably seated, the TMS coil is placed over their scalp (over the prefrontal cortex for most psychiatric indications) and electromagnetic pulses are released (each one with an audible "click"). The coil's electromagnetic field passes through the scalp and skull, focally inducing an electrical current in the underlying brain areas.

As with any treatment, finding the right dose is essential to treat a patient's symptoms and limit unwanted side effects. Clinicians determine a "motor threshold" to measure cortical excitability, and thus estimate the dose needed for a safe and effective treatment. The motor threshold is the least amount of electricity needed to contract the thumb's abductor pollicis brevis – extending the thumb. A percentage of the motor threshold is used as the dose for treatment (this percentage differs based on the device, indication, and method, but frequently is about 120% in conventional TMS).

The first TMS devices could only produce a single, brief pulse. Current devices on the market emit a series of pulses in repetition, what is known as repetitive TMS (rTMS). Increasing the amplitude or intensity of stimulation can increase the reach of the electrical current into the brain (only to a certain extent). However, the effects of rTMS

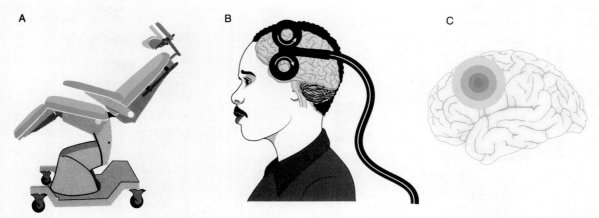

A   B   C

▲ **Figure 10–4** **TMS Set-Up. The TMS machine consists of a chair and figure-8 coil which is attached to a bank of capacitors plugged into the wall's outlet (A & B). The coil delivers a focal electromagnetic pulse to the brain (C), thus influencing underlying cortical activity. A typical course of rTMS for depression consists of treatments 5 days per week, for about 6 weeks (30–36 sessions).**

on cortical excitability depend on the frequency and duration of stimulation. Low frequency rTMS (1 Hz or less) focally inhibits the brain. High frequency rTMS (5 Hz and greater) increases cortical excitability. Theta burst stimulation (TBS) is a newer pattern of electromagnetic stimulation. The frequency mimics neuronal firing from the hippocampus, firing a triplet of pulses at 50 Hz, repeated at 5 Hz. Continuous theta burst (cTBS) is generally inhibitory, while intermittent theta burst (iTBS) is excitatory. Emerging interest in TBS is centered around its potential to deliver more pulses over a shorter amount of time, which significantly reduces the time patients must dedicate to treatment. Because theta burst is quicker and more efficient, recent studies have combined many treatments into a single day, and then delivered these accelerated treatments over one week, with remarkable and quick results.

Discussion of mechanism

As with other brain stimulation modalities, the exact mechanism of TMS remains unclear. When TMS is delivered to a specific region of the brain, the neurons under the coil are activated and the impulses are transmitted to deeper structures. If we think of the brain as a collection of electrical circuits, TMS allows us to strengthen or weaken aspects of those circuits depending on how well they are functioning. For example, high frequency TMS (excitatory) to the left prefrontal cortex (PFC) is the standard protocol for patients with depression. Functional neuroimaging trials have shown that the PFC of depressed patients is often hypoactive. TMS is thought to be enhancing the connections in a circuit where the left PFC is under-functioning.

Additionally, TMS exerts effects like other antidepressants, including ECT. TMS is known to increase monoamine turnover and increase expression of BDNF. Normalization of the hypothalamic-pituitary-adrenal (HPA) axis is commonly seen as well.

Safety

Many studies support good safety and tolerability of TMS for a variety of neuropsychiatric disorders. The incidence of side effects and serious adverse effects are minimal. Induction of an accidental seizure is the most severe adverse event reported in the literature, although this is a rare occurrence (overall risk less than 0.003%). All reported seizures have been self-limited and do not reoccur. Risk factors for seizure induction include targeting areas with higher epileptogenic potential (such as the motor cortex), treatments delivered at parameters outside of the suggested guidelines, treatment in the context of alcohol withdrawal, personal or family history of seizures or epilepsy, or treatment following significant

medication changes. The presence of one or more of any risk factor should be carefully considered. In the case of acute changes (alcohol withdrawal, medication dosing changes), delaying treatment or reassessing the motor threshold (dose) may be the best course of action. In patients with a history of seizures, the risks and benefits of treatment should be weighed before making the decision to treat.

Headache and stimulation site pain are commonly reported side effects. These can generally be treated with over-the-counter analgesics and tend to dissipate over the treatment course. Although there is not a significant association between TMS and hearing loss, it is recommended that patients and treaters wear earplugs during treatments due to the audible clicking that can be heard while in session. Hearing aids, and other devices capable of conducting electricity, should be removed prior to treatments if possible. TMS is generally considered safe in patients with cardiac pacemakers, VNS systems, and spinal cord stimulators if the TMS coil is not activated close to electronic components.

Psychiatric indications

TMS continues to gain approval for disorders across the neuropsychiatric spectrum. Of this growing group, patients with depression have been the most widely studied. Using evidence from functional neuroimaging trials and stroke patients, researchers focused on the left PFC and established positive effects with TMS for patients with depression. The most rigorous clinical trial of prefrontal TMS for depression to date was the OPT-TMS trial, led by George and colleagues. This short (3 week) randomized multi-site truly double-blind study demonstrated that active rTMS produced a significantly higher response and remission rate than did sham treatment (14.1 vs 5.1% remission rates and 15 vs 5% response rates). 30% of patients remitted in a follow up 3-week open label phase. Newer studies suggested that prolonged treatment can lead to improved response, even for those who do not have a significant response early in the treatment course. This trial along with an industry sponsored trial, were crucial in TMS gaining FDA approval and widespread clinical acceptance for the treatment of depression. Researchers continue to search for ways to optimize the treatment. Most recently, the FDA cleared a new accelerated protocol using TBS to treat patients with treatment-resistant depression. This novel protocol offers a shorter treatment duration (10 treatments per day for 5 days) and has demonstrated promising early results. This accelerated approach is now being tested on inpatient and emergency room settings.

Several manufacturers also gained approval for obsessive-compulsive disorder (OCD) in recent years. The approved devices use coils that stimulate more deeply and broadly than the typical figure eight coil. A developing hypothesis is the idea that brain stimulation paired with certain behaviors or tasks may enhance treatment outcomes. This paired behavioral approach is used when treating OCD patients with TMS. Patients construct an exposure hierarchy with a psychologist prior to beginning treatment, and TMS treatments are paired with exposure therapy.

Similarly, a manufacturer recently gained approval of a deep TMS device to assist with smoking cessation. This is a fast-growing area within TMS, along with investigations into other addictions. Often, TMS is paired with induced craving in these studies. Other indications of interest in this area include schizophrenia and PTSD. Although early evidence is promising in reducing specific symptoms associated with these disorders, more information is needed before any definitive statements can be made about these indications.

George MS, et al: Daily repetitive transcranial magnetic stimulation (rTMS) improves mood in depression. *Neuroreport* 1995;6(14): 1853–1856.

Li X, et al: Acute left prefrontal transcranial magnetic stimulation in depressed patients is associated with immediately increased activity in prefrontal cortical as well as subcortical regions. *Biol Psychiatry* 2004;55(9):882–890.

Stultz DJ, et al: Transcranial magnetic stimulation (TMS) safety with respect to seizures: a literature review. *Neuropsychiatr Dis Treat* 2020;16:2989–3000.

George MS, et al: Daily left prefrontal transcranial magnetic stimulation therapy for major depressive disorder: a sham-controlled randomized trial. *Arch Gen Psychiatry* 2010;67(5):507–516.

CRANIAL NERVE STIMULATION

▶ Vagus Nerve Stimulation

History

Electrical stimulation of the vagus nerve is another modality with roots that predate modern brain stimulation. Some of the earliest reports of this method can be found in the late nineteenth century; J.L. Corning, a neurologist in New York, documented his attempts to treat epilepsy using a fork-like device to mechanically compress and electrically stimulate the carotid sheath. Corning's method never gained traction, but the concept was revived in the twentieth century. Modern VNS was invented in the 1980s. In subsequent decades, neurologists and psychiatrists began using implanted wires around the vagus nerve in the neck to treat patients with epilepsy and depression (we call that form – invasive cervical VNS). For both epilepsy and depression, VNS worked particularly well in cases that previously failed to respond to medication.

The science behind VNS continues to grow. The vagus nerve may be stimulated in various locations, including as it exits an end-organ (i.e., the branch of the nerve innervating the stomach), along its cervical branch in the neck (invasively

with a wire around the nerve, or noninvasively through a handheld electromagnet), or noninvasively through a branch of the vagus in the ear (transcranial auricular VNS, taVNS). Animal models suggest VNS may be useful for other neuropsychiatric disorders and even many organ-specific diseases where the vagus is involved (e.g., heart failure). Scientists investigating VNS are starting to realize that paired models of stimulation (intermittent trains of stimulation paired with a behavioral task) may enhance therapeutic benefits.

Modern VNS

Invasive cervical VNS in its current form was developed in the 1980s by Jake Zabara as a treatment for epilepsy (and later discovered by George, Sackeim and Rush to have effects on depression). The device consists of a pulse generator connected via wire to an electrode cuff (see Figure 10–5). Surgical placement of the device is typically an ambulatory procedure performed by a surgeon. The pulse generator is implanted subcutaneously in the patient's left chest wall. The electrode cuff is tunneled under the skin superiorly where the cuff is wrapped around the left vagus nerve at the cervical level. After a 2-week recovery period, the device is turned "on" and programmed in the clinic by a psychiatrist or neurologist. The clinician uses a handheld infrared wand placed over the device to adjust the electrical parameters.

Recent years have seen an increased interest in noninvasive forms of VNS. One company developed a handheld apparatus that stimulates the vagus nerve when the device is held against the neck. The device, initially called gammaCore, has a similar appearance to an electric razor. In 2017, it was FDA approved for the treatment of cluster headaches. Methods of stimulating the vagus through the ear are also gaining traction. By placing electrodes over the skin of certain parts of the ear (typically the tragus and cymba conchae), it is possible to electrically stimulate the vagus nerve noninvasively. This method is known as transcutaneous auricular VNS (taVNS) and does not have any FDA approved indications to date.

Mechanisms

The vagus nerve has both afferent (traveling to the brain) and efferent fibers and can be stimulated in either direction. Invasive cervical VNS for depression or epilepsy is a "bottom-up" form of brain stimulation (in contrast to modalities like TMS and ECT that originate at the top of the brain and work their way down). Afferent signals are transmitted up the vagus nerve, through the nucleus tractus solitarius (in the medulla), locus coeruleus, and beyond to higher areas of the brain. Functional neuroimaging studies have confirmed the ability of VNS to modulate higher regions in the brain involved in depression (prefrontal cortex and limbic system). Evidence in several other areas has helped researchers understand how VNS works, but its exact mechanisms of action remain unclear.

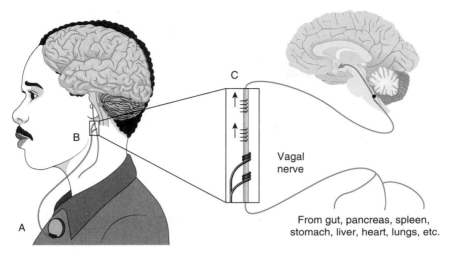

▲ **Figure 10–5** The modern invasive cervical VNS device consists of an implantable pulse generator (A & B) attached to an electrode cuff (C) that is wrapped around the left cervical bundle of the vagus nerve. The device electrically stimulates the nerve, sending signals centrally toward the brain.

A likely key mechanism of VNS for treating depression or epilepsy is its effects on norepinephrine. The vagus nerve connects with the locus coeruleus, one of the primary sources of norepinephrine in the brain. In fact, lesions of the locus coeruleus in rats inhibit the ability of VNS to suppress seizures. As we know, norepinephrine is also one of the targets of oral antidepressant therapies. Like other antidepressants, VNS also appears to modulate BDNF and the immune system. And like other antiepileptics, VNS appears to enhance GABA transmission and activity.

Adverse Effects

Invasive cervical VNS is a relatively safe modality, with an overall risk of adverse events of 2%. Adverse events related to invasive cervical VNS can be separated into events or complications associated with the surgery and those that are stimulation-related side effects. Wound infections, pain at the surgical site, and rarely vocal cord paralysis are possible surgical complications. Temporary asystole during the initial testing of the device is rare. (Luckily this happens during surgery with an anesthesiologist available.) Side effects related to stimulation are more common than those related to surgery. The most common side effects include hoarseness, dyspnea, and cough. Often, these side effects can be minimized or eliminated with adjustment of the stimulation parameters. Additionally, stimulation-related effects tend to decrease with time. Hypomania or mania remains a concern with VNS, as with other antidepressants (although the risk of their occurrence is rare).

Psychiatric Indications

Work with invasive cervical VNS for treatment-resistant depression was prompted by several lines of research, particularly brain imaging studies showing that invasive cervical VNS caused brain changes in emotion regulating regions. An open-label pilot trial found a 30% response rate at 10 weeks in a cohort of 59 patients, and unlike almost all other antidepressant treatments, the response and remission rates continued to improve at the 1-year mark. A follow up randomized, double-blinded trial found a nonsignificant improvement in depression at 10 weeks (15% response in the active group, 10% in the sham group). However, George and colleagues also compared a nonrandomized group of VNS patients with a group that received treatment as usual. After 12 months, the VNS group had a significantly higher response rate (27%) compared to the treatment as usual group (13%). The US FDA granted approval in 2005 based on this comparative study. Due to the lack of definitive proof and cost of the device, the US Centers for Medicare & Medicaid Services (CMS) in 2007 issued a noncoverage determination which has limited access to VNS for depression. However due to continued improvement in patients who were implanted with VNS and the scourge of depression, the Federal Government has stepped in to conduct an ongoing multicenter, randomized and controlled trial offering hope that this treatment will be easier to access in the future.

The vagus nerve is an essential part of the parasympathetic nervous system and carries crucial information between the central nervous system and the periphery. Given this cranial nerve's unique anatomy and function, VNS could potentially be harnessed as a potent anxiolytic agent. An open label, pilot trial from 2008 showed mild improvement in some patients with anxiety disorders. However, there have not been any controlled trials to date.

In addition to the psychiatric indications discussed above, VNS has a growing evidence base for several neurological disorders. VNS was approved for patients with epilepsy refractory to medications in 1997. More recently, a closed-loop invasive implanted cervical VNS system was approved for post-stroke motor rehabilitation. Noninvasive auricular VNS also has promising evidence in patients with pain and in neonates learning to feed.

▶ Trigeminal Nerve Stimulation

Overview

Trigeminal Nerve Stimulation (TNS) is another form of bottom-up stimulation, however much less studied than its counterparts. TNS can be driven from a handheld device that is portable, making it unique among the brain stimulation modalities. The mechanism of TNS is not well understood and there is only a small amount of evidence available. Due to the novelty of the method, TNS has less evidence than other modalities however it is FDA approved for attention deficit disorder.

Révész D, Rydenhag B, Ben-Menachem E: Complications and safety of vagus nerve stimulation: 25 years of experience at a single center. *J Neurosurg Pediatr* 2016;18(1):97–104.

Rush AJ, et al: Vagus nerve stimulation for treatment-resistant depression: a randomized, controlled acute phase trial. *Biol Psychiatry* 2005;58(5):347–354.

George MS, et al: A one-year comparison of vagus nerve stimulation with treatment as usual for treatment-resistant depression. *Biol Psychiatry* 2005;58(5):364–373.

McGough JJ, et al: Double-blind, sham-controlled, pilot study of trigeminal nerve stimulation for attention-deficit/hyperactivity disorder. *J Am Acad Child Adolesc Psychiatry* 2019;58(4):403–411.e3.

DEEP BRAIN STIMULATION

▶ Introduction

DBS is one of the most direct (invasive) forms of brain stimulation investigated for use in psychiatric disorders. In the 1980s, Benabid and colleagues were using brain stimulation to map the best location to remove the ventral intermediate nucleus of the thalamus for Parkinson disease and essential tremors. They found that if they injected current back into the brain, at high frequency (>100 Hz), the tremors immediately stopped. Pilot studies followed in short succession, leading to DBS being approved for both Parkinson disease, essential tremors, and epilepsy. Since

then, DBS has been explored as a treatment for depression and OCD.

Other ways to directly stimulate the brain exist but will not be discussed in depth in this section. Responsive neural stimulation is one of these methods. This approach uses a form of DBS and adds a microprocessor that can sense the brain's electrical signals and deliver stimulation in return. This device is approved for treatment-resistant epilepsy. Cortical brain stimulation is another similar method. Electrodes are placed directly on the surface of the cortex, between the skull and dura mater. This technique may be useful for conditions involving cortical gray matter (i.e., epilepsy with a cortical focus).

▶ Device & Mechanism

Similar to invasive cervical VNS, the DBS device has three components: the impulse generator, the extension, and the electrodes (Figure 10–6). Implantation of the device is usually an ambulatory procedure. A surgeon places the impulse generator subcutaneously in the chest wall, just below the patient's clavicle. The generator sends electrical impulses through the extension to the electrodes that are implanted in the subcortical regions of the brain. Electrodes are typically placed bilaterally. Some parts of this procedure can be performed under local anesthesia (compared to general), allowing the patient to participate in proper placement of the electrodes, for example, optimal placement of the electrodes to quiet a tremor.

The DBS device is programmed in the clinic by a specialized physician (neurologist or psychiatrist). Like VNS, the device is programmed externally. However, there are more variables to consider when programming DBS compared to VNS as there are many electrodes and brain locations. The implanted probe contains at minimum four electrodes that emit electrical signals. These four or more sites can be programmed to optimize the effect on the target site. Newer probes with more electrode sites allow even more precision in where to stimulate, thus enhancing the beneficial effects of stimulation. As with other brain stimulation modalities, clinicians can also program typical electrical parameters: voltage, pulse width, frequency, and wave forms. One can only imagine the infinite number of parameter combinations that could be used during treatment. There are now attempts to find biomarkers to help refine programming, and even using artificial intelligence programs to make a first pass approximation of where to start and likely useful combinations.

The mechanisms of action of DBS are unclear. The frequency of stimulation appears to be more important than other parameters in terms of therapeutic effects. Frequencies greater than 100 Hz are usually more effective, while pulse width may play a role in the part of the neuron that is activated. Chronic, high-frequency stimulation causes reversible inhibition of the stimulated site. Several theories about the mechanism of DBS exist. These theories implicate the inhibitory neurons and GABA as a means of blocking signal transmission through the neurons being targeted by the DBS electrodes.

Adverse Effects

Serious adverse effects associated with DBS are related to the neurosurgical procedure. These include bleeding and stroke (1–3%), as well as infection (4–5%). Infection may necessitate removal of the DBS system but is usually not life-threatening. Risk of death related to DBS is less than 1%.

Additionally, DBS may lead to neuropsychiatric side effects. There have been reports of patients developing paresthesias and involuntary movements. Others have developed cognitive side effects. Additionally, DBS entails a risk of mood changes, including disinhibition, gambling, or suicide. These issues can often be resolved with adjustments of the device's electrical parameters.

Psychiatric Indications

DBS is primarily used to treat neurological disorders (epilepsy, Parkinson disease, dystonia), but has been studied for various neuropsychiatric disorders. Media excitement surrounded the early use of DBS in patients with treatment-resistant depression. Helen Mayberg and colleagues pioneered this area, conducting the first pilot trial for treatment-resistant depression. Early results were promising and two large RCTs have been conducted since then. Unfortunately, both trials ended prematurely due to interim analyses showing no difference between the patients receiving active treatment compared to sham treatment. These two large trials were launched before there was good knowledge about DBS programming, speed of onset, patient selection and sham design. At least one of the commercial DBS manufacturers is launching a new study for treatment-resistant depression.

DBS has also been explored as a potential treatment for patients with OCD. Historically, ablative neurosurgery (anterior capsule or anterior cingulate) was an option for patients with severe, refractory OCD. An early pilot trial observed four patients experience a greater than 35% improvement in their symptoms, while two patients improved more than 25%. This led to a large randomized clinical trial, whose results showed no difference between active and sham treatment, but have yet to be published.

The history of DBS for psychiatric indications is a controversial one. Many positive reports have been published, but most of these were case studies and uncontrolled. The larger, randomized and sham-controlled trials have not shown positive results. While the evidence behind DBS in psychiatric disorders has been disappointing so far, the technique is already approved and improving the lives of those with more classically defined neurological disorders like epilepsy or Parkinson disease.

Benabid AL: Deep brain stimulation for Parkinson's disease. *Curr Opin Neurobiol* 2003;13(6):696–706.

Nair DR, et al: Nine-year prospective efficacy and safety of brain-responsive neurostimulation for focal epilepsy. *Neurology* 2020; 95(9):e1244–e1256.

Blumenfeld Z, Brontë-Stewart H: High frequency deep brain stimulation and neural rhythms in Parkinson's disease. *Neuropsychol Rev* 2015;25(4):384–397.

Dougherty DD, Deep brain stimulation: clinical applications. *Psychiatr Clin North Am* 2018;41(3):385–394.

Mayberg HS, et al: Deep brain stimulation for treatment-resistant depression. *Neuron* 2005;45(5):651–660.

TRANSCRANIAL DIRECT CURRENT STIMULATION

Overview & Mechanism

Transcranial direct current stimulation (tDCS) is a brain stimulation modality that may seem simpler than those previously discussed, but its effects on the brain and neuropsychiatric functions should not be ignored. Various forms of applying direct current to the brain were used in Europe starting in the 1800s and continued to garner interest into the twentieth century. Modern tDCS was revived by Dr. Walter Paulus in Gottingen, Germany at the turn of the century. Since then, investigations using tDCS have expanded into many neuropsychiatric domains.

tDCS has several advantages when compared to other forms of brain stimulation, due to its low cost, noninvasiveness, and portability. The device passes a weak electrical current through the brain between two electrodes. It commonly involves using two damp sponges as electrodes (attached to a source of electricity… most devices use a 9-volt battery) and placing them on the scalp over areas of interest. The current enters the brain through the anode and exits via the cathode. Historically researchers thought that the brain area under the anode would be activated, while the area under the cathode is inhibited. However, this is not always true – certain studies have shown the exact opposite. It is important to remember that electrical current flows between the electrodes. New research has found that the biggest tDCS effects are not under the electrodes, but somewhere in between them.

Transcranial *alternating* current stimulation (tACS) is a similar method of delivering electrical current to the brain. The difference between tACS and tDCS is in the name! tACS delivers an alternating, or oscillating, current to the brain (in contrast to constant direct current). Another related form of stimulation is called transcranial random noise stimulation (tRNS), which involves stimulating with a range of different frequencies.

Adverse Effects

tDCS is a relatively safe technique. Side effects depend on the site where electrodes are placed, the intensity of stimulation, and the duration of treatments. Most people receiving tDCS notice a mild tingling as stimulation begins but tend to desensitize over time. Skin burns are possible but, with proper monitoring and technique, can be avoided. Otherwise, side effects are minimal, but include headache (11%), nausea (3%), and insomnia (1%).

Potential Psychiatric Indications

While tDCS does not have any approved clinical indications to date, there is enough promising evidence to be excited about the future. Unlike the more powerful brain stimulation methods like ECT and TMS, tDCS and tACS cannot make a neuron depolarize, or your thumb twitch. They are thus true modulators, and not really brain stimulators. This means that they can help the brain complete a task that is already ongoing, much like a catalyst does for a chemical reaction. But on their own, tDCS and tACS do not have large effects. Thus, it is important to match stimulation with the symptom or task. Although our focus is on psychiatric indications, it is worth mentioning the work that has gone into motor and speech recovery in stroke patients where tDCS was paired with speech therapy. tDCS, in conjunction with speech therapy, was likely promoting plasticity during therapy – suggesting possible psychiatric indications. Pairing stimulation with a task is a common theme developing in brain stimulation.

Nitsche MA, et al: Shaping the effects of transcranial direct current stimulation of the human motor cortex. *J Neurophysiol* 2007;97(4):3109–3117.

Caulfield KA, George MS: Optimizing transcranial direct current stimulation (tDCS) electrode position, size, and distance doubles the on-target cortical electric field: Evidence from 3000 Human Connectome Project models. *bioRxiv*, 2021: p. 2021.11.21.469417.

Fridriksson J, et al: Transcranial direct current stimulation vs sham stimulation to treat aphasia after stroke: a randomized clinical trial. *JAMA Neurol* 2018;75(12):1470–1476.

Palm U, et al: tDCS for the treatment of depression: a comprehensive review. *Eur Arch Psychiatry Clin Neurosci* 2016;266(8):681–694.

Caulfield KA, et al: Transcranial electrical stimulation motor threshold can estimate individualized tDCS dosage from reverse-calculation electric-field modeling. *Brain Stimul* 2020; 13(4):961–969.

BRAIN STIMULATION IN CLINICAL PRACTICE

The astute reader may be wondering how physicians decide when to use each of the brain stimulation therapies discussed in the previous sections. Unfortunately, there is not a standardized pathway or algorithm for making these choices (although this could make for an interesting area of research). However, this section will provide general guidelines and helpful pearls for the medical student studying psychiatry. We will also briefly cover how psychopharmacology interacts, if at all, with brain stimulation therapies.

ECT, TMS, and VNS are the brain stimulation modalities with FDA approval for treatment-resistant depression. ECT (mania, psychosis, catatonia) and TMS (OCD, smoking cessation) are approved to treat other disorders, too (see Figure 10–6). Due to the rapid and robust response seen with ECT, it is generally reserved for highly acute cases where patients are suicidal, not eating/drinking, or for emergent situations. The potential memory deficits produced by treatment with ECT should be considered in populations who are cognitively vulnerable (i.e., dementia) or other specific situations (i.e., professionals who rely on their cognitive ability, such as physicians). Investigations of how psychopharmacology complements ECT treatments have shown that nortriptyline (a tricyclic antidepressant) and venlafaxine (a serotonin and norepinephrine reuptake inhibitor) in combination with ECT for depression have better outcomes (greater improvement during acute treatment and prolonged remission), Lithium is associated with better outcomes related to relapse (longer time to relapse), however, lithium

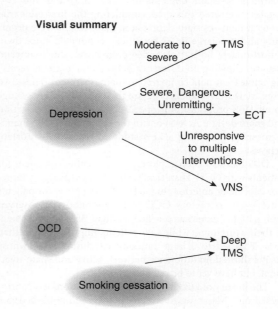

Visual summary

▲ **Figure 10–6** General Guidelines for Brain Stimulation Therapies. ECT, TMS, and VNS are approved for psychiatric indications. All three modalities are used for depression, although tend to be used in certain clinical contexts.

should not be used during the acute phase of ECT due to higher rates of delirium.

TMS is often reserved for less acute cases, although usually in situations where patients have not responded to multiple medications. VNS tends to be used for chronic, recurrent cases of treatment-resistant depression. We continue to learn how pharmacotherapy interacts with these newer forms of brain stimulation. Generally, most psychotropic medication can be used safely with TMS and VNS, and do not have major interactions that affect the outcomes associated with treatment. However, this is an ongoing area of research that may yield updates to this important question.

Sackeim HA, et al: Effect of concomitant pharmacotherapy on electroconvulsive therapy outcomes: short-term efficacy and adverse effects. *Arch Gen Psychiatry* 2009;66(7):729–737.

Prudic J, et al: Pharmacological strategies in the prevention of relapse after electroconvulsive therapy. *J ECT* 2013;29(1):3–12.

Lambrichts S, et al: Does lithium prevent relapse following successful electroconvulsive therapy for major depression? A systematic review and meta-analysis. *Acta Psychiatr Scand* 2021;143(4):294–306.

Hunter AM, et al: Concomitant medication use and clinical outcome of repetitive transcranial magnetic stimulation (rTMS) treatment of major depressive disorder. *Brain Behav* 2019;9(5): e01275.

11

Diagnostic Encounter for Children and Adolescents

Molly McVoy, MD
Barry Nurcombe, MD[†]

I. INTERVIEWING PARENT(S)/GUARDIAN(S)

INITIAL CONTACT

Children are usually brought to psychiatrists by their parents or caregivers. Parent(s)/guardian(s) should be made aware that a collaborative approach to diagnosis and treatment is essential and that their children older than 3 years of age should be prepared for the diagnostic encounter. The initial contact is usually made over the telephone by the parent or the referring agent. The importance of the impression made at that first contact cannot be underestimated. The initial intake staff members gather identifying information and a brief history of the presenting complaint. Emergency situations must be dealt with at once and urgent situations within 24 hours. Table 11–1 lists the situations, roughly in the order of frequency, that require immediate evaluation.

SEQUENCE OF INTERVIEWS

If the initial interview is prompted by a crisis, or if the family has come a long distance, the clinician should see the whole family together. Even if there is no crisis, some clinicians still favor interviewing the whole family first, whereas others prefer interviewing the parent(s)/guardian(s) first, before interviewing the child or the adolescent at a separate later interview. Even if the parents are separated or divorced, it is preferable to interview both parents, unless the tension between them would be unmanageable. Other clinicians prefer to interview an adolescent first, before interviewing the parents. In any case, the clinician should try to avoid having the child wait anxiously in the waiting room while lengthy parent interviews are conducted. At some point, the parents will need to be interviewed to obtain a detailed history (see "Interviewing Parents" section) and the family interviewed

together to throw light on family dynamics (see "Interviewing Families" section).

INTAKE QUESTIONNAIRES & CHECKLISTS

Important data can be collected even before the first interview. For example, the parent can complete a Child Behavior Checklist and a developmental history form. Teacher versions of the Child Behavior Checklist can also be obtained if the child's behavior in school is an important issue. Previous mental health evaluations, psychological reports, medical records, and school records are also available in some cases. Thus, the clinician can focus during the parent interview on the developmental issues and symptom patterns that emerge from the preliminary data.

PURPOSE OF THE PARENT/ GUARDIAN INTERVIEW

The initial parent interview serves several purposes. Most important, it helps the clinician form an alliance with the parent(s)/guardian(s), and it helps the parent(s)/guardian(s) prepare the child for the next interview. The clinician can use the parent interview to obtain a formal history of the child's presenting problem, medical history, early development, school progress, and peer relations, as well as information on the child's recreational activities and interests, home and family environment, and family history. The clinician can also gather from this interview information about parent–child relations and communication, the parent(s)' child-rearing techniques and methods of discipline used, and the family's values and aspirations. The clinician can gather information on the parents' current marital relationship, if married, and its developments, and can ascertain how the parents understand the child's problem and the kind of help they are seeking. If the child is not in the custody of their parents, an interview of the guardian of the child will provide similar information,

---

[†]Deceased.

Table 11–1 Situations Requiring Immediate Evaluation

Suicidality
Homicidal impulses
Dangerous assaultiveness
Dangerous risk-taking (e.g., running away from home)
Drug or alcohol intoxication
Psychotic thought disorder (e.g., hallucinations, delusions)
Impending parental breakdown related to the child's disruptive behavior
Recent trauma (e.g., as a result of rape or civilian catastrophe)
Recent loss with abnormal grief reaction
Acute school refusal
Suspension or expulsion from school
Police involvement
Physical deterioration in a patient known to have an eating disorder

in addition to establishing the circumstances that led to the child's current living situation.

SEQUENCE OF THE PARENT INTERVIEW

The parent interview proceeds through four key stages: (1) inception, (2) reconnaissance, (3) detailed inquiry, and (4) termination.

▶ Inception

The interviewer begins by greeting the parent(s)/guardian(s) in the waiting room and ushering them into the office, indicating where they should sit. The interviewer then tells the parent(s)/guardian(s) what he or she already knows and invites them to tell their story. The interviewer should also establish what relationship the parent(s) and/or guardian(s) have with the child.

▶ Reconnaissance

The interviewer should let the parent(s)/guardian(s) proceed at their own pace without interruption other than to facilitate the flow of associations or clarify issues. As the story unfolds, and if there is more than one adult in the room, the interaction between them is observed. Do they support each other? Does one parent do most of the talking? Do they interrupt or contradict each other? Which issues evoke the most emotion from them? Do they express warmth, humor, coolness, detachment, remoteness, tension, irritation, or hostility? If one parent becomes upset, how does the other respond?

▶ Detailed Inquiry

After the parent(s)/guardian(s) have finished their story, the areas listed in the next several sections are explored. These areas should be surveyed in a standard diagnostic inquiry, and particular areas should be explored in depth according to the diagnostic hypotheses triggered by the clinical pattern that is emerging.

A. The Problem

When did the problem first appear? Did its onset coincide with a physical or psychosocial stressor? How has the problem evolved? Is the problem persistent or intermittent? If intermittent, do exacerbations coincide with vicissitudes in physical health or the environment (e.g., family, school, peer relations)? What have the parent(s)/guardian(s) done about it? Are there any other problems in the child's behavior at home, at school, with siblings, or with peers?

B. Referral

Who referred the family? Why do they come now? How do they feel about it? Have they sought help before? If so, from whom, and how effective was the help? What kind of help do they expect now?

C. Medical History

Has the child had any significant physical illness, physical disability, surgeries, accidents, or hospitalizations? If so, at what age, what was the duration, and did any adverse psychological reactions occur? Has the child sustained any head injuries or had seizures, syncopes, headaches, eye symptoms, abdominal or limb pains, nausea or vomiting, or prolonged or frequent absences from school? Has the child had previous psychological disturbances? If so, what were the causes, treatment, and outcome? Is the child currently taking any medication? Does he or she have significant allergies?

D. Developmental History

1. Pregnancy—Is this a biological child of the parent/ guardian in your office? If so: What were the circumstances surrounding conception of the child (e.g., motivation, acceptance, convenience, emotional turmoil, reaction of in-laws)? What was the nature of the marital relationship during pregnancy? Did the parent(s)/guardian(s) have a sex preference? How was the mother's physical and emotional health during pregnancy? Did she have toxemia, eclampsia, kidney disorder, hypertension, or febrile illness? Were any X-rays taken during pregnancy? Did she take prescribed or over-the-counter medications, tobacco, alcohol, or illicit drugs during pregnancy, and if so, how much and how often? Did she experience excessive nausea, vomiting, or vaginal bleeding during pregnancy? How was she prepared for labor?

2. Delivery—Did the mother have a normal pregnancy? Was the child born at term? How long did labor last? What was the nature of the delivery? Did any complications occur? How soon did the mother see the infant after delivery? What were the mother's initial thoughts on seeing the infant?

3. Neonatal status—What was the infant's birth weight, maturity, and physical condition? Was the infant in intensive care? If so, for how long? What was the method of feeding? How well did the infant gain weight as a neonate? Did the infant have problems with asphyxia, cyanosis, jaundice, convulsions, vomiting, rigidity, or respiratory disorder?

4. Feeding—Was the child breastfed? If so, for how long? Was formula used? When were solids introduced? How well did the child gain weight? Did the child have problems with vomiting, diarrhea, constipation, colic, food allergies, or eczema? Did later conflicts over eating occur (e.g., refusal to eat, bulimia, hoarding)? What are the child's current eating habits?

5. Adoption and or placement—What were the circumstances surrounding the adoption or placement of this child in the parent/guardian's home (e.g., motivation, acceptance, support)?

6. Motor development—At what age (in months) did the child first hold his or her head erect, sit alone, stand, and walk alone? How is the child's coordination (gross and fine)? Is the child right- or left-handed? Does the child have repetitive movements or mannerisms?

7. Speech development—When did the child first use single words, two- and three-word phrases, and sentences? Did the child have trouble with faulty articulation or stammering? How mature is the child's current language, vocabulary, and syntax? Is the child able to carry a conversation?

8. Sphincter control—When did the child first learn to control his or her bladder and bowels? What method of training was used? How did the child respond to training (e.g., with resistance or acceptance)? Did the child regress during training? Has the child had problems with enuresis or encopresis?

9. Sleep—Has the child had sleep problems in the past? What are the child's current sleep habits (e.g., is the child a deep sleeper, restless, or insomniac)? Does the child have fears of the dark or of being alone? Does the child sleepwalk, rock head or body, have nightmares or night terrors, or resist going to bed?

10. Sexual development—Did the child display early sexual curiosity or sex play? Has the child received sex education? Has the child begun to menstruate, or have nocturnal emissions? Does the child masturbate? What is the child's gender-role identification? Is he or she interested in the opposite sex? Has the child experienced any sexual trauma?

E. Educational Progress

1. Academics & activities—What schools has the child attended? What grade is the child in now? Who are the child's teachers? How is the child's current academic performance? Does the child have any learning problems or any need for special education or tutoring? Does the child participate in school sports and activities?

2. Behavior—How are the child's relationships with peers and teachers? How does the child respond to school rules?

What is the child's capacity to concentrate? Does the child have problems with trua`ncy, fear of going to school, or school refusal? Has the child bullied others or been the victim of bullying? What is the child's attitude toward homework? Does the child exhibit any antisocial behavior at school? Does the child have any history of drug or alcohol use or abuse?

3. Ambitions & involvement—What are the child's ambitions? Is the child involved in social and recreational activities?

F. Home Environment

1. Physical arrangement—Where is the home located? What is the neighborhood like? What are the neighbors like? How is the home laid out? What are the sleeping arrangements? Does the home have inside and outside spaces for play? Are the parent(s)/guardian(s) satisfied with the domestic arrangements?

2. Schedule—What is the child's typical weekday and weekend schedule, from rising to retiring?

G. Parent–Child Relationships

1. Child's behavior—How was the child's early temperament (i.e., easy or difficult)? Has this changed with age? What is the child's general mood? What is the child's capacity for affection, tolerance for frustration, and proneness to tantrums? Is the child aggressive, resentful, fearful, or timid; depressed; sociable; and accepting of limits, rules, and discipline? How does the child respond to punishment (i.e., by being stubborn or compliant)?

2. Parenting methods—What methods do the parent(s)/guardian(s) use to set limits and discipline the child? Are these methods applied with consistency? How much time does the family spend together (i.e., father–child, mother–child, entire family)?

3. Attitudes & conflicts—What are the child's attitudes toward each parent (e.g., closeness, mutual understanding)? Do conflicts about dependence and independence exist between the child and parent(s)/guardian(s)?

H. Social Relationships

1. Siblings & peers—How are the child's relationships with siblings and peers? Does the child tend to be a leader, a follower, or a protector? Is the child overly dependent?

2. Games—Is the child able to win or lose at games? What are the child's favorite games?

3. Social behavior—Does the child exhibit any antisocial behavior? How are the child's relationships with authority figures?

4. Technology and social media use—What devices does the child have or have access to? What social media platforms does the child use? What are the expectations around technology and social media use?

I. Family Background

1. Parent(s)—What is each parent's age, occupation, and physical and mental health? What is each parent's drug and alcohol intake? What are the ages, health, and occupations of both sets of grandparents? What are each parent's family, educational, `and occupational backgrounds? Pay particular attention to the emotional climate of each parent's family of origin, the relationship between the parent(s)/guardian(s) and their parents, the parent(s)/guardian(s)' schooling, and their occupational histories. What is the family history of psychiatric disorders, mental retardation, learning problems, substance abuse, antisocial behavior, or physical illness?

2. Marital history—Were the parents married previously? How did they meet, and what was their courtship like? Were they both accepted by their respective in-laws? What were the early years of marriage like (e.g., sexual adjustment, division of labor, management of money, method of settling interparental disputes)? How effective is each parent's parenting ability? What is their capacity for affection? What is their motivation for childcare and childrearing?

3. Siblings—How old is each of the child's siblings? What is the current health of each sibling? How does each sibling do in school or in his or her occupation? What is each sibling's overall personality? How does each sibling relate to the child?

4. Family values—What is the family's ethnic or sociocultural background? Is there a relative emphasis on conformity or independence, authority or freedom, warmth or coolness, control or expression? What are the family's religious, moral and esthetic values? Does the family put an emphasis on education, piety, money, success, prestige, or gender differentiation?

5. Family & community—How involved is the family in school activities, religious organizations, cultural bodies, and civic affairs? What extended family support does the child/family have?

Termination—At the end of the parent interview (usually one or two 2-hour interviews), the information gathered is summarized. The parent(s)/guardian(s) should be invited to add anything they think is important and to correct any misinformation. The interviewer should then tell them when he or she wants to see the child and the family again.

Bostic JQ, King RA: Clinical assessment in children and adolescents. In: Martin A, Volkmar FR (eds). *Lewis' Child and Adolescent Psychiatry*, 4th edn. Philadelphia: Lippincott Williams & Wilkins, 2007, pp. 323–343.

Leckman JF, Taylor E: Clinical assessment and diagnostic formulation. In: Thapar A, Pine DS, Leckman JF, et al. (eds). *Rutter's Child and Adolescent Psychiatry*, 6th edn. Oxford: Blackwell, 2017.

Nurcombe B: The diagnostic encounter in child psychiatry: data gathering. In: Nurcombe B, Gallagher RM (eds). *The Clinical Process in Psychiatry*. New York: Cambridge University Press, 1986, pp. 460–506.

Simmons JE: *Psychiatric Examination of Children*, 2nd edn. Philadelphia: Lea & Febiger, 1974.

II. EVALUATING INFANTS

PURPOSE OF THE INFANT EVALUATION

The psychiatric evaluation of infants and their parent(s)/guardian(s) is designed to yield information concerning the following: the nature and development of the problem perceived by the parent(s)/guardian(s); the child's developmental history; the parent's history (e.g., early relationships, prior experience with children, knowledge of child development, marital relationship, and medical and psychiatric history); parent–child interaction; infant development and attachment; and the parent(s)/guardian(s)' perception of the infant.

Information on these matters is gathered by interviewing the parent, observing the infant, observing the interaction between parent and infant, and, if necessary, conducting standardized assessments.

INTERVIEWING THE INFANT'S PARENT(S)/GUARDIAN(S)

Infants and their parent(s)/guardian(s) are usually referred by a pediatrician because of disturbances in regulation (e.g., insomnia, excessive crying, feeding problems, head banging), social disturbances (e.g., interactional apathy or negativism, traumatic separation, excessive separation anxiety), psychophysiologic disturbances (e.g., failure to thrive, vomiting), or developmental delay.

It is debatable whether, at the first interview, the parent(s)/guardian(s) should be interviewed alone or together with the infant. The infant's presence is likely to generate historical information from the parent(s)/guardian(s) that might otherwise be missed. However, a number of interviews will be required, observation of parent–child interactions will always be necessary, and the aim of the interview will not be achieved unless a working alliance is formed.

The interview begins with introductory questions about family structure and dates of birth and quickly proceeds to a history of the problem. The following questions could be asked: When did the problem begin? How has it evolved? What is the problem now? What have the parent(s)/guardian(s) done about it? How do they account for it? Why do they come for help now? What do they want from the clinician?

Next, the clinician elicits the infant's developmental history, including the circumstances surrounding, and the reaction of both parent(s)/guardian(s) to, conception, pregnancy, delivery, and early infant care. The child's medical history will also be gathered.

As the alliance deepens, the clinician elicits information about the parent(s)/guardian(s)' relationships with their own parent(s)/guardian(s) and siblings, their prior experience of childcare, their knowledge of child development, their preconceptions about being a parent, and their expectations about the baby (and whether these expectations have been borne out). The history and current status of the marital relationship will also be explored. If other individuals provide a significant amount of the infant's care, they should also be interviewed.

The clinician seeks to identify critical dynamic sequences of behavioral interaction (e.g., the mother becomes anxious, disorganized, and angry if the baby refuses to eat), looking for connections between present emotional interactions and past significant relationships and events.

OBSERVING THE PARENT–INFANT INTERACTION

During the interview, parent(s)/guardian(s) should be encouraged to attend to the infant's needs, for example, consoling, changing, or feeding the infant, if necessary. Parent(s)/guardian(s) will also be asked to play with the child. Parent–child dyads can then be observed with regard to the quality of attachment, the vigilance of the parent(s)/guardian(s) concerning the infant's safety, the parent(s)/guardian(s)' attunement to and effectiveness in responding to the infant's need states, the quality of parent–child play, parental teaching ability, parental control, the affective tone of the interaction, and infant temperament. The clinician should remember that he or she is observing only brief samples of dyadic behavior. By seeking a working alliance and putting the parent(s)/guardian(s) at ease, the clinician can try to ensure that the samples of behavior observed are representative.

The next several sections describe specific observations about the parent/guardian–child interaction that the clinician can make during the infant evaluation.

1. Attachment—How close is each dyad? Are they, for example, detached or clinging, or able to separate sufficiently to allow the infant to explore? Does the infant seek body or eye contact with the parent/guardian? Does contact with the parent/guardian reassure the child, or is the infant inconsolable? Does the infant explore the surroundings recklessly, confidently, cautiously, or not at all? Does the infant get pleasure from the exploration? How does he or she respond to separation? How does the parent/guardian feel about it?

2. Protection—Is the parent/guardian vigilant, overprotective, or careless in regard to the infant's reckless, cautious, or confident exploration? Or does the parent/guardian strike a good balance, given the infant's apparent temperament? How does the parent/guardian feel about the infant's exploration?

3. Regulation of need states—Is the parent/guardian attuned to the infant's needs concerning hunger, discomfort, pain, or stimulation? Does the parent/guardian know when to stimulate the infant, when to back off, and when and how to console the infant? Does the parent/guardian make effective use of eye contact, soothing voice, smiling, facial movements, wrapping, touching, holding, rocking, nursing, and dorsal patting or rubbing in stimulating or consoling the infant? How does the infant respond to the parent/guardian's ministrations?

4. Play—Do parent/guardian and infant play together in a manner appropriate to the infant's developmental level? Do parent/guardian and infant enjoy the playful interaction?

5. Teaching—If the infant is old enough, ask the parent/guardian to teach him or her to stack blocks or solve a puzzle. Does the parent/guardian make effective use of modeling and language? Does the infant imitate the parent/guardian? Does the parent/guardian allow the infant sufficient opportunity for trial and error to solve a problem independently?

6. Control—Does each parent/guardian maintain calm, confident control of the infant, or is the parent/guardian helpless, passive, inconsistent, disorganized, explosive, punitive, or overly controlling? How effectively does the parent/guardian communicate in words? How does the infant respond? In response to the parent/guardian's attempts to control his or her behavior, is the infant heedless, provocative, negativistic, passive, disorganized, or biddable?

7. Emotion—What is the affective tone of the interaction? Is the infant generally happy, angry, sad, neutral, affectively "empty," or unresponsive? What is each parent's emotional state? Are the members of the dyads attuned to each other? If the infant becomes upset, is he or she able to regain equanimity in a reasonable time?

8. Temperament—Temperament refers to relatively enduring characteristics of the infant's behavioral response to the internal and external environments. Despite limitations in the duration and representativeness of the behavioral sample elicited, the clinician may be able to make observations concerning the infant's activity level, tendency to approach or withdraw from people, adaptability to new situations, affective intensity, mood, persistence with tasks or play, sensory threshold, and distractibility.

STANDARDIZED TESTING

Through standardized testing, the clinician can explore hypotheses generated from the history and observation of parent–infant interaction. Tests are available, for example, with regard to infant psychomotor development, parent–infant interaction, infant attachment, quality of the home environment, infant temperament, and the parent's working model of the infant. Although some of these tests are best regarded as research instruments, several may have clinical utility. Furthermore, parent(s)/guardian(s) can be involved in the data-gathering process of many of these tests, with potentially great educational benefit.

A. Developmental Level

Tests of infant development have only modest predictive validity with regard to tested intelligence in later childhood. There is increasing evidence that intellectual development is characterized by individual differences and discontinuity rather than a smooth progression. Early infant development tests must be applied too soon to tap those elements of intelligence (e.g., language-based cognitive skills) that are highly responsive to the home environment. Nevertheless, if the infant tests very low in some or all developmental domains, the clinician should be concerned.

1. Brazelton Neonatal Behavioral Assessment Scale— The Brazelton Neonatal Behavioral Assessment Scale (NBAS) was designed for use with the full-term neonate, but it has also been modified to apply to high-risk infants. The NBAS is usually administered 3 and 9 days after birth. It surveys reflexes and behavioral responses in such a way as to yield a profile of social interactiveness, state control, motoric behavior, and physiologic response to stress. It has modest predictive power with regard to later developmental measures.

2. Bayley Scales of Infant Development (2–30 months)— The Bayley Scales assess development in three domains: mental (perception, memory, problem solving, communication), psychomotor (gross and fine motor), and behavior (the affective responses of the infant). This test uses a structured play approach.

3. Infant Muller Scales of Early Learning (0–38 months)— The Infant Muller Scales of Early Learning assess gross motor development, visual reception, visual expression, language reception, and language expression. The scales are useful in following the progress of children who are thought to have specific areas of developmental delay.

4. Other instruments—The Transdisciplinary Play-Based Assessment and the Connecticut Infant–Toddler Developmental Assessment Program involve the parent(s)/guardian(s) with the clinical team in the collection of data on different domains of development.

B. Parent–Child Interaction

The Greenspan–Lieberman Observation System for Assessment of Caregiver Interaction During Semistructured Play and the Parent–Child Early Relationship Assessment rate interactive behavior from video samples of free or semistructured play. Parental detachment, emotional negativity, lack of vocal contact, lack of visual contact, and inconsistency, for example, can be detected, along with infant detachment, negative affect, inattention, and defects in motor and communication skills.

C. Infant Attachment

The best-known measure of infant attachment is the Strange Situation (12–24 months). In this technique, the infant–parent dyad is exposed to a series of brief episodes involving gradually increasing stress, as the parent/guardian stays with the child, leaves, returns, and leaves; a stranger joins the child; and the parent/guardian finally returns. The child's behavior during the two reunion episodes is classified as secure, insecure–avoidant, insecure–resistant, or disorganized. Disorganized behavior is particularly likely to be associated with serious environmental pathology and poor outcome.

D. Home Environment

The Home Observation for Measurement of the Environment (two versions: 0–3 years, 3–6 years) assesses the quality of intellectual stimulation in the home by rating the parent/guardian's involvement with and responsiveness to the child, the organization of the home environment, and the provision of a variety of play materials.

E. Infant Temperament

The Revised Infant Temperament Questionnaire asks the parent/guardian to rate the infant in nine domains of temperament and allows the infant to be categorized as easy, slow to warm up, difficult, intermediate low, or intermediate high. This instrument is a measure of parental perception of the infant and is influenced by the parent/guardian's personality.

F. The Parent's Working Model of the Child

The Working Model of the Child Interview is a research instrument with potential clinical applicability. It is a structured interview that explores topics such as the child's development, the parent's perception of the child's personality and behavior, and the parent–child relationship. The parent/guardian's responses are rated on a number of scales (e.g., coherence, richness, flexibility, intensity), and the parental model of the child is classified as balanced, disengaged, or distorted.

DIAGNOSTIC FORMULATION & TREATMENT PLANNING

The diagnostic hypotheses generated during the parent/guardian interview are tested and refined during the observation of parent–infant interaction and, when required, through the use of standardized tests. If no pediatric examination has been completed, or if specialized pediatric consultation is required, this will be requested. The current problem is classified, for example, according to the scheme developed by the National Center for Clinical Infant Programs (NCCIP; Table 11–2). Next a diagnostic formulation is completed and a treatment plan designed, and the diagnosis and plan

Table 11–2 The NCCIP Classification of Infant Disorders

Disorder of social development and communication
  Autism
  Atypical pervasive developmental disorder

Psychic trauma disorder
  Acute, single event
  Chronic, repeated

Regulatory disorder
  Hypersensitivity type
  Under-reactive type
  Active-aggressive type
  Mixed type
  Regulatory-based sleep disorder
  Regulatory-based eating disorder

Disorders of affect
  Anxiety disorder
  Mood disorder
    Prolonged bereavement
    Depression
    Labile mood disorder
    Mixed disorder of emotional expressiveness
    Deprivation syndrome

Adjustment reaction disorders

are discussed with the parent(s)/guardian(s) as the clinician seeks to consolidate the working alliance preparatory to the treatment phase.

Carter AS, Godoy L, Marakovitz SE, Briggs-Gowan MJ: Parent reports and infant–toddler mental health assessment. In: Zeanah CH (ed). *Handbook of Infant Mental Health*, 3rd edn. New York: Guilford Press, 2012, pp. 252–265.

Gilliam WS, Mayes LC: Clinical assessment in infants and toddlers. In: Martin A, Volkmar FR (eds). *Lewis' Child and Adolescent Psychiatry*, 4th edn. Philadelphia: Lippincott Williams & Wilkins, 2007, pp. 309–322.

Miron D, Lewis ML, Zeanah CH: Clinical use of observational procedures in early childhood relationship assessment. In: Zeanah CH (ed). *Handbook of Infant Mental Health*, 3rd edn. New York: Guilford Press, 2012, pp. 252–265.

III. INTERVIEWING CHILDREN

PURPOSE OF THE CHILD INTERVIEW

Depending on the child and the clinical circumstances, an interview with a child 4–11 years of age has a number of purposes. The interview can help the clinician ascertain how the child feels about being interviewed and what the child believes to be the purpose of the interview. It can also help to correct misapprehension and orient the child to the interview. The interview can be used to determine whether the child recognizes that a problem exists and, if so, what accounts for it. In terms of aiding the diagnosis, the interview can be used to complete a mental status examination; to explore the child's self-concept and perceptions of the key figures in his or her world (e.g., family, friends, authorities); to assess the child's intellectual, language, emotional, social, and moral development; and to gauge the effectiveness of the child's coping mechanisms. Finally, the interview can be used to establish a working alliance and to assess the child's capacity to benefit from treatment.

FACTORS AFFECTING THE CHILD INTERVIEW

Although the primary purpose of the interview is diagnostic, it is artificial to separate diagnosis from treatment. Adverse impressions formed early can impede or obstruct therapy; in contrast, if an alliance is formed early, the child will be more willing to return for treatment.

The type of interview that evolves depends on the child's developmental level, personality, and expectations; the environment in which the interview takes place; the interviewer's personality and interactive style; and the goals of the interview. For example, a preschool child is likely to express ideas and feelings through actions rather than words. In contrast, a mature 11-year-old child may be able to converse throughout the interview. Most children mix play with conversation. The clinician must, therefore, combine observation, play, and conversation in different degrees with children of different maturity levels.

The well-adjusted child is likely to be reticent about sharing very personal matters with a stranger, unless he or she accepts the need to do so. The psychologically disturbed child may be even more inhibited; initially, such children may express fantasies, secrets, or private fears indirectly. In contrast, some disorganized, emotionally needy younger children have such poor defenses that they release a torrent of psychopathologic material before they have established a trusting relationship with the examiner.

The child's expectation of the interview greatly influences its course. Children seldom come to a psychiatrist of their own accord, and the individuals who bring them may not have prepared them well. Children may enter the interview hostile, fearful, bewildered, apathetic, or even eager for help. Younger children commonly fear bodily invasion (e.g., injections) or are concerned that the physician will expose secret inferiorities or shameful memories. Some children are afraid that they will be induced to talk about matters so frightening that they have never talked about them before. Adolescents universally have a fear of being rendered helpless. Children with a history of antisocial behavior may expect a tricky cross-examination. Children with learning problems may be afraid of being exposed as dunces. The experienced interviewer can often anticipate these fears and deal with them early in the interview.

Office Environment

Although an experienced clinician can be surprisingly effective in unpromising surroundings, adequate space and equipment are helpful. Some clinicians have access to separate playrooms with extensive equipment and fittings, but many arrange their own offices to interview children.

An ideal room will be large enough to have a carpeted section for seated interviewing, a section with linoleum-tiled floor suitable for play, and a small table and chairs. Play equipment should be stored in a lockable cupboard that has additional space for materials associated with particular patients who are in therapy. Otherwise, the equipment is communal. An inquisitive child can be told that the play material belongs to the office and may not be taken away.

With regard to play equipment, it is preferable to err on the side of frugality. Clinicians should remember that equipment is a means to the development of a relationship and the expression of thoughts and feelings. The less clutter, the more the child must draw from inside. A list of basic equipment would include the following: easel, newsprint paper and felt pens, blocks, assorted toys of wild and domestic animals, Matchbox cars, dolls (representing parent(s)/guardian(s), brother, sister, baby, and grandparents, together with a nurse and a doctor), one or two stuffed animals, a rubber ball, a pack of playing cards, and a set of checkers. Clinicians can add to this list other items (e.g., puppets, toy pistols, board games, dolls' house furniture, plastic construction models), guided by their interest and what seems to work best for them. Clinicians should avoid games that preclude fantasy, such as chess or scrabble. Finger paints, poster colors, and Play-Doh are suitable only for fully equipped playrooms, but clinicians may wish to keep a soccer ball, a football, and a baseball and gloves for outdoor play.

Clinicians should not be anchored to the office. An occasional visit to a soda fountain, outdoor construction site, nursery, or gymnasium can be very useful, especially with highly active youngsters who find a restricted office environment tedious.

Style of the Interview

The goals of the interview shape its style. Sometimes it is essential to obtain from the child a detailed account of a past event, especially in medico-legal situations. Such situations are much less common than those in which clinicians can allow the interview to evolve as the interaction dictates.

Two polar interviewing styles are exemplified by the relatively **unstructured approach** and the highly **structured interview.** Structured interviewing may be valuable for research purposes, but it is not recommended for regular clinical interviewing.

A **semi-structured interview** involves the application of a flexibly and sensitively applied systematic approach. The interview should be organized in accordance with a hypothetico-deductive strategy, but it should not compromise a positive relationship for the sake of extracting information. In most cases, two or three 1-hour interviews are required in order to gather enough information to reach a reliable diagnosis.

Clinicians who wish to work with children should enjoy being with children. They should be sufficiently in touch with the past to be able to recapture and empathize with the sadness, anger, frustration, bewilderment, and enthusiasms of childhood. Clinicians should be warm, accepting, and supportive but neither overly identified with the child nor intolerant of children's natural messiness. Some interviewers are active, engaging, and direct. Some are very quiet, saying no more than is necessary to keep the child's conversation flowing. Some use humor to relax the anxious child. All should be unhurried, with no axe to grind; children are very perceptive of intolerance or irritation cloaked by a falsely bright exterior. The best interviewer is a kind of catalyst—able to attend when the child is freely associating or playing, able to interpolate a comment or question to restart a stalled interview, able to get down on the floor and play with the child when it is appropriate to do so, but capable of setting reasonable limits. Skillful clinicians inject only as much of themselves into the situation as necessary to allay the child's anxiety and promote his or her self-expression.

Clinicians should reflect on their personal responses to each patient. When these responses are dominant, inexorable, and overly generalized, they disrupt the empathic acceptance required for effective interviewing. They can vary from intellectualization and boredom when confronted by an inarticulate child, to the need to rescue a troubled child from what are perceived as villainous parent(s)/guardian(s). The rescuer is likely to set up an unproductive tug-of-war with parent(s)/guardian(s). Others are prone to reductionist thinking, avoiding close contact with the child and withdrawing into their particular theoretical preferences (e.g., neurobiology, systems theory, psychoanalytic theory, cognitive–behavioral theory).

CONDUCTING THE CHILD INTERVIEW

Guidelines

The interviewer should not wear a white coat; it signals needles to some children. Clothing should enable the interviewer to sit on the floor if needed. The interviewer should not whisper to the parent(s)/guardian(s) about the child in the child's presence. He or she should speak openly, or leave comments to a later time.

The interviewer should try to avoid taking notes during the interview. A few key phrases may be jotted down to provide reminders of the sequence of events. The interviewer then may dictate his or her memory of the interview as soon as it is finished.

Special Considerations

The cardinal aim of the first interview is to help the child relax with the interviewer and to lay the foundation of trust. Nothing should be allowed to compromise this aim, because without trust little can be achieved. If trust does develop, the interviewer will be able to clarify the purpose of the interview, ascertain whether the child perceives problems in his or her life, evaluate the child's affect and capacity to relate to the interviewer, and catch a glimpse of his or her family life. Further specific features of the child's history and mental status can often wait for a second or third interview, unless the child is especially cooperative at the initial interview, or unless the matter is urgent.

At the start of the interview, the interviewer should go into the waiting room and greet the parent(s)/guardian(s) and child. He or she should sit beside the child and offer an introduction. The interviewer should tell the child that together they will talk, draw, and play for about an hour and then should invite the child into the interview room. If the child is resistant, the interviewer should wait briefly to see if the parent(s)/guardian(s) can reassure the child. If this does not work, the parent(s)/guardian(s) may be asked to bring the child into the room, indicating that they will be leaving when the child is comfortable. Usually, the parent(s)/guardian(s) can leave after a short time, at a signal from the interviewer. If not, it is seldom necessary for the parent(s)/guardian(s) to be present for more than one or two interviews.

For the younger child, the interviewer will have set out suitable play materials in the interview room. The child of 9 or 10 years of age can be ushered to an appropriate chair. The interviewer can begin by asking older children why their parent(s)/guardian(s) asked them to come and how they feel about it. If the child cannot say, the interviewer should tell the child what he or she already knows and ask for the child's personal reaction to this information. If the child is younger, he or she may be invited to use the play equipment. The interviewer should not push the child. The play theme should emerge on its own. The interviewer may then gently test the child to see whether he or she is prepared to talk.

Questions to Ask

If the child is comfortable conversing with the interviewer, the topics listed in Table 11–3 can be touched on. These topics flow in a natural sequence from neutral to personal. The first seven topics, though informative, are essentially icebreakers. The last four topics require reflection and are likely to be more difficult for the child. However, the list should not be followed rigidly; rather, the topics can be explored in a discretionary manner. One child may be disposed to give a detailed account of peer and family relations, another will provide little on anything beyond neutral topics, and a third will prefer to play with toys and to converse intermittently about them.

Children are relatively more concrete than adolescents. They have difficulty understanding abstractions, taking an objective view of themselves or others, and accurately timing past events. Questions should not be framed in a leading or suggestive manner (a caution that applies particularly in medico-legal situations). Children are confused by complex or compound questions: One idea to one question is the best. The interviewer should avoid asking children "Why?" because it puts them on the defensive. Consider the following example:

Patient: The other kids pick on me.

Clinician: Why?

Patient: I don't know. They're mean.

The clinician might have asked the following questions: What do they say? What do they do? How do you feel about it? What do you do about it? When a child uses an unusual word or phrase, particularly if it has an "adult" quality, do not assume it has the same meaning for the child that it has for *you*. Inquire further.

The interviewer should avoid trying to ferret out the truth from a child who has been involved in antisocial behavior. Instead he or she should try to get in touch with the child's feelings about the situation and what led up to it. It can sometimes be useful to gently point out discrepancies or inconsistencies to an older child who is apparently fabricating a story.

When the interviewer introduces matters that have an anxiety-laden connotation, especially if they seem to imply that the child is "weird" or unique, it can be helpful to associate the issue with the difficulties of other children in similar circumstances. These are known as **buffer comments**. Consider the following example:

Clinician: I see a lot of kids here who have problems after their parent(s)/guardian(s) get divorced. Some of them can't help blaming somebody. I wonder if you ever felt like that.

Ending the Interview

At the end of the interview, the clinician should recapitulate with the child what they have both learned about the child's reasons for being seen and how he or she feels about it. If another interview is planned, the interviewer should indicate when it will be. Children should not be asked if they would like to return for another visit. The child may be taken back to the parent(s)/guardian(s) in the waiting room. Whispered hallway consultations with the parent(s)/guardian(s) should be avoided. If urgent consultation with the parent(s)/guardian(s) is needed at that time, the interviewer should conduct the discussion briefly in the interview room, preferably with the child present.

Table 11–3 Issues Covered During the Child Interview

Content Category	Issues Covered
Attendance	Reason for and feelings about attendance.
School	School, class, teacher. Best and least liked teachers. Reasons? Best and least liked subjects. Reasons? School grades and homework. Liking for other school activities. Reasons? Changes of school? Reasons?
Neighborhood	Neighborhood, social groups, clubs.
Recreation	Hobbies, talents. Best liked activity. Reasons? Sports.
Social relationships	Best friend. Reason best friend Is liked? Enemies. Reasons enemies are disliked? Experiences of persecution or scapegoating.
Leadership/ambitions	Opportunities and aspirations for leadership. Ambition with regard to occupation, marriage, and family.
Illness	Recent illnesses, experiences of hospitalization.
Domestic arrangements	House: layout, yard space, bedroom. Chores. Parents, siblings, pets. Family activities most enjoyed. Relationship between parents, alliances within the family, and conflicts within the family.
Fantasy	Dreams, good and bad. Three wishes. What would the child do with $1,000,000? Mutual story-telling. Drawings: of the family doing something together, of a person, of "something nice" and "something nasty."
Symptoms	Fears, anxiety, obsessions, compulsions, dissociative phenomena, depression, depersonalization. If indicated, hallucinations, ideas of reference, delusions, concerns about death, suicidal ideation, difficulty controlling anger, and antisocial behavior.
Insight	Understanding of the reason for attendance. Understanding of the nature of the problem. Desire for help.

INTERPRETING CHILDHOOD FEARS AND FANTASY

The interpretation of childhood play, fears and fantasy is a specialized skill requiring theoretical knowledge and supervised practical experience. It is important to know the normative fantasies of children of different ages. For example, 4-year-old children often have fantasy themes concerning omnipotence, loss of approval, bodily injury, and curiosity about body differences and functions. By 5–6 years of age, children have an emerging capacity for guilt following transgressions. The polarities of love and hate, kindness and cruelty, death and rebirth are often expressed in fantasy. By 7–8 years of age, children have a fear of injury, particularly in competitive interaction with peers. There are emerging fears of inferiority in comparative strength, speed, beauty, or intelligence, and a concern with rules and conformity. Gender-role differences are also important. By 9–10 years of age, children have a capacity for guilt and internal conflict, but morality tends to be black and white. Children may be normally preoccupied with the themes of television shows and cartoons, particularly those themes having to do with heroic invulnerability, pursuit and rescue, transgression and punishment. Gender-role differences become more imperative as adolescence approaches.

The clinician should not be surprised if an 8-year-old child prefers to draw with paper and pencil than with poster colors or finger paints. No particular importance should be attached to the observation that a 4-year-old enjoys constructing towers and knocking them over or that a 6-year-old recounts episodes of Spiderman. The trick is to recognize deviations from, distortions of, or immaturity in the normative phase-related themes discussed in this section.

Lewis M, King RA: Psychiatric assessment of infants, children, and adolescents. In: Lewis M (ed). Child and Adolescent Psychiatry: A Comprehensive Textbook. Philadelphia: Lippincott Williams & Wilkins, 2002, pp. 525–543.

Simmons JE: Psychiatric Examination of Children, 3rd edn. Philadelphia: Lea & Febiger, 1981.

▼ IV. INTERVIEWING ADOLESCENTS

PURPOSE OF THE ADOLESCENT INTERVIEW

The initial psychiatric interview of an adolescent has three general purposes: (1) establishing the possible diagnoses, (2) providing therapeutic intervention, and (3) creating a foundation for psychiatric treatment. The first purpose is to establish the possible diagnoses. The interview of the adolescent is only one part—perhaps the most important part—of the full diagnostic process, which also includes interviewing the parent(s)/guardian(s) and may include psychological testing, laboratory tests, a physical examination, and the gathering of information from outside sources.

The second purpose for the initial interview is to provide some form of therapeutic intervention. After a single conversation, this intervention is not likely to constitute a cure but may simply be a sense of relief for the adolescent to get something off his or her chest. The youngster may leave the appointment with a sense of satisfaction that somebody is making an effort to listen to his or her grievances or with a sense of hope that there will be a way to solve a particular problem over a period of time.

The third purpose of the initial interview is to create a foundation for a continuing course of psychiatric treatment. It is the time to start negotiating the alliance between the therapist and the adolescent. That is, the interviewer communicates that he or she will try to understand the youngster's point of view, even if he or she does not agree with it. The interviewer will promote the interests of the patient in both the short term (e.g., resolving an immediate impasse or conflict) and the long term (e.g., defining and encouraging goals and aspirations). At the same time the interviewer will help the adolescent acknowledge and accept his or her responsibilities to family and community.

FACTORS AFFECTING THE ADOLESCENT INTERVIEW

Although the diagnostic process can be both productive and enjoyable, it is frequently a difficult experience for both the interviewer and the interviewee. A physician who feels perfectly comfortable and competent in dealing with an adult patient may become frustrated and tongue-tied when he or she tries to develop a conversation with a 14-year-old adolescent. It is almost always possible to establish rapport and collect information from adolescents, despite the tension and suspicion that may be sensed by both parties.

The physical setting of the interview is important. The office does not need to be fancy, but it should be comfortable and pleasant, relatively soundproof, and located far enough from the waiting room to create a sense of privacy.

▶ Style of the Interview

The general manner in talking with adolescents should be relaxed and informal. It is good to have a sense of humor. Stuffiness creates distance; arrogance invites sarcasm; authoritarianism invites defiance. Being informal and friendly does not mean that the interviewer should become chummy and ingratiating. Teenagers want some degree of social distance between themselves and adults.

Should the interviewer initially meet with the parent(s)/guardian(s), with the teenager, or with the entire family together? It depends on the presenting problem and the circumstances of the interview, but the most common format is for the interviewer to go to the waiting room, introduce himself or herself to both the patient and the parent(s)/guardian(s), ask the patient to come with him or her to the office, and indicate that he or she will meet with the parent(s)/guardian(s) in a little while. The purpose, of course, is to communicate to the teenager that this meeting is for the teenager. It is helpful to know the parent(s)/guardian(s)' primary concerns ahead of time, which can be learned at the time the appointment is set up or perhaps through an intake questionnaire.

Some adolescents are cooperative, talkative, and quite aware of the purpose of the meeting. In that case, the patient may be perfectly willing to launch into a discussion of the reason for the evaluation. Other youngsters are embarrassed, guilty, or defensive. In that case, it is usually preferable initially to avoid the topics that are most difficult and to spend some time talking about subjects that are important but not as threatening. This part of the interview is an opportunity to take an interest in the patient's general life experience, not just in the immediate problem area. By the end of the meeting, the interviewer should know about the teenager's assets and successes as well as his or her problems.

Asking direct questions may not be the best way to elicit information. Teenagers become defensive almost automatically when they hear questions like "Where did you go?" and "Why did you do it?" Instead of asking, "Why did you steal that car?" the interviewer might say, "Tell me what you were thinking about when you were driving the car."

The interviewer may wish to propose other forms of communication, in addition to the usual dialogue. It might be helpful to ask the youngster to draw a picture of what happened or what he or she observed. The teenager may be able to communicate through dolls or puppets. Young adolescents may be more comfortable with play materials that are typically used with younger children. However, the interviewer should be careful not to insult a more mature teenager by suggesting that he or she use the dolls that are in the office.

Barker P: *Clinical Interviews with Children and Adolescents.* New York: WW Norton & Company, 1990.

Bernet W: Humor in evaluating and treating children and adolescents. *J Psychother Pract Res* 1993;2:307.

Katz P: Establishing the therapeutic alliance. *Adolesc Psychiatry* 1998;23:89.

Meeks J, Bernet W: *The Fragile Alliance.* Melbourne, FL: Krieger, 1990.

CONDUCTING THE ADOLESCENT INTERVIEW

It is advisable for the interviewer to develop and follow a fairly consistent format in interviewing adolescents. Such a format helps the interviewer remember to touch on a number of important areas in addition to the topic that is of most immediate interest. The interviewer should follow a regular format but be flexible and ready to improvise. As the interviewer moves from one topic to the next, he or she should use transitions and keep the youngster informed about why a particular subject is being discussed. For example, the interviewer could say, "Now I want to ask you some questions about your family, so that I know who everybody is."

▶ Starting the Interview

One way to start the interview is to ask the youngster whose idea it was to come for the appointment. That may lead to a discussion of the chief complaint and the present illness.

If the patient is defensive, the interviewer can invite the patient to tell about school, which is usually a nonthreatening subject. The patient can describe his or her schedule, comment on specific subjects studied, and talk about what he or she thinks is the best part and the worst part of school. A discussion of the patient's ideas about what he or she will be doing after high school graduation gives an indication of the patient's level of optimism and his or her ability to engage in long-range planning.

▶ Collecting Information

The interviewer might ask whether other children in the patient's school get in trouble and what happens to them, which is an opportunity for the youngster to talk about the various bad things that a child might do without necessarily attributing any of it to himself or herself. The discussion of other children in school leads naturally to the topic of peer relationships. Most teenagers can relate what they enjoy doing with friends and also what they may like to do by themselves.

Talking about enjoyable activities gives the adolescent an opportunity to tell about special interests, abilities, hobbies, music, and television. The interviewer can ask about the television shows that the youngster enjoys and ask whether he or she can relate what happened during specific episodes. Not only does this test the patient's memory and ability to organize a narrative, but the youngster may project his or her own issues and concerns onto favorite television shows. It is important to ask about technology and social media use with the adolescent. Asking what devices they have, what apps/social media platforms they use and how they engage with these technologies are increasingly important in adolescents' lives.

Another useful topic is the youngster's version of his or her health history, because he or she may have interesting and unusual notions about illnesses and operations he or she has had. The health history leads to other areas, such as substance abuse. The interviewer should ask specifically about use of tobacco, alcohol, marijuana, cocaine, hallucinogens, and inhalants. The health history also leads to a discussion of sexual activities and related issues, such as sexually transmitted diseases.

It is always important for the youngster to tell about his or her family: the names of family members, their ages, what kind of work they do, whether they have had serious illness or problems. It might be useful to ask what the parent(s)/guardian(s) do when the youngster has been particularly good or particularly bad. The interviewer could ask if the parent(s)/guardian(s) are unusually strict, which leads to questions about emotional abuse and physical abuse.

▶ Incorporating the Mental Status Examination

One way to blend the history and the mental status examination is to take an **inventory of affects**. The interviewer may ask the patient to tell about a time when he or she was particularly happy, a time he or she was worried, a time he or she was frustrated, and so on. The interviewer may ask about a time that something funny or silly happened or ask the patient to relate a favorite joke.

If the patient has been depressed, the examiner should ask about suicidal thoughts and behaviors, which are not unusual among adolescents. Sometimes it is preferable to be indirect, using questions such as, "Have you ever known anybody who was suicidal?" "Did your friend ever do anything to actually hurt himself?" or "Did anything like that ever happen to you?" Teenagers should be encouraged to tell a parent or other adult if they have persistent or serious suicidal thoughts. If suicidality is a serious concern, this would be a good time to tell the youngster about both confidentiality and the exceptions to confidentiality. Most youngsters find it reassuring (rather than threatening) to learn that the new doctor will keep them safe by discussing dangerous or risky impulses with their parent(s)/guardian(s).

Depending on the differential diagnoses that the interviewer is considering, it may be appropriate to ask the patient about psychotic processes such as delusions, hallucinations, thought insertions and removal, and ideas of reference. Because many adolescents like to demonstrate what they know about psychological phenomena, it is possible to ask a series of questions such as, "Do you know what a hallucination is?" "Can you give me an example of a hallucination?" "Have you ever known anybody who hallucinated?" and "Does that ever happen to you?"

Getting to the Point of the Interview

The interview should not end without addressing the issue or the behavior that led to the referral in the first place. Almost always, that topic will come up at some point during the interview—at the outset of the interview; during the discussion of the patient's school activities, friends, medical history, and family; or through questions related to mental status. Occasionally the patient is so defensive, embarrassed, or simply lacking in insight that he or she seems to avoid the basic reason for the evaluation. Perhaps the parent(s)/guardian(s) have brought the youngster because of their concerns about inappropriate sexual behaviors, bizarre obsessive preoccupations, or persistent antisocial conduct. In such cases, the patient may be strongly motivated to keep the interviewer busy discussing other topics. If the youngster seems to be avoiding the subject, the interviewer can bring it up by saying, for example, "Your mom told me on the phone that you have been taking three or four showers every day. Can you tell me about that?" The interviewer can explain that he or she needs to hear the whole story, including the adolescent's side of the story, in order to be of help.

Ending the Interview

After collecting this information, the clinician may want to summarize his or her understanding of the most significant topics. This summary communicates to the patient that the interviewer has tried to understand the situation from the patient's point of view and also allows the patient to make additions or corrections.

It is good to end the initial interview on a positive note. For example, the interviewer can comment positively on the youngster's plans for the future, make specific suggestions regarding the patient's presenting problems, or simply say that the interviewer has enjoyed the meeting.

The end of the initial interview is also an appropriate time to touch on the subject of confidentiality. Because the interviewer is about to meet with the patient's parent(s)/guardian(s), he or she might say, "We have talked about a lot of things today. Is there anything you said that I should not discuss with your folks?" This is a concrete way of communicating that the material discussed in therapy is generally confidential. The patient's answer may tell a lot about his or her relationship with the parent(s)/guardian(s), and it also

protects the therapist from making some blunders with the parent(s)/guardian(s) early in the relationship with the family. The interviewer can add that he or she would need to tell the parent(s)/guardian(s) if the patient appeared to be at risk for self-harm or for harming another person.

Kalogerakis MG: Emergency evaluation of adolescents. *Hosp Community Psychiatry* 1992;43:617.

STRUCTURED DIAGNOSTIC PROCEDURES

Clinical information regarding adolescents may also be collected through structured interviews and standardized inventories. These tools are commonly used in clinical research and epidemiologic studies, but they may be useful in clinical practice in some circumstances. These structured procedures are not required for a satisfactory diagnostic interview of an adolescent but may increase the sensitivity of the evaluation in some cases. See Chapter 34 for more information on structured interviews. Another instrument is the Child Behavior Checklist, a questionnaire regarding symptoms and behaviors that may be completed independently by the father, the mother, and the adolescent. The responses are compared to normative data, and the patient is scored along internalizing and externalizing symptom clusters.

Weist MD, Baker-Sinclair ME: Use of structured assessment tools in clinical practice. *Adolesc Psychiatry* 1997;21:235:.

V. INTERVIEWING FAMILIES

IMPORTANCE OF THE FAMILY INTERVIEW

The family (considered in its broadest sense to include the combined nuclear and extended family system) is the developmental matrix for every child's behavior: normal and symptomatic. This universal principle is the basis of family interviewing. The family interview provides a rapid and efficient method of diagnosis and treatment in child and adolescent psychiatry.

Family diagnosis is concerned with the prevailing condition of the family. Family assessment is the process of gathering information about that condition. Although the clinician endeavors to understand each individual, family interviewing concerns the patterns of interaction of those individuals.

The symptomatic behavior of the child or adolescent may not be the source of the family's problems, but rather its result. In children and adolescents, symptoms are shaped by the family matrix in which they start and are perpetuated. Symptoms in young people develop as their hereditary endowment is shaped by their experiences in the family environment. Pathologic behavior can be interpreted as a strategy for survival in a maladaptive family system.

These concepts are embodied in family systemic thinking in four ways: (1) symptoms reflect family relationship disturbances and not simply deviant behavior; (2) if the patient is approached as the exclusive repository of pathology, much diagnostic and therapeutic leverage is lost; (3) functional psychopathology can be fully understood only in context of the family; and (4) if the dysfunctional family matrix can be changed, the child's or adolescent's symptoms may change.

There is much debate in the field of family therapy concerning the classification of family psychopathology. A discussion of the various approaches is beyond the scope of this chapter.

PURPOSE OF THE FAMILY INTERVIEW

The family interview can provide important interactional data complementing individual interviews and contributing to diagnosis and treatment planning. The goals of the family interview are as follows: to gather a comprehensive history of the present illness, to observe and assess pathogenic family interactions, to determine whether the child's disturbed behavior stems from pathologic family interactions, to formulate a family diagnosis and design a treatment plan, to promote the family's understanding and motivation for treatment, and to negotiate a therapeutic alliance concerning the diagnosis and the treatment plan.

CONTENT OF THE FAMILY INTERVIEW

Table 11–4 lists the topics commonly covered in a family interview. It is desirable that all members of the family be present at the family interview. Clinicians may find this unfamiliar, but it is surprisingly easy to accomplish. Frequently a sibling will provide the key to a therapeutic dilemma, saving hours of diagnostic time. Table 11–5 lists the aspects of family interaction that can be observed in a family interview.

CONDUCTING THE FAMILY INTERVIEW

Haley has proposed four stages for the initial interview: (1) introduction, (2) problem identification, (3) family interaction, and (4) conclusion.

▶ Introduction

In the introduction, the clinician greets the family members, learns their names, and sets them at ease. The clinician gives recognition and status to every family member through direct

Table 11–4 Issues Covered During the Family Interview

Content Category	Issues Covered
Explicit information	What are the chief complaints of the family and the patient? ("Patient" denotes the identified patient; however, the symptomatic child often turns out to be quite adaptable and is the symptom bearer for an even more disturbed family system.) How do family members understand the present problem? How does the patient see it? Have organic factors been considered (hereafter, it will be assumed that these have been ruled out)? Why does the family come in at this time? What is the background of the problem? How has the family attempted to solve this problem in the past? What are the family's expectations of the interview? What are their motivations and resistances?
Background information	Perinatal and childhood development Current medical problems and medications Past medical and psychiatric illnesses and hospitalizations Family medical and psychiatric history Family demographics Family's employment, educational, housing, and financial status Legal problems of family and patient, past and present
The patient's relationships	With peers (Is the patient gregarious? Popular? Friendly? A loner? Combative?) With teachers and school personnel (Is the patient an academic success or failure? Compliant? Oppositional?) With siblings (Is the patient cooperative? Antagonistic?) With parents and extended family (Are family relationships close? Harmonious? Frictional? Distant? Hostile?) Are supportive aunts, uncles, or grandparents available?
Family's relationships	With the community, such as church and school (Is the family connected? Participative? Isolated? Aloof?) With extended family (Is the family cordial? Warm? Welcoming? Distant? Cold? Rejecting?) With friendship networks (Is the family rewarding? Congenial? Conflictual? Isolated?)

Table 11–5 Aspects of Family Interaction Observed in the Family Interview

Aspects of Family Interaction	Questions to Consider
Overall family communication	Are family members harmonious? Cooperative? Irritable? Immature?
Parental Interaction	Are the parents close? Encouraging Independence? Responsible? Congenial? Remote? Unstable? Frictional?
Parent-child Interaction	Are the parents appreciative? Accepting? Supportive? Respectful of privacy? Critical? Neglectful? Discouraging independence? Intrusive? Do exclusive alliances exist (e.g., overly close mother and overly dependent child, excluding father)?
Sibling Interaction	Interviews that include the patient's siblings can provide crucial data. Is the patient treated as the perfect child? Is the patient being scapegoated (i.e., blamed for the family's problems)? Do the siblings accept the blaming or try to defend the patient?
Extended family Interaction	Does the patient have a supportive aunt, uncle, or grandparent who resists the pathogenic atmosphere of the nuclear family? Is the mother so attached to her own mother that she Is more like a child herself? Is the father's anger toward a family member taken out on one of the children?

interaction with each of them. He or she explains the rationale for involving all members of the family, for example, by saying, "The more members of the family I see, the more they can help me to help Billy. Besides, I can get much more information more quickly." The clinician acknowledges family members' apprehensions and provides support. He or she avoids guilt-inducing statements by reframing the problem, for example: "Society is sometimes critical of these problems, but I can see you've done the best you could in the face of many difficulties." Finally, he or she observes the patterns of power and affiliation as they are revealed, for example, by where family members sit and who speaks out.

▶ Problem Identification

In the problem identification stage, the clinician elicits a statement of the problem from each member of the family. Labels attached to people are transformed into relationship questions (e.g., the statement "She's spoiled" elicits from the clinician, "I see—who spoils her the most?"). Statements that are too long or too short are controlled (e.g., with responses such as "Excuse me. I need to interrupt you, Mary, so I can hear what Tom has to say" or "I'm surprised, Mr. Smith. You must have noticed more than that"). At the end of this stage, the clinician elicits from a family member a summary of the problem (e.g., "Mr. Smith, would you summarize the problem as we've been discussing it?").

▶ Family Interaction

In the family interaction stage, the clinician has two members talk with each other about the problem (e.g., "Talk directly to your wife about this, instead of telling me"). The discussion may be interrupted to bring other family members into the conversation (e.g., "They seem to be stuck. Why don't you

help them out?"). The seating arrangement may be changed in order to alter interactive patterns (e.g., "Mom, I'd like you to sit by dad and give Billy a bit more space on the sofa"). The interviewer may reframe the family views of reality, for example, by emphasizing a family member's good intentions or recasting symptoms as having a positive function in the family (e.g., "What do you think might happen if they didn't have you to worry about?").

CONCLUSION

In the conclusion, the clinician provides a summary in such a way as to engender hope (e.g., "Most families have some periods of difficulty with their teenagers, and they get past them."). The clinician provides encouragement so as to increase motivation for treatment. Humor may be useful. The clinician invites questions to increase understanding, outlines a treatment plan, and arranges further sessions with key family members, as necessary.

Beavers WR, Hampson RB: *Successful Families: Assessment and Intervention*. New York: WW Norton & Company, 1990.

Eisler I, Lask J: Family interventions. In Thapar A, Pine DS, Leckman JF, et al. (eds). *Rutter's Child and Adolescent Psychiatry*, 6th edn. Oxford: Blackwell, 2017.

Gurman AS, Kniskern DP: *Handbook of Family Therapy*, Vol 2. Levittown, PA: Brunner/Mazel, 1991.

Kerr M, Bowen M: *Family Evaluation*. New York: Norton, 1988.

Ritvo EC, Glick ID: *The Concise Guide to Marriage and Family Therapy*. Washington, DC: American Psychiatric Press, 2002, pp. 1303–1327.

Sholevar GP: Family therapy. In: Martin A, Volkmar FR (eds). *Lewis' Child and Adolescent Psychiatry*, 4th edn. Philadelphia: Lippincott Williams & Wilkins, 2007, pp. 323–343.

Diagnostic Evaluation for Children and Adolescents

Barry Nurcombe, MD[†]
Michael G. Tramontana, PhD

Based on the diagnostic hypotheses (generated, tested, and refined during history taking), the mental status examination, and the observation of family interaction, the inquiry plan proceeds to physical examination and, if required, to laboratory testing, special investigations, consultations, and psychological testing.

Figure 12–1 summarizes the flow of clinical reasoning from history taking, mental status examination, and the generation of diagnostic hypotheses, through physical examination and special investigations, the refinement of the clinical pattern, secondary diagnostic hypotheses, psychological testing, and the diagnostic conclusion, to the diagnostic formulation and treatment plan.

▼ I. CHILD MENTAL STATUS EXAMINATION

PURPOSE OF THE CHILD MENTAL STATUS EXAMINATION

The child mental status examination is a set of systematic observations and assessments that provide a detailed description of the child's behavior during the diagnostic interview. Combined with the history and physical assessment, the mental status examination yields evidence that helps the clinician to refine, delete, or accept the diagnostic hypotheses generated during the diagnostic encounter and to decide whether special investigations are needed in order to test particular diagnostic hypotheses. Thus, the mental status examination is an integral part of the inquiry plan. In accordance with the diagnostic hypotheses and the inquiry plan, the mental status examination may be brief or comprehensive, but it always incorporates both standard and discretionary probes.

The mental status examination of the adolescent is similar to that of the adult (see Chapter 4). However, the examination of children is sufficiently different to warrant separate

discussion. Many of the observations required to complete the mental status examination are made in the course of the semistructured interview with the child. Other observations, such as the clinical tests that screen cognitive functions, are part of a standardized set of questions.

AREAS ADDRESSED BY THE MENTAL STATUS EXAMINATION

Table 12–1 lists the areas covered by the mental status examination. For the most part, the first five areas are noted as the interview proceeds, whereas the last five require special questions.

▶ Appearance

Note the following: height, weight, nutritional status; precocious or delayed physical maturation or secondary sexual characteristics; abnormalities of the skin, head, faces, neck, or general physique; personal hygiene and grooming; and style and appropriateness of dress.

▶ Motor Behavior

Observe the following: general level of physical activity (e.g., hyperkinesis, hypokinesis, bradykinesis), in comparison with others of the same age; abnormalities of gait, balance, posture, tone, power, and fine and gross motor coordination; abnormal movements (e.g., tremor, twitching, shivering, tics, fidgeting, choreiform movements, athetoid movements, motor overflow); mannerisms, rituals, echopraxia, or stereotyped movements; motor impersistence; or pronounced startle response.

▶ Voice, Speech, & Language

Listen for the following: accent; abnormality in pitch, tone, volume, phonation, or prosody (e.g., squawking, shouting, whispering, monotony, hoarseness, scanning, high-pitched voice); abnormality in the amount of speech (e.g., mute,

[†]Deceased.

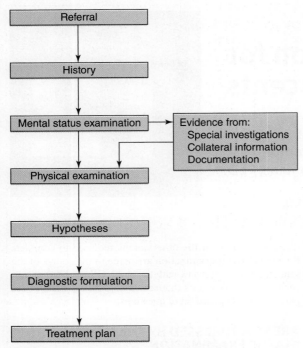

▲ **Figure 12–1** The process of clinical reasoning.

impoverished, voluble, loquacious) or its tempo (e.g., slowed, accelerated); abnormal rhythm (e.g., stuttering); abnormal articulation (e.g., dyslalia); unusual or inappropriate use of words (e.g., idioglossia, profanity); echolalia; abnormal syntax; and impairment in expressive or receptive language (e.g., difficulty finding words).

▶ Interaction with the Examiner

Note the patient's eye contact (e.g., eyes averted, unfocused, staring). Is the child friendly and cooperative, or resistant, oppositional, shy, or withdrawn? Is he or she assertive,

Table 12–1 Areas Covered by the Mental Status Examination

Appearance
Motor behavior
Voice, speech, and language
Interaction with the examiner
Mood and affect
Cognitive functions
Thought processes
Thought content
Fantasy
Insight

aggressive, impudent, sarcastic, cynical, fearful, clinging, inhibited, indifferent, clowning, invasive, coy, or seductive? Is the child a reliable informant?

▶ Mood & Affect

In demeanor and conversation, does the patient show evidence of a persistent abnormality of mood or of poor emotional regulation? For example, is there evidence of anxiety, tension, rage, depression, elevation of mood, silliness, apathy, or anhedonia? Is the child emotionally labile, or conversely, does he or she exhibit a restricted range of affect? Which topics evoke the most intense emotion?

▶ Cognitive Functions

Cognitive screening tests do not replace formal psychological testing. They serve as rapid clinical screens to determine whether formal testing is required. The following areas should be tested: attention, orientation, memory (immediate, recent, remote), judgment, abstraction, and intelligence (see Panels I–VI). Do not proceed with the tests described in the accompanying panels unless the patient has demonstrated a basic familiarity with numbers, letters, and words (see Table 12–2).

▶ Thought Processes

Is there evidence of abnormal tempo, with flight of ideas or acceleration, slowing, or poverty of thought processes? Does the stream of thought lack clear goal direction, with vagueness, incoherence, circumstantiality, tangential thinking, derailment, or clang associations? Is the normal continuity of associations disrupted by perseveration, circumlocution, circumstantiality, distractibility, or blocking? Is there evidence of impairment in logical or metaphorical thinking—for example, in a blurring of conceptual boundaries or abnormally concrete thinking?

▶ Thought Content

From the history given by the parents, the intake questionnaires and checklists, and free discussion with the child, the clinician will have generated hypotheses that can be tested by direct probes concerning clinical phenomenology. The following symptoms may not be routinely checked unless there are good hypothetico-deductive reasons for doing so:

Table 12–2 Prescreening Questions for Cognitive Testing

Area	Ask Patient To
Numbers	Count from 1 to 20
Letters	Recite the alphabet
Words	Point to his or her nose, mouth, chin, neck, and knees

I. ASSESSMENT OF ATTENTION

Clinician: "Listen carefully. I'm going to say some numbers, but sometimes I'll say a letter instead. Say Yes! each time you hear me say a letter instead of a number."
Recite the following at the rate of one item per second:

1 2 3 D 9 8 A 4 E Z 6 1 5 9 T 3 B 8 2 Q 7 3 2 J L 4 8 2 C

Evaluation:
Record number of errors of omission: _____
Record number of errors of commission: _____
Total: _____

Clinician: "Listen again. This time I'm going to say some letters, but sometimes I'll say a number instead. Say Yes! each time you hear me say a number instead of a letter."
Recite the following at the rate of one item per second:

B K L 4 O(oh) 6 P M 9 C N F O(oh) P 6 S 1(one) E G 3 J H U 0(zero) 9 6 W T 5

Evaluation:
Record number of errors of omission: _____
Record number of errors of commission: _____
Total: _____

Serial sevens. *Clinician:* "Can you subtract 7 from 100? What is 100 minus 7?" *If correct, say:* "Good. I want you to count backwards, taking 7 from 100, then 7 from 93, as far back as you can." *(Record response)*

Correct answer: 93, 86, 79, 72, 65, 58, 51, 44, 37, 30, 23, 16, 9, 2

Evaluation:
Record time (seconds) taken to reach final number: _____
Record number of errors: _____

If the subject cannot subtract 7 from 100, try serial threes.

Serial threes. *Clinician:* "Can you subtract 3 from 20? What is 20 minus 3?" *If correct, say:* "Good. I want you to count backwards, taking 3 from 20, then 3 from 17, as far back as you can." *(Record response)*.

Correct answer: 17, 14, 11, 8, 5, 2

Evaluation:
Record time (seconds) taken to reach final number: _____
Record number of errors: _____

II. ASSESSMENT OF ORIENTATION

Ask the patient the following questions:

Time:

"What is the day of the week?"
"What is the date?"
"What season is it?"
"What time is it?"
"How long have we been talking here?"

Place:

"What is this place?"
"What kind of place is this?"
"How did you get here?"
"How far is this place from your home?"

Person:

"Tell me your name."
"What school do you go to?"
"What grade are you in at school?"
"Who am I?"
"What is my job?"
"Why have you come to see me?"

Evaluation:

Record number of accurate responses: —————

III. ASSESSMENT OF MEMORY

Recent Memory

Clinician: "Now I will give you three things to remember, and in a few minutes I will ask you to recall what they are. John Smith, 500 Kings Highway, Green." *After five minutes, say:* "Please repeat those three things."

Evaluation (choose one):

Accurate
Needs prompting
Cannot repeat any
Refused

Clinician: "Now keep those things in your mind until I ask you for them again."

Immediate Memory

Clinician: "I want you to listen carefully and repeat these numbers after me." *Speak at the rate of one number per second. Continue upward until the patient fails. Record the last accurate repetition.*

8
4 3
3 9 6
4 2 1 9
8 5 1 9 2
9 3 5 2 8 6
7 5 8 3 9 2 4

Evaluation (record number):

Unable
Refused

(continued)

III. ASSESSMENT OF MEMORY (*Continued*)

Clinician: "Now please repeat these numbers backward." *Continue upward until the patient fails. Record the last accurate repetition.*

> 3
> 9 1
> 4 7 3
> 5 8 2 9

Evaluation (record number):
> Unable
> Refused

Clinician: "Now, what were those three things I asked you to remember?"

Correct answer: John Smith, 500 Kings Highway, Green

Evaluation (choose one):
> Refused
> None correct
> Parts of A *or* B correct, only
> Parts of both A *and* B correct
> C correct, only
> Two fully correct, only
> Two out of three correct
> Three correct

Remote Memory

Clinician:

> "What is your address?"
> "What is your telephone number?"
> "Where were you born?"
> "What is the date of your birthday?"
> "What is your mother's name?"
> "Where was she born?"
> "What is the date of your mother's birthday?"
> "What is your father's name?"
> "Where was he born?"
> "What is the date of your father's birthday?"

Evaluation:

> Record number of accurate responses: —————

IV. ASSESSMENT OF JUDGMENT

Clinician: "Suppose the teacher had her back to the class and someone else flicked a rubber band at you. What would you do?"

Wait for spontaneous answer and record it.

If no answer is given, offer the following prompts:
> "Ignore it?"
> "Raise your hand to tell the teacher?"
> "Go after the one that threw it?"

Clinician: "Suppose you were out walking and you saw smoke pouring out of the roof of a house on your street. What would you do?"

Wait for spontaneous answer and record it.

IV. ASSESSMENT OF JUDGMENT (*Continued*)

If no answer is given, offer the following prompts:
"Arouse someone in the house and tell them?"
"Ring a fire alarm?"
"Run home and tell your mother?"
"Ignore it?"

Clinician: "Imagine you were walking home from school and a girl in front of you dropped her purse without knowing it. What would you do?"

Wait for spontaneous answer and record it.
If no answer is given, offer the following prompts:
"Tell her or give it back?"
"Ignore it?"
"Look inside?"
"Keep it?"

V. ASSESSMENT OF ABSTRACTION

Clinician: "Tell me how these two things are alike:"

wood and coal
apple and peach
ship and automobile
iron and silver
baseball and orange
airplane and kite
ocean and river
penny and quarter

Clinician: "Do you know what a proverb is?" *(If not, discontinue.)* "Good. Tell me, in your own words, what these proverbs mean."

A stitch in time saves nine.
People in glass houses should not throw stones.
A rolling stone gathers no moss.

Clinician: "Tell me the meaning of the following words:" *Read out loud, ceasing after five consecutive items are incorrect:*

orange	roar	scorch
envelope	muzzle	brunette
straw	haste	peculiarity
puddle	lecture	priceless
tap	mars	regard
gown	skill	disproportionate
eyelash	juggler	shrewd
		tolerate

(continued)

V. ASSESSMENT OF ABSTRACTION (*Continued*)

Evaluation:

Number Correct	Vocabulary Age
5	6 years
6	6 years 8 months
7	7 years 4 months
8	8 years
9	8 years 8 months
10	9 years 4 months
11	10 years
12	10 years 8 months
13	11 years 4 months
14	12 years
15	13 years 3 months
16	14 years
17	14 years 3 months
18	14 years 6 months
19	14 years 9 months
20	Average adult

VI. DRAWING ABILITY

Clinician: Use a No. 2 pencil with eraser on 8 × 11 blank paper. Instruct the patient as follows: "On this piece of paper, I would like you to draw a whole person. It can be any kind of person, just make sure it's a whole person and not a stick figure or a cartoon figure." *For a young child who does not understand "person":* "You may draw a man or woman, a boy or girl." *(There is no time limit.)*

Evaluation: One point (3 months) is given for each item. Multiply the total number of correct items by 3. This is the patient's "drawing age" in months. Quote drawing age in years and months. Calculate the patient's "drawing quotient" as follows:

(Drawing age/Chronological age) × 100

Each feature present:

Head	Ear	Shoulders	Leg
Eye	Hair	Arm	Foot
Nose	Neck	Hand	Heel
Mouth	Trunk	Finger	Clothing

Details:

Pupil	Nostrils	Hands distinct from arms
Eyebrow	Two-dimensional nose	Arm joints
Eyelash	Hair more than on crown	Leg joints

Correct number off eatures:

Two eyes	Ten toes
Two ears	Two articles of clothing
Two hands	Four articles of clothing
Ten fingers	Costume complete

VI. DRAWING ABILITY (*Continued*)

Relatively correct location:
    Symmetrical features
    Ears in correct position
    Neck continuous with head
    Arms from shoulders

    Legs attached to trunk
    Opposition of thumb
    joints shown

Proportional size:
    Head more than circle
    Eye longer than high
    Body longer than head

    Fingers longer than wide
    Arms in proportion
    Legs in proportion

In profile:
    Eyes glance to front
    Forehead shown
    Chin projection shown
    Profile
    Correct profile

anxiety, separation anxiety, school refusal, panic attacks, phobias, obsessions, compulsions, impulsions, delusions, hallucinations, ideas of reference, ideas of influence, thought alienation, thought-broadcasting, depersonalization, déjà vu, derealization, suicidal ideation, impulses to injure the self or others, preoccupation with somatic functioning, somatic symptoms, stealing, fire setting, truancy, and fighting. In contrast, suicidal ideation, self-injury, assaultive impulses, substance abuse, physical or sexual abuse, risk taking, and antisocial behavior must always be inquired about when diagnostic evaluations are undertaken with adolescents.

▶ Belief Systems/Unstructured Fantasy

The child's way of thinking, belief systems, or fantasy can be elicited through play, drawing, and storytelling. By his or her unobtrusive interest, the clinician can facilitate the child's unstructured beliefs and encourage the child to express them. Table 12–3 lists a variety of techniques that can be used to elicit these worldviews of the child.

▶ Insight

Is the child aware that he or she has a problem? If so, how is the problem conceptualized? Does the child want help for the problem?

STRUCTURED INTERVIEWING

Semistructured playroom interviews with children 7–12 years of age have been found to have a test–retest reliability of 0.84 and an inter-rater reliability of 0.74, with regard to the detection of abnormality. However, interviewers who are unaware of the parents' perception of the child's problems tend to underestimate abnormality in comparison with parent reports of child behavior.

In order to compensate for the potential unreliability of unstructured or semistructured interviewing, a number of structured interviews have been introduced. As a rule, these interviews are too cumbersome for everyday clinical work; however, they are widely used to standardize subject selection in research studies. Arguably, semistructured and structured interviewing complement each other: The semistructured interview yields information mainly about the child's perception of self and environment, whereas the structured interview focuses on symptomatology. When reliable diagnostic categorization is the overriding consideration, structured interviews such as those described in this section are clearly preferable. It should be remembered, however, that with children younger than 10–12 years of age, the reliability of direct questions concerning symptomatology is affected by the fact that children are limited in their capacity to be objective about themselves. Furthermore, emotionally disturbed preadolescents tire if exposed to long, tedious interviews and may become careless in their answers. Table 12–4 provides more detailed information on these instruments.

A. Diagnostic Interview for Children and Adolescents (DICA)

DICA is a semistructured interview that uses a modular technique, organized by diagnostic syndrome. Parent, child, and adolescent versions are available. Clinical judgment is required at several decision points; otherwise, lay

Table 12–3 Techniques to Elicit Child's Belief Systems

After the child has drawn a person, ask him or her the following types of questions:
Is that person a man or a woman, a boy or a girl?
How old is he/she?
What is he/she doing in that picture?
What is he/she thinking about?
How does he/she feel about it?
What makes him/her happy?
What makes him/her sad?
What makes him/her mad?
What makes him/her scared?
What does he/she need most?
What's the best/worst thing about him/her?
Tell me about his/her family?
What will he/she do next?

Use the Kinetic Family Drawing test:
a. Ask the child to draw his or her family doing something together.
b. Note who the child puts in the family; the proximity of the figures; the coherence of or separations between group members; the relative importance and power of the family members; and their apparent emotions, attachments, rivalries, and so on.
c. Ask the child to explain the drawing, saying what the family members are doing, thinking, and feeling, and what the outcome will be. Base your questions, in part, on discretionary probes derived from the dynamic hypotheses you have generated.

Ask the child to draw "something nice" and "something nasty." Consider using the following questions as icebreakers:
What would you do if you had a million dollars?
If you had three wishes, what would they be?
If you were wrecked on a desert island, who (and what) would you like to have with you?
Ask the child to tell you about (good/bad) dreams he or she has had recently.
Ask the child for the earliest thing he or she can remember, and for his or her earliest memory about his or her family.

Table 12–4 Structured Interviews in Child and Adolescent Psychiatry

Instrument	Target Age (Years)	Time Needed (Minutes)	Reliability
Diagnostic Interview for Children and Adolescents (DICA)	6–17	60–90	Inter-rater and test–retest reliabilities are acceptable Parent–child agreement: 0–0.87 on specific items (k = 0.76–1.00 for anxiety and conduct disorders)
Diagnostic Interview Schedule for Children (DISC)	9–17	60–90	Inter-rater reliability: 0.94–1 for symptoms Test-retest reliability for parents: .9 (symptoms), 0.76 (syndromes); for children aged 14–18: 0.8 (symptoms), 0.36 (syndromes) Parent–child agreement: 0.27 (greatest for disruptive symptoms, less for depression or anxiety)
Schedule for Affective Disorders and Schizophrenia for School-Age Children (K-SADS)	6–18	180	Inter-rater reliability: .65–.96 (syndromes) Test-retest reliability: variable, 0.09–0.89 (symptoms), 0.24–0.7 (syndromes) Parent–child agreement: 0.08–1.00 (symptoms)
Child Assessment Schedule (CAS)	7–17	45–75	Inter-rater reliability: 0.73 (for content, less for diagnosis); higher for hyperactivity and aggression (0.8), less for anxiety (0.6)
Interview Schedule for Children (ISC)	8–17	90–120	Inter-rater reliability: 0.64–1.0 Parent–child agreement: 0.2–0.95 (symptoms), 0.32–0.86 (syndromes), lowest for subjective symptoms
Child & Adolescent Psychiatric Assessment (CAPA)	8–18	90–120	Not available

interviewers can administer DICA. A computerized version is available for recording and scoring results. DICA has reasonable validity comparing pediatric and psychiatric referrals (especially in academic and relationship problems).

B. Diagnostic Interview Schedule for Children (DISC)

DISC is a highly structured interview that is organized by topic, in a manner close to a natural free-flowing interview. It is mainly epidemiologic in purpose. Parent and child versions are available, and clinical judgment is not required. DISC has reasonable validity comparing pediatric and psychiatric referrals. Diagnoses are generated by computer algorithm.

C. Schedule for Affective Disorders and Schizophrenia for School-Age Children (K-SADS)

K-SADS is a semistructured instrument that has been used extensively in child psychiatry research. Parent, child, and epidemiologic versions are available. Clinical judgment is required. The same clinician interviews the parent and the child and attempts to resolve discrepancies in their reports. This interview was originally developed to identify children with affective disorder. It now emphasizes affective, anxiety, and schizophrenic disorders. It is scored manually, and diagnosis is reached from summary ratings. Pilot validity data come from follow-ups, treatment change, and biological correlate studies.

D. Child Assessment Schedule (CAS)

CAS is a semistructured interview that has been used with both children and adolescents. Parent and child versions are available. Interviewer training is required. Interview items are grouped by topic (e.g., school, peers, family), not syndrome. CAS does not cover posttraumatic stress disorder, dissociative disorder, or adolescent schizophrenia. Its pilot validity was estimated by comparing inpatients, outpatients, and normal subjects.

E. Interview Schedule for Children (ISC)

ISC was designed originally for a longitudinal study of depressed children and may be most useful for the diagnosis of depression. Parent and child versions are available. ISC requires clinical skill, judgment, and training.

F. Child and Adolescent Psychiatric Assessment (CAPA)

CAPA is intended for use in both clinical and epidemiologic settings. Parent and child versions are available. It starts with an unstructured discussion and proceeds to a systematic inquiry into a broad range of symptoms for which an extensive glossary is available. It contains psychosocial and

family functioning sections. Lay or clinician interviewers can administer it, and it is scored by computer algorithm.

Angold A, Costello AJ, Egger H: Structured interviewing. In: Martin A, Volkmar FR (eds). *Lewis' Child and Adolescent Psychiatry*, 4th edn. Philadelphia: Lippincott Williams & Wilkins, 2007, pp. 344–356.

Bostic JQ, King RA: Clinical assessment in children and adolescents. In: Martin A, Volkmar FR (eds). *Lewis' Child and Adolescent Psychiatry*, 4th edn. Philadelphia: Lippincott Williams & Wilkins, 2007, pp. 323–343.

Leckman JF, Taylor E: Clinical assessment and diagnostic formulation. In: Thapar A, Pine DS, Leckman JF, et al. (eds). *Rutter's Child and Adolescent Psychiatry*, 6th edn. Oxford: Blackwell, 2015.

Simmons JE: *Psychiatric Examination of Children*, 3rd edn. Philadelphia: Lea & Febiger, 1981.

▼ II. PHYSICAL EXAMINATION, LABORATORY TESTING, & SPECIAL INVESTIGATIONS

PHYSICAL EXAMINATION

Usually, a physical examination has already been completed by the child's pediatrician. If not, the clinician should refer the family to the primary physician. In some circumstances, however, it is important that the child psychiatrist complete the physical examination. Table 12–5 lists those aspects of the physical examination to which the clinician should pay particular attention.

Table 12–6 lists symptoms that could be referable to the central nervous system and indicate the need for a neurologic examination. The psychiatrist can perform a brief, routine neurologic screen during the interview by observing the

Table 12–5 Physical Examination Items Deserving Special Attention

Growth parameters: height, weight, and head circumference plotted on standard curves
Minor physical anomalies (associated with developmental problems such as hyperactivity):
Abnormally small or large head
"Electric" hair (fine, dry hair standing upright from the scalp)
Epicanthic folds (skin folds in the upper internal eyelid)
Hypertelorism (eyes deep-set and widely separated)
Low-set, malformed, asymmetrical ears with adherent earlobes
High palate
Furrowed tongue
In-curved little finger
Long third toe
Syndactyly
Gap between first and second toes
Other head, face, or body dysplasias that might indicate a congenital disorder (e.g., signs of fetal alcohol syndrome)

Table 12–6 Symptoms that Indicate the Need for Neurologic Examination

Headache
Visual impairment
Deafness
Tinnitus
Poor balance
Episodic disruption of consciousness
Memory defects
Intermittent confusion
Anesthesia
Paresthesia
Motor weakness
Impaired coordination
Abnormal movements
Recent loss of sphincter control

Table 12–8 Neurologic Soft Signs

Choreiform or athetoid movements, especially of the out-stretched fingers and hands
Dysdiadochokinesia (difficulty performing rapid alternating movements)
Dysgraphesthesia (difficulty interpreting a figure traced on the palm of the hand)
General clumsiness
Synkinesis (the tendency for other parts of the body to move in unison when one part is moving)

child's speech, gait, posture, balance, gross and fine motor tone, power and coordination, facial symmetry, and ocular movements and by checking for tics, tremors, clonus, or choreiform movements of the fingers and hands. Table 12–7 lists extensions to the routine screen that can be implemented by baring the child's feet and forearms.

Some child psychiatrists avoid physical examination. The clinician may worry that an upsetting physical examination will impede a positive relationship or tilt the spontaneous development of the child's transference. There may be some point to these considerations, but the potential

benefits of a nonintrusive physical examination outweigh its disadvantages.

Soft or nonfocal signs are phenomena thought to have no clear locus or origin, to be developmentally normal up to a certain age, and to reflect uneven neurologic maturation in older children. Table 12–8 lists commonly identified neurologic soft signs. Can these signs be consensually identified and elicited in a standard manner? Do they have significant test–retest and inter-rater reliability? Do they occur frequently enough in an at-risk population to make them worth eliciting? Are they singly or in clusters associated with disorders such as learning disability, attention-deficit/hyperactivity disorder, or schizophrenia? Do they predict which hyperkinetic children will respond to stimulant medication? For none of these questions is there a clear answer.

Towbin KE: Physical examination and medical investigation. In: Thapar A, Pine DS, Leckman JF, et al. (eds). *Rutter's Child and Adolescent Psychiatry*, 6th edn. Oxford: Blackwell, 2015.

SPECIAL INVESTIGATIONS

The routine use of special investigations for all referred adolescents is not justified. Before ordering a consultation, test, or special investigation, the clinician should consider whether it is a screen inquiry that has a reasonable chance of yielding important information in the clinical population in question (e.g., routine drug or pregnancy testing for hospitalized adolescents) or, in the case of a discretionary probe, whether the particular inquiry could conceivably rule out (or help to rule in) a diagnostic hypothesis. Table 12–9 lists the types of consultations and special investigations often used in child and adolescent psychiatry.

CLINICAL SITUATIONS LIKELY TO REQUIRE SPECIAL INVESTIGATIONS

The clinician must rule out physical disease by the judicious ordering of specific consultations, tests, or investigations in suspicious clinical situations. Table 12–10 lists the clinical situations in which organic causes must be ruled out.

Table 12–7 Extension of the Neurologic Examination

Domain	Functions or Abnormalities
Cranial nerves	Movement of eyes, face, and tongue Pupillary reflexes Visual fields Hearing
Motor power and tone	Shoulder Elbow Wrist Hand Knee Ankle
Reflexes	Biceps Triceps Supinator Patellar Ankle Plantar
Fundi	Papilledema Arteriovenous abnormalities Abnormal pigmentation

Note: Leave the examination of the reflexes and fundi to the end.

Table 12–9 Common Consultations and Special Investigations

Consultations
Pediatric consultation
Neurologic consultation
Other specialist consultations (e.g., speech pathology)
Special investigations
Laboratory testing (e.g., blood, urinalysis, electrolytes, liver function, thyroid function, urine drug screening, and genetic screening)
Acoustic and ophthalmologic examination
Electroencephalography
Neuroimaging
Psychological testing

▶ Acute or Sub-acute Disintegration of Behavior and Development

After a period of normal or relatively normal development, the child may fail to make developmental progress and lose recently acquired skills such as sphincter control, coordination, dexterity, attention and concentration, memory, language, capacity for problem solving, school performance,

Table 12–10 Clinical Situations Likely to Require Special Investigation

Acute or subacute disintegration of development and behavior, with loss of previously attained developmental milestones, deterioration in school performance, and the emergence of erratic aggressive behavior, clinging dependency, or confusion
Acute psychotic episode
Anorexia or weight loss
Attention-deficit, hyperactivity, and impulsivity, especially if of recent or sudden origin
Delay in speech and language development, loss of previously acquired speech and language, or the recent emergence of deviant speech or language
Depression, especially if associated with slowed thinking, deterioration of concentration, vagueness, and fatigue
Episodic or progressive lapses or deterioration of awareness with dreaminess; obtundation; defect in the sensorium; and perhaps, subjective depersonalization, derealization, and hallucinosis
Episodic violence out of proportion to the apparent precipitant, often with memory gaps or amnesia for the episode
General or specific learning problems (e.g., in reading, writing, or calculation)
Localized or generalized abnormal movements that may be associated with vocal abnormalities
Pervasive developmental impairment (especially if associated with an uneven profile of abilities)
Sleep disturbance or excessive drowsiness
Somatoform symptoms of recent onset that mimic a physical disorder but are not consistent with the typical pattern of physical disorder

emotional control, and social competence. In some cases, the child may demonstrate abnormal motor patterns, hallucinations, delusions, and disorganization of thinking. Table 12–11 lists organic causes that must be excluded.

▶ Acute Psychotic Episode

The child or adolescent may become mentally disorganized, socially inappropriate, affectively incongruent, or emotionally labile and report audiovisual hallucinations, illusions, ideas of reference, and delusions of persecution or grandeur. Sometimes the patient becomes mute, immobile, posturing, apparently self-absorbed, and assuming odd postures of the arms, head, and trunk. The following disorders must be excluded: substance-induced psychotic disorder (using urine and blood toxicology) and psychotic disorder due to general medical condition (which requires pediatric consultation and tests specific to hypothesized medical conditions such as hyperthyroidism, hypersteroidism, neurologic disorder).

▶ Anorexia or Weight Loss

The child or adolescent may lose weight markedly as a result of voluntary restriction of food intake. The following conditions should be ruled out: chronic systemic infection (especially tuberculosis); systemic malignancy (especially pancreatic, mediastinal, retroperitoneal, pulmonary, lymphatic, or leukemic malignancy); hypothalamic or pituitary tumor (using skull X-rays, computed tomography [CT] scan, tomogram of sella turcica, or magnetic resonance imaging [MRI]); diabetes mellitus (using urinalysis and glucose tolerance testing); hyperthyroidism (using thyroid function tests); and drug addiction (using toxicology screens).

▶ Headache

The chief causes of headache in childhood are migraine and tension headaches. Migraine is episodic and can be associated with vertigo, unexplained vomiting and abdominal pain, and, rarely, with hemiplegia, temporary episodic impairment of receptive or expressive language, and confusion. Tension headaches are commonly of daily occurrence and difficult to localize. Headaches due to raised intracranial pressure tend to be worse upon wakening or to wake the child, and tend to be associated with vomiting, papilledema, cranial nerve dysfunction, sluggish papillary reflexes, and visual impairment. Seizure-related headache can be ictal or postictal. Specialist consultation is required if the clinician suspects an organic cause of headache.

▶ Attention-Deficit, Hyperactivity, and Impulsivity

Before or after starting school, the child may demonstrate poor concentration, distractibility, and a tendency

Table 12–11 Excluding Organic Causes of Disintegration of Behavior and Development

Possible Organic Cause	Special Investigations
General systemic disease	
Thyroid disorder	Thyroid function tests
Adrenal insufficiency	Adrenal function tests
Porphyria	Examination for urinary porphyrins
Disseminated lupus erythematosus (LE)	Examination for LE cells
Wilson disease	Serum ceruloplasmin
Toxic factors	
Delirium due to systemic infection, electrolyte abnormality, or physiologic toxins	Electroencephalography; specific biochemical, bacteriologic, or virologic tests
Drugs (e.g., intoxication with sympathomimetic drugs, anticholinergic drugs, hallucinogens, or anticonvulsants; withdrawal from sedatives)	Urine drug screen, blood toxicology
Central nervous system disease	
Seizure disorder	Electroencephalography with nasopharyngeal electrodes, telemetry
Space-occupying lesion	Skull X-ray, CT scan, MRI
Herpes encephalitis	Electroencephalography, examination of cerebrospinal fluid, immunologic testing
Metabolic or subacute viral encephalitis	Electroencephalography, examination of cerebrospinal fluid, immunologic testing
Degenerative diseases	Urine amino acids, electroencephalography, MRI, Biopsy
Demyelinating disease	MRI
Leukemic infiltration of central nervous system	Examination of blood and cerebrospinal fluid

to impulsiveness, with or without hyperactivity and learning problems. Table 12–12 lists organic causes that must be excluded.

▷ Delay in Speech and Language Development

The child may manifest a relative delay in comprehending speech or in expressing and correctly enunciating words, phrases, and sentences. Table 12–13 lists organic causes that must be excluded.

▷ Depression

The child or adolescent may become underactive or overactive; insomniac or hypersomniac; impaired in thought tempo, concentration, and energy; readily provoked to tantrum or weeping; socially withdrawn; or preoccupied with thoughts of low self-esteem, guilt, and loss. The differential diagnosis includes virtually any physical disorder

Table 12–12 Excluding Organic Causes of Attention-Deficit, Hyperactivity, and Impulsivity

Possible Organic Cause	Special Investigations
Hyperthyroidism	Thyroid function tests (if there is other evidence of hyperdynamic cardiovascular function and sympathetic overactivity)
Plumbism	Urine lead levels, examination of blood for stippled cells, X-rays of long bones
Seizure disorder	Electroencephalography with nasopharyngeal leads
Sleep apnea	Otorhinolaryngologic examination, sleep electroencephalography and observation
Sydenham chorea	Blood antistreptolysin-O antibody titer

Table 12–13 Excluding Organic Causes of Speech and Language Development Delay

Possible Organic Cause	Special Investigations
Deafness	Acoustic testing
Palatal abnormality	Physical examination
Cerebral palsy	Neurologic examination
Mental retardation	Physical examination, psychological testing
Seizure disorder	Electroencephalography
Aphasia	Consult with speech pathology, neuropsychological testing
Developmental articulatory dyspraxia	Consult with speech pathology and pediatric neurology
Pervasive developmental disorder	See Table 30–4

that could sap energy, impair thinking, and disrupt the capacity to cope.

The following general systemic diseases should be excluded: malignancy, chronic infectious disease, viral infection (e.g., influenza, infectious hepatitis, infectious mononucleosis), hypothyroidism, hypoadrenalism, chronic anemia, and subnutrition (e.g., anorexia nervosa). Chronic intoxication with anticonvulsants or sedatives must be excluded (using urine drug screens and blood levels), as must degenerative central nervous disease (using central nervous system examination, specific tests for the systemic diseases being excluded, CT scan, or MRI).

It is often difficult to determine to what degree a child's depression is part of a pathophysiologic process or to what degree it represents a secondary psychological reaction to loss of function, hospitalization, restriction of freedom, lack of stimulation, or loneliness.

▶ Episodic or Progressive Lapses or Deterioration of Awareness

The patient, usually an adolescent, may experience recurrent episodes during which he or she has a sense of being abruptly altered, different, or unreal and of observing the self as a spectator. The adolescent may perceive that the world is unreal and different or that conversations and scenes have been experienced previously in precisely the same manner. The following organic causes must be excluded: seizure disorder (using electroencephalography), cardiac arrhythmia (using electrocardiology), narcolepsy (using electroencephalography), migraine, and hallucinogenic drug use (using urine drug screen).

▶ Episodic Violence

The child or adolescent may periodically lose control, assault others, or destroy property. Violent behavior may be unheralded, but it usually arises from an emotional context of tension with or without alcohol or drug intake and is disproportionate to the apparent provocation. The individual may or may not have a conduct disorder. The following disorders must be excluded: temporal lobe seizures (using electroencephalography with nasopharyngeal leads), herpes encephalitis (using electroencephalography, immunologic study, and examination of cerebrospinal fluid for viral culture and immunology), drug effects (e.g., alcohol, phencyclidine, hallucinogens, amphetamine; using urine drug screen), and idiosyncratic reaction to alcohol (using patient's history).

▶ General or Specific Learning Problems

The child or adolescent may manifest a general or specific difficulty in learning, particularly in reading, writing, written expression, calculation, or spatial skills. Table 12–14 lists organic causes that must be excluded.

Table 12–14 Excluding Organic Causes of Learning Problems

Possible Organic Cause	Special Investigations
Visual defect	Test visual acuity and visual fields; ophthalmoscopy
Deafness	Acoustic testing
Cerebral palsy	Neurologic examination
Mental retardation	Physical examination, psychological testing
Seizure disorder	Electroencephalography
Dementia due to intracranial space—occupying lesion or cerebral degeneration	Neurologic examination: skull x-rays, CT scan, MRI
Inability to pay attention in class because of debilitating illness, fatigue, hunger, pain, or drug use	None

▶ Localized or Generalized Abnormal Movements

The child or adolescent may manifest repetitive movements that may or may not be partly or wholly under control. The following disorders must be excluded: attention-deficit/hyperactivity disorder, tic disorder, Sydenham chorea (using antistreptolysin-O titer), Huntington's disease, Wilson's disease, paroxysmal choreoathetosis, dystonia musculorum deformans, cerebellar tumor or degeneration, and drug effects (e.g., caffeinism, extrapyramidal side effects of neuroleptic medication).

▶ Pervasive Developmental Impairment

During infancy or afterward, the child may manifest a severe arrest or retardation of language, intellect, and social development. Additional features may include unexplained episodes of panic or rage, marked resistance to environmental change, hyperactivity, repetitive motor phenomena, and deviant speech and language. The onset may be in early infancy (before 30 months) or afterward (up to about 7 years). Sometimes the child regresses from a state of relatively normal development to a state of developmental impairment. More often, the child's abnormal development becomes evident gradually. Several organic causes must be excluded (Table 12–15).

▶ Sleep Disturbance or Excessive Drowsiness

The child may present with hypersomnia, insomnia, nightmares, night terrors, restless sleep, or sleepwalking. Table 12–16 lists organic causes that must be excluded.

Table 12–15 Excluding Organic Causes of Pervasive Developmental Impairment

Possible Organic Cause	Special Investigations
Hearing impairment	Acoustic testing
Aphasia	Speech pathology consultation, language testing
Seizure disorder	Electroencephalography
Chromosomal anomaly	Chromosome analysis (especially if the child looks dysplastic)
Metabolic disorder	Tests for amino acids in the urine (especially phenylketonuria)
Intracranial lesion	Skull X-ray, CT scan, MRI (only if an intracranial space-occupying lesion or demyelinating disease is suspected)
Herpes encephalitis	Virologic studies of the cerebrospinal fluid, immunologic testing (if there has been an acute or subacute regression), electroencephalography

SOMATOFORM OR "FUNCTIONAL" SYMPTOMS

The child or adolescent may develop a set of symptoms that mimic physical disorder. Common functional (previously conversion) symptoms are loss of consciousness, loss

Table 12–16 Excluding Organic Causes of Sleep Disturbance or Excessive Drowsiness

Possible Organic Cause	Special Investigations
Seizure disorder	Electroencephalography (including polysomnography)
Delirium (e.g., in acute febrile illness or toxic states)	Electroencephalography
Narcolepsy	Electroencephalography
Intoxication with or withdrawal from sedative, opiate, anticonvulsant, neuroleptic, or antidepressant drugs	Urinary drug screen
Hypoglycemia	Blood sugar (e.g., insulinoma)
Sleep apnea	Polysomnography, otorhinolaryngologic examination
Any debilitating disease, especially disease associated with chronic hypoxia (e.g., congenital heart disease, pulmonary insufficiency, anemia)	None

Table 12–17 Excluding Disorders Likely to be Mistaken for Functional Neurological Symptom Disorder

Possible Organic Cause	Special Investigations
General Systemic Disease	
Disseminated lupus erythematosus (LE)	Examination for LE cells
Hypocalcemia	Blood calcium
Hypoglycemia	Blood sugar (e.g., insulinoma)
Porphyria	Urinary porphyrins
Central Nervous System Disease	
Multiple sclerosis	Neurologic examination, MRI
Movement disorders (chorea, dystonia musculorum deformans, Tourette's syndrome, Wilson's disease)	None
Spinal cord tumor	Neurologic examination, radiography, MRI
Intracranial space–occupying lesion (especially in brain stem, cerebellum, frontal lobe, or parietotemporal cortex)	Neurologic examination, skull radiography, CT scan, MRI
Seizure disorder	Electroencephalography
Migraine	None
Dystonic reactions produced by neuroleptic drugs	None

of phonation, motor impairment, abnormal movements, seizures, special sensory defect, anesthesia, pain, loss of balance, bizarre gait, or gastrointestinal complaints such as vomiting and abdominal pain. Functional Neurological Symptom Disorder (previously conversion disorder) can mimic many physical conditions. The inquiry plan should both exclude the hypothetical physical disorder and establish positive criteria for conversion (i.e., emotional trauma coinciding with onset; pattern of symptoms representing the patient's naive idea of pathology; contact with a model for the disease; pattern of symptoms fulfilling a communicative purpose; secondary gain for the patient in the form of nurturance, security, or avoidance of difficulty; and a pattern of symptoms and signs inconsistent with physical disease). Table 12–17 lists the physical disorders especially likely to be mistaken for a Functional Neurological Symptom Disorder.

Malas N, Ortiz-Aguayo R, Giles L, Ibeziako P: Pediatric somatic symptom disorders. *Curr Psychiatry Rep* 2017 Feb;19(2):11. doi: 10.1007/s11920-017-0760-3. PMID: 28188588.

van Geelen SM, Rydelius PA, Hagquist C: Somatic symptoms and psychological concerns in a general adolescent population: exploring the relevance of DSM-5 somatic symptom disorder. *J Psychosom Res* 2015 Oct;79(4):251–258. doi: 10.1016/j.jpsychores .2015.07.012. Epub 2015 Aug 8. PMID: 26297569.

Gillberg C: Part III: Assessment. In: Gillberg C (ed). *Clinical Child Neuropsychiatry*. New York: Cambridge University Press, 1995, pp. 295–322.

Neeper R, Huntzinger R, Gascon GG: Examination I: Special techniques for the infant and young child. In: Coffey CE, Brumback RA (eds). *Textbook of Pediatric Neuropathology*. Washington, DC: American Psychiatric Press, 1998, pp. 153–170.

▼ III. PERSONALITY EVALUATION

PURPOSE OF THE PERSONALITY EVALUATION

Questions that come to the attention of clinicians often relate to differential diagnosis (i.e., whether a patient is more appropriately assigned one *Diagnostic and Statistical Manual of Mental Disorders, Fifth Edition* [DSM-5] diagnosis as opposed to another). However, even in this age of managed care and associated limitations on testing, psychologists are still occasionally asked to perform evaluations that characterize the patient beyond this reductionistic level and that describe the patient's resources and liabilities, underlying conflicts, stress tolerance, and so on. Indeed, many psychologists take the position that in order to effectively assign a specific diagnostic label, it is frequently necessary to understand the functioning of the whole person.

TYPES OF PERSONALITY EVALUATIONS

Personality evaluation can be divided into three main areas. These include behavior rating scales used to assess a patient's overt behavior and, by extension, psychological functioning; projective tests ordinarily used to describe a patient's underlying concerns, issues, perceptions of other people, and self-attributions (the "content" of the mind, if you will); and structural tests used to characterize the patient's psychological structure, including coping resources, typical defensive tactics, capacity for intimacy, and reasoning capacity (the "form" of the mind). A fourth group of scales is used to assess the patient's functioning with respect to a specific diagnosis, such as depression. Table 12–18 summarizes these scales.

▶ Behavior Rating Scales

Behavior rating scales are used both by psychologists and by clinicians, including child psychiatrists. They describe a patient's functioning in everyday life, as a step toward understanding the patient. Perhaps the most well-known of such scales is Achenbach's Child Behavior Checklist. This scale requires a parent to respond to questions related to the child's social functioning and behavioral problems. On the basis of these responses, the child is rated on a number of symptom groupings, or factors, that can be divided into two categories: those that reflect internalizing psychopathology (e.g., sadness, withdrawal, anxiety) and those that reflect externalizing psychopathology (e.g., temper outbursts, demandingness, stubbornness). Such rating scales, although perhaps limited in the amount of information obtained from the respondent, are useful in that they provide psychologists with data derived from a careful observer, namely, the parent.

▶ Projective Tests

Projective measures assume that a subject projects unconscious issues, themes, and expectancies onto an ambiguous external stimulus, thereby providing the diagnostician with meaningful clinical data. Traditionally, such techniques have been organized on the basis of their assumed depth of exploration. For example, the Incomplete Sentences Test, which requires a patient to complete sentence stems such as "I like" or "My mother," is assumed to gather information of which the patient is reasonably conscious or aware. Alternatively, the Thematic Apperception Test may evoke material that is deeper and less obvious in meaning to the patient. However, the latter task is hampered by the fact that such information is generally quite symbolic in nature and hence is open to misinterpretation on the part of the examiner. Moreover, data derived from projective testing often have limited connection to the specific question being posed by the referral source, which often relates to distinguishing between competing diagnostic possibilities or characterizing a patient's psychological assets and liabilities.

Table 12–18 Types of Personality Evaluation

Evaluation Type	Function	Examples
Behavior rating scales	Describe an individual's functioning in everyday life	Achenbach's Child Behavior Check List
Projective tests	Characterize an individual's underlying concerns	Incomplete Sentences Test Thematic Apperception Test
Structural tests	Depict a person's personality	Rorschach Inkblot Test Minnesota Multiphasic Psychiatric Inventory-A (MMPI-A) Millon Adolescent Personality Inventory
Specific diagnosis scales	Assess an individual's functioning with respect to a specific diagnosis	Children's Depression Inventory Pediatric Anxiety Rating Scale

The reader may note that in discussing projective measures, we have yet to describe the Rorschach Inkblot Test. During the past 20 years or so, there has been much discussion of the nature of the Rorschach task. Various authors have noted that, in fact, there are two essential Rorschach functions. First, the Rorschach may serve as a projective measure, evoking material that leads us to define a person's idiosyncratic or specific concerns, fears, conflicts, or interests. For example, an abused teenage girl may provide the response "two men killing a little girl," emphasizing the degree to which this particular person fears or anticipates that aggressive males may victimize her.

Second, various authors have said that the real strength of the Rorschach task lies not in its projective function but in its use as a means of evoking behavior that can illuminate the patient's personality structure. For example, regardless of the particular content of a given protocol, one might assess the degree to which the outlines of a patient's perceptions match the outlines of the test stimuli, based on a consensus of others. Weakness in this regard may be interpreted as an impairment in perceptual accuracy or reality interpretation. Likewise, responses may be assessed with respect to unrealistic reasoning (e.g., "looks like a bat because it's green"). In general, most contemporary research and clinical work on the Rorschach relates to this use as a perceptual–cognitive task, as opposed to a stimulus to fantasy.

Structural Tests

I Minnesota Multiphasic Personality Inventory-Adolescent (MMPI-A) is frequently administered to young patients. A revision of the MMPI-2 for adolescents, this scale involves the original set of basic scales, which assess functioning along dimensions such as depression, hypochondriasis, rebelliousness, and social introversion. The test is published with information permitting scoring on various subscales that compose the basic scales. Finally, content scales are provided that are, for the most part, rationally derived groupings of items relating to matters such as obsessiveness, family problems, and school problems. MMPI-A administration and interpretation proceeds much like the relevant scale for adults. The patient is asked to complete almost 500 questions, and responses are then interpreted based on patterns of scale elevations.

The MMPI-A cannot be administered to children under the age of 13 years. Instead, an MMPI-like technique, the Personality Inventory for Children, may be administered. This test requires a knowledgeable adult, preferably the primary caregiver, to characterize the child by answering more than 400 questions. The responses can be scored to provide information in areas such as depression, somatic problems, delinquency, and withdrawal. Both the MMPI-A and the Personality Inventory for Children contain validity scales to evaluate the respondent's response set (i.e., attempts to provide an unrealistically positive or negative impression).

The Millon Clinical Multiaxial Inventory was originally published as an alternative to the MMPI, which was considered to be weak in several areas. For example, the MMPI has been criticized for neglecting factors such as personality styles and disorders that may lay the groundwork for the development of other disorders such as affective disorders or anxiety disorders. Millon's tests also offer a different definition of scale elevations. Millon has made the point that in view of the differing base rates for different forms of psychopathology, the traditional mode of interpreting personality scales is insufficient.

Specific Diagnostic Scales

In this era of managed care, an emphasis has been placed on the definition of very specific questions for the psychologist to address. Thus, scales assessing specific clinical entities are becoming used much more frequently than before. Traditional measures (e.g., the Beck Depression Inventory) are often used. So too are versions adapted for younger patients such as the Children's Depression Inventory.

Achenbach TM, Ruffle TM: The Child Behavior Checklist and related forms for assessing behavioral/emotional problems and competencies. *Pediatr Rev* 2000 Aug;21(8):265–271. doi: 10.1542/pir.21-8-265. PMID: 10922023.

Archer RP: *MMPI-A: Assessing Adolescent Psychopathology.* Mahwah NJ: Erlbaum, 1992.

Exner JE: *The Rorschach: A Comprehensive System.* New York: Wiley, 1993.

Handel RW: *An introduction to the Minnesota Multiphasic Personality Inventory-Adolescent-Restructured Form (MMPI-A-RF).* J Clin Psychol Med Settings 2016 Dec;23(4):361–373. doi: 10.1007/s10880-016-9475-6. PMID: 27752979.

Millon T: *Toward a New Personology.* New York: Wiley, 1990.

Strack S, Millon T: Contributions to the dimensional assessment of personality disorders using Mi'lon's model and the Millon Clinical Multiaxial Inventory (MCMI9-III). *J Pers Assess* 2007 Aug;89(1):56–69. doi: 10.1080/00223890701357217. PMID: 17604534.

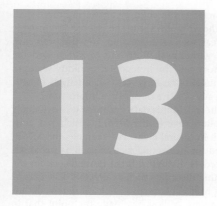

Diagnostic Formulation, Treatment Planning, and Modes of Treatment in Children and Adolescents

Barry Nurcombe, MD†
Andrés Martin, MD, MPH

DIMENSIONS OF THE DIAGNOSTIC FORMULATION

The diagnostic formulation summarizes and integrates the biopsychosocial, developmental, and temporal axes. The **biopsychosocial axis** refers to multiple systems, from molecular to socio-cultural, that interact constantly and are manifest in current objective behavior and subjective experience. The **developmental axis** is applied to different levels of the biopsychosocial axis in order to determine whether each level is developmentally normal, delayed, advanced, or deviant. The **temporal axis** refers to the ontogenesis of the individual from his or her origins to the present and beyond.

Biopsychosocial Axis

Current functioning is the expression of multiple biopsychosocial levels within the patient, as he or she interacts with the physical, family, socio-cultural, occupational, and economic environment. In order to evaluate present functioning, the clinician examines the levels and systems described in Table 13–1.

Developmental Axis

Each level of the biopsychosocial axis can be assessed with regard to what would be expected for that age. Some of these assessments (e.g., height, weight, head circumference) are very accurate. For others (e.g., intelligence), although a number of assessment instruments are available, existing measures represent a composite of skills potentially affected by extraneous factors (e.g., social class, motivation). For still others (e.g., coping strategies, working models of attachment), measurement techniques are relatively crude and the norms subjective.

Nevertheless, during interviewing and mental status examination, the clinician will scan the levels shown in

Table 13–2 for delay, precocity, or deviation from the normal and, when appropriate, order formal special investigations.

Temporal Axis

All individuals have come from somewhere, exist where they are now, and are headed somewhere. Using the temporal axis, the clinician explores the unfolding of a problem up to the present time and attempts to predict where the patient is headed. The mileposts in this evolution can be classified, somewhat arbitrarily, in the following sequence: (1) predisposition, (2) precipitation, (3) presentation, (4) pattern, (5) perpetuation, (6) potentials, and (7) prognosis.

1. Predisposition—What early biological or psychosocial factors have stunted or deflected normal development, or rendered the patient vulnerable to stress? Table 13–3 lists several examples.

Given the current state of knowledge, it is often difficult or impossible to reconstruct these factors and their effects on the growing organism, particularly with regard to inherited vulnerability or propensity (e.g., as hypothesized for depressive disorder). However, postnatal deprivation or trauma may be recorded, for example, in the patient's medical record.

2. Precipitation—A precipitant is a physical or psychosocial stressor that challenges the individual's coping capacity and causes him or her to exhibit the symptoms and signs of psychological maladjustment. Table 13–4 lists several examples. A temporal relationship exists between the precipitant and the onset of symptoms. Sometimes the precipitant (e.g., parental discord) later becomes a perpetuating factor. Sometimes the precipitant is a reminder of a previous traumatic experience. Sometimes the precipitant ceases, and the patient returns to normal coping. Sometimes the precipitant ceases, but maladaptive coping persists or even worsens. In that case, perpetuating factors must be operating (see later discussion).

Not all current patterns of psychopathology have precipitants. Some psychopathologies (e.g., autism) may have

---

†Deceased.

Table 13–1 The Biopsychosocial Axis

Level	Systems Assessed
Physical level	Peripheral organ systems Immune system Autonomic system Neuroendocrine system Sensorimotor system
Psychological level	Information-processing system Communication systems Social competence Internal working models of the self and others Unconscious conflicts, ego defenses, and coping style Patterns of psychopathology
Social level	Physical environment Family system (nuclear and extended) Socio-cultural systems (peers, adults, school)

Table 13–3 Predisposing Biological and Psychosocial Factors

Genetic vulnerability or propensity
Chromosomal abnormality
Intrauterine insult or deprivation
Perinatal physical insult
Postnatal malnutrition, exposure to toxins, or physical trauma
Physical illness
Neglect or maltreatment
Parental loss, separation, or divorce
Exposure to psychological trauma

evolved continuously since infancy or early childhood. The clinician should look for a precipitant when normal functioning is succeeded by the onset of psychopathology.

3. Presentation—The clinician should consider why the family is presenting at this time. Is it, for example, that the child's behavior worries them or disrupts family functioning? Has the family's capacity to tolerate the child's behavior deteriorated? If so, why?

4. Pattern—The current pattern represents the current biopsychosocial axis. The clinician should evaluate the patient's current physical, psychological, and social functioning. To the extent that abnormalities in physical functioning (e.g., somatoform symptoms), information processing (e.g., amnesia), communication (e.g., mutism), internal models (e.g., self-hatred), coping style (e.g., compulsive risk-taking), and social competence (e.g., social withdrawal)

can be defined as psychopathologic phenomena, the clinician will assemble configurations of symptoms and signs that form categorical syndromes (e.g., residual posttraumatic stress disorder, dysthymia) and dynamic patterns (e.g., introversion of aggression, unresolved conflict following trauma).

The clinician also evaluates the family, and the social, school, cultural, and economic environment in which the family lives. Table 13–5 lists the issues to consider in evaluating the quality of family interactions. The clinician also assesses the **acuity** of the problem pattern (i.e., its imminent danger to the patient and others), its **severity** (i.e., the levels of biopsychosocial functioning affected and the degree to which they are affected), and its **chronicity**.

5. Perpetuation—If the precipitating stress (e.g., parental conflict) does not dissipate, the child's maladaptation is likely to continue. If the stress is removed, the child is likely to spring back to normality. If not, the clinician must ask why not. The reason could be either within or outside the child.

Internal perpetuating factors can be biological or psychological. For example, overwhelming trauma can trigger a train of unreversed biochemical derangements, involving catecholamines, corticosteroids, and endogenous opiates, that cause the numbing and hyperarousal associated with the traumatic state. Unresolved trauma can also produce a

Table 13–2 The Developmental Axis

Level	Systems Assessed	Assessment Method
Physical level	Peripheral organ systems (e.g., height, weight, head circumference)	Growth charts
	Sensorimotor system	Developmental assessment, neuropsychological testing
Psychological level	Information processing	Intelligence testing, special testing for memory and other cognitive functions, educational attainment testing, neuropsychological testing
	Communication	Speech and language assessment, neuropsychological testing
	Social competence	Behavioral observation, psychological testing
	Internal working models	Interviewing, personality testing
	Conflicts, defenses, coping style	Interviewing, behavioral observation, personality testing
	Symptom patterns	Interviewing, checklists, structured interviews
Social level	Family system, peer relations, school functioning	Family interviews, observations, checklists

Table 13–4 Examples of Precipitating Factors

Physical
    Physical illness
    Surgery
    Accidental injury

Psychosocial
    Civilian catastrophe
    War
    Parental conflict, separation, or divorce
    Loss of a loved one
    Rejection
    Academic stress
    Hospitalization

personality that seeks compulsively to reenter traumatic situations, thus re-exposing the self to victimization and further trauma.

External perpetuating factors include the reinforcement of child psychopathology that occurs in dysfunctional family systems—for example, the protective parent who shields a delinquent child from punishment, or the anxious, enmeshed parent who unwittingly reinforces a child's separation anxiety and school refusal.

6. Potentials—In addition to addressing psychopathology and defects, the clinician should consider the child's physical, psychological, and social strengths. A child with a learning problem may be talented at sports, or be physically attractive, or have other talents. In treatment planning, the clinician must consider how strengths can be harnessed in order to circumvent or compensate for defects or problems.

7. Prognosis—The clinician should predict what is likely to happen with or without treatment, remembering that it is impossible to anticipate all the unfortunate and fortuitous happenstance that can block, divert, or facilitate a particular life trajectory.

THE DIAGNOSTIC FORMULATION: AN EXAMPLE

The clinician should summarize the diagnostic formulation in a succinct manner. Consider the following example:

Susan is a 14-year-old adolescent who has a 2-month history of the following symptoms, which were precipitated by her observation of a house fire in which the 4-year-old brother she was babysitting perished: traumatic nightmares, intrusive memories, frequent reminders, emotional numbing, avoidance of situations that remind her of the event, startle responses, irritability, depressive mood, social withdrawal, guilt, and suicidal ideation. She has acute posttraumatic stress disorder with complicated bereavement and secondary depression precipitated by psychic trauma.

Susan's physical health is good and her sensorimotor functioning is intact. She is of low average intelligence and approximately 2 years delayed in reading, language, and mathematical attainment. She has very low self-esteem, views herself as the family drudge, and is resentful of her father's alcoholism and domination of her mother and siblings. She has a close relationship with a married sister.

Susan's symptoms are reinforced by her mother's bereavement and the family's emotional insensitivity and poor communication. This is a large family, in which Susan has played the role of a parentified child, supporting the mother and taking responsibility for much of the housekeeping and child care. Susan was predisposed to develop a depressive trauma reaction by her longstanding (but suppressed) resentment at being the family drudge and at being the frequent target of her father's emotional abuse.

Susan has the following strengths and potentials: She has supportive friends; her older married sister is very helpful; and she enjoys childcare.

Without treatment, the current posttraumatic stress disorder is likely to continue. There is a risk of suicide.

GOAL-DIRECTED TREATMENT PLANNING

The purpose of treatment can range from short-term crisis management to long-term rehabilitation, remediation, or reconstruction. For that reason, the goals of treatment will vary according to the level of care the patient is receiving.

Table 13–5 Factors Involved in the Quality of Family Interactions

The quality of communication about important matters between family members. Do they express their messages clearly, and do they listen to and hear each other?

The capacity of family members to share positive and negative emotions. Are they able to praise and encourage each other? Can they express love? If they are angry with one another, can they say so without losing control?

The sensitivity of family members to each other's feelings. Are they aware when other family members are sad, upset, hurt, enthusiastic, or happy, and do they respond accordingly?

The capacity of the family to set rules and control behavior. Are they clear about rules and consistent in their following up of whether the rules are followed? If children must be disciplined, are penalties appropriate and timely?

The appropriateness and flexibility of family roles. Is it clear who does what in the family? If one family member is absent or indisposed, can other family members fill in?

The capacity of the family to solve problems and cope with crises. When the family is confronted with a problem, can family members work together to solve it?

The following levels of care are provided in child and adolescent mental health services: brief hospitalization, standard hospitalization, partial hospitalization, extended day programs, residential treatment, intensive outpatient care, and outpatient care. Brief hospitalization (1–14 days) is suited to crisis alleviation and the reduction of acuity. Standard hospitalization (2–4 weeks) aims at stabilization, as do partial hospitalization programs. Residential treatment programs, extended partial hospitalization programs, and outpatient treatment have more ambitious goals related to remediation, reconstruction, or rehabilitation.

COMPONENTS OF GOAL-DIRECTED TREATMENT PLANNING

The essence of goal-directed planning is the extraction of treatment foci from the diagnostic formulation and the expression of the foci as goals and objectives, with predictions of the time required for goal attainment. On the basis of the goals, treatment methods can be selected. On the basis of the objectives, goal attainment (i.e., treatment effectiveness) can be monitored until the goal is attained and treatment terminated (see Figure 13–1).

▶ Foci

Those problems, defects, and strengths that can be addressed, given the resources and time available, should be extracted from the diagnostic formulation. The clinician should not merely list behaviors in an unintegrated "laundry list." Pivotal foci, those internal or external factors that activate, reinforce, or perpetuate psychopathology, are especially important. For example, mother–child enmeshment may be the key

to a problem of separation anxiety. A behavioral program for separation anxiety applied in the school setting will fail unless the clinician addresses the mother's involvement in her child's fear of leaving home.

▶ Goals

Goals indicate what the clinician or clinical team aims to achieve, at the given level of care, on the patient's behalf (Table 13–6). A goal is a focus preceded by a verb. The focus "depressive mood," for example, becomes "Alleviate depressive mood" when rewritten as a goal. As described in the introduction to this section, goals are categorized according to whether they promote crisis alleviation, stabilization, reconstruction, remediation, rehabilitation, or compensation. Crisis alleviation, stabilization, reconstruction, and remediation foci are preceded by verbs such as "alleviate," "ameliorate," "remediate," "eliminate," "reduce the intensity of," "reduce the frequency of," "stabilize," or "counteract." Rehabilitation and compensation goals are preceded, for example, by "enhance," "augment," "facilitate," or "increase the intensity/frequency of." Behavioral goals are best suited to crisis alleviation and stabilization settings (e.g., inpatient hospitalization).

▶ Objectives

Goals assert what the clinician aims to do. Objectives indicate what the patient will (be able to) do, say, or exhibit at the end of that stage of treatment. Objectives should always be stated in behavioral terms. Goals and objectives may be intermediate (e.g., at the point of discharge from hospital) or terminal (e.g., at the end of outpatient treatment). Goals and objectives may be ambitious (e.g., "Resolve internal conflict regarding punitive father figure" or "The patient will be able to cooperate appropriately with his superior at work in

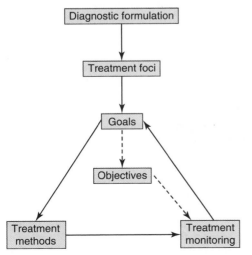

▲ **Figure 13–1** Goal-directed treatment planning.

Table 13–6 Categorization of Treatment Goals

Category	Example
Behavioral	Reduce the frequency and intensity of aggressive outbursts.
Educational	Remediate reading deficit.
Familial	Enhance quality of communication and emotional sensitivity between father and patient.
Medical	Stabilize diabetes mellitus.
Physical	Increase weight.
Psychological	Alleviate unresolved conflict concerning past physical abuse.
Social	Reduce the intensity and frequency of provocative behavior toward authority figures.

the performance of his assigned tasks") or advisedly limited (e.g., "Gain weight. At the end of hospitalization, the patient will weigh 79 pounds").

Whereas goals take the long, abstract view, objectives indicate when enough is enough, making the clinician or team accountable, and alerting them when treatment is not progressing as well as anticipated.

Target Date

For each set of goals and objectives, a time is predicted. For example, the goal "Alleviate depressive mood and suicidal ideation" may have the objective "The patient will express no suicidal ideation spontaneously or during mental status examination for a period of 1 week." The clinician may predict that such a stabilization objective will be attained, for example, in 3 weeks.

Therapy

For each goal, the clinician selects a therapy or a set of therapies, according to the following criteria: greatest empirical support, resource availability (i.e., clinical resources, time, finances), least risk, greatest economy (i.e., time, expense), and appropriateness to family values and interaction style.

The modes of therapy are discussed in the next section of this chapter. Do not confuse the term "objective" with a therapeutic strategy or tactic. An objective is the behaviorally stated endpoint of a phase of treatment. Treatment strategies or tactics (e.g., "Encourage father to attend patient's baseball games") represent the means of getting to the endpoint, that is, the adaptation of a particular intervention to the needs of the patient and family.

Treatment Monitoring

Objectives are the key to monitoring both the patient's progress and the treatment plan's effectiveness. Progress can be assessed by periodic milieu observations, mental status examinations, measurement of vital signs or other physical parameters, laboratory testing, standard questionnaires, rating scales, or psychological testing. To the extent that an objective can be measured, the measure should be stated (e.g., "The patient's score will drop to below 12 on the Conners Parent–Teacher Questionnaire"). Not all objectives can be measured numerically, and for some, subjective, qualitative monitoring is required. The clinician should not fall into the trap of deleting objectives that cannot be measured objectively. Some pivotal goals and objectives, particularly those related to psychodynamic or family systems issues, require qualitative monitoring, and ingenious assessments of dynamic issues can sometimes be planned. For example, the goal "Resolve conflict about past sexual abuse" could be monitored, for a particular patient, in terms of the frequency, duration, and acuity of dissociative episodes.

Revision

If progress stalls, the patient deteriorates, or unforeseen complications arise, the clinician or team will be alerted by the treatment monitors. Then a decision must be made. Continue? Change the goals? Modify the objectives? Reconsider the therapy? Periodic treatment monitoring (e.g., monthly for outpatient treatment, daily for inpatient or partial hospitalization) keeps the clinician or team accountable and prevents therapeutic drift.

Termination

When the objectives are reached, the patient is ready either to move on to the next phase or level of treatment or to terminate the treatment.

DISADVANTAGES & ADVANTAGES OF GOAL-DIRECTED TREATMENT PLANNING

Goal-directed treatment planning must be learned. It does not build on the naturalistic process of treatment planning (which usually starts from treatments rather than goals). It requires the clinician to be explicit about matters that are customarily avoided or blurred (e.g., target dates). Imposed on uncomprehending or resistant clinicians, goal-directed treatment plans are typically relegated to the status of irrelevant paperwork or to a mindless printout from a computerized treatment planning menu.

Goal direction has numerous advantages, however. It provides a common intellectual scaffolding with which a clinical team can plan. It serves notice to clinicians to monitor progress and review their plans if they are ineffective. It provides a useful basis for negotiating with families, obtaining truly informed consent, and facilitating or consolidating the treatment alliance. Finally, it is a potentially useful tool for utilization review and outcome research.

Nurcombe B: Goal-directed treatment planning and the principles of brief hospitalization. *J Am Acad Child Adolesc Psychiatry* 1989;27:26.

Nurcombe B, Gallagher RM: *The Clinical Process in Psychiatry.* New York: Cambridge University Press, 1986.

TYPES OF TREATMENT

A sophisticated, multifaceted, individually designed management plan requires a comprehensive biopsychosocial, temporal, and developmental diagnostic formulation. The diagnostic formulation should be shared with the patient and parents/guardian at a special interview, and the parents/guardians' and patient's collaboration should be sought in following the goal-directed treatment plan.

In almost every case, a combination of techniques will be used in child and adolescent psychiatry because the biopsychosocial needs of patients demand a multifaceted treatment plan. For example, an adolescent hospitalized for anorexia nervosa is likely to require a combination of the following forms of therapy: (1) pediatric treatment to correct subnutrition and fluid and electrolyte imbalance, follow nutritional progress, and treat medical complications; (2) behavior modification to counteract voluntary restriction of food intake; (3) nutritional education; (4) individual expressive psychotherapy to provide insight and promote conflict resolution; and (5) family therapy to help the family undo the parent–child enmeshment and hidden interparental conflict that are commonly associated with this disorder.

There are three broad modes of treatment in child and adolescent psychiatry: **physical**, **psychological**, and **social**. Within each mode there are modalities (e.g., medication); within each modality there are techniques or classes (e.g., selective serotonin reuptake inhibitor antidepressant medication); and within each technique there are specific subtechniques, therapies, or agents (e.g., fluoxetine). Research into the treatment of child and adolescent psychiatric disorders has far to go. Even though few if any specific treatments have been established, evidence is gathering that some empirical treatments (e.g., sertraline in obsessive–compulsive disorder) work better than placebo. As empirical information accrues, more of the indications for treatment described in the sections that follow are based on randomized clinical trials (RCTs) rather than on clinical experience alone. This chapter introduces readers to the broad range of modalities available. Subsequent chapters relate the details of treatment for particular conditions.

PSYCHOPHARMACOLOGY

A. General Principles of Psychopharmacology

1. Before commencing pharmacotherapy, the clinician should obtain from the patient a full psychiatric and medical history, a medication history, and a history of allergic reactions; ascertain what other drugs the patient is currently taking (including complementary or alternative medications), and ask whether the patient is using illicit drugs.

2. Psychopharmacologic treatment should always be part of a broader treatment plan derived from a comprehensive diagnostic formulation.

3. Parents/guardian and child should be involved in the treatment plan; informed consent for pharmacologic treatment must be obtained, and parents/guardian and child should be educated about the nature, side effects, risks, and benefits of the medication proposed (and of the alternative treatments, if any).

4. Psychopharmacologic treatment targets symptoms, not disorders. A natural corollary is that the clinician's focus should be on the child, not only the symptoms.

5. The clinician should ask the parents/guardian and child about misconceptions they may have of drug treatment in general or the particular pharmaceutical agent prescribed. For example, parents may be unnecessarily afraid that drug treatment will lead to addiction, whereas children may feel inferior if they must take medications at school. In light of direct-to-consumer advertising and in the universal availability of web-based access to medical information, the clinician needs to be attuned to the information (and misinformation) that patients and their families may have about psychiatric treatment in general, and about psychiatric drugs in particular.

6. The clinician should seek a working alliance with responsible, informed parents/guardian and an educated patient.

7. When necessary, after getting permission, the clinician should form a working alliance with the school.

8. A medical examination, appropriate special investigations, and laboratory tests (including pregnancy testing in female patients) are required in order to rule out contraindicated conditions.

9. Whenever possible, the clinician should quantify the targeted baseline symptom(s) and monitor progress with appropriate checklists or rating scales.

10. The clinician should select an appropriate drug according to the following criteria: least known risk and best evidence of efficacy. If possible, the clinician should follow U.S. Food and Drug Administration (FDA) guidelines, but if not, he or she should make a rational choice based on available scientific evidence. If the choice is nonstandard, the clinician should document a risk–benefit analysis and consider asking for a consultation from a colleague.

11. It is advisable to start with a low dosage and increase it gradually until the symptoms remit, no further improvement accrues, the upper recommended dosage is reached, or complications occur. Treatment should be continued at the lowest effective dosage.

12. The clinician should monitor side effects regularly, with appropriate measures (e.g., height and weight) or laboratory tests (e.g., electrocardiogram, lipid panel).

13. Side effects (e.g., the sedative effect of antidepressant medication) can sometimes be used to treat other symptoms (e.g., insomnia).

14. Whenever such testing is available, the clinician should monitor serum levels if unsure whether the patient is receiving an adequate dose, or if there is a possibility that a toxic level of drug has been reached.

15. The clinician should prescribe medication for as short a period as possible. When medication is an adjunctive part of treatment, for example, it may be possible to discontinue it when psychosocial therapies are in place.

"Drug holidays" are sometimes appropriate (e.g., for stimulants when the child is out of school during the summer).

16. Polypharmacy should be avoided. The clinician should use drug combinations only after single appropriate drugs have been given an adequate trial and found ineffective.

17. When withdrawing medication, the clinician should usually taper the dosage, unless it is known that abrupt cessation is not dangerous (e.g., for agents with long half-lives, such as fluoxetine or aripiprazole).

B. Classes of Psychopharmacologic Agents

The following classes of medication are used in child and adolescent psychiatry: psychostimulants, adrenergic agents, antidepressants, antipsychotics, mood stabilizers, anxiolytics, anticonvulsants, and miscellaneous agents.

▶ Psychostimulants

The best-known psychostimulants are methylphenidate and dextroamphetamine compounds. They are the drugs of choice for treating attention-deficit/hyperactivity disorder (ADHD) across the life cycle. In addition to very solid empirical evidence for their use in children and adolescents, there is a growing literature supporting their safety and efficacy in preschoolers and adults as well. Stimulants have very short half-lives and must be given in repeated doses. However, a wide array of slow-release forms of methylphenidate and dextroamphetamine are also available—as prodrugs, patches, osmotic pumps, or beaded pearls. Psychostimulants should also be used with caution if the patient has a history of psychosis, growth failure, or cardiac abnormality, or if the patient is pregnant. Common side effects are insomnia, irritability, and anorexia. Less common side effects are growth retardation, and hepatitis (with the now-abandoned agent pemoline). Patients taking psychostimulants should be monitored for involuntary movements, heart rate, and growth rate. Routine height and weight measurements are necessary. Electrocardiograms are not routinely recommended, but are prudent if there is a strong family history of arrhythmias.

▶ Adrenergic Agents

The most commonly prescribed adrenergic agents are clonidine and guanfacine. Both are presynaptic alpha-2 agonists whose net effect is to dampen the central sympathetic outflow. These agents are used either along with or in combination with stimulants in treating ADHD. Clonidine targets impulsivity and hyperactivity and has also been used in Tourette syndrome, opioid withdrawal, agitation, and posttraumatic stress disorder. Guanfacine targets inattention, impulsivity, and hyperactivity in ADHD. Clonidine should be used with caution if depression or a cardiovascular disorder is present. Its main side effects are sedation and orthostatic hypotension, but headache, dizziness, and depression are also possible. Guanfacine, though less sedating, has similar side effects. Both drugs have the potential to augment the sedating effects of other central nervous system (CNS) depressants and for a hypertensive rebound after abrupt discontinuation.

▶ Antidepressants

The antidepressants most often used in child and adolescent psychopharmacology are selective serotonin reuptake inhibitors (SSRIs) and tricyclic antidepressants (TCAs).

1. Selective serotonin reuptake inhibitors—The members of the SSRI class currently most often prescribed in the United States are fluoxetine, sertraline, citalopram, and escitalopram. Paroxetine and fluvoxamine have been largely abandoned because of side effects or twice-daily dosing, respectively. SSRIs are used for the treatment of depression, anxiety, and obsessive–compulsive disorder (OCD). Common side effects of the SSRIs include gastrointestinal symptoms, nervousness, restlessness, insomnia, and sexual dysfunction. Less common side effects include excitability and the induction of mania or hypomania. SSRIs may exacerbate suicidal ideation in a minority of patients, particularly during the early weeks of treatment. All antidepressants carry a black box label from the FDA alerting to this possibility and advising careful monitoring of suicidal ideation during treatment initiation. This potential side effect should be discussed openly with patients and families and weighted against the risks of leaving depression untreated (including the real risk of suicide). Before administering an SSRI, the clinician should record the patient's vital signs, height, and weight and test for pregnancy. Patients should be monitored at each visit for the emergence of mania and excitation. A medication trial of 6–8 weeks is required in order to allow full time to clinical effect. SSRIs with a long half-life (fluoxetine) may be discontinued without tapering, but others should be gradually lowered in order to prevent flulike discontinuation symptoms.

2. Tricyclic antidepressants—The most commonly prescribed TCAs are imipramine, nortriptyline, and clomipramine. These drugs are used to treat OCD and enuresis. Though formerly widely used in the treatment of depression in children and adolescents, empirical evidence for their effectiveness is lacking. There is ample empirical support for the use of TCAs in pediatric psychopharmacology (particularly in OCD), but these medications are regarded as a last resort for treatment-resistant conditions, given their many side effects. Side effects are largely anticholinergic as well as potentially cardiotoxic, with increased pulse rate, cardiac conduction slowing, arrhythmia, and heart block. Sudden death has been associated with high dosages of imipramine and desipramine, possibly because of cardiac conduction abnormalities. A baseline electrocardiogram (ECG) is always indicated, and ECG monitoring is required at intervals as the dosage is increased.

Antipsychotics

The most commonly prescribed antipsychotics used to be the phenothiazines (such as chlorpromazine) and butyrophenones (such as haloperidol). However, atypical antipsychotic drugs (e.g., risperidone, olanzapine, quetiapine, ziprasidone, aripiprazole) have largely replaced them. The atypicals are less likely to induce permanent movement disorders (e.g., tardive dyskinesia), but they commonly lead to increased appetite and weight gain, and eventually to metabolic abnormalities such as dysregulated lipid and glucose metabolism. Antipsychotics are indicated for the treatment of schizophrenia, bipolar disorder, delirium, agitation in autism and Tourette syndrome. They are contraindicated if the patient has a history of hypersensitivity, agranulocytosis, or neuroleptic malignant syndrome. They should be used with caution in pregnant patients and in patients who are also taking CNS depressants. Clozapine, an atypical and effective antipsychotic, is generally reserved for treatment-refractory cases of psychosis, given its side effects and the need to monitor for blood dyscrasia with frequent blood counts. Antipsychotic agents are described in more detail in Chapter 9.

Mood Stabilizers

Lithium is indicated for the treatment of bipolar disorder in adolescents and has been used in the treatment of bipolar disorder in children. It has also been used to alleviate violent behavior. Adolescent patients who exhibit psychosis should be monitored carefully for mood disorder, and a trial of lithium should be considered. Lithium can alleviate explosive aggression in patients with conduct disorder. Lithium is contraindicated if the patient has had a previous allergic reaction to the drug. It should be used with caution in pregnant patients and in patients who have severe dehydration; renal, cardiovascular, or thyroid disease; or diabetes mellitus. Lithium mobilizes calcium and may affect bone growth. Close monitoring of lithium levels (within a therapeutic range of 0.8–1.0 mEq/L) is necessary, as is periodic monitoring of renal and thyroid functions. Valproic acid appears to be as effective as lithium in juvenile mania, although clinical trials are very limited. Lithium and valproic acid may be combined with antipsychotic medication (e.g., risperidone, quetiapine, or olanzapine) in the treatment of mania. Lithium and valproic acid are described in more detail in Chapter 9.

Anxiolytics

The anxiolytics formerly most commonly prescribed in child and adolescent psychiatry were benzodiazepines and antihistamines. These drugs have been largely supplanted by the SSRIs.

Partly because of diagnostic confusion in the field of juvenile anxiety disorders and partly because of the paucity of controlled studies, knowledge concerning the indications for older anxiolytics is patchy. However, there is good evidence of the efficacy of SSRIs in anxiety disorders.

Martin A, Scahill L, and Kratochvil C. (Eds): *Pediatric Psychopharmacology: Principles and Practice*, 2nd edn. New York: Oxford University Press, 2011.

Pappadopulos EA, Guelzow ET, Wong C, et al: A review of the growing evidence base for pediatric psychopharmacology. *Child Adolesc Psychiatr Clin North Am* 2004;13:817–856.

Scahill LS, Oesterheld JR, Martin A: Pediatric psychopharmacology II: general principles, specific drug treatments, and clinical practice. In: Martin A, Volkmar FR (eds.). *Lewis's Child and Adolescent Psychiatry: A Comprehensive Textbook*, 4th edn. Baltimore: Lippincott Williams & Wilkins, 2007, pp. 754–789.

PSYCHOLOGICAL TREATMENT

Psychological treatments include a variety of techniques that can be divided into four main groups: (1) individual psychotherapy, (2) behavior modification, (3) social and cognitive–behavioral therapy, and (4) remedial therapies and education.

A. Individual Psychotherapy

The different forms of individual psychotherapy vary in accordance with four dimensions: (1) brief versus protracted; (2) supportive, directive, and reality-oriented versus expressive, exploratory, and oriented to unconscious material; (3) structured, interpretive versus unstructured, client-centered; and (4) play-oriented versus verbally oriented.

Supportive Psychotherapy

Supportive psychotherapy represents a loose collection of techniques without distinctive theoretical basis derived broadly from humanistic understanding and personal experience.

1. Aims—The aims of supportive psychotherapy are to (1) establish a close relationship; (2) define current problems; (3) consider and implement problem solutions; (4) avoid ego-alien, unconscious material; and (5) restore preexistent ego defenses.

2. Indications—Supportive psychotherapy is indicated for the treatment of adjustment disorders, temporary emotional crises due to situational stress, remitted psychotic disorders when the patient is in need of rehabilitative help, and substance use disorders.

3. Contraindications—Supportive psychotherapy should not be used to treat severe disorders that require more specific or more extensive therapy.

4. Dangers—Supportive psychotherapy is relatively safe except for the possibility of excessive dependency on the therapist. The development of an undesirably intense relationship with the therapist is a potential problem with any therapeutic technique, but it is more likely in intensive psychotherapy.

Client-Centered Therapy

Client-centered therapy is a form of play therapy or verbal psychotherapy in which the patient (client) is gently encouraged to explore personal feelings and attitudes. In client-centered therapy, the therapist empathically reflects the feelings, explicit or implicit, in the patient's play and verbal or nonverbal communications. The pace of therapy is determined by the patient. Therapy is usually brief to intermediate in duration.

1. Aims—The aims of client-centered therapy are (1) to establish an empathic, accepting relationship and (2) to encourage self-exploration by judicious reflection of feeling.

2. Indications—Client-centered therapy is indicated for the treatment of adjustment reactions and mild anxiety disorders in children and adolescents. It is also useful for treating problems of adolescence that involve career choice, academic commitment, or mild identity confusion.

3. Contraindications—Client-centered therapy should not be used to treat severe disorders, especially psychosis or prepsychosis, conduct disorder, and borderline personality.

4. Dangers—Client-centered therapy could lead to excessive or unresolved dependence in some cases. Otherwise, it is relatively safe.

Exploratory Psychotherapy

Exploratory psychotherapy is a form of play therapy or verbal psychotherapy in which the patient's unconscious conflicts, usually in a specified area, are resolved by interpretations baon the patient's play or verbal and nonverbal behavior. It is usually extended in duration (6–12 months) and moderately intensive (1–2 times per week).

1. Aims—The aims of exploratory psychotherapy are (1) to establish a relationship, (2) recognize transference feelings, (3) help the patient to become aware of unconscious wishes and defenses by judicious interpretation, and (4) help the patient to terminate the relationship.

2. Indications—Exploratory psychotherapy is indicated for treatment of anxiety, somatoform, and dissociative disorders; personality disorders and interpersonal difficulties related to neurotic conflict; and trauma spectrum disorders.

3. Contraindications—Exploratory psychotherapy is contraindicated if the patient's ego strength is too fragile to cope with the emergence of traumatic material in the context of a close therapeutic relationship, or if the patient has a psychotic or prepsychotic disorder.

4. Dangers—Exploratory psychotherapy could provoke an intense transference reaction with severe emotional turmoil.

Interpersonal Psychotherapy

Interpersonal psychotherapy is a brief form of psychotherapy that has been adapted for adolescents with major depression. Twelve weekly sessions are recommended, in accordance with a treatment manual. The interpersonal psychotherapist is an active, practical problem solver, focusing on the here-and-now. A variety of techniques are applied: psychoeducation, clarification, facilitating the expression of affect, communication analysis, problem solving, and decision analysis. Parents/guardian are involved in the initial and middle phases. Liaison with the school is encouraged.

1. Aims—In depression, the therapist aims first to provide education about the condition, then to relate depression to the interpersonal context. Problem areas are identified and a treatment contract set. In the middle stage of therapy, grief, role disputes and transitions, and interpersonal deficits are dealt with. The last four sessions focus on residual problems, reviewing progress, and relapse prevention.

2. Indications—Depressive disorders in adolescence.

3. Contraindications—As for exploratory psychotherapy.

4. Dangers—As for exploratory psychotherapy.

Child & Adolescent Psychoanalysis

Child and adolescent psychoanalysis is an extensive (e.g., 1–5 years) and intensive (e.g., 3–5 times per week) form of exploratory therapy in which a radical resolution of unconscious conflicts is sought through the exploration of a transference relationship between patients and analysts.

1. Aims—The aims of child and adolescent psychoanalysis are (1) to establish a relationship, (2) encourage spontaneous expression of thoughts and emotions (through play and conversation), (3) aid resolution of unconscious conflict by interpreting unconscious wishes and ego defenses, (4) support the patient in working through personal solutions to problems that have been rendered conscious in analysis, and (5) help the patient terminate the relationship.

2. Indications—Child and adolescent psychoanalysis is indicated for limited cases for the treatment of anxiety disorders, somatoform disorders, and some trauma spectrum disorders.

3. Contraindications—Child and adolescent psychoanalysis should not be used to treat psychotic disorder, pervasive developmental disorder, conduct disorder, severe personality disorder, or other disorders in patients who cannot tolerate intimacy. In addition, a patient has to have the capacity to engage verbally, limiting the age and developmental level this is appropriate for.

If psychoanalytic therapy is to succeed, the patient must have reasonable capacity to tolerate tension and intimacy, the ability to express emotions in words, the motivation to seek help, and considerable economic resources.

4. Dangers—The dangers of child and adolescent psychotherapy are similar to those associated with exploratory psychotherapy.

B. Behavior Therapy (Modification)

Behavior modification represents a group of loosely associated therapeutic techniques derived from the principles of learning and cognitive behavior therapy.

1. Aims

i. Systematic desensitization—Exposing the patient to progressively more anxiety-provoking stimuli, while at the same time teaching him or her to relax, or pairing the phobic stimuli with a pleasant activity (such as eating), or associating the phobic stimuli with pleasant fantasy.

ii. Reinforcement of coping responses—Rewarding responses that counteract, or are incompatible with, the problem behavior.

iii. Exposure—Forced entry into the phobic situation and the prevention of avoidance.

iv. Shaping—Rewarding progressive approximations to desired responses, especially in habit training.

v. Token reinforcement—Poker chips, stars on a calendar, and the like can be exchanged at stipulated times for reward (e.g., money, privileges). The tokens are used for immediate reinforcement of desirable behavior.

vi. Aversion—Interrupting undesirable behavior (e.g., self-destructive head banging) by applying a noxious stimulus (e.g., an electric shock) whenever the undesirable behavior is expressed.

vii. Time-out—Deprivation of anticipated reinforcement (e.g., attention) by consistently isolating the child when the undesirable behavior (e.g., tantrums) is expressed.

viii. Massed practice—Multiple repetitions of an undesired behavior (e.g., a habit spasm) in order to weaken its association with an underlying emotional state (e.g., anxiety).

ix. Substitution—Replacing an undesirable behavior (e.g., smoking) with a neutral one.

2. Indications—Behavioral therapy is indicated for treatment of phobic disorders, eating disorders, oppositional defiant disorder, and preschool management problems (e.g., tantrums), as well as for habit training (e.g., functional enuresis or encopresis).

3. Contraindications—Behavioral therapy should not be used to treat psychosis or in situations in which the patient has transference fears of, or is resistant to, being controlled.

4. Dangers—Behavioral therapy could lead to deterioration or aggravation of the psychiatric condition (reported after implosion) or to the appearance of new undesirable behavior (e.g., if desensitization is too limited in scope).

C. Social & Cognitive–Behavioral Therapy

Social and cognitive–behavioral therapy is a group of techniques that focus on intermediate cognitive responses as the primary target for intervention, with the aim of changing behavior.

1. Aims

i. Participant modeling—Combining the observation of a model that behaves in a desired way with the opportunity to practice the desirable behavior.

ii. Interpersonal problem-solving—Teaching the patient to infer the causes and consequences of interpersonal events and actions, and to consider alternative solutions to interpersonal dilemmas.

iii. Cognitive–behavioral therapy—Helping the patient to define and alter the self-defeating expectations and attitudes that underlie maladaptive behavior.

iv. Self-instruction training—Teaching the patient to reflect upon a problem rather than act impulsively.

2. Indications—Social and cognitive–behavioral therapy is used to encourage behavior that will counteract a phobia, to overcome social impulsiveness or inhibition, to counteract the pessimism that predisposes an adolescent to depression, to replace motor impulsiveness with reflectiveness, or to counteract obsessive–compulsive behavior. Cognitive behavior therapy has robust evidence in a wide range mood, anxiety and behavior disorders in children and adolescents.

3. Contraindications—Social and cognitive–behavioral therapy should not be used to treat psychosis.

4. Dangers—Social and cognitive–behavioral therapy could lead to deterioration or aggravation of the psychiatric condition or to the appearance of new undesirable behavior if the therapy is too limited in scope.

D. Remedial Therapies & Education

Remedial therapies and education represent a large group of remedial or rehabilitative programs designed to help the child or adolescent overcome chronic physical, educational, or social handicap or make the most of talents and potential strengths.

1. Aims—Remedial therapies and technologies have been developed for a variety of disabilities, including cerebral palsy, orthopedic handicap, blindness, deafness, aphasia, and learning disability.

These therapies may be provided in a separate institution (e.g., a school for the hearing impaired) or incorporated in a regular school program (i.e., in the case of mainstreaming). The contemporary trend is toward mainstreaming whenever possible.

2. Dangers—The child may be labeled and discriminated against in a separate (categorical) program, a disabled child's needs may overwhelm teachers and classmates in a mainstream program, or the child may not be accepted by unimpaired classmates.

SOCIAL TREATMENT

▶ Group Therapy

In group therapy, groups of six to eight children or adolescents, with a group leader, meet at intervals ranging from daily to once per week. Groups for preschool children emphasize social stimulation. Activity groups for latency-age children emphasize socialization. Groups for adolescents focus on mutual support and the sharing of common problems. Group therapy is often used as an adjunct to other forms of therapy (e.g., during hospitalization).

1. Aims—The aims of group therapy are (1) to provide social experience, (2) allow expression of feeling in an accepting environment, (3) foster awareness of common experience and allow the group to consider solutions to common problems, and (4) promote group cohesiveness (e.g., during hospitalization).

2. Indications—Group therapy is indicated during hospitalization of latency-age children or adolescents. It is useful for treating problems with social isolation and for helping adolescents who share the same problem (e.g., divorce, physical handicap, substance abuse).

3. Contraindications—Group therapy should not be used to treat disorders in patients who are disturbed by forced intimacy.

4. Dangers—Though it is not always possible, it is preferable for the group to be balanced, with a judicious combination of aggressive "instigators," compulsive "neutralizers," and dependent "followers." If there are too many aggressive children, the group can explode. If there are too many neutralizers or followers, group process can stagnate.

▶ Role Play

Role play is a subtechnique of group therapy, commonly used in hospital treatment, in which a recent social incident is reenacted. The role players usually are not the individuals who were involved in the incident, but those who were involved will help with the reenactment.

Role playing is used to help patients develop insight and consider common problems and alternative solutions. It can be used as a medium for cognitive–behavioral therapy.

▶ Casework for Parents/Guardian

Casework varies from intermittent contact with the patient's parents (in order to keep them informed about progress) to intensive therapy, for example, in regard to marital problems, child management, or health care.

1. Aims—Casework may be used to provide information, promote more consistent child management or health care, institute a behavior modification program at home, resolve marital problems, or prepare one or both parents/guardian for referral to another therapist.

2. Indications—Casework is indicated whenever the child is in intensive individual therapy, in order to keep parents/guardian aware and involved, and to facilitate behavior modification in the natural environment by enlisting the parents/guardian as agents of the therapeutic plan.

3. Contraindications—If parents/guardian are mutually antagonistic, they may need to be interviewed separately.

▶ Conjoint Family Therapy

Conjoint family therapy is a form of group therapy in which the identified patient's whole family receives treatment. The family members meet with a family therapist (sometimes with a male or female co-therapist) for intensive brief therapy (in order to facilitate crisis resolution) or for more extended periods of time (if radical changes in family interaction are proposed).

1. Aims—Conjoint family therapy is used to resolve family crises; to promote a common understanding of family problems; to consider alternative solutions to common problems, especially when the family has reached an impasse; to foster a common awareness of previously unexpressed family rules, roles, and expectations; and to alter longstanding maladaptive interaction patterns (e.g., coalitions, rifts, scapegoating, enmeshment, or skewing), promote clearer communication, and enhance the emotional sensitivity of family members.

2. Indications—Conjoint family therapy is indicated when the patient is recovering following hospitalization for severe mental illness and when the patient's problems are perpetuated by deleterious family interaction patterns.

3. Contraindications—Conjoint family therapy should be avoided or used with caution in the following situations: (1) when family members are excessively hostile or intrusive toward the patient; (2) when the parents are on the verge of separating; or (3) when the patient needs to become independent of the family system.

4. Dangers—Conjoint family therapy could result in the problem shifting to another family member, as the homeostasis of the family is changed when the designated patient improves. It could also aggravate a rift between the parents.

▶ Psychiatric Hospitalization

Psychiatric hospitalization involves the placement of a severely disturbed child or adolescent in a psychiatric inpatient unit that has special programs and a therapeutic milieu designed for children or adolescents. The special program coordinates psychiatric, pediatric, psychological, nursing, educational, and occupational care and therapies. The placement may be brief (e.g., 1–2 weeks), intermediate (2–4 weeks), or extended (longer than 1 month) depending on the patient's needs.

1. Aims—Psychiatric hospitalization aims to separate a patient temporarily from the family; to stabilize suicidal, self-injurious, aggressive, or disorganized psychotic behavior; or to institute treatment programs that require complex coordination and intensive monitoring.

2. Indications—Psychiatric hospitalization is warranted when suicidal, aggressive, or disruptive behavior that is beyond the control of the family is caused by treatable mental illness (especially schizophreniform disorder, schizophrenia, posttraumatic stress disorder, eating disorder, and severe mood disorder). It may also be warranted when the child's severe emotional disorder is perpetuated by complex family interaction pathology or when comprehensive diagnostic evaluation of a complex case is needed, especially for cases that require the coordination of a number of specialties (e.g., an adolescent who has a chronic physical illness associated with a serious psychiatric disorder and family interaction problems).

Specific disorders warranting hospitalization include the following: depressed mood and suicidality secondary to emotional stress; severe anxiety, somatoform, and dissociative disorders; severe eating disorder; substance use disorder; organic mental disorder (e.g., substance-induced delirium or hallucinosis); and pervasive developmental disorder (for diagnosis, behavioral analysis, and management planning in aggressive or self-injurious patients).

3. Contraindications—Psychiatric hospitalization should not be used to treat conduct disorder of the undersocialized, aggressive type without treatable comorbid psychiatric disorder or in some cases of personality disorder (especially of borderline type) in which there is a danger of reinforcing a patient's chronic sick role. Furthermore, it is contraindicated if hospitalization could cause alienation between the patient and his or her family.

4. Dangers—Psychiatric hospitalization may accentuate dependency and inadvertently train the child or adolescent to be a "patient." It may lead to scapegoating and permanent

Table 13–7 Safeguards Against the Dangers of Hospitalization

Clear but nonautocratic psychiatric leadership
Staff selected for defined but overlapping roles
Clarity of general aims and individual treatment goals
Good coordination of, and communication between, staff
A plan for post-discharge disposition
Family involvement in admission, diagnosis, management planning, and continuing treatment
An environment that, as far as possible, approximates that of the average child of that age (in schooling, social opportunity, and recreation) and that deemphasizes chronic invalidism
Partial hospitalization for less severely disturbed patients
Planned discharge to outpatient or partial hospital care as soon as possible
Good coordination between the regional inpatient unit and the community mental health agencies and clinicians

extrusion by an alienated family. Also, excessive pressure on inexperienced inpatient unit staff could lead to communication breakdown and deleterious effects on all patients. These dangers can be averted if the safeguards listed in Table 13–7 are implemented.

▶ Specialized Partial Hospitalization or Residential Units

Residential programs are based usually on an educational or behavioral (rather than a medical) model, with programs designed for children or adolescents who have special problems. Partial hospitalization programs are based on a psychiatric inpatient model, except that the patient returns home each night. In all cases, the child's or adolescent's problems are more severe or complex than can be dealt with in conventional outpatient treatment. Examples are given in Table 13–8.

Table 13–8 Examples of Partial Hospitalization Programs

Pediatric hospital units for infants and children who have experienced physical neglect or abuse affecting physical health
Preschool daycare programs for children with special physical, educational, or psychological needs (e.g., culturally disadvantaged children or children with pervasive developmental disorders)
Residential units for children and adolescents with severe physical handicaps or disorders
Residential units for adolescents with substance dependence (usually emphasizing behavior control)
Residential units for adolescents with conduct disorder (usually emphasizing behavior control)
Residential units for the mentally retarded
Boarding schools for adolescents with learning and emotional problems

▶ Other Placements Away from Home

Other placements may involve temporary or permanent placement of a child or adolescent in a foster or group home. Options include (1) foster placement as a temporary expedient, while the parents and child are in treatment, preparatory to the return of the child; (2) permanent foster placement, with or without view to adoption, after disintegration of the home of origin or when the parents are unable to provide adequate care; (3) group home placement for children and adolescents who are emotionally too overreactive to cope with the emotional vicissitudes of foster home placement; and (4) community group homes designed to promote independent-living skills for adolescents with intellectual disability and/or pervasive developmental disorders.

Josephson AM (ed): Current perspectives on family therapy. *Child Adolesc Psychiatr Clin North Am* 2001;10:395–662.

Leventhal BL, Zimmerman DP (eds): Residential treatment. *Child Adolesc Psychiatr Clin North Am* 2004;13:237–440.

Remschmidt H (ed): *Psychotherapy with Children and Adolescents.* Cambridge, UK: Cambridge University Press, 2001.

Weisz JR, Hawley KM, Doss AJ: Empirically tested psychotherapies for youth internalizing and externalizing disorders. *Child Adolesc Psychiatr Clin North Am* 2004;13:729–815.

Preventive Psychiatry and Wellness

14

Sidney H. Weissman, MD

THE ETIOLOGY OF PSYCHIATRIC DISORDERS

While we do not know the causes of most psychiatric disorders, we have learned that certain mental states, behaviors, and life experiences facilitate the experience of anxiety and depression which may lead to the development of a mental disorder that may become disabling. Further some individuals who grow up in unsupportive environments are more likely to develop behavioral disorders than those who do not. This knowledge has led to a two pronged psychiatric and mental health response. First, the development of behavioral responses in society and institutions to reduce potential triggers of mental health disorders, preventive psychiatry.

Second that individuals can develop personal behaviors which each of us can initiate and follow to reduce stress with potential reduction in anxiety and depression and mental disorders, Wellness Programs. These programs that facilitate the development of enhanced wellbeing and the reduction of work stress have been established in many institutions, for example schools, hospitals, and many workplaces.

ADVERSE FACTORS FOR DEVELOPING MENTAL DISORDERS

Before examining in more detail how to establish either preventive psychiatry or wellness programs we must first be aware of the factors which may increase the risk of developing a mental disorder. These vary from biological (e.g., chromosomal abnormality) to familial (e.g., parental depression and alcoholism; marital discord and domestic violence; familial physical abuse, sexual abuse, and neglect), socioeconomic (e.g., poverty or membership in a disadvantaged minority group) and catastrophic (e.g., civilian disaster or war).

Other personal and environmental factors may counterbalance these risks for individuals. An easy, likeable temperament, above-average intelligence, good support from a parental figure are potentially protective experiences. Additionally, for children, good schools, adequate community resources for skill-building, and good future employment prospects may offer protection for otherwise vulnerable individuals from psychiatric disorders. Protective factors may act by moderating the effects of risk factors or by promoting the development of alternative, compensatory processes that enhance personal effectiveness and self-esteem.

There is generally not a straight correlation between a given risk factor and the development of a psychiatric disorder. Most outcomes have multiple determinants. For example, psychopathology following child sexual abuse is associated with varied antecedent factors such as the quality of child relationships prior to the abuse, and the nature of the abuse adverse sexual abuse. Additional factors which adversely affect child psychological development include for example: whether the child has a sustained posttraumatic stress disorder.

An example of how preventive psychiatry works is in interventions programs that aim to reduce the incidence of psychopathology after child sexual abuse. Programs might focus on improving a number of areas of a child's life. Helping a family to identify a child's special needs in response to their trauma is one. Prevention that aims to both reduce and prevent child sexual abuse from occurring relies upon promoting community awareness. Making families and schools aware that children do not usually tell of being abused. However responsible adults can learn about child behaviors that indicate abuse may have occurred.

THE GOALS AND TYPES OF PREVENTION

Preventive psychiatry aims to eliminate, reduce the incidence of, or ameliorate the severity of general or specified psychopathology in a given population. It can also focus on particular groups that are at risk of developing psychiatric disorder or impairment.

Preventive intervention can be classified according to when in the course of the development of a psychiatric disorder an intervention is applied (Caplan, 1964). **Primary prevention** refers to intervention in normal populations to avert future mental ill health (e.g., school-based alcohol and drug education). **Secondary prevention** focuses on special at-risk groups in order to stave off or ameliorate development of psychopathology (e.g., the treatment of sexually abused children).

An alternative classification system of interventions defined by its goals and the needs of population served has been proposed by the Institute of Medicine (Mrazek & Haggerty, 1994). **Universal prevention** which is offered to the entire population of a particular area (e.g., good antenatal care). **Targeted prevention** which is directed at groups who are identified as being at risk by virtue of biological markers or symptom patterns (e.g., children with epilepsy, or highly aggressive preschool children). **Targeted selective prevention** which is aimed at individuals who are at increased risk by virtue of their membership of a vulnerable subgroup (e.g., the children of highly stressed, economically disadvantaged, single mothers), or because they are experiencing or about to experience a life transition or stressful event (e.g., change of schools or divorce).

Prevention can also be classified in accordance with the **level** and **timing** of intervention. The level of intervention refers to whether the intervention is aimed at an individual, the family, the peer group, the school, the workplace, or the community as a whole. Timing refers to the life phase of the individuals to whom the intervention is directed; for example, antenatal, infancy, preschool, middle childhood, adolescence, or adulthood.

Olds et al. (1986) successfully reduced the incidence of child maltreatment by developing a visiting nurse program to assist mothers who were at risk of abusing their children by virtue of adolescent pregnancy, poverty, and single parenthood. The program began antenatally and continued until the child was 2 years old. This was a primary, targeted, selective prevention of family-level type, begun in the antenatal/infancy period.

The structure of a preventive psychiatry program will be determined by a review of the needs of a specific population, the age and the vulnerabilities of the population to be served and the desired outcomes. A careful review of all elements of a program must be undertaken prior to developing a preventive program. It is particularly important to understand societal and cultural concerns when developing a community preventive program. A successfully designed program is developed when knowing that one community program may not fit another. After this assessment of needs and goals a review of the resources needed to implement the program must be made.

DEVELOPING EFFECTIVE PREVENTIVE PSYCHIATRY PROGRAMS

The first requirement in developing an effective preventive psychiatry program is to choose a problem that is serious and prevalent in a particular community. Next is to determine if the community is receptive to the idea of a prevention program and be willing and able to work with the program's initiators or, if not, could one change prevailing community attitudes? In conceiving a program, it is essential that it is suitable for the sociocultural or ethnic group which it will serve. To ensure this element it is probably essential to have a consultant familiar with the group the program will serve. Then one determines the resources and staff needed to implement the program. Finally, in addressing these concerns or questions, the planners of a program must consider its cost and the community's resources to implement a program.

In community-based programs planning and later implementation teams including members of the community are essential. Team members need varied skills (e.g., in particular intervention techniques, program design, or statistical analysis). When the planning steps are accomplished a specific intervention can be proposed to a community or organization. In general, targeted interventions aimed at a sub-group are more effective than universal interventions. Universal interventions often fail to reach those most in need and expend energy on those who do not need them. However, effective universal educational programs as first steps in a program can create a social environment favorable for targeted intervention. A program could be directed toward the individual, the family, or a social system such as a classroom, school, or workplace. Generally, directing a program to engage diverse groups is preferable. Parent education and involvement are essential to enhance the effect of a child-directed program.

Two other issues must be addressed prior to implementing a preventive psychiatry program. First a program assessment plan must be developed. Evaluation instruments need to be developed and an assessment plan to determine the effectiveness of the program. At this time a plan also needs to be developed as to how to report information for the program to the community?

In an ongoing program the community staff of the program must meet on a regular basis with members of the community or organization involved and keep them apprised of their work and ongoing planning.

COST-EFFECTIVENESS AND COST–BENEFIT ANALYSES PREVENTIVE PROGRAMS

The aim of psychiatric prevention is to provide or propose intervention in individual's lives in order to avert or limit the development of serious mental and behavioral problems. It is reasonable, therefore, to ask whether the cost of prevention (and its likelihood of success) is less or greater than the cost of the undesirable outcome. Durlak (1997) points out that there is no standard procedure for cost analysis: no agreement about what a cost is, or what is a benefit, or how to compare them. Furthermore, costs vary with the setting of implementation.

THE ETHICS OF PREVENTIVE INTERVENTION

When proposing a prevention program, it is important not to claim more benefit than it can deliver. Unfulfilled promises lead to the disillusionment of community or organization support. Researchers and administrators have the responsibility to ensure that the scarce amount of money available for prevention actions is appropriately spent.

THE FUTURE OF PREVENTIVE PSYCHIATRY

To date, no preventive programs have successfully reduced the incidence of the major DSM-5-TR categories of schizophrenia or bipolar disorder, The reduction of their incidence will require greater knowledge. Specifically of how genes effect and alter brain. Then how these alterations interact with an individual's environment to produce in some individuals major psychiatric disorders. Most preventive programs today target either risky behavior (e.g., smoking, drinking, drug use, unprotected sexual activity, school dropout, suicidal behavior) or parenting problems (e.g., coercive parenting or the prevention of cognitive delay in premature infants or socially disadvantaged preschool children,) and the prevention of psychopathology following psychological trauma.

Meta-analyses and reviews of the literature (e.g., Durlak and Wells, 1997; Reppucci et al., 1999; Carr, 2002) make it clear that a number of primary and secondary prevention programs are both clinically effective and cost-effective. The programs that work have definable characteristics (e.g., an empirically based theoretical model; clear goals and objectives; standardized interventions; effective staff training and supervision, and support. Universal programs with not clearly defined targets are often of insufficient intensity and duration to reach those most in need.

WELLNESS PROGRAMS

Let us now turn to wellness programs. Prior to the recent focus on promoting wellness programs because of the complex etiological factors which lead to psychiatric disorders the field attempted to primarily develop methods to reduce the development of serious mental disorders. This was accomplished through model programs created by utilizing a preventive psychiatry paradym. These programs focused on developing actions which would lead to change in individuals' behavior by professionally organized community-based activities or education. Wellness programs add a new dimension to preventive psychiatry's repertoire of actions.

One component of wellness programs addresses models that enhance an individual's experience of wellbeing which aids while adding to their resilience to stress (Weiss et al., 2021)

One model is derived from ancient eastern tradition which was introduced into western psychology in the 1980s and 1990s (Baer, 2003). An individual in a Wellness program learns how to alter their life experience by implementing daily life practices that reduce their experience of stress. The reduction in an individual's experience of stress leads to an enhancement in their psychological well-being, mental health, and resilience.

It creates in the individual a resilience in dealing with the "stresses of life." One learns to accomplish this by during a period of time each day concentrating only on one's physical movements, posture, and respiration. This activity leads to the nonjudgment of thoughts and emotions and at times the exclusion or blocking of feelings from both the external world and from one's inner world. This leads to an individual's experience of an inner calm that reduces their experience of stress.

This process is referred to as mindfulness. Mindfulness is formally defined as "the awareness that emerges through paying attention on purpose, in the present moment, and nonjudgmentally to the unfolding of experience moment by moment" (Kabat-Zinn, 2003). An individual working to accomplish and sustain this state is said to be engaged in Mindfulness. This process is at times facilitated by use of the principles of yoga. Not all of the principles of yoga are needed to attain mindfulness. One can obtain the inner experience of mindfulness alone or in a group. The ability to learn how to engage in mindfulness and attain its benefits can be learned in varying settings. These settings can be developed by individuals alone or in mindfulness programs within institutional wellness programs.

Hospital and other institutions are now developing wellness offices and programs. These have the responsibility to develop mindfulness training programs. They may be held at times either before, during or after the workday for employees to engage and develop individual mindfulness experiences. Wellness programs in hospital and other institutions additionally use the principles of preventive psychiatry. These principles are used to review the hospital workforce environment to learn of any situations which could cause students and workers' unneeded stress. After identifying any such areas, they will propose change in institutional procedures to alleviate them.

Using preventive psychiatry procedures, wellness staff will first identify work experiences and policies which could cause unneeded stress. Then they develop programs to reduce them. These programs are then presented to employees and management for implementation. The wellness staff then function as advisers for implementation. To implement broad based wellness programs some institutions have created wellness officers and staff.

The development of broad-based wellness programs is in its infancy. The full impact of wellness programs is yet to be fully determined in enhancing physician, student, and hospital worker well-being and resilience.

Achenbach TM: *Manual for the Child Behaviour Checklist/4–18 and 1991 Profile.* Burlington: University of Vermont, 1991.

Baer RA: Mindfulness training as a clinical intervention: A conceptual and empirical review. *Clin Psychol Sci Pract* 2003;10: 125–143.

Barton C, Alexander JF: Functional family therapy. In: Gurman AS, Kniskern DP (eds). *Handbook of Family Therapy*, New York: Brunner Mazel, 1981, pp. 403–443.

Caplan Prin*ciples of Preventive Psychiatry*. New York: Basic Books, 1964.

Carr A: *Prevention: What Works with Children and Adolescents?* Hove, UK: Brunner-Routledge, 2002.

Conduct Problems Prevention Research Group: Initial impact of the fast track prevention trial for conduct problems: I. The high-risk sample. *J Consult Clin Psychol* 1999;67:631–657.

Durlak JA: *Successful Prevention Programs for Children and Adolescents.* New York: Plenum, 1997.

Durlak JA, Wells AM: Primary prevention mental health programs for children and adolescents: A meta-analytic review. *Am J Community Psychol* 1997;25:115–143.

Fusar-Paul P, Correll C, Arango C, Berk M, Patel V, Ionandis J: 2021. Preventive psychiatry: A blueprint for improving the mental health of young people World psychiatry. https://www.scopus.com/inward/record.uri?eid=2-s20-

Henggeler SW, Schoenwald SK, Borduin CM, et al: *Multisystemic Treatment of Antisocial Behavior in Children and Adolescents.* New York: Guilford, 1998.

Kabat-Zinn J: Mindfulness-based interventions in context, past, present and future. *Clin Psych Sci Pract* 2003;101:144–156.

Landgraf JM, Koetz L, Ware JE: *The CHQ User's Manual*, 1st edn. Boston: The Health Institute, New England Medical Center, 1996.

Lipsey MW: Is delinquency prevention a cost-effective strategy? A California perspective. *J Res Crime Delinquency* 1984;21: 279–302.

Mrazek PJ, Haggerty RJ: *Reducing the Risk for Mental Disorder: Frontiers for Preventive Intervention Research.* Washington, DC: National Academy Press, 1994.

Nation M, Crusto C, Wandersman A, et al: What works in prevention: Principles of effective prevention programs. *Am Psychol* 2003;58:449–456.

Reppucci MD, Woolard JL, Fried CS: Social, community and preventive interventions. *Annu Rev Psychol* 1999;50:387–418.

Rotheram-Borus MJ, Duan N: Next generation of preventive interventions. *J Am Acad Child Adolesc Psychiatry* 2003; 42:518–526.

Sawyer MG, Kosky RJ, Graetz BW, et al: The national survey of mental health and wellbeing: The child and adolescent component. *Aust N Z J Psychiatry* 2000;34:214–220.

Spaccarelli S: Stress, appraisal, and coping in child sexual abuse: A theoretical and empirical review. *Psychol Bull* 1994;116: 340–362.

Stoewen D: Dimensions of wellness: Change your habits, change your life. *Can Vet J* 2017 (Aug):861–862.

Yates BT: Formative evaluation of costs, cost-effectiveness and cost benefit: Cost procedure, process, outcome analysis. In: Bickman L, Rog D (eds). *Handbook of Applied Social Research Methods.* Thousand Oaks, CA: Sage, 1998, pp. 285–314

Weiss J, Vu M. Hatch Q, Sohn V: Maintaining wellness and instilling resilience if general surgeons. *Surg Clin North Am* 2021 Aug;101(4):625–634.

Neurocognitive Disorders

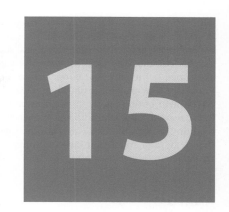

William M. Petrie, MD
Howard S. Kirshner, MD

INTRODUCTION

In everyday practice, psychiatrists serve as members of medical teams in providing treatment to patients who have delirium, dementia, or other cognitive disorders. Psychiatrists often see these patients in hospitals, nursing homes, and other institutional settings. A psychiatrist usually acts as a consultant to a primary care physician or to a hospital service. Psychiatrists help primary care physicians understand the degree to which medical illness contributes to psychiatric symptoms or cognitive symptoms such as confusion. Proper treatment of the medical problem may lead to substantial improvement in psychiatric or neurobehavioral symptoms. Psychotropic medication may be helpful in the management of the patient's illness. Psychiatrists must consider medical diagnoses, treatments, drug inter-actions, and side effects when they prescribe psychotropics as part of their role on the medical team.

Patients who have neurocognitive disorders are often unable to give a reliable history, and the history obtained from third parties usually does not totally reveal the diagnosis. The psychiatrist must rely heavily on data obtained from the physical examination and from laboratory tests, electroencephalogram (EEG) findings, and brain imaging. The medical model provides the most appropriate understanding of patient care in cases of delirium and dementia because the medical model stresses a biological etiology for the patient's symptoms. This approach helps the physician establish crucial links between the patient's medical pathology and the neurobehavioral or psychiatric symptoms. Once links have been established, the psychiatrist can recommend drug therapy and psychotherapy integrated in a comprehensive medical treatment plan.

Patients with delirium and the behavioral complications of dementia often require complicated therapeutic regimens. In some older patients, treatment is not well tolerated and may produce cognitive changes. This is particularly true when patients are receiving treatment for medical disorders. The clinician should understand the behavioral side effects of medical therapies. Removing drugs that produce confusion can help reestablish cognitive function.

Psychiatrists may attempt to treat agitation or hallucinations by adding psychotropics, but these drugs may worsen the patient's condition. Psychiatrists must be prepared to analyze the possibility of multiple drug interactions before launching into psychopharmacotherapy.

Physicians who treat cognitive disorders need to cross the traditional boundaries between psychiatry and neurology. More often than not, older patients have multiple disorders. Delirium, dementia, and affective disorder often coexist. The psychiatrist should not only treat depression and other correctable disorders, but also determine the existence of dementia and establish a prognosis, in order to plan appropriate treatment.

The physician must educate the patient and the family about the nature of the specific illness and the rationale for treatment. Disease processes that cause cognitive deficits may be very complex. Families are often exceedingly anxious because they anticipate the need to accept change in a meaningful relationship. They demand answers. Serious social and financial hardships add to a sense of dread about the future. Most families benefit from a thorough explanation of the patient's condition. Ultimately, the physician must be prepared to explain the contribution made by the various disease processes. The physician must know how to deliver bad news so that family members can take proper steps to prepare for the future. In the process, families expect the physician to respect the dignity of the cognitively impaired patient. Whenever possible, the psychiatrist must try to help the family salvage hope and meaning.

THE AGING BRAIN

Although organic mental disorders occur at any age, they are more common in older patients. As the number of elderly people increases, clinicians will more frequently encounter patients with these disorders. The diagnosis of cognitive disorders is more complex in older patients because physical problems interact with emotional and social factors. The psychiatrist must be familiar with the cognitive changes associated with normal aging before determining the impact of a neurological illness or a psychiatric disorder. Assessment of these patients requires meticulous attention to the mental status examination. If physicians are not thorough in the cognitive assessment of their geriatric patients, they may miss significant deficits, some of which may be treatable.

ANATOMY

Delirium, dementia, and memory disorders become more common with advancing age; as a person ages, the brain becomes more vulnerable to a variety of insults. Brain weight and volume attain their maximal values in the teenage years, and the brain loses both weight and volume as it ages. Significant atrophy of the brain has begun by age 60–70 in most people. By the 10th decade, the ratio of the brain to the skull cavity has fallen from 93% to 80%. When cortical neurons decrease in number, the cortical ribbon thins. Large neurons decrease in number, whereas the number of small neurons increases.

Normal aging and dementia affect specific areas of the brain, especially the association cortices of the frontal, temporal, and parietal lobes. The limbic system, the substantia nigra, the locus coeruleus, the hippocampus and the parahippocampal regions, and the deep frontal nuclei all exhibit a sizable loss of neurons. Despite the loss of neurons, the aged brain continues to undergo dynamic remodeling. In normal older people, dendrites in the hippocampal regions continue to show plasticity. When dendritic arborization fails, mental powers begin to decline.

The relationship between cognitive functions and the morphologic changes that occur as the brain ages is incompletely understood. The volume of the cerebral ventricles increases with age, but the range of ventricular size is greater in old age than in youth. Increases in the size of ventricles, sulci, and subarachnoid spaces are observed easily with modern imaging techniques.

On a microscopic level, lipofuscin granules collect in neurons of aging brains. Fibrous astrocytes increase in size and number. The hippocampus exhibits granulovacuolar changes. Senile plaques and neurofibrillary tangles may occur in the brains of normal older individuals. The number of plaques and tangles in normal brains is less than the number observed in the brains of patients with Alzheimer disease. The overlap between patients with seemingly normal cognition and those with mild Alzheimer disease, however, can be difficult to discriminate in an individual brain. Small infarcts and ischemic white matter lesions are observed in the brains of many normal older people, both at autopsy and in brain imaging studies. These vascular changes appear to lower the threshold for cognitive impairment in the elderly.

PHYSIOLOGY & NEUROTRANSMITTERS

Aging brains have a diminished capacity to respond to metabolic or psychological stress. The brain's demand for glucose decreases. EEG activity slows. Blood flow declines, and oxygen use diminishes. Glucose metabolism is crucial because it contributes to the synthesis of the neurotransmitters acetylcholine, glutamate, aspartate, gamma-aminobutyric acid (GABA), and glycine. Effects of slight abnormalities in glucose metabolism are obvious even in the resting state. The senile brain shows impaired transmitter synthesis and reduced transmitter levels.

Acetylcholine has been studied because of its role in memory. Older people exhibit a decrease in the synthesizing enzyme for acetylcholine, choline acetyltransferase. Uptake of circulating choline into the brain decreases with age. Decreased levels of acetylcholine in the hippocampus may relate to age-related declines in short-term memory. In Alzheimer disease, damage to the ascending cholinergic system plays an important role in the loss of memory and in other cognitive deficits.

Decreased catecholamines are linked more closely to affective changes than to cognitive changes in older people. Noradrenergic cell bodies in the locus coeruleus appear to decline in number with aging, but concentrations of norepinephrine appear to remain normal in target areas. The synthetic enzyme tyrosine hydroxylase decreases with aging, whereas the degradative enzyme monoamine oxidase increases. Research also suggests reduced serotonergic innervation in the aging neocortex.

Loss of dopaminergic innervation of the neostriatum is a prominent age-related change that corresponds with the loss of dopaminergic cell bodies from the substantia nigra. Age-related decreases in basal ganglia dopamine make older patients more sensitive to the side effects of neuroleptics. Dopaminergic innervation of the neocortex and the neostriatum are not affected.

Studies of the brains of older patients have revealed a decrease in norepinephrine, serotonin, acetylcholine, and dopamine receptors. A decrease in β-receptor density results in reduced cyclic adenosine mono-phosphate and decreased adaptability to the external environment.

In contrast, older patients exhibit an increase in benzodiazepine-GABA receptor inhibitory activity and an increased sensitivity to benzodiazepines.

The capacity of mitochondria declines with age. Mitochondrial oxidants may be the chief source of the mitochondrial lesions that accumulate with age. The brain becomes susceptible to injury by free radicals that damage mitochondrial DNA, proteases, and membranes. Free radicals are likely a major contributor to cellular and tissue aging.

MEMORY

Although some cognitive scientists use the term short-term memory to mean immediate attention span and long-term storage for longer retained memories, clinicians generally use the terms "immediate," "short-term," and "long-term" or remote memory. Immediate memory, also called "working memory," consists of registration and attention span, such as for seven digits forward. **Immediate memory** is retained for seconds only, unless the subject actively rehearses the information. Immediate memory retains information in reverberating neural circuits involving the frontal lobe. If it is not converted to short-term storage, information is lost. Memories are stored through a process called **consolidation**. Short-term memories are recalled through the hippocampi and related structures, and also the amygdala when emotion or fear are important to the memory. Long-term or remote memory is thought to be stored in the cortex and may not require the hippocampus for access. Short-term memory is a biochemical process that depends on protein synthesis and the development of dendritic connections. In the clinical setting, patients who have difficulty learning new material are described as having an **anterograde amnesia**.

Patients who have difficulty recalling information stored before the onset of an illness or injury have **retrograde amnesia**. The retention of material in long-term storage depends on that part of the cerebral cortex related to the specific sensory modality involved. Thus if both the occipital and occipital-parietal cortices are involved in an injury, visual memories may be impaired significantly.

IMPLICIT & EXPLICIT MEMORY

Cognitive neuroscience has provided strong support for the idea that multiple memory systems exist. One system divides memory into explicit and implicit types. **Explicit memory** is synonymous with declarative memory. Declarative memory reflects a conscious recollection of the past. The short-term memory discussed earlier, **episodic memory** of a person's own conscious experiences, is a form of declarative or explicit memory, but so is the recall of factual information, often called **semantic memory**. Declarative memories are consciously known and are therefore explicit. Explicit memory disorders are well recognized clinically. Lesions in the medial temporal lobes, midline diencephalon, or basal forebrain can impair declarative memory because relationships between sensory modalities are processed through the hippocampal diencephalic system.

Nondeclarative memory is sometimes called implicit memory. **Implicit memory** implies that a person may be able to know something without being aware of remembering it. Implicit memory is not usually tested clinically. Implicit memory does not involve the conscious recollection of recent experiences for the execution of tasks. Procedural learning (e.g., how to drive a car) is an example of implicit memory.

Apraxia can be seen as a deficit in implicit memory. Amnestic patients can learn certain skills or acquire problem-solving abilities, even though they have no memory of having learned the behavior.

The basal ganglia, cerebellum, and frontal lobes have been linked to procedural learning. Procedural learning does not involve the hippocampal diencephalic system. Procedural learning is most affected in subcortical dementias such as Huntington and Parkinson diseases.

Additional examples of implicit learning include classical conditioning (stimulus-response) and operant conditioning (reinforcing behaviors). Even people who do not have amnestic disorders learn by classical conditioning but may not be able to recollect the experience. People who have severe declarative memory disorders are quite capable of learning through stimulus-response and reinforcement paradigms. The cerebellum is heavily involved in this type of memory.

Yet another form of memory is **probabilistic learning**, in which we learn from past experiences to predict the future. This form of memory is also relatively independent of medial temporal lobe functions.

All memories are influenced heavily by emotions. Memory for emotionally arousing events is modulated by an endogenous memory-modulating system consisting of stress hormones and the amygdala. This system is an adaptive method of creating memory strength that is proportional to memory importance. In addition, some memory is state specific so that these memories can be recalled only during emotional states similar to the ones present when they were created.

Memory is highly complex and difficult to quantify at the bedside. It is equally important to recognize that in patients with memory syndromes, neuropsychological testing reveals normal perception, language, motor functions, and preserved intellectual skills.

THEORIES OF MEMORY

Recently, neural network theories of memory have been proposed. Distinct neural networks mediate different memory modalities. Neural networks are based on the idea that streams of information are combined by forming, strengthening, or pruning connections between neurons to form new representations that can later be retrieved. Evidence for this process comes from the fact that damage to specific areas of the association cortex affects individual sensory memory modalities. Currently research in functional brain imaging is being combined with these theories to provide a new source of information about how memory systems function.

COGNITION AND AGING

Changes in cognitive performance related to aging vary greatly. Information processing, particularly verbal speed and working memory, show the most pronounced changes.

The number of correct answers required for the same IQ score in a 70-year old, as compared to a 25-year old, is approximately 50%. On the other hand, some cognitive skills are resistant to aging. Vocabulary and ability to read quickly tend to remain preserved and can be used to estimate premorbid IQ in cognitively impaired senior citizens. Older people who possess highly developed cognitive abilities can mask memory defects for a time. This "cognitive reserve" is especially noted in topics related to the person's long-term reading. Even the Mini Mental State Exam, a relatively crude test of cognitive function, shows major effects of education on performance. These resistant aspects of cognition are often referred to as "crystallized intelligence," as compared to the "fluid intelligence" of memory and attention that is less resistant to aging. These studies encourage all of us to stay mentally active, continue reading in our professional disciplines, as we age.

After age 70, brain functions and capabilities decline more rapidly. Cognitive decline related to aging produces impaired memory, diminished capacity for complex ideas, mental rigidity, cautious responses, and behavioral slowing. Slowing of responses is the most consistent cognitive change. As a result, it takes longer to provide professional services to older people.

Physicians who spend sufficient time testing mental status in older individuals are more likely to obtain accurate results than physicians who rush through the examination. Given enough time, older people will complete the following tasks accurately: (1) random digits forward, (2) untimed serial arithmetic problems, (3) simple vigilance tests, (4) basic orientation, and (5) immediate memory. Unfamiliar stimuli, complex tasks, and time demands cause difficulty for older people. When older patients are asked to reorganize material (e.g., repeating digits backward), they often become anxious. Immediate memory continues to be normal in most patients, but if the memory task calls for split attention or reorganization, older people will have a harder time. Whenever the items to be remembered exceed primary memory capability, seniors show a decrement in memory acquisition and retrieval. Seniors have more difficulty remembering names and objects when they are not in a familiar routine. They do poorly on memory tasks that involve speed, unfamiliar material, or free recall. Although older people have difficulty organizing information, their memory performance improves if they control the rate of presentation. Practice also improves performance. Cognition does not operate in isolation from personality or social relationships. Because learning and memories occur within a range of contexts, a more useful test is one that emphasizes real-life memory.

Seniors usually perceive themselves as less effective than when they were younger, a perception that affects performance. The memory complaints of older adults are often related to low self-confidence or other personality variables. As a result, when seniors experience an increase in self-esteem and motivation, their objective performance also improves. Similarly, lack of confidence reduces cognitive expectations even further.

AMNESIA

Amnestic syndromes usually occur with specific structural or pathological bases. They may be present in disorders of the frontal or temporal lobe. They are caused by traumatic, infectious, vascular, inflammatory or other factors. Examination of memory in amnesia may be complex, with a focus on what is preserved as much as what is impaired.

Transient global amnesia (TGA) is a sudden temporary episode of memory loss that cannot be attributed to another neurological condition. Patients are alert and attentive, but with anterograde amnesia. TGA lasts less than 24 hours. The etiology of TGA remains unclear. While the event appears vascular, TGA patients do not seem to have a higher risk of stroke.

In other amnestic syndromes, psychiatric and stress-related factors should also carefully be examined.

Bartus RT, et al: The cholinergic hypothesis of geriatric memory dysfunction. *Science* 1982;217:408.

Budson AE, Price BH. Memory dysfunction. *N Engl J Med* 2005;352: 692–699.

Burke DM, McKay DG: Memory, language, and aging. *Phil Trans R Soc London B* 1997;352:1845–1856.

Cockburn J, Smith PT: The relative influence of intelligence and age on everyday memory. *J Gerontol* 1991;46:31–36.

Crum RM, Anthony JC, Bassett SS, Folstein MF: Population-based norms for the Mini-Mental State Examination by age and educational level. *JAMA* 1993;269:2386–2391.

Folstein MF, Folstein SE, McHugh PR: "Mini-Mental State": a practical method for grading the cognitive state of patients for the clinician. *J Psychiatry Res* 1975;12:189–198.

Hultsch DF, Dixon RA: Learning and memory in aging. In: Birren JE, Schaie KW (eds.) *The Handbook of the Psychology of Aging.* New York: Academic Press; 1990:258–274.

Kirshner HS: Mild cognitive impairment: To treat or not to treat. *Curr Neurol Neurosurg Rep* 2005;5:455–457.

Mangla A, Navi BB, Layton K, Kamel H: Transient global amnesia and the risk of ischemic stroke. *Stroke* 2014;45:389–393.

McCartney JR: Physician's assessment of cognitive capacity. Failure to meet the needs of the elderly. *Arch Intern Med* 1986;146:177.

Quinn J, Kaye J: The neurology of aging. *Neurologist.* 2001;7:98–112.

Sacks O: A neurologist's perspective on the aging brain. *Arch Neurol* 1997;54:1211–1214.

Salthouse TA: Are individual differences in rates of aging greater at older age? *Neurobiol Aging* 2012;10:2373–2381.

Shimamura AP, Berry JM, Mangels JA, et al: Memory and cognitive abilities in university professors. *Psychol Sci* 1995;6:387–394.

DELIRIUM

Delirium is one of the most dramatic presentations in psychiatry and neurology. Delirious patients become acutely agitated, disoriented, and unable to sustain attention, form memories, or reason. In the past, the term *delirium* was reserved for an agitated, hyperactive state, whereas *encephalopathy* applied to confusional states in which the level of consciousness was normal or depressed. Currently, no distinction is made between these two conditions. In fact, delirium is now synonymous with "acute brain syndrome," encephalopathy, acute confusional state, and toxic psychosis.

Delirium is an extremely common clinical problem in hospitalized patients. An estimated 30–50% of hospitalized elderly people become delirious, amounting to an overall incidence of about 10% of all hospitalizations. Delirium increases morbidity and mortality for any hospitalization, and the cost to society is enormous.

The definition of delirium from the The *Diagnostic and Statistical Manual of Mental Disorders*, Fifth Edition (DSM-5) follows, later. Delirium, like dementia, involves multiple cognitive functions, including attention, memory, reasoning, language, and executive function. In contrast to dementia, delirium typically develops relatively acutely and fluctuates more from hour to hour and day to day. Delirium involves alterations in level of consciousness, agitation and hypervigilance or drowsiness, disturbed perception (hallucinations, delusions), psychomotor abnormalities (restlessness, agitation), and autonomic nervous system hyperactivity (tachycardia, hypertension, fever, diaphoresis, tremor). All of these phenomena are less common in dementia.

GENERAL CONSIDERATIONS

▶ Epidemiology

The prevalence of delirium in general hospital patients is 10–30%. As many as 50% of surgical patients become delirious in the postoperative period. Delirium accompanies the terminal stages of many illnesses. It occurs in 25–40% of patients who have cancer and in up to 85% of patients with advanced cancer. Close to 80% of terminal patients will become delirious before they die.

Distinguishing delirium from depression in this population is important because physicians can treat both conditions and improve the quality of life for the terminally ill. Many patients today make living wills or assign loved ones a durable power of attorney for health care. By explaining the causes and treatment of delirium to family members, the physician empowers them to decide what is best for the patient.

Age is the most widely identified risk factor for delirium. Patients with dementia are at high risk for delirium. Forty-one percent of dementia patients have delirium on admission to the hospital. Twenty-five percent of patients who are admitted to the hospital with delirium will ultimately be diagnosed as having dementia. Other factors that predict delirium in hospitalized patients include prior brain disease; vision or hearing loss; presence of a fracture on admission; symptomatic infection; stress or major environmental change; neuroleptic,

anticholinergic, sedative medications or substance use or withdrawal; sleep deprivation; and use of restraints, a bladder catheter, or any surgical procedure during the admission.

The incidence of delirium in nursing homes is also quite high. Because the onset of delirium is more insidious in seniors than in young people, there is an even higher probability that delirium will be overlooked in nursing homes. Illnesses such as unrecognized urinary tract infection may cause delirium. More serious, life-threatening illnesses can also present with delirium. Hospital staff must be trained to recognize delirium at an early stage so that they can identify and promptly treat the primary medical condition. Common causes of delirium in older people include hypoxia, hypoperfusion of the brain, hypoglycemia, hypertensive encephalopathy, intracranial hemorrhage, CNS infection, and toxic-confusional states. Even when delirium is recognized and treated promptly, it predicts future cognitive decline. Many elderly patients who have been delirious never fully recover.

▶ Etiology

A variety of conditions lead to delirium. These conditions can be categorized into four major groups: (1) systemic disease secondarily affecting the brain, (2) primary intracranial disease, (3) exogenous toxic agents, and (4) withdrawal from substances of abuse. DSM-5 classifies delirium according to the presumed etiology. If delirium is due to a systemic medical condition or to primary intracranial disease, then the medical cause is listed in the Axis I diagnosis. Substance-induced delirium and substance withdrawal delirium are classified separately. Substance-induced delirium includes delirium caused by toxins and by drugs of abuse. If the etiology is not found, the diagnosis is delirium not otherwise specified. In most clinical situations, delirium is caused by multiple factors.

1. Systemic disease—Delirium can be caused by any type of systemic disease. When a medical condition causes delirium, the primary disease has caused either failure in cerebral blood flow or failure in cerebral metabolism. Cardiac conditions cause delirium by decreasing cerebral perfusion. Patients who have experienced cardiac arrest, cardiogenic shock, severe hypertension, or congestive heart failure are at risk of delirium. Organ failure syndromes such as renal, hepatic, and respiratory insufficiency can all cause delirium. Endocrine and metabolic disturbances affect brain metabolism. Hyponatremia and hypoglycemia may be the most prevalent causes in this category. Hypothyroidism is a common endocrine factor.

Central nervous system (CNS) causes of delirium include vasculitis, stroke, and seizure. Paraneoplastic phenomena in the brain (e.g., limbic encephalitis) may cause altered mental status in cancer patients.

Nutritional status also contributes to delirium; the most notable examples are vitamin B_1 deficiency in alcoholic patients, vitamin B_{12} deficiency, and pellagra. Infections may affect the nervous system directly, as in meningitis and encephalitis, but more often they cause delirium indirectly through toxins. In elderly patients who have generalized sepsis or even local infections such as urinary tract infections, altered mental status may precede both fever and leukocytosis. Mental status change may be the only manifestation of infection. In at least half of cases, the cause of delirium is multifactorial. Urinary tract infection, low serum albumin, elevated white blood cell count, and proteinuria are among the most significant risk factors. Other risk factors include hyponatremia, hypernatremia, severity of illness, dementia, fever, hypothermia, psychoactive drug use, and azotemia.

No matter what systemic illness causes delirium, the clinical consequences are stereotypical. The diverse insults that cause delirium appear to act via similar metabolic and cellular pathways. A cascade of pathology in central neurotransmitter systems destabilizes cerebral function. Factors include oxidative stress; reductions in dopamine, norepinephrine, and acetylcholine; changes in either direction in serotonin; depolarization of neurons; and effects of stress such as sympathetic discharges and activation of the hypothalamic-pituitary-adrenocortical system. Ultimately, dysfunctional second messenger systems may provide the cellular mechanism of metabolic delirium.

2. Primary intracranial disease—Delirium can be caused by lesions in a variety of brain regions. Vascular pathology is more likely to cause confusional states if lesions are present in the basal nuclei and thalamus. Bilateral lesions of the thalamus or caudate nuclei are especially associated with delirium. Delirium is also more likely to accompany strokes in patients with preexisting brain atrophy or seizures. In traumatic brain injury, deeper brain lesions are associated with longer periods of delirium. Frontal lobe syndromes can also mimic delirium.

3. Exogenous toxic agents—Delirium due to substances may occur as the result of substance abuse or as an undesirable effect of medical therapies. Patients with delirium may exhibit symptoms suggesting pathology in specific neurotransmitter systems. Delirium in substance abusers who overdose provides the best example of a neurotransmitter-specific delirium.

Stimulants act through dopamine and other catecholamine pathways. Stimulant overdoses can cause confusion, seizures, dyskinesia, and psychomotor agitation; however, the most common presentation is that of an agitated paranoid state. People who abuse stimulants are involved in violent acts more often than are those who abuse other substances. The dopamine excess observed in stimulant-induced delirium may provide a model to understand delirium in other general medical conditions. The effectiveness of dopamine-blocking agents such as haloperidol in the treatment of delirium suggests that excess dopamine relative to acetylcholine may produce delirium in general medical conditions and in stimulant-induced delirium.

D-Lysergic acid diethylamide (LSD), as well as other psychedelic agents which have become more popular, cause a different form of delirium through its action at serotonin receptors. This hallucinogen causes intensification of perceptions, depersonalization, derealization, illusions, hallucinations, and incoordination. Patients with delirium due to medical conditions may also experience illusions and hallucinations, usually visual. Serotonin systems also may be affected in these patients. Under certain circumstances patients who are taking selective serotonin reuptake inhibitor (SSRI) antidepressants, especially when combined with other serotonergic medications, develop the *serotonin syndrome*, of which delirium can be a prominent feature.

Disruption of pathways served by NMDA receptors (N-methyl-D-aspartate, a subtype of glutamate receptor) induces patients who are intoxicated with phencyclidine to display yet another symptom complex. Phencyclidine overdose is well recognized because of its tendency to produce assaultive behavior, agitation, diminished responsiveness to pain, ataxia, dysarthria, altered body image, and nystagmus. The NMDA receptor is also involved in the biological effects of alcoholism, such as intoxication and delirium tremens. Ethanol-induced upregulation of NMDA receptors may underlie withdrawal seizures. The NMDA receptor also mediates some of the more damaging effects of ischemia during a stroke. Stimulation of NMDA receptors can lead to permanent brain damage. For this reason, conditions that lead to NMDA stimulation should be treated promptly.

Activation of brain GABA receptors causes some manifestations of sedative or alcohol overdose. Sedative intoxication causes slurred speech, incoordination, unsteady gait, nystagmus, and impairment in attention or memory. Some manifestations of hepatic encephalopathy may be the result of excessive stimulation of GABA receptors. Delirium tremens occurs when insufficient stimulation of GABA receptors results from withdrawal from benzodiazepines or alcohol. Treatment with benzodiazepines improves delirium tremens.

Drugs that have anticholinergic properties are very likely to contribute to delirium. In hospitalized patients, symptoms of delirium occur when serum anticholinergic activity is elevated. Total serum anticholinergic activity also helps predict which patients in intensive care units become confused. Symptoms of anticholinergic delirium include agitation, pupillary dilation, dry skin, urinary retention, and memory impairment.

Physicians must be cautious when prescribing psychoactive drugs to seniors. One of the most common causes of delirium is iatrogenic. Common agents such as digoxin may induce cognitive dysfunction in older people, even with therapeutic digoxin levels. In the intensive care unit, antiarrhythmic agents such as lidocaine or mexiletine may cause confusion. Among the narcotics, meperidine is particularly likely to cause confusion and hallucinations.

Benzodiazepines, other narcotics, and antihistamines are also frequent contributors to delirium. In psychiatric patients, tricyclic antidepressants (TCAs) and low-potency neuroleptics are frequent contributors. Note that these drugs have anticholinergic properties, and agents such as benztropine or trihexyphenidyl, used to combat extrapyramidal effects, are also anticholinergic. The list of other drugs that may induce confusion is extensive.

The misuse of psychoactive drugs causes as many as 20% of geropsychiatric admissions. The chances of an adverse cognitive response increase as the number of drugs rises. Adverse drug reactions are a source of excess morbidity in elderly patients. A high index of suspicion, drug-free trials, and careful monitoring of drug therapy reduce this problem. Occasionally a specific antidote is available for a drug-induced delirium. Physostigmine may reverse anticholinergic delirium and is sometimes useful in treating TCA overdoses. Narcotic-induced delirium can be reversed with naloxone. Flumazenil is an imidazobenzodiazepine that antagonizes the effects of benzodiazepine agonists by competitive interaction at the cerebral receptor. Naloxone and flumazenil have short half-lives and may have to be readministered.

Boyer EW, Shannon W: The serotonin syndrome. *N Engl J Med* 2005;352:1112–1120.

Devinsky O, Bear D, Volpe BT: Confusional states following posterior cerebral artery infarction. *Arch Neurol* 1988;45: 160–163.

Diagnostic and Statistical Manual of Mental Disorders. Fifth Edition. Washington, DC: American Psychiatric Association, 2013.

Erkinjuntii T, et al: Dementia among medical inpatients. *Arch Intern Med* 1986;146:1923.

Fong TG, Tulebaev SR, Inouye SK: Delirium in elderly adults: diagnosis, prevention and treatment. *Nat Rev Neurol* 2009;5: 210–220.

Francis J, Martin D, Kapoor WN: A prospective study of delirium in hospitalized elderly. *JAMA* 1990;263:1097.

Gibson GE, et al: The cellular basis of delirium and its relevance to age-related disorders including Alzheimer's disease. *Int Psychogeriatr* 1991;3:373.

Gleckman R, Hibert D: Afebrile bacteremia. A phenomena in geriatric patients. *JAMA* 1982;248:1478.

Inouye SK: Delirium in older persons. *N Engl J Med* 2006;354: 1157–1165.

Inouye SK, Charpentier PA: Precipitating factors for delirium in hospitalized elderly persons. Predictive model and interrelationship with baseline vulnerability. *JAMA* 1996;275: 852–857.

Oh ES, Fong TG, Hshieh TT, Inouye SK: Delirium in older persons. Advances in diagnosis and treatment. *JAMA* 2017;318: 1161–1174.

Kirshner HS: Delirium and acute confusional states. In: Kirshner HS (eds). *Behavioral Neurology. Practical Science of Mind and Brain.* Boston: Butterworth Heinemann, 2002, pp. 307–324.

Kirshner HS: Delirium: a focused review. *Curr Neurol Neurosci Rep* 2007;7:479–482.

Kirshner HS: Vascular dementia: a review of recent evidence for prevention and treatment. *Curr Neurol Neurosci Rep* 2009;9:437–442.

Kumral E, Ozturk O: Delusional state following acute stroke. *Neurology* 2004;62:110–113.

Lipowski AJ: Delirium (acute confusional states). *JAMA* 1987;258: 1789.

Mach JR Jr et al: Serum anticholinergic activity in hospitalized older persons with delirium: a preliminary study [see comments]. *J Am Geriatr Soc* 1995;43:491.

McPherson JA, Wagner CE, Boehm LM, et al: Delirium in the cardiovascular ICU: exploring modifiable risk factors. *Crit Care Med* 2013;2:405–413.

Mesulam MM, et al: Acute confusional states with right middle cerebral artery infarction. *J Neurol Neurosurg Psychiatry* 1976;39:84.

Packard RC: Delirium. *Neurologist* 2001;7:327–340.

Padharipande PP, Girand TD, Jackson A: Long-term cognitive impairment after critical illness. *N Engl J Med* 2013;369: 1306–1316.

CLINICAL FINDINGS

▶ Basic Evaluation

Although the evaluation of delirium entails the analysis of very straightforward data, physicians often miss the diagnosis. The physician must obtain a careful history, perform a relevant physical examination, conduct a mental status examination, and review the patient's medications and laboratory tests. Physicians who do not conduct a careful physical examination may overlook asterixis, tremors, psychomotor retardation, and other motor manifestations of delirium. An organized mental status examination is the cornerstone of the assessment. The clinician who makes assumptions about the patient's cognitive status will make mistakes. This is particularly true in patients who are apathetic. After the physician has assessed the patient's mental status, he or she should carefully review laboratory data and the patient's medications.

▶ Signs and Symptoms

The essential feature of delirium is an alteration in attention associated with disturbed consciousness and cognition. One of the most disconcerting clinical characteristics of delirium is its fluctuating course. Symptoms are ever-changing. The patient's mental status varies from time to time. Cognitive deficits appear suddenly and disappear just as quickly. Patients may be apathetic at one moment, yet a short time later they may be restless, anxious, or irritable. Other patients become agitated and begin hallucinating without apparent change in the underlying medical condition. Waxing and waning of symptoms and perceptual disturbances may reflect the fact that the nondominant cortex is involved.

Common features of delirium include sleep disturbance and either decreased or agitated level of consciousness.

Delirium may first present as *sundowning* with daytime drowsiness and nighttime insomnia with confusion. As the patient becomes more ill, disorientation and inattention dominate the clinical picture. Nonetheless, consciousness does not always follow the course of the underlying illness. When the patient's sleep is disturbed and the affect is labile, delirium usually lasts longer. This cluster of symptoms points to involvement of the reticular activating system of the brainstem and ascending pathways in delirium. Symptoms usually resolve quickly when the underlying disorder is treated, but a degree of confusion can last as long as 1 month after the medical condition has resolved, and some patients are even left with a long-term dementia.

▶ Psychological Testing

The Mini Mental State Exam (MMSE) is often used to quantify cognitive impairment, but only specific items on the MMSE are useful for evaluating delirium. Delirious patients have the most difficulty with calculation, orientation, attention, memory, and writing. The other higher cortical functions and language are usually preserved. The MMSE may be normal in as many as one third of patients with clinical delirium. More specific delirium scales can be helpful. The Confusion Assessment Method is a rapid test designed to be administered by trained non-psychiatrists. The Delirium Rating Scale is a 10-item scale for assessment of delirium severity. One study found that patients whose delirious episode improved within 1 week had much lower Delirium Rating Scale scores at the time of psychiatric consultation than did patients whose delirium lasted more than 1 week. The Trail Making Test (Parts A and B) and clock drawing tests are psychomotor tasks that are sensitive and easy to administer. Unfortunately, these tests measure specific cognitive functions that may not be impaired in delirium. For the busy clinician, the MMSE is the most practical tool; however, the clock drawing test also provides useful information in a short time.

▶ Laboratory Findings

The vital signs are often abnormal. Common tests that often reveal the etiology of the delirium include complete blood count, sedimentation rate, electrolytes, blood urea nitrogen, glucose, liver function tests, toxic screen, electrocardiogram (ECG), chest X-ray, urinalysis, and others. Blood gases or appropriate cultures may be helpful. A computed tomography (CT) scan is sometimes necessary to diagnose structural damage. Prompt lumbar puncture will confirm the diagnosis of suspected intrathecal infection.

Imaging studies are needed when the neurologic examination suggests a focal process or when initial screening tests have not revealed a treatable cause of the delirium. Even in nonneurological causes of delirium, CT scans often reveal ventricular dilatation, cortical atrophy, and ischemic changes.

The right-hemisphere association cortex is often involved when some patients who are not paralyzed become delirious, suggesting a predisposing role for structural brain disease in the elderly with delirium. Subarachnoid hemorrhage, subdural hematoma, or right-hemisphere stroke can cause early mental status changes. Structural neurologic injury is sometimes the sole reason for delirium.

The EEG is useful in the evaluation of delirium when all other studies have been unrevealing. Generalized slowing is the typical pattern. A normal EEG is atypical but does not rule out delirium. Confusion and clouding of consciousness correlate partially with EEG slowing. In mild delirium, the dominant posterior rhythm is slowed. In more severe cases, theta and delta rhythms are present throughout the brain. Quantitative methods of EEG analysis supplement visual assessment in difficult cases. The severity of EEG slowing is correlated with the severity and duration of delirium and with the length of hospital stay. In more severe cases of metabolic or toxic delirium, triphasic waves replace diffuse symmetrical slowing. The appearance of periodic lateralized epileptiform discharges suggests a structural etiology. Rarely, the EEG reveals non-convulsive status epilepticus as the cause of the delirium. In sedative or alcohol withdrawal, the EEG may show low-voltage fast activity.

▶ Differential Diagnosis (Including Comorbid Conditions)

Distinguishing delirium from dementia can be difficult, because many clinical findings on mental status examination are similar. The most common differential diagnoses are as follows: whether the patient has dementia rather than delirium; whether he or she has a delirium alone; or whether the patient has a delirium superimposed on preexisting dementia. Regardless, the clinical history is the most important tool in the diagnosis. Delirium is an acute illness. Dementia is longstanding. Physical examination and mental status are also important. Tremor, asterixis, restlessness, tachycardia, fever, hypertension, sweating, and other psychomotor and autonomic abnormalities are more common in delirium than dementia. Positive neurobehavioral symptoms such as agitation, delusional thinking, and hallucinations are much more common in delirium than dementia. On the other hand, cortical disorders such as dysphasia (language impairment) or apraxia (motor impairment) are not as common in delirium as in dementia. Clinicians should remember, however, that the two conditions often coexist.

Patients with delirium frequently have altered perceptions. As a result, delirium is sometimes mistaken for a psychosis. It is usually possible to separate delirium from a psychosis because signs of cognitive dysfunction are more common in delirium than in psychotic disorders. Psychotic patients are not usually disoriented, and they can usually perform well on bedside tests of attention and memory. The EEG is normal in psychoses. When the laboratory evidence does not support a medical illness, the clinician should consider the possibility of a psychiatric cause. When a psychiatric illness causes symptoms of delirium, patients are said to have a *pseudodelirium*. A history of past psychiatric illness may help clarify whether a patient has delirium or a psychiatric illness with pseudodelirium (e.g., a dissociative fugue or trauma state).

In some clinical situations, the boundaries are blurred between delirium and purely psychiatric illness. Psychiatric illness causes certain populations to become prone to physical disease. As a result, delirium can be surprisingly prevalent in psychiatric patients. Delirium and depression often coexist in seniors because depressed older patients are prone to become dehydrated and malnourished. Psychiatric patients may misuse prescribed drugs or abuse street drugs. Psychiatrists must be alert for delirium in all psychiatric patients.

Treatment

The correct treatment of delirium entails a search for the underlying causes and an attempt to treat the acute symptoms. Close nursing supervision to protect the patient is essential. Staff should remove all dangerous objects. Brief visits from a familiar person and a supportive environment with television, radio, a calendar, and proper lighting help orient the patient. The physician should review the patient's medications for unnecessary drugs and stop them, or drugs or substances that the patient could be withdrawing from; he or she should also monitor the patient's laboratory test, especially electrolyte balance, hydration, renal and hepatic function, and nutrition.

Handling Treatment Resistance

When delirious patients become agitated, they may resist treatment, threaten staff, or place themselves in danger. Of equal importance, these patients have elevated circulating catecholamines, which causes an increase in heart rate, blood pressure, and ventilation. Hospital personnel must protect patient rights and apply the least restrictive intervention when dealing with an agitated patient. The use of mechanical restraints increases morbidity, especially if the restraints are applied for more than 4 days. A sitter, although expensive, can sometimes obviate the need for physical restraint. Specially designed beds can also reduce the need for restraints. The Health Care Financing Administration has recently introduced strict guidelines for the use of restraints in psychiatric settings.

When other methods fail to control agitated patients, chemical sedation is usually more effective and less dangerous than physical restraint. According to the practice parameters of the Society of Critical Care Medicine, haloperidol is the preferred agent for the treatment of delirium in the critically ill adult. Many clinicians prefer the atypical antipsychotic agents in elderly patients because of the lower incidence of extrapyramidal side effects. The U.S. Food and Drug Administration (FDA) has issued a warning because of the risk of cardiac complications and type 2 diabetes accompanying these agents, but similar warnings exist for haloperidol. Whether or not these warnings are meaningful during the short-term use of these agents in patients with delirium is unknown. Increasing data suggest that haloperidol and other high-potency neuroleptics had a higher mortality risk in elderly patients than the atypical antipsychotic agents such as olanzapine or quetiapine. In emergencies, haloperidol could be administered intravenously for a painless, rapid, and reliable onset of action that occurs in about 11 minutes. The dose regimen can be adjusted every 30 minutes until the patient is under control. For mildly agitated patients, 1–2 mg may suffice. Recent studies have shown that in an ICU setting the benefits of haloperidol are no better than placebo. Significant Q-T interval prolongation and torsades de pointes (an atypical rapid ventricular tachycardia) are possible complications of high-dose intravenous haloperidol. Droperidol was used in similar fashion in the past but is no longer available for this purpose because of the frequency of torsades. Hypotension may occur rarely. Acute dystonic reactions occur in less than 1% of patients. Other extrapyramidal side effects, however, such as Parkinsonism and tardive dyskinesia, are very common with this agent.

Treating Comorbid Anxiety

Patients admitted to the intensive care unit are often anxious and in pain, conditions that make delirium worse. Anxiety and delirium may be difficult to distinguish from one another. The interplay between confusion and anxiety may cause patients to become agitated when they are encouraged to engage in stressful activities such as weaning from mechanical ventilation. Benzodiazepines, if carefully monitored, can help in these situations. If benzodiazepines are given intravenously, they can cause respiratory depression or hypotension; however, this class of drugs can be easily titrated when monitoring is appropriate. As a result, benzodiazepines are effective in the treatment of delirium in selected patients. Neuroleptic agents such as haloperidol may act synergistically with benzodiazepines, resulting in control of agitation. The patient's level of consciousness and respiratory drive are usually maintained but should be monitored. Once sedation has been achieved, intermittent administration of a neuroleptic agent in combination with a benzodiazepine can usually maintain control.

Managing Side Effects

Physicians need to be aware of the side effects of benzodiazepines. Even when these medications are used as hypnotics, they may cause a decrease in the patient's MMSE score. Note that benzodiazepines are also employed to produce amnesia for uncomfortable procedures such as colonoscopy or transesophageal echocardiography. A variety of factors, including reduction in hepatic metabolism, modify the pharmacokinetics of many benzodiazepines in elderly patients. Lorazepam and oxazepam may be less affected by hepatic factors and are therefore preferred. Midazolam has been used as an intravenous infusion in intensive care settings because it is safe and has a short half-life.

Barbiturates are highly effective sedatives, but they depress the respiratory and cardiovascular systems. Given the efficacy of benzodiazepines, barbiturates should probably be reserved for agitated patients who have special indications for these drugs. Etomidate and propofol should be avoided for long-term use in agitated patients because of potentially serious side effects.

Managing Pain

Pain relief is important. Opiates are the cornerstone of analgesia, but they may also contribute to delirium. In acute settings, opiates with short half-lives are the most efficacious. The Society of Critical Care Medicine recommends morphine; however, the total daily dosage must be monitored carefully in situations in which as-needed dosing is permitted. Naloxone can reverse the effects of a morphine overdose, but the clinician must be aware of the 20-minute half-life of this antagonist. Morphine is contraindicated in patients who have renal failure. Meperidine has been associated with hallucinations and seizures and should not be given to patients with delirium.

Special Considerations

The determination of the effective dosage of sedatives and analgesics in patients who have multiple organ system insufficiency requires careful planning and monitoring. Because the liver and kidney eliminate these drugs, organ system failure usually affects their distributive volume and clearance. The physician must assess the patient's creatinine clearance and liver function. Malnourished patients may have reduced plasma binding. By reducing the size and frequency of doses, the physician can avoid toxic effects. In life-threatening delirium, consultation with the anesthesia service is recommended, and therapeutic paralysis with muscle relaxants and anesthetic agents can be considered.

Prognosis

Patients with delirium have longer hospital stays and higher mortality than lucid patients. About half of all patients with acute encephalopathies improve if they receive proper treatment. Of the remainder, half will die and half will prove to have early signs of dementia. The severity of the underlying illness determines whether the delirious person will live or die, and patients with the poorest cognitive status on admission have the poorest long-term outcome. Ideal management requires awareness of the causes of delirium and active preventive efforts. Very elderly patients and patients with sensory impairment are at highest risk. The alert physician who recognizes systemic illness early and avoids complicated drug regimens can help prevent delirium.

Adams R, Victor M: Delirium and other acute confusional states. In: *Principles of Neurology* (6th edn.). New York: McGraw-Hill; 1996.

Anderson-Ranberg NC, Poulsen LM, Perner A, Wetterslev J, et al: Haloperidol for the treatment of delirium in ICU patients. *N Engl J Med* 2022,387;2425–2435.

Ayd FJ: Intravenous haloperidol-lorazepam therapy for delirium. *Drug Ther Newslett* 1984;19:33.

Bowen BC, et al: MR signal abnormalities in memory disorder and dementia. *Am J Roentgenol* 1990;154:1285.

Ehlenbach WJ, Hough CL, Crain PK, et al: Association between acute care and critical illness hospitalization and cognitive function in older adults. *JAMA* 2010;303:763–770.

Ely EW, Inouye SK, Bernard GR, et al: Delirium in mechanically ventilated patients. Validity and reliability of the confusion assessment method for the intensive care unit (CAM-ICU). *JAMA* 2001;286:2703–2710.

Ely EW, Shintani A, Truman B, et al: Delirium as a predictor of mortality in mechanically ventilated patients in the intensive care unit. *JAMA* 2004;291:1753–1762.

Food and Drug Administration. FDA public health advisory: deaths with antipsychotics in elderly patients with behavioral disturbances. www.fda.gov/cder/drug/advisory/antipsychotics.htm

Hipp DM, Ely EW. Pharmacological and nonpharmacological management of delirium in critically ill patients. *Neurotherapeutics* 2012;9:158–175.

Inouye SK, Bogardus ST, Charpentier PA, et al: A multicomponent intervention to prevent delirium in hospitalized older patients. *JAMA* 1999;340:669–676.

Koponen H, et al: EEG spectral analysis in delirium. *J Nerv Neurosurg Psychiatry* 1989;52:980.

Ross CA, et al: Delirium: phenomenologic and etiologic subtypes. *Int Psychogeriatr* 1991;3:135.

Trzepacz PT, Dew MA: Further analyses of the delirium rating scale. *Gen Hosp Psychiatry* 1995;17:75.

Wang PS, Schneeweiss S, Avorn J, et al: Risk of death in elderly users of conventional vs. atypical antipsychotic medications. *N Engl J Med* 2005;353:2335–2341.

Witlox J, Eurelings LSM, de Jonghe JFM, et al: Delirium in elderly patients and the risk of postdischarge mortality, institutionalization, and dementia. A meta-analysis. *JAMA* 2010;304:443–451.

NEUROCOGNITIVE DISORDERS (DEMENTIA)

GENERAL CONSIDERATIONS

Slow evolution of multiple cognitive deficits characterizes dementia or major neurocognitive disorder (DSM-5). These are a wide variety of subtypes, described by their presumed etiologies. These etiologies depend on the causative disorder, such as Parkinson disease, Huntington disease or traumatic brain injury. The neurodegenerative disorders, such as Alzheimer disease, frontotemporal lobar degeneration (FTD), or Lewy body disease (LBD), are diagnosed primarily by cognitive, behavioral, and physical symptoms.

Neurocognitive disorders are now used in DSM-5 to describe dementias and other disorders for which cognitive impairment is the core feature. In addition, they are divided into mild and major cognitive disorders. **Mild neurocognitive disorder** now encompasses the concept of **Mild Cognitive Impairment (MCI)**. MCI carries a greatly increased risk of dementia, but not all cases progress to dementia, even within 10 years. Those with pure memory impairment ("amnestic MCI") are most likely to progress to AD.

The concept of a precursor of dementia reflects the growing awareness that neurodegenerative illnesses begin a pathological process, long before the appearance of major symptoms and decline. These mild neurocognitive disorders have been addressed by improved diagnostic information. Biological markers for Alzheimer disease appear long before symptoms manifest themselves. These include position emission tomography of β-amyloid using several ligands, and cerebrospinal fluid (CSF) levels of amyloid and tau.

However, these markers are not specific, meaning that not all people with markers of amyloid in the brain will definitely develop dementia, nor have they been proved adequately sensitive. Earlier diagnosis is fraught with increased error. At present, without a disease-modifying treatment, early diagnosis is not critical. As treatment advances, however, earlier diagnosis will become more and more important.

▶ Evaluation

Clinical diagnosis is ultimately an attempt to deduce the neuropathologic basis of the patient's problem. Most dementias are associated with destruction or degeneration of brain structures. The autopsy shows whether the damage is the result of degenerative disease, vascular disease, infection, inflammation, tumors, hydrocephalus, or traumatic brain injury. Multiple causes for dementia are often apparent at an autopsy. Because the autopsy comes too late to help the patient or the family, the clinician must be knowledgeable about the pathology that is most likely to be associated with a given clinical presentation.

Clinical diagnosis is based on the patient's history and mental status and on laboratory examination. Several basic tests are recommended in the evaluation of dementia. These include complete blood count with differential, electrolytes, liver function tests, blood urea nitrogen, creatinine, protein, albumin, glucose, vitamin B_{12}, vitamin D, urinalysis, and thyroid function tests. A brain imaging study, either CT or magnetic resonance imaging (MRI), is virtually always required. CT generally gives less information than MRI, which can provide quantitative analysis of hippocampal atrophy. In a

significant minority of cases, imaging does not clarify the diagnosis, but nonetheless provides comfort to the family and the clinician that "no stone has been left unturned," no treatable condition has been overlooked. Imaging studies are recommended in some practice guidelines, including those of the American Academy of Neurology. Optional tests include sedimentation rate, blood gases, folate, human immunodeficiency virus (HIV) screen, syphilis serology, testosterone level, heavy metals screen, PET (positron emission tomography) or SPECT (single-photon emission computed tomography) scanning. PET scanning can include either FDG uptake, a measure of regional metabolism in the brain, or new amyloid-binding ligands such as Pittsburgh Compound B or florbetapir (Amyvid), which can confirm a diagnosis of AD by detecting excessive amyloid deposition in the brain. Although the FDA has approved this new imaging ligand, Medicare has denied payment, pending further research to prove its usefulness. Genetic testing (for apolipoprotein E) and CSF assays of amyloid, tau, and neural thread protein are available but not recommended for widespread use.

CT and MRI scans are especially important in excluding focal lesions or conditions such as hydrocephalus, subdural hematoma, silent strokes, or brain tumors. The physician must be careful not to overinterpret findings. EEG was previously used more commonly in the evaluation of dementia; however, EEG slowing is difficult to interpret. Intermittent slowing is not related to MRI change or to decline in neuropsychological function. Runs of intermittent slowing increase in frequency with advancing age, but such episodes are brief and infrequent. Focal slow waves sometimes occur in temporal and frontal areas without significance. When any of these changes become prominent, pathology is usually present. Older people in good health may have an average occipital frequency that is a full cycle slower than young adults; however, they do not show EEG dominant frequencies below 8 hertz.

Occasionally, a dementia evaluation leads to the diagnosis of a treatable illness and permits curative treatment, especially when the dementia has toxic or metabolic etiologies. More commonly the physician establishes a plausible explanation of the clinical findings and suggests palliative care. Because families come to physicians for a diagnosis and a prognosis, the physician's explanation should include statements about what is likely to happen to the patient. The family needs an interpretation of the observed behavior and suggestions about ways to deal with it. The physician gives the family some understanding of what is happening and helps them in planning for future decline in the patient's status. The psychiatrist often manages the troubling behavior that occurs in the latter phases of many dementing illnesses. The psychiatrist also recognizes the needs of the caregiver and makes suitable suggestions to help the caregiver manage the patient and deal with the heavy burden of care.

DEGENERATIVE NEUROCOGNITIVE DISORDERS

Alzheimer disease, frontotemporal dementias, and diffuse Lewy body disease are primary degenerative processes occurring within the CNS. These syndromes are progressive and lead inevitably to severe disability and death. Other degenerative dementias are associated with diseases that affect other neurological systems; these include Huntington disease, Parkinson disease, progressive supranuclear palsy, corticobasal degeneration, and multiple system atrophy.

NEUROCOGNITIVE DISORDER DUE TO ALZHEIMER DISEASE

▶ Essentials of Diagnosis

The most widely applied criteria for the clinical definition of Alzheimer disease are those of the National Institute of Neurological and Communicative Disorders and Stroke and those of the Alzheimer Disease and Related Disorders Association. New guidelines for the diagnosis of Alzheimer disease were published in 2011 (for the first time since 1984). The diagnosis of probable Alzheimer disease requires the presence of dementia established by clinical examination, documented by standardized mental status assessment, and confirmed by neuropsychological tests. These tests must demonstrate deficits in two or more areas of cognition, with progressive worsening of memory and other cognitive functions in the absence of delirium. The new diagnosis criteria require two areas of cognitive dysfunction, but one no longer has to be memory loss. The onset must be between ages 40 and 90 years, and there must be no other brain disease that could account for the clinical observations (this implies a work-up, including the blood studies and brain imaging tests discussed earlier). The disorder must also be progressive and associated with disability in routine activities. Supportive features include family history, specific progressive deficits in cognitive functions, and laboratory data such as PET or SPECT scans. PET scans should employ ligands that bind to amyloid, such as the Pittsburgh Compound and florbetapir (^{18}F).

▶ General Considerations

Alzheimer disease is the most common form of dementia, accounting for over half of all dementias. Oddly enough, just 25 years ago, many textbooks considered Alzheimer disease to be rare, likely because the disease was confined to "presenile" cases (EOAD), younger than age 65, although some can occur in the 40s.

This early onset group has different phenotypic features including increased genetic contribution, more behavioral features and often greater parietal atrophy, more white matter abnormalities and less hippocampal volume loss.

Although memory problems dominate the early stages of the disorder, Alzheimer disease affects cognition, mood, and behavior. Cognitive impairment affects daily life because patients are unable to perform normal activities of daily living. Behavioral manifestations of the disease such as temper outbursts, screaming, agitation, paranoid ideations, disinhibited behavior, and severe personality changes are more troubling than the cognitive difficulties. It is these symptoms that lead to admission of AD patients of nursing facilities. No two patients with Alzheimer disease are exactly alike when it comes to the behavioral manifestations of the disorder. Only recently has this aspect of the disease received substantial attention.

A. Epidemiology

Alzheimer disease is the most common type of progressive dementia. Memory loss affects one in eight Americans by age 65. Alzheimer disease reaches 20% prevalence in 80-year-olds, as much as 48% prevalence in one study of community-dwelling elderly people over age 85, and afflicts more than 5 million Americans. It is present in one third of autopsies of elderly patients and is projected to affect 8–14 million by the year 2030. The disease affects women more often than men. The economic impact of Alzheimer disease has been estimated at more than $100 billion annually.

B. Etiology

In general, Alzheimer disease represents an imbalance between neuronal injury and repair. Factors contributing to injury may include free radical formation, vascular insufficiency, inflammation, head trauma, hypoglycemia, and aggregated β-amyloid protein. Factors contributing to ineffective repair may include the presence of the apolipoprotein E (ApoE) E4 gene, altered synthesis of amyloid precursor protein, and hypothyroidism. Some researchers hypothesize that β-amyloid causes chronic inflammation. Alzheimer disease also involves formation of tau-containing neurofibrillary tangles; most researchers feel that the tau protein changes (see later discussion) are a secondary phenomenon in AD, though they may be primary in frontotemporal dementia and other diseases. Tau has also been implicated in the propagation of abnormal protein from one brain area to another. By this theory, once the disease has begun propagating from neuron to neuron, treatments may be too late to cause improvement. Ultimately, the deficit of key neurotransmitters from pathways from the basal forebrain to the cerebral cortex, especially acetylcholine, plays a major role in the cognitive symptoms.

Plaques and tangles identify the illness at the microscopic level. Amyloid plaques occur in vast numbers in severe cases. Amyloid plaques were first recognized in 1892. PAS or Congo Red stains identify these structures. β-Amyloid peptide, which is concentrated in senile plaques, has been linked to Alzheimer disease. The β-amyloid protein, in the form of pleated sheets, appears early in the brain and in blood vessels in Alzheimer disease. Some studies suggest that β-amyloid is toxic to mature neurons in the brains of Alzheimer patients. Neurons in these areas begin to develop neurofibrillary tangles. Amyloid plaques and neurofibrillary tangles gradually accumulate in the frontal, temporal, and parietal lobes. The density of plaques determines postmortem diagnosis. Amyloid binding can now be imaged in research PET studies, using the Pittsburgh compound, florbetapir, and other ligands. The number of neurons and synapses is reduced. This is particularly true of acetylcholine-cholinergic-containing neurons in the basal nucleus of Meynert, which project to wide areas of the cerebral cortex. PET studies demonstrate a reduction in acetylcholinesterase and decreased binding of cholinergic ligands. Hirano bodies and granulovacuolar degeneration occur in the hippocampus and represent further degeneration.

Neocortical neurofibrillary tangles are rare in normal individuals; however, neuropil threads and neurofibrillary tangles appear at the onset of dementia. These intracytoplasmic filaments displace the nucleus and the cellular organelles. Neurofibrillary tangles contain an abnormally phosphorylated tau protein. The abnormal phosphorylation of tau protein probably causes defective construction of microtubules and neurofilaments. The neurofibrillary tangles in brains affected by Alzheimer disease abnormally express Alz-50, a protein antigen commonly found in fetal brain neurons. Neural thread protein is present in the long axonal processes that emerge from the nerve cell body and is found in association with neurofibrillary tangles. This protein may be involved in neural repair and regeneration.

Neurons bearing neurofibrillary tangles often project to brain regions that are rich in senile plaques containing β-amyloid. These plaques are found in areas innervated by cholinergic neurons. Cholinergic neurons in the hippocampus and the basal nucleus of Meynert degenerate early in Alzheimer disease, causing impairment of cortical and hippocampal neurotransmission and cognitive difficulty. The affected cortical areas become anatomically disconnected. One of the earliest areas to be disconnected is the hippocampus, which explains why memory disorder is one of the early manifestations of Alzheimer disease. As time goes on, there is a loss of communication between other cortical zones and subsequent loss of higher cognitive abilities.

These basal forebrain cholinergic projections not only mediate cognitive function but also mediate brain responses to emotionally relevant stimuli. In the late stages of Alzheimer disease, a wide range of behavioral changes occur, including psychosis, agitation, depression, anxiety, sleep disturbance, appetite change, and altered sexual behavior. These changes are mediated by cholinergic degeneration and by degeneration in other neural systems. Serotonergic neurons and noradrenergic neurons degenerate as the disease progresses.

Degeneration of these systems also contributes to some of the later cognitive and behavioral manifestations of the disorder. Because dopaminergic neurons are relatively immune to degeneration in Alzheimer disease, the performance of well-learned motor behaviors is preserved well into the late stages of the disease.

C. Genetics

Alzheimer disease has demonstrated genetic diversity. Chromosome 21 has been implicated for many years because it is well known that patients with Down syndrome are almost guaranteed to develop the histological features of Alzheimer disease if they live past age 40. Genetic mutations usually cause familial, autosomal dominantly transmitted, early-onset Alzheimer disease. Several mutations of the amyloid precursor protein gene on chromosome 21 have been described. These mutations increase the production of an abnormal amyloid that has been associated with neurotoxicity. Another form of early-onset disease has been localized to a variety of defects on chromosome 14. These mutations are associated with presenilin 1 and account for the majority of familial Alzheimer cases. A mutation on chromosome 1 is associated with presenilin 2. Both of these mutations also cause increased production of amyloid, in that the presenilins are now known to be secretase enzymes involved in the formation of β-amyloid peptide, a 40- to 42-amino-acid peptide, from the amyloid precursor protein.

The ApoE E4 allele is associated with the risk of late-onset familial and sporadic forms of Alzheimer disease. ApoE, a plasma protein involved in the transport of cholesterol, is encoded by a gene on chromosome 19. Disease risk increases in proportion to the number of ApoE E4 alleles. The population that is positive for ApoE E4 has a lower age at onset. The ApoE E2 allele may offer some protection. Although patients with the ApoE E4 allele may be more likely to have Alzheimer disease, a full diagnostic evaluation including imaging, laboratory tests, and neuropsychological evaluation is still indicated when the clinical situation warrants. It is premature to regard ApoE testing as a screening tool for Alzheimer disease, and it is not recommended for presymptomatic screening in family members of patients with AD. Another gene, SORL1, has recently been described as a marker for sporadic AD, as have other gene loci, and recently a gene protecting individuals against AD has been discovered. Genetic studies of AD have shown overlap with other neurodegenerative disorders.

▶ Clinical Findings

A. Signs and Symptoms

A subjective sense of memory loss usually appears first, followed by loss of memory detail and temporal relationships. All areas of memory function deteriorate including encoding, retrieval, and consolidation. Patients forget landmarks in their lives less often than other events. Amnesia for names and specific nouns is the earliest language abnormality in AD, and a mild anomic aphasia is often found in patients with early AD. Agnosia (failure to recognize or identify objects), more severe aphasia (language disturbance), apraxia, and visuospatial-topographical impairments such as getting lost while walking or driving occur later in the disease.

In the early stages of Alzheimer disease, a subjective memory deficit is difficult to distinguish from benign forgetfulness. Considerable research has examined patients with impaired memory but otherwise normal cognitive function, a disorder called "mild cognitive impairment." These patients are more likely to develop AD over time than are age-matched controls. Deficits in memory, language, concept formation, and visual spatial praxis evolve slowly. Later, patients with Alzheimer disease become passive, coarse, and less spontaneous. Many become depressed, and depression may worsen the patient's cognitive function. Depressed Alzheimer patients often exhibit degeneration of the locus coeruleus or substantia nigra.

More than half of patients with mild Alzheimer disease present with at least one psychiatric symptom, and one third present with two or more symptoms. After the initial stage of the disease, patients enter a stage of global cognitive deterioration. Denial or loss of self-awareness replaces anxiety, and cognitive deficits are noticeable to family and friends. In the final stages, patients become aimless, abulic (unable to make decisions), aphasic, and restless. At this stage, abnormal frontal lobe release signs, such as the snout, palmomental, and grasp reflexes, are common.

B. Psychological Testing

The clinical assessment and staging of Alzheimer disease have always been difficult. The MMSE is often used but sometimes seriously underestimates cognitive impairment. The Standardized MMSE has better reliability than the MMSE. The Blessed Dementia Scale uses collateral sources and correlates well with postmortem pathology. The inter-rater reliability of the Blessed Dementia Scale is low.

The Extended Scale for Dementia is a rating scale designed to distinguish the intellectual function of dementia patients from normal seniors. The Neurobehavioral Cognitive Status Examination (NCSE) is a tool that assesses a patient's cognitive abilities in a short amount of time. This instrument uses independent tests to estimate functioning within five major cognitive ability areas: language, constructions, memory, calculations, and reasoning. The Mattis Dementia Rating Scale (DRS) is useful in staging dementia. Both the NCSE and the DRS are sensitive, but they are more time consuming than the MMSE. In most clinical practices, the MMSE is used for assessment of dementia and for following the patient's progress, and common recommendations for drug therapy are based on the MMSE score. The Montreal Cognitive Assessment scale is another instrument helpful for cognitive and executive functions.

Comprehensive scales combine clinical judgment, objective data, and specific rating criteria. The Reisberg Brief Cognitive Rating Scale and the Global Deterioration Scale are brief comprehensive scales. The Clinical Dementia Rating Scale (CDR) is a more extensive instrument that includes subject interview, collateral interview, brief neuropsychological assessment, and interview impression. Patients with a CDR score of 0.5 are likely to have "very mild" Alzheimer disease. The CDR has a complicated scoring algorithm and is best reserved for research.

The Alzheimer disease assessment: Cognitive (ADAS COG) and the Behavioral Pathology in Alzheimer's disease (Behave-AD) instruments are used in clinical drug trials to determine pharmacologic efficacy in cognitive areas or behavioral areas, respectively.

The Consortium to Establish a Registry for Alzheimer's disease Criteria (CERAD) examination includes general physical and neurologic examinations as well as laboratory tests. Specified neuropsychological tests and a depression scale are also administered.

C. Laboratory Findings and Imaging

Although CT scans reveal atrophy in Alzheimer patients as a group, atrophy alone does not reliably predict Alzheimer disease in individual patients. Atrophy can be quantified using appropriate ratios and progresses on serial evaluation, but this information adds little to the patient's clinical care.

MRI region-of-interest techniques reveal reduced brain volume, especially in the hippocampal area, and higher CSF volume in patients with Alzheimer disease. Alzheimer disease may be associated with enlarged CSF spaces or atypical signal intensity in the medial temporal lobes. These findings imply that advancing Alzheimer disease is associated with increased brain water, where either the atrophy leads to an increase in CSF spaces, or there are associated ischemic changes in the deep cerebral white matter. Finally, volumetric studies may show hippocampal sclerosis in the brains of Alzheimer patients. Hippocampal atrophy may be relatively specific to Alzheimer disease and may be useful for early detection and differential diagnosis. Quantitative MRIs may help in the evaluation of hippocampal volume.

^{31}P–Nuclear magnetic resonance (NMR) spectroscopy profiles may be helpful in the evaluation of Alzheimer disease. ^{31}P-NMR profiles of Alzheimer disease patients show elevated ratios of phosphomonoesterase to phosphodiesters in the temporoparietal region.

In the early stage of dementia, functional brain imaging (i.e., PET and SPECT scans) is more sensitive than structural brain imaging (i.e., MRI and CT scan). PET scans reveal changes in temporoparietal metabolism that differentiate patients with Alzheimer disease from the normal elderly. PET scans reveal the following abnormalities in Alzheimer disease: (1) reductions in whole-brain metabolism (paralleling dementia severity), (2) hypometabolism in the association cortex exceeding that in the primary sensorimotor cortex, and (3) metabolic asymmetry in suitable cortical areas accompanying neuropsychological deficits. In Alzheimer disease, the visible metabolic deficits start in the parietal cortex. Frontal metabolism decreases as dementia progresses. Alzheimer disease spares the primary motor cortex, sensory cortices (except for the olfactory cortex), and basal ganglia. AD is not a "generalized" brain disease, but a neurodegeneration of specific brain structures and regions. Newer ligands used in PET imaging, including those binding to amyloid and those binding to tau, have also been helpful in diagnosis and especially in clinical trials of antiamyloid antibodies, but these are not typically paid for by Medicare or commercial insurance.

SPECT scans can reveal information about regional brain function at a much lower cost and degree of complexity than PET scans, but the spatial resolution is not as good. In more advanced Alzheimer disease cases, SPECT scans reveal decreased perfusion in the bilateral temporoparietal regions.

EEG abnormalities are not common early in Alzheimer disease, but they develop as the disease progresses. Diffuse slow-wave abnormalities occur first in the left temporal regions and become more frequent and longer as the disease progresses. EEG abnormalities that occur early in dementia suggest a coexisting delirium. Because dementia often presents first in association with delirium, infectious, toxic, or metabolic disturbances should be considered if the EEG slowing is severe.

Evoked potentials are an EEG technology that average many signals following a specific stimulus. In Alzheimer disease, the auditory P300 amplitude in the posterior parietal regions is suppressed on evoked potential maps. Other studies have not demonstrated clinically useful abnormalities of the P300 component in dementia. Compared to control subjects, Alzheimer disease patients show longer P100 latencies of pattern-reversal visual evoked potentials. The flash P100 distinguishes them only marginally. The long-latency auditory evoked potential helps differentiate between cortical and subcortical dementias. Patients with subcortical dementias exhibit prolonged latencies.

MILD NEUROCOGNITIVE DISORDER DUE TO ALZHEIMER DISEASE

In this disorder, there is definite impairment of recent memory, without gross deficits in other cognitive functions. The patient can usually still function at this stage. If another area of neuropsychological deterioration is present, such as deficits in executive function, visual-spatial function, or language, then other diagnoses are possible. Probable Alzheimer disease is diagnosed if there is evidence of a causative Alzheimer genetic mutation from either genetic testing or family history. Possible Alzheimer disease is diagnosed if there is no genetic mutation or family history factor

present, and there is evidence of (1) decline in memory and learning and (2) progressive gradual cognitive decline without plateaus, and if (3) no evidence exists of a mixed etiology (e.g., cerebrovascular or traumatic disease), or any other neurodegenerative disease.

▶ Differential Diagnosis (Including Comorbid Conditions)

Clinicians have traditionally used a battery of laboratory tests to differentiate Alzheimer disease from a variety of medical conditions that cause memory impairment. These tests include complete blood count, comprehensive metabolic panel, thyroid function tests, and vitamin B$_{12}$. In appropriate cases, the erythrocyte sedimentation rate, serological tests for syphilis, and even a lumbar puncture may be indicated. In many cases, a careful history and bedside mental status examination can reliably diagnose presumed Alzheimer disease and distinguish it from other forms of dementia. A detailed drug history is necessary because drugs, especially those with anticholinergic properties, can cause Alzheimer-like symptomatology. Other drugs implicated in causing memory deficits include anticholinergics, the antiepileptic drug topiramate, narcotic analgesics, and anxiolytics and hypnotics including benzodiazepines and zolpidem. Chemotherapeutic agents used to treat cancer also induce what patients refer to as "brain fog." A normal neurologic examination is entirely consistent with Alzheimer disease. Neurologic abnormalities are much more common in other dementing illnesses. The relationship between Alzheimer disease and depression is complex and is discussed later in this chapter.

The distinction between mild neurocognitive disorder and normal age-related memory loss may be difficult, especially if compounded by the patient's apprehension and anxiety. Nevertheless, a substantial portion of elderly without dementia have significant memory loss. It appears that 16–20% of elderly over age 70 have mild cognitive impairment (MCI), now synonymous with mild neurocognitive disorder. This group is at high risk to be diagnosed with Alzheimer disease, with more than half converting within 5 years. Patients with predominantly memory symptoms appear most at risk for this conversion.

Forgetfulness is a normal aspect of aging, usually first noted in the 50s. Episodic (memory for events), short-term memory, and associative memory (links between information) are particularly impaired in normal aging. Affording these individuals more time to respond will improve their performance. Many seniors will benefit from reassurance and assistance with improving their memory.

When Alzheimer disease is diagnosed, it should be through a careful diagnostic process and attention to clinical detail. The effect of diagnosis should be carefully assessed in the patient as well as family members, especially family members with common genetic ties.

▶ Treatment

The aim of pharmacotherapy in Alzheimer disease is as follows: (1) to prevent the disease in asymptomatic individuals, (2) to alter the natural course of the disease in those already diagnosed, and (3) to enhance patients' cognition and memory. As yet, no treatment has been shown to be effective in preventing the disease, though general health measures such as physical exercise; healthy diet; treatment of risk factors of heart disease and stroke, such as hypertension, diabetes, hyperlipidemia, and obstructive sleep apnea; and avoidance of tobacco and excessive alcohol are all suggested to delay or prevent the disease. These measures may slow deterioration in patients already diagnosed with AD. Mental exercise has also been touted, but the evidence for many of the commercial memory aids is lacking. Treatment to enhance memory in Alzheimer patients has focused on improving cholinergic activity. Cholinergic enhancement can occur through the administration of acetylcholine precursors, cholinesterase inhibitors, and combinations of AChE with precursors, muscarinic agonists, nicotinic agonists, or drugs facilitating AChE release. To date, only cholinesterase inhibitors and memantine (Namenda), a glutamatergic agent, have proved effective in clinical trials.

Historical attempts to treat dementia with ergoloid mesylates were of negligible benefit. In some early studies, ergoloid mesylates were more effective than placebo, but this was not confirmed in the few well-designed clinical trials.

Attempts to enhance acetylcholine transmission with precursors such as lecithin and choline failed to show benefit in Alzheimer disease. Cholinomimetic substances such as arecoline were more successful but have had limited use because of adverse side effects, short half-life, and narrow dose range. Physostigmine, an acetylcholinesterase inhibitor, has limited benefit because of its short half-life and significant side effects.

The first acetylcholinesterase inhibitor approved for use for in mild to moderate Alzheimer disease was tetrahydroaminoacridine (Tacrine). Tacrine frequently causes adverse side effects, particularly gastrointestinal hyperactivity. Elevation of liver transaminase is another significant side effect. Of the patients who take tacrine, 25% will experience elevations (up to three times the normal) in alanine aminotransferase levels. For these reasons, the use of tacrine has been abandoned.

Second-generation cholinesterase inhibitors such as donepezil are more specific for CNS acetylcholinesterase than for peripheral acetylcholinesterase. Donepezil has the advantage of daily dosing and does not cause significant hepatotoxicity. Donepezil has an orally dissolving tablet form and has been approved for mild, moderate, and severe AD. Dose increases to 23 mg have proven effective. Rivastigmine is another cholinesterase inhibitor that has a relative specificity for both acetylcholinesterase and butyrylcholinesterase, an effect shared only with tacrine. There is evidence that butyrylcholinesterase is present at high concentrations in the brains of patients with Alzheimer disease, but the relevance of this factor to its clinical effect is unknown. The drug has more gastrointestinal side effects than donepezil. It is given twice daily at doses of 1.5, 3, 4.5, and finally 6 mg, with dose advances made every 4 weeks.

This agent is also available in patches of 4.6-, 9.5-, and 13.5-mg strengths. The patch significantly reduces gastrointestinal effects.

A last cholinesterase agent, galantamine, has similar effects on the acetylcholinesterase enzyme, but may also increase presynaptic release of acetylcholine. This agent is available in both twice-daily and extended-release preparations. The daily doses are 8, 16, and 24 mg. The gastrointestinal side effects of this agent are intermediate between those of donepezil and rivastigmine, but individual patients may tolerate one better than another. It is available in a 16- and 24-mg extended release formulation.

Muscarinic M1 receptors are relatively intact in AD, despite the degeneration of presynaptic cholinergic innervation. Several muscarinic agonists have been studied in clinical trials, but none has been approved. Finally, stimulation of nicotinic receptors may have a protective effect in AD. Studies of nicotine patches have indicated potential in mild cognitive impairment.

Memantine, an antagonist at the NMDA receptor has also been approved for AD. The exact mechanism of action of this drug is not known; the NMDA effect could represent a neuroprotective effect on "excitotoxicity" of glutamate on surviving neurons, but this drug appears to have other beneficial effects on learning and memory. It has been approved for moderate to advanced AD, that is, patients with MMSE <20.

A "medical food" approved for AD is Axona, a containing medium-chain fatty acids, which can cross the blood-brain barrier and possibly enhance brain energy metabolism. Many patients experience diarrhea with this agent.

Treatment of behavioral complications of AD is problematic. Depression should always be treated, usually with an SSRI agent. Anxiety can be helped with trazodone at bedtime, but benzodiazepines tend to worsen the memory loss, increase the risk of falls, and may cause paradoxical agitation. Valproic acid has been found helpful in some but not all studies. Cholinergic agents and memantine appear to ameliorate behavioral disturbances in patients with AD. The same therapeutic considerations discussed under delirium are relevant in the treatment of psychosis in AD. Atypical antipsychotic agents are not greatly effective and have a black box warning due to elevated mortality in dementia. Low doses of olanzapine, risperidone, aripiprazole, or quetiapine may be used with increases in dosage or shifting to another agent if symptoms persist. In the CATIE trial, the benefit of those taking active drug compared to placebo was small. Patients and families must be warned of the serious potential risks of these agents, and treatment should be limited as much as possible, with reassessment and monitoring of adverse effects.

Therapeutic strategies intended to slow the progression of Alzheimer disease have not been very successful. Early studies suggested that the incidence of Alzheimer disease was reduced in postmenopausal women taking estrogen, but the Women's Health Initiative studies found the opposite: postmenopausal estrogen and progesterone hormone replacement therapy appears associated with a higher incidence of cognitive deficits and dementia. Use of nonsteroidal anti-inflammatory drugs has been inversely associated with incidence of dementia in population studies, but a therapeutic use of these agents in AD has not been proved. The Cox II inhibitor rofecoxib (Vioxx) was taken off the market because of increased cardiovascular events, and one of the two studies with this finding involved patients with AD. Antioxidants such as vitamin E and selegiline have shown a beneficial effect in some studies, but other studies have failed to establish any role for these agents. In particular, a study of mild cognitive impairment showed a very limited benefit for donepezil, and none whatsoever for vitamin E. Nicotine has been effective in one study of amnestic MCI. Attempts to treat Alzheimer disease with nerve growth factor have been limited by the inability of the substance to cross the blood-brain barrier.

The primary goal in most recent efforts to provide disease modifying treatments for AD has been monoclonal antibodies for amyloid beta. Aducanumab was given accelerated approval in 2021 in a controversial decision by the FDA, due to statistical and design issues with the drug. The evidence favored reduction in amyloid plaque on PET imaging, but there was no convincing clinical benefit. A more positive case was made for lecanemab, approved in 2023. Lecanemab also binds to amyloid protofibrils and produced 27% improvement over placebo after 18 months of treatment, in the form of reduced decline in cognitive tests. Both these agents required regular infusions and high cost. Amyloid imaging abnormalities were noted with both, as well as fatalities with lecanemab. Almost all patients were either mild cognitive impairment or mild dementia with evidence of amyloid beta imaging or CSF testing.

While the amyloid hypothesis is our most accepted at this time, there are some discrepancies, including dementia patients with high amyloid and no clinical disease. This is an area of ongoing intensive investigation. How long the monoclonal antibodies should be used and at what stage of the illness remains to be clarified. While cognitive improvement was noted in some patients, the more prominent effect was rather a slower decline than with placebo. Center for Medicare Services will play a role in determining how much of the high cost of these treatments will be borne by insurance.

Other approaches include electrical or transcranial magnetic stimulation of the brain, deep brain stimulation, stem cell transplant therapies, and other pharmacological agents. All of these studies are in an early stage.

Other non-drug formulations used by AD patients include coconut oil, curcumin, and *Ginkgo biloba*. None of these agents has been proved beneficial, and in the case of *Ginkgo*

biloba, a definitive clinical trial was negative. One responsibility of the physician treating AD patients is to advise against use of these agents, some of which can be harmful, despite the desperation of patients and families to find anything that might help.

Multiple studies have shown that addressing lifestyle factors can significantly delay the onset and slow the course of AD. These include physical activity and exercise, healthy diet, cognitive stimulation and social engagement. Cessation of smoking, reduction of alcohol intake and control of hypertension have also been significant.

▶ Prognosis

An early-onset form of Alzheimer disease occurs in some people in their 40s, 50s, or 60s. A prolonged, indolent, subtle deterioration in mental function characterizes the clinical course of illness. From the time of clinical diagnosis the course is variable, but survival is possible up to 20 years from clinical recognition. Early-onset cases tend to progress more rapidly. Ultimately, functional performance declines. The patient's ability to drive becomes impaired, and he or she becomes unable to manage personal finances or to produce a complete meal. In general, studies suggest that patients with MMSE below 20 are probably not safe drivers. Later, impairment of language and inability to recognize familiar people lead to agitation, restlessness, and wandering. Hallucinations and other disruptive behaviors may make management difficult. In the final stages of the disease, the patient is generally mute and completely devoid of comprehension. Death most often results from a comorbid illness such as pneumonia.

▶ LATE and PART, new neuropathogical findings underlying dementia in the elderly

Recently, two pathologies of late life dementia resembling Alzheimer disease have been identified. These are LATE (Limbic-predominant age-related TDP-43 encephalopathy and PART (Primary age-related tauopathy), LATE is a fairly common pathology in very elderly patients with dementia. Pathologically, it is often associated with hippocampal sclerosis. It has a very different pathology from the typical Alzheimer disease, but it can be admixed with changes of AD. PART is also a neuropathological description of neurofibrillary tangles but no amyloid plaques in elderly patients. It presents with memory loss, usually mild to moderate, and also executive function deficits. It may be more and more common with advancing age.

American College of Medical Genetics/American Society of Human Genetics Working Group on ApoE and Alzheimer Disease Consensus Statement. Statement on use of apolipoprotein testing for Alzheimer disease. *JAMA* 1995;20:1627.

Chartier-Harlin MC, et al: Early onset Alzheimer's disease by mutation at codon 17 of the beta-amyloid precursor protein gene. *Nature* 1991;353:844.

Cummings JL: Alzheimer's disease. *N Engl J Med* 2004;351:56–67.

Cummings JL, Kaufer D: Neuropsychiatric aspects of Alzheimer's disease: the cholinergic hypothesis revisited. *Neurology* 1996;47:876.

Cummings JL, Schneider E, Tariot PN, et al: Behavioral effects of memantine in Alzheimer disease patients receiving donepezil treatment. *Neurology* 2006;67:57–63.

Farlow MR, Evans RM: Pharmacologic treatment of cognition and Alzheimer's dementia. *Neurology* 1998;51(Suppl 1):S36.

Holmes C, Wilkinson D, Dean C, et al: The efficacy of donepezil in the treatment of neuropsychiatric symptoms in Alzheimer's disease. *Neurology* 2004;63:214–219.

Kirshner HS: Mild cognitive impairment: to treat or not to treat. *Curr Neurol Neurosug Rep* 2005;5:455–457.

Klunk WE, Engler H, Norberg A, et al: Imaging brain amyloid in Alzheimer's disease with Pittsburgh Compound-B. *Ann Neurol* 2004;55:306–319.

Knopman DS, DeKosky ST, Cummings JL, et al: Practice parameter: diagnosis of dementia (an evidence-based review). *Neurology* 2001;56:1143–1153.

McKhann GM, Knopman DS, Chertkow H, et al: The diagnosis of dementia due to Alzheimer's disease: recommendations from the National Institute of Aging-Alzheimer's Association workgroups on diagnostic guidelines for Alzheimer's disease. *Alzheimer's Dement* 2011;7:236–239.

Nelson PT, Dickson DW, Trojanowski JQ, et al: Limbic-predominant age-related TDP-43 encephalopathy (LATE): Consensus working group report. *Brain* 2019;142:1503–1527.

Petersen RC, Stevens JC, Ganguli M, et al: Practice parameter: early detection of dementia: mild cognitive impairment (an evidence-based review). *Neurology* 2001;56:1133–1142.

Rogaeva E, Meng Y, Lee JH, et al: The neuronal sortilin-related receptor SORL1 is genetically associated with Alzheimer disease. *Nat Genet* 2007;39:168–177.

Roses AD: Apolipoprotein E affects the rate of Alzheimer disease expression: β-amyloid burden is a secondary consequence dependent on APO E genotype and duration of disease. *J Neuropathol Exp Neurol* 1994;53:429.

Schneider LS, Olin JT: Overview of clinical trials of hydergine in dementia. *Arch Neurol* 1994;51:787.

Schneider LS, Tariot PN, Dagerman KS, et al: Effectiveness of atypical antipsychotic drugs in patients with Alzheimer's disease. *N Engl J Med* 2006;355:1528–1538.

Sink KM, Holden KF, Yaffe K: Pharmacological treatment of neuropsychiatric symptoms of dementia. A review of the evidence. *JAMA* 2005;293:596–608.

Small GW, Leiter F: Neuroimaging for diagnosis of dementia. *J Clin Psychiatry* 1998;59(Suppl 11):4.

Small GW, et al: Diagnosis and treatment of Alzheimer disease and related disorders. Consensus statement of the American Association for Geriatric Psychiatry, the Alzheimer's Association, and the American Geriatrics Society. *JAMA* 1997;278:1363.

Snitz BE, O'Meara ES, Carlson MC: Ginkgo Biloba for preventing cognitive decline in older adults. A randomized trial. *JAMA* 2009; 302:2663–2670.

Teylan M, Besser LM, Crary JF, et al: Clinical diagnoses among individuals with primary age-related tauopathy versus Alzheimer's neuropathology. *Lab Invest* 2019;99:1049–1055.

Van Dyck, CH, Swanson, CJ, Aisen, P, Bateman, RJ, et al: Lecanemab in early Alzheimer's disease. *N Engl J Med* 2023;288:9–21

Wang PS, Schneeweiss S, Avorn J, et al: Risk of death in elderly users of conventional vs. atypical antipsychotic medications. *N Engl J Med* 2005;353:2335–2341.

Winblad B, Kilander L, Eriksson S, et al: Donepezil in patients with severe Alzheimer disease: double-blind, parallel-group, placebo-controlled study. *Lancet* 2006;367:1057–1065.

Wolfe MS: Shutting down Alzheimer's. *Sci Am* May 2006;73–79.

Yankner BA, et al: Neurotoxicity of a fragment of the amyloid precursor associated with Alzheimer's disease. *Science* 1989; 245:417.

FRONTOTEMPORAL NEUROCOGNITIVE DISORDER (FRONTOTEMPORAL DEMENTIA)

► Essentials of Diagnosis

Frontotemporal dementias represent a cluster of related disorders associated with degeneration of the frontal and temporal lobes. These disorders differ from Alzheimer disease primarily in the presentation with focal symptoms such as frontal lobe dysfunction or aphasia, rather than memory loss. In the behavioral variants of this disorder, personality changes usually precede or overshadow the patient's cognitive problems. Many patients become apathetic and stop caring about hygiene or social involvement. Others become disinhibited or impulsive. Sexual inappropriateness is common. Executive functions such as planning and judgment may also be abnormal in some patients. Alternatively, patients may tend to exhibit anger, irritability, and even mania. In rare cases, the Klüver-Bucy syndrome may develop with hyperorality, hypersexuality, and a compulsion to attend to any visual stimulus; this syndrome is associated with bilateral temporal lobe pathology. These patients also have impaired visual object recognition. Other frontotemporal dementia patients present with progressive aphasia. In the United States, these patients have been referred to under the diagnosis "primary progressive aphasia." The term "frontotemporal dementia" is now considered a more general category, of which primary progressive aphasia is a major subtype, the other common one is "frontal" or "behavioral variant" FTD.

The variety of presentations is the result of the segmental nature of the pathology. Some areas of the frontal lobe may be devastated, whereas adjacent areas may be entirely normal. Therefore, any behavioral syndrome compatible with damage to a specific frontal region is possible.

GENERAL CONSIDERATIONS

Frontotemporal dementias represent about 10% of degenerative dementia, but onset before the age of 60 is virtually equal in incidence to AD. About 40% of patients with these disorders have a family history of dementia, which suggests dominantly inherited illness. Other risk factors include electroconvulsive therapy (ECT) and alcoholism. Pick disease is historically the most recognized frontal lobe dementia and is often familial. Currently, Pick disease is diagnosed only on the basis of characteristic silver-staining aggregations of tau protein at autopsy.

▶ Clinical Findings

A. Signs and Symptoms

Frontotemporal neurocognitive disorders (frontotemporal dementia) are pathologically heterogeneous conditions. Some patients with this type of presentation have Alzheimer pathology, and those represent primarily patients who present with fluent aphasia.

Pathological findings in frontotemporal neurocognitive disorders (dementias) include neurofibrillary lesions made of hyperphosphorylated tau proteins (tauopathies). Mutations of the tau gene in frontotemporal dementia has been linked to chromosome 17 (FT DP-17). Most common forms of sporadic frontotemporal dementia are associated with loss of tau protein expression. Transactive response (TAR) DNA–protein of 43 kDa (TDP-43) has also been observed in frontotemporal cases with ubiquitin inclusions. This is also present in amyotrophic lateral sclerosis and Alzheimer disease.

Research continues to delineate and characterize frontotemporal disorders and their variants. In addition to Alzheimer disease, frontotemporal dementia may overlap with progressive supranuclear palsy, corticobasal degeneration, Parkinson disease, and motor neuron disease.

Most FTD cases have a lobar atrophy pattern involving one or both frontal and temporal lobes. The microscopic pathology is variable. Some have intraneuronal, intracytoplasmic, silver-staining inclusions called Pick bodies; these cases are traditionally diagnosed as Pick disease. In some patients, neuropathologic evaluation shows no specific histopathologic changes, other than neuronal loss, microvacuolation of the neuropil, and gliosis. Many of these patients have abnormal tau proteins within neurofibrillary tangles. These disorders are often familial, and several gene mutations on the tau gene on chromosome 17 have been described. Some families have been described with features of progressive aphasia, frontotemporal dementia, and Parkinsonism. Other cases are tau-negative, but ubiquitin-positive. In other patients, frontal lobe dementia occurs simultaneously with lower motor neuron disease as in amyotrophic lateral sclerosis. The genetic and molecular biological characterization of these variants of frontotemporal dementia is an active field of research at present.

The primary progressive aphasia variant is now divided into three subtypes. The first, progressive nonfluent aphasia, is usually associated with the tau mutation. The second, semantic dementia, characterized by loss of single word comprehension, is most often related to an ubiquitinopathy. The third, logopenic primary progressive aphasia, in which naming and repetition suffer but simple fluency and comprehension are not compromised early on, is most often related to underlying Alzheimer disease.

Core features of frontal lobe dementias, especially the behavioral variant of FTD, include insidious onset and gradual progression. There is early decline in social interpersonal conduct. Emotional blunting and apathy also occurs early without insight. There is a marked decline in personal hygiene and significant distractibility and motor impersistence (failure to maintain a motor activity).

Personality change, lack of insight, and poor judgment dominate the early stages of frontal lobe dementias. Frontal lobe dementias cause patients to be apathetic when medial frontal damage occurs and disinhibited when basal-frontal dysfunction predominates. Social withdrawal and behavioral disinhibition may precede the onset of dementia by several years. Sometimes memory is impaired, but attention, language, and visuospatial skills are spared.

In patients whose frontal lobe dementia primarily affects frontal language, loss of spontaneity of speech is often the first noticeable symptom. Selective language defects may occur in the absence of significant cognitive decline. In these patients, the clinical picture resembles a progressive aphasia.

Most patients with frontal lobe dementias lack drive and motivation. Others are tactless or insensitive in the early stages of the illness. Some patients develop symptoms of Klüver-Bucy syndrome with hypersexuality and hyperorality, going on later to exhibit perseverative speech, apathy, or stereotyped behavior. The memory disorder of frontal lobe dementias is more prominent concerning recently acquired material. Remote memory remains intact until later in the disease. Behavioral symptoms are usually more prominent in frontal lobe dementias, whereas parietal lobe symptoms such as receptive aphasia and agnosia are less common.

B. Psychological Testing

On psychological testing, patients exhibit features consistent with frontal lobe dysfunction. Useful tests include the Wisconsin Card Sorting Test, the Stroop Test, the FAS test (in which the subject is asked to list words beginning with the letters F, A, and S and the response is timed), the Trail Making Test, and other tests designed to ferret out frontal lobe dysfunction. Some measures of aphasia should also be included in the neuropsychological test battery.

C. Laboratory Findings and Imaging

In classic cases of Pick disease or FTD, the patient's brain exhibits marked atrophy of the frontal and temporal lobes, resulting in a knifelike appearance of the gyri. MRI may show a dramatic frontal pole or temporal pole atrophy that clearly differentiates Pick and other frontal lobe dementias from the pattern of temporoparietal atrophy seen in Alzheimer patients.

In frontal lobe dementias, the EEG may remain normal despite severe pathology. PET and SPECT imaging also show the focal, lobar nature of the degeneration.

PET scans in patients with FTD disease show bilateral frontal hypometabolism without temporoparietal defects. These findings are not always observed in early disease. In some patients the findings may be unilateral. In cases with progressive aphasia, left frontal and temporal hypometabolism or hypoperfusion are evident.

At a microscopic level, cell loss is particularly marked in the outer layers of the cortex. Degenerating neurons may have Pick bodies. The structural changes of Alzheimer disease, including amyloid plaques and tangles, are entirely lacking. Frontal lobe dementias are not associated with Lewy bodies; however, areas of spongiform degeneration, similar to those found in Creutzfeldt-Jakob disease, may be observed. The pathology is patchy: Some frontal lobe areas remain normal. From a histopathologic point of view, frontal lobe dementia (Pick disease) is characterized by gliosis, microvacuolation, neuronal atrophy loss, and 40–50% loss of synapses in three superficial cortical laminae of the frontal convexity and anterior temporal cortex. The deeper laminae are little changed.

Differential Diagnosis

Other conditions can present with frontal lobe behaviors and dementia, for example, vascular dementias, normal pressure hydrocephalus, Huntington disease, and mass lesions. Butterfly gliomas are particularly likely to present with pure frontal lobe behaviors and dementia. Frontal lobe dementias can also be confused with personality disorder, mania, and depression. This is particularly true early in the course of the illness when the cognitive involvement is minimal.

Treatment

Treatment of frontal lobe dementias is limited to psychosocial interventions, such as protecting the patient from his or her indiscretions, and symptomatic psychiatric treatment. At times an associated depression occurs. Treatment of this depression as well as other behavioral symptoms with SSRIs can be helpful. Psychostimulants, such as methylphenidate, may help motivate apathetic patients, but they may aggravate the disturbed behavior. Carbamazepine may be helpful for Klüver-Bucy syndrome by reducing the frequency of behaviors. Olanzapine or other antipsychotics may be helpful when extreme disinhibition occurs. In patients with memory disorder, donepezil may be helpful, but no treatment trials have confirmed a benefit of either anticholinesterase medications or memantine in frontotemporal dementias, and it is not clear that degeneration of the cholinergic system is prominent in this condition. Occasional patients seem to develop increased behavioral disturbance with cholinesterase inhibitors. Memantine has been thought helpful in FTD, mostly on anecdotal evidence, but a recent multicenter trial did not demonstrate any significant benefit. Other, new therapeutic agents for FTD are currently in clinical trials, but none is available as yet.

Prognosis

Frontotemporal dementias often have primarily a presenile onset. Progression is quite variable but, generally speaking, slow. Memory functions may be retained until later in the illness. Patients with frontal lobe dementias can later develop motor neuron disease, although the clinical features of motor neuron disease may accompany or occasionally precede the onset of dementia.

Boxer AL, Knopman DS, Kaufer DI, et al: Memantine inpatients with frontotemporal lobar degeneration: a multicenter, randomized, double-blind, placebo-controlled trial. *Lancet Neurol* 2013;12:149–156.

Diehl J, Grimmer T, Drzezga A, et al: Cerebral metabolic patterns at early stages of frontotemporal dementia and semantic dementia. A PET study. *Neurobiol Aging* 2004;25:1051–1056.

Gorno-Tempini ML, Brambati SM, Ginex V, et al: The logopenic/phonological variant of primary progressive aphasia. *Neurology* 2001;71:1227–1234.

Grossman M, Mickanin J, Onishi K, et al: Progressive nonfluent aphasia: language, cognitive, and PET measures contrasted with probable Alzheimer's disease. *J Cogn Neurosci* 1996;8:135–154.

Heutink P, Stevens M, Rizzu P, et al: Hereditary frontotemporal dementia is linked to chromosome 17q21-q22; a genetic and clinicopathological study of three Dutch families. *Ann Neurol* 1997;41:150–159.

Hodges JR, Davies RR, Xuereb JH, et al: Clinicopathological correlates in frontotemporal dementia. *Ann Neurol* 2004;56: 399–406.

Hodges JR, Patterson K: Semantic dementia: a unique clinicopathological syndrome. *Lancet Neurol* 2007;6:1004–1014.

Hodges JR, Patterson K, Oxbury S, Funnell E: Semantic dementia. Progressive fluent aphasia with temporal lobe atrophy. *Brain* 1992;115:1783–1806.

Huey ED, Putnam KT, Grafman J: A systematic review of neurotransmitter deficits and treatments in frontotemporal dementia. *Neurology* 2006;66:17–22.

Kertesz A, Munoz DG: Primary progressive aphasia and Pick complex. *J Neurol Sci* 2003;206:97–107.

Kirshner HS: Frontotemporal dementia and primary progressive aphasia: An update. *Curr Neurol Neurosci Rep* 2010;10:504–511.

Kirshner HS: Primary progressive aphasia and Alzheimer's disease: brief history, recent evidence. *Curr Neurol Neurosci Rep* 2012;12: 709–714.

Kirshner HS, Tanridag O, Thurman L, Whetsell WO, Jr.: Progressive aphasia without dementia: two cases with focal, spongiform degeneration. *Ann Neurol* 1987;22:527–532.

Lebert F, Stekke W, Hasenbroekx C, et al: Frontotemporal dementia: a randomized, controlled trial with trazodone. *Dement Geriatr Cogn Disord* 2004;17:355–359.

Leyton CE, Villemagne VL, Savage S, et al: Subtypes of progressive aphasia: application of the international consensus criteria and validation using β-amyloid imaging. *Brain* 2011;134:3030–3043.

Mesulam MM: Primary progressive aphasia. *Ann Neurol* 2001; 49:425–432.

Mesulam MM: Primary progressive aphasia—a language-based dementia. *N Engl J Med* 2003;349:1535–1542.

Neary D, et al: Frontotemporal lobar degeneration: a consensus on clinical diagnostic criteria. *Neurology* 1998;51:1546.

Rascovsky K, Hodges JR, Knopman D: Sensitivity of revised diagnostic criteria for the behavioral variant of frontotemporal dementia. *Brain* 2011;134:2456–2477.

Schwartz JR, Miller BL, Lesser IM, Darby AL: Frontotemporal dementia: treatment response to serotonin selective reuptake inhibitors. *J Clin Psychiatry* 1997;58(5):212–216.

Sonty SP, Mesulam MM, Thompson CK, et al: Primary progressive aphasia: PPA and the language network. *Ann Neurol* 2003;53: 35–49.

NEUROCOGNITIVE DISORDER WITH LEWY BODIES

▶ Essentials of Diagnosis

Lewy bodies are cytoplasmic inclusions seen in the neurons of the substantia nigra and other pigmented nuclei in patients with Parkinson disease (PD). In recent years, similar neuronal inclusions have been discovered in cortical neurons in patients with dementia. Neurocognitive disorder with Lewy bodies (Lewy body dementia) refers to patients who present with dementia symptoms before or simultaneously with motor disturbances suggestive of PD. Patients with Lewy body disease typically demonstrate fluctuating cognitive impairment, with active confusion and hallucinations, in addition to deterioration of memory and higher cortical functions. This fluctuating, delirium-like presentation distinguishes this disorder from Alzheimer disease. Associated features include early hallucinations, usually visual rather than auditory; mild extrapyramidal signs; or repeated and unexplained falls. Autonomic findings are common, and diffuse Lewy body disease may present as part of the multiple system atrophy or Shy-Drager syndrome. Another associated phenomenon is rapid eye movement (REM) sleep behavior disorder, in which patients act out dreams, shouting, flailing limbs, sometimes striking bed partners. This sleep disorder can predate the dementia by decades. The illness progresses at a variable rate to an end stage of severe dementia. Vascular dementias and other physical illness must be excluded.

▶ General Considerations

The prevalence of diffuse Lewy body disease may have been underestimated in the past because of the difficulty of making the neuropathologic diagnosis. Lewy bodies may occur in the cortex or in subcortical regions. They may also be intermixed with plaques and tangles. When Lewy bodies occur together with the pathology of Alzheimer disease, the term Lewy body variant of Alzheimer disease is used. This condition is also referred to as the common form of Lewy body disease. The pure form of Lewy body disease lacks Alzheimer's pathologic features. This form is sometimes referred to as diffuse Lewy body disease. Both disorders are included in the more general term Lewy body dementia. Diffuse Lewy body disease may underlie the dementia associated with Parkinson disease, but many such cases also have Alzheimer disease pathology at autopsy.

A. Epidemiology

The disease represents approximately 15% of dementias seen at autopsy. The age at onset is somewhat earlier than Alzheimer and shows a greater degree of variability. There is substantial overlap with Alzheimer disease, and many patients exhibit mixed pathology. The mean age at onset is 68 and at death is 75 years. Men are affected more often than women.

B. Genetics

The ApoE E4 allele is overrepresented in patients with Lewy body disease. The mutant allele of *CYP2D6B* is a risk factor for both Parkinson disease and Lewy body disease. This gene encodes an enzyme that is involved in detoxifying environmental toxins. The mutation eliminates the active form of the enzyme.

▶ Clinical Findings

A. Signs and Symptoms

In the early stages of neurocognitive disorder with Lewy bodies, memory loss, inattention, and difficulty in sustaining a train of thought are characteristic. Psychiatric signs are prominent in many patients with diffuse Lewy body disease and may be the first indication of the disorder. Psychiatric symptoms include personality change, depression, hallucinations, or delusions. Weight loss is common. Extrapyramidal signs are less severe in diffuse Lewy body disease than in Parkinson disease. Bradykinesia, rigidity, and gait difficulty are more common than tremors. Sometimes extrapyramidal signs are limited to the patient's gait. The anatomic location of the Lewy bodies explains some characteristics of the disorder. Diffuse Lewy body disease affects both cholinergic and dopaminergic systems.

B. Psychological Testing

Patients with diffuse Lewy body disease present with both cortical and subcortical neuropsychological findings. The subcortical features distinguish the condition from Alzheimer disease along with the fluctuating, delirium-like changes in mentation and the early hallucinations. Although not a pure subcortical dementia, diffuse Lewy body disease has prominent subcortical features.

The primary symptoms of subcortical dementias include forgetfulness, slowed thinking, and apathy. In addition, the patient's ability to manage information efficiently is reduced. Executive functions are also diminished. Memory is more disturbed for free recall than recognition. Patients with subcortical dementias are unable to profit from feedback because of poor concentration and inability to maintain set. They have difficulty sequencing and conceptualizing ideas. Another symptom is perseveration. Memory problems and visual spatial disturbances are also common but are not as severe as in Alzheimer disease. Subcortical dementias differ from Alzheimer disease in that the former are not associated with aphasia, recognition deficits, and denial of illness.

C. Laboratory Findings and Imaging

The hallmark of diffuse Lewy body disease is extensive Lewy body formation in the neocortex. The severity of dementia is related to the density of cortical Lewy bodies. Lewy bodies are usually found in the pigmented neurons of the substantia nigra in Parkinson disease. Cortical Lewy bodies are much easier to overlook. Staining with antiubiquitin antibodies simplifies identification and increases the recognition of diffuse Lewy body disease. In contrast, Alz-50 immunoreactivity is small or nonexistent.

The EEG can be helpful in distinguishing between diffuse Lewy body disease and Alzheimer disease. Diffuse slowing and frontal intermittent delta activity are common in Lewy body disease. Significant slowing and frontal intermittent rhythmic delta are not usually present in early Alzheimer disease; however, slowing of the background EEG does occur in vascular dementias. Vascular dementias, particularly those caused by stroke, are likely to demonstrate focal EEG changes consistent with the underlying structural damage. Focal EEG findings are not consistent with either diffuse Lewy body disease or Alzheimer disease. Even though the EEG may provide useful information, EEG alone cannot reliably differentiate vascular dementias from Alzheimer disease or diffuse Lewy body disease. MRI and CT are not greatly different from AD, but PET shows a different pattern of glucose hypometabolism.

▶ Differential Diagnosis

A noninvasive diagnostic test does not exist for Lewy body disease. The most distinctive feature of the disease is the delirium-like episodes with psychotic features that occur and then remit spontaneously. Diffuse Lewy body disease shares some features with progressive supranuclear palsy, frontotemporal dementia, Parkinson disease, Alzheimer disease, and normal pressure hydrocephalus. The dementia caused by the later stages of small vessel disease may also bear a striking resemblance to Lewy body dementia. Late-life psychosis, delirium, syncope, and drug toxicity must also be considered.

▶ Treatment

Because diffuse Lewy body disease affects neocortical dopamine systems, typical neuroleptic treatment of the psychiatric symptoms is usually not successful and can produce significant extrapyramidal side effects. Severe and often fatal neuroleptic sensitivity may occur in some elderly patients with dementia of the Lewy body type. Neuroleptic sensitivity may be manifested as neuroleptic malignant syndrome. Although the typical neuroleptics are not well tolerated, atypical neuroleptics such as olanzapine, clozapine, or quetiapine may produce significant antipsychotic effects with fewer side effects. However, increased mortality has been reported with antipsychotic use and these drugs carry a Black Box Warning. The drug pimavanserin (Nuplazid) is approved for hallucinations in Parkinson disease, but not for Lewy body dementia.

The response to L-dopa is less dramatic than in other Parkinson syndromes, though early in the course it may have benefit in the motor part of the disorder. Higher doses of L-dopa often produce or aggravate psychosis, and this is even more true of dopamine agonist drugs such as pramipexole or ropinirole. In contrast, depression is treatable and responds readily to antidepressant agents, often with a corresponding improvement in cognition. Antidepressants that cause orthostasis should be avoided. Some patients may need fludrocortisone to support blood pressure. Anticholinesterase agents may be of benefit for the memory disorder of Lewy body dementia; rivastigmine in both oral and patch preparations has been approved by the FDA for the treatment of patients with Parkinson disease and dementia. Neuroprotective agents such as vitamin E or selegiline may be tried, but there is no proof of their benefit.

▶ Prognosis

The neurocognitive disorder with Lewy bodies has quite a variable course but generally progresses more rapidly than Alzheimer disease. The average time from diagnosis to death is approximately 6 years. The disease often presents as a psychiatric condition because of the strange and complex hallucinations and delusions. The psychiatric symptoms occur much earlier in the course of diffuse Lewy body disease than in Alzheimer disease. Cardinal features of fully developed Lewy body dementia include delirium, hallucinatory-delusional states, disturbed behavior, akinesia, rigidity, and orthostatic hypotension. Aphasia is notably absent. Although the cognitive impairment is progressive, there is marked daily variability. As the disease progresses, parkinsonian signs may become more severe. Involuntary movements, myoclonus, quadriparesis in flexion, and dysphagia (difficulty swallowing) occur in the final stages.

Bonanni L, Thomas A, Onofrj M: Diagnosis and management of dementia with Lewy bodies: third report of the DLB consortium. *Neurology* 2006;66:1455.

Emre M, Aarsland D, Albanese A, et al: Rivastigmine for dementia associated with Parkinson's disease. *N Engl J Med* 2004;351:2509–2518.

Filley CM: Neuropsychiatric features of Lewy body disease. *Brain Cogn* 1995;28:229–239.

Karla S, Bergeron C, Lang AE: Lewy body disease and dementia. *Arch Intern Med* 1996;156:487.

McKeith I, et al: Neuroleptic sensitivity in patients with senile dementia of Lewy body type [see comments]. *Br Med J* 1992; 305:673.

McKeith I, Del Ser T, Spano P: Efficacy of rivastigmine in dementia with Lewy bodies: a randomized, double-blind, placebo-controlled international study. *Lancet* 2000;356: 2031–2036.

Schmidt ML, et al: Epitope map of neurofilament protein domains in cortical and peripheral nervous system Lewy bodies. *Am J Pathol* 1991;139:53.

SUBCORTICAL DEMENTIAS (NEUROCOGNITIVE DISORDERS)

▶ Essentials of Diagnosis

Patients with subcortical dementias have a diagnosed disorder of deeper brain structures in the presence of a relatively unaffected cerebral cortex. These patients have problems with arousal, attention, mood, motivation, language, and memory. Subcortical dementias may occur in Parkinson disease, Huntington disease, progressive supranuclear palsy, cortical basal ganglia degeneration (now called corticobasal degeneration), Hallervorden-Spatz disease, idiopathic basal ganglia calcification, the spinocerebellar degenerations, and normal pressure hydrocephalus. Subcortical dementias have also been identified in inflammatory, infectious (especially AIDS [acquired immunodeficiency syndrome] dementia complex), vascular, and demyelinating illness.

▶ General Considerations

The concept of subcortical dementias unifies conceptually those conditions affecting the relationship of deeper structures to the cortex. In subcortical dementias, cerebral cortical functioning is relatively intact, but the basal ganglia are dysfunctional or disconnected. Subcortical dementias are not entirely homogeneous entities, and specific features will depend on the pathologic causes. Thus the features of the cognitive disorder observed in Parkinson disease are not exactly the same as those seen in Huntington disease or in progressive supranuclear palsy.

A. Epidemiology

Estimates of the prevalence of dementia in Parkinson patients depends on the population studied and criteria used. Estimates ranging from 30% to 50% have frequently been reported, but if neuropsychological testing criteria are used, prevalence may reach 90%. The overall prevalence rate of Parkinson disease with dementia is estimated to be about 40 per 100,000.

The prevalence of Huntington disease is about six per 100,000. Dementia is a ubiquitous feature of Huntington disease, but the severity of impairment varies greatly among patients.

There are other degenerative diseases of the basal ganglia frontal circuits that lead to subcortical dementia. Progressive supranuclear palsy, the disease in which subcortical dementia was first described, is less common than Parkinson disease. It is a tauopathy and has overlap with frontotemporal dementia. Striatonigral degeneration and corticobasal degeneration can also cause subcortical dementia, though corticobasal degeneration also affects cortical structures and often presents with language and cognitive deficits. Corticobasal degeneration is also associated with tau protein abnormalities and often overlaps with the frontotemporal dementia syndrome. Parkinsonism and apraxia of one upper limb are associated symptoms. These entities are more widely recognized with improved diagnostic techniques.

B. Etiology

Subcortical dementias involve primarily the thalamus, basal ganglia, and related brainstem nuclei with relative sparing of the cerebral cortex. Patients with basal ganglia disease or with disease affecting basal ganglia frontal circuits develop subcortical dementias.

Parkinson disease is always associated with neuronal loss in the substantia nigra, leading to destruction of dopaminergic connections to the basal ganglia. As a result, subcorticocortical pathways function defectively. Striatal dopamine depletion disrupts the normal pattern of basal ganglia function in Parkinson disease and, consequently, interrupts normal transmission of information through frontostriatal circuitry. Dopaminergic transmission, along the nigrostriatal pathway, may be implicated in sustaining various cognitive and motor processes.

In addition, neuronal loss occurs throughout the CNS. Patients with dementia due to Parkinson disease have significant cell loss in many other CNS structures, particularly in the basal nucleus of Meynert. The depletion of acetylcholine in the cortex is less severe than in Alzheimer disease. There is significant damage to the locus coeruleus, secondary loss of cortical norepinephrine, and cell loss in the raphe nucleus leading to serotonin depletion. This may explain the anxiety and depression so commonly associated with Parkinson disease.

C. Genetics

Huntington disease has an autosomal-dominant mode of inheritance. An excess number of CAG trinucleotide repeats in the 5′-translated region of chromosome 4 causes

Huntington disease. A DNA test can detect the gene before symptoms appear. Virtually 100% of patients with more than 40 repeats of the gene will manifest the disease at some point in their lives; however, the age at which the disease manifests itself is quite variable. Huntington disease exhibits an earlier onset in successive generations of a pedigree, especially when transmitted through the father. There is greater variability of repeat length with paternal transmission, and the gene tends to have ever-increasing CAG repeats. The change in repeat length with paternal transmission is correlated significantly with decreasing age at onset between the father and offspring.

The genetics of progressive supranuclear palsy has recently been clarified. Studies suggest that progressive supranuclear palsy is an autosomal recessive condition that maps to a polymorphism in the tau gene. It has been reported that a genetic variant of tau, known as the A0 allele, was represented excessively in patients with progressive supranuclear palsy in comparison to control subjects. A highly significant overrepresentation of the A0/A0 genotype and a decrease in the frequency of the A0/A3 genotype were found in patients with progressive supranuclear palsy. The presence of the tau A0/A0 genotype is a risk factor for developing the disorder, whereas A3 may be protective. PSP, made famous by the comedian and actor Dudley Moore, is also a tauopathy.

Hallervorden-Spatz syndrome is a rare, autosomal recessive neurodegenerative disorder in which iron accumulates in the basal ganglia. Recently, the eponym has been controversial because of the background of the named authors, and the disorder is referred to as "neurodegeneration with brain iron accumulation (NBIA)" or pantothenate kinase-associated neurodegeneration (PKAN). Extrapyramidal signs are dominant and include dystonia. Mental deterioration occurs as the disease progresses. MRI reveals marked overall low signal from the globus pallidus.

The genetics of Parkinson disease are extremely complex and reflect the fact that the disorder has multiple etiologies. Several genes have been discovered in families with more than one member with PD; to date, these genetic types of PD account for less than 10% of the cases. There may be genetic factors influencing susceptibility to Parkinson disease. In addition, it has long been believed that Parkinson represents an interaction between genetic and environmental factors. A large twin study also suggests that genetic influences are less important in patients with disease beginning after the age of 50 years. In contrast, genetic influences are larger in earlier-onset disease.

Several purely genetic forms of Parkinson disease have been identified. The g209a mutation in the alpha-synuclein gene has been associated with autosomal dominant Parkinson disease in a number of families. Other gene loci have been reported. Different mutations in the microtubule-associated tau protein gene have been identified in several families with hereditary frontotemporal dementia and Parkinsonism (ftdp-17) linked to chromosome 17q21–22. Another gene, Gstp1-1, expressed in the blood-brain barrier, may influence response to neurotoxins and explain the susceptibility of some people to the parkinsonism-inducing effects of pesticides. The dopamine receptor gene has also been implicated in Parkinson disease. Autosomal recessive juvenile parkinsonism and early-onset parkinsonism with diurnal fluctuation are other forms of Parkinson disease with relatively clear genetic causes.

▶ **Clinical Findings**

In contrast to cortical dementias such as Alzheimer disease, subcortical dementias are relatively circumscribed syndromes. The principal features of subcortical dementias include slowed mentation, impairment of executive function, recall abnormalities, and visuospatial disturbances. Recall is better than in Alzheimer disease, and overall memory impairment is not as severe. At each functional stage, patients with subcortical dementias are less intellectually impaired than are patients with Alzheimer disease. Subcortical dementias do not involve aphasia, agnosia, or apraxia.

Subcortical dementias may constitute a group of partially treatable forms of dementia. Subcortical dementias create a cognitive picture similar to that of major affective disorder. Moreover, if the patient becomes depressed, his or her cognitive abilities are reduced even further. Psychiatric consultation may be obtained to treat depression and apathy. Depression aggravates the memory and language impairments associated with subcortical dementias. Antidepressants may improve cognition in subcortical syndromes. Specific subtypes of cognitive impairment are related directly to the neuropathology of each disease. In progressive supranuclear palsy, behavioral and cognitive changes resemble those associated with lesions of the frontal lobes.

Symptoms of subcortical dementias may respond to psychotropic medication. Mood disorders are extremely common in subcortical dementias and may respond to antidepressants. Sometimes the cognitive deficits improve along with the mood disorder. The response of psychotic symptoms to neuroleptics is more variable. The choice of neuroleptic must be thought out more carefully. Antipsychotics may be required to control psychotic symptoms and agitation; however, many of these patients have associated movement disorders, and antipsychotics may affect motor symptoms in either a positive or a negative manner depending on the specific movement disorder.

The dementias associated with Parkinson disease and Huntington disease are discussed in detail in the sections that follow. Normal pressure hydrocephalus and AIDS dementia complex also present as subcortical dementias but will be discussed in later sections.

NEUROCOGNITIVE DISORDER DUE TO PARKINSON DISEASE

▶ Clinical Findings

A. Signs and Symptoms

Cognitive changes, particularly mild impairment in memory, executive functions, attention, and information processing, occur early in Parkinson disease. The time required to make decisions is prolonged. These effects are more noticeable if the primary symptoms are bradykinesia and rigidity. Patients who complain primarily of tremor have fewer cognitive abnormalities.

Some Parkinson patients have only a subcortical dementia. Others are more seriously mentally impaired, and these patients appear to have either cortical Lewy bodies or plaques and tangles, suggesting Alzheimer disease. These patients also differ from others with the disorder in that they present a more marked severity of the extrapyramidal syndrome with predominant bradykinesia and an earlier deteriorating response to L-dopa treatment. The presence of dysphasia or other cortical deficits early in the course of the illness suggests the presence of coexisting Alzheimer disease. These patients are also more likely to develop a significant depression early in the course of the illness. In the presence of depression, Parkinson patients are more likely to develop a cognitive disorder that persists even when the depression is treated.

B. Psychological Testing

Very early in the disease course, Parkinson patients demonstrate mild impairment on tests sensitive to information processing speed, maintaining set, and visuospatial discrimination. Neuropsychological tests suggest that an underlying perceptual motor deficit exists in Parkinson disease. Personality changes occur early, whereas recall abnormalities and apathy tend to occur later. These subtle cognitive difficulties might underlie the mental inflexibility and rigidity associated with Parkinson disease and could be attributed to destruction of the ascending dopaminergic and mesocorticolimbic pathway.

Parkinson patients whose disease develops relatively late in life are prone to develop comorbid dementing illness such as Alzheimer disease, diffuse Lewy body disease, or vascular dementia. Neuropsychological testing can help determine whether these patients are developing a mixed syndrome.

C. Laboratory Findings and Imaging

PET scans using [18F]fluorodeoxyglucose will often show hypofrontality in nondemented Parkinson patients or in those with mild subcortical dementia. The presence of bilateral temporoparietal deficits in addition to hypofrontality suggests the coexistence of either Lewy body disease or Alzheimer disease.

PET scans can be used to examine glucose metabolism through the use of [18F]fluorodeoxyglucose and to examine dopamine metabolic patterns through the use of [18F]fluorodopa. [11C]Raclopride can be used to examine dopamine D_2 receptor binding; this ligand is not routinely available in clinical practice. These techniques hold promise for future diagnostic clarification.

In Parkinson patients, SPECT scans demonstrate decreased frontal lobe blood flow that is more significant on the left side than on the right. Basal ganglia decrements are also visible. These changes appear to be particularly accentuated in the early stages of Parkinson disease with subcortical dementia. SPECT binding studies demonstrate decreased basal ganglia binding in demented Parkinson patients compared to nondemented Parkinson patients. Bilateral temporoparietal deficits probably indicate concomitant Alzheimer disease.

NMR spectroscopy indicates an increase in cerebral lactate in patients with Parkinson disease, especially in those with dementia. Finally, evoked potential studies indicate some difference between Parkinson patients with and without dementia. Reaction time is prolonged in both groups of patients. The event-related P300 evoked potential is normal in nondemented Parkinson patients but is prolonged in demented Parkinson patients. Visual evoked potentials show an increased latency of P100 in demented Parkinson patients compared to nondemented Parkinson patients.

▶ Differential Diagnosis

Parkinson disease with subcortical dementia must be distinguished first from Parkinson disease with coexisting Alzheimer or diffuse Lewy body disease. Functional imaging may help. Other conditions to consider include vascular dementias and other parkinsonian syndromes such as progressive supranuclear palsy.

▶ Treatment

Many medications affect cognition in Parkinson disease patients. As a rule, anticholinergic medication impairs cognition, whereas dopaminergic medication may mildly enhance it. The dosage of dopaminergic medication is important, because at higher dosages patients may become confused or hallucinate. Levodopa-carbidopa or direct dopamine agonists such as pramipexole and ropinirole are the standard initial treatments for PD. Neuroleptics may cause significant rigidity in patients with PD or diffuse Lewy body dementia. Atypical neuroleptics are usually preferred in these patients because standard neuroleptics cause extrapyramidal side effects, tardive dyskinesia, and neuroleptic malignant syndrome. Clozapine or quetiapine may be preferred neuroleptics for patients with subcortical dementias because these atypical agents may improve psychotic symptoms without adverse motor effects. Pimavanserin is a new antipsychotic with a novel pharmacology, inverse agonism (total blockade of the serotonin 2A receptor. It is approved for psychosis in Parkinson disease and is of theoretical value in Lewy body dementia and other dementias. Currently it is approved only for psychosis or hallucinations in patients with Parkinson disease.

ECT has been used in the management of psychiatric complications in Parkinson disease. Not only do affective symptoms respond, but motor symptoms improve. Unfortunately, patients with dementia due to Parkinson disease may develop post-ECT delirium. Nonetheless, ECT remains an occasionally used treatment for intractable depression associated with Parkinson disease. The dosage of antidepressant or number of ECT treatments should be considered together with antiparkinsonian therapies. Demented parkinsonian patients often experience side effects after taking antiparkinsonian medication. As a result, the clinician should be inclined to treat the motor symptoms conservatively in order to minimize cognitive side effects. The use of rivastigmine for dementia associated with Parkinson disease is effective in improving cognitive symptoms.

▶ Prognosis

Patients with PD with neurocognitive disorder are older, have a longer duration of disease, and a later age at onset than those who do not become demented. Age is the biggest risk factor. The development of dementia is strongly related to the age at which the patient developed motor manifestations. In some patients, cortical Lewy bodies cause the dementia. Although most patients with Parkinson disease do not have Alzheimer disease, some Parkinson patients have dementia that is due to the coexistence of Alzheimer disease. The dual diagnosis of Parkinson and Alzheimer disease is associated with a particularly poor prognosis.

The cognitive deficits evident in early Parkinson disease do not progress to dementia in all patients. When dementia does develop, the symptoms are quite heterogeneous. Patients with Parkinson dementia have a great deal of difficulty with tasks that involve visual and spatial orientation. Intellectual ability begins a global decline in Parkinson disease with dementia, but memory is more severely impaired than are language and other cortical functions. Episodic memory (i.e., memory for items relating to date and time) is especially distorted. Although the patient can drive an automobile, decline in spatial memory may make following directions difficult, and slowed reaction time makes driving dangerous.

The association between depression and Parkinson disease has been recognized for more than 150 years. Depression affects up to 50% of Parkinson patients and is more pronounced during the early stages of the illness. Affective disorder aggravates the poor concentration and impaired information processing associated with Parkinson disease.

The treatment of depression tends to improve some of these cognitive deficiencies.

Christine CW, Aminoff MJ: Clinical differentiation of Parkinsonian syndromes: prognostic and therapeutic relevance. *Am J Med* 2004;117:412–419.

Cummings JL: Depression and Parkinson's disease: a review. *Am J Psychiatry* 1992;149:443.

Eskandar EN, Cosgrove GR, Shinobu SA: Surgical treatment of Parkinson's disease. *JAMA* 2001;286:3056–3059.

Feany MB: New genetic insights into Parkinson's disease. *N Engl J Med* 2004;351:1937–1940.

Freed CR, Greene PE, Breeze RE, et al: Transplantation of embryonic dopamine neurons for severe Parkinson's disease. *N Engl J Med* 2001;344:710–719.

Hawkins T, Berman BD: Pimavanserin A novel therapeutic option for Parkinson's disease psychosis. Neurol Clin Pract 2017;7(2):157–162.

Lang AE, Lozano AM: Parkinson's disease. First of two parts. *N Engl J Med* 1998;339:1044–1053.

Lang AE, Lozano AM: Parkinson's disease. Second of two parts. *N Engl J Med* 1998;339:1130–1143.

Miyasaki JM, Martin W, Suchowersky O, et al: Practice parameter: Initiation of treatment for Parkinson's disease: an evidence-based review: report of the Quality Standards Subcommittee of the American Academy of Neurology. *Neurology* 2002;58:11–17.

Nutt JG, Wooten GF: Diagnosis and initial management of Parkinson's disease. *N Engl J Med* 2005;353:1021–1027.

Oken MS: Deep-brain stimulation for Parkinson's disease. *N Engl J Med* 2012;367:1529–1538.

Schapira AH, Olanow CW: Neuroprotection in Parkinson disease. Mysteries, myths, and misconceptions. *JAMA* 2004;291:358–364.

The Deep-Brain Stimulation for Parkinson's Disease Study Group. Deep-brain stimulation of the subthalamic nucleus or the pars interna of the globus pallidus in Parkinson's disease. *N Engl J Med* 2001;345:956–963.

Lewy Body Dementia

Aarsland D, Perry R, Brown A, et al: Neuropathology of dementia in Parkinson's disease: a prospective, community-based study. *Ann Neurol* 2005;58:773–776.

Cummings JL: Lewy body diseases with dementia: pathophysiology and treatment. *Brain Cogn* 1995;28:266–280.

Poewe W: Treatment of dementia with Lewy bodies and Parkinson's disease dementia. *Mov Disord* 2005;12:S77–S82.

Progressive Supranuclear Palsy

Daniel SE, deBruin VM, Lees AJ: The clinical and pathological spectrum of Steele-Richardson-Olszewski syndrome (progressive supranuclear palsy): a reappraisal. *Brain* 1995;118: 759–770.

Litvan I, Campbell G, Mangone CA, et al: Which clinical features differentiate progressive supranuclear palsy (Steele-Richardson-Olszewski syndrome) from related disorders? A clinicopathological study. *Brain* 1997;120:65–74.

Multisystem Atrophy

Mark MH: Lumping and splitting the Parkinson Plus syndromes: dementia with Lewy bodies, multiple system atrophy, progressive supranuclear palsy, and cortical-basal ganglionic degeneration. *Neurol Clin* 2001;19:607–627.

Wenning GK, Colosimo C, Geser F, Poewe W: Multiple system atrophy. *Lancet Neurol* 2004;3:93–103.

Corticobasal Degeneration

Bergeron C, Pollanen MS, Weyer L, et al: Unusual clinical presentations of cortical-basal ganglionic degeneration. *Ann Neurol* 1996;40:893–900.

Gibb WRG, Luthert PJ, Marsden CD: Corticobasal degeneration. *Brain* 1989;112:1171–1192.

Litvan I, Cummings JL, Mega M: Neuropsychiatric features of corticobasal degeneration. *J Neurol Neurosurg Psychiatry* 1998;65:717–721.

NEUROGOCNITIVE DISORDER DUE TO HUNTINGTON DISEASE

▶ Clinical Findings

A. Signs and Symptoms

Huntington disease often has a delayed onset, with a mean age at onset of about 40 years. Progressive cognitive decline is a cardinal feature of Huntington disease; however, mild deficits in cognitive function are an early finding. Severe mental deterioration is apparent later in the disease. The onset is proportional to the number of CAG repeats in the Huntington disease allele, although the degree of cognitive deficit is not proportional to the number of CAG repeats but rather to chronicity of the illness.

Huntington disease usually presents with choreiform movements, but it can present as incipient dementia or depression. As the disease progresses, all patients become demented. The cognitive changes are quite varied, even in the late stages of the illness.

The dementia develops slowly and is consistent with damage to pathways linking the frontal areas to the striatum. Prominent complaints are apathy, slow information processing, and problems in maintaining attention. Difficulty with attention and concentration is more pronounced than in Parkinson disease. Compared to patients with Alzheimer disease, those with Huntington disease have less memory impairment. Cortical symptoms such as aphasia, agnosia, and apraxia are less common in Huntington than in Alzheimer disease.

Most patients with Huntington disease develop prominent psychiatric symptoms. Depression is the most common symptom, but up to 10% of patients have symptoms resembling bipolar disorder. Irritability, personality change, and other behavioral problems are also common. Frontal lobe impairment results in poor judgment that may lead to embarrassing or even illegal activities. A paranoid psychosis is common in Huntington patients.

B. Psychological Testing

Huntington patients initially show difficulty with attention tasks. Other early deficits include psychomotor speed and the ability to shift set. Go/no-go tasks are impaired early as are other tasks that require internal cues. Huntington patients are unable to maintain divided attention and to perform tasks in which multimodal sensory information is provided. When compared to Alzheimer patients, Huntington patients demonstrate greater impairment on the initiation/perseveration subscale of the DRS. Alzheimer patients demonstrate greater impairment on the memory subscale than do Huntington patients. Constructional apraxia becomes apparent at moderate and severe levels of dementia in Huntington patients but appears relatively early in Alzheimer patients.

C. Laboratory Findings and Imaging

At autopsy, there is a marked decrease in small cholinergic neurons in the striatum, with low levels of choline acetyltransferase. The disease also damages the small cells containing GABA. Consequently the basal ganglia have decreased concentrations of GABA. Acetylcholine-containing neurons in the basal nucleus of Meynert are preserved. The dopaminergic system is also spared. In Huntington disease, brain imaging reveals atrophy in the caudate nucleus, reflecting this loss of neurons.

CT scans and MRI show atrophy of the basal ganglia years before the development of symptoms. The putamen is less affected than the caudate. PET scans show striatal hypometabolism in the brains of Huntington patients early in the course of the disease. Asymptomatic carriers can be identified with 86% sensitivity and 100% specificity. Glucose metabolism decreases at a rate of about 2% per year. Raclopride binding is decreased by about 6% per year and correlates with the number of CAG repeats. The easy availability of the genetic test for Huntington disease has made brain imaging less crucial in this disease.

▶ Differential Diagnosis

Huntington disease must be differentiated from other choreiform disorders. The existence of a specific genetic test has aided greatly in diagnosis. The most compelling question of differential diagnosis is whether to perform this test on asymptomatic individuals who have not yet developed the disease; in general, this should be reserved for genetics clinics with counseling readily available.

Treatment

Patients with Huntington disease may experience an improvement in chorea from neuroleptics but may concurrently experience cognitive decline. Affective disorder is extremely common in HD patients. Mood-stabilizing agents, particularly lithium, can be helpful. Ten percent of patients become psychotic. Clozapine can be used effectively in psychotic Huntington patients. Other patients show prominent obsessive–compulsive features. Clomipramine may be effective for associated obsessive–compulsive disorder. An interesting finding is that psychiatric illness is increased significantly in patients who are at risk for the disease but in whom later genetic testing reveals the absence of the HD gene. This finding emphasizes the need for considerable counseling and social support in this disease.

Prognosis

The prognosis of HD is universally fatal. The later the onset of Huntington disease, the greater the probability that cognitive decline will be minimal; however, 60% of Huntington patients develop features typical of subcortical dementia. Initially chorea predominates, but later the patient becomes rigid. Striatal damage progresses at a rate that is determined by the length of the CAG repeat. If the patient is affected by psychiatric illness, particularly affective disorder, there is a high prevalence of suicide. The relationship between the severity of chorea and dementia is robust, particularly regarding memory loss. The degree of cognitive disability is ultimately related to the chronicity of the illness but not to the length of the CAG repeat.

Foroud T, et al: Cognitive scores in carriers of Huntington's disease gene compared to noncarriers. *Ann Neurol* 1995;37:657.

Furtado S, Sucherowsky O: Huntington's disease: recent advances in diagnosis and management. *Can J Neurol Sci* 1995;22:5–12.

Pillon B, et al: Severity and specificity of cognitive impairment in Alzheimer's, Huntington's, and Parkinson's diseases and progressive supranuclear palsy. *Neurology* 1991;41:634.

Walling HW, Baldassae JJ, Westfall TC: Molecular aspects of Huntington's disease. *J Neurosci Res* 1998;54:301–308.

VASCULAR NEUROCOGNITIVE DISORDER

Essentials of Diagnosis

Vascular dementias are a varied group of disorders. The true incidence of dementia cases that represent pure vascular dementia is unknown. Because of the variety of types of vascular diseases, the diagnosis of this disorder has been problematic. Cases with mixed vascular disease and Alzheimer disease are likely the second most common dementia, after AD itself.

Table 15–1 California Criteria for Ischemic Vascular Dementia (IVD)

1. Dementia established by clinical examination
2. Progressive worsening of cognitive function
3. Evidence of at least two strokes by clinical or neuroradiological criteria
4. Evidence of at least one hemisphere infarct by CT or MRI (T1-weighted)
5. Diagnosis of definite IVD requires neuropathology

Data from Chui HC, Victoroff JI, Margolin D, et al. Criteria for the diagnosis of ischemic vascular dementia proposed by the State of California Alzheimer's Disease Diagnostic and Treatment Centers. *Neurology*. 1992 Mar;42(3 Pt 1):473–480.

Diagnostic subclassifications and the concept of vascular dementia are very much in flux. The Hachinski ischemic score is used primarily to exclude vascular dementia when studying Alzheimer disease. Table 15–1 shows the California Criteria for ischemic vascular dementia. The criteria from the National Institute of Neurological Disorders and Stroke and from the European Association Internationale pour la Recherche et l'Enseignement en Neurosciences are more specific in regard to etiology and are more flexible (Table 15–2).

General Considerations

Because such a large number of possible etiologic mechanisms exist, the clinical features related to vascular dementia differ from one patient to another. Vascular dementias have many causes: small vessel disease, multi-infarct dementia,

Table 15–2 NINDS-AIREN Criteria

1. Documented dementia
2. Evidence of cerebrovascular disease by clinical history, clinical examination, or brain imaging
3. Three dementia and cerebrovascular disease must be "reasonably related."

The diagnosis of vascular dementia, by these criteria, also must include a decline in memory and at least two domains of intellectual ability, with resultant impairment of activities of daily living. Single strokes are permitted, if the other criteria apply. The NINDS-AIREN criteria also emphasize typical clinical features of impairment of multiple cognitive domains, usual presence of focal neurological signs, gait abnormalities, mood changes, psychomotor slowing, and extrapyramidal signs. Against vascular dementia are: early onset and progressive worsening of a deficit in memory or other cognitive functions, in the absence of focal lesions and CT or MRI scans; absence of focal neurological signs, other than cognitive ones; and absence of infarcts on brain imaging studies.

Reproduced from Roman GC, Tatemichi TK, Erkinjuntti T, et al. Vascular dementia: diagnostic criteria for research studies. Report of the NINDS-AIREN International Work Group. *Neurology*. 1993;43(2):250–260.

strategic strokes, cerebral hypoperfusion, vasculitis, subarachnoid hemorrhage, genetic causes, and cerebral amyloid angiopathy. Recent neuroimaging studies have revealed that vascular dementias may be more common than previously supposed.

Factors in cerebrovascular disease leading to vascular dementia include (1) volume of lesion (e.g., one large lesion or several small lesions), (2) number of cerebral injuries, (3) location of cerebral injury (e.g., cortical lesions produce a different form of dementia than do subcortical lesions; strokes in strategic locations may produce dementia), (4) white-matter ischemia due to small vessel disease, and (5) co-occurrence of vascular disease and Alzheimer disease or another dementing process.

Vascular dementias may be more amenable to prevention and treatment than is Alzheimer disease. Generally, the risk factors for vascular dementias are the same as those for strokes: hypertension, diabetes mellitus, advanced age, male sex, smoking, and cardiac disease.

SMALL VESSEL DISEASE

Small vessel disease can cause a subcortical neurocognitive disorder. Personality and mood changes are frequent. Psychomotor retardation and poor judgment accompany memory deficits. Binswanger disease is an extreme form of this condition and is characterized by pseudobulbar signs, abulia, and significant mood and behavior change. Binswanger disease is associated with multiple small areas of hemispheric softening and demyelination. It occurs mainly in hypertensive males. In most cases, there is not only atherosclerosis of the extracranial arteries but also fibrous and muscular thickening of the small vessels.

▶ Clinical Findings

Small vessel disease can cause cortical and subcortical lesions. Imaging studies can identify these lesions, often referred to as leukoaraiosis, or ischemic deep white-matter disease. Imaging studies identify excessive CNS water caused by damage to the capillaries and postcapillary venules: Collagen is deposited in the media and adventitia and may eventually block the lumen of the arteriole, ultimately affecting the regulation of blood flow in the brain parenchyma. The result is a characteristic pathologic change in the nervous system: rarefaction of the white matter. This finding on MRI scans is extremely common in elderly people, whereas Binswanger disease is rare in autopsy series. To qualify as a stroke, white-matter lesions must be clearly dark on CT or on T1-weighted MRI. Most ischemic changes in the white matter are bright on T2 and FLAIR but not clearly dark on T1. The correlates of ischemic white-matter changes with behavioral and cognitive measures have been controversial. The presence of these lesions correlates both with age and with vascular risk factors

such as hypertension. In some series, cognitive decline has correlated with the degree of white-matter ischemic change, but many normal people have some degree of white-matter change. Neurologists and psychiatrists spend a great deal of time explaining the significance of "ischemic white-matter changes" on MRI to patients and families. Anxiety, depression, and overall severity of neuropsychiatric symptoms are also associated with white-matter ischemia.

The effects of small vessel disease are synergistic with lacunar infarcts. PET research has shown that reduction in cortical metabolism is related to the severity of subcortical pathology. Pathology in the subcortical nuclei greatly influences the metabolism of the frontal cortex.

MULTI-INFARCT DEMENTIA

Lacunar infarcts are small, punctate lesions usually found in the deep white matter, basal ganglia, and brainstem. Multiple lacunar strokes or a few larger strokes can lead to multi-infarct dementia. Hypertension is the greatest risk factor. Previous strokes or myocardial infarction often precede dementia; as compared to Alzheimer disease, most patients have had abrupt, strokelike events. Previous strokes and cortical atrophy are also correlated with dementia.

▶ Clinical Findings

Multi-infarct dementia advances in stepwise fashion. The clinical signs and symptoms of the disease are associated with changes in MRI, CT scan, and EEG. The Hachinski Scale is a rating scale based on clinical course and illness features that is intended to assess the probability of multi-infarct dementia. Mean Hachinski ischemic scores of 10 predict the presence of infarcts in 93% of patients. Small, localized strokes in brain areas that are functionally important cause well-recognized conditions such as Weber or Wallenberg syndromes; however, these lesions may not cause dementia. In patients with multi-infarct dementia, the deep middle cerebral artery territory supplied by the lenticulostriate branches is most likely to be affected. Bilateral infarcts are very common.

A subcortical dementia can sometimes develop in patients with strokes. Paramedial mesencephalic and diencephalic infarcts cause cognitive and affective disorder closely resembling that associated with subcortical degenerative disorders. In these cases, CT scans or MRI sometimes delineate clinical anatomic relationships that account for specific constituents of the syndrome. Dementia resulting from small deep infarctions may involve disease in the same cholinergic projections from the deep frontal nuclei to the cerebral cortex involved in Alzheimer disease. Multiple lesions are thought to have a cumulative effect on mental function, and they also lower the threshold for dementia in patients with early changes of Alzheimer disease.

NEUROCOGNITIVE DISORDER DUE TO STRATEGIC STROKES

Strategic single infarcts in specific areas of the brain can cause dementia. Patients who have strokes in the left supramarginal or angular gyrus may develop profound difficulties with comprehension. Strategic strokes in the frontal lobes or in the nondominant parietal lobe can lead to significant reduction in cognitive abilities. Right temporal lesions can be associated with acute confusional states. One or more strategically placed strokes can therefore lead to dementia. The most common single strokes associated with dementia would be major middle cerebral artery strokes on either side, posterior cerebral strokes that affect the hippocampus, and frontal lobe strokes. Up to a third of patients who have survived a stroke have dementia 1 year after the initial event.

Stroke patients are prone to affective disorder that can affect recovery. About 40% of stroke patients develop post-stroke depression. Post-stroke depression has been associated with poor prognosis. In some studies, depression correlates with infarctions in the left hemisphere and frontal more than posterior location. These studies are mainly in the early weeks after a stroke, and the right hemisphere stroke patients may have a more delayed depression that is equally profound, yet may be difficult to diagnose because of the flat affect that many of these patients develop. Systemic vascular disease, drug therapy, and psychological reactions to disability contribute to post-stroke depression. Subcortical atrophy may predispose to the development of post-stroke depression. Patients with ventricular enlargement may be more likely than those without atrophy to develop major depression following a left frontal or left basal ganglia lesion. As mentioned earlier, left-hemisphere injury leads to early depression; right-hemisphere lesions and preexisting subcortical atrophy predispose to delayed onset of depression, and occasionally to mania.

▶ Clinical Findings

Each brain hemisphere has a different biochemical response to injury. PET scan findings suggest the biochemical response of the two hemispheres to stroke may be different. Right-hemisphere stroke increases serotonin-receptor binding. This does not occur following comparable left-hemisphere stroke. The lower the serotonin binding within the left hemisphere, the more severe the depression is likely to be. This finding suggests that the right, not the left, hemisphere produces biochemical "compensation" for damage by increasing serotonin binding in the non-injured regions. After a stroke, depression may be a result of the failure to up-regulate serotonin receptors. Other factors influencing the differences between hemispheres in post-stroke depression undoubtedly include the dominance of the right hemisphere for emotions, such that damage to the right hemisphere causes emotional flatness or apathy, and

the presence of neglect of deficit in right-hemisphere stroke patients (see later), which often results in a delayed onset of poststroke depression. Nondepressed patients experience less cognitive impairment than do depressed patients. Structural neurologic damage may produce either classic affective disorder or disorders of affective expression and personality that bear little resemblance to classic affective disorder. Stroke patients with depression often respond to antidepressant treatment. In addition, there is evidence that SSRI treatment may improve motor recovery from stroke.

A. Right-Hemisphere Lesions

The expression and understanding of affect are right-hemisphere functions. Evaluation of mood disorders in patients with right-hemisphere damage requires consideration of alterations of affective communication. Depression may be underdiagnosed in patients with right temporoparietal lesions. These patients are often unable to understand nuances of affect. Common cognitive complications of right parietal dysfunction include denial of illness, hemi-inattention (lack of attention to one side of the body), constructional apraxia, and spatial discrimination. Patients with right posterior lesions may not verbally acknowledge depressed feelings. They may appear emotionally flat, or indifferent. A late-onset depression may occur in these patients.

Right frontal lobe damage causes expressive aprosodia (impairment in the normal variations of speech), an inability to express nuances of affect. Affective explosiveness, a temporal lobe function, is preserved. Depressed patients with expressive aprosodia do not appear depressed during a psychiatric interview.

B. Left-Hemisphere Lesions

With left-hemisphere lesions, language impairment complicates the diagnosis of affective disorder. Patients with Broca aphasia exhibit nonfluent speech, impaired writing, defective naming, and (usually) hemiparesis (one-sided paralysis). Verbal acknowledgment of a depressed mood may be difficult to elicit. In spite of diagnostic difficulties, the incidence of depression in patients with unilateral left frontal lobe damage is striking. The putative mechanism is interruption of catecholamine axons to, and arborization in, the cerebral cortex. Comprehension deficits in patients with posterior aphasia make accurate diagnosis of affective disorder difficult. Clinically, posterior aphasia can resemble either dementia or affective disorder. Speech is fluent and associated neurologic deficits often subtle; however, neologisms and paraphasic errors punctuate the speech of patients with Wernicke aphasia. In addition, Wernicke patients exhibit impaired reading, writing, naming, repetition, and comprehension. Patients with left posterior lesions display exaggerated affect because the main remaining vehicle of communication is affective expression. When their speech is not understood, they may become angry or even paranoid.

Left parietal dysfunction can mimic Alzheimer disease because it produces ideomotor apraxia, right-left disorientation, finger agnosia, amnestic aphasia, dyslexia (inability to read, spell, and write words), dysgraphia (difficulty in writing), and acalculia (inability to do simple arithmetic calculations). Right parietal dysfunction causes left spatial neglect and "dressing apraxia." These patients do not usually have as great a memory impairment as do Alzheimer disease patients. Some visuospatial disruption attends normal aging. Neuropsychological evaluation distinguishes normal elders from those with parietal disorder or dementia.

Clinical deterioration may occur in brain-disordered patients without a new lesion. Erratic recovery and poor cooperation during rehabilitation suggest affective disorder. Pathologic laughing or crying (known as pseudobulbar affect), depressive propositional language, and perhaps abnormal dexamethasone suppression test suggest depression. Bilateral hemispheric dysfunction may cause excessive crying.

C. Subcortical lesions

The importance of white matter lesions, which have become much more evident since the advent of MR imaging, to cognitive decline has been controversial. Extensive white matter lesions do appear to affect executive function, as will be discussed below in the context of neuropsychological testing.

▶ Differential Diagnosis

A. Differentiating Frontal Lobe Disorder from Depression

Several characteristics differentiate frontal lobe disorder from depression. Frontal patients are apathetic and not deeply depressed. Frontal personality changes are more dramatic than are those in depression. Frontal lobe systems are responsible for affect modulation. When these systems disconnect from brainstem centers, pseudobulbar affect develops. Patients who feel a fleeting emotion may be unable to inhibit a prolonged affective display such as crying. The phrase "emotionally incontinent" is sometimes applied to these patients because of their inability to inhibit emotional expression. Frontal patients often have impaired insight and judgment. They are perseverative concerning some social responses, yet they may be unable to initiate others. As a result, they can appear bizarre in social settings.

CEREBRAL HYPOPERFUSION OF WATERSHED AREAS

Hypotension, decreased volume of body fluids, cardiac arrhythmias, and other causes of hypoperfusion can cause ischemia in the watershed areas between the major sources of cerebral arterial supply. Significant watershed strokes can lead to serious disconnection syndromes. Lesions circling Broca's area cause a transcortical motor aphasia. Transcortical motor aphasia displays elements of Broca aphasia with intact repetition. Patients with transcortical motor aphasia have decreased speech production. Mild forms of the disorder can be identified by poor performance on the FAS test and on other frontal lobe tests.

Watershed lesions surrounding Wernicke's area cause transcortical sensory aphasia. This syndrome is similar to Wernicke aphasia, but repetition remains intact. The most severe form of watershed infarct causes isolation of the speech area. In this condition the entire language apparatus is disconnected from other brain structures. Echolalia is the only form of speech of which the patient is capable. Mixed transcortical aphasia, or isolation of the speech area syndrome, is also seen in advanced Alzheimer disease.

Bilateral strokes in the posterior parts of the hemispheres can result in complex neurobehavioral deficits such as visual agnosia, prosopagnosia (inability to recognize familiar faces), or auditory agnosias. These deficits are often explained by disconnections between sensory input and centers that interpret the information. Unilateral left posterior cerebral artery territory strokes are associated with alexia without agraphia, and severe memory disorder. These cognitive deficits can contribute to vascular dementia.

NEUROCOGNITIVE DISORDER DUE TO CEREBRAL VASCULITIS

Autoimmune vasculitis is an uncommon cause of dementia. Systemic vasculitis that affects the CNS occurs most often in conjunction with collagen vascular disease (such as polyarteritis nodosa). The most common autoimmune disease associated with stroke is systemic lupus erythematosus, but this disease is associated with antineuronal antibodies that cause delirium and antiphospholipid antibodies associated with stroke; a true vasculitis is rare. Renal involvement with hypertension can also be a risk factor for stroke. Antiphospholipid antibodies can also be associated with stroke syndromes in patients who do not have lupus. CNS vasculitis can occur in isolation (e.g., granulomatous angiitis or isolated CNS vasculitis). Infectious diseases such as neurosyphilis and Lyme disease can cause CNS vasculitis, which can be extremely difficult to diagnose but should be considered in the presence of any rapidly progressing dementia.

NEUROCOGNITIVE DISORDER DUE TO SUBARACHNOID HEMORRHAGE

Subarachnoid hemorrhage causes intense vasospasm, which can lead to significant ischemia. This ischemia can cause a dementing syndrome that persists after the subarachnoid hemorrhage has resolved.

NEUROCOGNITIVE DISORDER DUE TO CEREBRAL AUTOSOMAL DOMINANT ARTERIOPATHY WITH SUBCORTICAL INFARCTS & LEUKOENCEPHALOPATHY (CADASIL)

CADASIL is an inherited arterial disease of the brain recently mapped to chromosome 19p13.1. Features of the disorder include recurrent subcortical ischemic events, progressive or stepwise subcortical dementia, pseudobulbar palsy, migraine with aura, and severe depressive episodes. Attacks of migraine with aura occur earlier in life than ischemic events. The diagnosis should be considered in patients with recurrent small subcortical infarcts leading to dementia that also have transient ischemic attacks, migraine with aura, and severe depression. Demented patients exhibit frontal, temporal, and basal ganglia deficits on SPECT scans despite the relative absence of focal neurologic findings.

CEREBRAL AMYLOID ANGIOPATHY

Cerebral amyloid angiopathy is the term given to a condition in which amyloid is deposited on the walls of small arteries and arterioles, weakening the blood vessels and leading to an increased incidence of intracerebral hemorrhage. Amyloid angiopathy can also interfere with blood flow in small vessels and contribute to deep white-matter ischemic changes. The hemorrhages are lobar, may be recurrent, and often occur in patients without hypertension. Cerebral amyloid angiopathy often occurs within the context of Alzheimer disease and is a cause of mixed vascular-Alzheimer dementia.

▶ Clinical Findings

A. Signs and Symptoms

See discussions of individual dementias.

B. Psychological Testing

The neuropsychological deficits in vascular dementias tend to be variable and depend on both the underlying pathology and the location of the lesion. Although memory is almost always affected, executive, subcortical, and frontal lobe functions may exhibit significant deterioration, usually more so in Alzheimer disease. For example, patients with vascular dementia have more difficulty with generating lists of words starting with a specific letter (letter fluency) than with semantic categories, such as animals or flowers. The opposite pattern is typical of AD. The Trails A and B test are also impaired early in vascular dementia, later in AD. Patients with vascular dementias generally have better language function and better memory than do those with Alzheimer disease (unless the language areas are directly affected by strokes).

Neuropsychological findings in vascular dementias depend heavily on the volume and location of the infarct.

Usually, multiple forms of vascular pathology contribute concurrently to the overall findings of vascular cognitive impairment.

C. Laboratory Findings and Imaging

A variety of clinical laboratory findings may be indicated in the investigation of vascular dementias. A complete blood count, sedimentation rate, blood glucose and hemoglobin A1C, fasting lipid panel, and ECG are obtained routinely. Often a carotid Doppler, vascular imaging with CT or MR angiography, transthoracic or transesophageal echocardiogram, and Holter monitor (recording ambulatory ECG) add to the investigation. In some cases, coagulation screen, lupus anticoagulant, anticardiolipin antibodies, and autoantibody screens may be necessary. Cerebral angiography may be necessary to diagnose cerebral vasculitis but is not routinely obtained. If an infection or inflammation is suspected, then a spinal tap may be helpful.

MRI is the most helpful radiologic tool in the diagnosis of vascular dementias, but CT scans may be helpful in some cases. Patchy diffuse white-matter lucency on CT scan or hyperintensity on MRI suggests leukoaraiosis. Normal scans may show lesions that are punctate or partially confluent. The aging brain becomes susceptible to an assortment of changes in the periventricular and subcortical white matter. These changes are radiolucent on CT scans and hyperintense on T2-weighted MRI. White-matter changes are common in patients with chronic hypertension. Examination of affected tissues reveals dilated perivascular (Virchow-Robin) spaces, mild demyelination, gliosis, and diffuse neuropil vacuolation. The associated clinical abnormalities are usually not serious, but defects of attention, mental processing speed, and psychomotor control may be evident, although usually only through neuropsychological testing. As a result, significant overlap occurs between the scans of normal patients and those who have clinically significant vascular disease. These changes also appear in early Alzheimer disease, making the interpretation of early disease more difficult. Leukoaraiosis is associated with increased age, hypertension, limb weakness, and extensor-plantar responses. Some patients have extensive deep white-matter brain lesions without detriment to cognitive, behavioral, or neurologic functioning.

Pathology becomes evident when periventricular capping and plaquelike hyperintensities become confluent. When these changes are at their most severe, the diagnosis of Binswanger disease can be suspected. Lesions that distinguish patients with vascular dementias include definite infarctions, dark on T1- and bright on T2-weighted MRI scans. Irregular periventricular hyperintensities extending into the deep white matter and large confluent areas of deep white-matter hyperintensity likely contribute, but these alone cannot be used to diagnose vascular dementia. These abnormalities are associated with extensive arteriosclerosis, diffuse white-matter rarefaction, and even necrosis. In general, the hyperintensities associated with Alzheimer disease are smaller. A common error is to diagnose vascular dementia rather than Alzheimer disease solely on the basis of T2 hyperintensities on MRI.

A relationship exists between the extent of MRI abnormality and dementia, in population studies, but not in individual patients. MRI white matter abnormalities relate to advanced age and vascular risk factors, and loosely to degree of cognitive impairment. In CADASIL, MRI reveals prominent signal abnormalities in the subcortical white matter and basal ganglia. Cognitive impairment is linked to signal abnormalities and hypoperfusion in the basal ganglia.

^{31}P-NMR spectroscopy profiles may be helpful in the evaluation of vascular dementias. Patients with vascular dementias exhibit elevations of the phosphocreatine/inorganic orthophosphate ratio in temporoparietal and frontal regions.

PET scans may be helpful in diagnosing vascular dementias. They may demonstrate focal areas of hypometabolism that correspond roughly to areas of impairment discovered on neuropsychological testing. Hypometabolism, even without atrophy, is visible on anatomic images. Areas of hypometabolism seen on PET scans conform to cortical high signal intensity on MRI. In addition, cerebral metabolism is reduced globally because isolated lesions have extensive and distant metabolic effects. The pattern of hypometabolism observed in vascular dementias is distinct from that observed in Alzheimer disease. Vascular dementias are associated with multiple defects in the cortex, deep nuclei, subcortical white matter, and cerebellum. Dementia increases as global and frontal hypometabolism evolve. Consequently, PET scans detect more widespread brain involvement than do structural imaging modalities such as CT or MRI. In Alzheimer disease, hypometabolism can involve areas that appear structurally normal on MRI, but in vascular dementia the two imaging modalities correlate better. SPECT scans of patients with vascular dementias show varying degrees of irregular uptake in the cerebral cortex, similar to that seen in PET scans. In SPECT studies of individuals affected with CADASIL, cerebral blood flow reduction matched with MRI signal abnormalities.

EEG often shows focal slowing corresponding to areas of cerebral ischemia or infarction. These areas of slowing may be demonstrated visually on EEG brain maps. Computer-analyzed EEGs use mathematical formulas to break the EEG into power distributions across frequencies. This technique reveals decreased alpha power and increased theta power and delta power that parallel the degree of dementia. The ratio of high-frequency to low-frequency electrical activity in the left temporal region is decreased. Compared to Alzheimer disease, vascular dementias are associated with lower EEG frequency and reduced synchronization. Somatosensory evoked potentials show prolonged central conduction time and a reduction of the primary cortical response amplitude in multi-infarct dementia but not in Alzheimer disease.

▶ Treatment

Prevention is important in vascular dementias. Lifestyle modification, exercise, diet, and risk factor management are the best way of preventing vascular dementia, as they are for avoidance of any dementing illness. Control of hypertension is probably the single most important preventive measure; however, caution must be taken not to lower the blood pressure too much and thus cause hypoperfusion. Control of diabetes, cholesterol and lipid management, and abstinence from cigarettes are also important. Sleep apnea is an independent risk factor for stroke and should be identified and treated. Treatment of atrial fibrillation can prevent embolic strokes. Although anticoagulants are highly effective for preventing cardioembolic strokes, their effectiveness in non-cardioembolic strokes is uncertain. Antiplatelet agents, including aspirin, clopidogrel, or aspirin and extended-release dipyridamole, have been shown to reduce the incidence of second strokes. These agents are likely beneficial also in patients with vascular dementia. Diagnosis and surgical or endovascular treatment of carotid disease is also important in patients with transient ischemic attack (TIA) and stroke secondary to carotid artery stenosis. Pentoxifylline has been tested but has demonstrated limited efficacy. A similar drug, cilostazol, is used extensively in Japan and appears to have a lower bleeding risk than aspirin. In cases of either systemic or cerebral vasculitis, high-dose corticosteroids may prevent further cognitive loss. As yet, no specific agent has been approved for vascular dementia itself, though clinical trials have supported efficacy of anticholinesterase medications.

▶ Prognosis

Vascular dementias shorten life expectancy. Three-year mortality is almost three times greater in the elderly than in age-matched controls. About one third of patients die from dementia itself; the others die from cerebral vascular disease, cardiac disease, or other, unrelated conditions.

CADASIL: *Lancet Neurol* 2008;7:310–318.

Chabriat H, et al: Clinical spectrum of CADASIL: a study of 7 families. Cerebral autosomal dominant arteriopathy with subcortical infarcts and leukoencephalopathy [see comments]. *Lancet* 1995;346:934.

Chui HC, Victoroff JI, Margolin D, et al: Criteria for the diagnosis of ischemic vascular dementia proposed by the State of California Alzheimer's Disease Diagnostic and Treatment Centers. *Neurology* 1992;42:473–480.

Dichgans M, Mayer M, Uttner I, et al: The phenotypic spectrum of CADASIL: clinical findings in 102 cases. *Neurology* 1998;44:731739.

Dichgans M, Markus HS, Stalloway S, et al: Donepezil in patients with subcortical vascular cognitive impairment: a randomized double-blind trial in CADASIL. *The Lancet Neurology* 2008;7:310–318.

Gorelick PB, Erkinjuntti T, Hofman A, et al: Prevention of vascular dementia. *Alzheimer Dis Assoc Disord* 1999;13:S131–S139.

Gorelick PB, Bowler JV: Advances in vascular cognitive impairment. *Stroke* 2010;e9–e98.

Hachinski VC, Iliff LD, Zilkha E, et al: Cerebral blood flow in dementia. *Arch Neurol* 1975;32:632–637.

Hachinski VC, Potter P, Merskey H: Leuko-araiosis. *Arch Neurol* 1987;44:21–23.

Kavirajan H, Schneider LS: Efficacy and adverse effects of cholinesterase inhibitors and memantine in vascular dementia: a meta-analysis of randomized clinical trials. *Lancet Neurol* 2007;6:782–792.

Kirk A, Kertesz A, Polk MJl: Dementia with leukoencephalopathy in systemic lupus erythematosus. *Can J Neurol Sci* 1991;18:344–348.

Kirshner HS: Vascular dementia: a review of recent evidence for prevention of treatment. *Curr Neurol Neurosci Rep* 2009;9:437–442.

Kirshner HS, Bradshaw MJ: The inflammatory form of cerebral amyloid angiopathy or "Cerebral amyloid angiopathy-related inflammation" (CAARI). *Curr Neurol Neurosci Rep* 2015;2015(8):54.

Leys D, Henon H, Mackowiak-Cordoliani M-A: Poststroke dementia. *Lancet Neurol* 2005;4:752–759.

Mayeux R: Risk of dementia after stroke in a hospitalized cohort: results of a longitudinal study. *Neurology* 1994;44:1885–1891.

Moore PM, Richardson B: Neurology of the vasculitides and connective tissue diseases. *J Neurol Neurosurg Psychiatry* 1998;65:10–22.

Robinson RG, Starkstein SE: Mood disorders following stroke: new findings and future directions. *J Geriatr Psychiatry* 1989;22:1.

Rockwood K, Bowler J, Erkinjuntti T, et al: Subtypes of vascular dementia. *Alzheimer Dis Assoc Disord* 1999;13:S59–S65.

Roman GC, Tatemichi TK, Erkinjuntti T, et al: Vascular dementia: diagnostic criteria for research studies. Report of the NINDS-AIREN International Work Group. *Neurology* 1993;43:250–260.

Verhey FRJ, Lodder J, Rozendaal N, Jolies J: Comparison of seven sets of criteria used for the diagnosis of vascular dementia. *Neuroepidemiology* 1996;15:166.

Vermeer SE, Longstreth WT, Koudstaal PJ: Silent brain infarcts: a systematic review. *Lancet Neurol* 2007;6:611–619.

Viswanathan A, Greenberg SM: Cerebral amyloid angiopathy in the elderly. *Ann Neurol* 2011;70:871–880.

Zhang WW, et al: Structural and vasoactive factors influencing intracerebral arterioles in cases of vascular dementia and other cerebrovascular disease: a review. Immunohistochemical studies on expression of collagens, basal lamina components and endothelin-1. *Dementia* 1994;5:153.

NEUROCOGNITIVE DISORDER DUE TO CEREBRAL INFECTION & INFLAMMATION

▶ Essentials of Diagnosis

Infectious processes can cause a sustained, progressive loss of intellectual function. The diagnosis of dementia due to cerebral infection or inflammation is made when the infectious process can be established as a causal agent of the dementia.

▶ General Considerations

Neurosyphilis is the classic dementia due to an infectious process. More recently, the AIDS dementia complex has become the most common form of infectious dementia. Other viral causes of dementia include herpes simplex, COVID-19, progressive multifocal leukoencephalopathy, and subacute sclerosing panencephalitis. Any severe encephalitis can cause a subsequent dementia. Creutzfeldt-Jakob disease is an uncommon cause of rapidly developing dementia caused by a prion, a novel infectious entity that produces a spongiform encephalopathy.

NEUROCOGNITIVE DISORDER DUE TO HIV INFECTION AND OTHER INFECTIOUS AGENTS

Dementia due to HIV disease is often referred to as the AIDS dementia complex, which eventually affects about 15% of AIDS patients.

▶ Clinical Findings

A. Signs and Symptoms

Early in HIV infection, patients are likely to experience an acute encephalitis or aseptic meningitis. In HIV-infected patients, impaired memory and reduced psychomotor speed are more common than is global intellectual deterioration. HIV-induced neuropsychological impairment does not correlate with subjective complaints, neurologic signs, reduced T4 lymphocytes, CSF abnormalities, EEG slowing, atrophy on brain CT scan, or nonspecific hyperintensities on brain MRI. Dementia, cancer of the CNS, and opportunistic infection present later in HIV infection.

AIDS dementia complex is characterized by a clinical triad of progressive cognitive decline, motor dysfunction, and behavioral abnormality. Early symptoms include memory difficulty and psychomotor slowing. Behavioral symptoms include apathy and social withdrawal. It can be difficult to distinguish the AIDS dementia complex from depression, and the pattern of dementia is subcortical. Eventually, cognitive and motor impairment progresses, leading in the final stages to global dementia and paraplegia. Although the AIDS dementia complex may present at any stage of HIV infection, it usually appears relatively late in the course of the disease. Before the introduction of protease inhibitors, the mean survival time in patients with AIDS dementia complex was 7 months.

B. Psychological Testing

Patients with the AIDS dementia complex have a neuropsychological profile consisting of decreased motor speed, decreased memory, and failure on frontal lobe tasks. The HIV Dementia Scale tests specific abilities including timed motor tasks, frontal lobe function, and memory. The test is easy to administer and may be used to follow the patient's progress and response to treatment. Physical findings in the HIV dementia complex include hyperreflexia and hypertonia.

C. Laboratory Findings and Imaging

In the AIDS dementia complex, HIV probably enters the CNS through macrophages that cross the blood-brain barrier. These macrophages infect microglia. In the AIDS dementia complex, the HIV virus can be detected in macrophage- and glial-activated cells in the white matter and deep gray matter. Activated macrophages and microglia probably cause dementia through the secretion of neurotoxins that cause neuronal depopulation and a loss of dendritic arborization. The most common neuropathologic finding is a diffuse destruction of white matter and subcortical gray matter.

Sixty percent of patients show a slightly elevated spinal fluid protein. There may also be an elevated IgG fraction and oligoclonal bands. CSF lymphocytosis may occur; the CD4/CD8 ratio mirrors that of the peripheral blood. HIV can usually be isolated directly from the CSF.

Brain imaging is essential in the evaluation of patients with the AIDS dementia complex because infection with the human immunodeficiency virus-type 1 (HIV-1) predisposes the individual to a number of opportunistic CNS infections and tumors. In order to diagnose the AIDS dementia complex, the clinician must exclude these opportunistic infections, including progressive multifocal leukoencephalopathy, toxoplasmosis, tuberculosis, and cryptococcosis. On MRI and CT scans, the brains of patients with the AIDS dementia complex demonstrate atrophy. MRI shows scattered white-matter abnormalities.

▶ Differential Diagnosis

Diagnostic uncertainty may exist in severe cases. Progressive multifocal leukoencephalopathy produces focal white-matter abnormalities due to multiple foci of demyelination. PET brain imaging techniques help to distinguish opportunistic infections from intracerebral lymphoma.

▶ Treatment

The presentation of neurocognitive disorders due to HIV infection has changed with the dramatic advances in antiretroviral therapy (ART). The symptoms are not as severe but may still affect daily function, quality of life, and treatment adherence. Early initiation of ART prior to advanced immunosuppression is likely beneficial to the central nervous system. ART appears to suppress CSF HIV RNA and inflammation, although neurocognitive impairment may not parallel peripheral response.

▶ Prognosis

In the early stages of the illness, the AIDS patient experiences forgetfulness, lapses in concentration, and social withdrawal.

Cognitive and motor slowing are prominent. The memory problem is mild compared to that observed in Alzheimer disease. Patients retain a relatively good sense of self-awareness and rarely experience the denial of illness that often occurs in other dementias. As the disease progresses, patients become unable to perform activities of daily living. Motor function is affected simultaneously. Patients become unable to walk or require a walker and personal assistance. In the final stages of the disease, patients are nearly vegetative.

NEUROCOGNITIVE DISORDERS DUE TO OTHER VIRUSES

Herpes simplex encephalitis damages the temporal lobes. The disease can present initially with confusion or psychiatric symptomatology. Later the patient develops a severe headache, fever, often seizures, and confusion. MRI and CSF examination are helpful for early diagnosis. A specific EEG pattern is associated with the disorder. Early recognition is essential so that antiviral therapy can be initiated. If the disease progresses, the patient may be left with rather severe cognitive deficits. Klüver-Bucy syndrome, an amnestic syndrome, or global dementia are common residuals of herpetic encephalitis.

Progressive multifocal leukoencephalopathy generally occurs in older immunocompromised patients. It may also occur in the later stages of AIDS. This disorder proceeds extremely rapidly, and death usually occurs within months. Subacute sclerosing panencephalitis is a rare disease of late childhood caused by measles virus. It has become extremely rare since the measles vaccine was introduced. Sporadic encephalitis is another uncommon cause of dementia.

More recently, the world-wide pandemic of COVID-19 has resulted in short-term and long-term cognitive impairment. New-onset dementia has been a consequence of the virus. In addition, it appears that COVID-19 also accelerates the progression of other forms of dementia.

NEUROSYPHILIS

Neurosyphilis, caused by the virus *Treponema pallidum,* was historically a major cause of dementia, but it is a rare diagnosis in the current era. Neurosyphilis presents as a vascular occlusive disease. The meninges may appear thickened and inflamed. Neuroimaging may show infarction, arteritis, cortical lesions, or meningeal enhancement. The basal areas of the brain are preferentially affected, leading to frontal and temporal lobe dysfunction.

▶ Clinical Findings

A. Signs and Symptoms

Neurosyphilis frequently causes psychiatric symptoms such as labile affect, depression, or mania. Patients are usually moderately demented but experience a preponderance of personality disturbances. The Argyll Robertson pupil (the pupil accommodates but does not react to light) is observed occasionally, but many patients become demented without exhibiting this sign. Tabes dorsalis, with posterior column sensory loss and lightening pains, is an associated finding in some patients.

B. Laboratory Findings

A variety of screening tests are used to establish the possibility of syphilitic infection. Once the infection is suspected, a spinal tap is indicated. The diagnosis of neurosyphilis is made by performing the Venereal Disease Research Laboratory (VDRL) test on the patient's CSF.

▶ Treatment

The principal mode of treatment for neurosyphilis is intravenous penicillin. The decision to re-treat a patient who has already had a course of penicillin is difficult to make and is usually based on the patient's clinical response, CSF cell count, and protein concentration. Even after successful treatment of the infection, the patient may continue to have significant deficits. VDRL titer may be an indicator of continued *T. pallidum* activity in patients without obvious clinical deterioration.

▶ Prognosis

Neurosyphilis can occur decades after the original infection. It is not uncommon for an elderly woman to present with this disorder, having been infected many years earlier by her spouse. Early symptoms include fatigue, personality change, and forgetfulness. Neurosyphilis is a great imitator and can produce almost any psychiatric or cognitive disorder. Late in the disease the patient becomes confused and disoriented. Myoclonus, seizures, and dysarthria are common.

NEUROCOGNITIVE DISORDERS DUE TO LYME DISEASE

Lyme disease is a multisystemic illness that can affect the CNS, causing neurologic and psychiatric symptoms. It is caused by the spirochete *Borrelia burgdorferi,* which enters the host after a bite by a deer tick.

▶ Clinical Findings

Lyme disease may involve either the peripheral or the central nervous system. Dissemination to the CNS can occur within the first few weeks after skin infection. Like syphilis, Lyme disease may have a latency period of months to years before symptoms of late infection emerge. A broad range of psychiatric reactions have been associated with Lyme disease, including dementia, psychosis, and depression.

NEUROCOGNITIVE DISORDER DUE TO PRION DISEASE

An unusual infectious agent, known as a prion, leads to Creutzfeldt-Jakob disease (CJD), a condition associated with a rapidly progressive dementia. There are three forms of Creutzfeldt-Jakob disease: infectious, sporadic, and inherited. Formerly, the infectious variety was usually iatrogenic; however, the addition of sheep brain to cow feed in Britain has led to an outbreak of an atypical variant of the disease, bovine spongiform encephalopathy ("mad cow disease") among beef eaters in Britain.

▶ Clinical Findings

A. Signs and Symptoms

The majority of patients with CJD present with myoclonus, exaggerated startle responses, seizures, and pyramidal signs. Although most cases are sporadic, 10–15% are familial. The Gerstmann-Straussler syndrome is a rare familial dementia caused by a prion and related to Creutzfeldt-Jakob syndrome. It resembles a cerebellar degeneration. Spongiform encephalopathy accompanies both Gerstmann-Straussler syndrome and Creutzfeldt-Jakob disease. Mutation in the prion protein (PrP) gene occurs in Gerstmann-Straussler syndrome. Fatal familial insomnia is another rare inherited dementia caused by the prion. Patients with this disorder experience a complete lack of sleep in the year or two prior to death. PrP gene analysis is potentially useful for diagnosis and genetic counseling.

B. Laboratory Findings

Creutzfeldt-Jakob disease is the only dementia that can be distinguished by characteristic electrical patterns. EEG shows triphasic bursts, sometimes correlating with myoclonic jerks. PrP genetic analysis can be helpful in some cases of prion disease. MRI also shows lesions early in the course, often affecting the basal ganglia and cortex; in relatively acute cases, diffusion-weighted MRI shows bright lesions resembling strokes in the cortex and basal ganglia.

▶ Prognosis

Prion disease is uniformly fatal. The time between diagnosis and death is generally less than 2 years, often a matter of a few months. There are no treatments. Because the "mad cow" variant of the disease has been transmitted through careless production and processing of meat, primary prevention of this type is possible. Sporadic cases occur throughout the world.

Geraci AP, Di Rocco A, Simpson DM: Neurologic complications of AIDS. *Neurologist* 2001;7:82–97.

Heaton RK, Franklin DR, Ellis FR, et al: HIV-associated neurocognitive disorders before and during the era of combination antiretroviral therapy: differences in rates, nature and predictors. *J Neurovirol* 2011;17:3–16.

Navia BA, Cho ES, Petito RW: The AIDS dementia complex: II. Neuropathology. *Ann Neurol* 1986;19:517.

Price RW: Management of AIDS dementia complex and HIV-1 brain infection. Clinical-virological correlations. *Ann Neurol* 1995;38:563.

Prusiner SB: Genetic and infectious prion diseases. *Arch Neurol* 1993;50:1129.

Simpson DM, Berger JR: Neurologic manifestations of HIV infection. *Med Clin North Am* 1996;80:1363–1394.

NEUROCOGNITIVE DISORDER DUE TO ANOTHER MEDICAL CONDITION

These neurocognitive syndromes are described by evidence from history, physical examination, or laboratory findings that the condition is a pathophysiological consequence of another medical condition. These include structural disorders such as brain tumors, subdural hematomas or normal pressure hydrocephalus, or metabolic disorders, such as dialysis dementia, hepatic encephalopathy, hypothyroidism, or hypoxia.

VITAMIN B$_{12}$ DEFICIENCY

Vitamin B$_{12}$ deficiency causes subacute combined degeneration, in turn causing demyelination in the posterior columns and loss of pyramidal cells in the motor strip. Often a peripheral neuropathy is present. Slow information processing, confusion, memory changes, delirium, hallucinations, delusions ("megaloblastic madness"), depression, and psychosis have been observed in patients with vitamin B$_{12}$ deficiency.

Anemia is not necessary for the syndrome to develop. Sometimes a familial pattern occurs. Antiparietal-cell antibodies are often present. Current state-of-the-art testing uses serum cobalamin levels as a screening test and serum or urine homocysteine and methylmalonic acid determinations as confirmatory tests. Homocysteine abnormalities are associated with neurologic deficits and psychiatric symptomatology. A Schilling test can be used to determine gastrointestinal absorption of vitamin B$_{12}$ but the test is rarely used anymore.

Depression and dementia respond rapidly to the administration of vitamin B$_{12}$ when the condition is diagnosed in its early stages. Vitamin B$_{12}$ deficiency is treatable with monthly injections, daily oral supplements, or an intranasal gel. If the condition is not diagnosed in the early stages, neurologic, psychiatric, and cognitive impairment may persist and become irreversible. The prevalence of low cobalamin levels is significantly increased in Alzheimer disease. Contrary to widely accepted beliefs, subnormal serum vitamin B$_{12}$ levels are a rare cause of reversible dementia.

Older people frequently have mildly decreased thyroid function. This does not cause an irreversible dementia. In some people, hypothyroidism exacerbates a depression. Thyroid deficiency can also hasten a severe melancholic depression that causes a patient to appear demented. Consequently, thyroid function tests (including thyroid stimulating hormone level) should be obtained. On exceedingly rare occasions, hyperthyroidism or hypothyroidism cause a delirium that can be mistaken for dementia. Patients with vascular dementias often have hypothyroidism. The reason for this association is unclear, but thyroid replacement can improve the performance of patients who have this condition. Finally, the condition known as "Hashimoto encephalopathy" is rarely associated with antithyroid antibodies, even in euthyroid patients, and it can present with encephalopathy, seizures, and ultimately, dementia. Hashimoto encephalopathy is treatable with corticosteroids and immunosuppressive therapies.

Patients who are undergoing dialysis may experience impaired mental functioning that can be secondary to a parathyroid hormone abnormality and its effect on calcium metabolism. Patients who have been on dialysis for extended periods may experience a general decline in intellectual function that is usually mild. True dialysis dementia has become rare since aluminum was eliminated from the dialysate.

Many toxins can cause dementia. Organic solvents inhaled in the workplace cause cognitive deficits. Organic solvents can occasionally cause dementia when used as intoxicants. Carbon monoxide and heavy metals are other toxins that affect mental function. Appropriate history, physical examination, and toxicology evaluation are necessary for the diagnosis of toxin-induced dementias.

Dementia can be caused by the direct or indirect effect of cancer. Patients with cancer develop dementia as a result of intracranial tumors, cerebral metastases, carcinomatous meningitis, progressive multifocal leukoencephalitis, opportunistic infections, and paraneoplastic effects ("limbic encephalitis"). Tumors can lead to noncommunicating hydrocephalus by obstructing the outflow of CSF. Some patients develop progressive dementia as a complication of whole-brain radiotherapy.

NORMAL PRESSURE HYDROCEPHALUS

Normal pressure hydrocephalus causes a relatively distinct syndrome consisting of gait difficulty, sometimes called gait apraxia, urinary incontinence, and dementia. Normal pressure hydrocephalus may be idiopathic, but it may follow a subarachnoid hemorrhage, meningitis, or other entity that can cause altered spinal fluid dynamics. Normal pressure hydrocephalus is the most common type of hydrocephalus diagnosed in people over age 60 years. It occurs when the CSF pressure inside the ventricles is higher than that in the subarachnoid space, and the ventricles expand.

Clinical Findings

The clinical diagnosis of hydrocephalus as a cause of dementia is confusing because many conditions can cause similar symptoms. Nonetheless, a timely diagnosis is important because dementia caused by normal pressure hydrocephalus can sometimes be reversed if the diagnosis is made early enough.

A. Signs and Symptoms

The patient presents the classic triad of dementia, incontinence, and gait disturbance. The dementia is of the subcortical type and often develops at a rapid pace. The patient's gait becomes magnetic in quality, and he or she is likely to experience frequent falls.

B. Psychological Testing

Patients with normal pressure hydrocephalus are impaired on tests designed to detect frontal lobe involvement. The pattern of dementia suggests a subcortical process. Successful ventriculoperitoneal shunt placement improves the patient's cognitive function in 50–67% of cases, in published series.

C. Laboratory Findings and Imaging

The clinical picture associated with vascular dementias can closely resemble that associated with normal pressure hydrocephalus. Unfortunately, MRI findings in patients with normal pressure hydrocephalus overlap those seen in patients who have small vessel disease. Both conditions are associated with increased ventricular size and significant periventricular hyperintensity, as shown on T2-weighted MRI. Normal pressure hydrocephalus differs from small vessel disease in that in the former the MRI can show a large cerebral aqueduct when the pulsation of CSF creates a flow void.

When radioisotope-labeled albumin (RISA) is injected into the lumbar sac (the RISA cisternogram test), it usually diffuses readily over the cerebral convexities. Patients with normal pressure hydrocephalus have abnormal CSF dynamics: Radioactivity appears in the ventricles but is absent over the convexities. Although this test may sometimes be useful, it is not often used today.

Cerebral fluid drainage procedures are sometimes used to help predict whether surgery will be successful. If the patient's gait improves after removal of a large amount of CSF, then the patient is judged to be a better candidate for surgery. Lack of improvement militates against surgery.

Differential Diagnosis

Normal pressure hydrocephalus can be difficult to distinguish from vascular dementias and Alzheimer disease. Although imaging tests help, there is some overlap between the findings of normal pressure hydrocephalus and other forms of dementia. Tests of spinal fluid dynamics help clarify the matter, but ultimately, improvement after shunt placement clarifies the issue. Unfortunately, clinical experience with shunt placement may not be as favorable as that seen in published reports. Improvement may be more transient.

Treatment

Dementia from normal pressure hydrocephalus may respond to shunting, the treatment of choice; however, shunting is associated with significant morbidity. Thus the procedure should probably be carried out only in cases in which the indications are clear and in which the dementia has not progressed to an irreversible degree.

Prognosis

Patients whose normal pressure hydrocephalus has a defined etiology, such as previous head trauma or subarachnoid hemorrhage, respond more reliably to shunting than patients with idiopathic hydrocephalus. Variables associated with a positive outcome from CSF shunting include CSF pressure, duration of dementia, and gait abnormality preceding dementia.

NEUROCOGNITIVE DISORDER DUE TO TRAUMATIC BRAIN INJURY (TBI)

Essentials of Diagnosis

Dementia due to traumatic brain injury refers to a wide range of alterations in thinking, mood, and behavior resulting from specific neurologic damage associated with brain trauma. The severity of the injury is an important determinant of outcome. Specific vulnerabilities such as age, preexisting neurologic or psychiatric disease, and social support determine the ultimate prognosis.

General Considerations

A. Epidemiology

In the United States, 1.7 million TBIs occur annually with 1.4 million emergency room visits and more than 50,000 deaths. Two percent of the population lives with a TBI-associated disability. TBIs are most common among young adult males and most often are the result of automobile accidents. Older adults also represent a significant risk group. Falls are the most common cause of injury in children and older adults. Older adults are more likely than younger adults to have a severe injury. The military has been another source of TBIs, and these have been associated with posttraumatic stress disorder and other psychiatric disorders.

B. Etiology

Head trauma severe enough to cause brief loss of consciousness or posttraumatic amnesia can produce long-lasting cognitive and behavioral changes.

The principal mechanisms underlying traumatic brain injury have been well established. Forces of deceleration and acceleration act within the cranial compartment to produce injury. The swirling movement of brain tissue causes diffuse injury to axons and contusions to cortical areas adjacent to jagged bone. Because the hippocampus is found near the sphenoid ridge, it is especially susceptible to damage when the brain is set in sudden motion. Memory mechanisms fail, and both anterograde and retrograde amnesia follow. The length of posttraumatic amnesia is closely related to the overall severity of diffuse brain damage. The frontal lobes are also susceptible to contrecoup injury. Closed head trauma causes both diffuse and focal brain injury. Subarachnoid hemorrhage and subdural hematoma may produce additional damage, and cerebral edema further complicates the picture.

Beyond structural changes, biochemical alterations also develop. For example, free acetylcholine may appear in large quantities in the CSF, or anoxic damage may produce an increase in CSF lactate.

In recent years the term "chronic traumatic encephalopathy" has been applied to patients in whom repeated minor head injuries lead to dementia. This has been described both in military veterans and in professional athletes such as football players.

▶ Clinical Findings

A. Signs and Symptoms

Fatigue, headache, and dizziness may occur shortly after a mild head trauma. Later a postconcussive disorder may develop. The most significant features of postconcussive syndrome are slowing of information processing, impaired attention, and poor memory.

More severe head injuries are rated according to the Glasgow coma scale. This is a measure of consciousness that analyzes eye opening response, verbal response, and motor response. Head trauma is categorized on this scale as mild, moderate, or severe. The Glasgow coma scale gives a rough judgment regarding prognosis.

Recovery from moderate and severe head trauma is an extremely long process. Recovery is most rapid during the first year or two, and it can continue for many years. In the initial stages of recovery, progress can be followed with the Rancho Los Amigos scale. In the later stages of recovery, measurement of recovery is based on clinical indicators such as return to work.

Recovery from head trauma is also affected by secondary brain injury. Intracranial hematomas, brain edema, and vasospasm affect prognosis by causing occlusion of intracranial vessels, thus producing secondary strokes. Infection, seizures, or metabolic imbalance may affect the postinjury course. Traumatic brain injury produces physical disability ranging from sensory and motor deficits to posttraumatic epilepsy.

In addition, there is usually some deterioration in cognitive ability. Emotional or behavioral deviation usually produces the most significant disability. Some individuals show personality disturbance characterized by anxiety, depression, or irritability. Others may demonstrate a classic frontotemporal syndrome with memory impairment, apathy, lack of motivation, and indifference to the environment. Physicians must consider these emotional difficulties when providing treatment and rehabilitation to these patients.

Chronic traumatic encephalopathy (CTE) has been widely publicized in recent years in the context of multiple concussions in professional football players, though the phenomenon has been recognized for many years in boxers and other victims of multiple traumatic brain injuries. The disorder is still being studied in terms of early symptoms, which often involve depression as well as cognitive deficits, followed by frank dementia.

B. Psychological Testing

Neuropsychological test data are used to develop treatment strategies tailored for an individual's strengths and deficits. Neuropsychological testing can sometimes reveal subtle changes in information processing in patients who otherwise appear normal. A commonly used test is the paced auditory serial addition task. During this exercise, subjects listen to digits presented at a standard rate and add each digit to the one immediately preceding. Head trauma patients are both slower and less accurate than are normal subjects.

Patients with mild to moderate postconcussive disorder may become irritable, or even aggressive, and exhibit blunt affect, apathy, or lack of spontaneity. The effects of mild to moderate head trauma can be subtle, and both patients and practitioners may make light of the cognitive impairment associated with mild head trauma despite sometimes devastating consequences.

In more severe forms of head trauma, neuropsychological testing can be used to measure the extent of secondary injury. To some extent this helps establish the prognosis. Neuropsychological testing can then be used to measure progress. Because cognitive rehabilitation is an important part of recovery, neuropsychological testing can help the psychologist focus on the particular areas of deficit.

C. Laboratory Findings and Imaging

The EEG is sensitive to brain changes following trauma. Local suppression of the alpha rhythm may extend bilaterally. In more severe injury, EEG discharges become progressively slower and delta activity may predominate. The EEG is not a reliable guide to prognosis, and other clinical features must be considered. An EEG that becomes normal early in the course of the illness usually predicts good recovery following head trauma. MRI is invaluable in detecting areas of structural damage.

Treatment

Recovery from head trauma is a dynamic process rather than a static one. As a result, treatment evolves during the course of recovery. In mild head trauma, treatment consists in determining the neuropsychological deficit and giving appropriate counseling. In addition, symptomatic treatment of headaches, dizziness, and mood alteration is useful. Intervention with the patient's employer may help foster understanding and help encourage work conditions that are more conducive to success.

In moderate or severe head trauma, the goals of treatment change as the patient recovers. The early stages of treatment may be directed mainly to suppressing violent outbursts and improving sleep. Later, therapy is tailored to improving memory, impulsiveness, irritability, and affective disorder. Both pharmacotherapy and psychotherapy are useful in this regard. Carbamazepine is generally useful for impulsiveness and may be combined with an atypical neuroleptic. Sleep disturbance may respond to trazodone. The affective disorders respond to SSRIs and other antidepressants. In general, these agents should be started at low doses, with gradual increases. Head trauma patients tend to be sensitive to medication side effects.

Complications/Adverse Outcomes of Treatment

Depression and anxiety are common in outpatients with traumatic brain injuries. These symptoms add to the morbidity of closed head trauma because depressed or anxious patients perceive themselves as more severely disabled. Death by suicide is a risk after head injury, as well as in chronic traumatic encephalopathy.

Alcohol and substance abuse also worsen the outcome of traumatic brain injury. Alcohol intoxication is present in up to one half of patients hospitalized for brain injury. Two thirds of rehabilitation patients have a history of substance abuse preceding their injuries. Untreated substance abuse adversely affects cognitive status in rehabilitation patients.

Repeated head trauma in boxers produces dementia pugilistica. In its fully developed form, the disorder consists of cerebellar, pyramidal, and extrapyramidal features, along with intellectual deterioration. The syndrome may progress even after the boxer has retired from the sport. This syndrome is a particularly severe form of the disorder now called chronic traumatic encephalopathy, increasingly discussed in football players.

Prognosis

Periods of unconsciousness may last several hours yet still be compatible with complete recovery. The longer the patient is unconscious, the poorer the outcome. As the patient recovers

from severe head trauma, a period of confusion may follow lasting from hours to months. Some patients pass through a period of extremely disturbed behavior that poses severe management problems. The patient may be abusive, aggressive, or uncooperative. The patient may appear delirious during this time with vivid auditory and visual hallucinations. When head trauma is associated with prolonged unconsciousness, recovery is usually followed by some degree of dementia. Recovery from mild to moderate head trauma is more variable and difficult to predict.

Dekosky ST, Blennow K, Ikonomovic, Gandy S: Acute and chronic traumatic encephalopathies: pathogenesis and biomarkers. *Nat Rev Neurol* 2013;9:192–200.

Levin HS, et al: Serial MRI and neurobehavioral findings after mild to moderate closed head injury. *J Neurol Neurosurg Psychiatry* 1992;55:255.

McKee AC, Stein TD, Kiernan PT, Alvarez VE: The neuropathology of chronic traumatic encephalopathy. *Brain Pathol* 2015;25:350–364.

Olmez I, Moses H, Sriram S, et al: Diagnostic and therapeutic aspects of Hashimoto's encephalopathy. *J Neurol Sci.* 2013;331:67–71.

NEUROCOGNITIVE DISORDERS & DEPRESSION

Depressed seniors often deny mood disorder and focus on memory problems, complaining of memory loss disproportionate to their actual decrement in memory functioning. Because depressed seniors commonly exhibit impaired attention, perception, problem solving, or memory, psychometric testing may not distinguish depression from Alzheimer disease. This lack of diagnostic clarity has led to the term **pseudodementia**. This term creates unrealistic expectations for a psychiatric cure for dementia. Cognitive disorder seen during late-life affective disorder is real and not simulated. **Depressive neurocognitive dysfunction** is a more accurate term. In most cases, depression is a factor worsening dementia rather than the sole cause.

Essentials of Diagnosis

The cognitive decline encountered in depressed older people is more abrupt and precipitous than in demented patients. The history often reveals previous depression. The combined effects of age and depression produce a pattern of deficits distinct from that found in younger depressed patients and less severe than that in Alzheimer patients. The actual memory impairment is modest in depressed patients, but the level of subjective complaint is high. In contrast, organically impaired patients have more memory loss and less subjective complaints. The cognitive dysfunction encountered in depressed patients is probably secondary to decreased arousal with associated deficits in motivation and attention. Depressed patients do well on simple tasks but poorly on tasks requiring sustained attention or concentration. Following drug treatment, their performance improves. Patients' cognitive complaints correlate with depressive symptoms rather than with MMSE scores. This depressive dementia, however, is not a pseudodementia, as it does encompass genuine cognitive dysfunction. In addition, depression can accompany early stages of dementing illness. Depression should be seen as a treatable component of cognitive impairment in dementia, rather than as an either-or, depressive pseudodementia or true dementia.

▶ Clinical Findings

A. Signs and Symptoms

Patients with depressive neurocognitive disorder often exhibit early morning awakening, anxiety, weight loss, psychomotor retardation, and decreased libido. Patients with dementia present with disorientation, and their daily activities are more seriously impaired. Despite these differences, there is no definitive diagnostic tool. Cognitive decline in depressed older people commonly has a multifactorial etiology. In fact, depression may be the presenting symptom of a degenerative disorder.

B. Laboratory Findings

Sleep studies distinguish depression from dementia with about 85% accuracy. Depressed seniors experience shorter REM latency, higher REM sleep percentage, less non-REM sleep disturbance, and early morning awakening. Patients with Alzheimer disease experience less REM sleep. Computerized techniques, including amplitude frequency measures and spectral analyses, permit new approaches to the examination of delta sleep. Many depressed patients show lower delta wave intensity during the first non-REM period than during the second period. Actigraphy can be used to assess patients' sleeping and walking periods.

Several studies have shown an association between depressive neurocognitive disorder and degenerative dementia. The longer the follow-up, the more likely it is that depressive neurocognitive disorder will evolve into degenerative dementia. Elderly depressed patients also display a remarkable increase in prevalence of cortical infarcts and leukoencephalopathy. Depressed patients tend also to have basal ganglia lesions, sulcal atrophy, large cerebral ventricles, and subcortical white-matter lesions. Nevertheless, Alzheimer disease patients have more prominent cortical atrophy compared to those with major depression.

C. Imaging

PET scans distinguish dementia from late-life depression more clearly than does structural imaging (i.e., CT scan and MRI). The temporoparietal pattern observed in patients with primary degenerative dementia is not observed in those with affective disorder. In severely depressed patients, PET scans show left-right prefrontal asymmetry in resting-state cerebral metabolic rates. Successful drug therapy reduces the asymmetry. In depression, the decrease in glucose metabolism is more pronounced in prefrontal areas, and these changes persist despite clinical improvement, suggesting that the abnormality is not state dependent.

▶ Differential Diagnosis

Both mania and depression can present as pseudodelirium. Vegetative signs are not helpful in distinguishing depression from delirium. Laboratory investigations are required. Mania may present with symptoms of dementia, but delirium is more common. About one quarter of manic patients over age 65 years have no history of affective illness. Cognitive changes often persist even after the patient has "switched" into depression.

▶ Treatment

Treatment with lithium, carbamazepine, or valproate resolves both mania and cognitive impairment. Antidepressant medication for affective disorder is usually effective; however, side effects are troublesome in older patients. Previous treatment response should help guide therapy. Unfortunately, one third of the seniors hospitalized for mania experience a permanent decline in their MMSE scores. This suggests that late-life mania is related to structural changes in the brain.

Because tricyclic antidepressants are likely to cause adverse drug reactions in seniors, SSRIs or serotonin–norepinephrine reuptake inhibitors (SNRIs) are generally preferred. Occasionally, monoamine oxidase inhibitors, alprazolam, and bupropion are useful. For mild depression, SSRIs are first-line agents. Psychostimulants such as methylphenidate and dextroamphetamine present yet another treatment option. These drugs appear to be of particular benefit when used in the short term for the treatment of depression that complicates medical illness.

Lithium is effective in treating bipolar disorder, but its side effect of impairing renal function limits its use. In elderly patients, lithium has a very narrow therapeutic index. Lithium toxicity can occur quickly, damaging already-compromised kidneys. Valproate may be preferred if the patient has a new-onset illness and has not previously been exposed to treatment. If lithium is used, very close monitoring is required.

When other therapies have failed, ECT may reverse pseudodementia or pseudodelirium dramatically. ECT is safe and effective, even in patients older than 80 years or in those with poststroke depression. Common complications of ECT in the elderly include severe confusion, falls, and cardiorespiratory problems.

NEUROCOGNITIVE DISORDERS WITH PSYCHOSIS AND BEHAVIORAL SYMPTOMS

As dementia worsens, behavioral problems emerge. Problem behavior often stems from the inability of staff to understand patients' needs. It is important to identify the cause of the dementia before initiating pharmacologic treatment. Patients can exhibit behavioral disturbances because they are hungry, thirsty, bored, constipated, tired, sexually aroused, or in pain. Patients with dementia, like all of us, need to feel valued, and they benefit from opportunities to develop self-esteem. An initial psychosocial approach to these problematic patients should assess whether these needs are being met.

A multidisciplinary team setting is the most appropriate format for setting treatment goals that are then communicated to the family. It is essential to involve the family in order to educate them and to initiate social interventions. Patients and family members need to believe that a meaningful life is possible despite dementia. This is particularly true if family members are taught to validate the patient's emotional experience. Very little can be gained by approaches aimed at reorientation or enforcing confrontation with reality. Support groups help family members learn not only to cope with the negative outcomes but also to understand their loved one in the context of the illness.

Drug therapy of abnormal behaviors associated with dementia is problematic. First, the anticholinesterase agents and memantine have been demonstrated to improve behavior to some degree. Psychotropic medications must be used cautiously. The Omnibus Reconciliation Act of 1990 introduced specific restrictions on the use of psychotropic medication in the care of nursing home residents. Nonetheless, pharmacotherapy is often essential for treatment of the behavioral disorders that accompany dementia. Psychiatrists are frequently asked to treat agitation in demented patients. Antipsychotics, antidepressants, and sedative-hypnotics are used widely for this purpose; however, data from double-blind clinical trials are limited.

Antipsychotics are effective in some patients with dementia-related psychosis. In many other patients they are of absolutely no benefit and may even be harmful. Although atypical agents have a lower incidence of extrapyramidal side effects including tardive dyskinesia, these newer agents all carry a black box warning regarding an increase in death rate in treated patients. A review of 17 placebo-controlled studies involving four of the atypical antipsychotics showed that the death rate for elderly patients with dementia was about 1.6–1.7 times that of placebo.

There is no evidence that atypical agents offer convincing benefits in this population. Despite many millions of dollars spent by pharmaceutical companies on double-blind placebo-controlled trials, these agents demonstrate limited or no efficacy when compared to placebo. In a large government-funded study (CATIE) of atypical antipsychotics in Alzheimer disease, only 30% of those taking the active medications improved, compared to 21% of those taking placebo. Atypical antipsychotic medications, however, were more often associated with troubling side effects, such as sedation, confusion, and weight gain, compared to placebo. All antipsychotics should be used in the lowest possible dose and for the shortest possible duration. Antipsychotic agents should be reduced periodically or discontinued in order to determine ongoing need. Dementia is a progressive and dynamic process. Patients who required therapy at an early stage of the illness may no longer benefit at a later stage.

Short-acting benzodiazepines control agitation and may be used on occasion in the short term to treat agitation or as a hypnotic in severely demented patients. They can be used in conjunction with antipsychotics. Benzodiazepines are effective for only a minority of patients, and they cause drowsiness, paradoxical agitation, memory loss, an increased risk of falling, and potential habituation. Their use should be reserved for the management of short-term crisis situations in which a rapid response is necessary.

Trazodone has been used to control aggression in demented patients on the theory that aggression is related to serotonergic depletion. Patients generally receive a mild benefit with nighttime doses of 50–100 mg/day. Because some elderly patients experience gait disturbances immediately after the nighttime dose, fall precautions must be taken. Buspirone reduces agitation in dementia in dosages of 20–40 mg/day. Some patients respond preferentially to valproic acid. These patients often have manic symptoms associated with agitation, including pressured speech, flight of ideas, and sleeplessness.

There are few placebo-controlled studies of the drugs used to treat agitation in older people, but the use of psychopharmacology is common in patients who have failed conventional treatment. Carbamazepine or valproate may be best for patients with manic symptoms, buspirone for patients with anxiety, and antidepressants for patients who appear depressed. Because these medications often are given to dementia patients for prolonged periods, studies are needed to define their long-term clinical efficacy.

Some behaviors such as wandering, purposeless repetitive activity, stealing, and screaming are not amenable to pharmacologic intervention. These behaviors must be dealt with by environmental design such as the wander-guard system (a wristband alarm system) and appropriate soundproofing. Clinicians can reduce the occurrence of sundowning by promoting daytime activity, preventing daytime napping, and enforcing a regular sleep schedule. The medical treatment of sundowning can be frustrating; however, sedatives are sometimes helpful.

Burke WJ: Neuroleptic drug use in the nursing home: the impact of OBRA. *Am Fam Phys* 1991;43:2125.

Cummings JL, Schneider E, Tariot PN, et al: Behavioral effects of memantine in Alzheimer disease patients receiving donepezil therapy. *Neurology* 2006;67:57–63.

Flint AJ, van Reekum R: The pharmacologic treatment of Alzheimer's disease: a guide for the general psychiatrist [see comments]. *Can J Psychiatry* 1998;43:689.

Schneider LS, Dagerman KS, Insel P: Risk of death with atypical antipsychotic drug treatment for dementia. Meta-analysis of randomized placebo-controlled trials. *JAMA* 2005;294: 1934–1943.

Schneider L, Tariot P, Dagerman K, et al: Effectiveness of atypical antipsychotic drugs in patients with Alzheimer's disease. *N Engl J Med* 2006; 355:1525–1538.

Sink KM, Holden KF, Yaffe K: Pharmacological treatment of neuropsychiatric symptoms of dementia. A review of the evidence. *JAMA* 2005;293:596–608.

Wang PS, Schneeweiss S, Avorn J, et al: Risk of death in elderly users of conventional vs. atypical antipsychotic medications. *N Engl J Med* 2005;353:2335–2341.

SUBSTANCE/MEDICATION INDUCED NEUROCOGNITIVE DISORDER

KORSAKOFF SYNDROME

Korsakoff syndrome, now usually referred to as the **Wernicke-Korsakoff syndrome**, is a severe anterograde learning defect associated with confabulations. These patients have difficulty encoding and consolidating explicit memory. Storage is mildly impaired, but retrieval and new learning are severely impaired. When Korsakoff patients process new material, they forget information at a normal rate, but learning new material is extremely difficult; in severe cases, new learning is impossible. Retrograde memory is also impaired in Korsakoff syndrome, especially back to the onset of illness and perhaps a period earlier. The most remote memories prior to the onset of illness are spared. As a result, Korsakoff patients retain more distant memories dramatically more proficiently than they learn new material.

Korsakoff patients have little impairment in implicit memory, and their ability to perform motor procedures remains intact. They may retain the capacity to complete complex motor tasks. Typically general intelligence, perceptual skills, and language remain relatively normal. The cardinal symptom of Korsakoff syndrome is confabulation. Although remote memory for events before the neurologic insult is often surprisingly intact, Korsakoff patients are unable to organize memories in a temporal context. Because they distort the relationships between facts, Korsakoff patients have remote memory deficits.

Korsakoff syndrome commonly follows an episode of Wernicke encephalopathy. This neurologic condition is manifested by confusion, ataxia, and nystagmus; thiamine deficiency is its direct cause. If thiamine is given during the acute stage of Wernicke encephalopathy, Korsakoff syndrome can be prevented. The administration of glucose-containing fluid must be avoided, for it will hasten Korsakoff syndrome unless the patient has been adequately dosed with thiamine and recovery has begun. Alcohol abuse causes the conditions that lead to Korsakoff syndrome, but malnutrition alone can cause the disorder, for example, in hyperemesis gravidarum or in patients with surgery for morbid obesity. The lesions caused by thiamine deficiency occur in the hippocampus, the mammillary bodies, and the anterior and dorsal nucleus of the thalamus and disrupt the Papez circuit.

DRUGS & TOXINS

Patients prescribed sedatives, hypnotics, and anxiolytics can develop substance-induced amnestic disorders. Amnestic syndromes usually follow intense, continuous use of these drugs, but recovery usually occurs when the patient stops using the offending agent. Toxins can also cause amnestic disorders. Neurotransmitters involved in memory include acetylcholine, catecholamines, GABA, and glutamic acid. Disruption of these transmitter systems by drugs or toxins also disrupts specific memory functions. Drugs having this effect include benzodiazepines, anticonvulsants, and antiarrhythmics. Amnesia is a characteristic of all the benzodiazepines, with the effect depending on the route of administration, dose, and pharmacokinetics of the specific drug. The amnestic effects of benzodiazepines are sometimes used for therapeutic purposes during surgical procedures. Toxins that affect memory include organophosphates, carbon monoxide, and organic solvents. Chronic exposure to these and other neurotoxins may also affect memory. The patient's ability to recover memory functions depends on the substance, the length of exposure, and other comorbidities.

CONCLUSION

The psychiatrist must use the medical model skillfully to participate fully in the care of patients who have delirium, dementia, or other cognitive disorders. The dual diagnosis of neurologic and affective disorders is more the rule than the exception. In many patients, affective state and optimal cognitive functioning are mutually dependent. The diagnostic skills obtained through the practice of general psychiatry have tremendous value. Treatment of affective disorders and other psychiatric conditions contribute significantly to the patient's ultimate cognitive outcome.

In the care of patients who have delirium and dementia, the boundary between neurology and psychiatry is blurred; the specialties of neuropsychiatry and behavioral neurology have evolved to meet the needs of patients with these disorders. Specific neurologic disorders cause specific neurobehavioral disorders and psychiatric symptoms. Although diagnosis does not determine a cure, it does suggest an appropriate clinical treatment plan. The cost-effective treatment of neuropsychiatric disorders requires a basic understanding of the neurological underpinnings to the disorders. The psychiatrist must have a thorough understanding of the effects of normal aging, delirium, and dementia. Eventually research will uncover prevention techniques based on diet, exercise, antioxidants, or other yet-undiscovered compounds. Until then, the medical model remains the most useful method for the treatment of these mental disorders.

Substance-Related and Addictive Disorders*

Peter R. Martin, MD

CLASSIFICATION OF SUBSTANCE-RELATED AND ADDICTIVE DISORDERS

The substance-related disorders are classified into two categories: (1) substance-use disorders and (2) substance-induced disorders. The substance-use disorders are characterized according to severity based on the number of relevant symptoms that the patient exhibits. The *Diagnostic and Statistical Manual of Mental Disorders,* fifth edition (DSM-5) specifies substance-use disorders that result from the self-administration of several different drugs of abuse.

The specific criteria for diagnosis of substance-use disorders draw heavily on the concept of the **dependence syndrome**. This important advance in our thinking about these disorders frames the interactions among the pharmacologic actions of the drug, individual psychopathology, and the effects of the environment in a clinically meaningful construct that is generalizable to all drugs of abuse. This concept is derived from the clinical observation that patients may have maladaptive behavior as a result of drug use without the presence of overt neurophysiologic adaptive changes such as tolerance or withdrawal (also referred to as **neuroadaptation**). Neuroadaptation is not necessarily dysfunctional if there is no concomitant inappropriate desire (**craving**) to continue the use of the drug (**drug seeking**). For example, driving while drunk may have devastating consequences, particularly in the sporadically drinking young driver who has not acquired tolerance to ethanol. In another example, the patient who receives morphine for pain relief for a limited period postsurgically clearly exhibits neuroadaptation but is not likely to develop the dependence syndrome.

Fundamental to the concept of the dependence syndrome is the priority of drug seeking over other behaviors in the maintenance of dysfunctional drug use. Lesser weight is attributed to the presence of tolerance or withdrawal. In general, two (or more) individual criteria from among the 11 criteria enumerated in DSM-5, which easily fall into the following three symptom clusters, need to be part of the clinical presentation to support the diagnosis of substance-use disorder: (1) **loss of control** (i.e., the substance is taken in larger amounts or over a longer period than intended, or there are unsuccessful efforts to reduce use); (2) **salience to the behavioral repertoire** (i.e., a great deal of time is spent in substance-related activities at the expense of important social, occupational, or recreational activities that are reduced or given up, or there is continued substance use despite knowledge of having a persistent or recurrent physical or psychological problem likely to have been caused or exacerbated by the substance); and (3) **neuroadaptation** (i.e., the presence of tolerance or withdrawal or craving manifested by a strong desire or urge to use a specific substance).

Diagnosis of a substance-use disorder by the presence of a given number of symptoms provides at best an incomplete picture of various clinically important features of the illness, such as severity, course, and prognosis, as well as indicated treatment for this heterogeneous patient population. The issue of illness severity is addressed in DSM-5 by **severity specifiers**, that is, moderate substance-use disorder with two to three criteria and severe with four or more criteria. In order to augment diagnostic sensitivity and also maintain the primacy of drug-seeking behavior, a person can be diagnosed as having a substance-use disorder without ever having exhibited tolerance or withdrawal. In DSM-5, substance-use disorder is formally subtyped according to whether or not there is physiologic dependence (i.e., the presence of tolerance or withdrawal). Finally, to better characterize individual

*This work was supported in part by the National Institute on Alcohol Abuse and Alcoholism (RO1 AA014969) and the National Institute on Drug Abuse (RO1 DA015713 and T32 DA021123).
**Please note that the DSM-5 text revision (DSM-5-TR), the first published revision of the DSM-5 since its publication in 2013, has only very minor changes of relevance to substance use disorders and are mentioned as appropriate in the text.

patients, certain descriptive terms, or **course specifiers**, have been added to distinguish among different clinical courses of substance-use disorder. For example, a patient may be in remission (which may be early or sustained, full or partial), on agonist therapy (e.g., methadone or buprenorphine, a partial μ-opioid receptor agonist–antagonist), or in a controlled environment (e.g., locked hospital ward).

It may be exceedingly difficult to establish whether psychopathology in a given individual who has a substance-use disorder is a consequence of drug use or is due to an additional psychiatric diagnosis. There is a broad overlap between substance-induced disorders and other psychiatric syndromes considered in this book. For example, diverse psychiatric signs and symptoms, including those of delirium (see Chapter 14), psychotic disorders (see Chapters 15 and 16), mood disorders (see Chapter 17), anxiety disorders (see Chapter 18), sexual dysfunction (see Chapter 24), and sleep disorders (see Chapter 26), can have their onset during intoxication or withdrawal. Dementia, amnestic disorder, and flashbacks (recurrences of the intoxicating effects of the drug that may occur years after use) associated with hallucinogen use may persist long after the acute effects of intoxication and withdrawal have abated. Accordingly, it is helpful to determine, preferably by longitudinal observation or by history, the timing of the onset of psychopathology with respect to the initiation of drug use, and whether it is still present when drug use has ceased, recognizing that the duration of abstinence can be a determining variable.

Pharmacotherapy of a complicating psychiatric disorder is most appropriate if it is an independent (i.e., a primary) disorder, but is less likely to be effective if it is a consequence (i.e., a secondary disorder) of a substance-use disorder. The distinction between whether a complicating psychiatric disorder is primary or secondary to substance-use disorder is not easily made, particularly if both disorders started early in life or are historically closely intertwined. Nevertheless, the use of medications with dependence liability per se (e.g., benzodiazepines, methylphenidate, barbiturates, anticholinergics) for the treatment of a coexisting psychiatric disorder may be severely detrimental to the patient. Moreover, some medications may do more harm than good, e.g., administering a selective serotonin reuptake inhibitor (SSRI) to patients with externalizing disorders may result in mood instability and poor impulse control, increasing the likelihood of relapse. On the other hand, anticonvulsants for the treatment of mood instability may have beneficial effects on drug use and also on other psychopathology associated with drug use disorders. Nevertheless, treatment of a secondary disorder is unlikely to be successful if the co-occurring substance-use disorder is not adequately addressed.

The classification approach employed in DSM-5 is not always adequate to describe fully how the dependence syndrome may be modified by diverse factors such as complex drug-use patterns (i.e., more than one drug via different routes of administration), disabilities resulting from drug use (e.g., mood disorders, brain dysfunction, medical complications), or various personality disorders and the sociocultural context of drug use. Physicians cannot ignore these more difficult issues as they communicate with each other and with other health care professionals or as they serve as legal consultants, perform disability assessments, and help develop health care policy.

▶ Use of Psychoactive Substances

Throughout history, members of almost every society have used indigenous psychoactive substances (e.g., opium, stimulants, cannabis, tobacco) for widely accepted medical, religious, or recreational purposes. In more recent times, a wide range of substances (e.g., central nervous system [CNS] depressants and stimulants, hallucinogens, and dissociative anesthetics), synthesized de novo or structurally modified from naturally occurring psychoactive compounds, have also become available for self-administration.

Descriptors of the magnitude and context of psychoactive drug use (e.g., excessive use, abuse, misuse, addiction) represent difficult value judgments. Even if such terms are defined explicitly, they are not likely to be readily generalizable from one society (or group within the society) to another. To demonstrate the arbitrary nature of these terms, one needs only to examine the changes in perceptions of drug use in the United States since the 1960s.

▶ Maladaptive Patterns of Drug Use

Maladaptive patterns of use involve the self-administration of psychoactive agents to alter one's subjective state and experience of the environment, under inappropriate circumstances or in greater amounts than generally considered acceptable within the social constraints of one's culture. Medical diagnosis of substance-related disorders requires meaningful diagnostic criteria that are generalizable across cultures and drugs of abuse. Definition of maladaptive patterns of use in terms of their consequences, presumably less influenced by value judgments, has provided the conceptual basis for DSM-5 diagnostic criteria. Accordingly, considerable weight is placed on behavioral factors rather than on purely medical complications of use or physiologic effects. This conceptual advance, theoretically consistent with the biopsychosocial model of health care, is readily amenable to prevention and has important implications for treatment. The diagnostic focus has shifted from the drug per se to the interactions of drug, individual, and societal factors. Such a perspective is quite different from the traditional medical model of considering drug use as merely a bad "habit" until organ damage is diagnosable, or the social model in which even use sufficient to cause physical complications is not considered an illness.

▶ General Considerations

A. Epidemiology

Surveys conducted by various government agencies at fixed intervals since the 1960s have monitored changes in population attitudes, the prevalence of different types of drug use, health consequences, estimated costs to society, and treatment outcome. Cross-sectional epidemiologic studies are valuable to the clinician, because knowledge of the prevalence of drug-related problems suggests the likelihood that these problems will be encountered in the patient population. For example, a physician may be assisted in the management of an overdose or other drug-related emergency by knowing "what's on the street" at that point in time. Longitudinal population studies of cohorts of drug users are particularly informative with respect to understanding antecedents of substance-use disorders, dose–response relationships for consequences of use, and determinants of effective treatment outcome.

1. Prevalence of drug use—Patterns of drug use change over time, as do the criteria employed to identify problematic use, and contemporaneous prevalence rates can vary according to the epidemiologic survey quoted. Epidemiologic surveys in the United States documented epidemics of marijuana abuse in the 1960s, heroin in the 1970s, and cocaine in the 1980s. Although no single drug captured society's imagination in the 1990s, opioid dependence, particularly nonmedical use, has been on the rise in the past two decades, and along with methamphetamine was perceived to have reached "epidemic" proportions in the new millennium to the present. Furthermore, epidemiologic studies have documented an upward trend in the usage of all drugs and alcohol during the 1970s, followed by a downward trend in the 1980s; this trend reversed and then stabilized in the 1990s and has again been on the rise in the new millennium. An ongoing epidemic of overdose deaths from opioids combined with central nervous system depressants like alcohol and benzodiazepines and stimulants like methamphetamine, climbing precipitously since the 2010s in the United States, is unprecedented and has reduced the life expectancy in the population. Knowledge about the prevalence of **drug use** is highly predictive of the proportion of the population that will develop a **drug use disorder** (see later discussion).

Although Americans use alcohol more often than they do any other drug, younger individuals tend to combine alcohol with multiple illicit drugs. Older cohorts (age 35 years and older) frequently use alcohol alone, or with prescribed drugs of abuse. According to the 2021 National Survey on Drug Use and Health (Table 16–1), 133 million Americans (47.5% of the population aged 12 years and older) reported being current drinkers of alcohol (at least one drink in the past month). An estimated 60.0 million (21.5%) were binge drinkers (five or more drinks within a couple of hours of

Table 16–1 Prevalence of Substance Use in Last Month (Per 100 Persons Aged 12 Years or Older)

Drug	Prevalence (%)
Alcohol	47.5
• Binge drinker*	21.5
• Heavy drinker**	5.8
Tobacco	22.0
An illicit drug	14.3
• Marijuana	13.0
• Cocaine	0.7
• Methamphetamine	0.6
• Hallucinogens	0.8
• Heroin	0.2
Nonmedical use of psychotherapeutic drugs	1.5
• Pain relievers	0.9
• Tranquillizers	0.5
• Stimulants	0.4
• Sedatives	0.1

*Defined as having five or more drinks on the same occasion on at least 1 day in the 30 days prior to the survey.

**Defined as binge drinking on at least 5 days in the past 30 days. Adapted from Substance Abuse and Mental Health Services Administration. Results from the Substance Abuse and Mental Health Services Administration (2022). Key substance use and mental health indicators in the United States: Results from the 2021 National Survey on Drug Use and Health (HHS Publication No. PEP22-07-01-005, NSDUH Series H-57). Center for Behavioral Health Statistics and Quality, Substance Abuse and Mental Health Services Administration.

each other at least once in the past 30 days), and 16.3 million (5.8%) were heavy drinkers (five or more drinks on the same occasion on at least 5 different days in the past 30 days). An estimated 61.6 million persons (22.0%) reported use of the other legal drug, tobacco.

An estimated 40.0 million (14.3% of the U.S. population aged 12 or older) used an illicit drug during the month prior to the survey. Marijuana is the most prevalent illicit drug by far, used by 36.4 million in the past month. An estimated 9.0 million people (3.2%) were current users of illicit drugs other than marijuana. Most (4.3 million) used psychotherapeutic drugs nonmedically. An estimated 2.4 million used pain relievers, 1.2 million used tranquilizers, 1.1 million used stimulants, and 227,000 used sedatives. An estimated 1.8 million persons were current cocaine users; hallucinogens were used by 2.2 million persons; and 589,000 were current heroin users. National data have consistently shown that substance-use and use disorders are most prevalent among the young (age 18–34 years) and that the highest rates are observed in young men.

2. Prevalence of substance-use disorders—According to the National Comorbidity Survey, the first survey to be administered in the early 1990s using a structured psychiatric interview (Composite International Diagnostic Interview) to a nationally representative household sample of over 8000 respondents, the lifetime prevalence rate of a substance-use disorder (except for use of nicotine or caffeine) was 19.5 per 100 persons 18 years and older. Drugs covered by this survey included alcohol, tobacco, sedatives, stimulants, tranquilizers, analgesics, inhalants, marijuana/hashish, cocaine, hallucinogens, heroin, nonmedical use of prescription drugs, and polysubstance use. Alcohol abuse or dependence (combined as alcohol use disorder in DSM-5) was identified in 13.2% of the population during their lifetime, and drug abuse or dependence in 8% of the population. According to the 2021 National Survey on Drug Use and Health, an estimated 24.0 million persons (8.6% of persons 12 years and older) were classified as having drug use disorder in the past year (Table 16–2). Of these, 7.3 million had both alcohol and drug use disorders; 16.7 million had only a drug use disorder; and 22.2 million had only an alcohol use disorder. Of the 20.1 million persons classified as having an illicit drug use disorder, 2.9 million met criteria for misuse of prescription psychotherapeutics, including 1.9 million for disordered use of pain relievers; 2.5 million for misuse of opioids; and 3.4 for misuse of central nervous system stimulants. Most other illicit drugs were used in combination with alcohol, marijuana, cocaine, or opioids and by a relatively small proportion of the population who met criteria for substance-use disorder. Of note, due to legislative changes in some jurisdictions, marijuana is not considered among the illicit drugs as it was previously.

3. Risk of co-occurring psychiatric diagnoses—According to the National Institute of Mental Health Epidemiologic Catchment Area Survey, in which 20,291 persons representative of the U.S. community and institutional population were interviewed, the odds of having a mental disorder were 2.7 times greater if one also had a substance-use disorder (excluding nicotine or caffeine) in comparison with no drug-use disorder. Drug-use disorders occurred at higher rates in individuals who had alcohol use disorder (21.5%) than in those who did not (3.7%). Alcohol use disorders were more prevalent among those who met criteria for drug use disorder (47.3%) than among those who did not (11.3%). Specific psychiatric diagnoses, such as major depressive disorder, schizophrenia, anxiety disorders, and especially bipolar affective disorder and antisocial personality disorder, have been associated with substance-use disorders in epidemiologic studies, leading to theories of related pathogenesis. For example, according to the 2021 National Survey on Drug Use and Health, persons with a major depressive episode (MDE) in the previous year were twice as likely (44.7% vs. 20.7%) as those without MDE to have used an illicit drug in the past year. Similar patterns were observed for specific illicit drugs in the previous year, such as marijuana, cocaine, heroin, hallucinogens, inhalants, methamphetamine, as well as for the misuse of prescription psychotherapeutics (pain relievers, stimulants, and tranquilizers or sedatives). However, persons with MDE in the past year had similar rates of heavy alcohol use (8.7% vs. 6.2%) as those without MDE. The rate of daily cigarette use was 1.3 times greater in those who had MDE in the last year.

Persons with MDE were more likely than those without MDE to have a drug use disorder (25.5% vs. 7.3%) and alcohol use disorder (22.7% vs. 10.3%). Among persons with substance-use disorder, 39.1% had at least one MDE in the past year compared with 22.4% who did not have at least one MDE. An important caveat for interpreting these associations is that for many individuals with substance-use disorders and MDE, the depressive episode can, and often does, represent the depressed phase of an unrecognized bipolar illness, not major depressive disorder.

Such associations suggest that the clinician should have a high index of suspicion for substance-use disorders when dealing with clinical populations diagnosed with mental disorders. The clinician should also be circumspect about prescribing psychoactive medications with dependence liability to these patients.

B. Etiology

The etiology of substance-use disorders has been conceptualized in terms of an integration of biological, psychological, and social theories. A recent advance has been recognition of shared clinical features, similar biopsychosocial

Table 16–2 Prevalence of Substance-Use Disorders During the Previous Year (Per 100 Persons Aged 12 Years or Older)*

Substance-Use Disorder	Prevalence (%)
Any substance-use disorder	16.5
• Alcohol abuse or dependence, no illicit drug-use disorder	7.9
• Illicit drug abuse or dependence, no alcohol use disorder	6.0
• Alcohol and illicit drug abuse or dependence	2.6
—Marijuana abuse or dependence	5.8
—Cocaine abuse or dependence	0.5
—Opioid abuse or dependence	2.0

*Prevalence rates obtained using DSM-IV criteria in which construct substance-use disorder is dichotomized as abuse (mild substance-use disorder) or dependence (moderate/severe substance-use disorder). Adapted from Substance Abuse and Mental Health Services Administration. Results from the Substance Abuse and Mental Health Services Administration (2022). Key substance use and mental health indicators in the United States: Results from the 2021 National Survey on Drug Use and Health (HHS Publication No. PEP22-07-01-005, NSDUH Series H-57). Center for Behavioral Health Statistics and Quality, Substance Abuse and Mental Health Services Administration.

underpinnings, and frequent co-occurrence of substance-use disorders and so-called behavioral addictions, such as pathological gambling, problematic hypersexuality, and obesity or other eating disorders. In DSM-5, such behavioral addictions are termed non-substance-related addictive disorders. Gambling disorder is the only accepted entity in this category to date.

1. Individual vulnerabilities—The major goal of any etiologic theory is to explain why, in the face of widespread availability of drugs and alcohol, certain individuals develop a substance-use disorder, and others do not. This is a gargantuan task because these are complex and multifaceted disorders. Substance-use disorders are heterogeneous disorders that represent the final common pathway for a variety of behavioral difficulties in diverse sociocultural contexts. Also, circumstances or causes that result in these disorders may differ among individuals. Equally difficult to understand is why in some patients, substance-use disorders continue inexorably to death despite treatment, whereas in others, drug use can be decreased or stopped (either spontaneously or with treatment). Therefore, substance-use disorders are perhaps most usefully conceptualized in terms of multiple simultaneous variables interacting over time.

The fact that not all individuals who self-administer psychoactive agents, during given developmental stages or life circumstances, progress to repeated out-of-control and problematic use has led to the search for factors that determine individual vulnerability. Biological factors that may contribute to the development of substance-use disorders include interindividual differences in (1) susceptibility to acute psychopharmacologic effects of a given drug; (2) metabolism of the drug; (3) cellular adaptation within the CNS to chronic exposure to the drug; (4) predisposing personality characteristics (e.g., sensation seeking, poor impulse control, difficulty delaying gratification, or antisocial traits); and (5) susceptibility to medical and neuropsychiatric complications of chronic drug self-administration. Psychological factors—such as the presence of co-occurring psychopathology (e.g., depression, anxiety, attention-deficit/hyperactivity disorder, psychosis, pathological gambling, eating disorders, or problematic hypersexuality); medical illnesses (e.g., chronic pain, essential tremor); or past or present severe stress (e.g., resulting from crime, battle exposure, sexual trauma, or economic difficulties)—have received considerable attention as potential causes for "self-medication." The possibility exists that susceptibility to psychological stressors and substance-use disorders may have similar etiologies. For example, some of the etiologic factors that predispose an individual to depression following major losses (e.g., dysregulation of noradrenergic neurotransmission or the hypothalamic–pituitary–adrenal axis) may also contribute to the development of substance-use disorders. Similarly, prefrontal cortical dysfunction due to impaired connectivity of regulatory brain circuits

manifested clinically by impulsiveness or poor decision making is observed in individuals diagnosed with either pathological gambling or cocaine dependence. Finally, social factors also contribute to the initiation of drug use and progression of substance-use disorders. Such social factors include peer group attitudes toward and shared expectations of the benefits of drug use (such as enhanced pleasurable activities with drug use); the availability of competing reinforcers to substance use in the form of educational, recreational, and occupational alternatives; and the availability of drugs during vital developmental stages.

The fact that individuals often use more than one drug simultaneously, or give a history of having used different drugs at different times during their lifetime, has led to an emphasis on the similarities rather than the differences among abused substances with respect to the ontogeny of drug-use behaviors. Further, the stepwise development of different substance-use disorders over time suggests common mechanisms of susceptibility and generalizable diagnostic criteria and treatment strategies. Likewise, the co-occurrence and parallel life courses of substance-use disorders and other out-of-control and self-destructive behaviors, such as pathological gambling, problematic hypersexuality, and overeating have pointed to shared abnormalities of fundamental brain reward (drive) mechanisms that may be generalized beyond drug self-administration.

i. Drug-seeking behavior—Conceptualization of substance-use disorders in terms of the biopsychosocial model, rather than as simply the physiologic consequences of chronic drug use, has led to recognition of the central role of conditioning and learning. The behavioral perspective provides a framework for understanding the entire spectrum of psychoactive substance use, from its initiation to its progression to compulsive drug use, as well as the acquisition of tolerance and physical dependence; it also explains how co-occurring psychopathology so frequently influences the clinical course of substance-use disorders. Psychopharmacologic processes that initiate, maintain, and regulate drug-seeking behavior include (1) the positive reinforcing and discriminative effects of drugs, (2) the environmental stimuli associated with drug effects (which facilitate drug seeking), and (3) the aversive effects of drugs (which extinguish drug seeking) (Figure 16–1). These processes change over the life cycle and the course of the disorder and are modulated by social, environmental, and genetic factors such as the individual's personal history, the presence of psychopathology (e.g., anxiety, depression, thought disorders), and the individual's previous exposure to (expectancy of) psychoactive drugs. For example, a youngster may first use alcohol/drugs (initiation of use, Figure 16–1) for novelty or to allow them to overcome shyness to approach a member of the opposite sex at a dance (Reinforcers, Figure 16–1); if this is effective, drug seeking will continue and the youngster may repeatedly engage in this behavior in many other social situations

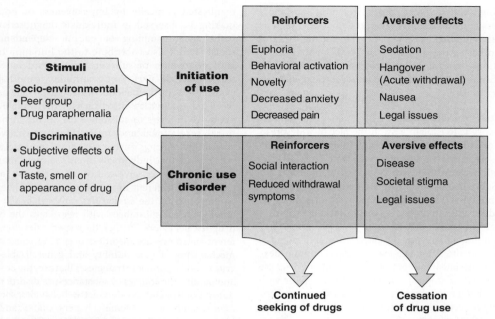

▲ **Figure 16–1** The characteristics of drug-seeking behaviors change over the clinical course of drug use disorders. Reinforcers and aversive effects are different at the initiation of drug use and at the point when the individual has been using the drug over many years and has developed a drug use disorder. This is related to plastic changes in brain reward circuits and psychosocial characteristics of the individual which typically occur with extended periods of use of the drug in question. (Adapted from Munson P, Mueller RA, Breese GR. *Principles of Pharmocology: Basic Concepts and Clinical Applications.* New York: Chapman & Hall; 1995.)

until neuroadaptive brain changes develop that make this a routine activity in their behavioral repertoire. On the other hand, this same youngster might become very ill and need to be taken to the hospital emergency room due to vomiting or passing out or might get into legal difficulties like driving while intoxicated (Aversive effects, Figure 16–1); any of these untoward consequences may lead to vowing to never use again (Cessation of drug use, Figure 16–1). In contrast, a middle-aged individual who has been drinking for decades and has developed a chronic use disorder may only find social support in their local bar and this contributes to continued drinking (Reinforcers, Figure 16–1). Continued drinking may keep them from developing the shakes and other distressing withdrawal symptoms should alcohol drinking stop. However, this individual may be able to reduce their use if the physician warns them of the adverse effects on health of continued alcohol or if they are incarcerated due to a crime committed while intoxicated (Aversive effects, Figure 16–1). The neural mechanisms and behavioral factors that influence psychoactive drug use are amenable to detailed analysis using drug self-administration models in laboratory animals, in which the neuropharmacology and neuroanatomy of the brain systems that mediate reward can be explored.

ii. **Drug intoxication**—Individual factors that affect the quality and magnitude of intoxication also influence drug reinforcement, and ultimately, the development of substance-use disorders. Among these are variables such as initial tolerance, previous experience with the drug, the social context of administration, and presence of disorders that affect CNS responses to the drug or disorders of other organs that determine the brain concentration of the drug. Direct adverse consequences of acute intoxication are predictable from the pharmacologic actions of the drug. For example, CNS depressants have a spectrum of dose-related effects from initial disinhibition at low doses to stupor and coma at higher doses. Similarly, CNS stimulants enhance arousal, attention, and performance at low doses but can lead to psychomotor agitation, psychotic disorganization, and convulsions at higher doses. Often the most serious consequences of these agents are indirect effects, namely, impaired performance or judgment, which can cause automobile or work-related accidents, drug-related violence, or unprotected sexual activity. Finally, the route of drug administration can greatly influence intoxication. For example, both intravenous administration and smoking result in rapid entry of the drug into the brain with intense but relatively short-lived euphoria; for highly reinforcing drugs (e.g., cocaine, opioids), this can result in compulsive use in a binge-like manner. Nasal insufflation, subcutaneous administration ("skin popping"), and oral ingestion result in relatively slower access to the drug's site of action in the brain, with greater variability in drug bioavailability and less reinforcement.

iii. Neural mechanisms—Investigation of the neural pathways that mediate the powerful (positive) reinforcing effects of drugs of abuse have implicated dopamine, opioid, glutamate, and gamma-aminobutyric acid (GABA) systems within a midbrain-forebrain-extrapyramidal reward circuit with its focus in the nucleus accumbens. The connections of the ventral midbrain and forebrain, commonly called the medial forebrain bundle, are a major conduit for hypothalamic afferents and efferents and also support (more than any other brain region) the repeated self-administration of current through electrodes (an intracranial self-stimulation model of addiction). This system modulates, or filters, signals from the limbic system that mediate basic biological drives and motivational variables, convert emotion into motivated action and movement via the extrapyramidal system, and may also be the neuronal substrate for the rewarding effects of drugs of abuse. It has been hypothesized that the mesocorticolimbic dopamine system may be critical in mood arousal associated with the anticipation of reward, and that all addictive drugs have a psychostimulant (dopaminergic) action as a common underlying mechanism that contributes to reinforcement. Therefore, drugs of abuse activate neural pathways evolved to guide an organism through the challenges of the environment by reinforcing behavior essential for the survival of the species. If drugs of abuse are repeatedly administered, these reward circuits may cease to shape survival behavior effectively.

iv. Behavioral mechanisms—The effects of drugs that mediate their positive reinforcing influence are desirable changes in mood (euphoria), alleviation of negative affective states (e.g., anxiety, depression), functional enhancement (e.g., improved psychomotor or cognitive performance), and alleviation of withdrawal symptoms. It is difficult to understand why certain psychoactive drugs with profound aversive effects can nonetheless maintain drug-seeking behavior and have dependence liability. Aversive effects of drugs counteract the tendency toward self-administration and may limit drug use if they result in dose-dependent toxicity. For example, initial exposure to nicotine in the form of cigarettes often results in distressing symptoms, such as coughing, nausea, and lightheadedness, which may terminate smoking. Similarly, severe gastritis in the chronic alcoholic patient may result in attempts to cut down drinking or limit continued alcohol ingestion. It is now recognized that the stimulus properties of most drugs of abuse, a major determinant of drug-seeking behavior, are complex and multifaceted. Specifically, their pharmacologic profiles include both positive reinforcing and aversive components, and their effects are modified readily by associated environmental stimuli and individual differences among drug users.

If a drug is repeatedly administered under given circumstances (situation, time, place), environmental stimuli can become associated with effects of the drug by means of classical (Pavlovian) conditioning. Subsequently, the circumstances under which the drug was administered (without actual presentation of the drug) comprise certain environmental (conditioned) stimuli that can modify drug-seeking behavior, subjective state, or psychophysiologic responses (conditioned reinforcement). For example, patients who have abstained from intravenous heroin for many years can experience a desire to use heroin when they return to the location where they previously used or when they view a film that portrays others who are injecting drugs intravenously. Using positron emission tomography (PET), researchers have shown that in dependent patients, dopaminergic activation accompanies the presentation of relevant cues from the environment or the anticipation of drug (without its administration). Moreover, similar patterns of brain activation are demonstrable using functional magnetic resonance imaging (fMRI) when a subject is presented cues related to highly rewarding behaviors that do not involve drug self-administration, such as gambling, sexual activity, and food. The importance of conditioned stimuli in the response to drugs is also demonstrated readily in laboratory animals by tolerance after a drug is tested in an environment in which it was administered previously that is greater than in a distinctly different environment.

2. Neuroadaptation—Neuroadaptation refers to the neuronal changes and consequent clinical signs and symptoms that result from repeated drug administration independent of drug-seeking behavior or use-related organ damage. It encompasses the biological substrata of tolerance and physical (as opposed to psychological) dependence.

i. Tolerance—After repeated exposure to many psychopharmacologic agents, individuals require a larger dose to produce intoxication of the magnitude that was experienced when the drug was first administered. Conversely, less intoxication results from doses of the drug that were used initially. This phenomenon, called tolerance, is a pharmacologic characteristic shared by many of the substances of abuse considered in DSM (particularly the CNS depressants and the opioids). Tolerance allows and may encourage progressively greater doses to be self-administered. (After repeated exposure to CNS stimulants, reverse tolerance, or a greater pharmacologic effect, may be observed.) Tolerance is an adaptive physiologic response of the intact organism that opposes the pharmacologic effects of the drug. The mechanistic underpinnings reside in molecular changes at the cellular level and in interactions between the organ systems of the body. The components of tolerance include (1) increased capacity for clearance of a drug by metabolizing enzymes in the liver (pharmacokinetic or metabolic tolerance), (2) reduced response from the same drug concentration (functional or pharmacodynamic tolerance), and (3) accommodation to drug effects through learning (behavioral or learned tolerance). Tolerance to one CNS depressant usually results in some cross-tolerance to other (sometimes chemically unrelated) CNS depressants. Tolerance accelerates dose-related complications of drug use.

Acquired tolerance should be distinguished from sensitivity to a given drug on first administration and from acute tolerance that develops over the course of a single exposure to the drug. Differences in the population in initial or acute tolerance to a given drug are innate characteristics of the CNS that may influence individual vulnerability to the development of psychoactive substance-use disorders.

ii. Dependence—Traditionally, dependence refers to the neuronal changes (neuroadaptation) that develop after repeated exposure to a given agent, the clinical syndrome characterized by out-of-control drug use, and the serious biopsychosocial consequences that accompany these neuronal changes. At present, dependence can be defined only indirectly in terms of (1) the presence of tolerance or the emergence of a withdrawal syndrome (immediate and protracted) upon drug discontinuation (physical dependence) and (2) the craving or drug-seeking behavior manifested because of conditioned stimuli (psychological dependence). The dependence syndrome represents the elements of psychological dependence, including drug seeking and psychosocial consequences of drug use. Physical dependence usually develops in concert with tolerance, and controversy remains over whether physical dependence and tolerance are simply different manifestations of the same neuronal changes. The reacquisition of both tolerance and physical dependence are accelerated following repeated cycles of drug administration and withdrawal, suggesting certain similarities between these phenomena and learning and memory. Furthermore, the reinforcing and aversive effects of drugs may differ considerably at different stages in progression of a substance-use disorder (see Figure 16–1).

iii. Withdrawal—Upon discontinuation of chronic administration of many psychoactive agents (or administration of a specific antagonist), a withdrawal (abstinence) syndrome emerges as drug concentrations (or receptor occupancy) at the pharmacologic sites of action decline. This syndrome is characterized by a spectrum of signs and symptoms that are generally opposite to those of intoxication and whose severity is related to the cumulative dose (dosage and duration of administration). For example, withdrawal from CNS depressants results in CNS hyperexcitability, whereas withdrawal from psychostimulants causes CNS depression. For most drugs of abuse, the withdrawal syndrome also involves homeostatic responses. These represent reversal of the neuroadaptive changes that occurred with long-term drug administration, resulting in significant activation of the autonomic nervous system in the equivalent of a stress response.

iv. Cellular & molecular mechanisms of neuroadaptation—Advances in neuroscience, such as the development of specific receptor antagonists, electrophysiological and brain imaging techniques, and molecular methods to measure subtle cellular alterations including gene expression, have enhanced our fundamental understanding of neuroadaptation. Neuroadaptation can be conceptualized not only in terms of the intact organism (of relevance to understanding the clinical signs and symptoms of withdrawal), but also at the level of neuronal signal transduction, which can be studied in vitro and in animal models. Changes in synaptic membrane composition, receptor function, and post receptor intracellular events including gene regulation have all been proposed as the basis of neuroadaptation to psychoactive drugs of abuse. For example, acute alcohol exposure fluidizes cell membranes, but chronic alcohol exposure results in alterations in the lipid composition that render synaptic membranes more rigid and alters the environment and affinities of neurotransmitter receptors. The inhibition by cocaine of dopamine reuptake leads to increased intrasynaptic dopamine, subsequent depletion of presynaptic dopamine due to reduced synthesis of the neurotransmitter, and eventual upregulation (enhanced sensitivity) of postsynaptic dopamine receptors. Finally, in rats, chronic morphine administration increases G proteins, cyclic adenosine monophosphate–dependent protein kinase, and the phosphorylation of a number of proteins, including transcription factors which regulate gene expression. Emerging evidence points to such functional changes occurring specifically in neurons of the reward pathways following administration of many of the drugs of abuse, as well as natural reinforcers. Such a common pathway of responses is akin to the molecular-level alterations that occur during learning and memory. Keys to molecular changes during acute drug administration and during neuroadaptation have clear implications for the pharmacotherapy of alcohol/drug use disorders and withdrawal.

C. Genetics

The clinical features and course of alcohol use disorder have been studied more extensively than have those of other substance-use disorders. Alcohol use disorder provides a heuristically useful paradigm for understanding the genetic factors that contribute to the development of most substance-use disorders. In fact, recent studies show shared genetic factors associated with alcohol and other drug use disorders. As discussed earlier in this chapter, individual vulnerabilities to substance-use disorders span biological, psychological, and social domains. These domains are tightly interrelated and can influence one another, such that it may be difficult to unravel the role(s) of single variables. Furthermore, substance-use disorders in family members disrupt family life in countless ways, thereby affecting developmental processes in children within the family. It is not surprising, therefore, that higher than normal rates of alcohol or drug use disorders, as well as of other forms of psychopathology, exist among children of these families. In addition to these environmental factors, genetic factors also play a role in the familial predisposition to substance-use disorders. However, it is recognized that **interactions** of the genetic and environmental factors associated with substance-use disorders may be more important than either of these factors alone.

1. Inheritance of alcohol use disorder—Findings from twin and adoption studies demonstrate the relative contributions of genetic and environmental factors in predisposition to alcohol use disorder. For example, the concordance rate for severe alcohol use disorder is substantially higher in monozygotic (0.70) than dizygotic (0.33) twins, whereas concordance rates are no different for less severe forms of the disorder (0.8 for both monozygotic and dizygotic twins). Adoption studies show that adopted-away men with alcoholic biological parents have an increased likelihood of developing alcoholism regardless of whether they are raised in an alcoholic or nonalcoholic environment. In general, the severity of parental alcoholism tends to influence the prevalence of alcoholism in adopted-away sons; patients with the most severe alcoholism have the highest rates of alcohol use disorder in their offspring. These studies suggest that the relative contributions of environmental and genetic factors in development of alcoholism may vary with the severity or type of alcohol use disorder.

2. Heterogeneity of alcohol use disorder—As discussed earlier in this chapter, groups of alcoholic patients are heterogeneous. The challenge in genetic studies of alcohol use disorder has been to identify homogenous subgroups of alcoholic patients. Clearly defined phenotypes in patients (and their families) could then be studied in depth to identify predictors of etiology, longitudinal course, and response to treatment. One heuristically useful classification is based predominantly on age at onset of alcohol use disorder: onset after age 25 (type 1) and onset before age 25 (type 2). Reliably different clusters of alcohol-related problems and personality traits tend to occur with these two subtypes of alcohol use disorder. In general, patients with type 2 alcoholism are characterized by thrill seeking, impulsiveness, and aggressiveness, whereas those with type 1 alcoholism have a greater tendency to become anxious and depressed due to their drinking. Type 2 alcoholism tends to be more recalcitrant to treatment than is type 1 alcoholism.

Both genetic predisposition and an alcoholic rearing environment were required for adopted-away sons of fathers with type 1 alcoholism to express type 1 alcoholism. In contrast, adopted-away sons of fathers with type 2 alcoholism were significantly more likely to manifest this type of alcohol use disorder than were the offspring of fathers without type 2 alcoholism, whether or not they were raised in an alcoholic family. This observation indicates that the genetic loading for alcohol use disorder is influenced profoundly by the environment in the case of late-onset alcohol use disorder, whereas environmental background is relatively less important for early-onset alcoholism.

3. Women & addiction—There are distinct differences between the genders in the inheritance, clinical presentation, and the longitudinal course of alcohol use disorder. It is particularly important to understand alcohol use disorders in women because of the adverse effects of drinking on the developing fetus, and the disruptive effects of alcohol on the mother–child relationship. Both these consequences of alcohol consumption in women can perpetuate the transmission of alcohol use and other psychiatric disorders from one generation to the next via mechanisms that are not strictly genetic but rather environmental or epigenetic.

Women have lower rates of alcohol use disorder compared to men, although these rates are rising at a disquieting pace. Lower rates of alcohol use disorder result in part from the smaller amounts of alcohol consumed by women in general, for several psychosocial and biological reasons. Even though women start drinking later than men, they tend to develop, at about the same age as men, more serious physical complications. These observations suggest greater intrinsic toxicity of ethanol to the liver, brain, and possibly other organ systems of women compared to men. This "telescoping" of the clinical course in women is characteristic of the clinical courses of most other drug use disorders as well. Established gender-related differences in predisposition to co-occurring psychopathology (e.g., depression and somatic anxiety) may complicate and exacerbate alcohol use disorder. Daughters of fathers with type 1 alcoholism are at increased risk for alcoholism but not for other psychopathology; daughters of fathers with type 2 alcoholism are at higher risk only for somatization disorder.

4. Genetic factors in development of alcohol use disorder—Although genetic studies suggest that genetic factors are important contributors to the development of alcohol use disorder, the mechanisms involved are only now beginning to be elucidated. This is an exciting area of research, but its clinical relevance is not yet apparent. Because there is likely a complex cascade of events between the genetic underpinnings of alcohol use disorder and the eventual manifestation of symptoms, this clinical diagnosis is probably not the best phenotype for use in genetic analyses. A preferable phenotype for genetic analyses might be an intermediary measure of the neuropsychiatric functioning involved in the pathway between genotype and the outcome of interest (endophenotype). For example, it has been suggested that children of alcoholic fathers are less sensitive to the intoxicating effects of ethanol than are children of nonalcoholic fathers. Presumably, these children would have to drink more than would children of nonalcoholic fathers to become intoxicated and, thus, be more likely to develop alcohol use disorder. The abilities of researchers to match subjects retrospectively in terms of lifetime exposure to, and experience with, alcohol are important limitations of these studies. Such limitations can be overcome only by carefully conducted longitudinal investigations beginning in childhood. Early notions that difference in innate tolerance to ethanol or susceptibility to alcohol use disorder were based on differences in ethanol metabolism have not been firmly established. More recently, researchers have focused on molecular underpinnings of interindividual differences in, for example, the GABA$_A$, mu-opioid, and glutamate receptor genotypes or brain biogenic amine metabolism as predisposing to development of alcohol use disorder. Specifically, considerable preclinical and human data implicate low brain serotonergic activity in stimulating alcohol consumption and in producing the aggressive and impulsive behavior often associated with type 2 alcoholism. In addition, an impaired ability to allocate significance to targeted stimuli, as manifested by reduced amplitude of the late positive component of event-related electroencephalographic (EEG) potential, has been identified in children of fathers with type 2 alcoholism and is considered a genetic factor predisposing to alcohol use disorder. Early-onset alcoholics may be more prone to develop brain damage because of alcohol consumption, or else they may be cognitively impaired before beginning drinking, especially with respect to attention and motor control. This line of reasoning is supported by relationships found between adult alcohol use disorder and early delays in motor development, suggesting that frontocerebellar deficits play a causal role. Of note, similar findings have been observed in individuals with all drug use disorders and in impulsive characteristics of behavioral addictions.

5. Inheritance of substance-use disorders other than alcoholism—It is unknown whether the genetic mechanisms that predispose individuals to alcohol use disorder also influence the development of other substance-use disorders. Common causality is suggested (though difficult to prove) because many (particularly younger) individuals tend to combine alcohol and other drugs of abuse, often indiscriminately.

The twin and adoption studies described earlier in this chapter provide guidelines for how to study this question in patients with other drug use disorders. For example, in one adoption study of genetic and environmental factors in drug use disorders, drug abuse in adult adoptees was associated in equivalent proportions with (1) antisocial personality in the adoptees, related to a biological background of antisocial personality; (2) no antisocial personality in the adoptees but with a biological background of alcoholism; and (3) neither antisocial personality nor alcoholism in either the adoptee or the biological background, but psychosocial factors such as divorce and psychiatric illness in the adopting family environment. Such studies show that interactions between genetic and environmental factors are as important in the development of other substance-use disorders as they are for alcoholism. A shared underlying mechanism seems most likely to involve endophenotypes related to attention, impulse control, executive functioning, related abnormalities of brain functioning, or the presence of, or vulnerability to, affective disorders, anxiety, or related psychopathology.

Bevilacqua L, Goldman D: Genetics of impulsive behaviour. *Philos Trans R Soc B Biol Sci Royal Soc* 2013;368(1615):20120380.

Kwako LE, Schwandt ML, Ramchandani VA, Diazgranados N, Koob GF, Volkow ND, Blanco C, Goldman D: Neurofunctional domains derived from deep behavioral phenotyping in alcohol use disorder. *Am J Psychiatry* 2019;176(9):744–753.

Martin PR: Gambling. *Historical Vocabulary of Addiction*. Cordoba, Argentina: INHN Publisher; 2021, pp. 90–96.

McLellan AT, Koob GF, Volkow ND: Preaddiction—a missing concept for treating substance use disorders. *JAMA Psychiatry* 2022;79((8):749–751.

Volkow ND, Michaelides M, Baler R: The neuroscience of drug reward and addiction. *Physiol Rev* 2019;99(4):2115–2140.

▶ Clinical Findings

A. Signs & Symptoms

1. Alcohol & Other CNS Depressants

i. Intoxication—Alcohol and other CNS depressant intoxication proceeds in stages that depend on dosage and time following administration. Apparent CNS stimulation, which occurs early in alcohol or CNS depressant intoxication or at low dosages, results from depression of inhibitory control mechanisms. The most sensitive parts of the brain are the polysynaptic structures of the reticular activating system and the cortex, depression of which causes euphoria and dulling of performance that depends on training and previous experience. Excitation resulting from intoxication is characterized by increased activity, verbal communication, and often aggression (Table 16–3). Euphoric feelings or calming effects are typically the expressed reason for drug self-administration. Higher blood concentrations of alcohol or other CNS depressants cause mild impairment of motor skills and slowing of reaction time, followed by sedation, decreased motor coordination, impaired judgment, diminished memory and

Table 16–3 Signs and Symptoms of CNS Depressant Intoxication and Withdrawal

Intoxication	Withdrawal
Anxiolysis	Anxiety or psychomotor agitation
Disinhibition (e.g., inappropriate sexual or aggressive behavior, impaired judgment, mood liability)	Tremor
	Insomnia
	Autonomic hyperactivity (e.g., tachycardia, hypertension, sweating, hyperthermia, arrhythmia)
Somnolence, stupor, or coma	
Impaired attention or memory	Craving
Slurred speech	Sensory distortions or hallucinations (e.g., transient visual, tactile, or auditory)
Incoordination	
Unsteady gait	Nausea or vomiting
Nystagmus	Seizures
	Delirium

other cognitive deficits, and eventually diminished psychomotor activity and sleep. At still higher concentrations, alcohol and most CNS depressants can induce stupor, and ultimately coma and death, by progressive depression of midbrain functions and interference with spinal reflexes, temperature regulation, and the medullary centers controlling cardiorespiratory functions. Death due to benzodiazepine overdose is very unlikely unless combined with alcohol or other CNS depressants.

The dose–response curve of ethanol has been studied in greater depth than has any other CNS depressant. Sensitivity to alcohol intoxication varies widely within the population. For example, at blood ethanol concentrations of 50, 100–150, and 200 mg/100 mL, it is estimated that approximately 10%, 64%, and almost all of the general population, respectively, would be overtly intoxicated. In contrast, at a blood ethanol concentration of 300 mg/100 mL, some alcoholic individuals may appear only mildly intoxicated even though their psychomotor performance and judgment are impaired significantly. According to the Council of Scientific Affairs of the American Medical Association, blood alcohol concentrations of 60, 100, and 150 mg/100 mL increase an individual's relative probability of causing an automobile accident 2-, 6-, and 25-fold, respectively. Legal limits of blood ethanol concentration for automobile drivers are 80 mg/100 mL (the term in common use is 0.08) for most states in the United States and in most countries in Western Europe, and between 0 and 50 mg/100 mL for Scandinavian and Eastern European countries. There is ongoing pressure to lower levels of legal impairment in many states in the United States.

ii. Drug-seeking behavior—The classic sedative–hypnotic actions of ethanol, barbiturates, and benzodiazepines correlate well with their shared ability to modulate GABA-induced chloride anion fluxes in vitro. However, the ability of alcohol to interact with a number of different receptor types, including inhibiting subtypes of NMDA receptors that mediate long-term potentiation and cannabinoid receptors, implicated in reward learning, appetite regulation, mood regulation, pain modulation, and cognition, suggests that our understanding of the mechanisms of action of CNS depressant drugs remains incomplete. These drugs can act as anxiolytics; however, benzodiazepines are unique among CNS depressants because of their ability to reduce anxiety while causing relatively little sedation. It is believed that the reinforcing actions and abuse potential of CNS depressants reside primarily in their anxiolytic and tension-reducing properties. In animal models, established GABA efferents from the nucleus accumbens to the substantia innominata–ventral pallidum can influence the expression of cocaine- or opioid-induced behavioral stimulation. This may explain why alcohol and other CNS depressants are often used by addicted individuals along with cocaine or opioids.

iii. Neuroadaptation—Adaptive neuronal changes resulting from the continued presence of alcohol or other CNS depressants involve a decrease in inhibitory functions of the nervous system. Although the molecular basis of such neuronal adaptation has not been elucidated fully, the clinical consequences are well characterized and include the development of tolerance and dependence, which usually proceed in parallel. Although pharmacokinetic differences among CNS depressants may alter the duration of time the agent is present at its site of pharmacologic action, and subtle molecular differences may influence the precise interactions of the different agents with their binding site(s) and the neuronal receptors occupied, the neuroadaptive changes that eventually result from chronic ingestion of alcohol, benzodiazepines, barbiturates, or nonbarbiturate hypnosedatives are for practical purposes much the same.

The development of tolerance to, and dependence on, CNS depressants can occur after only a few days of repeated ingestion. As with all drugs, tolerance and dependence are determined by dosage and frequency of use. For example, a drug dosage that initially caused sedation and anxiolysis may in time be insufficient to induce sleep or reduce anxiety; thus, higher dosages are needed to attain these therapeutic goals. Tolerance may not develop at the same rate to all actions of a CNS depressant. For example, whereas sedation usually diminishes after the first few days of treatment with most benzodiazepines, anxiolytic effects may persist for months without a need to increase the dosage. Euphoric effects may not be as predictable, which can cause rapid increases in dosage if the drug is being self-administered for this purpose. In general, for alcohol and other CNS depressants there is no marked elevation of the lethal dosage with repeated use, and respiratory depression may be superimposed on chronic consumption after a severe, acute overdose.

iv. Withdrawal—Cessation of alcohol or CNS depressant intake after prolonged use is associated with a syndrome of neuronal hyperexcitability with increased noradrenergic and adrenocortical activity. This syndrome is initially characterized by anxiety, apprehension, restlessness, irritability, and insomnia with clinically apparent tremors and hyperreflexia (see Table 16–3). Moderately severe cases progress to signs of autonomic hyperactivity with tachycardia, hypertension, diaphoresis, hyperthermia, and muscle fasciculations. Often patients experience anorexia, nausea, or vomiting with subsequent dehydration and electrolyte disturbances. Paroxysmal EEG discharges may precede generalized tonic–clonic seizure activity. The most severe cases develop delirium (agitation, disorientation, fluctuating level of consciousness, visual and auditory hallucinations, and intense autonomic arousal).

Among the CNS depressants, the most severe and potentially dangerous withdrawal syndrome results from barbiturates and nonbarbiturate hypnosedatives; alcohol withdrawal is of intermediate severity; and withdrawal from benzodiazepines poses the least risk. The onset, severity, and duration of the withdrawal syndrome in a given class of CNS depressants are determined by the rate of elimination of the drug and its metabolites from the body. In the alcohol withdrawal syndrome, generalized tonic–clonic seizures typically occur 12–48 hours after the last drink, and delirium tremens begins at 48–72 hours. The signs of acute alcohol withdrawal typically abate by 3–5 days after the last drink, but subtle brain abnormalities may persist for an undetermined period. Among the barbiturates, nonbarbiturate hypnosedatives, and benzodiazepines, withdrawal usually begins within 12 hours and is most severe for rapidly eliminated compounds (e.g., amobarbital, methyprylon, triazolam). For slowly metabolized compounds (e.g., phenobarbital, diazepam, clonazepam), the syndrome may be delayed for several days after drug discontinuation. More protracted effects of withdrawal from CNS depressants have not been well studied, but residual problems related to cognitive impairment, anxiety and depressive symptoms, and insomnia has emerged as an area of concern.

2. Stimulants: Cocaine & Amphetamines

i. Intoxication—The main clinically relevant pharmacologic action of cocaine and amphetamine-related stimulants is the blockade of reuptake of the catecholamine neurotransmitters norepinephrine and dopamine. The consequences of noradrenergic reuptake blockade include tachycardia, hypertension, vasoconstriction, mydriasis, diaphoresis, and tremor. The effects of dopamine reuptake blockade include self-stimulation, anorexia, stereotyped movements, hyperactivity, and sexual excitement. As a result, many of the signs and symptoms of cocaine and amphetamine intoxication are similar (Table 16–4). CNS stimulation and a subjective "high" are accompanied by an increased sense of energy, psychomotor agitation, and autonomic arousal.

The psychoactive effects of most amphetamine-like substances last longer than those of cocaine. Furthermore, because cocaine has local anesthetic actions, the risk of its causing severe medical complications such as cardiac arrhythmia and seizures is greater than for amphetamine-like stimulants. Amphetamine-related compounds therefore remain popular in the stimulant-abusing population.

ii. Drug-seeking behavior—The most striking pharmacologic characteristic of cocaine is its tremendous reinforcing effect. Women who are cocaine dependent have higher rates of primary major depression than do cocaine-dependent men, consistent with drug use as a form of self-medication. Men with cocaine dependence have higher rates of co-occurring antisocial personality disorder than do cocaine-dependent women. Studies in animal models have shown that animals will self-administer cocaine in preference to food, leading to emaciation and death (in contrast to other highly reinforcing agents such as opioids). Dopamine seems to be the main neurotransmitter involved in the positive reinforcement of cocaine.

iii. Neuroadaptation—Although not well understood, neuroadaptation appears to occur in response to chronic stimulant use. Users develop acute tolerance to the subjective effects of cocaine, which can play a major role in dose escalation and subsequent toxicity. Sensitization appears to play a role in cocaine-induced panic attacks, paranoia, and lethality.

iv. Withdrawal—In humans, discontinuation of cocaine leads to dysphoria (a "crash"). Hypersomnolence and anergia are also common (see Table 16–4). In rats, termination of repeated cocaine administration produces interoceptive stimuli that are similar to the discriminative stimulus effects of pentetrazol, a drug that is anxiogenic in humans. As a result, the typical cycle of use consists of binges, each followed by a "crash" (lasting 9 hours to 4 days), followed by withdrawal (lasting 1–10 weeks), during which craving and relapse are common.

3. Opioids

i. Intoxication—The characteristic pharmacologic action of opioids is analgesia. Centrally, opioids are activating at low dosages and sedating at higher dosages. Other major features of intoxication are feelings of euphoria or dysphoria, feelings of warmth, facial flushing, itchy face, dry mouth, and pupil constriction (Table 16–5). Intravenous use can cause lower abdominal sensations described as an orgasm-like "rush." This is followed by a feeling of sedation (called the "nod") and dreaming. Severe intoxication may cause respiratory suppression, areflexia, hypotension, tachycardia, apnea, cyanosis, and death.

ii. Drug-seeking behavior—Addiction to opioids (particularly heroin) can be severe and often leads individuals to dysfunctional behavior to support their habit. Animals tend to repeat opioid self-administration and prolong its effects.

Self-administered opioid compounds affect the endogenous opioid systems of the body. Endogenous opioid peptides are distributed throughout the brain and form three

Table 16–4 Signs and Symptoms of Stimulant Intoxication and Withdrawal

Intoxication	Withdrawal
Stimulation (euphoria, hypervigilance, anxiety, tension, anger, impaired judgment)	Depression (dysphoria)
Psychomotor agitation (stereotyped behaviors, dyskinesias, dystonias)	Psychomotor retardation
	Fatigue (increased need for sleep)
	Increased appetite
Energy (decreased need for sleep)	Craving
Anorexia (nausea or vomiting, weight loss)	
Autonomic arousal (tachycardia, hypertension, pupillary dilation, perspiration, or chills)	
Chest pain, cardiac arrhythmias, respiratory depression	
Confusion	
Seizures	

Table 16–5 Signs and Symptoms of Opioid Intoxication and Withdrawal

Intoxication	Withdrawal
Activation or "rush" (early or with low dosages) and sedation/apathy or "nod" (late or with high dosages)	Depressed mood and anxiety
	Dysphoria
	Craving
Euphoria or dysphoria	Piloerection ("goose flesh")
Feelings of warmth, facial flushing, or itching	Lacrimation or rhinorrhea
	Hyperalgesia, joint and muscle aches
Impaired judgment, attention, or memory	Diarrhea and gastrointestinal cramping, nausea, or vomiting
Analgesia	Pupillary dilation and photophobia
Constipation	
Pupillary constriction	Insomnia
Drowsiness	Autonomic hyperactivity (e.g., tachypnea, hyperreflexia, tachycardia, hypertension, sweating, hyperthermia)
Respiratory depression, areflexia, hypotension, tachycardia	
Apnea, cyanosis, coma	
	Yawning

major functional systems defined by their precursor molecules: β-endorphin from pro-opiomelanocortin, enkephalins from proenkephalin, and dynorphin from prodynorphin. Endogenous opioids modulate nociceptive responses to painful stimuli, stressors, reward, and homeostatic adaptive functions (hunger, thirst, and temperature regulation). Rats will self-administer opioid peptides into the ventral tegmental area and nucleus accumbens, suggesting that these regions may be responsible, at least in part, for the reinforcing properties of opioids (and cocaine). Other regions supporting rewarding effects for opioids are the hippocampus and hypothalamus. Endogenous opioid tone contributes to the maintenance of normal mood and a nondopaminergic system of opioid reward.

There are three main types of opioid receptor: μ, δ, and κ. These G protein–coupled proteins inhibit adenylyl cyclases in various tissues and cause their pharmacologic actions by reducing cyclic adenosine monophosphate (cAMP) levels. The μ-opioid receptor appears to be important for the reinforcing actions of opioids, whereas the δ-opioid receptor may play a role in the opioid motor stimulation that is dopamine (D_1 receptor) dependent. Like other substances of abuse, opioids can increase dopamine release in the nucleus accumbens as measured by in vivo microdialysis in awake, freely moving animals; however, the reinforcing effect of opioids in the nucleus accumbens can be independent of dopamine release. The reinforcing actions of opioids may involve both a dopamine-dependent (i.e., ventral tegmental area) and a dopamine-independent (nucleus accumbens) mechanism.

iii. Neuroadaptation—Neuroadaptation occurs in response to regular opioid use. For example, when chronically abused by humans, heroin rapidly loses its aversive properties and

increases its reinforcing ones. The tolerance that develops when opioids are administered repeatedly appears to be receptor selective. It has been theorized that μ receptors couple less well to G proteins in rat locus coeruleus neurons that have been chronically treated with morphine. Tolerance occurs both to specific opioid effects such as analgesia and motor inhibition and to the generally depressant properties of opioids, whereas the psychomotor effects are potentiated.

iv. Withdrawal—Withdrawal of opioids is characterized by hyperalgesia, photophobia, goose flesh, diarrhea, tachycardia, increased blood pressure, gastrointestinal cramps, joint and muscle aches, and anxiety and depressed mood (see Table 16–5). Spontaneous withdrawal results in intense craving because of the reduction of dopamine release in the nucleus accumbens, but the degree of physical dependence does not predict the severity of craving. The motivational (affective) properties of withdrawal are independent of the intensity and pattern of the physical symptoms. Because opioids can counteract withdrawal dysphoria and the reduction of dopaminergic transmission, these changes may contribute to maintenance of opioid addiction. This intense need to continue using opioids makes individuals particularly vulnerable to high potency synthetic opioids such as fentanyl that are now readily available and are responsible for most drug overdose deaths in the United States.

4. Cannabinoids

i. Intoxication—The subjective effect of marijuana intoxication varies from individual to individual. It is determined in part by highly variable pharmacokinetics, dosage, route of administration, setting, experience and expectation, and individual vulnerability to certain psychotoxic effects. Typically, intoxication is characterized by an initial period of "high" that has been described as a sense of well-being and happiness (Table 16–6). This euphoria is followed frequently by a period of drowsiness or sedation. The perception of time

Table 16–6 Signs and Symptoms of Cannabis Intoxication and Withdrawal

Intoxication	Withdrawal
Euphoria, drowsiness, or sedation	Insomnia, irritability, dysphoria, aggressiveness
Sensation of slowed time	
Auditory or visual distortions, dissociation	Depression/craving
	Strange, vivid dreams
Impaired judgment, motor coordination, attention, or memory	Tremor/shakiness, muscle twitches
	Headache
Slowed reaction time	Mild fever, chills
Conjunctival injection	Anorexia, nausea, weight loss
Tachycardia	
Increased appetite	
Anxiety, acute panic reactions, paranoia, illusions, or agitation	

is altered, and hearing and vision distorted. The subjective effects of intoxication often include dissociative reactions. Impaired functioning occurs in a variety of cognitive and performance tasks, including memory, reaction time, concept formation, learning, perception, motor coordination, attention, and signal detection. At dosages equivalent to one or two "joints" (marijuana cigarettes), processes involved in the operation of motor vehicles or airplanes are impaired. The impairment persists for 4–8 hours, long after the user perceives the subjective effects of the drug. The impairment produced by alcohol is additive to that produced by marijuana. Tolerant individuals may exhibit somewhat less performance decrement.

Physically, dilation of conjunctival blood vessels and tachycardia may be noted. Blood pressure remains relatively unchanged unless high dosages are used, in which case orthostatic hypotension ensues. Increased appetite is often attributed to marijuana but has not been observed consistently in controlled studies. At higher dosages, acute panic reactions, paranoia, hallucinations, illusions, thought disorganization, and agitation have been observed. With extremely high dosages, an acute toxic psychosis is accompanied by depersonalization and loss of insight.

ii. Drug-seeking behavior—In chronic cannabinoid users, the degree of drug-seeking behaviors and if a use disorder may result are controversial in part because of the long-lasting biological effects of these highly lipid-soluble drugs. In some patients, drug-seeking behavior appears to be manifested primarily as drug craving. The psychological and physiologic mechanisms underpinning this craving are not understood. Laboratory animals do not self-administer the drug. The recognition and characterization of the endogenous cannabinoid system has led to important advances in our understanding of cannabinoid the degree of drug-seeking behaviors and if a use disorder may result. Moreover, there is a growing body of evidence that the endogenous cannabinoid system may contribute to psychopathologic states such as anxiety, depression and psychosis and might participate in the motivational and dopamine-releasing effects of several drugs of abuse other than cannabinoids. Finally, chronic cannabinoid use has increasingly become associated with enduring psychotic illnesses and panic disorder even after drug use has ceased.

iii. Neuroadaptation—Neuroadaptation in response to cannabinoid use has been more difficult to document than in some of the other drugs of abuse. Tolerance to cannabinoids appears to develop in animals and in humans, although it does not seem to be as profound as with some other drugs. It occurs mostly with heavy use. Chronic use of exogenous cannabinoids activates the same receptors as do endogenous cannabinoids, the CB1 and CB2 cannabinoid receptors. These G protein–coupled receptors play an important role in many processes, including metabolic regulation, craving, pain, anxiety, mood, bone growth, and immune function. The functioning of cannabinoid receptors can now be studied directly using agonists or antagonists, or indirectly by manipulating endocannabinoid metabolism, and this will likely help elucidate processes of neuroadaptation and other physiological effects of cannabinoids.

iv. Withdrawal—Cannabinoid withdrawal does not produce well-characterized withdrawal symptoms, perhaps because cannabinoids are so lipophilic that they are very slowly eliminated from the body. The DSM-5 is the first version of DSM to include cannabis withdrawal because converging evidence from basic laboratory and clinical studies indicates that a withdrawal syndrome consistently follows discontinuation of chronic heavy use of cannabis, or treatment with cannabinoid receptor antagonists. Some patients report insomnia, vivid or strange dreams, irritability, dysphoria, aggressiveness, depression/cravings, anorexia, weight loss, hand tremor/shakiness, mild fever/chills, or slight nausea with discontinuation of use. These symptoms occur primarily in patients who smoke very potent preparations.

5. Tobacco

i. Intoxication—Tobacco intoxication is not a DSM-5-TR diagnosis. However, smoking or chewing tobacco has multiple effects via its main psychoactive substituent nicotine. For example, many users report improved mood, skeletal muscle relaxation, and diminished anxiety and appetite. In addition, cognitive effects including enhanced attention, problem solving, learning, and memory have been reported.

ii. Drug-seeking behavior—Users of tobacco products frequently exhibit substance-seeking behavior. Smokers often describe strong cravings for tobacco, especially in particular situations such as after eating or while experiencing stress. The degree of craving differs among individuals, and the ability to discontinue tobacco products varies greatly.

iii. Neuroadaptation—Nicotine is thought to be the chief substance in tobacco that causes neuroadaptation. Tolerance to nicotine has been shown in both laboratory animals and humans. Dependence is indicated by the difficulty of discontinuing use of nicotine products due to withdrawal symptoms and particularly, intense cravings, despite a desire to quit.

The primary pharmacologic actions of nicotine appear to occur via nicotine binding to acetylcholine receptors in the brain and autonomic ganglia. Several subtypes of nicotinic cholinergic receptors are found in the CNS. Activation of these receptors appears to cause the reinforcing effects and diminished appetite associated with nicotine. Some of the reinforcing actions of nicotine may be due to the effects of nicotine on dopamine pathways projecting from the ventral tegmental area to the limbic system and the cerebral cortex. Stimulation of peripheral nicotine receptors causes many of the autonomic effects associated with nicotine use. Short-term use of tobacco appears to increase cerebral blood flow, whereas long-term use has the opposite effect. Aspects of neuroadaptation to nicotine may also be secondary to release of hormones such as β-endorphin, adrenocorticotropic hormone, cortisol, epinephrine, norepinephrine, endocannabinoids, and vasopressin.

iv. Withdrawal—Withdrawal symptoms often occur with abrupt discontinuation of nicotine intake: craving, anxiety, depression, irritability, headaches, poor concentration, sleep disturbances, elevated blood pressure, and increased heart rate. In some cases, craving lasts for years under appropriate circumstances. Management of withdrawal symptoms behaviorally or pharmacologically has been used to prevent relapses in those trying to quit smoking.

6. Hallucinogens & Volatile Inhalants

i. Intoxication—Intoxication with hallucinogens causes effects that vary greatly and may last 8–12 hours. Flashbacks are possible after termination of use (Table 16–7). The cardinal features of hallucinogen intoxication include visual hallucinations and disturbance of thoughts and perception in multiple sensory modalities. These features can lead to devastating consequences if they occur in dangerous situations (e.g., when driving or standing in precarious areas such as on a balcony). Other features include sensory changes (e.g., colors, shapes), synesthesia (the perception in one modality when a different modality has been stimulated), delusions, paranoia, derealization, depersonalization, cognitive impairment, coordination problems, behavioral changes, euphoria (or dysphoria), nausea, tremors, time distortion, dizziness, weakness, and giddiness. A "bad trip" involves striking dysphoria and sensory disturbances. Visual hallucinations with perception of various light patterns, and incorrect movement perception or object recognition have been reported. Augmented sensory perception (particularly tactile), which can be pleasurable (thus the term "ecstasy" for MDMA), often occurs with methamphetamine use. Other symptoms such as ataxia, dizziness, nausea, perspiration, and bruxism can occur with use. Many complications are related to hallucinogen use (e.g., panic reactions, seizures, exacerbation of psychiatric illnesses). Suicidal or homicidal tendencies may be enhanced. There is emerging clinical research of psychedelic medications under highly controlled

circumstances for treatment of depression, drug use disorders and posttraumatic stress disorder, among other psychiatric conditions.

Anticholinergic drugs of abuse include antihistamines and the belladonna alkaloids such as scopolamine and atropine. Anticholinergic drugs are characterized by "dreamlike" states, feelings of euphoria, heightened social interaction, and sedation. At high dosages, disorientation or paranoia may occur. These substances are sometimes used with mild opioids (called "Juice and Beans" or "T's and Blues" on the streets) to enhance the euphoric effect.

Arylcyclohexylamines, such as PCP (phencyclidine), act as dissociative anesthetics. A closely related agent ketamine has received much recent interest for its rapidly acting antidepressant effects. Behavioral alterations of PCP may include paranoia, mood shift, agitation, catalepsy, and violence. PCP may be smoked, snorted, or injected. It causes reddening of the skin, pupillary changes, dissociation, delusions, amnesia, dry skin, dizziness, poor coordination, excitement, and nystagmus. Increased blood pressure and tachycardia may also occur.

Intoxication by volatile inhalants generally lasts only several minutes. Confusion, sedation, and euphoria may often result from use. Physical effects include analgesia, respiratory depression, hypotension, and ataxia. Nitrous oxide is associated with euphoria and laughter ("laughing gas").

ii. Drug-seeking behavior—Psychedelic substances do not typically cause a use disorder, and regular use is not common. Animals generally do not self-administer these drugs (except for MDMA-like compounds), and frequent users generally do not report craving. Tolerance to LSD occurs after only days of use; however, the intoxicating effects return after a few days without use. Other indolamines are cross-tolerant with LSD, but the phenylethylamine hallucinogens are not. Tolerance to anticholinergic drugs can also occur but usually requires prolonged use.

iii. Neuroadaptation—Little is known about neuroadaptation to the actions of hallucinogens. Phenylalkylamines and indolamines are serotonin receptor agonists, which probably relates to their clinical effects. Phosphatidylinositol hydrolysis is stimulated after receptor binding and leads to enhanced excitability of certain neurons in the limbic system, cerebral cortex, and brainstem.

The phenylisopropylamines inhibit reuptake of catecholamine and indolamine neurotransmitters and may be transported into serotonin neurons. It is hypothesized that the serotonergic action of these drugs accounts for their hallucinogenic effects (as with other hallucinogens), whereas the effect on catecholamines causes arousal.

Anticholinergic drugs such as scopolamine and atropine act as antagonists of muscarinic receptors. These receptors are found in the cerebral cortex, and several subtypes have been reported. Stimulation may excite or inhibit neuronal activity including effects on serotonin receptors.

Table 16–7 Signs and Symptoms of Hallucinogen Intoxication

Marked anxiety or depression
Perceptual changes (e.g., intense perceptions, depersonalization, derealization, illusions, hallucinations, synesthesias)
Thought disorders (e.g., ideas of reference, paranoia, impaired reality testing)
Impaired judgment
Autonomic arousal (e.g., pupillary dilation, tachycardia, sweating, palpitations, blurring of vision)
Motor impairment (ataxia, tremors, incoordination, nystagmus)

Arylcyclohexylamines, such as PCP, act as antagonists to the N-methyl-D-aspartate class of glutamate receptors, which are themselves ion channels. PCP also binds to σ-type opioid receptors and inhibits catecholamine reuptake.

iv. Withdrawal—Withdrawal symptoms are not common with these drugs; however, the anticholinergic substances may cause tachycardia, sweating, depression, anxiety, or psychomotor agitation after use has been discontinued.

B. Psychological Testing

Alcohol and other substances of abuse can cause both transient and enduring damage to the brain. Neuropsychological testing is important in the overall assessment of some patients with substance-related disorders. Most of these tests are readily available, noninvasive, and inexpensive. They require the full participation of the patient; therefore, they may not be as objective as blood chemistries or radiologic procedures. Neuropsychological tests are preferably conducted at least 3 weeks after the most recent substance use so that lasting brain dysfunction can be detected. Although these tests are useful, many factors influence them, including medication, co-occurring medical conditions or psychiatric disorder, and compliance with testing.

Intelligence tests such as the Wechsler Adult Intelligence Scale (WAIS) are useful in determining the patient's global behavioral and adaptive potential. The WAIS is predictive of the patient's likely success in activities such as work and school. Other intelligence tests may be more appropriate for specific patient populations. Different aspects of cognition may be evaluated by specific tests. For example, the Wechsler Memory Scale is useful for patients who have possible substance-induced memory impairment.

Neuropsychological batteries such as the Halstead-Reitan Neuropsychological Test Battery and the Luria-Nebraska Neuropsychological Battery can provide comprehensive information about many aspects of brain functioning. In alcoholic patients, the Halstead-Reitan Battery frequently reveals impairment on many of the individual tests such as Tactual Performance, Categories (visual–spatial abstracting), Trails B (perceptual motor speed), and Tactual Performance Test-Location (incidental memory for spatial relationships).

Some assessment tools have been developed for evaluation of presence of harmful substance use (as opposed to possible causes or consequences thereof). One of the major difficulties in using such measures is in distinguishing use from use disorder. The four-question CAGE assessment is used to screen patients for alcoholism. CAGE stands for an acronym reflecting (1) the subjective need to **cut down**, (2) being **annoyed** at other people when they comment on one's drinking, (3) feelings of **guilt** over use, and (4) the need for an "**eye opener**." Generally, two out of four yes answers are considered positive. Sensitivity and specificity are high for most populations. The more complex Michigan Alcoholism Screening Test (MAST) is often used in the assessment of alcohol intake and the consequences of consumption. It has 25 differentially weighted items in a true–false format. Sensitivity, specificity, and validity testing have all been favorable. Shorter 10- and 13-item forms are available with reasonably good validity. A reliable test of the consumption and consequences of drug use disorders is the Drug Abuse Screening Test (DAST). It has 28 items (unlike the MAST, not differentially weighted), in a true–false format. Another useful instrument is the Alcohol Dependence Scale. This scale has 25 multiple-choice items and is concerned primarily with the loss of ability to control drinking.

Because co-occurring psychiatric illnesses and social difficulties are common in those who have substance use disorder, other psychological tests may be of value in certain patients. An example is the Addiction Severity Index (ASI), a semistructured interview designed to address seven problem areas in patients who use substances: medical status, employment and support, drug use, alcohol use, legal status, family/social status, and psychiatric status. The ASI provides an overview of recent (past 30 days) and lifetime problems related to substance use. The Minnesota Multiphasic Personality Inventory, a commonly used assessment tool with more than 500 items (with results formatted into 10 clinical scales and 3 validity scales), provides typical personality profiles for substance-use disorder patients. (See also Chapter 6, *Psychological and Neuropsychological Assessment*.)

C. Laboratory Findings

Several laboratory findings are of use in the evaluation and care of substance-use disorder patients. Urine drug screens and blood alcohol levels provide objective information as to what drugs are in the patient's system, at what concentration. The relative degree of intoxication or withdrawal at specific drug levels can provide clues as to the patient's level of tolerance and dependence. A complete evaluation considers whether particular drugs are detectable in urine and the length of time that they are detectable. This will vary according to many factors, including dosage, duration of use, and individual metabolic and renal clearance rates. Average upper limits on urine detection times are provided in Table 16–8.

Many other blood chemistries are useful. The acute toxic effects of alcohol on the liver are evaluated with liver function tests, such as AST (Aspartate Aminotransferase) and ALT (Alanine aminotransferase). GGT (γ-glutamyl transpeptidase) was considered the most sensitive monitor of ongoing alcohol consumption until superseded by carbohydrate-deficient transferrin (CDT) and phosphatidylethanol (PEth) as markers for monitoring abstinence. Alcohol-induced hepatitis classically presents with a AST:ALT ratio of about 2:1. Viral hepatitis screens can help differentiate causes of abnormalities in hepatic function. Severe chronic liver dysfunction is reflected by impaired synthetic function, malnutrition and impaired hemostasis. Serum amylase is valuable in the detection of pancreatitis.

Table 16–8 The Upper Limit of Urine Detection

Drug	Limit
Alcohol	12 hours
Amphetamine	2 days
Cannabis	4 weeks
Cocaine	8 hours (4 days for metabolites)
Opioids	3 days
Phencyclidine (PCP)	8 days
Benzodiazepines	3 days
Barbiturates	1 day (short-acting); 3 weeks (long-acting)
Codeine	2 days

A complete blood cell count can monitor bone marrow functioning: mild, macrocytic anemia is often observed in alcohol use disorder patients. Low potassium and bicarbonate are consistent with drug-related diarrhea. Chloride deficiencies are associated with chronic vomiting. Although total body stores of magnesium may be difficult to assess, alcohol-induced magnesium wasting can lead to detectable extracellular deficiencies. Protein, albumin, elevated international normalized ratio (INR), potassium, and phosphorus are helpful indicators of nutritional status.

D. Neuroimaging

Intellectual impairment is perhaps the earliest complication of chronic alcoholism. It is difficult to determine whether subtle neuropsychological impairments are consequences of chronic alcohol consumption. Computed tomography or magnetic resonance imaging studies of patients with 2–36 weeks of abstinence have shown that a large proportion of alcoholic patients have detectable cerebral and cerebellar atrophy and ventricular dilation. Recently, functional measures of brain activity have corroborated these neuroanatomic findings.

E. Course of Illness

1. Alcohol & other CNS depressants—The CNS depressants include brewed or distilled alcoholic beverages and various pharmaceutical agents prescribed for the treatment of insomnia, anxiety, depression, and, less frequently, for seizure control or as muscle relaxants. No CNS depressant (e.g., alprazolam, zolpidem, eszopiclone, zaleplon) has been developed that is totally free of abuse liability and the potential for a withdrawal syndrome, problems shared with alcoholic beverages.

Alcoholic beverages are readily available at affordable cost with minimal legal restrictions. Accordingly, there is widespread use of alcohol in diverse recreational and work-related circumstances, and traumatic injuries sustained while under the influence of elevated blood alcohol are among the most common public health problems today. Youngsters with little experience with drinking are particularly vulnerable as they first begin to participate in high-risk activities such as sports, sexuality, and driving. Heavy drinkers, who often have blood alcohol concentrations that impair judgment and motor skills or use other drugs in combination with alcohol, are particularly at risk for alcohol-related violence, traumatic injury, and death.

The benzodiazepines are currently (as barbiturates were previously) among the most widely prescribed and often misused medications for insomnia, anxiety and nonspecific physical symptoms. With continued use, individuals develop tolerance and need higher doses to achieve symptomatic relief. If the physician does not educate the patient and provide careful prescription monitoring and assist in tapering the prescribed dose, the patient may eventually receive high doses of these medications with attendant side effects such as mood disorder, cognitive dysfunction, social difficulties, impaired work performance, and traumatic injury due to falls or vehicular accidents. The term benzodiazepine-induced neurological dysfunction (BIND) has recently been coined to represent a constellation of functionally limiting neurologic symptoms (both physical and psychological) that are the consequence of neuroadaptation and/or neurotoxicity to benzodiazepine exposure. Additional problems may develop when a patient combines alcohol, other psychoactive medications, or illicit drugs (e.g., marijuana, opioids) with the prescribed dose of CNS depressant, seeks other physicians to provide additional prescriptions (so-called doctor shopping), or engages in illegal activities such as forging prescriptions. The combination of alcohol with other CNS depressants greatly increases the risk associated with its use and is a common clinical cause of severe drug overdose. Cessation of drug use leads to undesirable, and potentially harmful, withdrawal symptoms (such as seizures). Thus, drug-seeking behavior and repeated drug use are often continued to prevent these effects. Fulminant withdrawal occasionally occurs in patients who discontinue CNS depressant use because of illness or other unforeseen circumstances such as hospitalization for a motor vehicle accident.

2. Stimulants: cocaine & amphetamines—The alkaloid cocaine is derived from *Erythroxylum coca*, a plant indigenous to South America, where since time immemorial its leaves have been chewed for their stimulating effects. Because the only contemporary medical use for cocaine is as a local anesthetic, the drug is almost always purchased illegally by users. Amphetamine and amphetamine-like stimulants may be obtained by prescription for the treatment of obesity, attention-deficit/hyperactivity disorder, and narcolepsy. As a result, prescribed stimulants are commonly diverted into the illegal market. An epidemic of cocaine use started in the late 1970s, preceded by a period in which it was thought not to be particularly dangerous. Cocaine's significant dependence liability came to be recognized later, resulting in a diminution in use of the drug in the late 1980s. Abuse of amphetamine-like compounds has continued unabated because of their widespread availability and relatively low cost. Recently, use of illegally manufactured methamphetamine derivatives has reached epidemic proportions, reminiscent of the cocaine epidemic of the 1980s. Methamphetamine, including a crystallized, smokeable form called "ice," is representative of a group of "designer drugs." These ring-substituted derivatives of amphetamine and methamphetamine, synthesized in clandestine laboratories, derive their popularity from their mixed stimulant and hallucinogenic effects.

Cocaine and other stimulants are almost always used with other psychoactive substances, most commonly alcohol but also other CNS depressants or opioids. Alcohol is considered a gateway drug for cocaine and other stimulant use. It can accentuate the "high" obtained from stimulants, alleviate some of the adverse effects (e.g., "wired" feelings), and is a readily available (i.e., legal) substitute. Heroin (sometimes called "speedball") is another drug that is commonly combined with cocaine and other stimulants and is reported to increase euphoria.

Methods of use include inhalation via the nostrils ("snorting"), subcutaneous or intravenous injection, and smoking ("free basing"). Nasal insufflation is the most common and least dangerous method, but it does not provide the ecstatic sensation associated with smoking or injection. These latter routes of administration give the drug rapid access to the brain, thereby increasing its reinforcing effect and toxicity.

3. Opioids—Opioid use and addiction has occurred for centuries, and many opioid compounds are abused throughout the world. Opioid use disorder may start with initially appropriate use for medical analgesia or as experimental use of illicit substances. The use of long-acting oral forms (e.g., morphine sulfate, MS Contin and oxycodone, OxyContin), developed for presumed safe treatment of chronic pain, quickly surpassed that of illicit heroin or morphine in most Western countries. Urban dwellers in the Northeast were initially the most frequent abusers of heroin, whereas in rural regions, oral formulations of morphine and oxycodone became the primary opioids of abuse. Prescription opioids have emerged as a significant cause of morbidity and mortality due to accidental overdoses over the past decade. As physician prescriptions became tightly monitored due to fear of overdose deaths, addicted individuals were compelled to use illicit and affordable street sources like heroin for their opioids. Most recently, illicit preparations of the high potency synthetic opioid fentanyl have become widely available and are used either alone or in combination with stimulants. Medical professionals with easy access to opioids are at increased risk to develop opioid use disorder. In Asia, opium use is still widespread.

Unrefined opium is often smoked using a water pipe. Intravenous heroin (mainlining) and morphine are popular because of the sudden (less than a minute) "rush" produced. Subcutaneous injection is sometimes used, especially if veins

have become unusable because of frequent injections. Refined opioids can also be self-administered by nasal insufflation, a method often preferred by new users. Long-acting oral opioid preparations are typically used with medical prescription or ground up and injected. Although the euphoric state of opioid intake is short, its sedative and analgesic effects can continue for hours. Street drugs are frequently "cut" (mixed or combined) with other substances, such as caffeine, powdered milk, quinine, and strychnine, to dilute the concentration of the active ingredient. These other substances can lead to altered clinical effects and medical difficulties beyond those associated with the opioid; however, the unpredictable potency of these street preparations can often lead to accidental overdose.

4. Cannabinoids—Marijuana is the common name for the plant *Cannabis sativa*. Other names for the plant or its products include hemp, hashish, charas, bhang, ganja, and dagga. The highest concentrations of the psychoactive cannabinoids are found in the flowering tops of both male and female plants. Most commonly the plant is cut, dried, chopped, and then incorporated into cigarettes. The primary psychoactive constituent of marijuana is delta-9-tetrahydrocannabinol, although many other active cannabinoids are known. The hemp plant synthesizes at least 400 of these chemicals.

Since the 1960s, marijuana has been the most used illicit substance. It has recently been legalized in many U.S. states first for medical purposes and more recently for personal recreational use. Marijuana has been the first illicit drug, other than alcohol, used by youngsters. For the first time in history, the use rate in females appears to be higher than in males. The likelihood of having used cocaine and other illicit drugs increases with the extent of marijuana use in all age groups. The epidemiology of marijuana use, therefore, can be viewed as a predictor of illicit drug-related problems in the population.

5. Tobacco—Tobacco is a substance commonly used in many countries and across age groups, from early teens to the elderly. Cigarette smoking is the most common method of use, although cigar smoking, pipe smoking, and smokeless tobacco (snuff) use each have had varying levels of popularity at different times and among different groups. Primarily because of educational programs, the use of tobacco products has declined over the past 30 years in North America. Nevertheless, the use of tobacco products continues to be a significant public health problem and has increased recently in some subpopulations, such as teenage girls.

According to studies that alter the nicotine and tar content of cigarettes, user satisfaction appears to be related to nicotine content, suggesting that this agent is responsible for the reinforcing effects. Heated debates, litigation, changes in laws, and greater enforcement of existing laws regulating the cigarette industry have evolved as the adverse public health effects of smoking have become more widely appreciated. A recent challenge has been initiation or transition to non-tobacco vaporized preparations of nicotine ("vaping") which can be useful for tapering nicotine, but may come with its own mostly unknown toxicity.

6. Hallucinogens & volatile inhalants—Hallucinogens are subdivided into two major categories: the indolealkylamines (such as d-lysergic acid diethylamide [LSD], dimethyltryptamine [DMT], psilocin, psilocybin, diethyltryptamine [DET]), the phenylethylamines (such as trimethoxyphenyl ethylamine [mescaline], 3,4-methylenedioxy methamphetamine [MDMA; called "ecstasy" on the streets], 2,5-dimethoxytryptamine [DOM, STP], and 3,4-methylenedioxy amphetamine [MDA]). Other hallucinogens include peyote (mescaline, from Mexican cactus), *Myristica fragrans* (nutmeg), and morning-glory seeds (similar in effect to LSD). Arylcyclohexylamines include phencyclidine (PCP; called "angel dust," "crystal," "weed," and "hog" on the streets) and ketamine. Ketamine is most commonly used as an anesthetic in veterinary medicine; however, it is currently being examined for efficacy in treatment of depression and anxiety. PCP has no current medical uses.

Volatile inhalants include aromatic, aliphatic, and halogenated hydrocarbon compounds such as gasoline, industrial solvents (e.g., acetone, toluene), paints, glues, refrigerants (e.g., Freon), and paint thinners (e.g., turpentine). Nitrous oxide (an anesthetic) and amyl nitrite (a vasodilator; called "poppers" on the streets) are included.

Native Americans used psychedelic drugs such as mushrooms (psilocybin and psilocin) and peyote before the Spanish exploration of Mexico. Hoffman described the hallucinogenic effects of LSD in 1943. Scopolamine (and other belladonna alkaloids), mescaline (a plant product), and amphetamine designer drugs have similar effects. Hallucinogens in the United States were most popular in the 1960s and early 1970s, with a dramatic decline shortly afterward. The use of these drugs has continued, however, at a constant level since the late 1970s. An increase of use, particularly of the designer drugs, has been noted among teens and young adults. A recent disturbing trend involves the use of several of these drugs by large numbers of youngsters during all-night dance parties ("raves"). Some Native Americans and other groups continue to use plant hallucinogens in their mystic ceremonies. PCP is used most in urban areas.

Users of volatile inhalants are most often in their preteen and teenage years. Professionals such as dentists, who have easy access to substances such as nitrous oxide, are also at increased risk of use. The use of volatile inhalants was perhaps greatest in the late 1970s and early 1980s.

Connor JP, Stjepanović D, Budney AJ, Le Foll B, Hall WD: Clinical management of cannabis withdrawal. *Addiction* 2022; 117(7):2075–2095.

Ostroumov A, Dani JA: Convergent neuronal plasticity and metaplasticity mechanisms of stress, nicotine, and alcohol. *Annu Rev Pharmacol Toxicol* 2018;58(1):547–566.

Volkow ND, Boyle M: Neuroscience of addiction: relevance to prevention and treatment. *Am J Psychiatry* 2018;175(8):729–740.

▶ **Differential Diagnosis**

Patients are unlikely to present to physicians complaining of difficulties with the use of psychoactive substances. Rather, they present for treatment of the complications of substance use. Such patients are unlikely to offer information that they use psychoactive agents, much less admit to problematic drug use. They may deny that they have a drug problem when questioned. The nonspecificity and wide variety of symptoms that accompany these psychoactive substances, as well as the unreliability of patient reports, make the diagnosis of these disorders difficult. The physician must approach with a high index of suspicion patients who exhibit signs and symptoms consistent with a substance-use disorder. Only if the physician is open to the diagnosis will it be made appropriately.

Because of the many clinical manifestations of substance-use disorder, the physician must consider it in the differential diagnosis of myriad medical and psychiatric illnesses. For example, a withdrawal-induced delirium must be differentiated from the many other causes of delirium, ranging from CNS infection and metabolic disturbance to medication toxicity. Similarly, numerous medical problems must be eliminated before a physician can assume that all the signs and symptoms exhibited by a drug-abusing patient are the result of a substance of abuse (even if one or more drugs have been used). For example, an intoxicated substance abuser may have fallen and incurred a closed head injury or be in diabetic ketoacidosis.

Numerous similar presentations can be cited. For example, patients with hyperthyroidism or bipolar affective disorder may have similar initial clinical features to those on stimulants, and vice versa. Patients with psychosis (e.g., schizophrenia, bipolar affective disorder, or major depressive disorder with psychotic features) may exhibit signs and symptoms like those of a person withdrawing from CNS depressants, or vice versa.

A common problem is the differential diagnosis of the anxious or depressed alcoholic patient. The physician must determine whether the patient has a primary mood or anxiety disorder with subsequent substance abuse or a substance-induced mood disorder. In such circumstances, the only way the physician can differentiate the cause(s) of the depressed mood or anxiety is by taking a careful history or by observing the patient's response to treatment. On the other hand, the correct diagnosis may require discussion with others who have known the patient over time.

In the differential diagnosis of substance abuse, the physician must be aware that the patient could be in denial, in which case the reported history may be intentionally or unintentionally inaccurate or incomplete. Denial may be followed by unexpected medical or psychiatric problems or concomitant drug abuse.

Chennapan K, Mullinax S, Anderson E, Landau MJ, Nordstrom K, Seupaul RA, Wilson MP: Medical screening of mental health patients in the emergency department: a systematic review. *J Emerg Med* 2018;55(6):799–812.

Rich JS, Martin PR: Chapter 33 – Co-occurring psychiatric disorders and alcoholism. In: Sullivan EV, Pfefferbaum A (eds). *Handb Clin Neurol*. Elsevier, Waltham MA USA 2014. pp. 573–588.

▶ Treatment

A. Other Interventions

The treatment of substance-use disorders is perhaps influenced more by the widely held societal attributions of responsibility for causation of the problem than by an understanding of etiology. Such attributions can lead to a broad range of responses, the most extreme being to view the addict as either a patient or a criminal, and as moral or immoral, innocent or guilty, victim or perpetrator.

A corollary of this viewpoint is to regard rehabilitation from substance-use disorder as belonging either in the realm of medicine or in the criminal justice system. However, the social control mechanisms used for prevention or deterrence are not so easily dichotomized. There are distinct inconsistencies and tensions between the medical (i.e., prevention) and legal (i.e., deterrence) systems as evidenced by the lack of a straightforward relationship between the pharmacologic properties and health risks of a drug, and whether it is considered legal or illegal (the term "illicit" is often used) within criminal law. Drugs such as alcohol and nicotine (as smoked in tobacco)—which cause the greatest expense by far for the health care system—are freely available. Whether other drugs that present societal problems should be legally controlled is heatedly debated, with current trends for legalization of marijuana in more states being a prime example. In general, the more alternatives available to the law for controlling dysfunctional drug use, the less legal regulation is required. Attitudinal changes in society have contributed to the reemergence over time of "epidemics" of drug use. This is currently the case with respect to prescription opioid analgesics, but it has been observed in the past century for most other psychoactive drugs. For example, there are historical examples of failed attempts at prohibition of caffeine and nicotine; the chief focus of legal suppression during the twentieth century has been, in turn, alcohol, heroin, cannabis, cocaine, and methamphetamine.

The treatment of substance-use disorders is a multistage process. Generally, patients must go through detoxification, rehabilitation, and relapse prevention (aftercare). Emphasis is currently on similarities (e.g., common neurobiological mechanisms of drug-seeking behavior and underlying psychopathology) rather than differences (as was the case in the past) among substances of abuse. Thus, patients who abuse different drugs can receive treatment in the same programs, and abstinence from all substances of abuse is promoted. In addition, the treatment of co-occurring psychiatric and medical problems is begun simultaneously with treatment of the substance-use disorder. One problem affects the other. This has resulted in the emergence of "dual diagnosis" treatment units, which provide general psychiatric care for those who have both addiction and a co-occurring disorder. The pharmacologic treatment of concomitant psychiatric disorder requires careful diagnosis and the avoidance of potentially addicting psychoactive substances (e.g., treatment of panic attacks with alprazolam).

The biopsychosocial model is a useful guide to the treatment of substance-use disorder. As a result, both pharmacologic and psychosocial approaches, combined in a so-called pharmacopsychosocial strategy, are implemented.

B. Psychotherapeutic Interventions

Whereas detoxification (treatment of withdrawal) differs among individual drugs of abuse because of differing pharmacologic profiles, long-term management is more similar than different for the numerous substances of abuse (Table 16–9).

The quality of outside social support and the reliability and stability of the patient's social circumstances are the chief determinants of whether inpatient or outpatient treatment is indicated. After initial detoxification (usually inpatient, but outpatient if appropriate), a rehabilitation program is initiated. Substance-abuse education (of the patient and family) is very helpful and can be achieved in formal or informal settings. Coping skills and relaxation training are of great value to many patients who have clinical anxiety. Inpatient and outpatient treatment should include appropriately selected

Table 16–9 Nonpharmacologic Modalities of Substance-Use Disorder Treatment

Education
12-Step support program facilitation (e.g., Alcoholics Anonymous, Narcotics Anonymous, Cocaine Anonymous)
Enhancement of coping strategies
Relaxation training
Family therapy
Lifestyle change (avoiding drug use trigger situations)
Psychotherapy (usually cognitive, relational, or supportive, in a group or individual setting)
Vocational and physical rehabilitation
Recreational therapy
Exercise
Sexual education
Health and nutritional counseling
Spiritual growth
Aftercare

psychotherapy (e.g., social/milieu, insight-oriented, behavioral, individual, cognitive, and group, in various combinations). Patients should participate in self-support groups.

Health maintenance issues must be addressed with an emphasis on smoking cessation, hygiene, exercise, sleep cycle, diet, sex education (e.g., preventing the transmission of human immunodeficiency virus [HIV] and other sexually transmitted diseases). Nonaddictive medications for conditions such as chronic pain should be used. Physicians should coordinate the care of each patient. An examination of spirituality should be encouraged if appropriate for the needs of the patient. Research is emerging on the beneficial effects of aerobic exercise and maintenance of the sleep cycle on mood, brain functioning, and diminishing drug cravings.

Aftercare is at least as important as the initial treatment program. Participation in organized aftercare groups following formal treatment keeps patients engaged with the professionals and peer groups with whom care was initiated and allows them to monitor their relative progress. Individuals with a disorganized family situation or no outside support benefit from structured living facilities such as halfway houses. Lifestyle changes may be needed, the patient removing himself or herself from people and circumstances that promote drug use or stimulate craving. Vocational rehabilitation can be valuable. Twelve-step programs (e.g., Alcoholics Anonymous and Narcotics Anonymous) and other mutual support groups are helpful.

The psychiatric treatment of co-occurring conditions, such as depression, anxiety disorder, bipolar affective disorder, and chronic pain disorder, is essential in preventing relapse, for example, if the patient has been using addictive drugs as misguided self-medication. Appropriate pharmacologic and psychosocial therapies should be prescribed, but potentially addicting medication avoided. It is important that the physician recognizes it may be counterproductive to treat comorbid psychiatric symptoms that will disappear or diminish with abstinence. Education should be provided about commonly used medications that are mood altering and can lead to relapse (e.g., anxiolytics or opioid analgesics).

C. Psychopharmacologic Interventions

The following sections describe some of the well-accepted pharmacologic approaches for the treatment of withdrawal from drugs of abuse (Table 16–10). Pharmacologic strategies for the long-term treatment of substance-use disorder,

Table 16–10 Pharmacological Treatment of Withdrawal Syndromes from Substances of Abuse

Substance	Agent and Dosage	Other Treatment
Alcohol	Diazepam, 10–20 mg/1–2 hours (typical dosage required, 60 mg)	Thiamine, 100 mg intramuscularly or 50 mg twice daily by mouth, and multivitamin tablets for 3 days
Other CNS depressants	Phenobarbital, 120 mg/hour (typical dosage, 900–1500 mg)	
Stimulants	Not usually needed	Anxiolytics or neuroleptics acutely for agitation or toxic psychosis
Opioids	Currently, the goal is to treat withdrawal by initiating maintenance doses of either buprenorphine (16–24 mg daily) or methadone (eventually 60–140 mg daily, slowly titrated) Alternatively, if patient does not want maintenance, detoxification can be accomplished: 3–5 days of clonidine 0.1–0.3 mg every 4–6 hours (check BP prior to each dose, hold for BP ≤ 90/60); methadone dosed at 10–20 mg by mouth every 12 hours initially, or buprenorphine dosed at 4–12 mg under tongue daily initially, both taper over a 5- to 10-day period to reduce withdrawal symptoms (1 mg buprenorphine is equivalent to 5 mg methadone, 5 mg of heroin, 15 mg of morphine, 100 mg of meperidine)	Ibuprofen for muscle cramps, loperamide for loose stools, and promethazine for nausea or vomiting
Nicotine and tobacco	Nicotine patch started at 7–21 mg per day based on addiction severity with slow taper over 3 months Nicotine gum started at 2–4 mg every 1–3 hours based on addiction severity with slow taper over 3 months Varenicline by mouth at 1 mg twice per day for 3 months	Clonidine acutely can minimize withdrawal discomfort
Cannabinoids	Not usually needed	Anxiolytics or neuroleptics acutely for agitation or severe anxiety
Hallucinogens	Not usually needed	Anxiolytics or neuroleptics acutely for toxic psychosis

Table 16–11 Pharmacological Maintenance Strategies for Substance-Use Disorders After Detoxification Completed

Substance	Agent and Dosage
Alcohol	Disulfiram 125–500 mg daily Naltrexone 25–100 mg daily; intramuscular Vivitrol (an injectable suspension containing 380 mg of naltrexone in a microsphere formulation in a single-dose vial) administered monthly Acamprosate 666 mg three times per day Topiramate 25–150 mg twice per day (not FDA approved)
Other CNS depressants	None approved or recommended; anticonvulsants may be effective
Stimulants	None approved or recommended; anticonvulsants or antidepressants may be effective
Opioids	Methadone by mouth at 30–140 mg/day Buprenorphine 4–32 mg under the tongue (available as buprenorphine/naloxone [4/1] to prevent diversion); intramuscular formulation is now available, administered monthly Intramuscular formulation of naltrexone (Vivitrol) at 380 mg monthly once opioids have been discontinued
Nicotine and tobacco	Antidepressants often used; nicotine substitution use various formulations (e.g., patch, lozenges); varenicline by mouth at 1 mg twice per day for maintenance over 3 months
Cannabinoids	None approved or recommended
Hallucinogens	None approved or recommended

independent of co-occurring psychopathology, is an exciting new field of research. Its clinical utility remains adjunctive to psychosocial approaches and will not be discussed in detail here (Table 16–11). The physician must not focus on only treating psychopathology before being sure that it is not a complication of drug use. Inappropriate treatment is very unlikely to be effective and may harm the patient.

1. Alcohol & other CNS depressants—Cross-tolerance and cross-dependence among alcohol and other CNS depressants indicates shared cellular and molecular mechanisms of action and provide the rationale for pharmacologic treatment of CNS depressant withdrawal. Once the obvious clinical signs of withdrawal are apparent, the strategy is to administer a CNS depressant that has a longer elimination half-life than the drug from which the patient is being withdrawn. A long-acting benzodiazepine such as diazepam (or chlordiazepoxide) is the treatment of choice for alcohol withdrawal. The slowly eliminated barbiturate phenobarbital is optimal for other CNS depressants (see Table 16–10). Hourly doses are administered until withdrawal symptoms are eliminated (for treatment of alcohol withdrawal) or until the patient manifests signs of mild intoxication (for other forms of CNS depressant withdrawal). Physicians sometimes use a tapering dose of the abused benzodiazepine for detoxification; however, the phenobarbital loading-dose strategy appears to be the better treatment option. Benzodiazepine tapers are generally very slow (about 10% per week) because of the risk of significant withdrawal reactions and are often associated with poor compliance or an exacerbation of the use disorder. In those relatively few individuals with benzodiazepine-induced neurologic dysfunction who have been prescribed benzodiazepines for extended periods, tapering must be collaborative between prescriber and patient and can require a year, or even more.

All drugs currently used for the treatment of CNS depressant withdrawal are liable to reactivate use disorder. When prescribing these medications, careful patient education is needed concerning risks and benefits, and particularly about the potential for dependence. Problems can occur if patients are not monitored carefully, or if they take more of the medication(s) than prescribed. The treating physician may not be aware that the patient is obtaining prescriptions (from other doctors) of the same (or similar) drug(s). This underlines the need to check controlled substance monitoring databases for patients with whom the physician is working. A major challenge for pharmacologists is to develop agents that ease CNS depressant withdrawal without risking development of a drug use disorder. Some anticonvulsants (e.g., carbamazepine) can effectively be used to manage withdrawal without risk of addiction.

Patients in alcohol detoxification should be prescribed thiamine and other vitamins to prevent the neurologic, hematopoietic, and cognitive effects of chronic drinking. The goal is to institute a nutritional diet. The FDA has approved the administration of naltrexone to prevent alcohol craving and relapse (see Table 16–11). Aversion therapy with disulfiram has also been used; however, its long-term effectiveness has not been established, and patients must be carefully educated and monitored because of the potential for serious reactions if disulfiram is combined with alcohol (see section "Adverse Outcomes of Treatment"). Randomized placebo-controlled studies have shown that acamprosate, topiramate and various other anticonvulsants are efficacious in the treatment of alcohol use disorder. Acamprosate is now FDA approved for the long-term treatment of relapse in alcohol-dependent patients. However, there is little research to help the physician select one or another of these medications.

2. Stimulants: cocaine & amphetamines—The treatment of stimulant intoxication is usually supportive. Anxiolytics are the primary treatment but neuroleptics may be needed for severe agitation. Psychostimulants can be highly addictive, and chronic users must understand the causes of relapse and design strategies for relapse prevention. Pharmacologic agents such as anticonvulsants (e.g., carbamazepine) and antidepressants can help prevent relapse, but controlled studies have been inconclusive. In animal models, environmental manipulation such as inflicting punishment, increasing the amount of effort required to obtain the drug, or offering alternative reinforcers decrease its self-administration. Such behavioral observations have guided clinical treatment approaches, such as contingency management. Only if the patient can maintain abstinence beyond the withdrawal period can extinction and ultimate abstinence follow. Therefore, treatment should address the conditions that lead to relapse, reducing the effects of conditioned cues that trigger craving. Such conditions involve the persons with whom, or situations in which, the individual has used stimulants, together with the availability of stimulants in the neighborhood. Rewards should be provided contingent on abstinence.

After stimulant overdose, further treatment may be needed. In the case of amphetamines, the patient's urine can be acidified with ammonium chloride to increase excretion of the substance. Benzodiazepines are the first choice but α-adrenergic antagonist can be used to decrease elevated blood pressure, and antipsychotic medication may be needed to alleviate CNS overstimulation.

Cocaine overdoses are more complicated because of the greater potential for cardiac arrhythmia, respiratory failure, and seizures. Phentolamine or chlorpromazine (as it has some α-adrenergic–antagonist action) can be useful in reducing CNS and cardiovascular problems. Artificial respiration or cardiac life support may be needed. Severe anhedonia and depression are associated with dysfunctional brain-reward pathways due to chronic use (e.g., after methamphetamine use) and can necessitate antidepressant treatment.

3. Opioids—Opioid withdrawal can be treated in several ways, depending on whether the goal is abstinence or maintenance treatment with agonists (methadone or buprenorphine) or antagonists. Often, a slow taper of methadone (a long-acting opioid agonist that requires special licensure for use in opioid maintenance treatment) is used for gradual detoxification over weeks to months. In other circumstances, the abused opioid is discontinued abruptly and clonidine, lofexidine, methadone, or buprenorphine are used short-term to reduce withdrawal symptoms. Clonidine and lofexidine have the advantage of not being an opioid and not having addicting properties, but it may not provide as smooth a withdrawal. Baseline readings of blood pressure and regular monitoring are advised. Methadone, a pure μ-opioid agonist, or buprenorphine, a partial μ-opioid agonist, alleviate the symptoms of withdrawal, but each has significant dependence liability. Proper hydration and supportive care can be combined with other agents, such as ibuprofen for muscle cramps, loperamide for loose stools, and promethazine for nausea.

Methadone maintenance programs (1–2 years or longer) are used in some locations to reduce the risk of reverting to the drug and promoting crime cultures (see Table 16–11). Some patients on methadone maintenance use other drugs such as alcohol and cocaine and sell the methadone they receive to support their drug use. Buprenorphine maintenance is another accepted pharmacologic means of relapse prevention that was first approved for the office-based treatment of opioid dependence by trained physicians through the Drug Abuse Treatment Act of 2000. Regulations have recently been greatly relaxed to allow prescribing for opioid use disorder by all physicians. Naltrexone has been demonstrated to be effective in various formulations for treatment of opioid use disorder. In the treatment of chronic pain, which is often associated with opioid dependence, nonaddictive medication (e.g., anticonvulsants and certain antidepressants) and other treatments (e.g., physical therapy, nerve blocks) should be used when appropriate to minimize the likelihood of relapse.

4. Cannabinoids—The treatment of cannabinoid intoxication usually requires no more than a safe, calm environment. Anxiolytic medication is used only in cases of severe agitation or anxiety. Educational programs and lifestyle changes, for example, exercise, are important for prevention, particularly among younger people.

5. Tobacco—Nonpharmacologic approaches are frequently used to help tobacco users quit smoking. Weight gain and mood lability may need to be addressed. Strategies may need to be developed to help users endure the day without tobacco use. Clonidine can help reduce withdrawal symptoms. Nicotine-containing products such as dermal patches and gum can be used to taper smokers from nicotine. Antidepressants have been helpful in some patients. A significant advance to promote long-term abstinence from nicotine is varenicline (see Table 16–10).

6. Hallucinogens & volatile inhalants—Detoxification from low dosages of hallucinogens can often be achieved in a safe, structured environment with emotional support. Anxiolytics and possibly neuroleptics (such as haloperidol or olanzapine, but not phenothiazines because of possible side effects) may be needed. If respiratory suppression occurs, emergency oxygen may be required. The primary treatment for arylcyclohexylamine overdose is removal from sensory stimulation, and possibly treatment with benzodiazepines or neuroleptics.

▶ Co-occurring Disorders

Psychoactive substance-use disorder can contribute to or result from various forms of psychopathology. Physicians are most likely to encounter patients with substance-use disorders when they present for the treatment of a complicating or associated physical or emotional illness. Medical and psychiatric complications of drug use are attributable either to the direct pharmacologic actions of the substance (e.g., overdose, organ toxicity, metabolic consequences) or to the indirect effects of drug self-administration on lifestyle. The indirect effects include use of other than the primary drug of abuse (including tobacco), inappropriate use of prescribed medications such as analgesics or anxiolytics, malnutrition, trauma, infection, neglect, or lack of compliance with the medical regimen for coexistent illnesses. The treatment of severe medical complications takes precedence if the illness is life threatening or incapacitating. However, if the underlying substance-use disorder and emotional concomitants are not recognized and addressed, treatment may be for naught.

Agabio R, Trogu E, Pani PP: Antidepressants for the treatment of people with co-occurring depression and alcohol dependence. *Cochrane Database Syst Rev* 2018;4(4):CD008581.

Rich JS, Martin PR: Co-occurring psychiatric disorders and alcoholism. In: Sullivan EV, Pfefferbaum A (eds). *Handbook of Clinical Neurology*. Elsevier, Waltham MA USA 2014, pp. 573–588.

Swinford-Jackson SE, O'Brien CP, Kenny PJ, Vanderschuren LJMJ, Unterwald EM, Pierce RC: The persistent challenge of developing addiction pharmacotherapies. *Cold Spring Harb Perspect Med* 2021;11:a040311.

▶ Complications

A. Alcohol

The medical complications of chronic alcoholism derive from the pharmacologic effects of ethanol, the changes in intermediary metabolism resulting from its biotransformation to acetaldehyde in the liver, and the toxic effects of this metabolite in various body tissues (Table 16–12). Moreover, poor nutrition, which is frequently associated with chronic alcohol consumption can complicate those related to alcohol alone.

Ethanol metabolism leads to conversion of pyruvate to lactate and to the formation of acetoacetate, acetone, and β-hydroxybutyrate. These chemicals can interfere with the renal tubular secretion of uric acid, causing increases in blood urate and exacerbating gout.

Heavy drinking after a period of not eating can cause severe, sometimes fatal, hypoglycemia. This is the result of the combination of low hepatic glycogen stores and inhibition by ethanol of gluconeogenesis. Fatty liver can be caused by single episodes of ethanol binging. Chronic fatty liver, probably in combination with nutritional deficiencies, progresses to alcoholic hepatitis and finally cirrhosis and increased likelihood of hepatoma. It has been shown that obesity (nonalcoholic steatohepatitis, NASH) and alcohol consumption act

Table 16–12 Medical Complications of Alcoholism

Metabolic and malnutrition
Gout
Hyperlipidemia and fatty liver
Hypoglycemia
Weight loss or obesity
Immune compromise (opportunistic infections)
Impaired protein synthesis
Mineral and electrolyte imbalances
Vitamin deficiencies
Decreased blood clotting

Gastrointestinal
Esophagitis
Gastritis or ulcer
Pancreatitis
Liver disease (alcoholic hepatitis, cirrhosis, hepatoma)
Malabsorption
Altered drug and carcinogen metabolism
Increased cancer incidence

Endocrine
Pancreatic insufficiency (glucose intolerance)
Increased adrenocorticotropin (ACTH), glucocorticoid, or catecholamine release
Inhibited testosterone synthesis (male hypogonadism)
Inhibition of antidiuretic hormone (ADH), oxytocin release

Neurologic
Dementia
Amnesia
Cerebellar degeneration
Fetal alcohol effects
Neuropathy

Cardiovascular
Hypertension
Stroke
Arrhythmias
Coronary heart disease

synergistically to increase the risk of fibrosis progression, hepatic carcinogenesis and mortality, while genetic polymorphisms can strongly influence disease progression. Ethanol can induce an isozyme of cytochrome P450 to convert some chemicals to hepatotoxic metabolites. Alcoholic cirrhosis continues as a major preventable cause of death among individuals aged 24–44 years in large urban areas.

The diuresis associated with drinking alcoholic beverages is caused primarily by inhibition of antidiuretic hormone (ADH) release from the posterior pituitary. Alcohol also increases the release of adrenocorticotropic hormone, glucocorticoids, and catecholamines. The synthesis of testosterone is inhibited, and its hepatic metabolism increased. Men with chronic alcoholism often have signs of hypogonadism and feminization (e.g., gynecomastia).

Ethanol stimulates the secretion of gastric and pancreatic juices. This effect on gastric juices and the direct irritant action of concentrated solutions of ethanol help to explain why one of every three heavy drinkers has chronic gastritis. High dosages of ethanol can cause vomiting independent of any local irritation. Alcohol abuse is associated with acute and chronic pancreatitis and esophagitis. An increased incidence of carcinoma of the pharynx, larynx, and esophagus has been found among heavy users of alcoholic beverages. Nutritional problems are common among alcoholic patients and are manifested by weight loss or obesity, impaired protein synthesis, altered amino acid metabolism, immune incompetence, mineral and electrolyte imbalance, and vitamin deficiencies.

B. Stimulants: Cocaine & Amphetamines

Physical consequences of stimulant abuse include sleep problems, chronic fatigue, severe headaches, and, depending on the route of administration, nasal sores and bleeding, severe dental caries, chronic cough and sore throat, nausea, and vomiting (Table 16–13).

Stimulant abuse can lead to seizures, cerebrovascular accidents, cerebrovasculitis, hyperpyrexia with rhabdomyolysis, and dystonia. Possible mechanisms for neuropsychiatric complications include cerebrovascular vasoconstriction, neurotransmitter depletion, and a reduction of the limbic seizure threshold by repeated subconvulsant stimulation.

Cocaine abuse is particularly dangerous because of the devastating cardiovascular effects that can occur in healthy

and young individuals: angina pectoris, myocardial infarction, syncope, aortic dissection, pulmonary edema, and sudden arrhythmic death. Similar cardiovascular morbidity has been observed for amphetamine-related drugs. Note that infectious complications of cocaine/stimulants are similar to those due to opioids (below) when used intravenously.

C. Opioids

Opioid abuse can lead to many serious medical complications in addition to dependence (Table 16–14). For example, injuries can result from sedation, especially if an individual drives or uses dangerous machinery while taking opioid medication. The analgesic effect can block natural mechanisms that alert the user of physical injury. Decreased respiratory drive, vomiting, and death (from respiratory suppression) can occur with overdose. Shared needle use in intravenous users increases the risk of HIV infection, hepatitis, brain abscess, thrombophlebitis, pulmonary emboli, pulmonary infection, infective endocarditis, septic arthritis, and other infectious diseases. Substances added to opioid street preparations (e.g., strychnine) can lead to peripheral neuropathy, myelopathy, and amblyopia. Deaths from opioid overdoses, alone or in combination with stimulants and CNS depressants, have climbed in the last two decades, greatly exacerbated recently by ready availability of very high potency synthetic opioids like fentanyl.

D. Cannabinoids

A controversial amotivational syndrome has been described in the literature, wherein chronic marijuana users have been noted to exhibit apathy; dullness; impairment of judgment, concentration, and memory; and loss of interest in personal appearance and conventional goals. Well-controlled clinical studies have not provided strong evidence that an amotivational syndrome is a direct consequence of marijuana use;

Table 16–13 Medical Complications of Stimulant Abuse

General health
Chronic fatigue
Sleep problems
Nasal congestion, ulceration, or bleeding
Chronic cough or sore throat
Nausea or vomiting
Sexual disinterest
Intravenously or sexually transmitted hepatitis or HIV
Traumatic injuries and overdose

Neurologic
Seizure
Cerebrovascular accident
Hyperpyrexia and rhabdomyolysis
Headaches
Dystonias
Cerebrovasculitis

Cardiovascular
Arrhythmia
Angina pectoris
Myocardial infarction
Syncope
Pulmonary edema
Aortic dissection
Infective endocarditis

Table 16–14 Medical Complications of Opioid Abuse

General health
Chronic fatigue
Sleep problems
Nausea or vomiting
Sexual disinterest
Traumatic injuries

Pulmonary
Pulmonary edema
Overdose
Respiratory depression
Death

Infectious diseases
Intravenously or sexually transmitted hepatitis or HIV
Thrombophlebitis
Pulmonary emboli or abscess
Infective endocarditis

however, such symptoms would be of particular concern to school-aged adolescents. Over recent years, the association between marijuana use and development of psychotic illnesses has become quite convincing. There is evidence of alterations in heart rate; blood pressure; and reproductive, immunological, and pulmonary function. Cannabinoid-induced testosterone suppression is an issue of concern. It has become apparent that chronic marijuana use has widespread physiological consequences.

E. Tobacco

Much has been written and debated about the adverse effects of tobacco use. It is generally accepted that users have significantly increased risk of many serious illnesses: pulmonary disease (e.g., emphysema, lung cancer); cardiovascular disease (e.g., coronary artery disease); peripheral vascular disease, particularly with chronic use; dental disease (e.g., oral cancer, especially with smokeless tobacco); nicotine stomatitis and stained teeth; and diminished birth weight in the babies of mothers who smoke. Some researchers have estimated that as many as 25% of deaths in the United States are associated with tobacco use. Exposure to high doses of nicotine, as is found in some insecticides, can cause diarrhea, nausea, vomiting, irritability, headache, convulsions, tachypnea, coma, or death.

F. Hallucinogens & Volatile Inhalants

The acute effects of hallucinogens include sympathomimetic actions such as high blood pressure and seizures, particularly with use of phenylisopropylamine compounds. Anticholinergic substances can cause amnesia, hallucinations, dry mouth, constipation, bronchodilation, tachycardia, urinary retention, diminished penile erection, photophobia, increased intraocular pressure, and blurred vision (from dilated pupils). Long-term complications include flashbacks that seem to be stimulated by stress and fatigue.

PCP use can lead to paranoid hallucinations, violent behavior, and self-injury. Medical effects include hypersalivation, catalepsy, perspiration, rigidity, myoclonus, stereotyped movements, hyperreflexia, cardiac arrhythmia, hypertension, and convulsions.

Intoxication with volatile inhalants can be associated with dizziness and syncope. Cardiac arrhythmia, pulmonary edema, liver damage, asphyxiation, and renal dysfunction can occur. Neurotoxic effects can lead to severe dementia in young adults.

Bataller R, Arab JP, Shah VH: Alcohol-associated hepatitis. *N Engl J Med* 2022;387(26):2436–2448.

Ciccarone D: The rise of illicit fentanyls, stimulants and the fourth wave of the opioid overdose crisis. *Curr Opin Psychiatry* 2021;34(4).

Volpicelli JR, Menzies P: Rethinking unhealthy alcohol use in the United States: a structured review. *Subst Abuse Res Treat* 2022;16. https://doi.org/10.1177/11782218221111832.

▶ Adverse Outcomes of Treatment

A. Unrecognized or Untreated Medical Complications

Patients with alcohol and drug dependence are often inappropriately triaged to treatment facilities lacking the medical expertise needed to manage medical complications. This may be because intoxicated patients cannot provide adequate histories or because of hostile attitudes among treating professionals. All substance-use disorder patients deserve a meticulous history, physical examination, and appropriate laboratory examination to rule out common medical complications. Medical and surgical consultation and joint management are often necessary for more complex cases. In addition, it is important to recognize addictive disorders in patients who have the medical disorders typically complicating alcohol or drug abuse and correctly diagnose patients who are recalcitrant to usually effective treatments. These points are discussed in greater detail in the section "Differential Diagnosis."

B. Unrecognized or Untreated Other Psychiatric Disorders

It can be disastrous if a treatable psychiatric disorder is overlooked in a substance-abusing patient. Many jurisdictions artificially separate the psychiatric care of patients with addictions from those with other psychiatric disorders. Some 12-step support groups proscribe the use of all psychopharmacologic agents, even if they have no known abuse liability and are potentially beneficial. This is to some degree the result of a mistrust of psychiatrists, who until recently believed that the care of patients with substance-use disorders was outside their bailiwick or treated other psychiatric disorders without addressing co-occurring addictions. It is now commonly accepted that all psychiatrists should develop the expertise needed for the diagnosis and appropriate treatment or referral of substance-use disorder patients and should seek collaborative relationships with community resources such as 12-step programs.

▶ Drug Interactions

Disulfiram inhibits aldehyde dehydrogenase (involved in alcohol metabolism), and its effects in the drinker are largely if not entirely due to accumulation of acetaldehyde. Taken alone, disulfiram causes little or no effect. With alcohol, it causes intense flushing of the face and neck, tachycardia, hypotension, nausea, and vomiting. It has caused death. Disulfiram also significantly inhibits microsomal drug-metabolizing enzymes and increases the elimination half-life of many drugs such as phenytoin, warfarin, thiopental, benzodiazepines, and caffeine. In treating alcoholism, physicians must use disulfiram with caution and combine it with psychosocial treatment.

Although alcohol can alter absorption of some drugs (e.g., it increases the absorption of diazepam), the basis for most pharmacokinetic ethanol–drug interactions involve the alcohol dehydrogenase pathway and/or liver microsomal enzymes. Microsomal drug metabolism (cytochrome P450) is inhibited in the presence of high concentrations of ethanol. Therefore, when ethanol and prescribed drugs are taken together, the drug's effect may be augmented (in the case of phenytoin and warfarin) or the effect of alcohol prolonged (in the case of chloral hydrate, chlorpromazine, or cimetidine). Microsomal induction after long-term alcohol consumption contributes to accelerated ethanol metabolism at high blood ethanol concentrations. Increased drug metabolism and activation of xenobiotics (e.g., carcinogens) following microsomal induction results in lower-than-therapeutic blood levels (in the case of barbiturates, phenytoin, isoniazid, meprobamate, methadone, and warfarin) or increased production of toxic metabolites (in the case of acetaminophen). Although most recently launched drugs have been developed by the pharmaceutical industry to minimize drug interactions via microsomal enzyme metabolism, pharmacodynamic interactions are still widespread. Common mechanisms for pharmacodynamic ethanol–drug interactions include increased drug effects when an individual is intoxicated with ethanol, because of additive CNS depression (in the case of antihistamines, other CNS depressants, opioids, antipsychotics, and antidepressants); or diminished drug effects when the individual has not been drinking, because of the presence of cross-tolerance to other CNS depressants.

Metabolism of methadone can be altered by the coadministration of medications that induce cytochrome P450 (e.g., rifampin, antiretrovirals, phenytoin, barbiturates, carbamazepine), thereby complicating dosing during methadone maintenance.

▶ **Prognosis**

The prognosis and course of illness in substance-use disorders depends on numerous factors involving a complex interaction of biological, psychological, and environmental elements. The specific substance(s) used, the duration and dosage of substance-use, co-occurring psychiatric and medical disorders, coping skills, developmental history, socioeconomic status, social support, genetic predispositions, treatment choices, and other aspects are all important. The prognosis for individuals with substance-use disorders can be greatly complicated by an antisocial lifestyle. In addition, the intravenous use of drugs (as well as sex-for-drugs transactions) increases the risk and the spread of life-threatening illnesses such as acquired immunodeficiency syndrome (AIDS) and hepatitis.

The outcome of substance-related problems is enhanced by relapse prevention using nonpharmacologic approaches involving psychotherapy and self-help groups (such as Alcoholics Anonymous). Appropriate adjunctive pharmacologic treatments can be effectively combined with psychosocial treatments with an emphasis on healthy lifestyle, including exercise, sleep, diet, and relationships to prevent relapse.

It is important to treat co-occurring psychiatric illnesses. Most substance-use disorder patients have another psychiatric illness, particularly affective, anxiety, and personality disorders, which can worsen prognosis if not addressed. Complete psychiatric evaluation and treatment is therefore essential in patients with substance and related disorders.

A. Alcohol & Other CNS Depressants

Disulfiram, naltrexone, and acamprosate are the only medications approved by the FDA to prevent alcohol relapse. Naltrexone is a μ-opioid receptor antagonist. Acamprosate (calcium bis acetyl homotaurinate), a chemical analog of L-glutamic acid, affects GABAergic and glutamatergic neurotransmission. Both naltrexone and acamprosate can reduce relapse by approximately half that of placebo control subjects over a 2- to 3-month period (down to a rate of about 20–25%). Moreover, the type of psychotherapy used with naltrexone appears to influence treatment outcome, as lower rates of relapse were reported in patients using supportive therapy compared to coping skills therapy.

More recently investigators have studied whether combining these medications improves alcoholism treatment outcome. Naltrexone or acamprosate as well as the combination of the two were significantly more effective than placebo in one study. Naltrexone treatment tended to be superior to acamprosate regarding time to first drink and time to relapse in this study. Naltrexone/acamprosate combined was most effective with significantly lower relapse rates than placebo and acamprosate alone; however, the combination was not significantly better than naltrexone alone. More recently, beneficial effects of anticonvulsants such as topiramate and oxcarbazepine have been demonstrated, but these medications are not FDA approved for alcohol use disorder. There is some evidence for combining naltrexone with an appropriate psychopharmacologic agent in alcohol use disorder patients with co-occurring mood disorder or PTSD. Despite some demonstrated benefits from these medications, they should preferably be used in conjunction with psychosocial therapies.

B. Stimulants: Cocaine & Amphetamines

Users of stimulants such as cocaine and amphetamines tend to use the drug nearly daily (in low or high dosages) or intermittently (e.g., weekend binges). Binge use of stimulants often leads to dependence. Daily users often rapidly increase the dosage taken. Intravenous use or smoking of cocaine can lead to dependence in a matter of weeks or months. Dependence takes longer to develop in individuals who nasally insufflate the drug. Preliminary studies indicate that cognitive–behavioral therapy is more effective than interpersonal psychotherapy in preventing relapse in cocaine-dependent patients (with abstinence rates over a 3-week period of 60% and 33%, respectively). Behavioral treatment (contracting, counseling, community reinforcement) increases abstinence to about 40% in a 3- to 4-month period compared to 5% in those who participate in drug counseling only. In addition, preliminary trials suggest that some patients with cocaine dependence benefit from anti-depressants and anticonvulsants (e.g., carbamazepine).

C. Opioids

Opioid dependence is often characterized by short periods of abstinence followed by relapse. Even after years of forced abstinence by incarceration, many subjects relapse after being released from prison. Relapse often occurs when patients fail to inform their physician about their addictions and opioids are prescribed for medical ailments. Psychosocial therapies for opioid dependence are often helpful. Agonist substitution with methadone is well established as benefiting the most severely addicted patient population when provided in methadone maintenance programs. Buprenorphine, approved for admin-istration by appropriately trained physicians in office-based practice, provides an alternative to methadone in treatment of opioid dependence. However, it is not yet established for which patients methadone or buprenorphine is the preferred treatment modality, and choices are made based on availability and resources. On the other hand, similar benefits have been found for standard outpatient counseling or psychotherapy in patients on methadone maintenance (for opioid use disorder) compared to those in therapeutic communities. Subjects who remain in combined treatment have lower relapse rates than do those who drop out. Psychodynamic therapy and cognitive therapy have been of greater benefit than standard drug coun-seling alone. Interestingly, limited monthly interactions with a psychotherapist, when combined with methadone mainte-nance, appear to be as effective as more intensive and frequent interpersonal psychotherapy alone.

D. Cannabinoids

Cannabis dependence occurs slowly in those who develop patterns of increasing dosage and frequency of use. The plea-surable effects of cannabis often diminish with regular heavy use. In patients with marijuana dependence, manual-guided individual treatment and group therapy appear to have similar beneficial effects. Marijuana use drops about 50% in response to these treatment modalities. Lifestyle change is vital in recovery.

E. Tobacco

Tobacco smokers usually start in their early teen years, often in social settings. Children are at increased risk if their par-ents or close friends smoke. Since the 1970s, smoking has decreased in the U.S. population but less in females than in males. The greatest prevalence rate of smoking is in the psy-chiatric population, especially among patients with schizo-phrenia or depression. Smoking is very reinforcing, and although some people can stop smoking "cold turkey," overall failure rates of treatment are high (over 70% at 1 year).

F. Hallucinogens & Volatile Inhalants

The onset of hallucinogen use depends on availability, social and cultural setting, and expectations. Use is often experi-mental and intermittent, but chronic or heavy use can lead to long-term consequences such as flashbacks, mood lability, personality disturbances, and dementia.

Aharonovich E, Scodes J, Wall MM, Hasin DS: The relationship of frequency of cocaine use to substance and psychiatric disorders in the U.S. general population. *Drug Alcohol Depend* 2021;227:108933.

Vaillant GE: A 60-year follow-up of alcoholic men. *Addiction* 2003;98(8):1043–1051.

CONCLUSION

The substance-related disorders exact an immense toll on the mental and physical well-being of many individuals. Consequently, they jeopardize the integrity of the family and other social forces represented by the health care sys-tem, the law, and the economy. Because of the prevalence of substance-related disorders, and because they can mas-querade as diverse medical and other psychiatric disor-ders, their recognition and initial treatment are relevant to all physicians—in particular, to psychiatrists. Substance-related disorders are heterogeneous in terms of the inter-actions between the manifest psychopathology of the individual patient and the psychopharmacologic actions of a given drug, within the relevant sociocultural context. This perspective is useful in seeking an etiologic understanding of these disorders, conducting a clinical assessment, plan-ning for the initial treatment of the direct consequences of drug use, and developing and implementing a comprehen-sive treatment strategy for patients. Recent perspectives of addictive disorders have broadened to include other out-of-control, self-destructive, so-called behavioral addictions, the first example of which to be incorporated in DSM 5 is gambling disorder, which for many individuals seem to be woven into the fabric of substance-use and co-occurring psychiatric disorders.

Future directions in substance-use disorder treat-ment research are likely to focus on understanding issues of co-occurring psychiatric conditions, developing new psychopharmacologic treatment options, and combining pharmacotherapy and psychotherapy and lifestyle changes in the management of these disorders. Agents that can help reduce drug craving and relapse are of particular interest, as are genetically based interindividual differences in these disorders. Overall, considerably more research is needed on the optimal combination of treatment modalities to prevent relapse in substance-use disorder patients and improve prognosis.

Alcohol Use Disorder

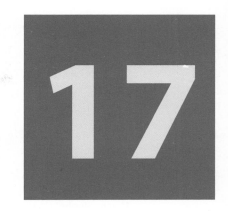

Kristopher A. Kast, MD
Jolomi Ikomi, MD
Stephanie S. O'Malley, PhD

▶ General Considerations

A. Epidemiology

1. Prevalence—In 2021, the prevalence of alcohol use in the United States was 47.5% among individuals >12 years of age, with roughly half of current drinkers reporting binge alcohol use and 12.3% reporting heavy alcohol use (NSDUH 2021). The prevalence of alcohol use disorder (AUD) was 12.1% (NSDUH 2021), a higher rate than pre-DSM-5 epidemiologic data that reported 8.5% of adults experienced a DSM-IV diagnosis of alcohol abuse (4.7%) or alcohol dependence (3.8%) in the preceding 12 months (Figure 17–1) using data from the National Epidemiological Survey of Alcohol and Related Conditions (NESARC). The lifetime prevalence for an AUD has consistently been reported as ~30% (Grant et al. 2015).

Alcohol-related deaths have increased steadily at a rate of 2.2% per year across preceding decades, with a more recent abrupt increase by 25.5% during the COVID-19 pandemic. This translates into >100,000 alcohol-related deaths in 2021, rising from ~79,000 in 2019 (CDC 2023; White et al. 2022). This follows an unprecedented increase in alcohol sales during the pandemic, likely associated with increased alcohol consumption by vulnerable individuals with preexisting comorbidity, as well as a marked increase in alcohol-related traffic deaths (Slater et al. 2022; Acuff et al. 2022; USDOT 2022).

2. Demographics—There has been a noteworthy decline in underage alcohol use from 28.8% of 12- to 20-year-olds in 2002 to 15.1% in 2021 (NSDUH 2021). However, the young adult population has consistently demonstrated the greatest AUD prevalence across epidemiologic studies, with 26.7% of 18- to 29-year-olds meeting DSM-5 AUD criteria in the 2012–13 NESARC-III cohort, compared to only 2.3% of those aged > 65 years (Grant et al. 2015).

Recent epidemiologic findings also suggest a closing "gender gap" between men and women with AUD, driven by increasing rates of young women (aged 12–20 years) with binge alcohol use now exceeding the rate of male peers (9.3% vs. 7.4%, respectively; NSDUH 2021). This increase is especially concerning given the risk for negative health and reproductive/perinatal outcomes for women at lower doses of alcohol compared to men, including hepatic, cardiovascular, and cancer-related disease (White 2020).

There are also variations in prevalence of alcohol use by race and ethnicity (Table 17–1). Native American populations have experienced elevated rates of AUD compared with the general population; Asian American populations experienced lower rates; and Black, Latinx, native Hawaiians, and Pacific Islander Americans have rates comparable to national averages (NSDUH 2016). However, even for populations with relatively similar rates of AUD, there are disparities in medical and psychiatric sequelae. For example, Black Americans experience higher mortality from AUD than White Americans despite similar prevalence, with socioeconomic factors and other social determinants of health possibly contributing to this disparity (Jackson et al. 2015).

Individuals immigrating to the United States generally have lower risk of any substance use disorder (SUD) than native-born Americans, though this risk increases to match the general population over 10 years of residence (Breslau et al. 2007). However, among disadvantaged immigrant populations (undocumented Mexican groups being most frequently studied), alcohol use is elevated compared to control populations in the home country. In one sample, 42.3% of Mexican migrants reported at-risk alcohol use (Zhang et al. 2015).

Cultural norms for low-risk alcohol use also differ internationally, leading to geographic differences in reported AUD prevalence despite standardized diagnostic criteria. Among European countries, estimated prevalence of AUD in 2010 ranged between <1% in Italy and Spain and >12% in Latvia—though per capita consumption only varied threefold. Further, reported use in countries with religious prohibition against alcohol consumption leads to markedly elevated per capita consumption rates, most likely representing underreporting of individual use (Rehm 2017).

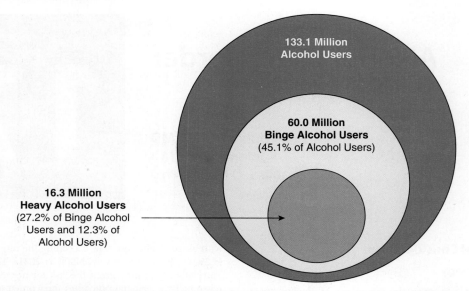

133.1 Million
Alcohol Users

60.0 Million
Binge Alcohol Users
(45.1% of Alcohol Users)

16.3 Million
Heavy Alcohol Users
(27.2% of Binge Alcohol
Users and 12.3% of
Alcohol Users)

Note: Binge Alcohol Use is defined as drinking five or more drinks (for males) or four or more drinks (for females) on the same occasion on at least 1 day in the past 30 days. Heavy Alcohol Use is defined as binge drinking on the same occasion on 5 or more days in the past 30 days; all heavy alcohol users are also binge alcohol users.

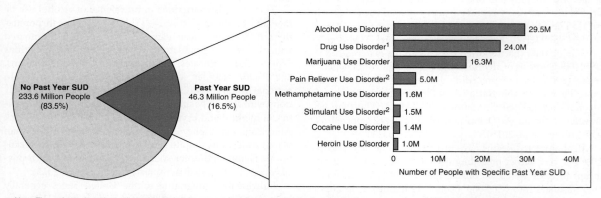

No Past Year SUD
233.6 Million People
(83.5%)

Past Year SUD
46.3 Million People
(16.5%)

Alcohol Use Disorder — 29.5M
Drug Use Disorder[1] — 24.0M
Marijuana Use Disorder — 16.3M
Pain Reliever Use Disorder[2] — 5.0M
Methamphetamine Use Disorder — 1.6M
Stimulant Use Disorder[2] — 1.5M
Cocaine Use Disorder — 1.4M
Heroin Use Disorder — 1.0M

Number of People with Specific Past Year SUD

Note: The estimated numbers of people with substance use disorders are not mutually exclusive because people could have use disorders for more than one substance.

[1]Includes data from all past year users of marijuana, cocaine, heroin, hallucinogens, inhalants, methamphetamine, and prescription psychotherapeutic drugs (i.e., pain relievers, tranquilizers, stimulants, or sedatives).

[2]Includes data from all past year users of the specific prescription drug.

▲ Figure 17–1 12-month prevalence of alcohol use, binge use, heavy use, and alcohol use disorder compared to other substance use disorders in the general population, as per the NSDUH 2021.

3. Risk of psychiatric comorbidity—Results from NESARC showed that 1.1% of adults reported SUD and AUD combined, whereas 7.35% and 0.9% reported AUD alone and other substance use disorder alone, respectively. Yet individuals using a combination of drugs and alcohol had a much higher rate of treatment seeking than those using drugs or alcohol alone, which may indicate a need for more integrated alcohol and other substance treatment services. There is also a strong association between having an AUD and any psychiatric disorder (most commonly mood and anxiety disorders, but also posttraumatic stress disorder and attention deficit disorder). In addition, rates of personality disorders, most commonly antisocial personality disorder and borderline personality disorder, are higher among those with AUD (Castillo-Carniglia et al. 2019).

Table 17–1 12-Month Prevalence of Alcohol Use Disorder Among Individuals Aged 12 Years or Older by Race–Ethnicity, as per NSDUH 2021

Race–Ethnicity	Alcohol Use Disorder (Standard Error)
General population	10.6% (0.24)
American Indian or Alaskan native	15.6% (2.55)
Native Hawaiian or other Pacific Islander	14% (3.65)
White	11% (0.31)
Hispanic or Latinx	10.3% (0.57)
Black or African American	10.1% (0.61)
Asian	6% (0.75)
Multiracial	14.7% (1.87)

B. Etiology

1. Neurobiology—The neurobiological basis of AUD remains an ongoing area of research, which involves multiple neuronal pathway systems. Alcohol causes direct activation and excitation of neurons in the ventral tegmental area (VTA). It does this via direct release of dopamine in the mesolimbic pathway, which is associated with positive reinforcement and reward following alcohol consumption. Animal studies show that there is a dose-dependent release of dopamine in the nucleus accumbens following alcohol self-administration. However, dopamine denervation within the nucleus accumbens does not abolish alcohol consumption, indicating involvement of other pathways. Opioid mechanisms have also been implicated in the development of AUD. Alcohol ingestion causes release of endorphins from the nucleus accumbens. Direct inhibition of this action could explain the attenuating effect of naltrexone, an opioid antagonist, on alcohol consumption.

Other biochemical systems that have been studied are N-methyl-D-aspartate (NMDA), gamma-aminobutyric acid (GABA), serotonin, and endocannabinoids, as well as neuropeptide Y. Manipulation of these systems has been shown to have some degree of effect on alcohol-seeking behavior in animal models and possible AUD in humans. Acamprosate, another pharmacologic intervention for preventing AUD relapse, modulates NMDA-receptor transmission and may indirectly affect GABA-receptor transmission (Kalk et al. 2014).

2. Environmental—Multiple environmental risk factors are associated with the development of AUD.

i. **Early age onset**—Early age (adolescent) onset of drinking is associated with higher risk of development of AUD and its consequences later in life. Poor parental monitoring may contribute to early onset of drinking. There may also be a genetic vulnerability for early-onset drinking (Prescott & Kendler 1999).

ii. **Availability**—There is a higher prevalence of AUD in societies, cultures, and neighborhoods where alcohol is more readily available, related to social norms or fewer legal or zoning restrictions. In families where alcohol is readily available, children are more likely to model alcohol use behavior from their parents and are more likely to develop an AUD (Hawkins et al. 1992).

iii. **Societal conflict, trauma, and economic deprivation**—Lack of structure, housing, and basic needs has been associated with higher rates of crime, delinquency, and conduct/antisocial disorder. There is a higher rate of alcohol use among individuals within this population. Trauma history is also a risk factor.

iv. **Peer pressure**—There is a higher risk of development of AUD in children who associate with peers who drink.

3. Personality traits

i. **Personality disorders**—AUDs are more prevalent in individuals diagnosed with any personality disorders, most especially conduct/antisocial, histrionic, and dependent personality disorders.

ii. **Impulsivity and risk-taking behavior**—Impulsivity, as defined by acting in an unplanned manner without thinking through possible consequences of one's actions, is associated with higher rates of aggression, anger outbursts, suicide, and addictive behavior. These individuals are more likely to try alcohol at an earlier age, have more frequent relapses, and suffer more alcohol-related consequences.

C. Genetics

Genetics heavily influence the risk of alcoholism in individuals. Heritability and family studies have shown that genetic factors account for about 40–60% of the risk of developing an AUD. Hundreds of genetic markers have been associated with AUD, though as with other substance use disorders AUD is polygenic and non-Mendelian with multiple contributing genetic alleles, each with relatively small effect size on the phenotype (Prom-Wormley et al. 2017). Polygenic risk scores bundling multiple at-risk genetic markers into a single construct have been associated with development of AUD in genome-wide association studies studies, though also with relatively small effect size.

Specific genotypes associated with risk and protection have been identified, the most noteworthy being polymorphisms of genes involved in alcohol metabolism. The genetic polymorphisms of the two liver enzymes alcohol dehydrogenase (ADH2) and the mitochondrial acetaldehyde dehydrogenase (ALDH2) system remain the most clearly understood. There are six different isoenzymes of ALDH, with ADLDH2 being found in the mitochondria. The ALDH2-1 allele produces the active form of the enzyme, whereas ALDH2-2 produces the inactive form. Individuals with a homozygous ALDH2-2 are unable to break down acetaldehyde and experience aversive reactions (facial flushing, nausea, and autonomic dysregulation) after consumption of small amounts of alcohol. As a result, they are less likely to drink or to drink heavily. This homozygous ALDH2-2 or its milder heterozygous allele is more common in some east Asian populations, which may account for a lower prevalence of AUD (Prom-Wormley et al. 2017). Regarding ADH, a homozygous ADH2 or a milder heterozygous form could possibly lead to higher conversion of alcohol to acetaldehyde, which would eventually lead to aversive responses to alcohol and thus protection against AUD.

Acuff SF, Strickland JC, Tucker JA, et al: Changes in alcohol use during COVID-19 and associations with contextual and individual difference variables: a systematic review and meta-analysis. *Psychol Addict Behav* 2022 Feb;36(1):1–19. PubMed PMID: 34807630

Breslau J, Aguilar-Gaxiola S, Borges G, et al: Risk for psychiatric disorder among immigrants and their US-born descendants: evidence from the National Comorbidity Survey Replication. *J Nerv Ment Dis* 2007;195(3):189–195.

Castillo-Carniglia A, Keyes KM, Hasin DS, et al: Psychiatric comorbidities in alcohol use disorder. *Lancet Psychiatry* 2019; 6(12):1068–1080. doi:10.1016/S2215-0366(19)30222-6

Grant BF, Goldstein RB, Saha TD, et al: Epidemiology of DSM-5 alcohol use disorder. *JAMA Psychiatry* 2015;72(8):757–766. doi:10.1001/jamapsychiatry.2015.0584

Hawkins JD, Catalano RF, Miller JY: Risk and protective factors for alcohol and other drug problems in adolescence and early adulthood: implications for substance abuse prevention. *Psychol Bull* 1992;112(1):64–105.

Jackson CL, Hu FB, Kawachi I, et al: Black-White differences in the relationship between alcohol drinking patterns and mortality among US men and women. *Am J Public Health* 2015; 105 Suppl 3(Suppl 3):S534–543. doi:10.2105/AJPH.2015.302615

Kalk NJ, Lingford-Hughes AR: The clinical pharmacology of acamprosate. *Br J Clin Pharmacol* February 2014;77(2):315–323. https://doi.org/10.1111/bcp.12070.

National Center for Statistics and Analysis, National Highway Traffic Safety Administration: Overview of motor vehicle crashes in 2020 [Internet]. Washington: U.S. Department of Transportation; 2020 Mar [cited 2022 June 20]. 43 pp. Available from: https://crashstats.nhtsa.dot.gov/Api/Public/ViewPublication/813266

Prescott CA, Kendler KS: Age at first drink and risk for alcoholism: a noncausal association. *Alcohol Clin Exp Res.* 1999; 23(1):101–107.

Prom-Wormley, Elizabeth C, Ebejer J, et al: The genetic epidemiology of substance use disorder: a review. *Drug Alcohol Depend* November 1, 2017;180:241–259. https://doi.org/10.1016/j.drugalcdep.2017.06.040.

Rehm J, Room R: The cultural aspect: how to measure and interpret epidemiological data on alcohol-use disorders across cultures. *Nordic Stud Alcohol Drugs.* 2017;34(4):330–341.

SAMHSA, Center for Behavioral Health Statistics and Quality: 2021 National Survey on Drug Use and Health. Table 5.6A—Alcohol use disorder in past year: among people aged 12 or older; by age group and demographic characteristics, numbers in thousands, 2021. [cited 2023 Jan 11]. Available from: https://www.samhsa.gov/data/sites/default/files/reports/rpt39441/NSDUHDetailedTabs2021/NSDUHDetailedTabs2021/NSDUHDetTabsSect5pe2021.htm#tab5.6a

Slater ME, Alpert HF, Surveillance Report #119: Apparent per capita alcohol consumption: national, state, and regional trends, 1977–2020. Sterling (VA): NIAAA, Division of Epidemiology and Prevention Research; 2022 Apr. 66 p. Contract No.: HHSN275201800004C. https://pubs.niaaa.nih.gov/publications/surveillance119/CONS20.htm

U.S. Department of Health and Human Services, Centers for Disease Control and Prevention (CDC) [Internet]. National Center for Health Statistics Mortality Data on CDC WONDER. Multiple cause of death, 2018–2021. 2023. Available from: https://wonder.cdc.gov/controller/saved/D157/D324F825

White A: Gender differences in the epidemiology of alcohol use and related harms in the United States. *ARCR* 2020;40(2):01. doi:10.35946/arcr.v40.2.01

White AM, Castle IP, Powell PA, et al: Alcohol-related deaths during the COVID-19 pandemic. *JAMA* 2022 May 3;327(17): 1704–1706. PubMed PMID: 35302593

Zhang X, Martinez-Donate AP, Nobles J, et al: Substance use across different phases of the migration process: a survey of Mexican migrants flows. *J Immigr Minor Health* 2015;17(6):1746–1757.

▶ Clinical Findings

A. Signs & Symptoms

Patients with a history of AUD can present in various clinical settings such as outpatient, the emergency room, or the general hospital (Table 17–2). Clinical presentation varies widely; problems may sometimes be vague/nonspecific or even seemingly unrelated to alcohol. Initial screening can be accomplished using brief screening measures, followed by more in-depth history. A detailed history and examination are vital in making a diagnosis of AUD.

B. Alcohol Screening Questions

AUD is a major public health concern, associated with high rates of morbidity and mortality as well as a global health and economic burden. As a result, the U.S. Preventive Services Task Force recommends that clinicians screen adults for hazardous use with one of two brief validated screens (AUDIT-C or NIAAA SASQ) and provide brief behavioral interventions to those who screen positive. There are several validated screening tools available in clinical practice, with varying degrees of efficacy.

1. The NIAAA single alcohol screening question (SASQ)—The SASQ has similar sensitivity and specificity to other longer screening tools, with the advantage of requiring only a single question: "How many times in the past year have you had (4 for women, or 5 for men) or more drinks in a day?" Any response greater than zero requires further assessment. The SASQ can be woven easily into a clinical interview, as there is no scoring (unlike other screens).

2. The AUD identification test (AUDIT)—The AUDIT is also recommended by the USPSTF as an initial screening tool (in the abbreviated version) for identifying current at-risk

Table 17–2 Clinical Features of Alcohol Use Disorders

History	Clinical Signs and Symptoms
Presentation	Intoxication, withdrawal symptoms, intense cravings, physical and psychosocial consequences of chronic alcohol consumption.
Chemical dependence history	Coexisting drug use. History of nicotine dependence.
Psychiatry history	Primary psychiatric disorder or a substance-induced psychiatric disorder (anxiety, mood disorder, psychosis), personality disorders, insomnia
Trauma history	History of domestic violence, sexual or physical abuse, posttraumatic stress disorder
Medical history	Multisystemic Cardiovascular—hypertension, cardiomyopathy, elevated triglycerides Gastrointestinal—gastritis, stomach and duodenal ulcers, liver cirrhosis/physical stigmata of chronic liver disease, pancreatitis Endocrine—feminizing syndromes in males (due to reduced testosterone), menstrual irregularities in females Hematology—anemia, macrocytosis, thrombocytopenia Oncology—stomach, esophageal, liver, and breast cancer Neurology—paresthesia, neuropathy, cognitive impairment, Wernicke-Korsakoff syndrome, tremor, ataxia Musculoskeletal evidence of body injury (multiple causes, such as fall risk, vehicular accidents) Sexual—erectile dysfunction in males
Family history	History of family member with drug and alcohol use disorder as well as mental illness
Social	Low academic achievement, legal issues, marital discord/divorce

drinking and can detect hazardous and harmful drinking as well as AUD. The full AUDIT is a 10-question screening tool with ratings from 0 to 4. A value of 8 or higher is indicative of hazardous alcohol use. A revised and more concise three-item version, AUDIT-C, is used more frequently in clinical practice. The three questions asked and scoring guidelines are presented in Table 17–3. The AUDIT-C is a reliable tool, with 57–97% sensitivity and 78–96% specificity for identifying at-risk drinking within different ethnicities and genders. A limitation of the AUDIT is its lack of efficacy in detecting AUD in the older population (Reinert & Allen 2007).

3. CAGE—The four-item CAGE questionnaire asks respondents: (1) Have you ever felt you need to Cut down on your drinking? (2) Have people Annoyed you by criticizing your drinking? (3) Have you ever felt bad or Guilty about

your drinking? (4) Have you ever had a drink first thing in the morning to steady your nerves or to get rid of a hangover (Eye-opener)? The CAGE questionnaire has the advantage of being very brief (less than a minute to administer) and easy to memorize. It is scored from 0 to 4 with a score of 1 for every positive answer. A cutoff of ≥2 is suggestive of an AUD. The CAGE questionnaire is reliable, with a sensitivity of 77–94% and a specificity of 79–97%. A limitation of the CAGE questionnaire is its inability to distinguish between current and past drinking disorders (Fiellin et al. 2000).

C. Laboratory Investigations

The diagnostic value of laboratory tests to help detect AUD is limited by the short half-life of alcohol as well as the low specificity of the available biomarkers. Despite these limitations,

Table 17–3 AUDIT-C Questions, Response Options, and Scoring Values

Question	Response Options (Response Score)				
How often do you have a drink containing alcohol?	Never (0)	Monthly or less (1)	2–4 times a month (2)	2–3 times a week (3)	≥4 times a week (4)
How many drinks containing alcohol do you have on a typical day when drinking?	1 or 2 (0)	3 or 4 (1)	5 or 6 (2)	7 to 9 (3)	≥10 (4)
How often do you have six or more drinks on one occasion?	Never (0)	Less than monthly (0)	Monthly (2)	2–3 times per week (3)	≥4 times a week (4)

Total score ranges from 0 to 12. A score of ≥4 identifies 86% of alcohol use disorders criteria in men, whereas a score ≥2 identifies 84% of alcohol use disorder criteria in women.

laboratory test results help raise a level of suspicion or supplement findings seen in clinical/mental state examination. They are of value in giving patients objective feedback, which can motivate patients to seek assistance with their drinking or make conscious positive changes such as reduction in drinking. Laboratory tests are also useful for monitoring treatment response (Conigrave et al. 2003).

1. Blood or breath alcohol level—A high blood alcohol level (BAL) or breath alcohol concentration at the time of presentation can be informative. For example, a BAL greater than 35 mmol/dL in an alert patient likely reflects high tolerance to alcohol as seen in individuals with an AUD. The clinical use of a BAL test, however, is limited by the very short period alcohol is detectable in the blood (<10–12 hours) and even shorter in breath. Newer devices that allow for multiple random breath alcohol level testing throughout the day or for breath alcohol testing prior to operating a motor vehicle may be used by diversion courts or professional monitoring programs, including physician health programs, for enhanced detection of relapsed alcohol use in high-risk populations.

2. Serum gamma-glutamyltransferase (GGT)—This is a liver enzyme involved in amino acid metabolism. An elevated serum GGT (levels > 35 U/L) can be indicative of heavy drinking. GGT is limited by its low sensitivity and multiple false positives from other causes (such as pregnancy, smoking, diabetes, medications, and obesity).

3. Alanine and aspartate aminotransferase ratio—These liver enzymes are both elevated in AUD but may also be elevated because of hepatocellular injury from various causes, so they are not specific markers. An aspartate aminotransferase to alanine aminotransferase ratio greater than 2 is more indicative of liver damage secondary to heavy alcohol use.

4. Carbohydrate-deficient transferrin test (CDT)—CDT measures structural changes in transferrin, which can occur following heavy alcohol consumption. The plasma half-life of CDT is about 14 days, and so levels remain elevated for 2–3 weeks following abstinence from alcohol. Like GGT, CDT has a relatively low sensitivity, with false positives seen in cases of transferrin deficiency and hepatocellular carcinoma. However, CDT has a higher specificity than serum GGT.

5. Mean corpuscular volume (MCV)—The red blood cell MCV is often enlarged in patients with history of AUD. An MCV greater than 100 fL is suggestive of heavy drinking. It has a low sensitivity and specificity compared to CDT and GGT and is elevated in several conditions, such as vitamin B_{12} and folic acid deficiency; in those taking medications such as methotrexate, anticonvulsants, or chemotherapeutic drugs; and in those with endocrinopathies such as hypothyroidism. Because of the long half-life of erythrocytes, values may remain abnormal for up to 3 months after abstinence. MCV is more useful in conjunction with other tests or in monitoring treatment response.

6. Ethyl glucuronide (EtG) and ethyl sulfate (EtS)—EtG is a water-soluble direct metabolite of alcohol and can be detected in several body fluids, tissues, and hair. It is detectable in the human body shortly after the consumption of alcohol and for longer periods than can be measured with blood or breath alcohol. A single drink on the previous evening should be detectable the next morning. The duration of positivity depends on the amount of alcohol consumed and the assay cutoff used. A cutoff of 100 ng/mL is more sensitive but could potentially be influenced by extraneous sources of alcohol (e.g., extreme use of hand sanitizers); a cutoff of 200 ng/mL reduces this risk with little loss of sensitivity. This cutoff can detect moderate alcohol consumption that occurred 24 hours earlier. Heavier drinking may be detected up to 48 hours later in some people. A commercially available immunoassay uses a cutoff of 500 ng/mL; although less sensitive, this test has the advantage of real-time feedback. EtG is a direct metabolite of ethanol metabolism and hence is more specific than other biochemical markers of alcohol consumption, which mainly measure end-organ damage. Because of this unique quality of EtG, it has been used in forensic psychiatry for cases of driving under the influence, as well as in judging driving ability (Wurst et al. 2003), and its use in clinical practice has been recommended (Jatlow & O'Malley 2010).

EtS is also a direct metabolite of ethanol, which has been used and studied to a lesser extent than EtG.

7. Phosphatidylethanol (PEth)—PEth is detected in the blood after consumption of about 1000 g of alcohol over about a 2-week period. Some advantages of the PEth test are its high sensitivity and specificity compared to many other biomarkers, its long window for assessment (2 weeks), and its use in patients with liver disease (values are less affected by liver disease). This test is increasingly used in early abstinence monitoring (Schrock et al. 2017).

D. Neuroimaging

Neurodegenerative alcohol-related brain changes are seen on radiology studies, showing volume loss and shrinkage of brain tissue. These changes have a predilection for the white matter. Alcohol-related brain changes seen on computed tomography (CT) and magnetic resonance imaging (MRI) scans include shrinking of the frontal lobe (due to neurodegeneration of the superior and inferior frontal cortex), ventricular enlargement with widening of cortical sulci, and shrinkage of the thalamus, inferior colliculus, and mammillary bodies (which are seen more specifically in Wernicke-Korsakoff syndrome). The cerebellum is also affected, with volume deficits and shrinkage, which is more profound in the anterior superior vermis. Functional MRI studies show frontocerebellar circuitry disruption as the principal mechanism underlying symptoms such as ataxia, cognitive impairment, and visuospatial impairment in individuals with chronic AUD (Sullivan & Pfefferbaum 2005).

There is also a difference in imaging findings based on gender, with women showing more brain-related radiological changes (Pfefferbaum et al. 2001; Sullivan & Pfefferbaum 2005). With abstinence, there is improvement in neuroimaging scans, but some changes may not reverse entirely (Mann et al. 1995).

Course of Illness

The mean age of first alcohol use is 13–14 years (Faden 2006), though there is some variability based on sociocultural practices and norms (Schuckit 2009), and more recent epidemiologic data show down-trending underage alcohol use over time (NSDUH 2021). Onset of hazardous drinking begins usually between late teens and early 20s. By 18 years of age, approximately 60% of teenagers in the United States have experienced drunkenness and 30% have experienced a hazardous event because of alcohol use. The best predictors of transition from heavy drinking in adolescence to alcohol dependence is a history of conduct disorder (Vaillant 1983) and behavioral problems in adolescence as well as early onset of drinking (Grant & Dawson 1997). Predictors of alcohol-related consequences in patients with AUD are positive family history, coexisting drug use, and greater frequency and intensity of drinking (Schuckit et al. 2000). Many people with an AUD during adolescence or young adulthood, however, experience natural remission without treatment.

The longitudinal course of AUD can vary depending on sex of the individual. Women have less body water, lower hepatic metabolism of ethanol, and experience a higher BAL at a given dose of ethanol compared to men.

Irrespective of gender, chronic alcohol use is associated with morbidity and mortality because of medical sequelae (liver disease, cancer, acid reflux disease), psychological sequelae (anxiety, depression, and suicide), and accidents, as well as use of other substance use (nicotine and other drugs), all which lead to decreased life expectancy in these patients, as outlined above. Most individuals with AUD, however, have periods of recovery, and some return to nonhazardous drinking while others achieve sustained abstinence. This suggests that people with AUD may have a natural remission that occurs even without treatment, with reported rates of up to 70% of individuals with lifetime AUD (Tucker et al. 2020). Factors associated with natural remission include severe medical illness, new job, life partner, parenthood, and maturation with age.

Arnone M, Maruani J, Chaperon F, et al: Selective inhibition of sucrose and ethanol intake by SR 141716, an antagonist of central cannabinoid (CB1) receptors. *Psychopharmacology (Berl)* 1997;132:104–106.

Conigrave KM, Davies P, Haber P, et al: Traditional markers of excessive alcohol use. *Addiction*. 2003;98 Suppl 2:31–43.

Faden VB: Trends in initiation of alcohol use in the United States 1975 to 2003. *Alcohol Clin Exp Res* 2006;30:1011–1022.

Fiellin DA, Reid MC, O'Connor PG: Outpatient management of patients with alcohol problems: *Ann Intern Med* 2000;133:815–827.

Flórez G, Saiz PA, García-Portilla P, et al: Topiramate for the treatment of alcohol dependence: comparison with naltrexone. *Eur Addict Res* 2011;17:29–36.

Grant BF, Dawson DA: Age at onset of alcohol use and its association with DSM-IV alcohol abuse and dependence: results from the National Longitudinal Alcohol Epidemiologic Survey. *J Subst Abuse* 1997;9:103–110.

Grant BF, Dawson DA, Stinson FS, et al: The 12-month prevalence and trends in DSM-IV alcohol abuse and dependence: United States, 1991–1992 and 2001–2002. *Drug Alcohol Depend* 2004;74:223–234.

Hasin DS, Stinson FS, Ogburn E, et al: Prevalence, correlates, disability, and comorbidity of DSM-IV alcohol abuse and dependence in the United States: results from the National Epidemiologic Survey on Alcohol and Related Conditions. *Arch Gen Psychiatry* 2007;64:830–842.

Hawkins JD, Catalano RF, Miller JY. Risk and protective factors for alcohol and other drug problems in adolescence and early adulthood: implications for substance abuse prevention. *Psychol Bull* 1992;112:64–105.

Higuchi S, Matsushita S, Murayama M, et al: Alcohol and aldehyde dehydrogenase polymorphisms and the risk for alcoholism. *Am J Psychiatry* 1995;152:1219–1221.

Jatlow P, O'Malley SS. Clinical (nonforensic) application of ethyl glucuronide measurement: are we ready? *Alcohol Clin Exp Res* 2010;34:968–975.

Kreek MJ, Nielsen DA, Butelman ER, et al: Genetic influences on impulsivity, risk taking, stress responsivity and vulnerability to drug abuse and addiction. *Nat Neurosci* 2005;8:1450–1457.

Mann K, Mundle G, Strayle M, et al: Neuroimaging in alcoholism: CT and MRI results and clinical correlates. *J Neural Transm Gen Sect* 1995;99:145–155.

Mason BJ, Quello S, Goodell V, et al: Gabapentin treatment for alcohol dependence: a randomized clinical trial. *JAMA Intern Med* 2014;174:70–77.

Pfefferbaum A, Rosenbloom M, Deshmukh A, et al: Sex differences in the effects of alcohol on brain structure. *Am J Psychiatry* 2001;158:188–197.

Prescott CA, Kendler KS. Age at first drink and risk for alcoholism: a noncausal association. *Alcohol Clin Exp Res* 1999;23:101–107.

Reinert DF, Allen JP. The AUD identification test: an update of research findings. *Alcohol Clin Exp Res* 2007;31:185–199.

Sass H, Soyka M, Mann K, et al: Relapse prevention by acamprosate. Results from a placebo-controlled study on alcohol dependence. *Arch Gen Psychiatry* 1996;53:673–680.

Schröck A, Thierauf-Emberger A, Schürch S, et al: Phosphatidylethanol (PEth) detected in blood for 3 to 12 days after single consumption of alcohol—a drinking study with 16 volunteers. *Int J Legal Med* 2017;131(1):153–160. https://doi.org/10.1007/s00414-016-1445-x.

Schuckit M, Smith TL, Landi NA: The 5-year clinical course of high-functioning men with DSM-IV alcohol abuse or dependence. *Am J Psychiatry* 2000;157:2028–2035.

Schuckit MA. Genetics of the risk for alcoholism. *Am J Addict* 2000;9:103–112.

Stinson FS, Grant BF, Dawson DA, et al: Comorbidity between DSM-IV alcohol and specific drug use disorders in the United States: results from the National Epidemiologic Survey on Alcohol and Related Conditions. *Drug Alcohol Depend* 2005;80:105–116.

Sullivan EV, Pfefferbaum A: Neurocircuitry in alcoholism: a substrate of disruption and repair. *Psychopharmacology (Berl)* 2005;180:583–594.

Tucker J, Chandler SD, Witkiewitz K: Epidemiology of recovery from alcohol use disorder. Alcohol research. *Curr Rev* 2020; 40(3):2. https://doi.org/10.35946/arcr.v40.3.02.

U.S. Preventive Services Task Force, Curry SJ, Krist AH, et al: Screening and behavioral counseling interventions to reduce unhealthy alcohol use in adolescents and adults: US Preventive Services Task Force Recommendation Statement. *JAMA* 2018;320(18):1899–1909. doi:10.1001/jama.2018.16789

Vaillant GE: Natural history of male alcoholism V: is alcoholism the cart or the horse to sociopathy? *Br J Addict* 1983;78:317–326.

Weiss F, Porrino LJ: Behavioral neurobiology of alcohol addiction: recent advances and challenges. *J Neurosci* 2002;22:3332–3337.

Wurst FM, Skipper GE, Weinmann W: Ethyl glucuronide—the direct ethanol metabolite on the threshold from science to routine use. *Addiction* 2003;98 Suppl 2:51–61.

▶ Differential Diagnosis

A. Alcohol Intoxication

1. Opioids, sedative/hypnotic intoxication—Patients with opioid or sedative/hypnotic intoxication may also present with euphoria, altered mental status, reduced psychomotor coordination, diminished reflexes, hypothermia, decreased respiration, coma, and death via overdose. Pupillary constriction (miosis) is seen in opioid intoxication. Alcohol level and urine drug test are quick assessment tools to help further differentiate these substances.

2. Lithium toxicity—Patients present with slurred speech, altered mental status, ataxia, and impaired neurocognition. Neuromuscular excitation (including tremulousness and hyperreflexia), alcohol level, and serum lithium levels will help differentiate this from alcohol intoxication.

3. Medical conditions—Hypo-/hyper-glycemia, hypothyroidism, cerebrovascular accidents, head injuries, hepatic encephalopathy, diabetic ketoacidosis, and metabolic derangements could all present with altered mental state, impaired motor coordination, and eventually coma. Careful medical assessment is required to ensure alternative etiologies are ruled-out in a patient presenting with possible alcohol intoxication driving altered mental status.

B. Alcohol Withdrawal

1. Opioid, sedative/hypnotic withdrawal—Opioid withdrawal and most especially sedative/hypnotic withdrawal can present very similarly to alcohol withdrawal. Symptoms such as restlessness, psychomotor agitation, and autonomic dysfunction may be present in these withdrawal states. Sedative/hypnotic withdrawal, like alcohol withdrawal, can also present with withdrawal tremors, psychosis, seizures, and delirium. Urine drug screen and the patient's history of opioids or sedative/hypnotic use will help differentiate this from alcohol withdrawal. Mixed withdrawal states are not uncommon and require stabilization of each underlying cause to prevent medical sequelae. For sedative/hypnotic withdrawal, GABAergic medications (usually benzodiazepines or barbiturates) will stabilize both the alcohol and the sedative/hypnotic withdrawal states, while opioid withdrawal requires stabilization with additional agents (buprenorphine or methadone for most situations).

2. Stimulant intoxication—This state may also present with hypertension/tachycardia, seizures, psychomotor activation, and delirium or psychosis. Urine drug screen and the patient's history of recent stimulant ingestion is helpful in differentiating this state, though benzodiazepine therapy may also be helpful in stimulant intoxication states.

3. Medical conditions—Endocrine disorders such as thyroid storm may present with autonomic dysfunction, seizures, and agitation, as seen in alcohol withdrawal. Essential tremors or other causes of hand tremors such as cerebellar disease or neuromuscular disorders should be kept in mind when assessing for alcohol withdrawal.

Further, thiamine deficiency is common in chronic heavy alcohol use due to impaired absorption and poor nutritional intake, increasing the risk of delirium or encephalopathy due to thiamine deficiency (i.e., Wernicke encephalopathy, WE). Two or more Caine criteria (evidence of nutritional deficiency, extraocular movement abnormalities, ataxia, mild amnesia, or other altered mental status) suggest increased risk of WE and empiric high-dose parenteral thiamine repletion should be considered.

4. Alcohol-related psychosis.

Psychotic-spectrum symptoms induced by alcohol, including hallucinations, may occur independently of delirium and during any phase of alcohol use (intoxication, withdrawal, and early abstinence). It is important to assess for co-occurring delirium/encephalopathy when distinguishing alcohol-related psychosis from alcohol withdrawal-related delirium (formerly delirium tremens), as the treatment approach differs. Alcohol related psychosis in the absence of alcohol withdrawal delirium may be managed with supportive behavioral interventions or antipsychotic medications for severe distress unresponsive to non-pharmacologic interventions.

C. Heavy Drinking

For most substances, no amount of use is considered safe, and single episodes of intoxication may risk severe consequences (e.g., myocardial infarction with first cocaine use). Alcohol is a notable exception, where specific definitions of heavy use have been identified and are known to increase risk of adverse health outcomes based on epidemiological data. At-risk, unhealthy, or heavy alcohol use is defined as 5 or more standard (containing 14 g of ethanol) drinks within 24 hours for men and 4 or more drinks for women, or more than 14 drinks per week in men or 7 drinks in women or anyone 65 years or older. More nuanced definitions of heavy alcohol use have also been outlined by the WHO drinking risk levels, including very high risk (>7.15 drinks/day for men, >4.3 drinks/day for women), high risk (4.3–7.14 vs. 2.87–4.29 drinks/day for men and women), medium risk (2.87–4.29 vs. 1.44–2.86 drinks/day for men and women), low risk (<2.86 vs. <1.43 drinks/day for men and women). Reductions in WHO drinking risk level have been shown to result in improvements in how individuals feel and function and in the outcome of treatment.

1. Associated medical conditions—Chronic heavy alcohol use is commonly associated with medical comorbidities, such as have been mentioned earlier. Patients may present with signs of chronic liver disease that are not necessarily a result of AUD. Detailed history and laboratory investigations will be helpful in determining the etiology of hepatic dysfunction.

D. Psychiatric Comorbidity

Psychiatric disorders that are comorbid with AUD can be alcohol-induced disorders (such as mood, anxiety, psychosis, and sleep disorders) or primary psychiatric disorders. There is a higher rate of AUD among all primary psychiatric disorders, with bipolar disorders, antisocial personality disorder/conduct disorder, and specific phobias having the strongest association, although the most frequent comorbidities are depressive and anxiety disorders (Hasin et al. 2007). Prospective observation of individuals presenting with a major depressive episode during AUD treatment shows that the majority will experience depressed mood for ~1 week, with ~40% experiencing remission of depressive symptoms and ~60% experiencing recurrent major depressive disorder (MDD) over 1 year of follow-up, with prior history of MDD during abstinent periods predicting a greater likelihood of recurrent MDD during follow-up (Nunes et al. 2006). Notably, even alcohol-induced depressive disorder was associated with a relatively high rate of transition to primary MDD in that cohort, with 32% of these individuals being diagnosed with independent MDD during 1 year of follow-up.

Differentiating between alcohol-induced disorders and primary psychiatric disorders can be difficult. Subtle differences such as less severe illness and shorter duration of illness may point more toward alcohol-induced disorders, and the persistence of illness during periods of sobriety suggests a primary disorder. Often, a presenting mood, anxiety, or psychotic syndrome during acute intoxication, withdrawal, or early abstinence is considered alcohol-induced pending prospective monitoring of symptom remission with abstinence

more than 1 month. If symptoms persist beyond the expected course, then a primary psychiatric disorder may be diagnosed. However, waiting to initiate effective pharmacotherapy or psychotherapeutic interventions until more than 1 month of recovery may risk prolonged duration of symptom burden and under-treatment of a primary disorder, so a decision to initiate treatment sooner may be made in collaboration with the patient.

Hasin DS, Stinson FS, Ogburn E, et al: Prevalence, correlates, disability, and comorbidity of DSM-IV alcohol abuse and dependence in the United States: results from the National Epidemiologic Survey on Alcohol and Related Conditions. *Arch Gen Psychiatry* 2007;2064:830–842.

Nunes EV, Liu X, Samet S, et al: Independent versus substance-induced major depressive disorder in substance-dependent patients: observational study of course during follow-up. *J Clin Psychiatry* 67:10, October 2006.

Witkiewitz K, Falk DE, Litten RZ, et al: Maintenance of World Health Organization risk drinking level reductions and posttreatment functioning following a large alcohol use disorder clinical trial. *Alcohol Clin Exp Res* 2019;43(5):979–987. doi:10.1111/acer.14018

► Treatment

A. Other Interventions

1. Medically supervised withdrawal (detoxification)—The DSM criteria for alcohol withdrawal can be seen in the essentials for diagnosis section above. The alcohol withdrawal syndrome is a constellation of signs and symptoms that occur because of reduction or discontinuation of alcohol use in an individual with AUD. This leads to an imbalance between excitatory and inhibitory neurotransmission, causing excessive activity of the glutamate (NMDA) pathway and reduced activity within the GABA pathway, resulting in the clinical features seen in alcohol withdrawal. These symptoms, which can range from mild or moderate to severe, can be documented using the Clinical Institute Withdrawal Assessment of Alcohol scale (CIWA-Ar; Sullivan et al. 1989). The scale is used to rate the severity of 10 clinical signs of alcohol withdrawal: nausea/vomiting, headache, anxiety, paroxysmal sweats, tactile disturbances, visual disturbances, auditory disturbances, tremors, agitation, and disorientation/clouding of sensorium. A score of more than 15 is classified as severe withdrawal, 8–15 is moderate, and less than 8 is classified as mild withdrawal. Symptoms of mild to moderate withdrawal can be managed effectively in an outpatient setting with careful monitoring, with or without medications (Mayo-Smith 1997). In cases of more severe symptoms of withdrawal, patients are best managed in an inpatient setting with close monitoring and medication management. Inpatient medically supervised withdrawal is indicated in patients with delirium tremens, severe withdrawal symptoms, pregnancy, and severe medical comorbidities and where close outpatient follow-up is not possible. Inpatient treatment is strongly advised when there is a prior history of delirium tremens and seizures (Saitz & O'Malley 1997).

B. Psychopharmacologic Interventions

1. Management of Alcohol Withdrawal

i. Benzodiazepines—The mechanism of action of benzodiazepines is facilitation of inhibitory neurotransmitter GABA at the $GABA_A$ receptors.

Benzodiazepines remain the gold standard of treatment for alcohol withdrawal. They are effective in relieving symptoms and preventing delirium tremens and alcohol withdrawal seizures, which occur in 5–10% of untreated individuals. There are several different medications within this class. The longer-acting drugs such as chlordiazepoxide and diazepam have better outcomes than shorter-acting drugs in preventing seizures and result in a smoother detoxification process. Lorazepam, which has shorter half-life, has value in patients with hepatic dysfunction, where reduced metabolism and drug accumulation resulting in toxicity is a concern.

These medications are administered based on two protocols: fixed-schedule dosing and symptom-triggered dosing. In fixed-schedule dosing, the medication is given at specified doses and at specified times and tapered gradually, whereas in symptom-triggered dosing, medication is given only in response to clinical findings. Both protocols are effective; however, a risk of the fixed-schedule dose protocol is increased length of hospital stay because of overmedication. Comparison of both protocols showed an average duration of treatment of 9 hours in the symptom-triggered group versus 68 hours in the fixed-schedule group. Amount of medication administered is also considerably higher in the fixed group compared to the symptom-triggered group (Mayo-Smith 1997). Symptom-triggered dosing, on the other hand, requires intense monitoring by clinicians well trained in the use of the CIWA-Ar protocol to prevent progression of alcohol withdrawal symptoms. Despite the benefits of a symptom-triggered dosing approach in lower-risk patients, individuals at high risk of severe withdrawal may be undertreated using this approach. A fixed-schedule load and taper is usually preferred for individuals at higher risk of a severe withdrawal course.

Adverse effects of benzodiazepines include sedation, drowsiness, impaired motor coordination that may lead to falls and injuries, cognitive impairment, and disinhibition. Benzodiazepine use may also lead to a sedative/hypnotic use disorder, and treatment with these medications for AUD is not recommended outside of acute withdrawal stabilization.

ii. Barbiturates—Barbiturates are also $GABA_A$ receptor agonists, like benzodiazepines. However, barbiturates inhibit the frequency of neuronal firing more reliably than do benzodiazepines because they increase the duration chloride channels remain open, decrease activation of AMPA glutamate

receptors, and also decrease activity of voltage-dependent sodium channels. Some individuals with severe alcohol withdrawal experience a benzodiazepine-resistant syndrome despite high doses of benzodiazepine therapy. In these cases, phenobarbital is increasingly used with good effect for higher-risk patients and in emergency department and ICU settings, and it has the advantage of allowing weight-based dosing rather than empiric titration to symptom remission, as is required for benzodiazepine treatment (Martin & Katz 2016; Nisavic et al. 2019).

iii. Anticonvulsants—These medications suppress seizures. There are many different medications in this class of drugs, and they have varied mechanisms of action, most of which involve altering sodium or calcium channels or by GABA facilitation.

Carbamazepine and valproic acid have both shown to be as effective as the benzodiazepines for the treatment of mild to moderate alcohol withdrawal, but because of their significant side-effect profile, their use as first-line agents is limited. Gabapentin has been shown to be as effective as lorazepam in the treatment of alcohol withdrawal in the outpatient setting. It also reduces drinking during alcohol withdrawal treatment compared to placebo, which may be as a result of its anxiolytic effect. Because of the safety and mild adverse drug profile of this drug, it should be considered in the outpatient treatment of mild alcohol withdrawal (Myrick et al. 2009). However, not all antiepileptic medications are effective for alcohol withdrawal treatment. For example, phenytoin does not effectively treat alcohol withdrawal.

The nature and severity of adverse effects depend on the drugs used. Gabapentin has a mild side effect profile, with sedation being the most prominent. Carbamazepine and valproic acid have more extensive adverse effects (e.g., electrolyte and hematological effects) and should be monitored more closely.

iv. Sympatholytics—Centrally acting alpha agonists such as clonidine or dexmedetomidine and beta-blockers such as propranolol reduce sympathetic activity that can be elevated in alcohol withdrawal.

Excessive activity of the sympathetic system occurs during alcohol withdrawal and hence these medications may have a role in treatment, particularly as adjunctive agents in ICU settings; however, they are not helpful in preventing progression to seizures or delirium tremens.

Beta-blockers can have the deleterious effect of masking the autonomic symptoms seen in alcohol withdrawal, preventing the clinician from observing warning signs of progression to a more severe state of withdrawal if patients are receiving only symptom-triggered treatment. These medications are better used as adjunct therapy as opposed to monotherapy.

v. Neuroleptics—These agents cause reduction in psychotic symptoms by binding and activity at the central serotonin and dopamine receptors. They may help alleviate some of the symptoms of alcohol withdrawal such as agitation and hallucinations. They do not treat progression to or reverse symptoms of delirium tremens or alcohol withdrawal seizures.

Neuroleptics should be used with caution, as they could reduce the seizure threshold in humans, which would further worsen patient outcome.

vi. **Ethyl alcohol**—Self-administration of alcohol relieves the symptoms of alcohol withdrawal and is the primary mode of self-treatment outside a health care setting. In the past, alcohol was sometimes administered orally or intravenously, especially in trauma and surgical patients, to treat alcohol withdrawal during forced abstinence in the hospital. Benzodiazepine or barbiturate treatment is clearly the preferred approach due to the adverse health effects of ethyl alcohol, and this approach is not recommended.

vii. **Thiamine**—Thiamine is a coenzyme for carbohydrate metabolism. It can be given orally or parentally.

Thiamine is recommended as an adjunctive treatment to replenish thiamine stores, which are commonly deficient in patients with chronic alcoholism. Thiamine administration is protective against the development of WE and Korsakoff dementia, but should be administered early on in treatment, ideally at the time of presentation for care. Parenteral thiamine is used initially in patients with elevated risk for WE to more rapidly replete central nervous system (CNS) thiamine stores, followed by oral supplementation. Oral supplementation alone is usually insufficient to treat patients at risk for WE; see the Caine criteria referenced above for risk factors associated with WE.

Adverse events include nausea and very occasional allergic response. There can be induration at the injection site when thiamine is given intramuscularly.

2. Pharmacotherapy for Relapse Prevention and Maintenance

—The APA Practice Guideline recommends the use of naltrexone or acamprosate for individuals with moderate or severe AUD, and this guideline suggests the use of topiramate or gabapentin for individuals who prefer these agents or do not respond to the first-line therapies (APA 2018). Disulfiram may also be used in select patients who recognize and understand the risks associated with alcohol use on this medication, which includes a potentially life-threatening disulfiram-ethanol reaction. These medications have shown some benefit in the treatment of AUD and, except for topiramate and gabapentin, are Food and Drug Administration (FDA)-approved for treatment of AUD in the United States. Selecting the appropriate medication for the patient is based on the history and clinical presentation and clinician judgment as well as individual patient's goals. Adjunct counseling along with medication management improves long-term outcome.

i. **Disulfiram**—Disulfiram's primary mode of action is by inhibiting aldehyde dehydrogenase, which is a liver enzyme that catalyzes the oxidation of acetaldehyde, a toxic by-product of alcohol metabolism. Accumulation of acetaldehyde leads to the "disulfiram–alcohol reaction," which is characterized by facial flushing, dizziness, blurry vision, nausea, headaches, vomiting, chest pain, palpitations, weakness, hypotension, and tachycardia. In some cases, more severe reactions such as seizures, congestive heart failure, respiratory depression, myocardial infarction, and even death may occur. The risk of this potentially life-threatening reaction if a patient experiences relapse to alcohol use has limited the use of disulfiram outside of highly selected and supervised patient populations.

Disulfiram may be helpful in highly motivated patients committed to abstinence from alcohol. Knowledge of the disulfiram–alcohol reaction is intended to serve as a deterrent to drinking and to support abstinence. Because of adherence problems, disulfiram is generally recommended in combination with supervised dosing in which a spouse or other support system is involved to ensure direct observation of medication ingestion. The recommended initial daily dose is 250 mg.

Patients should be abstinent from alcohol, educated about the disulfiram–alcohol interaction, and advised to avoid other ethanol-containing products for more than 2 weeks after a dose, either ingested or absorbed through the skin, that may interact with disulfiram. Contraindications to disulfiram include severe cardiopulmonary compromise, liver failure/cirrhosis, pregnancy (due to association with birth defects), and cognitive disorders (inability to understand the risks associated with the disulfiram–alcohol reaction). Other side effects of this medication include hepatotoxicity, hepatitis, depression, and psychosis.

ii. **Naltrexone**—Naltrexone is a nonselective opioid antagonist that was approved for the treatment of AUD in 1994. Unlike disulfiram, it is not an aversive agent; instead it blocks the effects of alcohol-related release of endogenous opioids, hence attenuating the positive/rewarding effects of alcohol. Advantages of this drug are its anticraving effect and its mild adverse effect profile as well as the lack of abuse potential. Naltrexone is available in oral and extended-release forms.

Placebo-controlled trials examining the efficacy of naltrexone have shown it to be more effective than placebo in reducing return to heavy drinking as well as abstinence maintenance. Naltrexone has also been shown to have better efficacy in patients reporting significant cravings, a family history of alcohol dependence, comorbid smoking (Fucito et al. 2012), and possibly those with the Asp variant of the OPRM1 mu receptor gene. The FDA-approved dose for oral naltrexone is 50 mg daily, but 100 mg daily is also used.

Adverse effects are primarily gastrointestinal and sedative (i.e., daytime sleepiness). At higher doses than used for alcohol dependence treatment, naltrexone can have hepatotoxic effects. Naltrexone can precipitate opioid withdrawal in those currently dependent on opioids, and naltrexone will block the effectiveness of opiates for analgesia. Abstinence from opioids for 7–14 days is usually requiring prior to the first dose to prevent precipitated opioid withdrawal.

iii. Extended-release naltrexone—Vivitrol is the only extended-release preparation of naltrexone (XR-naltrexone) approved for treatment of AUD in the United States and was developed to address problems with adherence to oral naltrexone. It is a polylactide-co-glycolide (PLG)–based long-acting naltrexone formulation that releases the drug over a 4-week period. Approved for the treatment of alcohol dependence in 2006, vivitrol is given as a single monthly dose of 380 mg.

A study comparing placebo versus XR-naltrexone at 190 mg and 380 mg showed better reduction in heavy drinking days (Garbutt et al. 2005); among the subgroup that was abstinent 4 or more days before treatment, 380 mg XR-naltrexone significantly enhanced rates of abstinence from alcohol as well as heavy drinking (O'Malley et al. 2007). It is well tolerated, with minimal adverse reactions, and has good adherence rates with 64% of patients receiving at least six injections and 73% receiving at least four injections within a 24-week period (Garbutt et al. 2005). Head-to-head comparison of XR-naltrexone and oral naltrexone has shown increased adherence to XR-naltrexone compared to the oral formulation, suggesting an advantage for the long-acting injectable (Stewart et al. 2021).

Administered as an intramuscular gluteal injection, the side effect profile of XR-naltrexone is similar to that of oral naltrexone, with the exception of injection-site reactions. These reactions can sometimes be severe, and proper injection technique is important. There were two reported cases of eosinophilic pneumonia in the study carried out by Garbutt et al. (2005). This resolved with treatment and discontinuation of the medication. Unlike oral naltrexone, XR-naltrexone does not undergo first-pass metabolism, and hence there may have a reduced risk of hepatotoxicity.

iv. Acamprosate—Acamprosate has been considered an NMDA glutamate receptor antagonist, which works to restore balance to the glutamate-GABA system, which is dysregulated in chronic alcohol use, though the mechanism of action for its relapse-prevention effects remains unclear. The FDA approved acamprosate for the treatment of AUD in 2004, based on the results of large-scale multisite European studies across several countries.

A double-blind placebo-controlled trial on 272 patients who recently completed alcohol detoxification showed acamprosate to have significant advantage over placebo in the maintenance of abstinence as well as a longer latency period in return to drinking for those who relapsed (Sass et al. 1996). Similar multisite studies carried out in the United States did not show acamprosate to have any significant benefit when compared to placebo, perhaps because of differences in the severity of alcohol dependence compared to the European studies (Anton et al. 2006). Further, naltrexone was more effective than acamprosate in a large multisite randomized-controlled trial focused on abstinence outcomes (Anton et al. 2006).

Despite this, acamprosate remains a viable option for the treatment of alcohol dependence, especially in patients with hepatic compromise, as it has no hepatotoxic adverse effects and is renally cleared.

Acamprosate is excreted renally and so is contraindicated in patients with poor kidney function. The primary adverse events associated with acamprosate are gastrointestinal. Dosing for this medication is 666 mg taken three times per day.

v. Topiramate—Topiramate is an anticonvulsant medication that has shown efficacy in reducing alcohol consumption. Its primary mode of action is complex, and may involve decreasing dopamine-mediated mesolimbic signaling via suppression of excitatory glutamate activity and augmentation of inhibitory GABA activity (Johnson et al. 2003).

Topiramate requires gradual titration of the dose over the course of several weeks to avoid adverse effects. At a dose of 200–300 mg daily, topiramate is more effective than placebo in improving quality-of-life measures as well as abstinence, reducing drinking, cravings for alcohol, and serum GGT (Blodgett et al. 2014).

The more commonly occurring side effects seen with topiramate include anorexia, cognitive impairment, paresthesia, and taste perversion.

vi. Gabapentin—Gabapentin is FDA approved for the treatment of epilepsy as well as neuropathic pain. It modulates GABA neurotransmission via blockage of voltage-gated calcium channels at selective presynaptic sites.

A 12-week double-blind, placebo-controlled, randomized trial of 150 individuals with a history of alcohol dependence showed reduction in heavy drinking days, cravings, and dysphoric symptoms associated with chronic alcohol consumption with a gabapentin dose of 900–1800 mg per day (Mason et al. 2014). A subsequent randomized-controlled trials, with some evidence for gabapentin's effect being modulated by a history of alcohol withdrawal symptoms (Anton et al. 2020).

Fatigue is the most common adverse effect. Gabapentin is excreted renally, so it can be used in patients with liver disease.

3. Other non–FDA-approved medications—Other medications have been studied that have shown some promise for the treatment of AUD.

i. Baclofen—Baclofen is a GABA$_B$ receptor agonist. At a dose up to 30 mg daily, there is some evidence for increased abstinence, improvement in anxiety, and fewer cravings. At 10 mg daily, this medication has few side effects, but higher doses can be associated with sedation and potential nonprescribed use liability. Baclofen does not show hepatotoxic side effects, so it could be used in more severely affected patients with hepatic impairment (Addolorato et al. 2000). Additional research is needed before recommending this agent, as some trials and meta-analyses have not shown efficacy (Minozzi et al. 2018). There is notable evidence for baclofen efficacy in patients with hepatic cirrhosis, with some trials showing improvement in abstinence and relapse prevention (Mosoni et al. 2018).

Common side effects seen are sedation and drowsiness.

iii. Ondansetron—Ondansetron is a 5-HT$_3$ receptor antagonist that attenuates the reinforcing effects of alcohol, which are mediated by serotonin and dopamine in the cortico-mesolimbic system.

Ondansetron reduces alcohol intake and has an anticraving effect. It has better efficacy in type B (early-onset) and is ineffective in type A AUD (late-onset) (Johnson et al. 2000; Kranzler et al. 2003). There is limited evidence to support its regular use in clinical practice.

Ondansetron produces cardiac side effects such as QT prolongation and, in rare cases, extrapyramidal side effects.

iv. Varenicline—Varenicline is an nicotinic acetylcholine α4β2 receptor partial agonist, which is approved for the treatment of nicotine dependence. As a partial agonist, varenicline has a greater affinity for the α4β2 nicotinic receptor than does nicotine, but it stimulates less dopamine release and attenuates the effects of nicotine. Alcohol activation of nicotinic receptors has partly been implicated in the positive rewarding effects of alcohol. Varenicline has been shown to reduce alcohol consumption and seeking in both animal (Steensland et al. 2007) and human models (McKee et al. 2009).

A placebo-controlled multisite study (Litten et al. 2013) found that varenicline reduced measures of drinking intensity (e.g., percent days heavy drinking, drinks per drinking day) and alcohol craving; this effect occurred among smokers and nonsmokers. Another multisite study of individuals with AUD and smoking found evidence of efficacy in reducing alcohol consumption men, but not women and increased smoking abstinence (O'Malley et al. 2018).

The primary adverse events associated with varenicline are nausea, dizziness, and vivid dreaming. Although generally well tolerated, there have been concerns for increased psychiatric symptoms and cardiovascular events in postmarketing studies. A black box warning was removed in 2016 after incorporating findings from a large multisite international trial demonstrating no significant increase in neuropsychiatric adverse events attributable to varenicline relative to nicotine patch or placebo. The FDA safety communication that varenicline may be associated with a small increase in risk of certain cardiovascular events was updated in 2012 with additional meta-analytic data, and the 2018 ACC consensus statement continues to recommend varenicline as a first-line pharmacotherapy for individuals with coronary artery disease and tobacco use.

C. Psychotherapeutic Intervention

Behavioral interventions, including brief advice, can be effective in management of AUD. In medical settings, screening and brief advice can include feedback about the diagnosis, vital signs and laboratory values, advice about health risks of alcohol, education about low-risk drinking, and referral to a specialist. Brief interventions last less than 15 minutes and have been carried out in multiple treatment settings, even in the emergency room. They have been shown to reduce alcohol consumption and alcohol-related consequences (D'Onofrio et al. 2012). The National Institute on Alcohol Abuse and Alcoholism (NIAAA) Clinician's Guide provides guidance about assessing and intervening in alcoholism.

More intensive evidence-based interventions have been extensively studied, including cognitive–behavioral therapy (CBT), motivational enhancement therapy (MET), and twelve-step facilitation treatment (TSF). CBT incorporates a functional analysis of drinking and teaches cognitive and behavioral skills for coping with craving and high risk situations. MET makes use of motivational interviewing to help resolve patient's own ambivalence as well as encourage reductions in drinking. TSF is a behavioral platform that encourages participation in mutual support groups such as Alcoholics Anonymous and SMART Recovery. Project MATCH (Matching Alcoholism Treatments to Client Heterogeneity), which was a large-scale study comparing psychotherapeutic interventions for patients with AUD, showed that CBT, MET, and TSF were effective, and none was superior to the others at 1-year follow-up. Other interventions include mindfulness interventions to help people tolerate and resist urges to drink (Garland & Howard 2018), contingency management that incorporates monitoring and rewards for abstinence, and family and couples therapy to improve communication and support. Digital platforms show promise for extending the reach of treatment and for delivering interventions in real time in response to craving or high-risk situations.

Addolorato G, Caputo F, Capristo E, Colombo G, Gessa GL, Gasbarrini G: Ability of baclofen in reducing alcohol craving and intake: II—Preliminary clinical evidence. *Alcohol Clin Exp Res* 2000;24:67–71.

The American Psychiatric Association Practice Guideline for the Pharmacological Treatment of Patients with Alcohol Use Disorder. American Psychiatric Association Publishing, 2018. https://doi.org/10.1176/appi.books.9781615371969.

Anton RF, O'Malley SS, Ciraulo DA, et al: Combined pharmacotherapies and behavioral interventions for alcohol dependence: the COMBINE study: a randomized controlled trial. *JAMA* 2006;295:2003–2017.

Anton RF, Latham P, Voronin K, et al: Efficacy of gabapentin for the treatment of alcohol use disorder in patients with alcohol withdrawal symptoms: a randomized clinical trial. *JAMA Intern Med* March 9, 2020. https://doi.org/10.1001/jamainternmed.2020.0249.

Blodgett JC, Del Re AC, Maisel NC, Finney JW: A meta-analysis of topiramate's effects for individuals with alcohol use disorders. *Alcohol Clin Exp Res* 2014;38(6):1481–1488. https://doi.org/10.1111/acer.12411.

D'Onofrio G, Fiellin DA, Pantalon MV, Chawarski MC, Owens PH, Degutis LC, Busch SH, Bernstein SL, O'Connor PG. A brief intervention reduces hazardous and harmful drinking in emergency department patients. *Ann Emerg Med.* 2012; 60(2):181-192. doi: 10.1016/j.annemergmed.2012.02.006. Epub 2012 Mar 28. PMID: 22459448; PMCID: PMC3811141.

Fucito LM, Park A, Gulliver SB, Mattson ME, Gueorguieva RV, O'Malley SS: Cigarette smoking predicts differential benefit from naltrexone for alcohol dependence. *Biol Psychiatry* 2012;72: 832–838.

Garbutt JC, Kranzler HR, O'Malley SS; V. S. Group: Efficacy and tolerability of long-acting injectable naltrexone for alcohol dependence: a randomized controlled trial. *JAMA* 2005;293: 1617–1625.

Garland EL, Howard MO: Mindfulness-based treatment of addiction: current state of the field and envisioning the next wave of research. *Addict Sci Clin Pract* 2018;13(1):14. doi:10.1186/s13722-018-0115-3

Johnson BA: Update on neuropharmacological treatments for alcoholism: scientific basis and clinical findings. *Biochem Pharmacol* 2008;75:34–56.

Johnson BA, Roache JD, Javors MA, et al: Ondansetron for reduction of drinking among biologically predisposed alcoholic patients: a randomized controlled trial. *JAMA* 2000;284:963–971.

Johnson BA, Koob GF, Schuckit MA, et al: Understanding and treating alcohol dependence. *Alcohol Clin Exp Res* 2006;30: 567–584.

Kranzler HR, Pierucci-Lagha A, Feinn R, et al: Effects of ondansetron in early- versus late-onset alcoholics: a prospective, open-label study. *Alcohol Clin Exp Res* 2003;27: 1150–1155.

Martin K, Katz A: The role of barbiturates for alcohol withdrawal syndrome. *Psychosomatics* August 2016;57(4):341–347. https://doi.org/10.1016/j.psym.2016.02.011.

Mason BJ, Quello S, Goodell V, Shadan F, Kyle M, Begovic A: Gabapentin treatment for alcohol dependence: a randomized clinical trial. *JAMA Intern Med* 2014;174:70–77.

McKee SA, Harrison EL, O'Malley SS, et al: Varenicline reduces alcohol self-administration in heavy-drinking smokers. *Biol Psychiatry*. 2009;66:185–190.

Minozzi S, Saulle R, Rösner S: Baclofen for alcohol use disorder. *Cochrane Database Syst Rev* November 26, 2018;11:CD012557.

Mosoni C, Dionisi T, Vassallo GA, et al: Baclofen for the treatment of alcohol use disorder in patients with liver cirrhosis: 10 years after the first evidence. *Front Psychiatry* 2018;9:474. https://doi.org/10.3389/fpsyt.2018.00474.

Myrick H, Malcolm R, Randall PK, et al: A double-blind trial of gabapentin versus lorazepam in the treatment of alcohol withdrawal. *Alcohol Clin Exp Res* 2009;33:1582–1588.

Nisavic, Mladen, Shamim H. Nejad, et al: Use of phenobarbital in alcohol withdrawal management—a retrospective comparison study of phenobarbital and benzodiazepines for acute alcohol withdrawal management in general medical patients. *Psychosomatics* October 2019;60(5):458–467. https://doi.org/10.1016/j.psym.2019.02.002.

O'Malley SS, Garbutt JC, Gastfriend DR, Dongj Q, Kranzler HR: Efficacy of extended-release naltrexone in alcohol-dependent patients who are abstinent before treatment. *J Clin Psychopharmacol* 2007;27:507–512.

O'Malley SS, Zweben A, Fucito LM, et al: Effect of varenicline combined with medical management on alcohol use disorder with comorbid cigarette smoking: a randomized clinical trial. *JAMA Psychiatry* February 1, 2018;75(2):129–138. doi: 10.1001/jamapsychiatry.2017.3544. PMID: 29261824; PMCID: PMC5838706.

Saitz R, O'Malley SS: Pharmacotherapies for alcohol abuse. Withdrawal and treatment. *Med Clin North Am.* 1997;81:881–907.

Sass H, Soyka M, Mann K, Zieglgänsberger W. Relapse prevention by acamprosate. Results from a placebo-controlled study on alcohol dependence. *Arch Gen Psychiatry* 1996;53:673–680.

Steensland P, Simms JA, Holgate JK, Richards JK, Bartlett SE: Varenicline, an alpha$_4$beta$_2$ nicotinic acetylcholine receptor partial agonist, selectively decreases ethanol consumption and seeking. *Proc Natl Acad Sci U S A* 2007;104:12518–12523.

Stewart H, Mitchell BG, Ayanga D, Walder A: Veteran adherence to oral versus injectable AUD medication treatment. *Ment Health Clin* May 2021;11(3):194–199. https://doi.org/10.9740/mhc.2021.05.194.

Sullivan JT, Sykora K, Schneiderman J, Naranjo CA, Sellers EM: Assessment of alcohol withdrawal: the revised Clinical Institute Withdrawal Instrument for Alcohol Scale (CIWA-Ar). *Br J Addict* 1989;84:1353–1357.

▶ Complications

A. Medical

The medical complications of chronic alcohol consumption are listed in the medical history section of Table 17–2. Chronic heavy alcohol consumption can cause widespread multisystemic end-organ damage. Heavy alcohol drinking is hepatotoxic, causing acute hepatic injury (hepatitis) and steatosis. Chronic repeated hepatic injury from heavy alcohol use can eventually lead to chronic steatosis, which could progress to hepatic cirrhosis. Heavy alcohol consumption is one of the most common causes for hepatic cirrhosis in the United States. Heavy alcohol consumption along with tobacco use are preventable causes of hypertension and cardiovascular disease. Additional health consequences of chronic heavy alcohol use are esophagitis and gastritis, with the potential for life-threatening upper gastrointestinal hemorrhage, as well as acute pancreatitis. Carcinomas of the esophagus, stomach, pharynx, larynx, liver, and colon have also been linked to alcohol consumption. Chronic alcohol use is associated with malnutrition from poor eating habits as well as depletion of glycogen stores by alcohol, which can cause hypoglycemia, electrolyte imbalance, seizures, cardiac arrhythmias, and immunodeficiency. Additional adverse effects on the pulmonary, endocrine, hematologic, and musculoskeletal systems have been described.

Alcohol use in pregnancy is associated with fetal alcohol spectrum disorders, affecting organ development, cognitive, and behavioral outcomes for the developing fetus. No amount of alcohol intake is recommended during any trimester of pregnancy.

There is also significant risk associated with combining alcohol use with specific medications, including sedative/hypnotics and opioids, given additive sedation effects and risk of precipitating an overdose.

B. Wernicke Encephalopathy and Korsakoff Syndrome

WE is an acute neuropsychiatric emergency characterized by a triad of ophthalmoplegia, mental status changes, and gait disturbances resulting from depletion of intracellular thiamine. In developed countries, about 90% of the cases of WE are a result of thiamine depletion due to heavy alcohol consumption (Thomson & Marshall 2006).

WE is an acute emergency. Once it is identified, treatment should be started immediately even if patient is intoxicated. High-dose parenteral thiamine accompanied by magnesium is the treatment of choice and should be administered before administration of intravenous glucose, to prevent sudden progression to irreversible brain injury. With adequate treatment, ophthalmoplegia resolves within hours and ataxia within days, but mental changes may persist for weeks. About 20% of undiagnosed or undertreated WE will result in death. The remaining 80% will go on to progress to the chronic irreversible Korsakoff syndrome. Korsakoff syndrome is characterized by marked anterograde amnesia, which is initially accompanied by confabulation; however, confabulation is lost as disease progresses.

C. Social

Heavy alcohol use has been related with lost housing, poverty, loss of social support network, and estrangement from friends and family.

D. Adverse Outcomes of Treatment

1. Pharmacotherapy—Pharmacological treatment as well as side effects of alcohol maintenance medication has been discussed earlier. Most notable is the adverse disulfiram-alcohol reaction produced in patients taking daily disulfiram.

The response, characterized by facial flushing, wheezing, and autonomic dysfunction, has been associated with some cases of mortality, especially in patients with cardiopulmonary compromise.

2. Failure to recognize comorbid disorders—Heavy alcohol consumption is associated with several psychiatric and medical disorders (APA 2018). Medical or behavioral treatment centers may focus on their area of expertise and may not identify and intervene for comorbid pathology. This may be the cause of primary care and medical specialties identifying and treating ongoing medical disorders but not recognizing the primary AUD, which leads to delay of treatment and disease progression. The converse is when patients attending alcohol specialty clinics have coexisting medical disorders that may go undiagnosed, and treatment may be delayed. A thorough history from the patient, relatives, and the patient's other treatment providers as well as laboratory and psychological testing is vital to help prevent this.

▶ Prognosis

The course of AUD has been discussed earlier in this chapter. As outlined, many patients with AUD will undergo remission, most of them with natural remission. This remission may be complete abstinence or an asymptomatic low-risk drinking pattern. Heavy drinking, nicotine dependence, coexisting drug use, mental illness, and personality disorders are associated with a worse prognosis for achieving remission (APA 2018). Female gender, older age group, and marriage are all factors associated with better prognostic outcomes.

The American Psychiatric Association Practice Guideline for the Pharmacological Treatment of Patients with Alcohol Use Disorder. American Psychiatric Association Publishing, 2018. https://doi.org/10.1176/appi.books.9781615371969.

Thomson AD, Marshall EJ: The natural history and pathophysiology of Wernicke's encephalopathy and Korsakoff's psychosis. Alcohol Alcohol. 2006;41:151–158.

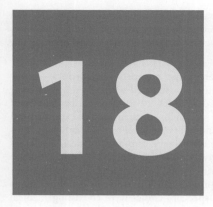

Opioid Use Disorders

Ellen L. Edens, MD, MPE
Ismene L. Petrakis, MD

OPIOID-RELATED DISORDERS CLASSIFICATION AND DIAGNOSIS

▶ What's in a Name? Opiate versus Opioid

It may seem trivial to distinguish between an opiate and an opioid, the terms being frequently used interchangeably by the medical community. However, there are significant differences between the classes that have some practical impact (results of urine drug testing, for instance, can be more easily interpreted using knowledge of the differences). Put simply, although all opiates are also opioids, not all opioids are opiates. An opioid is any natural or synthetic chemical that has opium-like effects like those of morphine. All opioids bind to opioid receptors in the central nervous system (CNS). Opiates, on the other hand, are a specific type of opioid derived directly from the opium poppy and include opium, codeine, morphine, and thebaine. Ingestion of an opiate will produce an opiate-positive result using immunoassay urine drug screens. Other nonopiate opioids have been either modified from an opiate (semisynthetic) or created de novo (synthetic). Semisynthetic opioids demonstrate variable sensitivity in toxicology testing, whereas fully synthetic opioids, including fentanyl and methadone, will not be positive with an opiate screen and require additional tests. The term "narcotic"—derived from the Greek "narkotikon" meaning "to numb"—is a generally outdated and nonspecific term referring to illicit drugs, often opioids, that induce sleep, numbness, or stupor.

▶ Opioid Use Disorder

According to the *Diagnostic and Statistical Manual of Mental Disorders,* 5th edition (DSM)-5, and similar to other substance use disorders, an opioid use disorder (OUD) is diagnosed when—due to using an opioid—at least two of the 11 criteria are present within the past year. Unlike many other substance use disorders, however, DSM-5 takes special consideration when an opioid is being prescribed for a medical condition (e.g., to suppress cough or relieve pain), given the expected **neuroadaptation** (i.e., tolerance and withdrawal) that develops after prolonged prescription opioid therapy. In this case, DSM-5 excludes tolerance and withdrawal from the criterion list, requiring at least two of nine (rather than of 11) criteria to support a diagnosis of an OUD. Without being able to rely on the signals of tolerance or withdrawal for diagnosis, clinicians must concentrate on the following three symptom clusters for diagnostic clarity: (1) **loss of control** (i.e., the substance is taken in larger amounts or over a longer period than was intended, or there are unsuccessful efforts to control use), (2) **salience to the behavioral repertoire** (i.e., a great deal of time is spent using or recovering from use, important activities are given up because of use, or use is continued despite great physical, psychological, occupational, or interpersonal consequence or risk), and (3) **craving** (strong desire to use opioid). Severity is determined by symptom count with the presence of 2–3 symptoms required for mild disorder, 4–5 for moderate, and 6+ for severe OUD. It is worth noting that this exclusion, based upon who is providing the opioid and for what, was added not due to strength of research evidence but by expert workgroup consensus. The clinical and research fields continue to struggle to distinguish those for whom long term opioid therapy for chronic pain is no longer benefiting and yet tapering or discontinuing opioids is difficult from those with an OUD.

▶ Opioid Intoxication

Opioid intoxication is potentially life threatening—especially among individuals with limited tolerance to opioids. Diagnosis requires both a history of recent opioid ingestion as well as concomitant signs including euphoria, pupillary constriction (unless severe overdose with anoxia and pupillary dilation), slowed respiratory rate, drowsiness, slurred speech, and inattention.

Opioid Withdrawal

Uncomplicated acute opioid withdrawal, although described as extremely unpleasant, is generally not life threatening. Symptoms include dysphoric mood, nausea or vomiting, muscle aches, lacrimation or rhinorrhea, pupillary dilation, piloerection or sweating, diarrhea, yawning, fever, and insomnia, and typically appear within minutes or days following cessation of an opioid or administration of an opioid antagonist (e.g., naltrexone) or partial agonist (e.g., buprenorphine). In addition to acute withdrawal, there is growing awareness that many individuals exposed to long-term opioid use experience **protracted** withdrawal symptoms beyond the expected time frame of acute opioid withdrawal symptoms (4–10 days, up to 21 days for methadone). Symptoms such as anxiety, depression, sleep disturbance, irritability, cognitive impairment (including impaired attention and executive control), and fatigue can last for weeks or months beyond acute withdrawal. The challenge of the treatment provider is to determine to what extent such protracted symptoms are substance-induced and likely to subside, and which indicate a possible co-occurring disorder (SAMHSA, 2022).

Other Opioid-Induced Disorders

DSM-5 includes the following opioid-induced disorders: depressive disorder, anxiety disorder, sleep disorder, and sexual dysfunction. Opioids may also be associated with delirium due to opioid intoxication or withdrawal. Opioid-induced psychiatric disorders are diagnosed when symptoms consistent with the disorder predominate in the clinical picture.

Unspecified Opioid-Related Disorders

Occasionally an individual will have significant distress or impairment in social, occupational, or other important areas due to opioid use but not meet criteria for an OUD. In this case, a diagnosis of unspecified opioid-related disorder may be given.

General Considerations

A. Epidemiology

1. Prevalence of opioid use—Although trends in illegal drug use are expected to be dynamic, rarely have such dramatic shifts occurred as has been witnessed in opioid use in the first decades of the twenty-first century (Compton & Jones, 2019; Jalal et al., 2018). The turn of the century was dominated by an increase in prescribed opioids for the management of chronic pain, which led to a concomitant rise in prescription opioid misuse and addiction (Okie, 2010). In response to this, state legislatures and licensing boards implemented measures to curb the flood of opioid prescriptions being used. Today, all 50 U.S. states and the District of

Columbia have ability to track opioid prescriptions through state **prescription drug monitoring programs** (PDMPs) to prevent multiple prescribers with overlapping prescriptions. Some states have implemented policies requiring providers to check a state PDMP prior to prescribing controlled substances, to ensure that PDMPs are used. The Centers for Disease Control (CDC) recommends checking the state PDMP prior to every opioid prescription and at least once every 3 months when prescribing opioids for chronic pain (Dowell, Ragan, Jones, Baldwin, & Chou, 2022). Additionally, many state licensing boards now require education on the treatment of pain and/or addiction and clinical guidelines have been released by various agencies to set standards for the use of opioid in the management of chronic pain (Dowell et al., 2022; Sandbrink et al., 2023). Perhaps because of such efforts, after a steady increase in overall national opioid prescription dispensing rates peaking in 2012 at 81.3 prescriptions per 100 persons, the overall national opioid dispensing rate fell to its lowest in 15 years in 2020 to about 43.3 prescriptions per 100 persons. While this is a national trend, certain regions of the country continue to have higher prescribing rates than others.

Unfortunately, simultaneous to this downward trend in prescription opioid prescribing in the United States, opioid use transferred and expanded to include nonprescribed or illegal opioid use with devastating results. As the supply of prescription opioids shrank over the second decade of the century, heroin use initially increased (Jones, Logan, Gladden, & Bohm, 2015) and then shifted from a largely heroin-based market to a fentanyl-based market. Fentanyl is roughly 50 times as potent as heroin, with analogues having even greater potency. This shift to fentanyl and synthetic derivatives is the major contributor to the current rise in fatal and nonfatal opioid deaths (Hedegaard, Minino, Spencer, & Warner, 2021) which, in 2021, topped 100,000 deaths (Spencer, Minino, & Warner, 2022) and contributed to an unprecedented downturn in life-expectancy among the U.S. population (Dowell et al., 2017).

According to the 2021 National Survey of Drug Use and Health (SAMHSA, 2022), 9.2 million people ages 12 and older had past year opioid misuse (either using a prescription opioid or heroin). Most of these report using prescription opioids alone (88.1%; although there is growing concern about illegal, counterfeit "pressed pills" that mimic scheduled opioids but are not) or in combination with heroin (6.2%). Heroin-only use is relatively rare (5.7% of those who misuse opioids). It is not possible to compare the 2021 national rates of opioid use to prior years given changes to survey data collection brought on by the COVID-19 pandemic.

2. Prevalence of OUD—It is difficult to accurately gauge the prevalence of OUD among those who use and misuse opioids. Population-level surveys often miss people at high risk either due to underreporting, declining participation, or not including people experiencing homelessness, incarceration, or hospitalization. And administrative claims data may miss a diagnosis due to underreporting in the claim or be less representative of populations with less insurance and more mistrust of the healthcare system. So, while recent population survey data indicate over 2 million people in the United States have an OUD, the rates are likely as much as three to four times higher (Keyes et al., 2022). Trends also suggest that, while rates of OUD are remaining stable or even declining since 2016, the mortality associated with opioid use and OUD has increased exponentially in recent years and admission for OUD treatment is increasing (Arfken, Owens, & Greenwald, 2020).

3. Prevalence of opioid overdose—In recent years, the number of opioid overdose deaths, both intentional and unintentional, has seen an exponential rise, primarily attributed to the proliferation of **fentanyl** and other **high potency synthetic opioids** in illicit drug supplies. Since the beginning of the 21st century, the United States has witnessed the tragic loss of nearly 600,000 lives due to opioid-related overdoses, with over 100,000 deaths occurring in the year leading up to April 2021. These distressing trends can be delineated into three distinct waves, each characterized by specific contributing factors (CDC, 2022b).

The first wave originated with the surge in opioid prescriptions during the late 1990s and early 2000s. This era saw a significant increase in the prescribing and availability of opioids, setting the stage for widespread misuse and addiction.

The second wave emerged around 2010, marked by a notable rise in heroin-related incidents. As opioid prescriptions became more closely regulated, individuals turned to heroin as a cheaper and more accessible alternative, fueling a new way of addiction and overdose deaths.

The third wave commenced in 2013, as the problem escalated with the influx of synthetic opioids, particularly illicitly manufactured fentanyl. These potent synthetic opioids began appearing in drug supplies, leading to a drastic spike in overdose fatalities and an already alarming death toll.

Of those who die by opioid overdose, the majority are classified as unintentional, with 5–7% recorded as intentional. Because it is difficult to accurately assess intent, the actual numbers are likely higher. Many people who develop a substance use disorder also have another mental illness including mood disorders, PTSD, anxiety disorders, or chronic pain which are independently associated with increased suicide risk. Among people with an OUD or those who use or are prescribed opioids, routine evaluation of co-occurring disorders and suicide risk is warranted.

4. Co-occurring psychiatric diagnoses—Similar to other substance use disorders, OUD co-occurs with other psychiatric illnesses at higher rates than seen in the general population (Jones & McCance-Katz, 2019). Common co-occurring disorders include mood, anxiety, psychotic, cognitive, eating, sleep, and personality disorders as well as attention-deficit/

hyperactivity disorder (ADHD), chronic pain, and posttraumatic stress disorder (PTSD). PTSD, in particular, appears to have a complex relationship to OUDs. Trauma exposure is necessary for a diagnosis of PTSD and is simultaneously associated with the development of chronic pain, an independent risk factor for developing OUD (Bilevicius, Sommer, Asmundson, & El-Gabalawy, 2018). A 2012 study of returning veterans from the Middle East wars found those veterans with co-occurring mental health diagnoses were more likely than those without such diagnoses to receive a prescription for an opioid analgesic. Of the psychiatric diagnoses examined, PTSD conferred the highest probability of receiving an opioid prescription. Furthermore, veterans with PTSD were more likely than those without mental health diagnoses to receive high doses of opioids and concurrent sedative-hypnotics, obtain early refills, and suffer adverse opioid-related outcomes (Seal et al., 2012). Among those in treatment for OUDs, PTSD is associated with more severe addiction, higher rates of depression, attempted suicide, and psychosocial problems (Meshberg-Cohen, Ross MacLean, Schnakenberg Martin, Sofuoglu, & Petrakis, 2021). Several clinical practice guidelines for PTSD now recommend trauma-focused psychotherapy treatment as the first-line treatment for PTSD. If medication is preferred to treatment PTSD, specific guidance for treating individuals with PTSD and co-occurring OUDs have been written and disseminated by SAMHSA to promote optimal care for patients with both disorders and to highlight the importance of proactively screening and treating both disorders in a clinical setting (SAMHSA, 2012).

B. Etiology

Current formulations of addiction predominantly cut across substance type, emphasizing common factors contributing to addiction. From conception, genetic and environmental factors interact and influence the risk of both using drugs and, subsequently, developing addiction. Recognized risk factors for drug-seeking include young age, male sex, history of trauma, co-occurring psychiatric disorders, and psychological factors such as high sensation-seeking. Once exposed, it is difficult to predict who will or will not progress to addiction. Acute effects of the drug (pleasant or aversive), drug metabolism, and developmental stage of the individual at time of use (young age being a strong predictor) are among the influencing factors for regular drug use and later addiction. Quantity, frequency, and route of administration (IV or inhalation confer highest risk) of opioid use may also influence the development of addiction. With chronic exposure, neuroadaptation occurs to produce withdrawal symptoms when the opioid is discontinued. This negative reinforcement fuels the person to continue taking and seeking opioids to avoid the discomfort of withdrawal. Craving, or intense desire to seek and use drugs, may also emerge with chronic use, and serves to maintain the cycle of addiction. Substance use disorders remain among the most highly heritable medical disorders, with roughly half of the variation in disease liability attributable to heritable influences. Two large-scale studies of male twins examining opioid addiction reported between 23% and 54% of the variation in opioid addiction was attributable to genetic factors (Kendler, Karkowski, Neale, & Prescott, 2000; Tsuang et al., 1998). Lastly, a personal past history of a substance use disorder is among the strongest predictors of future risk and all persons being considered for a trial of opioid therapy for longer than a few days should be asked about a history of substance use disorder.

C. Genetics

Genetic factors contribute to the development of addiction, and vulnerability may be nonspecific. Using approaches such as twin, family and adoption studies suggest there are significant genetic underpinning for drug addiction in general and heritability of OUD has been estimated to be at about 50% (reviewed in Berrettini, 2017). Studies, including linkage studies, genetic association studies, and genome-wide association studies, have begun to identify and locate associated genes in OUD. Important areas of genetic vulnerability for OUD include (1) genetic variations that code for proteins in the pathway where opioids have their direct action, particularly those that lead to individual differences in biochemical and behavioral responses; (2) genes encoding proteins involved in metabolism; (3) genes encoding proteins involved in treatment agents; and (4) nonspecifically in genes that affect traits such as impulsivity and stress response (which is beyond the scope of this chapter; for more comprehensive review, see Wang, Chen, Lee, and Cheng, 2019).

Some promising findings include variance in alleles in the μ-opioid receptor gene (OPRM1), which regulates OPRM1 expression, in potassium-ion-channel genes (KCNC1 and KCNG2) and in a glutamate receptor auxiliary protein (CNIH3). Regarding metabolism, methadone dose may be regulated by variants in cytochrome P450 2B6 (CYP2B6), a methadone-metabolizing enzyme, and by a variance in OPRM1. Interestingly, δ-opioid-receptor gene single-nucleotide polymorphisms may also be important in the pharmacogenetic response to methadone compared to buprenorphine (Berrettini, 2017).

Most recently, a meta-analysis for OUD found genetic variation in 19 genes that was associated with OUD risk; OPRM1 and FURIN were two genes identified in the analysis of OUD alone. Further, the study found genetic links to other such as chronic pain, the inability to work because of a sickness or a disability, and other psychiatric disorders such as anxiety, depression, and PTSD (Deak et al., 2022).

▶ Clinical Findings

A. Signs & Symptoms

1. Opioid intoxication and overdose—Opioid intoxication and overdose are potential medical emergencies due to diminished respiratory drive and reduced level of consciousness. Miosis (pinpoint pupils), slowed respiratory rate (hypoxemia/hypercarbia), slurred speech, pruritus, constipation, sedation, and psychomotor slowing are all signs and symptoms of intoxication.

2. Opioid withdrawal—Symptoms of opioid withdrawal emerge after stopping or dramatically reducing opioid use following a period of prolonged use and can be conceptualized as rebound hyperactivity in the biologic systems suppressed by the agonists. Symptoms of withdrawal can be seen after as little as 2–3 weeks of daily opioid use (Jaffe JH, 1975) and, in mild form, often manifest as flulike symptoms (anorexia, fatigue, rhinorrhea, lacrimation, insomnia, irritability, anxiety, yawning, piloerection). In more severe or advanced withdrawal, nausea, diarrhea, vomiting, abdominal pain and cramping, hot or cold flashes, musculoskeletal pain and spasms, increased blood pressure and elevated temperature, and mydriasis are seen. The **Clinical Opioid Withdrawal Scale** (COWS), a validated and easily accessible 11-item clinician-administered instrument designed to assess a patient's level of opioid withdrawal, is often used to determine the presence of and extent of opioid withdrawal (Wesson & Ling, 2003). This scale is particularly useful in guiding the initiation of buprenorphine, which traditionally has required someone with physiologic dependence and recent use to be in moderate withdrawal before the initial dose.

The time course of a patient's withdrawal after last use of an opioid depends largely on the half-life of the opioid being used and on the individual factors affecting absorption and elimination (Table 18–1). Regardless of which opioid is used, the acute symptoms of withdrawal are often followed by a more **protracted abstinence syndrome**, with disturbances of mood and sleep that can persist for months (Martin & Jasinski, 1969). It is hypothesized that these negative emotional symptoms accompanying abstinence (profound dysphoria, irritability, anxiety, heightened emotional pain, sleep disturbances, and intense desire/urges to obtain and use opioids) is the key motivational component of addiction, rather than merely the desire to relieve symptoms of withdrawal (Shurman, Koob, & Gutstein, 2010) and is a promising target for drug development (Koob, 2021).

3. Opioid addiction and sequelae—Unlike with alcohol, where there are measures of frequency and quantity of use that allow us to estimate risk, *any* nonprescribed opioid use in the past year warrants an assessment of DSM-5 criteria for an OUD. The classic "3 Cs" of addiction include (1) loss of control, (2) craving, and (3) continued use despite negative consequences, which roughly corresponds to the DSM-5 syndrome. As noted earlier, DSM-5 OUD includes some combination of a general loss of control over opioid use (using more than intended, difficulty cutting down or limiting use), repeated negative consequences of use (including interpersonal/social, psychiatric, and medical consequences, loss of activities once enjoyed, excessive

Table 18–1 Properties of Various Opioids

Opioid	Mechanism of Action	Available Formulations	Pregnancy Category/ DEA-Schedule	Expected Positive Urine Screen	Dose Equivalent to Oral Morphine 30 mg	Detection Time in Urine[a]	Half-life	Onset & Peak of Withdrawal Symptoms After Last Dose	Metabolism
Opiates-natural (from opium)									
Codeine	μ-Opioid receptor agonist	Oral	CII	Opiates immunoassay—positive; GC/MS or LC/MS/MS—codeine, possibly morphine & hydrocodone	200 mg	1–3 days	2.5–4 h	12 h/48–72 h	CYP2D6, morphine is active metabolite
Morphine	μ-Opioid receptor agonist; κ-opioid receptor agonist	Oral, parenteral (SC, IM, IV), intrathecal, rectal	CII	Opiates immunoassay—positive; GC/MS or LC/MS/MS—morphine, possibly hydromorphone on GC/MS	N/A	1–3 days	2–4 h	6 h/36–72 h	CYP2D6; phase II glucuronidation
Semisynthetic Opioids (derived from opium)									
Buprenorphine	Partial μ-opioid receptor agonist; κ-opioid receptor antagonist; δ-opioid receptor antagonist	Transmucosal (sublingual), parenteral (IM, IV), transdermal	CIII—requires special DEA license when prescribing for opioid addiction	Buprenorphine immunoassay—positive; GC/MS or LC/MS/M—buprenorphine, norbuprenorphine	N/A	3–7 days	20–44 h	24–48 h/ 72–96 h	CYP3A4
Heroin	μ-Opioid receptor agonist	N/A	CI	Opiates immunoassay—positive; GC/MS or LC/MS/M—6-acetyl morphine (<24 h), morphine	N/A	1–3 days	60–90 min	3–4 h/ 36–72 h	Rapid deacetylation to 6-MAM, morphine
Hydrocodone	μ-Opioid receptor agonist	Oral	CII	Opiates immunoassay—positive; GC/MS or LC/MS/MS-hydrocodone, possibly hydromorphone	30 mg	1–3 days	4–5 h	6 h/48–72 h	CYP2D6; CYP3A4
Hydromorphone	μ-Opioid receptor agonist	Oral, parenteral (SC, IM, IV), Rectal	CII	Opiates immunoassay—positive; GC/MS or LC/MS/MS-hydromorphone	7.5 mg	1–3 days	2.5 h	6 h/48–72 h	Phase II glucuronidation

Drug	Mechanism	Route	Schedule	Drug testing	Equianalgesic dose			Metabolism
Oxycodone	μ-Opioid receptor agonist; κ2b-opioid receptor agonist	Oral	CII	Oxycodone immunoassay—positive; opiates immunoassay—possibly positive, particularly at high doses; GC/MS or LC/MS/MS—oxycodone, possibly oxymorphone	20 mg	1–3 days	3.5–4 h	6 h/48–72 h	CYP3A4; CYP2D6
Oxymorphone	μ-Opioid receptor agonist	Oral, parenteral (SC, IM, IV)	CII	Opiates or oxycodone immunoassay—positive; GC/MS or LC/MS/MS—oxymorphone	10 mg	1–3 days	7–11 h	6 h/48–72 h	Phase II glucuronidation
Synthetic Opioids (human-made)								
Fentanyl	μ-Opioid receptor agonist	Transdermal, transmucosal (intranasal, buccal, sublingual)	CII	GC/MS or LC/MS/MS—fentanyl, norfentanyl	12.5 mcg/h	1–3 days	4 h	6–36 h/24–48 h	CYP3A4
Methadone	μ-Opioid receptor agonist; NMDA-receptor antagonist	Oral	CII—requires administration in federally regulated methadone clinic if prescribed for opioid addiction	Methadone immunoassay—positive; GC/MS or LC/MS/MS—methadone	Complex; a slow conversion to/initiation of methadone is required	1–7 days	8–59 h	24–48 h/72–96 h	CYP3A4; CYP2B6; CYP2C19; CYP2C9 (minor); CYP2D6 (minor); chronic dosing may induce its own metabolism
Tramadol	μ-Opioid receptor agonist; norepinephrine and serotonin reuptake inhibition	Oral	CIV	GC/MS or LC/MS/MS—tramadol	225 mg	1–3 days	6–8 h	12–20 h/3–7 days	CYP2B6; CYP2D6; CYP3A4

[a]Detection times are approximate and depend on individual metabolism and the dose of the drug.

time spent on addiction-related activities, repeated use in high-risk situations), the presence of cravings, and physiologic dependence (tolerance or withdrawal). Symptoms of tolerance and withdrawal are often present with prolonged opioid use, but neither are necessary to make a diagnosis of an OUD, nor are they sufficient in the case of medically prescribed opioid use.

If looking for a reliable test of the consumption and consequences of drug use disorders, the **Drug Abuse Screening Test** (DAST) can be used. The DAST has 28 items, each weighted equally, in a true–false format, and can aid in identifying the presence of a drug use disorder.

Physical and laboratory signs (see later discussion) may accompany ongoing opioid use, addiction, and medical sequelae. Addiction to opioids increases the likelihood of drug injection. Injecting opioids bypasses first-pass metabolism, increasing bioavailability and, therefore, allowing more efficient use of the drug. In addition, drug injection produces a rapid and intense effect known as a "rush." Frequently, the median cubital vein of the nondominant arm is used for injecting; however, because of venous scarring or the stigma of drug injection, veins in the hand, foot, or other less obvious areas may preferred. There are several cutaneous signs that may signal addiction and intravenous drug use. These include needle puncture marks, track marks (hyperpigmented linear scars located along veins), hand edema (from injecting into fingers and hands), thrombophlebitis, abscesses, truncal piloerection (sign of opioid withdrawal), and jaundice (due to viral hepatitis often acquired through nonsterile injection of opioids).

4. Screening and identification of addiction in setting of prescription opioids—Current guidelines recommend nonopioid therapies be used for subacute and chronic pain (Dowell et al., 2022) and that opioids only be considered if expected benefits in pain and function are anticipated to outweigh potential harms. There is, at this time, no validated, reliable screening tool to predict which patients will experience harm and which will benefit from opioid therapy—though ample evidence exists that risk of serious harm increases as the dosage of opioids rises, without a clearly defined threshold below which no risk is present (Chou et al., 2020; Sandbrink et al., 2023). Once the decision has been made to initiate opioids for chronic pain, however, clinicians have a responsibility to engage in thorough discussions with patients, addressing realistic benefits and well-known risks associated with opioid use, including OUD, overdose, and death.

Diagnosing an OUD in the context of long-term opioid therapy for chronic pain can be difficult. As noted previously, DSM-5 OUD excludes the criteria of tolerance and withdrawal in the context of prescribed opioids. Yet other criteria may be equally problematic. For example, is someone having a hard time tapering opioids because of an inability to cut back on use or loss of control, or because of poorly controlled pain? Is a patient's depression worsening because of an opioid addiction or, again, because of underlying pain? One of the criteria is spending a great deal of time in activities necessary to obtain, use, or recover from the effects of opioids—but what does this mean for patients who are using opioids as prescribed around the clock long term, even for decades?

Therefore, shifting the central question from "*Does my patient have an addiction?*" to "*Do the risks of continued opioid prescribing outweigh the benefits or could equal or greater benefit be achieved at a lower dose?*" can be an extremely helpful first step in determining whether a trial of opioids for chronic pain should be continued or not. It is recommended to monitor all patients on long-term opioid therapy through routine drug testing, most commonly urine. Moderate quality evidence suggests that increased drug screens and more follow-up after new prescriptions is associated with fewer suicide attempts (Sandbrink et al., 2023). Other risk-mitigation strategies include routinely reviewing the state PDMP and provision of naloxone to reverse opioid overdose.

When, in the context of long-term opioid therapy, the risks appear to outweigh the benefits, it is important to apply a rational, patient-centered approach to treatment. Misapplication of the 2016 CDC Opioid Prescribing Guidelines (Dowell, Haegerich, & Chou, 2016) inadvertently led to some systems adopting stringent and harmful policies including rapid opioid tapers and abrupt discontinuation without collaboration with patients. Such actions are not recommended as they have contributed to significant harm including worsening pain outcomes, serious opioid withdrawal, increased suicidal ideation and behavior, overdose and death (Dowell et al., 2022). Rather, when risks outweigh benefits, several treatment options exist: (1) switch to a medication for OUD, if diagnosis is present (i.e., methadone through an opioid treatment program (OTP), buprenorphine, or IM naltrexone); (2) initiate a patient-centered opioid taper—either to discontinuation or to lowest effective dose—while optimizing nonopioid pain care treatments; (3) offer a switch to a partial agonist opioid therapy (e.g., buprenorphine) to provide immediate safety benefit and potential improvement in function and pain relief (Becker, Frank, & Edens, 2020; Edens, 2020).

B. Psychological Assessment and Measurement-based Care

1. Initial assessment—Once an OUD has been identified and diagnosed, it's important to follow up with a thorough substance use evaluation identifying: (1) acute or urgent safety *risks* including withdrawal, overdose, and suicidal thinking; (2) age of *initiation* of any use, regular use, and problematic use; (3) *patterns* of use, including quantity of frequency of use, and questions of when, where, how (route of administration), and with whom the patient uses; and (4) *treatment* history, including periods of *abstinence* and details surrounding prior or current *relapse*.

Neuropsychological tests can be useful in determining the extent of lasting brain dysfunction, require patient participation, and are preferably conducted at least 3 weeks after the most recent substance use. Although these tests may be useful, many factors influence them, including medication, co-occurring medical conditions or psychiatric disorder, and compliance with testing.

2. Monitoring progress—While psychological assessment has long played a central role in the field of psychology, providing valuable insights into individuals' psychological functioning, in more recent years, measurement-based care has emerged as an evidence-based practice, representing a specialized form of applied psychological assessment (Resnick, Oehlert, Hoff, & Kearney, 2020). Measurement-based care involves the systematic use of standardized instruments, questionnaires, or scales that capture patients' self-reported experiences and perceptions related to their mental health and well-being. These measures are administered at regular intervals throughout the course of treating, allowing clinicians to gather objective data on patients' progress and outcomes.

The **Brief Addiction Monitor, revised** (BAM-R) is an assessment tool designed to provide a comprehensive snapshot of an individual's substance use and related behaviors. The BAM-R consists of several key components including substance use patterns, consequences and problems related to substance use, motivation to change, social support, and recovery environment. It is a 17-item scale that offers a valuable tool for health professionals and to quickly assess and monitor an individual's progress, tailor treatment plans, and identify areas that require intervention or additional support (Cacciola et al., 2013).

C. Laboratory Findings

In patients presenting with evidence or history of opioid addiction, the following laboratory tests are often performed:

- Urine drug of abuse screens. The panel of drugs tested in routine urine toxicology can vary depending on the laboratory used. It is important, therefore, to be familiar with local procedures. The most commonly tested classes of drug in a urine drug screen include amphetamines, barbiturates, benzodiazepines, cannabis, cocaine, opiates, and phencyclidine (PCP). The "NIDA 5," a frequently used U.S. federal drug panel determined by the National Institute of Drug Abuse (NIDA), includes amphetamines, cocaine, marijuana, opiates, and PCP. Notably, many, if not most, routine urine tests do not include and will not detect synthetic opioids including fentanyl, methadone, and buprenorphine, which will require a special lab order. Oxycodone also usually requires a separate test, although, at high doses, it may result in an opiate positive finding. If needed, therefore, these tests should be ordered separately if not included in the local panel. Increasingly, local facilities are adding oxycodone and fentanyl onto routine opioid screens, given the rising prevalence.

- Complete blood count and differential. Leukocytosis is common (in detoxification), and white blood cell counts greater than 14,000/mm^3 are not unusual. In the context of human immunodeficiency virus (HIV) infection, however, white blood cell counts may be low.

- Liver panel

- Electrolytes

- Thyroid

- Syphilis serology

- HIV

- Hepatitis panel

- Urinalysis

- Pregnancy test in women

- Electrocardiogram. If considering methadone, which can prolong the QTc interval, a baseline ECG is essential.

- Chest X-ray

- Tuberculin skin test

- Though not routinely ordered, obtaining hormonal (e.g., testosterone) levels may be useful in patients complaining of erectile dysfunction, a common complaint with long-term opioid use.

D. Neuroimaging

Brain imaging techniques—both structural and functional—have allowed for a significant understanding of complex behavioral disorders including addiction. Acute and chronic effects of opioids include neurovascular disorders, leukoencephalopathy, and atrophy (Cadet, Bisagno, & Milroy, 2014), perhaps in part because μ-opioid agonists are vasoconstrictors on vascular smooth muscle and are thought to induce vasospasms and subsequent ischemia. Autopsy results of those who die from heroin overdose show a high percentage of cerebral edema; a smaller percentage have ischemia in the globus pallidus. These abnormalities are thought to be related to cerebral hypoxia. Some of these findings may be due to the impurities and not directly related to opioid use, as injection opioid use is associated with a higher incidence of acute cerebral ischemia than other routes of administration. There is evidence from neuroimaging of brain morphology alterations in substance use disorders in general, suggestive of adaptation which in the future may lead to better understanding of the disorder. Further, addiction has been conceptualized as dysregulation of reward processes mediated by the limbic system. Functional imaging techniques have confirmed heightened neural activation in OUD (Pando-Naude et al., 2021). Much of this work is not specific to opioid addiction and is beyond the scope of this chapter (Moningka et al., 2019).

E. Course of Illness

The course of OUD is variable and influenced by factors such as types of opioids used, route of administration, length of time misusing, and setting of use. To illustrate the power of environment and setting, Lee Robins' famous 1974 study of 900 returning Vietnam veterans found that, although 35% had tried heroin in Vietnam and 20% were addicted to it, only 1% reported addiction 1 year later and 2% reported 2 years later. Moreover, although half of the veterans who had been addicted to heroin in Vietnam used heroin on their return to the United States, only one-eighth of the men became readdicted to heroin. Thus, the great majority of U.S. service members who used heroin or developed heroin addiction while stationed in Vietnam during the Vietnam War were able to quit completely or use intermittently and sparingly after return to the United States, where heroin was less available and less pure (Robins, Davis, & Nurco, 1974; Robins, Helzer, Hesselbrock, & Wish, 2010). Among those who continued a pattern of addiction upon return, however, the course was characterized by significant social problems including arrests and unemployment, not unlike another important naturalistic study of people who used heroin. In that study, 581 incarcerated males who were addicted to heroin were compulsorily enrolled between 1962 and 1964 in the California Civil Addict Program, a mandated drug treatment program for heroin-addicted criminal offenders. At 33-year follow-up, close to half of the initial study participants were dead, 20% tested positive for heroin (with 10% refusing urine drug screening and 14% incarcerated), and 40% reported past-year heroin use (Hser, Hoffman, Grella, & Anglin, 2001). From these two landmark studies, therefore, we can confidently conclude that the course of OUD is variable, yet potentially severe and even deadly. Frustratingly for clinicians, what we are less certain of is how to predict who will have a relatively benign or malignant course.

Two large U.S. population studies, the National Survey of Drug Use and Health (NSDUH) and the National Epidemiologic Survey on Alcohol and Related Conditions (NESARC), have also provided valuable insights into the course of OUD. Both studies confirm that many individuals with OUD first use opioids for nonmedical reasons in their teenage or young adult years, most often obtaining it from friends or family. These studies also highlight the high prevalence of co-occurring mental health conditions as well as the significant treatment gap that exists between people who need treatment and people who can access it (Saha et al., 2016; Saini, Johnson, & Qato, 2022). Optimistically, however, longitudinal data from NSDUH and NESARC have provided evidence that recovery and remission from OUD are achievable with treatment, the mainstay of which is medications that have been shown to reduce opioid use, prevent relapse, and improve overall outcomes for individuals with OUD. An important caveat to these national epidemiologic studies is the exclusion of the incarcerated persons, where substance use disorders are disproportionately high and theoretically contain the more severe cases, with more psychosocial barriers to treatment and recovery.

▶ Differential Diagnosis

Other substance use disorders should be included in the differential diagnosis when seeing a patient with suspected opioid addiction. In the intoxicated patient, one should consider alcohol, benzodiazepines, and PCP intoxication as well as other medical causes of altered mental status such as traumatic brain injury, anticholinergic overdose, or hypoglycemia. History of opioid ingestion and urine drug testing are the most useful in determining the etiology of intoxication. Patients in opioid withdrawal typically have good insight into their condition, and the diagnosis is determined by history. However, other intoxication and withdrawal syndromes may mimic opioid withdrawal.

Diagnosing OUDs becomes most challenging in patients with chronic pain conditions who are prescribed opioids. Given that tolerance and withdrawal commonly develop upon repeated exposure to opioids, these symptoms cannot be included in the diagnosis of a DSM-5 OUD—yet, in clinical practice, it is not uncommon to see these symptoms incorrectly equated with prescription opioid misuse. As previously mentioned, it is important to weigh the overall risks and benefits of continued opioid therapy for the management of chronic pain conditions, recognize that daily exposure to opioids is a risk factor for developing OUD and monitor all patients on long-term opioid therapy accordingly, and to transition to medications for OUD if two of the nine remaining DSM-5 OUD criteria (excluding tolerance and withdrawal) are present.

▶ Treatment

A. Psychotherapeutic Interventions

The most robust evidence for treatment of OUDs is medication. However, there are times when nonmedication behavioral or talk therapies may be helpful to address ambivalence, improve treatment adherence, or target co-occurring mental health conditions. **Contingency management** (CM) is a behavioral approach involving giving patients tangible rewards to reinforce positive behaviors. Studies conducted in OTPs and outpatient substance use treatment programs have demonstrated that incentive-based interventions are highly effective in promoting abstinence from opioids, other substances of abuse (e.g., stimulants), medication adherence, and treatment engagement and retention (Kidorf, King, Gandotra, Kolodner, & Brooner, 2012; Prendergast, Podus, Finney, Greenwell, & Roll, 2006). Though monetary rewards are most often thought of and appear most effective when considering treatment with CM, a common example of CM is rewarding patients with take-home methadone doses after so many days of negative urine drug panel testing in an OTP setting. A 2021 systematic review and meta-analysis that included 74 randomized clinical trials and more than 10,000 adults receiving medications for OUD (MOUD) further supported contingency management's overall medium to large effect size in addressing co-use of stimulants, abstinence from opioids, adherence to treatment, and other health behaviors such as smoking cessation (Bolivar et al., 2021). The authors urged policy makers—and the Centers for Medicare and Medicaid Services specifically—to allow funds to include CM in the treatment of people with substance use disorders.

Defined broadly, **cognitive–behavioral therapy for substance use disorder** (CBT-SUD) may include any behavioral or cognitive–behavioral intervention designed to help patients overcome addiction through promoting treatment engagement, retention, or reducing substance use. As such, CBT may describe heterogeneous treatments involving positive or negative reinforcements, motivational and cognitive elements, and skills building (McHugh, Hearon, & Otto, 2010). More narrowly, CBT-SUD incorporates several key ingredients: functional analysis of the patient's substance use, training in recognizing and coping with cues, cravings, thoughts about using substances, planning for emergencies and identified high-risk situations, development of drug refusal skills, and practice of skills within sessions (McHugh et al., 2010). CBT is a mainstay of psychotherapy in addiction treatment programs. Compared to MOUD, however, its effect is limited in opioid addiction and is typically considered adjunctive to pharmacotherapy rather than a standalone treatment. A randomized controlled trial involving patients prescribed buprenorphine for OUD in a primary care setting showed no additional benefit of CBT as compared to physician management with buprenorphine alone. Patients with significant comorbidities including cocaine, alcohol, or benzodiazepine dependence and untreated major depression or psychosis were excluded from the study (Fiellin et al., 2013).

Motivational enhancement therapy (MET) is a specific application of motivational interviewing (MI), a style of counseling that addresses patient ambivalence and enhances a patient's intrinsic motivation to facilitate change. It is explicitly nonconfrontational. MET is provided in four sessions typically over 12 weeks. Research has shown MET to be most effective for patients with alcohol, nicotine, and cannabis use disorders. One large study showed MI promoted treatment retention in individuals receiving methadone for OUD (Saunders, Wilkinson, & Phillips, 1995). Another study successfully incorporated brief motivational interventions into opioid programming to reduce cocaine and heroin use (Bernstein et al., 2005). The few numbers of studies and lack of reviews indicate the insufficient evidence to recommend MI or MET for people seeking treatment for opioid use (DiClemente, Corno, Graydon, Wiprovnick, & Knoblach, 2017).

Acceptance and commitment therapy (ACT) is a mindfulness-based therapy that encourages patients to observe their thoughts without judgment, accept even sometimes painful feelings and sensations that arise, and identify and commit to value-based behaviors. Although a form of CBT, it also differs in its emphases on noticing and accepting thoughts and feelings rather than working to change them. Research is limited, although there are some data showing augmentation of opioid negative urines in individuals treated with methadone and aid in discontinuing methadone if that is a goal (Stotts et al., 2012). There has been more recent interest in using ACT for people with OUDs and co-occurring psychiatric conditions, such as chronic pain (Smallwood, Potter, & Robin, 2016) or depression (Saedy, Kooshki, Jamali Firouzabadi, Emamipour, & Rezaei Ardani, 2015).

Twelve-step facilitation (TSF) is a brief (12–15 sessions) manualized therapy designed to introduce central tenets of Alcoholics Anonymous (AA), including acceptance that willpower is not enough to achieve sobriety, that group process must supplant self-centeredness, and that spiritual renewal is a key to long-term recovery. The TSF counselor assesses the client's alcohol or drug use, advocates abstinence, explains the basic 12-step concepts, and actively supports and facilitates initial involvement and ongoing participation in AA. TSF was originally developed for Project MATCH, an 8-year, national clinical trial of alcohol use disorder treatment matching funded by the NIAAA, and appears comparable in efficacy to cognitive–behavioral and motivational enhancement therapies for people who use drugs (Nowinski, 1995). TSF has also been studied among individuals with opioid addiction, including those taking methadone in an OTP setting, and has been found comparable to other therapies in promoting remission (Ball, 2007). It has also been found to improve cocaine use outcomes in an OTP setting (Carroll, Nich, Shi, Eagan, & Ball, 2012).

B. Psychopharmacologic Interventions

1. Intoxication and overdose—Because opioids reduce respiratory drive and diminish level of consciousness, opioid intoxication and overdose are medical emergencies requiring close monitoring and intervention. Emergency management includes assessment of airway access, providing ventilation if needed, an assessment of cardiac function, IV fluids, and administration of naloxone. Naloxone, a μ-opioid antagonist that is administered intravenously or subcutaneously, is first-line treatment of acute overdose, as it rapidly reverses the respiratory depression and sedation caused by opioid intoxication. Opioids with a high receptor affinity (e.g., buprenorphine) require greater naloxone concentrations and/or continuous infusion to antagonize opioid effects than opioids with lower affinity (Dahan, Aarts, & Smith, 2010). Continued monitoring of the patient is essential, as the half-life of naloxone is short compared to longer-acting opioids (e.g., buprenorphine and methadone) and, therefore, repeated dosing may be required to prevent return of sedation and respiratory compromise. Given the current abundance of fentanyl and other high-potency synthetic opioids being sold in illicit markets, the risk of opioid overdose is very high for all people using nonprescribed opioids—with risk further increased in young people, people recently leaving prison or other settings in which abstinence is required, people who mix sedatives (e.g., benzodiazepines) with opioids, people who mix stimulants with opioids, and people with other significant medical comorbidities such as obstructive sleep apnea (SAMHSA, 2018).

In 1996, recognizing the growing problem of opioid overdose and the time-sensitive nature of naloxone administration, the first community-based programs began offering naloxone and other opioid overdose prevention services to persons who use drugs, their families, friends, and service providers (e.g., homeless shelters and substance use treatment programs). These services include education regarding overdose risk factors, recognition of signs of opioid overdose, appropriate responses to an overdose, and administration of naloxone. Since that time, hundreds of local, state, and federal agencies, including the U.S. Veteran Healthcare Administration (Oliva, Richardson, Harvey, & Bellino, 2021), have developed overdose prevention and naloxone distribution programs. Just as one would keep a fire extinguisher readily available for use in a time of emergency, naloxone should be stored in a pocket, purse, or cabinet for rapid access in an emergency. Originally approved as a prescription in 2015 by the U.S. Food and Drug Administration (FDA), over the counter naloxone nasal spray was approved in 2023.

2. Opioid withdrawal—Symptoms of acute opioid withdrawal can be managed medically to reduce suffering and significant associated morbidity. Though rarely life threatening, opioid withdrawal is associated with intense discomfort, strong cravings to use opioids, and low completion rates—which is a set up for risk of subsequent overdose and high mortality. Without coupling to ongoing medication treatment for OUD, medical-managed opioid withdrawal in patients with OUD is generally insufficient, ineffective, and associated with very high rates of relapse (Kakko, Svanborg, Kreek, & Heilig, 2003; Weiss et al., 2011) and death. Therefore, it is essential to clarify the goals of opioid withdrawal before and during the process, including initiation of MOUD with linkage to ongoing treatment. Generally, goals of opioid withdrawal include: (1) relief of suffering during the transition from physical dependence to nondependence, (2) initiation of MOUD, (3) identification and management of co-occurring medical and psychiatric problems, and (4) engagement in ongoing SUD treatment (Capata, 2021). Given the relapsing and remitting nature of addiction and the high rate of death associated with a return to use after reduced tolerance, medically managed opioid withdrawal in people with OUD should not be initiated without a predetermined plan for ongoing medication and treatment.

Pregnant women with on OUD are recommended to start opioid agonist medications, rather than undergo a medically supervised withdrawal that is associated with high relapse rates and death ("Committee Opinion No. 711: Opioid Use and Opioid Use Disorder in Pregnancy," 2017). Occasionally, a taper or discontinuation of prescribed opioids for patients with chronic pain without evidence of addiction may be considered. When doing so, it is recommended that the person agrees with the taper and that it proceeds cautiously to avoid transition to nonprescribed opioid use and emergence of an OUD. Rapid opioid tapers without collaboration with patients have contributed to significant patient harm and is not recommended (Dowell et al., 2022).

Medically managed opioid withdrawal may take place in any setting—including outpatient, partial-hospital, or inpatient settings. The initial evaluation of opioid withdrawal and OUD should include route of opioid use, last opioid use, type and quantity of opioid, use of other substances, and interest in various medication options (Torres-Lockhart, Lu, Weimer, Stein, & Cunningham, 2022). There are three dominant approaches to managing opioid withdrawal medically: (1) **opioid agonist medications**, including methadone, buprenorphine, and, in Canada only and approved as a third-line treatment, slow-release oral morphine, (2) **nonopioid medications** for opioid withdrawal, or (3) in patients prescribed long term opioids for the management of pain who do not have evidence of OUD, a **gradual reduction** of prescribed opioids or transition to buprenorphine. Especially with the rise of fentanyl and other high potency synthetic opioids, two approaches may be used together (e.g., nonopioid medications during the initiation of opioid withdrawal followed by initiation of an opioid agonist). Many individuals with opioid withdrawal symptoms and an OUD diagnosis have previous treatment experience and preferences. If patients express a preference for MOUD treatment and there are no contraindications, it is possible to manage opioid withdrawal using the same medication. This approach simplifies the transition to long-term treatment. Conversely, people who prefer MOUD treatment with opioid antagonists, such as extended-release (XR) injectable naltrexone, should generally be provided nonopioid medications targeting opioid withdrawal symptoms to prevent delays in initiating XR naltrexone treatment (Torres-Lockhart et al., 2022).

The long-acting opioid agonists, methadone and buprenorphine, are considered first-line treatment for opioid withdrawal. Factors such as patient preferences, prior OUD treatment, and medication availability should guide the choice of which medication to use. In the United States, prescribing regulations for methadone and buprenorphine are governed by laws passed by Congress. Either can be administered for opioid withdrawal in emergency departments and other nonopioid detoxification settings. In the inpatient setting, methadone and buprenorphine can be administered as long as needed for treatment of a concomitant medical problem. However, in outpatient settings, only buprenorphine can be prescribed. Methadone is dispensed to treat OUD through a highly regulated, SAMHSA-certified, facility known as an OTP.

Methadone is a long-acting high-affinity μ- and δ-opioid receptor agonist. The starting dose of methadone should consider the potential risks of respiratory depression and sedation and is typically 20–30 mg. Methadone should be initiated at the initial signs of withdrawal and additional doses of 5–10 mg can be given every 4–6 hours, with a recommended maximum of 30 mg on day 1. In patients with significant physiologic dependence, 30 mg should be adequate for even the most severe withdrawal. Because deaths in opioid-intolerant individuals have occurred at a dose of 40 mg, lower doses are initially given in the range of 10–20 mg to individuals with an unclear degree of physiologic dependence. After 1–2 hours of observation, withdrawal symptoms may be reassessed and, if needed, additional medication up to 30 mg provided. Further dosing should be held if intoxication or sedation is observed. Once the dose requirement for methadone has been established, methadone may be given daily and, if it's going to be used for ongoing OUD treatment, increased each 3–5 days to a dose that suppresses cravings and nonprescribed opioid use. If methadone is being used to treat withdrawal with a goal to stop opioid agonists, it should be tapered over 3–5 days in 5- to 10-mg increments. The half-life of methadone is subject to individual variability, averaging 24 hours but ranging between 4 and 130 hours (Eap, Buclin, & Baumann, 2002) resulting in cumulation of blood levels and associated death from respiratory depression if methadone doses are too rapidly increased early in treatment.

Buprenorphine is a partial agonist at the μ-opioid and antagonist at the δ- and κ-opioid receptors and is frequently used to manage opioid withdrawal with less restrictive regulations. Unlike methadone, buprenorphine may be prescribed out of a physician's office. The availability of this medication has greatly increased access to care for persons with OUD. For almost two decades, however, prescribing buprenorphine required physicians to complete additional training and apply for a special waiver to prescribe. In late 2022, the MAT Act (Mainstreaming Addiction Treatment) was signed into law eliminating this requirement. All practitioners with a current Drug Enforcement Agency (DEA) registration that includes schedule III authority are now allowed to prescribe buprenorphine for OUD in their practice if permitted by state law. As part of the same legislation, the MAT Act requires new or renewing DEA registrants to attest to either (1) a total of eight hours of training on opioid or other substance use disorder, (2) board certification in addiction medicine or addiction psychiatry, or (3) graduation within 5 years from health profession schools that included at least 8 hours of SUD curriculum (SAMHSA, 2023b).

Before initiating buprenorphine, people should discontinue all nonprescribed opioids and be exhibiting symptoms of mild to moderate withdrawal. Buprenorphine is a partial agonist with a very high affinity for the μ-opioid receptor.

If the person has physiologic dependence but is not yet in withdrawal, buprenorphine will displace the full μ-opioid agonist and lead to **precipitated opioid withdrawal**, an often dramatic and uncomfortable outcome. Most people who use drugs are keenly aware of their personal withdrawal time course, and it is good practice to obtain their prior experiences. This information, along with an objective assessment of the COWS (a minimum score of 7–13 is generally recommended), can aid in timing the initial dose. Once moderate opioid withdrawal symptoms have emerged, an initial dose of buprenorphine 4 mg/naloxone 1 mg (2/0.5 mg if physical dependence is low or significant medical concerns that might warrant lower initial dose) is recommended. In the sublingual buprenorphine/naloxone formulation, naloxone is biologically inactive. Its purpose is solely to prevent diversion and injection of buprenorphine—when buprenorphine/naloxone is injected, naloxone becomes active and can precipitate withdrawal. After 2–4 hours, in the absence of sedation, a second dose of 4/1 mg (or 2/0.5 mg if that was initially used) may be provided if withdrawal symptoms remain. Buprenorphine 8 mg is generally the recommended target dose for day 1, with 12 mg being a maximum. If withdrawal symptoms are expected to continue beyond the maximum dose on day 1, nonopioid medications targeting specific symptoms should be provided. Over the next 2 days, the dose should be increased to 12/3–16/4 mg/day, with a daily maximum generally not exceeding 24 mg a day. Many clinicians are noting that, with the prevalence of fentanyl and other high potency synthetic opioids in the current market, people are coming to treatment settings with higher degrees of tolerance and physiologic dependence than seen with other, earlier full agonist opioids (e.g., heroin, nonprescribed oxycodone, etc.). There is little research to guide clinicians in how to manage the changing landscape—and alternative buprenorphine initiation protocols are emerging (Blevins, 2023). Nonetheless, the standard buprenorphine initiation protocol described above remains the most well studied and clinical experience supports this method of initiation in people who use fentanyl and other high potency synthetic opioids.

Once initiated, the goal of treatment is to continue one of the three FDA-approved treatments for OUD. If a taper to discontinuation is desired, however, a buprenorphine taper is best performed over a long period of time in conjunction with ongoing treatment. Occasionally, patients have compelling reasons to need a moderate or even a short taper, for example, because of impending incarceration where MOUD may not be continued. In these cases, a taper over 3–14 days may be initiated. Nonopioid medications (see below paragraph on these medications) may be used concurrently for symptoms that persist and to minimize discomfort. Medically managed opioid withdrawal without linkage to MOUD is generally ineffective, with high relapse rates and associated death. Every effort should be made to engage patients in ongoing treatment for opioid addiction, with medications being most effective and first line (2004).

Though largely beyond the scope of this chapter, it's important for healthcare providers to be aware of alternative medication treatment options available outside the United States. Widely used in Europe and now recommended as a third-line treatment for OUD in Canada, **slow-release oral morphine**, prescribed by specialists in primary care and administered daily by community pharmacies, is showing promise for those who have not tolerated or responded to methadone or buprenorphine yet remain at high risk of poor outcomes, including overdose and death (Bruneau et al., 2018). Other countries are using injectable hydromorphone or even injectable, inhaled, or smoked diacetylmorphine to treat OUD (Humphreys et al., 2022). There is increasing interest in alternative opioid agonist medications in the United States as well, though none are currently legally available.

For people who prefer treatment with the opioid antagonist intramuscular XR naltrexone, symptomatic management of opioid withdrawal with **nonopioid medications** can be used to minimize discomfort and promote treatment retention. Alpha-2 adrenergic agonists, such as clonidine or lofexidine, are the primary medications used, targeting the autonomic hyperactivity and associated anxiety seen in opioid withdrawal. Lofexidine was FDA approved in 2018 and was the first nonopioid treatment for opioid withdrawal symptoms (Urits et al., 2020). While it has been shown to have weaker side effects (less sedation and hypotension) than clonidine, the high cost limits its use compared to clonidine. In addition to α-2 adrenergic agonists, symptomatic treatment of gastrointestinal symptoms is commonly treated with loperamide, a peripheral μ-opioid agonist with limited CNS activity to manage diarrhea. Dicyclomine, an anticholinergic medication that relaxes smooth muscle and inhibits cramping, is often used for abdominal cramping. Antihistamines (e.g., hydroxyzine or diphenhydramine) or sedating antidepressants (e.g., trazodone or doxepin) are used for insomnia and restlessness. Nonsteroidal anti-inflammatory drugs may be used for muscle aches. Promethazine or metoclopramide are often used for nausea and vomiting and muscle relaxants (e.g., methocarbamol) can help with muscle spasms. Initiation of XR naltrexone to treat OUD is recommended after full resolution of opioid withdrawal, which can take 7–10 days.

3. Medications for OUD—The goal of any medically-supervised opioid withdrawal in the context of an OUD is to initiate medication treatment and engage people in long-term treatment. Appropriately prescribed and dosed pharmacologic treatment has been shown to improve patient survival, decrease nonprescribed opioid use and associated criminal activity, improve birth outcomes among pregnant women, lower a person's risk of contracting HIV or hepatitis C, and increase treatment retention (SAMHSA, 2023a). Because of this, the SAMHSA clinical guidelines on treatment of opioid addiction are unequivocal in writing, "absent

a compelling need for the complete avoidance of all opioids, long-term maintenance treatment … is to be preferred in most instances to any form of detoxification or withdrawal treatment" (2004). There are three approaches to long-term pharmacologic management of opioid addiction which include prescribing an opioid (1) agonist, (2) partial agonist, or (3) antagonist medication.

i. Methadone has decades of demonstrated efficacy in reducing opioid consumption; criminal behavior; psychosocial and medical morbidity, including rates of HIV infection; and mortality (Heikkinen et al., 2022; Russolillo, Moniruzzaman, & Somers, 2018). Methadone administration for the treatment of opioid addiction is highly regulated in the United States with facilities required to obtain SAMHSA certification and referred to as OTPs. Pharmacologically, methadone is a long-acting medication (half-life ~24 hours) that fully agonizes the high-affinity μ- and δ-opioid receptors. Two enantiomeric forms exist: *levo*-methadone and *dextro*-methadone. *levo*-Methadone accounts for most the opioid agonist effects of the drug and has no effect on the electrocardiographic QT interval. *dextro*-Methadone, on the other hand, is an N-methyl-D-aspartate (NMDA) antagonist. In most countries, including the United States, the racemic mixture is the only formulation available (Soyka & Zingg, 2009). Given its long action and the slow accumulation in solid organs, caution is required in the early phases of induction or during dose increases to prevent overdose; initial daily dose should not exceed 30 mg. In addition, patients should be cautioned regarding cardiac effects, including the risk of QTc prolongation and potentially fatal arrhythmias. Baseline and follow-up ECGs are recommended, particular for those on doses greater than 100 mg daily. Common side effects of methadone are like other opioids and include constipation, sweating, nausea, lightheadedness, insomnia, and sedation. Because it is metabolized primarily through the CYP3A4 and CYP2B6 pathways, caution is advised when combined with potent CYP3A4 inducers (e.g., carbamazepine, rifampin) or inhibitors (e.g., protease inhibitors, ketoconazole, grapefruit juice). Chronic opioid use is generally well tolerated, though constipation, sweating, sleep abnormalities, hyperalgesia and changes in endocrine function may be ongoing (Arout, Edens, Petrakis, & Sofuoglu, 2015; Brennan, 2013).

ii. Buprenorphine is a partial agonist at the μ-opioid receptor. Because of the partial μ-opioid agonism, there is a ceiling to the effect on respiratory suppression that can provide some protection from respiratory depression and death in overdose. Most often, buprenorphine/naloxone, rather than buprenorphine alone, is prescribed as treatment for OUD. The purpose of the addition of naloxone—biologically inactive in sublingual form—is to reduce diversion and injection. Generally, buprenorphine monotherapy is reserved for pregnant women or those in a controlled environment such as a hospital. Both formulations are DEA schedule III and can be prescribed in an office-based setting. Just as with a medically supervised withdrawal, buprenorphine/naloxone is typically initiated once a patient is in mild to moderate withdrawal. It is administered in sublingual form (because of poor oral bioavailability) and should be held under the tongue until it dissolves completely. The half-life of buprenorphine is long, about 37 hours, allowing for once-daily or even as much as three-times-weekly dosing. The target dose for day 1 is 8 mg, with higher doses used on subsequent days until withdrawal symptoms and cravings are controlled. The typical daily maintenance dose is between 12 and 24 mg (average 16 mg) but may be up to 32 mg. Common potential adverse effects include constipation, nausea or vomiting, sedation, and worsening opioid withdrawal (if taken too close to last opioid ingestion). Buprenorphine, like methadone, is metabolized through CYP3A4 and should be used with caution when potent CYP3A4 inducers or inhibitors are co-prescribed (McCance-Katz, Sullivan, & Nallani, 2010).

iii. **Naltrexone** is the third FDA-approved medication for treating OUD. It is available in both oral and extended-release IM formulation. Naltrexone blocks the action of agonist or partial-agonist opioids and removes the rewarding effects of using opioids. Data on the effect of naltrexone on opioid cravings are mixed (Dijkstra, De Jong, Bluschke, Krabbe, & van der Staak, 2007; Krupitsky et al., 2011). A 2011 Cochrane review of 13 studies showed that oral naltrexone did not perform better than placebo or no pharmacological treatments and is not recommended for treatment of OUD. The extended-release injectable form of naltrexone, approved for treatment of OUD in 2010, however, has shown more promising results (Tanum et al., 2017). A 24-week randomized trial conducted in Russia—a country that does not provide alternative agonist therapies—showed significantly decreased cravings, greater treatment retention, and more opioid-free days compared to placebo (Krupitsky et al., 2011). A U.S. trial of 570 patients randomized to receive either IM naltrexone or buprenorphine-naloxone found that patients struggled to be initiated onto an opioid antagonist. For those who were successfully inducted, however, 24-week relapse rates, opioid negative urines, and days abstinent from opioids were similar between buprenorphine and IM naltrexone (Lee et al., 2018). Injectable naltrexone is now considered a second-line MOUD (Perry et al., 2022).

C. Harm Reduction

In response to what the CDC calls an opioid overdose epidemic, the federal and state governments have enacted prevention strategies to combat these disturbing trends. In addition to encouraging safe opioid prescribing practices, other strategies designed to reduce harm include prescribing **naloxone** to reverse opioid overdoses—like prescribing epinephrine in the unlikely but potentially deadly event of anaphylaxis, expanding access to **sterile syringe programs**, and providing **fentanyl test strips** to people who use drugs so they can test their own supply of opioid before using it. Though largely unavailable and still considered illegal in the United States, **safe consumption sites** are emerging in large cities such as New York and San Francisco as a way for people who use drugs to do so in a monitored setting with immediate access to opioid overdose treatment.

D. Other Interventions

Mutual (or peer) support programs including 12-step (e.g., Narcotics Anonymous [NA] and SMART Recovery can be helpful to many people with OUD entering treatment. **Narcotics Anonymous** is a self-help organization that follows the 12-step model of recovery as outlined by AA in 1939 (Company, 1939). NA is frequently attended by individuals with cocaine, heroin, other opioid, methamphetamine, alcohol, cannabis and other illicit drug use. Long-term members tend to rate themselves as spiritual, if not religious, and many have served as sponsors to other members. NA is free, anonymous, and readily available throughout the country in a variety of community settings (Galanter, Dermatis, Post, & Santucci, 2013). **SMART** (Self-Management and Recovery Training) **Recovery** is a global online and in-person mutual support organization offering an alternative to those for whom 12-step programs aren't accessible or desired. SMART Recovery uses facilitated meetings and topics to cover their four-point program: (1) building and maintaining motivation to change; (2) coping with urges to use; (3) managing thoughts, feelings, and behaviors in an effective way; (4) living a balanced, positive, and healthy life ("Why SMART," 2022).

Acupuncture, including body, auricular, and electro acupuncture, is sometimes used to treat opioid and other drug cravings as well as symptoms of opioid withdrawal. Two large rigorous trials in patients with alcohol- and cocaine-addiction showed no benefit of acupuncture on treatment retention or abstinence (Bullock et al., 2002; Margolin et al., 2002). Yet, other studies have showed significant reductions in craving in response to acupuncture (Chang & Sommers, 2014) and an exploratory review noted promising results when using different outcomes such as opioid withdrawal and cravings, rather than abstinence or treatment retention (White, 2013).

Family interventions may be needed because, frustratingly for loved ones, drug addiction is often complicated by a perceived lack of need for treatment by the addicted individual. The **Community Reinforcement and Family Training (CRAFT)** approach is a brief, typically 12- to 20-session, psychotherapy intervention designed to engage the addicted individual's significant other—be it parents, partners, or children—with a goal to ultimately engage the addicted person and to improve overall family function. A 2010 systematic review found four high-quality randomized controlled trials with a total sample of 264 concerned significant others. CRAFT significantly outperformed both Al-Anon/Nar-Anon (three times more engagement) and the Johnson Institute intervention (two times more engagement) over a 6-month period, engaging over two-thirds of individuals with addiction in an average of four to six treatment sessions (Roozen, de Waart, & van der Kroft, 2010).

Co-occurring Disorders

The most common co-occurring medical disorders among individuals with OUD are infectious—both viral (e.g., HIV, hepatitis C and B virus) and bacterial (e.g., endocarditis), particularly among people who injection drugs. Patients should routinely be consented and screened for the presence of HIV and hepatitis. Hepatitis C (HCV) can now be treated and cured with oral direct-acting antivirals and the World Health Organization has called for the elimination of HCV as a public health threat by the year 2030. To achieve this goal, 90% of people with HCV should be diagnosed, and 80% treated, including people who use drugs (Falade-Nwulia et al., 2020). Substance use treatment clinic settings and addiction specialty prescribers should be trained and equipped to screen, diagnose, and treat HCV (Roder et al., 2021). The other common comorbidity is chronic pain, which can complicate the treatment of OUD (Volkow, Jones, Einstein, & Wargo, 2019). Current guidance recommends nonpharmacologic and non-opioid therapies for the management of chronic pain, even among people on MOUD. Many of these treatments are familiar to mental health providers, including cognitive and behavioral therapies (Barry et al., 2019), antidepressants, and antiepileptics—and providers who treat people with substance use disorders should develop comfort talking with patients about strategies for managing chronic pain.

Co-occurring mental health disorders are also common among individuals with OUD and confer risk for poorer psychosocial functioning, increased suicidal behavior, and worse treatment outcomes (Jones & McCance-Katz, 2019). The most frequent co-occurring mental health condition is another substance use disorder (including tobacco, alcohol, cannabis, stimulant, and benzodiazepine). Mood, anxiety, and trauma-related disorders also commonly co-occur with opioid addiction. According to NESARC, more than half of individuals meeting criteria for an OUD also met criteria for a mood disorder, an anxiety disorder, or both (Conway, Compton, Stinson, & Grant, 2006; Grella, Karno, Warda, Niv, & Moore, 2009). In addition, NESARC's longitudinal design allowed for the recognition that mood and anxiety disorders were predictive of incident nonmedical prescription opioid use and of development of prescription opioid addiction, though the reverse was not true (i.e., lifetime prescription opioid addiction did not predict an incident mood or anxiety disorder (Martins et al., 2012). A history of conduct disorder in childhood or adolescence has been identified as a significant risk factor for substance-related disorders, including OUD (Carpentier, Knapen, van Gogh, Buitelaar, & De Jong, 2012). PTSD is also seen with increased frequency among people who use opioids; indeed, one study found PTSD to be present in one third of those with OUD—the most of any substance use disorder. Treatment of OUD produced

similar addiction-related improvements among those with and without a co-occurring PTSD diagnosis. However, those with PTSD were lower functioning at baseline and continued to have poorer functioning at 2 years, perhaps suggesting that PTSD symptoms remained despite addiction treatment (Mills, Teesson, Ross, & Darke, 2007). There is also a high degree of comorbidity between PTSD, OUD and chronic pain complicating the treatment of all three (Lopez-Martinez, Reyes-Perez, Serrano-Ibanez, Esteve, & Ramirez-Maestre, 2019). Treatment targeting both opioid addiction and co-occurring substance, mood, anxiety, and stress-related disorders should be provided to individuals with comorbidities.

▶ Complications

There are many serious medical and public health consequences of opioid addiction. Of particular concern is the high risk of lethal and nonlethal opioid overdose. Overdose risk has risen exponentially over the past several decades—with more than 100,000 overdose deaths in 2021. In addition, opioid use substantially increases the risk of infectious disease, with as many as 80–90% of people who inject opioids screening positive for hepatitis B or C. HIV risk, endocarditis, pulmonary embolism, thrombophlebitis, and other sequelae are all significantly elevated among those who inject drugs. Pregnant women with opioid addiction are at increased risk of poor outcomes including miscarriage, stillbirth, or preterm or low-birth-weight infants. Mothers prescribed methadone or buprenorphine throughout pregnancy have improved outcomes, and ongoing medication treatment is strongly recommended. Neonatal abstinence syndrome is an expected and treatable condition that follows prenatal exposure to opioid agonists ("Committee Opinion No. 711: Opioid Use and Opioid Use Disorder in Pregnancy," 2017). Other complications of chronic opioid use include constipation, pruritus, urinary retention, sedation, endocrine and immunologic dysfunction, and hyperalgesia (Benyamin et al., 2008).

▶ Adverse Outcomes of Treatment

Because treatment retention and receipt of MOUD is a strong predictor of remission from OUD symptoms, it's important to minimize side effects of medication treatments. Methadone, being a full opioid agonist, is potentially addictive and fatal in overdose. Though unquestionably safer, buprenorphine as a partial agonist, can still be associated with overdose—particularly when combined with other sedating medications. There is also concern that long-term opioid therapies may negatively affect cardiac and endocrine function and play a complicated role in the maintenance of chronic pain.

▶ Drug Interactions

Methadone and buprenorphine are both metabolized via cytochrome P450 isoenzymes, particularly CYP3A4, and therefore are affected by drugs that either induce or inhibit these isoenzymes. **CYP 3A4 inhibitors** may lead to elevated plasma levels of buprenorphine and methadone and subsequent oversedation, reduced respiratory drive, and even death. Conversely, removal of inhibiting medications can increase buprenorphine and methadone metabolism, leading to withdrawal symptoms. Potent inhibitors of this isoenzyme include the azole antifungals (e.g., ketoconazole, itraconazole). Of importance given the overlap of HIV and OUDs, several protease inhibitors (e.g., ritonavir, nelfinavir) also inhibit CYP 3A4, and caution is advised when using them concomitantly with opioids. The addition of **CYP3A4 inducers** to a medication regimen may lead to withdrawal symptoms in methadone- or buprenorphine-maintained individuals, and discontinuation of inducers can lead to elevated opioid levels. CYP3A4 inducers include nonnucleoside reverse transcriptase inhibitors (e.g., nevirapine, efavirenz), antiepileptics (carbamazepine, phenytoin, oxcarbazepine, phenobarbital), antibiotics (rifampin, rifabutin, rifapentine) (Baciewicz, Chrisman, Finch, & Self, 2013), St. John's wort, and even cocaine (McCance-Katz, Rainey, & Moody, 2010; McCance-Katz, Sullivan, et al., 2010). Drug interactions are not limited to the cytochrome P450 system and may be influenced by changes in absorption, protein binding, or renal clearance. In addition, interactions between sedating medications (such as benzodiazepines or alcohol) and methadone or buprenorphine are of particular concern and are frequently involved in lethal and nonlethal overdose.

▶ Prognosis

Left untreated, the prognosis for people with OUD is very poor. People with severe OUD are at risk for injuries, infections, incarceration, overdose, and death—either from overdose or by suicide. The mortality rate is 10-fold for people with OUD compared to the average US population. In 2021, life expectancy declined in the US for the second year in a row—an unprecedented statistic attributed to increased overdose deaths, along with COVID-19 (CDC, 2022a). Psychotherapy alone has extremely poor outcomes, as do medically assisted opioid withdrawal programs without initiation of MOUD. With MOUD however, OUD is treatable, and prognosis and course are dramatically improved. MOUD has been shown to decrease opioid use, opioid-related deaths, transmission of infectious disease, and incarceration and is associated with improved social functioning and treatment retention (NASEM, 2019). Among pregnant women, MOUD improves not only the health of the mother but also outcomes for newborns ("Committee Opinion No. 711: Opioid Use and Opioid Use Disorder in Pregnancy," 2017). Sadly, only one in four people who need MOUD, receive it, despite often high levels of contact with the healthcare or prison systems, with adolescents and older adults showing the greatest treatment gap (Mauro, Gutkind, Annunziato, & Samples, 2022).

CONCLUSION

Opioid addiction and overdose are now a public health problem of epidemic proportions associated with enormous costs to the economy, family structure, and individual lives. Untreated, it bears significant and mounting morbidity and mortality risks, leading to an unprecedented decline in life-expectancy in the U.S. population in the past decade. On the side of hope, opioid addiction is the substance use disorder with the widest and most effective treatment options. With the rising concern over synthetic opioid use, OUD, and overdose deaths, government regulations around prescribing MOUD are loosening and healthcare systems are working to increase treatment access. Adequately trained providers to treat OUD will continue to be in demand.

Center for Substance Abuse Treatment. *Clinical Guidelines for the Use of Buprenorphine in the Treatment of Opioid Addiction.* Rockville (MD): Substance Abuse and Mental Health Services Administration (US); 2004. Report No.: (SMA) 04-3939. PMID: 22514846.

Arfken, C. L., Owens, D. D., & Greenwald, M. K. (2020). US national treatment admissions with opioids and benzodiazepines. *Drug Alcohol Rev, 39*(7), 862-869. doi:10.1111/dar.13129

Arout, C. A., Edens, E., Petrakis, I. L., & Sofuoglu, M. (2015). Targeting opioid-induced hyperalgesia in clinical treatment: neurobiological considerations. *CNS Drugs, 29*(6), 465-486. doi:10.1007/s40263-015-0255-x

Baciewicz, A. M., Chrisman, C. R., Finch, C. K., & Self, T. H. (2013). Update on rifampin, rifabutin, and rifapentine drug interactions. *Curr Med Res Opin, 29*(1), 1-12. doi:10.1185/03007995.2012.747952

Ball, S. A. (2007). Comparing individual therapies for personality disordered opioid dependent patients. *J Pers Disord, 21*(3), 305-321. doi:10.1521/pedi.2007.21.3.305

Barry, D. T., Beitel, M., Cutter, C. J., Fiellin, D. A., Kerns, R. D., Moore, B. A., ... Schottenfeld, R. S. (2019). An evaluation of the feasibility, acceptability, and preliminary efficacy of cognitive-behavioral therapy for opioid use disorder and chronic pain. *Drug Alcohol Depend, 194*, 460-467. doi:10.1016/j.drugalcdep.2018.10.015

Becker, W. C., Frank, J. W., & Edens, E. L. (2020). Switching from high-dose, long-term opioids to buprenorphine: a case series. *Ann Intern Med, 173*(1), 70-71. doi:10.7326/L19-0725

Benyamin, R., Trescot, A. M., Datta, S., Buenaventura, R., Adlaka, R., Sehgal, N., ... Vallejo, R. (2008). Opioid complications and side effects. *Pain Physician, 11*(2 Suppl), S105-120. Retrieved from https://www.ncbi.nlm.nih.gov/pubmed/18443635

Bernstein, J., Bernstein, E., Tassiopoulos, K., Heeren, T., Levenson, S., & Hingson, R. (2005). Brief motivational intervention at a clinic visit reduces cocaine and heroin use. *Drug Alcohol Depend, 77*(1), 49-59. doi:10.1016/j.drugalcdep.2004.07.006

Berrettini, W. (2017). A brief review of the genetics and pharmacogenetics of opioid use disorders. *Dialogues Clin Neurosci, 19*(3), 229-236. doi:10.31887/DCNS.2017.19.3/wberrettini

Bilevicius, E., Sommer, J. L., Asmundson, G. J. G., & El-Gabalawy, R. (2018). Posttraumatic stress disorder and chronic pain are associated with opioid use disorder: results from a 2012-2013 American nationally representative survey. *Drug Alcohol Depend, 188*, 119-125. doi:10.1016/j.drugalcdep.2018.04.005

Blevins, D., Bramlette, E., Burns, A., DeVido, J., D'Onofrio, G., Herring, A., … Sanaty Zadeh, P. (2023). *Practice-Based Guidelines: Buprenorphine in the Age of Fentanyl*. Retrieved from https://pcssnow.org/wp-content/uploads/2023/05/PCSS-Fentanyl-Guidance-FINAL-1.pdf

Bolivar, H. A., Klemperer, E. M., Coleman, S. R. M., DeSarno, M., Skelly, J. M., & Higgins, S. T. (2021). Contingency management for patients receiving medication for opioid use disorder: a systematic review and meta-analysis. *JAMA Psychiatry, 78*(10), 1092-1102. doi:10.1001/jamapsychiatry.2021.1969

Brennan, M. J. (2013). The effect of opioid therapy on endocrine function. *Am J Med, 126*(3 Suppl 1), S12-S18. doi:10.1016/j.amjmed.2012.12.001

Bruneau, J., Ahamad, K., Goyer, M. E., Poulin, G., Selby, P., Fischer, B., … Misuse, C. C. R. I. i. S. (2018). Management of opioid use disorders: a national clinical practice guideline. *CMAJ, 190*(9), E247-E257. doi:10.1503/cmaj.170958

Bullock, M. L., Kiresuk, T. J., Sherman, R. E., Lenz, S. K., Culliton, P. D., Boucher, T. A., & Nolan, C. J. (2002). A large randomized placebo controlled study of auricular acupuncture for alcohol dependence. *J Subst Abuse Treat, 22*(2), 71-77. doi:10.1016/s0740-5472(01)00217-3

Cacciola, J. S., Alterman, A. I., Dephilippis, D., Drapkin, M. L., Valadez, C., Jr., Fala, N. C., … McKay, J. R. (2013). Development and initial evaluation of the Brief Addiction Monitor (BAM). *J Subst Abuse Treat, 44*(3), 256-263. doi:10.1016/j.jsat.2012.07.013

Cadet, J. L., Bisagno, V., & Milroy, C. M. (2014). Neuropathology of substance use disorders. *Acta Neuropathol, 127*(1), 91-107. doi:10.1007/s00401-013-1221-7

Capata, M., Hartwell, K.J.. (2021). Opioid antagonist treatment of opioid-related disorders.. In L. F. Brady KT, Galanter M, Kleber HD (Ed.), *The American Psychiatric Publishing Textbook of Substance Abuse Treatment* (6th ed.). Arlington, VA:: American Psychiatric Publishing.

Carpentier, P. J., Knapen, L. J., van Gogh, M. T., Buitelaar, J. K., & De Jong, C. A. (2012). Addiction in developmental perspective: influence of conduct disorder severity, subtype, and attention-deficit hyperactivity disorder on problem severity and comorbidity in adults with opioid dependence. *J Addict Dis, 31*(1), 45-59. doi:10.1080/10550887.2011.642756

Carroll, K. M., Nich, C., Shi, J. M., Eagan, D., & Ball, S. A. (2012). Efficacy of disulfiram and Twelve Step Facilitation in cocaine-dependent individuals maintained on methadone: a randomized placebo-controlled trial. *Drug Alcohol Depend, 126*(1-2), 224-231. doi:10.1016/j.drugalcdep.2012.05.019

CDC. (2022a, December 22, 2022). New report confirms U.S. life expectancy has declined to lowest level since 1996. Retrieved from https://www.cdc.gov/nchs/pressroom/nchs_press_releases/2022/20221222.htm

CDC. (2022b, June 1, 2022). Understanding the opioid overdose epidemic. Retrieved from https://www.cdc.gov/opioids/basics/epidemic.html

Chang, B. H., & Sommers, E. (2014). Acupuncture and relaxation response for craving and anxiety reduction among military veterans in recovery from substance use disorder. *Am J Addict, 23*(2), 129-136. doi:10.1111/j.1521-0391.2013.12079.x

Chou, R., Hartung, D., Turner, J., Blazina, I., Chan, B., Levander, X., McDonagh M, Selph S, Fu R, Pappas, M. (2020). In *Opioid Treatments for Chronic Pain*. Rockville (MD). Agency for Healthcare Research and Quality (US); 2020 Apr. Report No.: 20-EHC011. PMID: 32338848.

Committee Opinion No. 711: Opioid use and opioid use disorder in pregnancy. (2017). *Obstet Gynecol, 130*(2), e81-e94. doi:10.1097/AOG.0000000000002235

Company, W. P. (1939). *Alcoholics Anonymous: The Story of How Many More Than One Hundred Men Have Recovered from Alcoholism*. New York, NY: The Anonymous Press.

Compton, W. M., & Jones, C. M. (2019). Epidemiology of the U.S. opioid crisis: the importance of the vector. *Ann N Y Acad Sci, 1451*(1), 130-143. doi:10.1111/nyas.14209

Conway, K. P., Compton, W., Stinson, F. S., & Grant, B. F. (2006). Lifetime comorbidity of DSM-IV mood and anxiety disorders and specific drug use disorders: results from the National Epidemiologic Survey on Alcohol and Related Conditions. *J Clin Psychiatry, 67*(2), 247-257. doi:10.4088/jcp.v67n0211

Dahan, A., Aarts, L., & Smith, T. W. (2010). Incidence, reversal, and prevention of opioid-induced respiratory depression. *Anesthesiology, 112*(1), 226-238. doi:10.1097/ALN.0b013e3181c38c25

Deak, J. D., Zhou, H., Galimberti, M., Levey, D. F., Wendt, F. R., Sanchez-Roige, S., … Gelernter, J. (2022). Genome-wide association study in individuals of European and African ancestry and multi-trait analysis of opioid use disorder identifies 19 independent genome-wide significant risk loci. *Mol Psychiatry, 27*(10), 3970-3979. doi:10.1038/s41380-022-01709-1

DiClemente, C. C., Corno, C. M., Graydon, M. M., Wiprovnick, A. E., & Knoblach, D. J. (2017). Motivational interviewing, enhancement, and brief interventions over the last decade: a review of reviews of efficacy and effectiveness. *Psychol Addict Behav, 31*(8), 862-887. doi:10.1037/adb0000318

Dijkstra, B. A., De Jong, C. A., Bluschke, S. M., Krabbe, P. F., & van der Staak, C. P. (2007). Does naltrexone affect craving in abstinent opioid-dependent patients? *Addict Biol, 12*(2), 176-182. doi:10.1111/j.1369-1600.2007.00067.x

Dowell, D., Arias, E., Kochanek, K., Anderson, R., Guy, G. P., Jr., Losby, J. L., & Baldwin, G. (2017). Contribution of opioid-involved poisoning to the change in life expectancy in the United States, 2000-2015. *JAMA, 318*(11), 1065-1067. doi:10.1001/jama.2017.9308

Dowell, D., Haegerich, T. M., & Chou, R. (2016). CDC guideline for prescribing opioids for chronic pain—United States, 2016. *MMWR Recomm Rep, 65*(1), 1-49. doi:10.15585/mmwr.rr6501e1

Dowell, D., Ragan, K. R., Jones, C. M., Baldwin, G. T., & Chou, R. (2022). CDC clinical practice guideline for prescribing opioids for pain—United States, 2022. *MMWR Recomm Rep, 71*(3), 1-95. doi:10.15585/mmwr.rr7103a1

Eap, C. B., Buclin, T., & Baumann, P. (2002). Interindividual variability of the clinical pharmacokinetics of methadone: implications for the treatment of opioid dependence. *Clin Pharmacokinet, 41*(14), 1153-1193. doi:10.2165/00003088-200241140-00003

Edens, E. L., Abelleira, A., Barry, D., & Becker, W.C. (2020). You say pain. i say addiction. let's call the whole thing off. *Psychiatric Times, 37*(11), 47-51.

Falade-Nwulia, O., Gicquelais, R. E., Astemborski, J., McCormick, S. D., Kirk, G., Sulkowski, M., … Mehta, S. H. (2020). Hepatitis C treatment uptake among people who inject drugs in the oral direct-acting antiviral era. *Liver Int, 40*(10), 2407-2416. doi:10.1111/liv.14634

Fiellin, D. A., Barry, D. T., Sullivan, L. E., Cutter, C. J., Moore, B. A., O'Connor, P. G., … Schottenfeld, R. S. (2013). A randomized trial of cognitive behavioral therapy in primary care-based buprenorphine. *Am J Med, 126*(1), 74 e11-77. doi:10.1016/j.amjmed.2012.07.005

Galanter, M., Dermatis, H., Post, S., & Santucci, C. (2013). Abstinence from drugs of abuse in community-based members of Narcotics Anonymous. *J Stud Alcohol Drugs*, *74*(2), 349-352. doi:10.15288/jsad.2013.74.349

Grella, C. E., Karno, M. P., Warda, U. S., Niv, N., & Moore, A. A. (2009). Gender and comorbidity among individuals with opioid use disorders in the NESARC study. *Addict Behav*, *34*(6-7), 498-504. doi:10.1016/j.addbeh.2009.01.002

Hedegaard, H., Minino, A. M., Spencer, M. R., & Warner, M. (2021). Drug overdose deaths in the United States, 1999-2020. *NCHS Data Brief*(426), 1-8. Retrieved from https://www.ncbi.nlm.nih.gov/pubmed/34978529

Heikkinen, M., Taipale, H., Tanskanen, A., Mittendorfer-Rutz, E., Lahteenvuo, M., & Tiihonen, J. (2022). Real-world effectiveness of pharmacological treatments of opioid use disorder in a national cohort. *Addiction*, *117*(6), 1683-1691. doi:10.1111/add.15814

Hser, Y. I., Hoffman, V., Grella, C. E., & Anglin, M. D. (2001). A 33-year follow-up of narcotics addicts. *Arch Gen Psychiatry*, *58*(5), 503-508. doi:10.1001/archpsyc.58.5.503

Humphreys, K., Shover, C. L., Andrews, C. M., Bohnert, A. S. B., Brandeau, M. L., Caulkins, J. P., ... Timko, C. (2022). Responding to the opioid crisis in North America and beyond: recommendations of the Stanford-Lancet Commission. *Lancet*, *399*(10324), 555-604. doi:10.1016/S0140-6736(21)02252-2

Jaffe JH, M. W. (1975). Narcotic analgesics and antagonists. In G. A. Goodman LS (Ed.), *The Pharmacological Basis of Therapeutics* (5th ed., pp. 245-324). New York: Macmillan.

Jalal, H., Buchanich, J. M., Roberts, M. S., Balmert, L. C., Zhang, K., & Burke, D. S. (2018). Changing dynamics of the drug overdose epidemic in the United States from 1979 through 2016. *Science*, *361*(6408). doi:10.1126/science.aau1184

Jones, C. M., Logan, J., Gladden, R. M., & Bohm, M. K. (2015). Vital signs: demographic and substance use trends among heroin users—United States, 2002-2013. *MMWR Morb Mortal Wkly Rep*, *64*(26), 719-725. Retrieved from https://www.ncbi.nlm.nih.gov/pubmed/26158353

Jones, C. M., & McCance-Katz, E. F. (2019). Co-occurring substance use and mental disorders among adults with opioid use disorder. *Drug Alcohol Depend*, *197*, 78-82. doi:10.1016/j.drugalcdep.2018.12.030

Kakko, J., Svanborg, K. D., Kreek, M. J., & Heilig, M. (2003). 1-year retention and social function after buprenorphine-assisted relapse prevention treatment for heroin dependence in Sweden: a randomised, placebo-controlled trial. *Lancet*, *361*(9358), 662-668. doi:10.1016/S0140-6736(03)12600-1

Kendler, K. S., Karkowski, L. M., Neale, M. C., & Prescott, C. A. (2000). Illicit psychoactive substance use, heavy use, abuse, and dependence in a US population-based sample of male twins. *Arch Gen Psychiatry*, *57*(3), 261-269. doi:10.1001/archpsyc.57.3.261

Keyes, K. M., Rutherford, C., Hamilton, A., Barocas, J. A., Gelberg, K. H., Mueller, P. P., ... Cerda, M. (2022). What is the prevalence of and trend in opioid use disorder in the United States from 2010 to 2019? Using multiplier approaches to estimate prevalence for an unknown population size. *Drug Alcohol Depend Rep*, *3*. doi:10.1016/j.dadr.2022.100052

Kidorf, M., King, V. L., Gandotra, N., Kolodner, K., & Brooner, R. K. (2012). Improving treatment enrollment and re-enrollment rates of syringe exchangers: 12-month outcomes. *Drug Alcohol Depend*, *124*(1-2), 162-166. doi:10.1016/j.drugalcdep.2011.12.008

Koob, G. F. (2021). Drug Addiction: Hyperkatifeia/Negative reinforcement as a framework for medications development. *Pharmacol Rev*, *73*(1), 163-201. doi:10.1124/pharmrev.120.000083

Krupitsky, E., Nunes, E. V., Ling, W., Illeperuma, A., Gastfriend, D. R., & Silverman, B. L. (2011). Injectable extended-release naltrexone for opioid dependence: a double-blind, placebo-controlled, multicentre randomised trial. *Lancet*, *377*(9776), 1506-1513. doi:10.1016/S0140-6736(11)60358-9

Lee, J. D., Nunes, E. V., Jr., Novo, P., Bachrach, K., Bailey, G. L., Bhatt, S., ... Rotrosen, J. (2018). Comparative effectiveness of extended-release naltrexone versus buprenorphine-naloxone for opioid relapse prevention (X:BOT): a multicentre, open-label, randomised controlled trial. *Lancet*, *391*(10118), 309-318. doi:10.1016/S0140-6736(17)32812-X

Lopez-Martinez, A. E., Reyes-Perez, A., Serrano-Ibanez, E. R., Esteve, R., & Ramirez-Maestre, C. (2019). Chronic pain, posttraumatic stress disorder, and opioid intake: a systematic review. *World J Clin Cases*, *7*(24), 4254-4269. doi:10.12998/wjcc.v7.i24.4254

Margolin, A., Kleber, H. D., Avants, S. K., Konefal, J., Gawin, F., Stark, E., ... Vaughan, R. (2002). Acupuncture for the treatment of cocaine addiction: a randomized controlled trial. *JAMA*, *287*(1), 55-63. doi:10.1001/jama.287.1.55

Martin, W. R., & Jasinski, D. R. (1969). Physiological parameters of morphine dependence in man–tolerance, early abstinence, protracted abstinence. *J Psychiatr Res*, *7*(1), 9-17. doi:10.1016/0022-3956(69)90007-7

Martins, S. S., Fenton, M. C., Keyes, K. M., Blanco, C., Zhu, H., & Storr, C. L. (2012). Mood and anxiety disorders and their association with non-medical prescription opioid use and prescription opioid-use disorder: longitudinal evidence from the National Epidemiologic Study on Alcohol and Related Conditions. *Psychol Med*, *42*(6), 1261-1272. doi:10.1017/S0033291711002145

Mauro, P. M., Gutkind, S., Annunziato, E. M., & Samples, H. (2022). Use of medication for opioid use disorder among US adolescents and adults with need for opioid treatment, 2019. *JAMA Netw Open*, *5*(3), e223821. doi:10.1001/jamanetworkopen.2022.3821

McCance-Katz, E. F., Rainey, P. M., & Moody, D. E. (2010). Effect of cocaine use on buprenorphine pharmacokinetics in humans. *Am J Addict*, *19*(1), 38-46. doi:10.1111/j.1521-0391.2009.00001.x

McCance-Katz, E. F., Sullivan, L. E., & Nallani, S. (2010). Drug interactions of clinical importance among the opioids, methadone and buprenorphine, and other frequently prescribed medications: a review. *Am J Addict*, *19*(1), 4-16. doi:10.1111/j.1521-0391.2009.00005.x

McHugh, R. K., Hearon, B. A., & Otto, M. W. (2010). Cognitive behavioral therapy for substance use disorders. *Psychiatr Clin North Am*, *33*(3), 511-525. doi:10.1016/j.psc.2010.04.012

Meshberg-Cohen, S., Ross MacLean, R., Schnakenberg Martin, A. M., Sofuoglu, M., & Petrakis, I. L. (2021). Treatment outcomes in individuals diagnosed with comorbid opioid use disorder and Posttraumatic stress disorder: a review. *Addict Behav*, *122*, 107026. doi:10.1016/j.addbeh.2021.107026

Mills, K. L., Teesson, M., Ross, J., & Darke, S. (2007). The impact of post-traumatic stress disorder on treatment outcomes for heroin dependence. *Addiction*, *102*(3), 447-454. doi:10.1111/j.1360-0443.2006.01711.x

Moningka, H., Lichenstein, S., Worhunsky, P. D., DeVito, E. E., Scheinost, D., & Yip, S. W. (2019). Can neuroimaging help combat the opioid epidemic? A systematic review of clinical and pharmacological challenge fMRI studies with recommendations for future research. *Neuropsychopharmacology*, 44(2), 259-273. doi:10.1038/s41386-018-0232-4

NASEM. (2019). *Medications for Opioid Use Disorder Save Lives* (M. Mancher & A. I. Leshner Eds.). Washington, DC: National Academies Press.

Nowinski, J., Baker, S, Carroll, K. (1995). *Twelve Step Facilitation Therapy Manual: A Clinical Research Guide for Therapists Treating Individuals with Alcohol Abuse and Dependence*. U.S. Department of Health and Human Services, National Institute on Alcohol Abuse and Alcoholism.

Okie, S. (2010). A flood of opioids, a rising tide of deaths. *N Engl J Med*, 363(21), 1981-1985. doi:10.1056/NEJMp1011512

Oliva, E. M., Richardson, J., Harvey, M. A., & Bellino, P. (2021). Saving lives: the veterans health administration (VHA) rapid naloxone initiative. *Jt Comm J Qual Patient Saf*, 47(8), 469-480. doi:10.1016/j.jcjq.2021.06.004

Pando-Naude, V., Toxto, S., Fernandez-Lozano, S., Parsons, C. E., Alcauter, S., & Garza-Villarreal, E. A. (2021). Gray and white matter morphology in substance use disorders: a neuroimaging systematic review and meta-analysis. *Transl Psychiatry*, 11(1), 29. doi:10.1038/s41398-020-01128-2

Perry, C., Liberto, J., Milliken, C., Burden, J., Hagedorn, H., Atkinson, T., ... Group, V. A. D. G. D. (2022). The management of substance use disorders: synopsis of the 2021 U.S. Department of Veterans Affairs and U.S. Department of Defense Clinical Practice Guideline. *Ann Intern Med*, 175(5), 720-731. doi:10.7326/M21-4011

Prendergast, M., Podus, D., Finney, J., Greenwell, L., & Roll, J. (2006). Contingency management for treatment of substance use disorders: a meta-analysis. *Addiction*, 101(11), 1546-1560. doi:10.1111/j.1360-0443.2006.01581.x

Resnick, S. G., Oehlert, M. E., Hoff, R. A., & Kearney, L. K. (2020). Measurement-based care and psychological assessment: using measurement to enhance psychological treatment. *Psychol Serv*, 17(3), 233-237. doi:10.1037/ser0000491

Robins, L. N., Davis, D. H., & Nurco, D. N. (1974). How permanent was Vietnam drug addiction? *Am J Public Health*, 64 Suppl 12 (12 Suppl), 38-43. doi:10.2105/ajph.64.12_suppl.38

Robins, L. N., Helzer, J. E., Hesselbrock, M., & Wish, E. (2010). Vietnam veterans three years after Vietnam: how our study changed our view of heroin. *Am J Addict*, 19(3), 203-211. doi:10.1111/j.1521-0391.2010.00046.x

Roder, C., Nguyen, P., Harvey, C., Wardrop, M., Finlay, J., Ogunleye, L., ... Wade, A. J. (2021). Psychiatrists can treat hepatitis C. *J Viral Hepat*, 28(12), 1763-1764. doi:10.1111/jvh.13622

Roozen, H. G., de Waart, R., & van der Kroft, P. (2010). Community reinforcement and family training: an effective option to engage treatment-resistant substance-abusing individuals in treatment. *Addiction*, 105(10), 1729-1738. doi:10.1111/j.1360-0443.2010.03016.x

Russolillo, A., Moniruzzaman, A., & Somers, J. M. (2018). Methadone maintenance treatment and mortality in people with criminal convictions: a population-based retrospective cohort study from Canada. *PLoS Med*, 15(7), e1002625. doi:10.1371/journal.pmed.1002625

Saedy, M., Kooshki, S., Jamali Firouzabadi, M., Emamipour, S., & Rezaei Ardani, A. (2015). Effectiveness of acceptance-commitment therapy on anxiety and depression among patients on methadone treatment: a pilot study. *Iran J Psychiatry Behav Sci*, 9(1), e222. doi:10.17795/ijpbs222

Saha, T. D., Kerridge, B. T., Goldstein, R. B., Chou, S. P., Zhang, H., Jung, J., ... Grant, B. F. (2016). Nonmedical prescription opioid use and DSM-5 nonmedical prescription opioid use disorder in the United States. *J Clin Psychiatry*, 77(6), 772-780. doi:10.4088/JCP.15m10386

Saini, J., Johnson, B., & Qato, D. M. (2022). Self-reported treatment need and barriers to care for adults with opioid use disorder: the US National Survey on Drug Use and Health, 2015 to 2019. *Am J Public Health*, 112(2), 284-295. doi:10.2105/AJPH.2021.306577

SAMHSA. (2012). *Pharmacologic Guidelines for Treating Individuals with Post-Traumatic Stress Disorder and Co-occurring Opioid Use Disorders*. (SMA12-4688).

SAMHSA. (2018). *SAMHSA Opioid Overdose Prevention Toolkit*. (SMA18-4742). Rockville, MD Substance Abuse and Mental Health Services Administration Retrieved from https://store.samhsa.gov/product/Opioid-Overdose-Prevention-Toolkit/SMA18-4742

SAMHSA. (2022). *Key Substance Use and Mental Health Indicators in the United States: Results from the 2021 National Survey on Drug Use and Health*. (HHS Publication No. PEP22-07-01-005, NSDUH Series H-57). Center for Behavioral Health Statistics and Quality, Substance Abuse and Mental Health Services Administration Retrieved from https://www.samhsa.gov/data/report/2021-nsduh-annual-national-report

SAMHSA. (2023a, April 25, 2023). Medications for Substance Use Disorders.

SAMHSA. (2023b, June 6, 2023). Waiver Elimination (MAT Act). Retrieved from https://www.samhsa.gov/medications-substance-use-disorders/waiver-elimination-mat-act

Sandbrink, F., Murphy, J. L., Johansson, M., Olson, J. L., Edens, E., Clinton-Lont, J., ... Group, V. A. D. G. D. (2023). The use of opioids in the management of chronic pain: synopsis of the 2022 updated U.S. Department of Veterans Affairs and U.S. Department of Defense Clinical Practice Guideline. *Ann Intern Med*, 176(3), 388-397. doi:10.7326/M22-2917

Saunders, B., Wilkinson, C., & Phillips, M. (1995). The impact of a brief motivational intervention with opiate users attending a methadone programme. *Addiction*, 90(3), 415-424. doi:10.1046/j.1360-0443.1995.90341510.x

Seal, K. H., Shi, Y., Cohen, G., Cohen, B. E., Maguen, S., Krebs, E. E., & Neylan, T. C. (2012). Association of mental health disorders with prescription opioids and high-risk opioid use in US veterans of Iraq and Afghanistan. *JAMA*, 307(9), 940-947. doi:10.1001/jama.2012.234

Shurman, J., Koob, G. F., & Gutstein, H. B. (2010). Opioids, pain, the brain, and hyperkatifeia: a framework for the rational use of opioids for pain. *Pain Med*, 11(7), 1092-1098. doi:10.1111/j.1526-4637.2010.00881.x

Smallwood, R. F., Potter, J. S., & Robin, D. A. (2016). Neurophysiological mechanisms in acceptance and commitment therapy in opioid-addicted patients with chronic pain. *Psychiatry Res Neuroimaging*, 250, 12-14. doi:10.1016/j.pscychresns.2016.03.001

Soyka, M., & Zingg, C. (2009). Feasability and safety of transfer from racemic methadone to (R)-methadone in primary care: clinical results from an open study. *World J Biol Psychiatry*, *10*(3), 217-224. doi:10.1080/15622970802416057

Spencer, M. R., Minino, A. M., & Warner, M. (2022). Drug overdose deaths in the United States, 2001-2021. *NCHS Data Brief*(457), 1-8. Retrieved from https://www.ncbi.nlm.nih.gov/pubmed/36598401

Stotts, A. L., Green, C., Masuda, A., Grabowski, J., Wilson, K., Northrup, T. F., ... Schmitz, J. M. (2012). A stage I pilot study of acceptance and commitment therapy for methadone detoxification. *Drug Alcohol Depend*, *125*(3), 215-222. doi:10.1016/j.drugalcdep.2012.02.015

Tanum, L., Solli, K. K., Latif, Z. E., Benth, J. S., Opheim, A., Sharma-Haase, K., ... Kunoe, N. (2017). Effectiveness of injectable extended-release naltrexone vs daily buprenorphine-naloxone for opioid dependence: a randomized clinical noninferiority trial. *JAMA psychiatry*, *74*(12), 1197-1205. doi:10.1001/jamapsychiatry.2017.3206

Torres-Lockhart, K. E., Lu, T. Y., Weimer, M. B., Stein, M. R., & Cunningham, C. O. (2022). Clinical management of opioid withdrawal. *Addiction*, *117*(9), 2540-2550. doi:10.1111/add.15818

Tsuang, M. T., Lyons, M. J., Meyer, J. M., Doyle, T., Eisen, S. A., Goldberg, J., ... Eaves, L. (1998). Co-occurrence of abuse of different drugs in men: the role of drug-specific and shared vulnerabilities. *Arch Gen Psychiatry*, *55*(11), 967-972. doi:10.1001/archpsyc.55.11.967

Urits, I., Patel, A., Zusman, R., Virgen, C. G., Mousa, M., Berger, A. A., ... Viswanath, O. (2020). A comprehensive update of lofexidine for the management of opioid withdrawal symptoms. *Psychopharmacol Bull*, *50*(3), 76-96. Retrieved from https://www.ncbi.nlm.nih.gov/pubmed/32733113

Volkow, N. D., Jones, E. B., Einstein, E. B., & Wargo, E. M. (2019). Prevention and treatment of opioid misuse and addiction: a review. *JAMA Psychiatry*, *76*(2), 208-216. doi:10.1001/jamapsychiatry.2018.3126

Wang, S. C., Chen, Y. C., Lee, C. H., & Cheng, C. M. (2019). Opioid addiction, genetic susceptibility, and medical treatments: a review. *Int J Mol Sci*, *20*(17), 4294. doi:10.3390/ijms20174294

Weiss, R. D., Potter, J. S., Fiellin, D. A., Byrne, M., Connery, H. S., Dickinson, W., ... Ling, W. (2011). Adjunctive counseling during brief and extended buprenorphine-naloxone treatment for prescription opioid dependence: a 2-phase randomized controlled trial. *Arch Gen Psychiatry*, *68*(12), 1238-1246. doi:10.1001/archgenpsychiatry.2011.121

Wesson, D. R., & Ling, W. (2003). The clinical opiate withdrawal scale (COWS). *J Psychoactive Drugs*, *35*(2), 253-259. doi:10.1080/02791072.2003.10400007

White, A. (2013). Trials of acupuncture for drug dependence: a recommendation for hypotheses based on the literature. *Acupunct Med*, *31*(3), 297-304. doi:10.1136/acupmed-2012-010277

Why SMART. (2022). Retrieved from https://www.smartrecovery.org/why-smart/

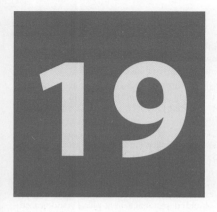

Stimulant Use Disorders

Elizabeth K.C. Schwartz, MD, PhD
Sean D. Regnier, PhD
William W. Stoops, PhD
Robert F. Leeman, PhD
Mehmet Sofuoglu, MD, PhD

▶ Introduction

Cocaine and amphetamines are stimulant drugs that activate the central nervous system (CNS), with resulting strong rewarding effects (e.g., euphoria, "rush" and "high") that contribute to high misuse liability. Most clinical characteristics pertain to all stimulant drugs, with certain exceptions such as the longer duration of action of methamphetamine compared to the brief action of cocaine. Given this commonality, unless otherwise noted, all discussion in this chapter pertains to stimulant drugs as a class. Specific comments will be focused primarily on cocaine, followed by methamphetamine, given that these drugs have received the most research attention. Brief specific mention will be made of other stimulants that are commonly abused, such as methylenedioxmethamphetamine (MDMA, commonly known as "ecstasy").

▶ Essentials of Diagnosis

Substance use disorder (SUD) criteria described in the *Diagnostic and Statistical Manual*, Fifth Edition (DSM-5) (American Psychiatric Association [APA], 2013) are applicable to cocaine and other stimulants. The stimulant use disorder criteria reflect neuroadaptation to prolonged and heavy substance use (i.e., tolerance and withdrawal) and effects of substance use on psychosocial functioning. Neither tolerance nor withdrawal are essential for a diagnosis of stimulant use disorder. When occurring within the same 12-month period, presence of two or three of the criteria in the following list indicate mild disorder; four or five indicate moderate disorder; and six or more of these criteria indicate severe SUD. This represents a change from the DSM-IV (APA, 2000), which differentiated between substance abuse (thought to be a less severe diagnosis) and dependence. Indeed, several of the studies cited in this chapter referred to recruitment of participants meeting criteria for stimulant abuse or dependence. To be consistent with the DSM-5 criteria, DSM-IV stimulant abuse will be referred to as mild stimulant use disorder, whereas DSM-IV stimulant dependence will be referred to as moderate-to-severe stimulant use disorder.

Stimulant intoxication is typically characterized by euphoria, increased energy, hyper-vigilance, restlessness, anxiety, increased sociability, and a range of biopsychosocial problems (see Signs & Symptoms). Though the same criteria apply to all addictive substances, DSM-5 offers guidance regarding the withdrawal syndromes resulting from cessation of use of each type of substance. For stimulants, withdrawal symptoms tend to be psychological such as anxiety, fatigue, depression, difficulty maintaining concentration, anhedonia, increase in appetite, increased sleep and craving (APA, 2013; Kampman et al., 2001). Physical complaints tend to be minor and include tremors, chills and musculoskeletal pain (APA, 2013; Kampman et al., 2001).

▶ General Considerations

A. Epidemiology

According to 2021 estimates, approximately 1.8 million Americans used cocaine within the past month, a 20% increase from 2015. Over 1.5 million people used methamphetamine in the past month, a twofold increase from 2015. Use of both drugs is more common among males than females. Though increasing over the past few years, cocaine use has declined by about 25% since 2007 (2.4 million). About 1.3 million Americans age 12 or older met past-year criteria for cocaine use disorder (Substance Abuse Mental Health Services Administration [SAMHSA], 2022).

Substance use/misuse, generally, and stimulant use/misuse, specifically, are costly to society and public health. The cost of illegal drug use to U.S. society has been estimated to be $193 billion dollars per year (National Drug Intelligence Center, 2011). Health care costs related to SUDs are one reason for this high cost to society. In 2021, methamphetamine was highly likely to be associated with emergency room visits. Methamphetamine was implicated in about 31%

of illicit-drug–related emergency department visits in the United States, compared to 31% associated with marijuana and 24% tied to heroin and fentanyl use, and 13% associated with cocaine use (SAMHSA, 2021). Cocaine overdoses increased 26.5% from June 2019 to May 2020 (CDC, 2020). One in every five drug overdose deaths involves cocaine (Hedegaard et al., 2020).

B. Etiology

1. Initial onset—Environmental factors including religiosity and family background (e.g., a one- or two-parent family; family history of SUD) have an impact on the likelihood of initial cocaine use (Kendler et al., 2007). A frequently-reported finding is that an early age of substance use onset increases risk of future SUD and other health-related risk behaviors (DuRant et al., 1999). Further, there is empirical evidence to support the "gateway theory" in that early use of alcohol, cigarettes, and marijuana increases risk of subsequent harder drug use (Fiellin et al., 2013). At this time, it is not clear to what extent early age of onset is a proxy for genetic and other risk factors or if the added risk relates mainly to increased exposure to substance-related toxicity over time.

Environmental factors may interact with person-level variables to contribute to the development of a SUD. There is evidence that impulsive, risk-taking tendencies are associated with an earlier age of onset (Nees et al., 2012). Although novelty or sensation seeking (the seeking out of intense, hedonic experiences; Zuckerman, 1994) relates more closely to likelihood of initial cocaine use (Belin et al., 2008), impulsivity (i.e., the tendency to act rapidly, without forethought or consideration of the consequences of one's actions; Brewer & Potenza, 2008; Moeller et al., 2001) relates more closely to development of addiction following initial use (Belin et al., 2008).

2. Pharmacology of stimulants—One of the main actions of stimulants in the CNS is to increase synaptic levels of monoamines (dopamine, serotonin, and norepinephrine) by blocking the monoamine transporters (e.g., cocaine, methylphenidate) or releasing monoamines by inhibition of the vesicular monoamine transporter 2 (VMAT-2) (e.g., methamphetamine) (Moszczynska and Callan 2017). Increased synaptic dopamine levels in the mesolimbic dopamine pathway are believed to mediate the reinforcing effects of stimulants (Haber, 2014). The mesolimbic dopamine pathway originates from the ventral tegmental area of the midbrain with connections to several cortical and limbic structures including the prefrontal cortex, amygdala, and nucleus accumbens (Haber, 2014). Serotonergic activation mediates stimulant effects on mood (Ruhe et al., 2007) (Müller and Homberg, 2015). Norepinephrine, on the other hand, mediates cognitive arousal and cardiovascular activation in response to stimulants (Sofuoglu & Sewell, 2009), as well as stress response including stress-induced drug use/relapse (Sinha et al., 2003). In addition to monoamines, many other mechanisms mediate stimulant effects in the CNS, including increased release of glutamate, gamma-aminobutyric acid (GABA), acetylcholine, oxytocin, corticotropin releasing factor (CRF), and additional stress hormones (Koob and Volkow, 2016; Sofuoglu, DeVito et al., 2021). Increased sociability that is associated with acute intoxication may be mediated at least in part by acute release of oxytocin (Dumont et al., 2009). In addition, cocaine blocks voltage-gated sodium ion channels, which underlies its anesthetic effects (Matthews & Collins, 1983).

Chronic stimulant use is associated with many neuroadaptations in the CNS. Most notably, chronic stimulant use may lead to hypofunction of dopaminergic activity, thought to contribute to dysphoria and drug craving (Koob et al., 1997). While prolonged stimulant exposure induces neuroadaptation and neuroplastic changes in many areas of the brain, those in the ventral tegmental area are thought to be particularly relevant (Korpi, den Hollander et al., 2015). Recent data also demonstrate that microglia, the immune cells of the CNS, play a role in the rewarding properties of stimulants (Bachtell, Jones et al., 2017). Cocaine and methamphetamines activate the toll-like receptor 4 immunosurveillance receptor complex on microglia, which causes multiple downstream effects, including reward inhibition by reducing dopamine release in the nucleus accumbens (Northcutt et al., 2015).

Stimulants are absorbed readily, both through mucous membranes and the respiratory tract (Fowler et al., 2001). The onset of action of stimulants is fast but depends on the form used. Cocaine can be used intranasally (by snorting), inhaled in free base form (as crack-cocaine), or injected intravenously. Methamphetamines can be used orally, via inhalation, or intravenously (Courtney and Ray, 2014). Rapid delivery of addictive substances enhances their reinforcing effects. A short duration of effect could lead to repeated use (e.g., cocaine binges). Delay to onset of action and duration of action by type of stimulant and route of administration are summarized in Table 19–1 (Meredith et al., 2005; NIDA

Table 19–1 Delay to Onset of Action and Duration of Action by Type of Stimulant and Route of Administration

Type of Stimulant	Route of Administration	Time Until Onset of Action	Duration of Action
Cocaine	Smoked	Within seconds	15–30 minutes at most
	Intravenous	Within seconds	15–30 minutes at most
	Nasal	20–30 minutes	1–3 hours
Amphetamine	Smoked	Within seconds	8–12 hours
	Intravenous	Within seconds	
	Nasal	5 minutes	
	Oral	20–30 minutes	

[National Institute on Drug Abuse], 1998). In addition to the speed of delivery, both frequency and amount of cocaine synergistically increase progression to cocaine use disorder (Liu et al., 2020).

3. Progression to substance use disorder—The progression of addiction is characterized by initial impulsive patterns of use (i.e., use without ample consideration of the consequences). For those who do not curb their use as a result of experience of negative consequences, patterns of use may escalate into a compulsive drug use pattern (Everitt et al., 2008). Compulsive patterns of use occur despite a tendency for the drug's hedonic value to dissipate over time because of tolerance. Many people who use drugs describe this experience as continued "wanting" even though "liking" has decreased (Robinson & Berridge, 1993). Compulsive use at the expense of important activities and responsibilities has been described as the hallmark of cocaine use disorder (Sofuoglu & Kosten, 2006). Among amphetamines, methamphetamine use is mostly associated with compulsive use patterns, with basic research demonstrating that extended daily access to methamphetamine is associated with development of compulsive drug seeking patterns. Among those who try cocaine, about 21% develop a use disorder in comparison with cigarette smoking (68%) alcohol (23%), and marijuana (9%) (Lopez-Quintero et al., 2011). There are several important predictors that can accelerate this development, including conduct disorder and childhood abuse (Sartor et al., 2014).

C. Genetics

SUDs are among the most heritable psychiatric disorders (Pierce et al., 2018). For cocaine, studies have found that about 70% of the risk to become addicted is estimated to be heritable (Fernàndez-Castillo et al., 2022). However, the specific genes responsible for increased risk have not been identified. A number of potential candidate genes have been identified, but findings to date cannot be considered definitive (Uhl et al., 2008). Whereas the mu opioid receptor gene (OPRM1) variation has been associated with likelihood of moderate-to-severe methamphetamine use disorder (Ide et al., 2006), delta opioid receptor gene (OPRD1) polymorphisms relate to moderate-to-severe cocaine use disorder among African Americans (Crist et al., 2013). These initial findings suggest a considerable role for genetics in stimulant use disorder. However, given the importance of the environment, genetic effects are most appropriately considered in terms of gene–environment interactions, as with other addictive substances (Kendler et al., 2007).

▶ Clinical Findings

A. Signs & Symptoms

Several acute psychological and physical effects are associated with stimulant use. Stimulant intoxication typically includes enhanced energy, decreased fatigue, euphoria, hyperalertness, grandiosity, alertness, and sociability. In addition, stimulant use may be accompanied by adverse psychological effects, including dysphoria, anxiety, restlessness, stereotypical behavior, psychomotor agitation, and impaired judgment (Meredith et al., 2005; Williamson et al., 1997). Agitation is a particular problem with methamphetamine use and in extreme cases can present a challenge to health care providers attempting to treat stimulant users (Richards et al., 1999). Both cocaine and methamphetamine can cause psychotic symptoms. Substance-induced psychotic disorder is common among those who use methamphetamines, with a prevalence estimated to be 36.5% (Lecomte, Dumais et al., 2018). Methamphetamine psychosis, which can include paranoia, hallucinations, and stereotyped compulsive behaviors (McKetin 2018), is typically brief but can last for longer than 6 months, or can even present during times of abstinence without relapse (Grant et al., 2012; Zweben et al., 2004). People who use methamphetamines experience more positive psychotic symptoms (such as delusions and hallucinations) than those who use cocaine (Alexander et al., 2017). Heavy stimulant use can produce a state of confusion and excitement, referred to as stimulant delirium (Ruttenber et al., 1997). This state is also characterized by loss of consciousness, disorientation, and disturbances of perception including auditory and visual hallucinations. Delirium is indicative of stimulant overdose (Shanti & Lucas, 2003).

Physiologically, acute intoxication effects are mediated by increased blood pressure and heart rate, which can be dramatic, particularly at higher doses (Afonso et al., 2007). Other physiologic signs and symptoms include dilated pupils, perspiration, and chills. Stimulant use is often linked to reports of less need for sleep, despite evidence of dysfunctional sleep patterns, including poor sleep quality (Garcia & Salloum, 2015). Stimulant use is also tied to reduction in appetite (Williamson et al., 1997), which may relate to acute gastric effects of stimulant use, including delayed emptying of the stomach (Boghdadi & Henning, 1997). Seizures, which typically do not last long, are also relatively common in relation to stimulant use, even among those without medical conditions that predispose to seizures (Neiman et al., 2000). Cardiac-related adverse effects such as chest pain are also relatively common and may lead to a need to seek medical attention (McCord et al., 2008; Turnipseed et al., 2003). Most dramatically, these effects can lead to myocardial infarction even in younger people who use stimulants (Qureshi et al., 2001). Smoked cocaine and methamphetamine lead to acute respiratory effects, including shortness of breath and cough (Tashkin, 2001). Among those with asthma, common symptoms such as wheezing may be made worse (Tashkin, 2001).

As discussed earlier, cessation of stimulant use can lead to withdrawal, which is typically psychological. Medical treatment is not typically required but is warranted in cases such as those involving particularly strong agitation, paranoia or hallucinations (see Treatment section).

B. Psychological Testing

Prior research on chronic stimulant use has found an association with impairment in various cognitive functions, including memory, attention, visuomotor performance, and risk-reward decision making (Rogers & Robbins, 2001). More recently, the long-term effects of stimulant use on cognitive performance have been disputed when compared to healthy controls and normative data (Frazer et al., 2018a, 2018b; Hart et al., 2011). Some decision-making differences have been noted, however. People who use cocaine (Fillmore et al., 2002; Grant et al., 2000; Li et al., 2006) and methamphetamine (Monterosso et al., 2005; Rogers et al., 1999) have been found to have inordinately high propensities for risk taking and difficulties with response inhibition. Particularly relevant to the addictions are findings that individuals with moderate-to-severe cocaine use disorder (Coffey et al., 2003; Garcia-Rodriguez et al., 2013) and those who use amphetamines (Clark et al., 2006) have been found to devalue long-term rewards in favor of immediate gains, a tendency called delay discounting (Bickel et al., 2007). Cognitive functioning is likely to affect clinical outcomes. For instance, patients with moderate-to-severe cocaine use disorder who dropped out of treatment before completion performed worse than those who completed treatment on the Stroop task, a measure of ability to direct attention and avoid interfering stimuli (Streeter et al., 2008). Additionally, delay discounting is predictive of treatment outcome. Those who discount more steeply often have difficulty achieving extended abstinence (Washio et al., 2011), suggesting that these patients may require more intensive treatment.

C. Laboratory Findings

The primary metabolite of cocaine is benzoylecgonine (BE). Urine tests to detect BE have had strong sensitivity and specificity, and cross-reactivity with other drugs has not been found to be a problem (Carney et al., 2012). Thus, BE can be assessed in urine accurately and reliably in order to determine the presence of cocaine; however, BE tests do not yield accurate information about the frequency or amount of use (Cone & Dickerson, 1992). Urine and blood tests for other stimulants have been more challenging. Cross-reactivity has traditionally been a concern with both endogenous substances and other drugs leading to false positives for amphetamines (Kirschbaum et al., 2011; Schütz et al., 1998; Stout et al., 2003). Thus, specificity has tended to be a greater issue than sensitivity (Kupiec et al., 2002). Issues with false positives have led some to recommend high cutoff rates, which leads to increased specificity but could compromise sensitivity (Savoca et al., 2004). A study of ELISA (enzyme-linked immunosorbent assay) of urine showed excellent sensitivity and good specificity for amphetamine (Kirschbaum et al., 2011). Thus, although progress has been made, clinicians should approach urine testing for stimulants with some caution, particularly for stimulants other than cocaine.

D. Neuroimaging

Neuroimaging studies have provided evidence regarding changes in general brain activity and neurochemistry due to stimulant use, along with effects on brain function and structure. These findings are clinically relevant because they parallel clinical characteristics commonly observed among those who have used stimulants heavily over a long-term period (e.g., tendencies toward impulsive behavior).

1. General brain activity—Cocaine intoxication has been associated with reduced glucose metabolism throughout the brain, which is thought to be indicative of decreased overall brain activity (London et al., 1990). This reduced neural activity may increase the likelihood of impulsive, risky behavior (Bond, 1998). Overall, neuroimaging findings have enhanced our understanding of neural mechanisms underlying impulsive, risky actions under the influence of heavy stimulant use.

2. Neurochemistry—Findings from several early studies demonstrated that dopamine release occurs following stimulant use (Schlaepfer et al., 1997). In one study, amphetamine-triggered dopamine release in healthy participants was found to be associated with drug "wanting" but not with mood elevation (Leyton et al., 2002), which supports a contention that dopamine relates more closely to the salience of drug cues and to craving than to hedonic effects tied to drug "liking" (Berridge and Robinson, 2016). A subsequent study involving participants with moderate-to-severe cocaine use disorder identified limbic regions (i.e., the amygdala and hippocampus) as particularly important sites for cocaine cue-induced dopamine activity that related strongly to craving for the drug (Fotros et al., 2013). Consistent with tolerance development to stimulant effects following chronic use, dopamine release following cocaine administration has been found to be greater in nonaddicted compared to addicted individuals (Volkow et al., 1997).

The relationship between the serotonergic system and stimulant use disorder has also gained attention. Most studies on this topic suggest that serotonin affects cocaine use disorder by interacting with dopamine signaling via specific serotonin receptor subtypes (Howell & Cunningham, 2015). Finally, a small human study showed that heavy MDMA use was tied to toxic effects on serotonin neurons (Reneman et al., 2001), which supports the conclusion that stimulant use affects serotonergic activity.

3. Brain function—Neuroimaging findings have contributed to knowledge regarding activity in frontal and striatal regions associated with chronic stimulant use. Regarding frontal activity, individuals with cocaine use disorder have displayed hypo-activation in the orbitofrontal cortex when completing a Stroop interference task conducted during functional magnetic resonance imaging (fMRI) (Goldstein et al., 2007b). Compared to controls, participants with mild cocaine use disorder exhibited reduced regional responsivity in the orbitofrontal and prefrontal cortices in response to differences in monetary value across trials in a cognitive task (Goldstein et al., 2007a). Compared to controls, participants with mild cocaine use disorder had stronger activation in the right orbitofrontal cortex (OFC) and weaker activation in areas of the prefrontal cortex (PFC) (dorsolateral and medial regions) during the Iowa Gambling Task (IGT) (Bolla et al., 2003). Underactivity in frontal regions among those with heavy stimulant users may underlie impulsive response and risk-taking proclivities in this group (Leeman et al., 2012).

Prolonged stimulant use has also been tied to changes in striatal activity. Increased ventral striatal activity was found during the reward anticipation phase of a cognitive task among those with moderate-to-severe cocaine use disorder (Jia et al., 2011), which may suggest hypersensitivity to reward anticipation. Relatively diminished D_2-like receptor availability has been found in the striatum among those with stimulant use disorder (Volkow et al., 2003), and dorsal striatal hyperactivity has also been localized among those with moderate-to-severe cocaine use disorder (Volkow et al., 2006). These findings dovetail with the empirically supported view that escalation of drug addiction is tied to relative shifts in activity from the ventral to the dorsal striatum in parallel with a shift from substance use being impulsive to more compulsive (Everitt & Robbins 2016). Finally, a recent systematic review and metanalysis of 31 neuroimaging studies found that those with stimulant use, compared to healthy controls, had reduced dopamine release, striatal dopamine transporter availability, and striatal D2/D3 receptor availability, which the authors interpreted to reflect downregulation of pre- and postsynaptic components of the striatal dopamine system (Ashok et al., 2017).

4. Brain structure—Both white and gray matter changes have been observed with chronic stimulant use. Stimulant use and stimulant use disorder have been associated with poorer white matter integrity, including lower volume, reduced myelination, and axon caliber (Ersche et al., 2013; Lane et al., 2010; Lim et al., 2002, 2008; London et al., 2015; Moeller et al., 2005, 2007; Pando-Naude et al., 2021)., Some of these findings suggest that these changes are linked to risk-taking, impulsivity (Verdejo-Garcia et al., 2008), and cognitive deficits (London et al., 2015). In moderate-to-severe cocaine use disorder, reduced fractional anisotropy (FA) was associated with higher scores on a self-report measure of impulsivity (Lim et al., 2008) and disadvantageous decision making on a cognitive task of risk-taking (Lane et al., 2010). White matter integrity has potential clinical ramifications in that better white matter integrity has been tied to longer periods of abstinence in cocaine treatment (Xu et al., 2010).

In addition to white matter findings, decreased gray matter volume has been observed among individuals with stimulant use disorder (Hirsiger et al., 2019; Pando-Naude et al., 2021). Decreased gray matter concentrations have been found in frontal regions among individuals with ongoing cocaine use (Franklin et al., 2002; Ide et al., 2014), which are likely related to compromised executive functioning. Compromised executive function has clinical ramifications. A recent investigation demonstrated that poor executive function on a battery of neuropsychological tasks was predictive of subsequent early drop out from residential treatment for cocaine use disorder (Verdejo-Garcia et al., 2012). A recent study found that reducing cocaine use is associated with recovery in prefrontal cortex gray matter structures that correlates with improved cognitive performance (Hirsiger et al., 2019), demonstrating that these structural changes and clinical impairments may be reversible if substance use can be reduced or discontinued.

Other more specific alterations include reduced hippocampal volume, specific to females, in methamphetamine use and abstinence (Du et al., 2015), and, in individuals who use cocaine, lower volume in the claustrum, which may be involved in incentive salience (Graf et al., 2020; Pando-Naude et al., 2021).

Summary—Imaging findings have suggested neural activity tied to acute stimulant use. These findings include overall reduced brain metabolism during stimulant intoxication and evidence of dopamine release triggered by substance use. These results may help to explain impulsive behavior that often occurs during stimulant intoxication and the rewarding effects of stimulant use. Neuroimaging results have also suggested possible factors mediating compromised cognition associated with long-term stimulant use. These findings include dysfunction in frontal and striatal activity and poorer structural brain integrity among those who have used stimulants chronically, which may be reversible following reduction of substance use.

▶ Course of Illness

Chronic stimulant use has been associated with psychological and medical complications including neurological (Neiman et al., 2000), cardiac (Mouhaffel et al., 1995), and sexual (Palha & Esteves, 2008) issues (see Table 19–2 for a summary of consequences of stimulant use) (Darke et al., 2017). After accidental overdose, cardiovascular disease is the second leading cause of death among people who use methamphetamines (Darke et al., 2017), as high catecholamine levels are cardiotoxic, and methamphetamine binds with high affinity to dopamine and norepinephrine transporters in the cardiovascular system (Kevil et al., 2019). Cocaine use has been implicated in renal failure (Fernandez et al., 2005) and interacts with hypertension in that cocaine use appears to accelerate the decline in kidney function among hypertensive individuals (Vupputuri et al., 2004). Although cocaine use has not been implicated in long-term decline in endocrine function, results support

Table 19–2 Common Consequences of Stimulant Use

Category	Type of Consequence	Specific Consequences
Physical	Cardiac	Chest pain, myocardial infarction, cardiomyopathy, arrhythmias, atherosclerotic plaque build-up, heart failure, and myocarditis.
	Respiratory	Exacerbation of asthma, lung injury, pneumonia
	Neurological	Cerebral vasoconstriction, cerebrovascular disease and stroke, seizures, movement disorders, headache
	Renal	Renal failure: cocaine use interacts with decline in renal function.
	Endocrine	Recent evidence for reduced cortisol levels with methamphetamine use
	Sexual dysfunction	Delayed ejaculation in men, irregular menses in women
	Dental	Tooth decay with methamphetamine use
	Skin	Skin abrasions with methamphetamine use
	Other	Weight loss
		Sleep disturbance
		Injuries from methamphetamine lab explosions
		Toxin inhalation from fumes given off by methamphetamine "cooking" process
		Prenatal exposure linked to lower birth weight, shorter body length, preterm birth, placental displacement, and smaller head circumference
Psychological	Cognitive effects	Difficulty inhibiting impulses and risk-taking behavior, although these tendencies may also predate substance use; particularly concerning among adolescents and young adults
	Stimulant-induced psychosis	Symptoms can include paranoia, auditory hallucinations, and stereotyped compulsive behavior. Those with methamphetamine use more often experience delusions and hallucinations, compared to those who use cocaine
	Psychiatric/mood effects	Increased risk for suicide
Psychological/ physical	Withdrawal	Primarily psychological (e.g., anxiety, depression, difficulty maintaining concentration), although some physical (e.g., tremors, chills, and musculoskeletal pain)
		Changes in sleep patterns associated with difficulty achieving abstinence

reduced cortisol levels associated with methamphetamine user, which was taken as evidence for dysregulation of the hypothalamic–pituitary–adrenal (HPA) axis, possibly due to sympathetic reduction in natural cortisol production (Carson et al., 2012). Weight loss has been attributed to the appetite-suppressive effects of stimulant use, and sleep disturbance is also reported often by those who use stimulants frequently (Williamson et al., 1997).

Respiratory complications depend in part on the route of cocaine use. Chronic stimulant smoking is believed to increase the risk of lung injury and conditions such as pneumonia and exacerbation of asthma symptoms (Gotway et al., 2002; Tashkin, 2001). Nasal stimulant use has been associated with problems such as reduced blood flow to the nasal septum and sinus inflammation (Boghdadi & Henning, 1997).

Besides obvious differences in respiratory complications in those who smoke crack cocaine, other differences in risk profile have been found based on route of administration. For instance, people who use crack cocaine have been found to engage in more crime and report more frequent social and health problems than people who use cocaine intranasally (Ferri & Gossop, 1999). Both crack cocaine use and intravenous cocaine use have been linked to increased risk for infections such as human immunodeficiency virus (HIV) and hepatitis (Booth et al., 2000; Butler et al., 2017; Lexau et al., 1998).

Well-known negative effects associated with methamphetamine use are poor oral hygiene, dry mouth, and tooth decay (Hamamoto & Rhodus, 2009). Skin-related adverse effects are also common with methamphetamine use. Some individuals who use methamphetamine over the long term report a feeling as if small insects are crawling under their skin (often referred to colloquially as "crank bugs"). In an attempt to ameliorate this feeling, methamphetamine users will often pick, resulting in skin abrasions that can become irritated or infected (NIDA, 2006). Other negative effects that are unique to methamphetamine concern the clandestine laboratories that have been set up to produce the drug (commonly known as "meth labs"). Malfunctioning equipment has led to burns and explosions that have damaged property and led to injuries. In addition, inhalation of toxic fumes given off during the process of "cooking" has negative health consequences, particularly for young children residing in homes where "meth labs" are located (Messina et al., 2014). Given that MDMA and other designer stimulants are especially popular with young people, cognitive decline is a particular concern given the critical cognitive development that occurs in the adolescent and young adult years (Zakzanis & Young, 2001).

Differential Diagnosis (Including Comorbid Conditions)

Given psychosis symptoms that sometimes accompany acute stimulant intoxication and mood-altering effects of stimulant use, primary diagnoses to be considered alongside stimulant use disorder include schizophrenia and bipolar disorder (McKetin et al., 2006; Schuckit, 2006a). In addition to effects tied to acute use, ongoing use of stimulants may also lead to psychosis symptoms. For instance, chronic methamphetamine use can cause cognitive and psychotic symptoms similar to those seen in primary psychotic disorders (Wearne & Cornish, 2018), and chronic MDMA use can sometimes lead to a pattern of paranoid psychosis that is difficult to distinguish from paranoid schizophrenia (Buchanan & Brown, 1988). Thus, clinicians must be aware of the possibility that psychotic symptoms may relate to one extent or another to intoxication effects and/or to effects of chronic stimulant use.

Another consideration is that these and other psychological symptoms of stimulant use may relate in larger part to a comorbid condition, as the majority of individuals with a stimulant use disorder have a comorbid psychiatric disorder (MacLean & Sofuoglu, 2018). Among those seeking treatment for stimulant use disorder, the primary psychiatric disorders that have been observed include schizophrenia, attention-deficit/hyperactivity disorder (ADHD), anxiety, and mood disorders (Ford et al., 2009; MacLean & Sofuoglu, 2018). Stimulants are often prescribed for ADHD, thus abuse potential is an important clinical consideration (Dodson, 2005).

Unfortunately, patients with comorbid primary psychiatric and SUDs tend to fare worse in terms of their course and treatment outcomes for both the stimulant use disorder and the comorbid psychiatric disorder, compared to individuals without co-occurring illness (Gonzales et al., 2011; Schwartz et al., 2022). Cocaine use is clearly associated with an increased risk for suicidal ideation and suicide attempt, underscoring the importance of identifying and treating co-occurring depression (Abdalla et al., 2019; Bohnert et al., 2017; Pavarin & Fioritti, 2018). It is important that all patients with comorbid psychiatric illness be identified accurately and engaged in treatment that addresses their multiple conditions. Cessation of drug use may enable more clear and definitive assessment for comorbid conditions. It can be challenging clinically to determine which symptoms relate primarily to an underlying psychiatric condition or cognitive impairment and which symptoms relate more closely to heavy substance use (Schuckit, 2006a).

In addition to comorbidity with primary psychiatric conditions, co-use and multiple SUDs (and perhaps behavioral addictions as well) are important considerations when treating individuals with stimulant use disorder. According to a recent meta-analysis, cocaine is commonly used with other substances including cannabis (64%) and alcohol (77%) (Liu et al., 2018). Those who use stimulants typically use other substances for one of two main reasons. In some cases, other drugs are taken to accentuate the high from the stimulant. An example is the co-use of opioids, referred to as "speedballing." Another reason is to temper intoxication or withdrawal through the use of depressants such as alcohol, benzodiazepines, or cannabis, which, although not typically classified primarily as a depressant, has a number of depressant properties (Turkanis & Karler, 1981). According to the National Epidemiologic Study of Alcohol and Related Conditions (NESARC), lifetime opioid use (heroin and nonmedical use of other opioids) is associated with elevated risk of cocaine use disorder, compared to nonopioid drug use (Wu et al., 2011). Accordingly, concurrent cocaine use is an issue in many methadone maintenance programs, with cocaine and opioid co-use associated with a greater likelihood of attrition from treatment (Magura et al., 1988) and worse treatment outcomes (Hubbard et al., 1997; Williamson et al., 2006). Co-use of cocaine and opioids has increased the risk of cocaine overdose deaths (Kariisa et al., 2019). Alcohol and cocaine co-use is also common and comes with unique risks because their co-use leads to an additional metabolite. Cocoethylene (also known as benzoylmethylecgonine or ethyl cocaine) has pharmacologic actions like cocaine, except that it has a longer duration of action. The main risk associated with coaethylene formation is that it will enhance the toxic effects of cocaine (Baker et al., 2007). Notably, cocoethylene is as effective as cocaine in inhibiting dopamine reuptake (Hearn et al., 1991).

Treatment

This section begins with a brief discussion of treatment for stimulant intoxication and then withdrawal. We then continue with a discussion of psychopharmacologic, psychotherapeutic, and other types of interventions for chronic stimulant use/stimulant use disorder. Findings pertaining to interventions for various stimulant drugs are considered; however, the majority of clinical trials conducted have concerned cocaine use disorder.

A. Treatment of Acute Intoxication

More often than not, stimulant intoxication does not require formal treatment. Typically, it is sufficient to simply monitor patients in a quiet, safe environment until symptoms subside. In some cases, benzodiazepines (typically lorazepam or diazepam) may be indicated for severe intoxication symptoms including intense agitation (Greene et al., 2008). Administration of antipsychotics should be limited to intoxication coupled with extreme paranoia or other signs of psychosis (Kosten, 2002). Benzodiazepine use is preferred because antipsychotics can lead to a decrease in seizure threshold and increased hypothermia associated with stimulant overdose (Delbridge & Yealy, 1995). In rare cases, physiological symptoms such as tachycardia, hypertension, chest pain, and seizures may accompany stimulant intoxication, in which case additional treatment will likely be required. Use of pure beta-adrenergic blockers for acute treatment of cocaine-associated chest pain and myocardial infarction should be avoided because of concerns about possible coronary spasms (McCord et al., 2008).

B. Treatment of Withdrawal

Similar to stimulant intoxication, stimulant withdrawal typically does not require formal medical treatment. The best course of action is usually to allow patients to eat and sleep in a safe, quiet environment (Schuckit, 2006b). Again, paralleling intoxication, a benzodiazepine such as lorazepam may be used to treat intense agitation. Benzodiazepines may also be helpful for patient safety, or sleep difficulties, given that sleep changes during stimulant withdrawal are associated with difficulty achieving abstinence (Garcia & Salloum, 2015). Presence of depression that fulfills the criteria for depressive disorder may need to be treated by an antidepressant or psychotherapy, particularly when accompanied by suicidal ideation (Schuckit, 2006b). Although stimulant withdrawal is often not medically significant, relapse risk is high; thus, patients should be monitored and referred to longer-term addiction treatment.

C. Psychopharmacologic Interventions

Progress has been made with regard to basic science and clinical neurosciences of stimulant use disorder (see earlier discussion); however, these findings have not translated into considerable advances for treatment approaches. As a result of negative and inconsistent efficacy findings, there are, at present, no FDA-approved pharmacotherapies for the treatment of stimulant use disorder.

In this subsection, we present highlights of clinical research findings pertaining to several classes of pharmacotherapy: dopamine agonists; medications for neuroadaptations from long-term stimulant use; medications for cognitive deficiencies; vaccines; gender-specific treatments; and other pharmacotherapies. We conclude with a brief discussion of tests of combination pharmacotherapy and medications for individuals with comorbid conditions. Pharmacotherapies that have shown promise for treating stimulant use disorder are summarized in Table 19–3, including probable mechanisms of action and brief summaries of evidence supporting their efficacy.

1. Dopamine agonist approaches—Paralleling methadone treatment for opioid use disorder, the primary strategy of agonist treatment is to substitute a safer, long-acting drug for a risky, short-acting drug. Following the pharmacological action of stimulants, agonist treatment for stimulant use disorder has targeted synaptic dopamine levels mainly (Herin et al., 2010). There have been several trials yielding promising results for long-acting, prescription psychostimulants in the treatment of stimulants use disorder (Tardelli et al., 2023),

supported by results from a recent meta-analysis including 38 trials (Tardelli et al., 2020). In short-term, randomized clinical trials (RCTs), dextroamphetamine reduced cocaine (Grabowski et al., 2004; Shearer et al., 2003) and methamphetamine use (Longo et al., 2010; Shearer et al., 2001). Dextroamphetamine disrupts storage of dopamine within intracellular vesicles and reverses the dopamine transporter, with the net result of increased synaptic dopamine release. More recently, RCTs for cocaine use disorder testing sustained-release dexamfetamine among those also taking medication for opioid use disorder (Nuijten et al., 2016) and extended-release amphetamine salts combined with topiramate (Levin et al., 2020) both yielded positive results compared to placebo. Like cocaine, methylphenidate increases synaptic dopamine by inhibiting transporter reuptake. Thus far, methylphenidate has shown limited efficacy for moderate-to-severe cocaine use disorder (Levin et al., 2007; Schubiner et al., 2002), with some evidence for efficacy in one clinical trial for moderate-to-severe methamphetamine use disorder (Tiihonen et al., 2007). A recent systemic review and meta-analysis found low-strength evidence that methylphenidate may positively affect use-related outcomes for methamphetamine/amphetamine use disorder (Chan, Freeman et al., 2019). Based on these results, psychostimulants may be efficacious, however safety concerns must be considered, given the abuse liability of these drugs, and further studies are needed.

For treatment of stimulant use disorder, disulfiram could be considered an agonist because its use results in elevated synaptic dopamine levels. It appears to work by inhibiting dopamine-beta-hydroxylase (DBH), which is the enzyme that converts dopamine to norephinephrine. Among the agonist class, disulfiram initially had the most positive clinical trial results (Carroll et al., 2004; Petrakis et al., 2000; Pettinati et al., 2008). However, more recent results have not been as successful. In a recent, two-site, dose-ranging clinical trial among methadone-maintained patients with moderate-to-severe opiate and cocaine use disorder, none of the disulfiram doses yielded more cocaine-free urine tests than placebo (Oliveto et al., 2011). Another recent clinical trial testing placebo-controlled disulfiram and twelve-step facilitation (TSF) versus standard counseling in the same population also yielded negative results overall for disulfiram. One caveat was that disulfiram was associated with reduced cocaine use among patients without an alcohol use disorder history (Carroll et al., 2012), a finding for which there is precedent (Carroll et al., 2004; George et al., 2000; Petrakis et al., 2000). Another study showed that people using cocaine who had a genetic variation resulting in low dopamine beta hydroxylase were less likely to benefit from disulfiram than those with normal activity for this enzyme (Kosten et al., 2012). Finally, a recent systemic review and meta-analysis found no evidence that disulfiram can improve abstinence and instead may worsen rates of retention; however, the authors noted that due to the heterogeneity of the studies and patient populations, no firm conclusions could be drawn (Chan, Freeman et al., 2019).

Table 19–3 Pharmacotherapies That Have Shown Promise for the Treatment of Stimulant Dependence

Type of Pharmacotherapy	Agent	Mechanism of Action	Efficacy
Dopamine agonist approaches	Psychostimulants	Stimulate vesicle release, reverse dopamine transporter (DAT)	Some medications in this class, particularly methylphenidate, have shown evidence of reduction of cocaine and methamphetamine use in short-term clinical trials
	Disulfiram	Inhibition of dopamine-beta-hydroxylase	Best overall evidence of efficacy in decreasing cocaine use among agonists, but recent trials, and a metanalysis, have been negative. May be more effective among those without an alcohol use disorder history
	Modafinil, bupropion	Weak DAT inhibitors	Modafinil—initial findings promising but subsequent clinical trials and meta-analysis negative Bupropion—May be effective in medication adherent light methamphetamine users and in combination with contingency management for cocaine
Medications targeting neuroadaptations	Propranolol	β-Adrenergic blocker	Overall negative results, but some evidence it may be efficacious for cocaine users experiencing severe withdrawal
	Guanfacine	α2-Adrenergic receptor agonist	Human laboratory results showed reduced cue- and stress-induced cocaine craving, with potentially stronger utility among females, also found to enhance certain cognitive abilities
	Carvedilol	α- and β- adrenergic receptor antagonist	Human laboratory results showed reduced physiological response to cocaine and reduced self-administration
	N-Acetylcysteine (NAC)	Cystine–glutamate antiporter stimulation	Results suggesting safety and tolerability, positive efficacy results for cocaine in a small open-label trial, may be related to cognitive effects
	Vigabatrin	Irreversible GABA transaminase inhibitor	Safety and efficacy in small clinical trials for cocaine and methamphetamine. A recent multi-site study has yielded negative findings.
	Topiramate	GABA receptor agonist	Promising results including from a larger clinical trial indicating more cocaine-free urines with topiramate than placebo though cocaine use remained frequent and a meta-analysis showed low strength of evidence that topiramate may improve abstinence rates
	Tiagabine	GABA transporter inhibitor	Decreased cocaine use in a small clinical trial, but negative results in subsequent trials
	Naltrexone	Opioid receptor antagonist	Decreased craving and amphetamine use in a small clinical trial, and improved methamphetamine use outcome in combination with bupropion another small clinical trial, however negative results in other studies when used in long acting injectable form.
	Ketamine	Modulates glutamate signaling through NMDA receptor antagonism	Results of a single recent RCT found ketamine combined with mindfulness-based therapy showed efficacy, even at 6 months follow-up
Cognitive enhancers	Galantamine	Allosteric potentiator of acetylcholine receptor, acetylcholinesterase inhibitor	Improved working memory and sustained attention in abstinent cocaine users in one study, fewer cocaine-positive urines and less self-reported cocaine use in another study
Immunotherapy	TA-CD	Cocaine vaccine	Positive results overall in a clinical trial, but but only a minority of individuals with moderate-to-severe cocaine use disorder were able to generate an ample immune response, however results of a recent multisite clinical trial were negative
Gender-specific approaches	Micronized progesterone	Exact mechanism unknown; possible GABA agonist and sigma antagonist effects	In postpartum women with a history of cocaine use disorder, progesterone treatment reduced relapse rates
Other pharmacotherapy/ treatment for those with psychiatric comorbidities	Antidepressants and other psychotropic medications	Monoamine reuptake inhibition, other mechanisms	Some positive results in small clinical trials for some medications, but overall, results mixed, including when used for patients with psychiatric comorbidities. Antidepressants may be associated with higher drop-out rates, whereas antipsychotics may improve treatment retention

A number of other nonamphetamine agonist medications have been tested as well. Modafinil is a weak inhibitor of dopamine transporter with resulting increases in synaptic dopamine levels (Martinez-Raga et al., 2008). Initial clinical trials were promising for both methamphetamine (Shearer et al., 2009) and cocaine (Dackis et al., 2005; Shearer et al., 2009). Subsequent larger RCTs have been negative, however (Anderson et al., 2012; Dackis et al., 2012). A more recent meta-analysis of 11 studies found modafinil was not superior to placebo in reducing cocaine use disorder-related outcomes; however, a subgroup analysis of the studies carried out in the United States found increased cocaine abstinence rates with modafinil treatment (Sangroula et al., 2017). Finally, bupropion acts as a weak norepinephrine and dopamine reuptake inhibitor, enhancing levels of extracellular dopamine in the nucleus accumbens. Bupropion has not demonstrated evidence of efficacy for heavy cocaine or methamphetamine users. There is mixed evidence supporting its use with for methamphetamine reduction among lighter users (Shoptaw et al., 2008a, 2008b; Heinzerling et al., 2014; Anderson et al., 2015); however, medication nonadherence has been a noted limitation to studies. In combination with contingency management (CM), bupropion may have some efficacy in reducing cocaine use (Poling et al., 2006).

2. Medications targeting neuroadaptations associated with stimulant use disorder—Stimulant use disorder is associated with changes in the activity of several neurotransmitters including dopamine, norepinephrine, glutamate, and GABA. These changes are believed to underlie the reinforcing effects of stimulant use, and in some cases, low levels of these neurotransmitters are believed to contribute to withdrawal symptoms (Koob & Le Moal, 2008).

Medications targeting norepinephrine have demonstrated some promise for the treatment of stimulant withdrawal and for avoiding relapse (Sofuoglu & Sewell, 2009). In an initial double-blind, placebo-controlled trial, propranolol, a beta-adrenergic blocking agent, offered no significant advantage compared to placebo in cocaine-free urines, although participants on propranolol reported lessened withdrawal symptoms. However, among participants reporting particularly severe withdrawal at baseline, propranolol offered a significant advantage compared to placebo (Kampman et al., 2001). Following up on those results, among patients with moderate-to-severe cocaine use disorder who reported severe withdrawal, propranolol had a near-significant advantage in cocaine-free urines. Among highly adherent participants, this advantage was significant (Kampman et al., 2006). Regarding other adrenergic medications, human laboratory findings suggest possible benefits of guanfacine in abating cue- (Fox et al., 2012, 2014) and stress-induced cocaine craving, with potentially stronger utility among females (Fox et al., 2014). Among early abstinent patients with moderate-to-severe cocaine use disorder, guanfacine enhanced certain cognitive abilities including inhibitory control (Fox et al., 2015). Some evidence

supports clonidine's utility in reducing stress-induced cocaine craving (Jobes et al., 2011). While an earlier study supported carvedilol in reducing cocaine self-administration (Sofuoglu et al., 2000), a subsequent study found that it did not reduce cocaine use in individuals on methadone treatment for opiate use disorder who also had co-occurring cocaine use (Sofuoglu et al., 2016).

There is also increased interest in glutamate's role in stimulant use disorders based on preclinical findings (Adewale et al., 2006; Baptista et al., 2004) and neuroimaging results indicating reduced glutamatergic activity among those with moderate-to-severe cocaine use disorder (Martinez et al., 2014). N-Acetylcysteine (NAC), is thought to normalize extracellular glutamate levels in the nucleus accumbens and was also shown in preclinical research to reduce reinstatement of cocaine self-administration (Baker et al., 2003). Evidence supporting NAC's safety and tolerability was demonstrated in a small, placebo-controlled human trial (LaRowe et al., 2006), and positive results were shown in a small, open-label clinical trial for moderate-to-severe cocaine use disorder (Mardikian et al., 2007). NAC has also been found to reduce attentional bias to cocaine-related cues (Bolin et al., 2017). Clinical trial results in moderate-to-severe cocaine use disorder were negative for memantine, a noncompetitive N-methyl-D-aspartate (NMDA) glutamate receptor antagonist (Bisaga et al., 2000). Finally, ketamine regulates glutamate activity by antagonism of NMDA receptors, the principal glutamate receptor subtype involved in learned behavior, and it has demonstrated some promise in the treatment of cocaine use disorder. In a recent RCT, a single subanesthetic dose of ketamine infusion in conjunction with mindfulness-based relapse prevention therapy decreased cocaine cravings, risk of cocaine use, and relapse risk, and increased rates of abstinence at 6 months follow-up, compared to infusion of midazolam combined with MBRPT (mindfulness-based relapse prevention therapy) (Dakwar, Nunes et al., 2019).

Medications targeting GABA activity have also been investigated. GABA is the primary inhibitory neurotransmitter in the brain and has been shown to moderate dopamine activity (Tzschentke & Schmidt, 2000). GABA effects are mediated through GABAA receptors that mediate immediate inhibitory responses and GABAB receptors that moderate slower inhibitory responses (Blein et al., 2000). It is thought that enhancement of inhibitory GABA activity could lessen the impact of cocaine's prodopaminergic effects (Tzschentke & Schmidt, 2000). Vigabatrin, or gamma-vinyl-GABA (GVG), is an irreversible GABA transaminase inhibitor that has been demonstrated to attenuate cocaine- (Gerasimov & Dewey, 1999) and methamphetamine- (Gerasimov et al., 1999) induced dopamine release in preclinical studies. Small open-label trials among participants using methamphetamine or cocaine (Brodie et al., 2005; Fechtner et al., 2006) suggest that the drug is safe and provided suggestive evidence for its association with decreased drug use. In a subsequent RCT, a higher percentage of participants taking vigabatrin than placebo were abstinent from cocaine and alcohol (Brodie et al., 2009). However, a multisite clinical trial testing the efficacy of vigabatrin for cocaine use disorder was negative (Somoza et al., 2013).

A number of anticonvulsant medications with effects on GABA activity have also been explored. The anticonvulsant topiramate has agonist effects at the GABAA receptor among other effects associated with limitation of dopamine transmission (Shank et al., 2000). Topiramate has shown some promise. In a small double-blind, placebo-controlled trial, participants randomized to topiramate had more cocaine-free urines than those assigned to placebo (Kampman et al., 2004). Self-reported cocaine craving reduction reported in a small, open-label trial of topiramate suggests a possible mechanism for this effect (Reis et al., 2008). Results from a larger, placebo-controlled trial were similarly promising in that topiramate was associated with more abstinent days and cocaine-free urines compared with placebo, although use remained frequent in this sample (Johnson et al., 2013), and a later meta-analysis of five RCTs investigating topiramate for cocaine use disorder found that topiramate increases abstinence, although this finding was noted to have low strength of evidence (Chan, Kondo et al., 2019). The anticonvulsant tiagabine was associated with attenuated subjective stimulant effects and craving for cocaine following intravenous cocaine administration (Sofuoglu et al., 2005). In a small clinical trial, tiagabine was associated with decreased cocaine use compared to placebo, based on urine drug screening results (Gonzalez et al., 2003); however, in more recent trials, tiagabine was not associated with an advantage compared to placebo in reducing cocaine use (Winhusen et al., 2005, 2007).

Recently, the opioid antagonist naltrexone has gained interest in treatment of stimulant use disorder. Naltrexone may work by reducing the reinforcing effects of cue-induced cravings and modulating subjective drug effects (Ray et al., 2015, Roche et al., 2017). In a 12-week RCT of 80 participants with amphetamine dependence, those treated with naltrexone reported less craving and less amphetamine use, and had more amphetamine-negative urine samples (Jayaram-Lindström et al., 2008). However, in an RCT of 100 treatment-seeking patients with amphetamine dependence, extended release injectable naltrexone had no effect on any substance-related outcomes (Runarsdottir et al., 2017), and in a small RCT of 100 methamphetamine-dependent men who have sex with men, 12 weeks of monthly injectable naltrexone did not reduce methamphetamine use (Coffin et al., 2018).

3. Medications targeting cognitive deficits—Evidence suggests that chronic drug use tends to be associated with considerable cognitive impairments, particularly in working memory, inhibition of impulses and attention (Sofuoglu et al., 2013). People using stimulants often experience impairments during abstinence, which have been shown to persist for up to 6 months and may predict poor retention and treatment

outcome (Potvin et al., 2014; Woicik et al., 2009). Pharmacotherapy to ameliorate these cognitive issues is a potentially promising treatment strategy (Sofuoglu et al., 2013). Further, cognitive enhancement may offer the additional benefit of enhancing the abilities of individuals with stimulant use disorders to learn, recall, and put into action new coping strategies and skills they learn in treatment.

A number of medications with cognitive enhancement effects are possible candidates for use in stimulant use disorder treatment. These include long-acting amphetamines, modafinil, cholinesterase inhibitors (e.g., galantamine), partial nicotinic acetylcholine receptor (nAChR) agonists (e.g., varenicline), and glutamate agonists (Sofuoglu et al., 2013). Clinical trials have begun to test the efficacy of these medications for this indication. In a double-blind, placebo-controlled study, galantamine improved working memory and sustained attention among abstinent cocaine users (Sofuoglu et al., 2011). In an additional, double-blind study in a sample of patients with moderate-to-severe opioid and cocaine use disorder, those randomized to galantamine treatment submitted fewer cocaine-positive urines and self-reported less cocaine use than those in the placebo condition (Sofuoglu et al., 2011). In a more recent RCT galantamine reduced cocaine and opioid use among patients in methadone treatment (Carroll et al., 2017); however, in a separate study, galantamine did not improve cocaine use outcomes at 13 weeks in patients with cocaine use disorder (DeVito et al., 2019). Taken together and given the safety profile of galantamine, this medication deserves further study.

4. Immunotherapies—Vaccines or immunotherapies are a promising approach for the treatment of a number of addictive substances (Sofuoglu & Carroll, 2011). In the context of SUD treatment, vaccines develop antibodies that bind to addictive substances after they are taken. As a result, vaccines make the passage of drug molecules across the blood-brain barrier more difficult and thus reduce the amount of drug reaching the brain. This leads to a reduction in the drug's net rewarding effect. It is important to note that antibodies produced in response to a vaccine typically target a single addictive substance. Thus, efficacy for the treatment of poly SUD will likely be limited. Results from an initial placebo-controlled trial of a cocaine vaccine among methadone-maintained patients with moderate-to-severe opioid and cocaine use disorder were promising (Martell et al., 2009). However, in a multisite clinical trial, cocaine vaccine was no more effective than placebo in reducing cocaine use (Kosten et al., 2014).

5. Gender-specific treatment—Evidence suggests that the female sex hormones estradiol and progesterone may have a relationship to the types of effects one experiences from stimulant use. Among women with moderate-to-severe cocaine use disorder, those in the luteal phase of the menstrual cycle (associated with high progesterone) reported weaker subjective effects of cocaine in comparison with women in

the follicular phase (associated with high estradiol and low progesterone) (Sofuoglu et al., 1999). Consistent with these findings, treatment with oral progesterone was associated with attenuated subjective effects from cocaine administration (Evans & Foltin, 2006; Sofuoglu et al., 2002). Pregnancy, characterized by high levels of progesterone, tends to be associated with reduced substance use. Unfortunately, women have a high rate of relapse following childbirth (Yonkers et al., 2012). In concert with these findings, a double-blind, randomized, placebo-controlled clinical trial found that oral progesterone treatment reduced rates of relapse to cocaine use in among postpartum women with a history of cocaine use disorder (Yonkers et al., 2012), further supporting the potential efficacy of progesterone treatment.

6. Other psychopharmacologic interventions—A Cochrane review of 14 studies found that antipsychotics had no effect on cocaine use disorder-related outcomes, but did decrease treatment drop-out rates (Indave et al., 2016). A subsequent systematic review and meta-analysis similarly found that antipsychotics may improve treatment retention (Chan, Kondo et al., 2019). Human laboratory findings have indicated that risperidone and aripiprazole may reduce subjective effects and behaviors associated with methamphetamine use (Lile et al., 2005; Rush et al., 2003). A small, short-term, open-label clinical trial of risperidone showed reduced methamphetamine use and psychiatric symptoms (Meredith et al., 2009); however, there have been no conclusive clinical trial findings to support use of antipsychotic medications for stimulant use disorder. Regarding the use of serotonergic drugs, there have been some positive results for cocaine. For instance, in a small, randomized, double-blind clinical trial, the reuptake inhibitor citalopram was associated with fewer cocaine-positive urines than placebo (Moeller et al., 2007). Also, in a small, randomized, double-blind trial, a higher dose of the receptor antagonist ondansetron was associated with some results indicative of possible efficacy for moderate-to-severe cocaine use disorder (Johnson et al., 2006). Overall, however, accumulated results from a Cochrane review (Pani et al., 2011), an umbrella review (Ronsley, Nolan et al., 2020), and a systematic review and meta-analysis (Chan, Kondo et al., 2019) suggest that antidepressant medications do not consistently improve any major outcome related to cocaine use disorder and instead are associated with higher drop-out rates. With regard to amphetamine use disorder, evidence is limited, but there are some findings suggesting possible efficacy for certain serotonergic medications for treatment of patients in withdrawal (see Hill & Sofuoglu, 2007).

7. Combination pharmacotherapy—Given a lack of definitive results for monotherapies, testing combination pharmacotherpy may be a promising option. For example, a recent trial tested the efficacy of a combination of extended-release amphetamine with topiramate versus double placebo for moderate-to-severe cocaine use disorder. The

combination was associated with a greater likelihood of at least 3 weeks of urine-confirmed abstinence. The combination was particularly efficacious for those with heavy baseline use (Mariani et al., 2012). In a separate study, the combination of bupropion and extended-release injectable naltrexone to treat methamphetamine use disorder in a group of adults with moderate or severe methamphetamine use disorder was explored. The combination reduced drug use (which the authors defined as having three out of four methamphetamine-negative urine samples) compared to placebo; however, response rate was low in both groups overall (Trivedi et al., 2021). Further studies are needed to test these and other appropriate combinations, including trials testing factorial designs (i.e., randomization to both active medications, one or the other paired with placebo or double placebo).

8. Treatment for individuals with stimulant use disorder and comorbidities—Treatment for individuals with SUDs and comorbidities is particularly challenging. Thus, it is not surprising that clinical trials testing treatments for comorbid stimulant use disorder have had mixed success. In a double-blind, placebo-controlled trial for individuals with moderate-to-severe cocaine use disorder and bipolar disorder, the antiepileptic lamotrigine was not associated with significant differences from placebo in cocaine-free urines or mood symptoms; however, self-reported money spent on cocaine was greater for those assigned to lamotrigine (Brown et al., 2012). In stimulant users with depression, imipramine (Nunes et al., 1995) and desipramine (McDowell et al., 2005) were associated with reduced cocaine use and craving and fewer depressive symptoms. In contrast, fluoxetine treatment has not been demonstrated to be efficacious for depressive symptoms or for cocaine use (Schmitz et al., 2001). Among those with concurrent cocaine use and depression, a combination of cognitive behavioral therapy with desipramine led to greater treatment retention and abstinence (Carroll et al., 1995). Methylphenidate treatment for stimulant use concurrent with ADHD was associated with improvement in ADHD symptoms but no notable change in cocaine (Schubiner et al., 2002) or amphetamine use (Konstenius et al., 2010). Methylphenidate was, however, found to reduce cocaine use among participants with comorbid ADHD in another clinical trial (Levin et al., 2007).

Summary—Although there is no definitive evidence to support any particular pharmacotherapy for the treatment of stimulant use disorder, there have been some favorable results. Potentially promising future directions include cognitive enhancers and further research on combination pharmacotherapy.

B. Nonpharmacological Interventions

The lack of an FDA-approved medication for stimulant use disorder has created a special interest in nonpharmacological interventions. There is significant evidence supporting use of nonpharmacological interventions for stimulant use disorder. A benefit to nonpharmacological interventions is that, unlike some pharmacotherapies that are selective in their efficacy, they can treat a range of addictive behaviors. They can also be combined with pharmacotherapy and, when successful, enhance patients' engagement with treatment and facilitate long-term behavior change (Carroll et al., 2004). We briefly describe and summarize evidence for two popular modalities: cognitive–behavioral therapy and CM.

1. Cognitive–behavioral therapy (CBT)—The objective of CBT is to teach strategies and enhance coping ability to prevent substance use. One of the underlying assumptions of CBT is that SUD and other psychiatric conditions are perpetuated by faulty, maladaptive cognitions (e.g., "I have to use when I am with this particular friend"). Therapists work with patients to challenge these cognitions and develop strategies to change them. Another key tenet of CBT is the development of specific, concrete skills that patients can utilize to identify and avoid high-risk situations and to cope effectively should they end up in a high-risk situation. Often these skills are practiced during sessions, and therapy sometimes involves "homework" to put a skill into action in the real world. A beneficial aspect of CBT is its versatility, as sessions can be adapted to the needs of individual clients (Kadden, 1992). Multiple studies have yielded evidence favoring CBT over control conditions for cocaine use (e.g., Maude-Griffin et al., 1998; Magill et al., 2019; Rawson et al., 2002); however, other studies have failed to show statistically significant advantages for CBT (e.g., Carroll et al., 1991, 1994; Crits-Cristoph et al., 1999). There have also been significant advances in the use of computerized CBT for SUD (Carroll et al., 2008; Kiluk et al., 2018). This approach allows for personalization of pace of treatment and the ability to repeat material. Findings support computer-based CBT over a standard care comparison for number of drug-free urines and duration of abstinence and have even shown improvements in long-term follow-up over standard clinician-delivered CBT.

2. Contingency management—CM has been widely considered the most effective psychosocial treatment of cocaine and methamphetamine use disorder (Bentzley et al., 2021; Brown & DeFulio, 2020; Dutra et al., 2008). The goal of CM is to reduce substance use through the provision of alternate reinforcers, which often take the form of vouchers contingent on verified abstinence (i.e., drug-free urines). Two main steps must be undertaken for CM to be implemented successfully. First, the goal behavior must be defined and detected reliably with frequent monitoring (e.g., three times per week). Second, tangible reinforcers must be provided immediately following observation of the goal behavior. An advantage to CM is that it can be readily combined with other therapies including CBT (Forronato et al., 2013, Petitjean et al., 2014),

and pharmacotherapies (Carroll & Rounsaville, 2007). Most CM studies have taken place in research settings. However, in 2021, The Biden-Harris Administration released their *Statement of Drug Policy Priorities for Year One*, indicating they will work through the Office of National Drug Control Policy of Drug Control Policy to "identify and address policy barriers related to contingency management interventions" and "explore reimbursement for motivational incentives and digital treatment for addiction" (ONDCP, 2021). In 2023, California began piloting its 24-week outpatient CM program (through Medi-CAL) across 24 counties (DCHS, 2022). Additionally, New Jersey's Department of Human Services awarded five contracts to treatment providers, worth $2 million to pilot a 16-week CM program for people with stimulant use disorder.

C. Other Interventions

TSF (Nowinski et al., 1992) is an alternate approach that has been used in stimulant use disorder clinical trials. TSF is an individual therapy based on spiritual, cognitive, and behavioral principles emphasized by organizations such as Alcoholics Anonymous (AA). A primary goal is to encourage active participation in self-help groups. Although there were doubts initially about whether TSF could be used effectively in conjunction with pharmacotherapy, given long-standing objections to this practice by organizations such as AA, there is evidence to suggest that TSF can be incorporated into pharmacotherapy clinical trials. An aforementioned disulfiram trial for moderate-to-severe cocaine use disorder (Carroll et al., 2012) is an example. TSF was associated with more self-reported abstinent days and more cocaine-free urine samples than standard counseling only.

▶ Complications/Adverse Outcomes of Treatment

In order to avoid complications and adverse outcomes, stimulant use disorder treatment requires comprehensive psychiatric and medical evaluations of all patients at the outset. Further, given that information provided by individuals with SUDs may be unreliable or incomplete, it is important that all patients receive a thorough physical examination including blood work and supervised urine drug testing. There is some risk of complications and adverse outcomes associated with treatment of acute intoxication and withdrawal (see Signs & Symptoms section earlier). In addition, the detoxification process has a degree of associated risk. During the detoxification phase, it is important for clinicians to be aware that polydrug use is common among those who use stimulants (Gouzoulis-Mayfrank & Daumann, 2006). Patients may have taken considerable amounts of multiple drugs at potentially lethal doses. Thus, it is important for medical professionals to be aware of dangers associated with possible drug combinations: cocaine with alcohol or heroin, for instance.

Prognosis

Long-term outcomes among individuals with SUDs make clear the severity of potential consequences but, at the same time, offer a degree of optimism about long-term prognosis. Mortality findings show clearly that stimulant use is associated with great risk. Compared to those who do not use, people who use methamphetamine had an age-, sex-, and race-adjusted standardized morality rate over four times that of others in a large longitudinal study of people hospitalized in California over a 15-year span. This same mortality rate was just under three times higher among those who use cocaine compared to those who do not (Callaghan et al., 2012). The overall lack of treatments with definitive evidence to support their efficacy suggests a degree of pessimism regarding prognosis. However, longitudinal research shows a considerable proportion of those who have received treatment through a variety of modalities are able to maintain long-term abstinence (Hubbard et al., 2003). For instance, at a 5-year posttreatment assessment, about one third of patients surveyed from 45 treatment programs in eight U.S. cities reported favorable past-year outcomes (Flynn et al., 2003). Duration of time spent in treatment has been identified as a predictor of long-term treatment success (Flynn et al., 2003; Hubbard et al., 2003), along with psychosocial predictors such as family support, religiosity, and motivation to change (Hubbard et al., 2003). Further longitudinal studies are needed to assess more definitively the likelihood of long-term recovery and predictors of favorable outcome.

Disclosures

Role of funding sources: This research was supported by the Veterans Administration Mental Illness Research, Education and Clinical Center (MIRECC) (MS and ES), and National Institute on Drug Abuse (T32DA035200).

Conflict of interest: The authors declare no conflicts of interest.

Abdalla RR, Miguel AC, Brietzke E, Caetano R, Laranjeira R, Madruga CS. Suicidal behavior among substance users: data from the second Brazilian National Alcohol and Drug Survey (Ii Bnads). *Braz J Psychiatry*. 2019;41:437–440.

Afonso L, Mohammad T, Thatai D. Crack whips the heart: a review of the cardiovascular toxicity of cocaine. *Am J Cardiol*. 2007;100:1040–1043.

Alexander PD, Gicas KM, Willi TS, et al: A comparison of psychotic symptoms in subjects with methamphetamine versus cocaine dependence. *Psychopharmacology*. 2017;234:1535–1547.

American Psychiatric Association. *Diagnostic and Statistical Manual of Mental Disorders*. 4th ed. Text Revision. Washington, DC: American Psychiatric Association; 2000.

Anderson AL, Li S-H, Biswas K, et al: Modafinil for the treatment of methamphetamine dependence. *Drug Alcohol Depend*. 2012; 120:135–141.

Anderson AL, Li SH, Markova D, Holmes TH, et al: Bupropion for the treatment of methamphetamine dependence in non-daily users: a randomized, double-blind, placebo-controlled trial. *Drug Alcohol Depend*. 2015;150:170–174.

Ashok AH, Mizuno Y, Volkow ND, Howes OD. Association of stimulant use with dopaminergic alterations in users of cocaine, amphetamine, or methamphetamine: a systematic review and meta-analysis. *JAMA Psychiatry*. 2017;74(5):511–519.

Bachtell RK, Jones JD, Heinzerling KG, Beardsley PM, Comer SD. Glial and neuroinflammatory targets for treating substance use disorders. *Drug Alcohol Depend*. 2017;180:156–170.

Baker DA, McFarland K, Lake RW, et al: N-Acetylcysteine-induced blockade of cocaine-induced reinstatement. *Ann N Y Acad Sci*. 2003;1003:349–351.

Baker J, Jatlow P, Pade P, et al: Acute cocaine responses following cocaethylene infusion. *Am J Drug Alcohol Abuse*. 2007;33:619–625.

Baptista MAS, Martin-Fardon R, Weiss F. Preferential effects of the metabotropic glutamate 2/3 receptor agonist ly379268 on conditioned reinstatement versus primary reinforcement: Comparison between cocaine and a potent conventional reinforcer. *J Neurosci*. 2004;24:4723–4727.

Belin D, Mar AC, Dalley JW, et al: High impulsivity predicts the switch to compulsive cocaine-taking. *Science*. 2008;320:1352–1355.

Bentzley BS, Han SS, Neuner S, Humphreys K, Kampman KM, Halpern CH. Comparison of treatments for cocaine use disorder among adults: a systematic review and meta-analysis. *JAMA Network Open*. 2021;4(5):e218049. https://doi.org/10.1001/jamanetworkopen.2021.8049

Berridge KC, Robinson TE. Liking, wanting, and the incentive-sensitization theory of addiction. *Am Psychol*. 2016;71(8):670.

Bickel WK, Miller ML, Yi R, et al: Behavioral and neuroeconomics of drug addiction: competing neural systems and temporal discounting processes. *Drug Alcohol Depend*. 2007;90:S85–S91.

Bisaga A, Aharonovich E, Cheng WY, et al: A placebo-controlled trial of memantine for cocaine dependence with high-value voucher incentives during a pre-randomization lead-in period. *Drug Alcohol Depend*. 2010;111:97–104.

Blein S, Hawrot E, Barlow P. The metabotropic GABA receptor: molecular insights and their functional consequences. *Cell Mol Life Sci*. 2000;57:635–650.

Boghdadi MS, Henning RJ. Cocaine: pathophysiology and clinical toxicology. *Heart Lung*. 1997;26:466–483.

Bohnert KM, Ilgen MA, Louzon S, McCarthy JF, Katz IR. Substance use disorders and the risk of suicide mortality among men and women in the US veterans health administration. *Addiction*. 2017;112(7):1193–1201.

Bolin BL, Alcorn III JL, Lile JA, et al: N-acetylcysteine reduces cocaine-cue attentional bias and differentially alters cocaine self-administration based on dosing order. *Drug Alcohol Depend*. 2107;178:452–460.

Bolla KI, Eldreth DA, London ED, et al: Orbitofrontal cortex dysfunction in abstinent cocaine abusers performing a decision-making task. *Neuroimage*. 2003;19:1085–1094.

Bond AJ. Drug-induced behavioural disinhibition—incidence, mechanisms and therapeutic implications. *CNS Drugs*. 1998;9:41–57.

Booth RE, Kwiatkowski CF, Chitwood DD. Sex related HIV risk behaviors: differential risks among injection drug users, crack smokers, and injection drug users who smoke crack. *Drug Alcohol Depend*. 2000;58:219–226.

Brewer JA, Potenza MN. The neurobiology and genetics of impulse control disorders: relationships to drug addictions. *Biochem Pharmacol*. 2008;75:63–75.

Brodie JD, Figueroa E, Laska EM, Dewey SL. Safety and efficacy of gamma-vinyl GABA (GVG) for the treatment of methamphetamine and/or cocaine addiction. *Synapse*. 2005;55:122–125.

Brodie JD, Case BG, Figueroa E, et al: Randomized, double-blind, placebo-controlled trial of vigabatrin for the treatment of cocaine dependence in Mexican parolees. *Am J Psychiatry*. 2009;166:1269–1277.

Brown HD, DeFulio A. Contingency management for the treatment of methamphetamine use disorder: a systematic review. *Drug Alcohol Depend*. 2020;216:108307. https://doi.org/10.1016/j.drugalcdep.2020.108307

Brown ES, Sunderajan P, Hu LT, et al: A randomized, double-blind, placebo-controlled trial of lamotrigine therapy in bipolar disorder, depressed or mixed phase and cocaine dependence. *Neuropsychopharmacology*. 2012;37:2347–2354.

Buchanan JF, Brown CR. "Designer drugs." A problem in clinical toxicology. *Med Toxicol Adv Drug*. 1988;3:1–17.

Butler AJ, Rehm J, Fischer B. Health outcomes associated with crack-cocaine use: systematic review and meta-analyses. *Drug Alcohol Depend*. 2017;180:401–416.

Callaghan RC, Cunningham JK, Verdichevski M, et al: All-cause mortality among individuals with disorders related to the use of methamphetamine: a comparative cohort study. *Drug Alcohol Depend*. 2012;125:290–294.

Carney S, Wolf CE, Tarnai-Moak L, Poklis A. Evaluation of two enzyme immunoassays for the detection of the cocaine metabolite benzoylecgonine in 1,398 urine specimens. *J Clin Lab Anal*. 2012;26:130–135.

Carroll KM, Rounsaville BJ, Gordon LT, et al: Psychotherapy and pharmacotherapy for ambulatory cocaine abusers. *Arch Gen Psychiatry*. 1994;51:177–187.

Carroll KM, Nich C, Rounsaville BJ. Differential symptom reduction in depressed cocaine abusers treated with psychotherapy and pharmacotherapy. *J Nerv Ment Dis*. 1995;183:251–259.

Carroll KM, Fenton LR, Ball SA, et al: Efficacy of disulfiram and cognitive behavior therapy in cocaine-dependent outpatients: A randomized placebo-controlled trial. *Arch Gen Psychiatry*. 2004;61:264–272.

Carroll KM, Ball SA, Martino S, et al: Computer-assisted delivery of cognitive-behavioral therapy for addiction: a randomized trial of CBT4CBT. *Am J Psychiatry*. 2008;165:881–888.

Carroll KM, Nich C, Shi JM, et al: Efficacy of disulfiram and twelve step facilitation in cocaine-dependent individuals maintained on methadone: a randomized placebo-controlled trial. *Drug Alcohol Depend*. 2012;126:224–231.

Carroll KM, Rounsaville BJ. A perfect platform: combining contingency management with medications for drug abuse. *The American journal of drug and alcohol abuse*, 2007;33(3):343–365. https://doi.org/10.1080/00952990701301319

Carroll KM, Nich C, DeVito EE, Shi JM, Sofuoglu M. Galantamine and computerized cognitive behavioral therapy for cocaine dependence: a randomized clinical trial. *J Clin Psychiatry*. 2017;79(1):7588.

Carson DS, Bosanquet DP, Carter CS, et al: Preliminary evidence for lowered basal cortisol in a naturalistic sample of methamphetamine polydrug users. *Exp Clin Psychopharmacol*. 2012;20:497–503.

Chan B, Freeman M, Kondo K, et al: Pharmacotherapy for methamphetamine/amphetamine use disorder—a systematic review and meta-analysis. *Addiction*. 2019;114(12):2122–2136.

Chan B, Kondo K, Freeman M, Ayers C, Montgomery J, Kansagara D. Pharmacotherapy for cocaine use disorder—a systematic review and meta-analysis. *J Gen Intern Med*. 2019;34:2858–2873.

Clark L, Robbins TW, Ersche KD, Sahakian BJ. Reflection impulsivity in current and former substance users. *Biol Psychiatry*. 2006;60:515–522.

Coffey SF, Gudleski GD, Saladin ME, Brady KT. Impulsivity and rapid discounting of delayed hypothetical rewards in cocaine-dependent individuals. *Exp Clin Psychopharmacol*. 2003;11:18–25.

Coffin PO, Santos GM, Hern J, et al: Extended-release naltrexone for methamphetamine dependence among men who have sex with men: a randomized placebo-controlled trial. *Addiction*. 2018;113(2):268–278.

Cone EJ, Dickerson SL. Efficacy of urinalysis in monitoring heroin and cocaine abuse patterns: implications in clinical trials for treatment of drug dependence. *NIDA Res Monogr*. 1992;128:46–58; discussion 59–63.

Courtney KE, Ray LA. Methamphetamine: an update on epidemiology, pharmacology, clinical phenomenology, and treatment literature. *Drug Alcohol Depend*. 2014;143:11–21.

Crist RC, Ambrose-Lanci LM, Vaswani M, et al: Case-control association analysis of polymorphisms in the delta-opioid receptor, OPRD1, with cocaine and opioid addicted populations. *Drug Alcohol Depend*. 2013;127:122–128.

Crits-Christoph P, Siqueland L, Blaine J, et al: Psychosocial treatments for cocaine dependence: National Institute on Drug Abuse Collaborative Cocaine Treatment Study. *Arch Gen Psychiatry*. 1999;56:493–502.

Dackis CA, Kampman KM, Lynch KG, et al: A double-blind, placebo-controlled trial of modafinil for cocaine dependence. *Neuropsychopharmacology*. 2005;30:205–211.

Dackis CA, Kampman KM, Lynch KG, et al: A double-blind, placebo-controlled trial of modafinil for cocaine dependence. *J Subst Abuse Treat*. 2012;43:303–312.

Dakwar E, Nunes EV, Hart CL, et al: A single ketamine infusion combined with mindfulness-based behavioral modification to treat cocaine dependence: a randomized clinical trial." *Am J Psychiatry*. 2019;176(11):923–930.

Darke S, Duflou J, Kaye S. Prevalence and nature of cardiovascular disease in methamphetamine-related death: a national study. *Drug Alcohol Depend*. 2017;179:174–179.

DCHS. (2022). *Medi-Cal Contingency Management Pilot Program Policy Design (draft)*. Retrieved from https://www.dhcs.ca.gov/Documents/Contingency-Management-Policy-Paper.pdf

Delbridge TR, Yealy DM. Wide complex tachycardia. *Emerg Med Clin North Am*. 1995;13:903–924.

DeVito EE, Carroll KM, Babuscio T, Nich C, Sofuoglu M. Randomized placebo-controlled trial of galantamine in individuals with cocaine use disorder. *J Subst Abuse Treat*. 2019;107:29–37.

Dodson WW. Pharmacotherapy of adult ADHD. *J Clin Psychol*. 2005;61:589–606.

Du J, Quan M, Zhuang W, et al: Hippocampal volume reduction in female but not male recent abstinent methamphetamine users. *Behav Brain Res*. 2015;289:78–83.

Dumont GJH, Sweep FCGJ, van der Steen R, et al: Increased oxytocin concentrations and prosocial feelings in humans after ecstasy (3,4-methylenedioxymethamphetamine) administration. *Soc Neurosci*. 2009;4:359–366.

DuRant RH, Smith JA, Kreiter SR, Krowchuk DP. The relationship between early age of onset of initial substance use and engaging in multiple health risk behaviors among young adolescents. *Arch Pediatr Adolesc Med*. 1999;153:286–291.

Dutra L, Stathopoulou G, Basden SL., Leyro TM., Powers MB, Otto MW. A meta-analytic review of psychosocial interventions for substance use disorders. *Am J Psychiatry*. 2008;165(2):179–187. https://doi.org/10.1176/appi.ajp.2007.06111851

Ersche KD, Williams GB, Robbins TW, Bullmore ET. Meta-analysis of structural brain abnormalities associated with stimulant drug dependence and neuroimaging of addiction vulnerability and resilience. *Curr Opin Neurobiol*. 2013;23(4):615–624.

Evans SM, Foltin RW. Exogenous progesterone attenuates the subjective effects of smoked cocaine in women, but not in men. *Neuropsychopharmacology*. 2006;31:659–674.

Everitt BJ, Belin D, Economidou D, et al: Review. Neural mechanisms underlying the vulnerability to develop compulsive drug-seeking habits and addiction. *Phil Trans R Soc Lond B Biol Sci*. 2008;363:3125–3135.

Everitt BJ, Robbins TW. Drug addiction: updating actions to habits to compulsions ten years on. *Annu Rev Psychol*. 2016;67:23–50.

Fechtner RD, Khouri AS, Figueroa E, et al: Short-term treatment of cocaine and/or methamphetamine abuse with vigabatrin: Ocular safety pilot results. *Arch Ophthalmol*. 2006;124:1257–1262.

Fernandez WG, Hung O, Bruno GR, et al: Factors predictive of acute renal failure and need for hemodialysis among ED patients with rhabdomyolysis. *Am J Emerg Med*. 2005;23:1–7.

Ferri CP, Gossop M. Route of cocaine administration: patterns of use and problems among a Brazilian sample. *Addict Behav*. 1999;24:815–821.

Fiellin LE, Tetrault JM, Becker WC, et al: Previous use of alcohol, cigarettes, and marijuana and subsequent abuse of prescription opioids in young adults. *J Adolesc Health*. 2013;52:158–163.

Fillmore MT, Rush CR, Hays L. Acute effects of oral cocaine on inhibitory control of behavior in humans. *Drug Alcohol Depend*. 2002;67:157–167.

Flynn PM, Joe GW, Broome KM, et al: Looking back on cocaine dependence: reasons for recovery. *Am J Addict*. 2003;12:398–411.

Ford JD, Gelernter J, Devoe JS, et al: Association of psychiatric and substance use disorder comorbidity with cocaine dependence severity and treatment utilization in cocaine-dependent individuals. *Drug Alcohol Depend*. 2009;99:193–203.

Farronato NS, Dürsteler-Macfarland KM, Wiesbeck GA, Petitjean SA. A systematic review comparing cognitive-behavioral therapy and contingency management for cocaine dependence. *J Addict Dis*. 2013;32(3):274–287. https://doi.org/10.1080/1055 0887.2013.824328

Fernàndez-Castillo N, Cabana-Domínguez J, Corominas R, Cormand B. Molecular genetics of cocaine use disorders in humans. *Mol Psychiatry*. 2022;27(1):624–639.

Fotros A, Casey KF, Larcher K, et al: Cocaine cue-induced dopamine release in amygdala and hippocampus: a high-resolution PET [^{18}F]fallypride study in cocaine dependent participants. *Neuropsychopharmacology*. 2013;38:1780–1788.

Fowler JS, Volkow ND, Wang GJ, et al: [(11)]Cocaine: PET studies of cocaine pharmacokinetics, dopamine transporter availability and dopamine transporter occupancy. *Nucl Med Biol*. 2001;28:561–572.

Fox HC, Seo D, Tuit K, et al: Guanfacine effects on stress, drug craving and prefrontal activation in cocaine dependent individuals: preliminary findings. *J Psychopharmacol*. 2012;26:958–972.

Fox HC, Morgan PT, Sinha R. Sex differences in guanfacine effects on drug craving and stress arousal in cocaine-dependent individuals. *Neuropsychopharmacology*. 2014;39:1527–1537.

Fox H, Sofuoglu M, Sinha R. Guanfacine enhances inhibitory control and attentional shifting in early abstinent cocaine-dependent individuals. *J Psychopharmacol*. 2015;29(3):312–23.

Franklin TR, Acton PD, Maldjian JA, et al: Decreased gray matter concentration in the insular, orbitofrontal, cingulate, and temporal cortices of cocaine patients. *Biol Psychiatry*. 2002;51:134–142.

Frazer KM, Manly JJ, Downey G, Hart CL. Assessing cognitive functioning in individuals with cocaine use disorder. *J Clin Exp Neuropsychol*. 2018;40(6):619–632. https://doi.org/10.1080/138 03395.2017.1403569

Frazer KM, Richards Q, Keith DR. The long-term effects of cocaine use on cognitive functioning: a systematic critical review. *Behav Brain Res*. 2018;348:241–262. https://doi.org/10.1016/j.bbr.2018.04.005

Garcia AN, Salloum IM. Polysomnographic sleep disturbances in nicotine, caffeine, alcohol, cocaine, opioid, and cannabis use: a focused review. *Am J Addict*. 2015;24(7):590–598.

García-Rodríguez O, Secades-Villa R, Weidberg S, Yoon JH. A systematic assessment of delay discounting in relation to cocaine and nicotine dependence. *Behav Processes*. 2013;99:100–105. https://doi.org/10.1016/j.beproc.2013.07.007

George TP, Chawarski MC, Pakes J, et al: Disulfiram versus placebo for cocaine dependence in buprenorphine-maintained subjects: A preliminary trial. *Biol Psychiatry*. 2000;47:1080–1086.

Gerasimov MR, Dewey SL. Gamma-vinyl gamma-aminobutyric acid attenuates the synergistic elevations of nucleus accumbens dopamine produced by a cocaine/heroin (speedball) challenge. *Eur J Pharmacol*. 1999;380:1–4.

Gerasimov MR, Ashby CR, Gardner EL, et al: Gamma-vinyl GABA inhibits methamphetamine, heroin, or ethanol-induced increases in nucleus accumbens dopamine. *Synapse*. 1999;34:11–19.

Goldstein RZ, Alia-Klein N, Tomasi D, et al: Is decreased prefrontal cortical sensitivity to monetary reward associated with impaired motivation and self-control in cocaine addiction? *Am J Psychiatry*. 2007a;164:43–51.

Goldstein RZ, Tomasi D, Rajaram S, et al: Role of the anterior cingulate and medial orbitofrontal cortex in processing drug cues in cocaine addiction. *Neuroscience*. 2007b;144:1153–1159.

Gonzales R, Ang A, Glik DC, et al: Quality of life among treatment seeking methamphetamine-dependent individuals. *Am J Addict*. 2011;20:366–372.

Gonzalez G, Feingold A, Oliveto A, et al: Comorbid major depressive disorder as a prognostic factor in cocaine-abusing buprenorphine-maintained patients treated with desipramine and contingency management. *Am J Drug Alcohol Abuse.* 2003;29:497–514.

Gotway MB, Marder SR, Hanks DK, et al: Thoracic complications of illicit drug use: an organ system approach. *Radiographics.* 2002;22:S119–S135.

Gouzoulis-Mayfrank E, Daumann J. The confounding problem of polydrug use in recreational ecstasy/MDMA users: a brief overview. *J Psychopharmacol.* 2006;20:188–193.

Grabowski J, Rhoades H, Stotts A, et al: Agonist-like or antagonist-like treatment for cocaine dependence with methadone for heroin dependence: two double-blind randomized clinical trials. *Neuropsychopharmacology.* 2004;29:969–981.

Graf M, Wong KLL, Augustine GJ. Neuroscience: a role for the claustrum in drug reward. *Curr Biol.* 2020;30(18):R1038-R40.

Grant S, Contoreggi C, London ED. Drug abusers show impaired performance in a laboratory test of decision making. *Neuropsychologia.* 2000;38:1180–1187.

Grant KM, LeVan TD, Wells SM, et al: Methamphetamine-associated psychosis. *J Neuroimmune Pharmacol.* 2012;7:113–139.

Greene SL, Kerr F, Braitberg G. Review article: amphetamines and related drugs of abuse. *Emerg Med Australas.* 2008;20:391–402.

Haber SN. The place of dopamine in the cortico-basal ganglia circuit. *Neuroscience.* 2014;282:248–257.

Hamamoto DT, Rhodus NL. Methamphetamine abuse and dentistry. *Oral Dis.* 2009;15:27–37.

Hart C, Marvin C, Silver R, et al: Is cognitive functioning impaired in methamphetamine users? A critical review. *Neuropsychopharmacol.* 2012;37:586–608. https://doi.org/10.1038/npp.2011.276

Hearn WL, Flynn DD, Hime GW, et al: Cocaethylene: a unique cocaine metabolite displays high affinity for the dopamine transporter. *J Neurochem.* 1991;56:698–701.

Heinzerling KG, Swanson AN, Hall TM, Yi Y, Wu Y, Shoptaw SJ. Randomized, placebo-controlled trial of bupropion in methamphetamine-dependent participants with less than daily methamphetamine use. *Addiction.* 2014;109(11):1878–1886.

Herin DV, Rush CR, Grabowski J. Agonist-like pharmacotherapy for stimulant dependence: Preclinical, human laboratory, and clinical studies. *Ann NY Acad Sci.* 2010;1187:76–100.

Hill KP, Sofuoglu M. Biological treatments for amfetamine dependence: recent progress. *CNS Drugs.* 2007;21:851–869.

Hirsiger S, Hänggi J, Germann J, et al: Longitudinal changes in cocaine intake and cognition are linked to cortical thickness adaptations in cocaine users. *Neuroimage: Clin.* 2019;21:101652.

Howell LL, Cunningham KA. Serotonin 5-Ht2 receptor interactions with dopamine function: implications for therapeutics in cocaine use disorder. *Pharmacol Rev.* 2015;67(1):176–197.

Hubbard RL, Craddock SG, Flynn PM, et al: Overview of 1-year follow-up outcomes in the Drug Abuse Treatment Outcome Study (DATOS). *Psychol Addict Behav.* 1997;11:261–278.

Hubbard RL, Craddock SG, Anderson J. Overview of 5-year followup outcomes in the Drug Abuse Treatment Outcome Studies (DATOS). *J Subst Abuse Treat.* 2003;25:125–134.

Ide S, Kobayashi H, Ujike H, et al: Linkage disequilibrium and association with methamphetamine dependence/psychosis of mu-opioid receptor gene polymorphisms. *Pharmacogenomics J.* 2006;6:179–188.

Ide JS, Zhang S, Hu S, et al: Cerebral gray matter volumes and low-frequency fluctuation of BOLD signals in cocaine dependence: duration of use and gender difference. *Drug Alcohol Depen.* 2014;134:51–62.

Indave BI, Minozzi S, Pani PP, Amato L. Antipsychotic medications for cocaine dependence. *Cochrane Database Syst Rev.* 2016;3.

Jayaram-Lindström N, Hammarberg A, Beck O, Franck J. Naltrexone for the treatment of amphetamine dependence: a randomized, placebo-controlled trial. *Am J Psychiatry.* 2008;165(11):1442–1448.

Jia ZR, Worhunsky PD, Carroll KM, et al: An initial study of neural responses to monetary incentives as related to treatment outcome in cocaine dependence. *Biol Psychiatry.* 2011;70:553–560.

Jobes ML, Ghitza UE, Epstein DH, et al: Clonidine blocks stress-induced craving in cocaine users. *Psychopharmacology.* 2011; 218:83–88.

Johnson BA, Roache JD, Ait-Daoud N, et al: A preliminary randomized, double-blind, placebo-controlled study of the safety and efficacy of ondansetron in the treatment of cocaine dependence. *Drug Alcohol Depend.* 2006;84:256–263.

Johnson BA, Ait-Daoud N, Wang XQ, et al: Topiramate for the treatment of cocaine addiction: a randomized clinical trial. *JAMA Psychiatry.* 2013;70:1338–1346.

Kadden R. *Cognitive-Behavioral Coping Skills Therapy Manual: A Clinical Research Guide for Therapists Treating Individuals with Alcohol Abuse and Dependence.* National Institute on Alcohol Abuse and Alcoholism; 1992.

Kampman KM, Volpicelli JR, Mulvaney F, et al: Effectiveness of propranolol for cocaine dependence treatment may depend on cocaine withdrawal symptom severity. *Drug Alcohol Depend.* 2001;63:69–78.

Kampman KM, Pettinati H, Lynch KG, et al: A pilot trial of topiramate for the treatment of cocaine dependence. *Drug Alcohol Depend.* 2004;75:233–240.

Kampman KM, Dackis C, Lynch KG, et al: A double-blind, placebo-controlled trial of amantadine, propranolol, and their combination for the treatment of cocaine dependence in patients with severe cocaine withdrawal symptoms. *Drug Alcohol Depend.* 2006;85:129–137.

Kariisa M, Scholl L, Wilson N, Seth P, Hoots B. Drug overdose deaths involving cocaine and psychostimulants with abuse potential—United States, 2003–2017. *Morb Mortal Wkly Rep.* 2019;68(17):388.

Kendler KS, Karkowski LM, Neale MC, Prescott CA. Illicit psychoactive substance use, heavy use, abuse, and dependence in a US population-based sample of male twins. *Arch Gen Psychiatry.* 2000;57:261.

Kendler KS, Myers J, Prescott CA. Specificity of genetic and environmental risk factors for symptoms of cannabis, cocaine, alcohol, caffeine, and nicotine dependence. *Arch Gen Psychiatry.* 2007;64:1313–1320.

Kevil CG, Goeders NE, Woolard MD, et al: Methamphetamine use and cardiovascular disease: in search of answers. *Arterioscler Thromb Vasc Biol.* 2019;39(9):1739–1746.

Kiluk BD, Nich C, Buck MB, et al: Randomized clinical trial of computerized and clinician-delivered CBT in comparison with standard outpatient treatment for substance use disorders: primary within-treatment and follow-up outcomes. *Am J Psychiatry.* 2018;175(9):853–863. https://doi.org/10.1176/appi.ajp.2018.17090978

Kirschbaum KM, Musshoff F, Wilbert A, et al: Direct ELISA kits as a sensitive and selective screening method for abstinence control in urine. *Forensic Sci Int.* 2011;207:66–69.

Kitamura O, Wee S, Specio SE, Koob GF, Pulvirenti L. Escalation of methamphetamine self-administration in rats: a dose-effect function. *Psychopharmacology (Berl).* 2006;186:48–53.

Konstenius M, Jayaram-Lindstrom N, Beck O, Franck J. Sustained release methylphenidate for the treatment of ADHD in amphetamine abusers: a pilot study. *Drug Alcohol Depend.* 2010;108:130–133.

Koob GF, Le Moal M. Addiction and the brain antireward system. *Annu Rev Psychol.* 2008;59:29–53.

Koob GF, Caine SB, Parsons L, et al: Opponent process model and psychostimulant addiction. *Pharmacol Biochem Behav.* 1997;57:513–521.

Koob GF, Volkow ND. Neurobiology of addiction: a neurocircuitry analysis. *Lancet Psychiatry.* 2016;3(8):760–773.

Korpi ER, Hollander B den, Farooq U, et al: Mechanisms of action and persistent neuroplasticity by drugs of abuse. *Pharmacol Rev.* 2015;67(4):872–1004.

Kosten T. Pathophysiology and treatment of cocaine dependence. *Neuropsychopharmacology.* 2002;1461–1475.

Kosten TR, Wu G, Huang W, et al: Pharmacogenetic randomized trial for cocaine abuse: disulfiram and dopamine beta-hydroxylase. *Biol Psychiatry.* 2013;73:219–224.

Kosten TR, Domingo CB, Shorter D, et al: Vaccine for cocaine dependence: a randomized double-blind placebo-controlled efficacy trial. *Drug Alcohol Depend.* 2014;140:42–47.

Kupiec T, DeCicco L, Spiehler V, et al: Choice of an ELISA assay for screening postmortem blood for amphetamine and/or methamphetamine. *J Anal Toxicol.* 2002;26:513–518.

Lane SD, Steinberg JL, Ma L, et al: Diffusion tensor imaging and decision making in cocaine dependence. *PloS One.* 2010 5:e11591.

LaRowe SD, Mardikian P, Malcolm R, et al: Safety and tolerability of *N*-acetylcysteine in cocaine-dependent individuals. *Am J Addict.* 2006;15:105–110.

Lecomte T, Dumais A, Dugre JR, Potvin S. The prevalence of substance-induced psychotic disorder in methamphetamine misusers: a meta-analysis. *Psychiatry Res.* 2018;268:189–192.

Leeman RF, Potenza MN. Similarities and differences between pathological gambling and substance use disorders: a focus on impulsivity and compulsivity. *Psychopharmacology.* 2012;219:469–490.

Levin FR, Evans SM, Brooks DJ, Garawi F. Treatment of cocaine dependent treatment seekers with adult ADHD: double-blind comparison of methylphenidate and placebo. *Drug Alcohol Depend.* 2007;87:20–29.

Levin FR, Mariani JJ, Pavlicova M, et al: Extended release mixed amphetamine salts and topiramate for cocaine dependence: a randomized clinical replication trial with frequent users. *Drug Alcohol Depend.* 2020;206:107700

Lexau BJ, Nelson D, Hatsukami DK. Comparing IV and non-IV cocaine users: characteristics of a sample of cocaine users seeking to participate in research. *Am J Addict.* 1998;7:262–271.

Leyton M, Boileau I, Benkelfat C, et al: Amphetamine-induced increases in extracellular dopamine, drug wanting, and novelty seeking: a PET/[11C]raclopride study in healthy men. *Neuropsychopharmacology.* 2002;27:1027–1035.

Li CSR, Milivojevic V, Kemp K, et al: Performance monitoring and stop signal inhibition in abstinent patients with cocaine dependence. *Drug Alcohol Depend.* 2006;85:205–212.

Lile JA, Stoops WW, Vansickel AR, et al: Aripiprazole attenuates the discriminative-stimulus and subject-rated effects of D-amphetamine in humans. *Neuropsychopharmacology.* 2005;30:2103–2114.

Lim KO, Choi SJ, Pomara N, et al: Reduced frontal white matter integrity in cocaine dependence: a controlled diffusion tensor imaging study. *Biol Psychiatry.* 2002;51:890–895.

Lim KO, Wozniak JR, Mueller BA, et al: Brain macrostructural and microstructural abnormalities in cocaine dependence. *Drug Alcohol Depend.* 2008;92:164–172.

Liu Y, Cheong JW, Vaddiparti K, Cottler LB. The association between quantity, frequency and duration of cocaine use during the heaviest use period and DSM-5 cocaine use disorder. *Drug Alcohol Depend.* 2020;213:108114.

Liu Y, Williamson V, Setlow B, Cottler LB, Knackstedt LA. The importance of considering polysubstance use: lessons from cocaine research. *Drug Alcohol Depend.* 2018;192:16–28.

London ED, Cascella NG, Wong DF, et al: Cocaine-induced reduction of glucose-utilization in human brain—a study using positron emission tomography and [fluorine-18]-fluorodeoxyglucose. *Arch Gen Psychiatry.* 1990;47:567–574.

London ED, Kohno M, Morales AM, Ballard ME. Chronic methamphetamine abuse and corticostriatal deficits revealed by neuroimaging. *Brain Res.* 2015;1628:174–185.

Longo M, Wickes W, Smout M, et al: Randomized controlled trial of dexamphetamine maintenance for the treatment of methamphetamine dependence. *Addiction.* 2010;105:146–154.

Lopez-Quintero C, Pérez de los Cobos J, Hasin DS, et al: Probability and predictors of transition from first use to dependence on nicotine, alcohol, cannabis, and cocaine: results of the National Epidemiologic Survey on Alcohol and Related Conditions (NESARC). *Drug Alcohol Depen.* 2011;115(1-2):120–130. https://doi.org/10.1016/j.drugalcdep.2010.11.004

MacLean RR, Sofuoglu M. Stimulants and mood disorders. *Curr Addict Rep.* 2018;5:323–329.

Magura S, Nwakeze PC, Demsky S. Research report pre- and in-treatment predictors of retention in methadone treatment using survival analysis. *Addiction.* 1998;93:51–60.

Mardikian PN, LaRowe SD, Hedden S, et al: An open-label trial of *N*-acetylcysteine for the treatment of cocaine dependence: a pilot study. *Prog Neuropsychopharmacol Biol Psychiatry.* 2007;31:389–394.

Mariani JJ, Pavlicova M, Bisaga A, et al: Extended-release mixed amphetamine salts and topiramate for cocaine dependence: a randomized controlled trial. *Biol Psychiatry.* 2012;72:950–956.

Martell BA, Orson FM, Poling J, et al: Cocaine vaccine for the treatment of cocaine dependence in methadone-maintained patients: a randomized, double-blind, placebo-controlled efficacy trial. *Arch Gen Psychiatry.* 2009;66:1116–1123.

Martinez D, Slifstein M, Nabulsi N, et al: Imaging glutamate homeostasis in cocaine addiction with the metabotropic glutamate receptor 5 positron emission tomography radiotracer [11C]ABP688 and magnetic resonance spectroscopy. *Biol Psychiat.* 2014;75:165–171.

Martinez-Raga J, Knecht C, Cepeda S. Modafinil: a useful medication for cocaine addiction? Review of the evidence from neuropharmacological, experimental and clinical studies. *Curr Drug Abuse Rev.* 2008;1:213–221.

Matthews JC, Collins A. Interactions of cocaine and cocaine congeners with sodium channels. *Biochem Pharmacol.* 1983;32:455–460.

McCord J, Jneid H, Hollander JE, et al: Management of cocaine-associated chest pain and myocardial infarction—a scientific statement from the American Heart Association Acute Cardiac Care Committee of the Council on Clinical Cardiology. *Circulation.* 2008;117:1897–1907.

McDowell D, Nunes EV, Seracini AM, et al: Desipramine treatment of cocaine-dependent patients with depression: a placebo-controlled trial. *Drug Alcohol Depend.* 2005;80:209–221.

McKetin R, McLaren J, Lubman DI, Hides L. The prevalence of psychotic symptoms among methamphetamine users. *Addiction.* 2006;101:1473–1478.

McKetin R. Methamphetamine psychosis: insights from the past. *Addiction.* 2018;113(8):1522–1527.

Meredith CW, Jaffe C, Ang-Lee K, Saxon AJ. Implications of chronic methamphetamine use: a literature review. *Harvard Rev Psychiatry.* 2005;13:141–154.

Meredith CW, Jaffe C, Cherrier M, et al: Open trial of injectable risperidone for methamphetamine dependence. *J Addict Med.* 2009;3:55–65.

Messina N, Jeter K, Marinelli-Casey P, West K, Rawson R. Children exposed to methamphetamine use and manufacture. *Child Abuse Negl.* 2014;38(11):1872–1883.

Moeller FG, Barratt ES, Dougherty DM, et al: Psychiatric aspects of impulsivity. *Am J Psychiatry.* 2001;158:1783–1793.

Moeller FG, Hasan KM, Steinberg JL, et al: Reduced anterior corpus callosum white matter integrity is related to increased impulsivity and reduced discriminability in cocaine-dependent subjects: diffusion tensor imaging. *Neuropsychopharmacology.* 2005;30:610–617.

Moeller FG, Hasan KM, Steinberg JL, et al: Diffusion tensor imaging eigenvalues: preliminary evidence for altered myelin in cocaine dependence. *Psychiatry Res.* 2007;154:253–258.

Monterosso JR, Aron AR, Cordova X, et al: Deficits in response inhibition associated with chronic methamphetamine abuse. *Drug Alcohol Depend.* 2005;79:273–277.

Mouhaffel AH, Madu EC, Satmary WA, Fraker TD. Cardiovascular complications of cocaine. *Chest.* 1995;107:1426–1434.

Moszczynska A, Callan SP. Molecular, behavioral, and physiological consequences of methamphetamine neurotoxicity: implications for treatment." *J Pharmacol Exp Ther.* 2017;362(3):474–488.

Müller CP, Homberg JR. The role of serotonin in drug use and addiction." *Behav Brain Res.* 2015;277:146–192.

National Drug Intelligence Center. *The Economic Impact of Illicit Drug Use on American Society.* Washington, DC: United States Department of Justice.

National Institute on Drug Abuse. *Methamphetamine Abuse and Addiction.* NIDA Research Report Series. Rockville MD: NIDA; 1998.

National Institute on Drug Abuse. *Methamphetamine Abuse and Addiction.* NIDA Research Report Series. 2006. http://www.drugabuse.gov/publications/research-reports/methamphetamine-abuse-addiction.

Nees F, Tzschoppe J, Patrick CJ, et al: Determinants of early alcohol use in healthy adolescents: The differential contribution of neuroimaging and psychological factors. *Neuropsychopharmacology.* 2012;37:986–995.

Neiman J, Haapaniemi HM, Hillbom M. Neurological complications of drug abuse: pathophysiological mechanisms. *Eur J Neurol.* 2000;7:595–606.

Northcutt, AL, Hutchinson MR, Wang X, et al: Dat isn't all that: cocaine reward and reinforcement require toll-like receptor 4 signaling. *Mol Psychiatry.* 2015;20(12):1525–1537.

Nowinski J, Baker S, Carroll KM. *Twelve Step Facilitation Therapy Manual: A Clinical Research Guide for Therapists Treating Individuals with Alcohol Abuse and Dependence.* US Dept. of Health and Human Services, Public Health Service, Alcohol, Drug Abuse, and Mental Health Administration, National Institute on Alcohol Abuse and Alcoholism; 1992.

Nunes EV, McGrath PJ, Quitkin FM, et al: Imipramine treatment of cocaine abuse: possible boundaries of efficacy. *Drug Alcohol Depend.* 1995;39:185–195.

Nuijten M, Blanken P, van de Wetering B, et al: Sustained-related dexamfetamine in the treatment of chronic cocaine-dependent patients on heroin-assisted treatment: a randomized, double-blind, placebo-controlled trial. *The Lancet.* 2016;387:P2226–2234.

Oliveto A, Poling J, Mancino MJ, et al: Randomized, double blind, placebo-controlled trial of disulfiram for the treatment of cocaine dependence in methadone-stabilized patients. *Drug Alcohol Depend.* 2011;113:184–191.

ONDCP. (2021). *The Biden-Harris Administration's Statement of Drug Policy Priorities for Year One.* Retrieved from https://www.whitehouse.gov/wp-content/uploads/2021/03/BidenHarris-Statement-of-Drug-Policy-Priorities-April-1.pdf?fbclid=IwAR2TBk34U_XRqlqK_pAYnUd_9f7zY3IbCQI9KxI6S5eYeRJdFzl9B09hZ84.

Palha AP, Esteves M. Drugs of abuse and sexual functioning. *Adv Psychosom Med.* 2008;29:131–149.

Pando-Naude V, Toxto S, Fernandez-Lozano S, Parsons CE, Alcauter S, Garza-Villarreal EA. Gray and white matter morphology in substance use disorders: a neuroimaging systematic review and meta-analysis. *Transl Psychiatry.* 2021;11(1):29.

Pani PP, Trogu E, Vecchi S, Amato L. Antidepressants for cocaine dependence and problematic cocaine use. *Cochrane Database Syst Rev.* 2011;CD002950.

Pavarin RM, Fioritti A. Mortality trends among cocaine users treated between 1989 and 2013 in Northern Italy: results of a longitudinal study. *J Psychoactive Drugs.* 2018;50(1):72–80.

Petitjean SA, Dürsteler-MacFarland KM, Krokar MC, et al: A randomized, controlled trial of combined cognitive-behavioral therapy plus prize-based contingency management for cocaine dependence. *Drug Alcohol Depend.* 2014;145:94–100. https://doi.org/10.1016/j.drugalcdep.2014.09.785

Petrakis IL, Carroll KM, Nich C, et al: Disulfiram treatment for cocaine dependence in methadone-maintained opioid addicts. *Addiction.* 2000;95:219–228.

Pettinati HM, Kampman KM, Lynch KG, et al: A double blind, placebo-controlled trial that combines disulfiram and naltrexone for treating co-occurring cocaine and alcohol dependence. *Addict Behav.* 2008;33:651–667.

Pierce RC, Fant B, Swinford-Jackson SE, Heller EA, Berrettini WH, Wimmer ME. Environmental, genetic and epigenetic contributions to cocaine addiction. *Neuropsychopharmacology.* 2018;43(7):1471–1480.

Poling J, Oliveto A, Petry N, et al: Six-month trial of bupropion with contingency management for cocaine dependence in a methadone-maintained population. *Arch Gen Psychiatry*. 2006; 63:219–228.

Potvin S, Stavro K, Rizkallah E, Pelletier J. Cocaine and cognition: a systematic quantitative review. *J Addict Med*. 2014;8(5):368–376.

Qureshi AI, Suri MF, Guterman LR, Hopkins LN. Cocaine use and the likelihood of nonfatal myocardial infarction and stroke: data from the Third National Health and Nutrition Examination Survey. *Circulation*. 2001;103:502–506.

Ray LA, Bujarski S, Courtney KE, et al: The effects of naltrexone on subjective response to methamphetamine in a clinical sample: a double-blind, placebo-controlled laboratory study. *Neuropsychopharmacology*. 2015;40(10) :2347–2356.

Reis A, Castro L, Faria R, Laranjeira R. Craving decrease with topiramate in outpatient treatment for cocaine dependence: an open label trial. *Rev Bras Psiquiatr*. 2008;30:132.

Reneman L, Booij J, de Bruin K, et al: Effects of dose, sex, and long-term abstention from use on toxic effects of MDMA (ecstasy) on brain serotonin neurons. *Lancet*. 2001;358:1864–1869.

Richards JR, Bretz SW, Johnson EB, et al: Methamphetamine abuse and emergency department utilization. *West J Med*. 170:198–202.

Robinson TE, Berridge KC. The neural basis of drug craving: an incentive-sensitization theory of addiction. *Brain Res Rev*. 1993; 18:247–291.

Roche DJO, Worley MJ, Courtney KE, et al: Naltrexone moderates the relationship between cue-induced craving and subjective response to methamphetamine in individuals with methamphetamine use disorder. *Psychopharmacology*. 2017;234:1997–2007.

Rogers RD, Robbins TW. Investigating the neurocognitive deficits associated with chronic drug misuse. *Curr Opin Neurobiol*. 2001;11:250–257.

Rogers RD, Everitt BJ, Baldacchino A, et al: Dissociable deficits in the decision-making cognition of chronic amphetamine abusers, opiate abusers, patients with focal damage to prefrontal cortex, and tryptophan-depleted normal volunteers: evidence for monoaminergic mechanisms. *Neuropsychopharmacology*. 1999;20:322–339.

Ronsley C, Nolan S, Knight R, et al: Treatment of stimulant use disorder: a systematic review of reviews. *PloS One*. 2020;15(6): e0234809.

Ruhe HG, Mason NS, Schene AH. Mood is indirectly related to serotonin, norepinephrine and dopamine levels in humans: a meta-analysis of monoamine depletion studies. *Mol Psychiatry*. 2007;12:331–359.

Runarsdottir V, Hansdottir I, Tyrfingsson T, et al: Extended-release injectable naltrexone (Xr-Ntx) with intensive psychosocial therapy for amphetamine dependent persons seeking treatment: a placebo-controlled trial. *J Addict Med*. 2017;11(3):197.

Rush CR, Stoops WW, Hays LR, et al: Risperidone attenuates the discriminative-stimulus effects of D-amphetamine in humans. *J Pharmacol Exp Ther*. 2003;306:195–204.

Ruttenber AJ, Lawler-Heavner J, Yin M, et al: Fatal excited delirium following cocaine use: epidemiologic findings provide new evidence for mechanisms of cocaine toxicity. *J Forensic Sci*. 1997;42:25–31.

Sangroula D, Motiwala F, Wagle B, Shah VC, Hagi K, Lippmann S. Modafinil treatment of cocaine dependence: a systematic review and meta-analysis. *Subst Use Misuse*. 2017;52(10):1292–1306.

Sartor CE, Kranzler HR, Gelernter J. Rate of progression from first use to dependence on cocaine or opioids: a cross-substance examination of associated demographic, psychiatric, and childhood risk factors. *Addictive behaviors*, 2014;39(2):473–479. https://doi.org/10.1016/j.addbeh.2013.10.021

Savoca R, Rentsch KM, Huber AR. Diagnostic efficiency of different amphetamine screening tests—the search for an optimal cutoff. *Clin Chem Lab Med*. 2004;42:1063–1065.

Schlaepfer TE, Pearlson GD, Wong DF, et al: Pet study of competition between intravenous cocaine and [C-11]raclopride at dopamine receptors in human subjects. *Am J Psychiatry*. 1997;154:1209–1213.

Schmitz JM, Averill P, Stotts AL, et al: Fluoxetine treatment of cocaine-dependent patients with major depressive disorder. *Drug Alcohol Depend*. 2001;63:207–214.

Schubiner H, Saules KK, Arfken CL, et al: Double-blind placebo-controlled trial of methylphenidate in the treatment of adult ADHD patients with comorbid cocaine dependence. *Exp Clin Psychopharmacol*. 2002;10:286–294.

Schuckit MA. Comorbidity between substance use disorders and psychiatric conditions. *Addiction*. 2006a;101:76–88.

Schuckit MA. *Drug and Alcohol Abuse: A Clinical Guide to Diagnosis and Treatment*. Boston: Springer; 2006b.

Schütz H, Erdmann F, Magiera E, Weiler G. Analytical confirmation of error in false positive amphetamine immunoassays and results. *Arch Kriminol*. 1998;201:93–96.

Schwartz EKC, Wolkowicz NR, De Aquino JP, MacLean RR, Sofuoglu M. Cocaine use disorder (CUD): current clinical perspectives. *Subst Abuse Rehabil*. 2022:25–46.

Shank RP, Gardocki JF, Streeter AJ, Maryanoff BE. An overview of the preclinical aspects of topiramate: pharmacology, pharmacokinetics, and mechanism of action. *Epilepsia*. 2000; 41:S3–S9.

Shanti CM, Lucas CE. Cocaine and the critical care challenge. *Crit Care Med*. 2003;31:1851–1859.

Shearer J, Wodak A, Mattick RP, et al: Pilot randomized controlled study of dexamphetamine substitution for amphetamine dependence. *Addiction*. 2001;96:1289–1296.

Shearer J, Wodak A, van Beek I, et al: Pilot randomized double blind placebo-controlled study of dexamphetamine for cocaine dependence. *Addiction*. 2003;98:1137–1141.

Shearer J, Darke S, Rodgers C, et al: A double-blind, placebo-controlled trial of modafinil (200 mg/day) for methamphetamine dependence. *Addiction*. 2009;104:224–233.

Shoptaw S, Heinzerling KG, Rotheram-Fuller E, et al: Bupropion hydrochloride versus placebo, in combination with cognitive behavioral therapy, for the treatment of cocaine abuse/dependence. *J Addict Dis*. 2008a;27:13–23.

Shoptaw S, Heinzerling KG, Rotheram-Fuller E, et al: Randomized, placebo-controlled trial of bupropion for the treatment of methamphetamine dependence. *Drug Alcohol Depend*. 2008b; 96:222–232.

Sinha R, Talih M, Malison R, et al: Hypothalamic-pituitary-adrenal axis and sympatho-adreno-medullary responses during stress-induced and drug cue-induced cocaine craving states. *Psychopharmacology*. 2003;170:62–72.

Sofuoglu M, Carroll KM. Effects of galantamine on cocaine use in chronic cocaine users. *Am J Addict*. 2011;20:302–303.

Sofuoglu M, Kosten TR. Emerging pharmacological strategies in the fight against cocaine addiction. *Expert Opin Emerg Drugs.* 2006;11:91–98.

Sofuoglu M, Sewell RA. Norepinephrine and stimulant addiction. *Addict Biol.* 14:119–129.

Sofuoglu M, Dudish-Poulsen S, Nelson D, et al: Sex and menstrual cycle differences in the subjective effects from smoked cocaine in humans. *Exp Clin Psychopharmacol.* 1999;7:274–283.

Sofuoglu M, Brown S, Babb DA, et al: Effects of labetalol treatment on the physiological and subjective response to smoked cocaine. *Pharmacol Biochem Behav.* 2000;65:255–259.

Sofuoglu M, Babb DA, Hatsukami DK. Effects of progesterone treatment on smoked cocaine response in women. *Pharmacol Biochem Behav.* 2002;72:431–435.

Sofuoglu M, Poling J, Mitchell E, Kosten TR. Tiagabine affects the subjective responses to cocaine in humans. *Pharmacol Biochem Behav.* 2005;82:569–573.

Sofuoglu M, DeVito EE, Waters AJ, Carroll KM. Cognitive enhancement as a treatment for drug addictions. *Neuropharmacology.* 2013;64:452–463.

Sofuoglu M, Poling J, Babuscio T, et al: Cavedilol does not reduce cocaine use in methadone-maintained cocaine users. *J Subst Abuse Treat.* 2016:63–69.

Sofuoglu M, DeVito EE, Kosten TR, et al: Neurobiology of stimulants. *The American Psychiatric Association Publishing Textbook of Substance Use Disorder Treatment* (2021).

Somoza EC, Winship D, Gorodetzky CW, et al: A multisite, double-blind, placebo-controlled clinical trial to evaluate the safety and efficacy of vigabatrin for treating cocaine dependence. *JAMA Psychiatry.* 2013;70:630–637.

Stitzer M, Petry N. Contingency management for treatment of substance abuse. *Annu Rev Clin Psychol.* 2006;2:411–434.

Stout PR, Klette KL, Wiegand R. Comparison and evaluation of DRI methamphetamine, DRI ecstasy, abuscreen online amphetamine, and a modified abuscreen online amphetamine screening immunoassays for the detection of amphetamine (AMP), methamphetamine (MTH), 3,4-methylenedioxyamphetamine (MDA), and 3,4-methylenedioxymethamphetamine (MDMA) in human urine. *J Anal Toxicol.* 2003;27:265–269.

Streeter CC, Terhune DB, Whitfield TH, et al: Performance on the Stroop predicts treatment compliance in cocaine-dependent individuals. *Neuropsychopharmacology.* 2008;33:827–836.

Substance Abuse and Mental Health Services Administration. (2022). Drug abuse warning network: findings from drug-related emergency department visits, 2021 (HHS Publication No. PEP22-07-03-002). Rockville, MD: Center for Behavioral Health Statistics and Quality, Substance Abuse and Mental Health Services Administration. Retrieved from https://www.samhsa.gov/data/.

Substance Abuse and Mental Health Services Administration. (2021). Key substance use and mental health indicators in the United States: results from the 2020 National Survey on Drug Use and Health (HHS Publication No. PEP21-07-01-003, NSDUH Series H-56). Rockville, MD: Center for Behavioral Health Statistics and Quality, Substance Abuse and Mental Health Services Administration. Retrieved from https://www.samhsa.gov/data/

Tardelli VS, Berro LF, Gerra G, et al: Prescription psychostimulants for cocaine use disorder: a review from molecular basis to clinical approach. *Addiction Biol.* 2023:28;e13271

Tardelli VS, Bisaga A, Arcadepani FB, et al: Prescription psychostimulants for the treatment of stimulant use disorder: a systematic review and meta-analysis. *Psychopharmacol.* 2020:237:2233–2255.

Tashkin DP. Airway effects of marijuana, cocaine, and other inhaled illicit agents. *Curr Opin Pulm Med.* 2001;7:43–61.

Tiihonen J, Kuoppasalmi K, Fohr J, et al: A comparison of aripiprazole, methylphenidate, and placebo for amphetamine dependence. *Am J Psychiatry.* 2007;164:160–162.

Trivedi MH, Walker R, Ling W, et al: Bupropion and naltrexone in methamphetamine use disorder. *N Engl J Med.* 2021;384(2):140–153.

Turkanis SA, Karler R. Electrophysiologic properties of the cannabinoids. *J Clin Pharmacol.* 1981;21:S449–S463.

Turnipseed SD, Richards JR, Kirk JD, et al: Frequency of acute coronary syndrome in patients presenting to the emergency department with chest pain after methamphetamine use. *J Emerg Med.* 2003;24:369–373.

Tzschentke TM, Schmidt WJ. Functional relationship among medial prefrontal cortex, nucleus accumbens, and ventral tegmental area in locomotion and reward. *Crit Rev Neurobiol.* 2000;14:131–142.

Uhl GR, Drgon T, Johnson C, et al: "Higher order" addiction molecular genetics: convergent data from genome-wide association in humans and mice. *Biochem Pharmacol.* 2008;75:98–111.

Verdejo-Garcia A, Lawrence AJ, Clark L. Impulsivity as a vulnerability marker for substance-use disorders: review of findings from high-risk research, problem gamblers and genetic association studies. *Neurosci Biobehav R.* 2008;32:777–810.

Verdejo-Garcia A, Betanzos-Espinosa P, Lozano OM, et al: Self-regulation and treatment retention in cocaine dependent individuals: a longitudinal study. *Drug Alcohol Depend.* 2012;122:142–148.

Volkow ND, Wang GJ, Fowler JS, et al: Decreased striatal dopaminergic responsiveness in detoxified cocaine-dependent subjects. *Nature.* 1997;386:830–833.

Volkow ND, Fowler JS, Wang G-J. The addicted human brain: insights from imaging studies. *J Clin Invest.* 2003;111:1444–1451.

Volkow ND, Wang GJ, Telang F, et al: Cocaine cues and dopamine in dorsal striatum: mechanism of craving in cocaine addiction. *J Neurosci.* 2006;26:6583–6588.

Vupputuri S, Batuman V, Muntner P, et al: The risk for mild kidney function decline associated with illicit drug use among hypertensive men. *Am J Kidney Dis.* 2004;43:629–635.

Wagner FA, Anthony JC. From first drug use to drug dependence: developmental periods of risk for dependence upon marijuana, cocaine, and alcohol. *Neuropsychopharmacology.* 2002;26:479–488.

Washio Y, Higgins ST, Heil SH, et al: Delay discounting is associated with treatment response among cocaine-dependent outpatients. *Exp Clin Psychopharmacol.* 2011;19(3):243–248. https://doi.org/10.1037/a0023617

Wearne TA, Cornish JL. A comparison of methamphetamine-induced psychosis and schizophrenia: a review of positive, negative, and cognitive symptomatology. *Front Psychiatry.* 2018;9:491.

White FJ, Kalivas PW. Neuroadaptations involved in amphetamine and cocaine addiction. *Drug Alcohol Depend.* 1998;51:141–153.

Williamson A, Darke S, Ross J, Teesson M. The effect of persistence of cocaine use on 12-month outcomes for the treatment of heroin dependence. *Drug Alcohol Depend.* 2006;81:293–300.

Williamson S, Gossop M, Powis B, et al: Adverse effects of stimulant drugs in a community sample of drug users. *Drug Alcohol Depend.* 1997;44:87–94.

Winhusen T, Somoza E, Ciraulo DA, et al: A double-blind, placebo-controlled trial of tiagabine for the treatment of cocaine dependence. *Drug Alcohol Depend.* 2007;91:141–148.

Winhusen TM, Somoza EC, Harrer JM, et al: A placebo-controlled screening trial of tiagabine, sertraline and donepezil as cocaine dependence treatments. *Addiction.* 2005;100:68–77.

Woicik PA, Moeller SJ, Alia-Klein N, et al: The neuropsychology of cocaine addiction: recent cocaine use masks impairment. *Neuropsychopharmacology.* 2009;34:1112–1122.

Wu LT, Woody GE, Yang CM, Blazer DG. How do prescription opioid users differ from users of heroin or other drugs in psychopathology: results from the National Epidemiologic Survey on Alcohol and Related Conditions. *J Addict Med.* 2011;5:28–35.

Xu J, DeVito EE, Worhunsky PD, et al: White matter integrity is associated with treatment outcome measures in cocaine dependence. *Neuropsychopharmacology.* 2010;35:1541–1549.

Yonkers KA, Forray A, Howell HB, et al: Motivational enhancement therapy coupled with cognitive behavioral therapy versus brief advice: a randomized trial for treatment of hazardous substance use in pregnancy and after delivery. *Gen Hosp Psychiatry.* 2012;34:439–449.

Zakzanis KK, Young DA. Memory impairment in abstinent MDMA ("ecstasy") users: a longitudinal investigation. *Neurology.* 2001;56:966–969.

Zuckerman M. *Sensation Seeking: Beyond the Optimum Level of Arousal.* Mahwah, NJ: Erlbaum; 1994.

Zweben JE, Cohen JB, Christian D, et al: Psychiatric symptoms in methamphetamine users. *Am J Addict.* 2004;13:181–190.

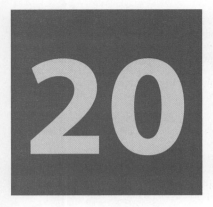

Tobacco Use Disorder

Judith Cooney, PhD
Christoffer Grant, PhD
Kristopher A. Kast, MD

Cigarette smoking is the leading cause of mortality in the United States, accounting for nearly 445,000 deaths, or one in five deaths per year (Centers for Disease Control and Prevention [CDC], 2009). This mortality rate continues to outpace deaths from alcohol and opioid use disorders combined, even with the recent rise in overdose deaths during the opioid crisis (CDC, 2021). Tobacco smokers tend to die prematurely, losing an average of about 14 years of life (CDC, 2009). Beyond mortality, smoking is linked to a large range of chronic and severe medical disorders that negatively impact health and function, including heart disease, cancer, pulmonary disease, infertility, sexual dysfunction. Encouragingly, U.S. smoking prevalence rates dropped from 50% in 1964 to 11.5–22% in 2021 (CDC, 2022; National Survey on Drug Use and Health [NSDUH], 2022). However, this prevalence still poses a large health and economic burden to smokers and to our society. Smoking prevalence rates are negatively correlated with education and socioeconomic status. Furthermore, smoking prevalence rates in individuals with psychiatric and substance use disorders are more than two to three times greater than rates among the general public (Lasser et al., 2000). Smokers with mental illness are large consumers of cigarettes, accounting for about 44% of all cigarettes smoked (Lasser et al., 2000).

▶ General Considerations

A. Epidemiology

Rates of tobacco use are reported by two national surveys collected by the CDC and Substance Abuse and Mental Health Services Administration (SAMHSA), the Behavior Risk Factor Surveillance System (BRFSS) and the NSDUH. The 2021 BRFSS reported 11.5% of all adults (age ≥ 18 years) smoke cigarettes (defined as persons who reported smoking at least 100 cigarettes during their lifetime and who, at the time of interview, reported smoking every day or some days), while the NSDUH reported 22% of adults used a tobacco product in the past month, including electronic nicotine delivery (vape) devices (CDC, 2022; NSDUH 2022). These rates have declined over the past 50 years, which is likely a response to improved education, treatment, and higher taxation. However, the difference between the BRFSS and NSDUH rates are partially attributable to detecting alternative forms of nicotine intake (e.g., e-cigarettes, smokeless tobacco, cigars, pipes, hookahs, bidis), which have increased in prevalence as regulations (e.g., indoor clean air laws) and taxation on cigarettes have increased.

In 2018, the U.S. Surgeon General issued an advisory on e-cigarette use among youth, responding to mounting epidemiologic evidence of unprecedented increases in use in this vulnerable population. In the most recent NSDUH data, 4.7% of Americans >12 years old used nicotine vaping devices in the past month (NSDUH, 2022). Of particular concern, recent surveys of youth suggest that electronic nicotine delivery devices (vapes) have been the most used tobacco product by individuals under 18 since 2014, with 11.3% of high school students reporting past month vaping in 2021 (MFS [Monitoring the Future Survey], 2019, NYTS [National Youth Tobacco Survey], 2019). And among all tobacco users age > 12 years, nicotine vaping is the second most common mode of delivery with 13.2 million users, behind cigarettes at 43.6 million users and ahead of cigars (10.3 million), smokeless (7.3 million), and pipe tobacco (1.3 million) (NSDUH, 2022). As the majority of nicotine intake is still accomplished with cigarettes, cigarette smoking is the focus of the bulk of this chapter (see Figure 20–1).

It is important to note that smoking rates are disproportionally stratified and are higher in groups with less education and lower income, as well as those with higher rates of psychiatric and substance diagnoses. Individuals with a psychiatric diagnosis (including mood, anxiety, psychosis, and substance use diagnoses) are nearly twice as likely to smoke cigarettes (41%) compared to those without a psychiatric diagnosis (22.5%) (Lasser et al., 2000). Smoking rates increase with more recent diagnosis and greater comorbidity of diagnoses. In addition, individuals with psychiatric diagnoses tend to be

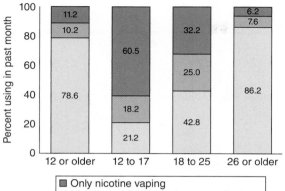

▲ **Figure 20–1** Type of nicotine product use among past-month nicotine users, as per NSDUH 2021.

heavier smokers (i.e., smoking more than 25 cigarettes per day), with rates from 15% to 30% compared with 10% of individuals with no history of psychiatric diagnosis.

Patients diagnosed with schizophrenia have particularly high levels of cigarette smoking. Previous reports have suggested that 80–90% of patients with schizophrenia are smokers, but more recent meta-analysis reveals the percentage to be around 62% (Chapman et al., 2009). Level of dependence appears to be related to increased negative, but not positive, symptoms (Patkar et al., 2002). Nicotine appears to have some effect on reducing positive symptoms by improving sensory gating (Lyon, 1999). This has implications for the treatment of patients with schizophrenia, in that addressing nicotine withdrawal in nonsmoking inpatient settings will be important to management of their symptoms. Providing nicotine replacement therapy (NRT) has been demonstrated to reduce agitation in the first 24 hours after forced abstinence (Allen et al., 2011).

A young cigarette smoker can begin to experience cravings within just 2 days of first inhaling. However, not all cigarette users who smoke regularly go on to develop nicotine dependence. Of persons who smoked daily for at least 1 month, between 66% and 71% met DSM-IV criteria for lifetime dependence (Hughes et al., 2006) and were more likely to be male, White, and have lower levels of education and personal income (Lopez-Quintero et al., 2011). Daily smokers smoke on average 15.1 cigarettes per day (CDC, 2011), a number that has steadily been declining. It is important to note that not all smokers smoke cigarettes daily.

Nicotine withdrawal is the effect felt by a person who has become nicotine dependent when they abruptly cease or cut down on their nicotine use. Withdrawal symptoms can begin in as little as 30 minutes and may last for weeks, although the acute effects are generally felt within the first 24 hours to 1 week. Withdrawal symptoms many manifest

themselves in a variety of ways from a mild craving to severe headaches (see DSM-5 criteria for Nicotine Withdrawal in Table 20–1).

B. Etiology & Course of Illness

The neurology of nicotine addiction has implicated several neural structures, transmitters, and receptors. Within about 10 seconds of smoking, nicotine crosses the blood-brain barrier and binds to the α4β2 nicotinic acetylcholine receptors (α4β2 nACHr) located in the ventral tegmental area. This results in increased dopamine levels in the nucleus accumbens, which is responsible for the rewarding effects of nicotine (Ray et al., 2008). In addition, there appears to be reduced gamma-aminobutyric acid (GABA) inhibitory tone as well as release of endogenous opioid peptides, which further increases dopamine.

Progression to tolerance and dependence occurs over time, and there are a host of complex factors that make persons vulnerable to initiating, maintaining, and developing dependence on nicotine. It begins as a social ritual influenced by peer groups, with a risk mitigating effect of parental oversight limiting access. Those initiated to cigarette smoking before age 17 are more than 50% as likely to become nicotine-dependent compared to those who are initiated after age 17, highlighting the public health risks of the rising nicotine vaping rates among adolescents. It is also clear, as noted earlier, that there are correlates with gender, ethnicity, and social inequality.

Over a period of years, the reinforcing effects of smoking begin to shift from positive reinforcement (i.e., experiencing the acute pleasurable effects of nicotine, enhancement of social contexts) to negative reinforcement (i.e., smoking to relieve withdrawal symptoms). The half-life of nicotine is relatively rapid (approximately 2 hours), meaning that dependence may occur in a short period of time because of the frequent need to resupply α4β2 nACHr agonism with inhaled nicotine. Although this progression occurs in most people in whom dependence occurs over time, it does not happen for everyone. It is unclear what differentiates those who go on to develop nicotine dependence from those who do not, or those who consider themselves social smokers or "chippers." Only 5–15% of smokers have five or fewer cigarettes a day, and the neurobiologic differences among this group are poorly understood, although they do tend to be younger, and many are in college, where this practice is more acceptable (Levinson et al., 2007). Some researchers theorize that this population of smokers is merely early in their dependence, whereas others maintain that confining cigarettes to certain settings or times of day is possible for a small subset of the population.

C. Genetics

Twin studies have documented the heritability of smoking initiation and nicotine dependence. Approximately 60% of the variability in smoking initiation is thought to

Table 20–1 Nicotine-Related Signs and Symptoms

	Signs	Symptoms
Poisoning (CDC) (may mimic nerve agent or organophosphate poisoning)	May include: Vomiting Diarrhea Tachycardia and hypertension Bradycardia and hypotension (in severe cases) Breathing difficulties Mental confusion Muscle twitches or convulsions Diaphoresis	May include: Physical symptoms: • Weakness • Nausea, abdominal cramping • Dizziness • Headaches • Gastrointestinal distress Mental symptoms • Restlessness, anxiety, depression
Dependence (Surgeon General)	May include: Highly controlled or compulsive use Stereotyped patterns of use Use despite harmful effects Relapse following abstinence Smoking more in morning Smoking even if ill in bed	May include: Physical symptoms: • Increased tolerance • Physical withdrawal symptoms at times (see below) Mental symptoms: • Recurrent cravings • Persistent desire or unsuccessful efforts to cut down or control use
Withdrawal (CDC and DSM-5)	May include: Diaphoresis Coughing, signs of cold Mental confusion Falling heart rate and blood pressure	May include: Physical symptoms: • Tingling in hands and feet • Nausea, abdominal cramps • Headaches • Sore throat Mental symptoms: • Increased appetite • Irritability, anxiety, depression • Difficulty concentrating • Insomnia

result from genetic influences. Twenty percent is thought to be due to shared environment and the remaining 20% due to individual specific variables (Sullivan & Kendler, 1999). There appears to be a partial overlap when it comes to susceptibility to nicotine dependence, where approximately 50% of the variability can be attributed to genetic vulnerabilities (Li, 2006).

Although evidence of contribution of specific genes is still limited, genotyping studies have indicated several specific genes including CHRNA5, which may be partially responsible for the initial pleasure experienced on smoking initiation. Other genome association studies have identified CHRNA3, CHRNB4, CHRNA6, CHRNB3, and CHRNA4 as playing a role in nicotine addiction and dependence (Prom-Wormley et al., 2017).

Gene polymorphisms may also play a role in treatment selection and likelihood of success. For example, variants of dopamine receptor DRD2 and DRD4 resulting in decreased dopamine in the mesolimbic system were associated with a modest but statistically significant increased risk of relapse in the short-term following a smoking cessation attempt (David et al., 2008). In addition, individuals with a specific polymorphism of CHRNA4, rs2236196, experience greater sensitivity to the effects of nicotine. Individuals with this polymorphism demonstrate improved treatment response to nicotinic nasal spray, likely due to the relatively fast-acting effect of this treatment modality as compared to the patch. Further evidence of specific polymorphisms predicting response to pharmacotherapy suggests that individuals with the CYP2B6*4 variant have an attenuated response to bupropion for smoking cessation compared to wild type (King et al., 2012; Tomaz et al., 2015).

At this point in time, the genetic influence on smoking cessation and maintenance is apparent. However, as with other complex polygenic disorders, the effect sizes of each genetic locus are relatively small (Prom-Wormley et al., 2017). In addition, the phenotypic expression of these genes and how these may influence treatment decision making is a complex area in need of considerable further research.

▶ Clinical Findings

A. Psychological Testing

In this section we report on specific brief, easy-to-administer tests that can assess for key smoking variables relevant to tobacco treatment.

1. Nicotine dependence—Individuals with higher levels of nicotine dependence may have greater difficulty in quitting, and therefore assessment of nicotine dependence may inform treatment intensity. The Fagerström Test of Nicotine Dependence (FTND; Heatherton et al., 1991) is a six-item inventory that measures aspects related to nicotine dependence. A shorter version, the Heaviness of Smoking Index (HSI; Heatherton et al., 1989) further condenses assessment to two items: time to first morning cigarette (within 30 minutes of awakening), and number of cigarettes smoked per day (25 cigarettes or more). The FTND and HSI have good internal consistency, are easy to administer, and are commonly used measures of severity of nicotine dependence and smoking severity.

2. Motivation to quit smoking—A smoker's current and proximal motivation for cessation directly affects type of treatments delivered and predicts treatment engagement and response. The Contemplation Ladder is a paper-pencil measure that provides a continuous measure of readiness to quit smoking, displayed on an 11-point Likert scale in the form of a ladder. Higher rungs on the ladder correspond with greater motivation for change. The Contemplation Ladder has demonstrated good predictive and concurrent validity in relation to an individual's likelihood of making a serious quit attempt within 6 months (Biemer & Abrams, 1991).

3. Past Quit Attempts—The longest length of past quit attempts (1 year or longer) and the length of recent quit attempts (5–14 days quit in most recent attempt) have been found to be indicators of a smoker's success in quitting (Farkas et al., 1996). Based on those data, the authors recommend four questions as valid brief assessments of past quit attempts:

1. How many serious quit attempts have you made in the past?
2. What was the longest amount of time that you were able to quit?
3. When was your most recent serious attempt to quit smoking?
4. How long were you abstinent in your most recent quit attempt?

4. Urges to Smoke—Assessment of urges to smoke inform treatment and detail expectancies of smoking. The Tiffany Questionnaire of Smoking Urges (QSU—brief; Cox et al., 2001) is a 10-item questionnaire that evaluates the structure and function of smoking urges. Subjects are asked to indicate on a 7-point Likert-type scale how strongly they agree or disagree with each statement on the questionnaire. The QSU scale characterizes urges to smoke in response to two separate affective systems: a negative affect related to relief of withdrawal, and positive affect related to expectancy of reinforcement.

B. Laboratory Findings

Biochemical verification of smoking and nicotine use is helpful to inform the level of tobacco use and to confirm self-reported smoking status in treatment. Breath carbon monoxide (CO) is a reliable and sensitive measure of recent smoking. Using a breath CO monitor to measure a smoker's expired air provides an easy, rapid, noninvasive, and relatively low-cost method for biochemical verification of smoking status. CO monitors are widely used in clinical and research settings. Breath CO readings of 8–10 parts per million (ppm) typically indicate smoking within the last 8–12 hours (Benowitz et al., 2002). However, because CO has a short half-life of 2–3 hours, breath CO readings are less valid in assessing for distal smoking or differentiating between short-term and long-term smoking abstinence. In the absence of smoking, elevated CO levels may be a result of passive smoking or environmental exposure to pollutants. Cotinine, a metabolite of nicotine, has a longer 16-hour half-life that allows for a useful measurement of ongoing smoking status. Salivary and blood cotinine levels are well correlated ($r = 0.82$–0.90; Jarvis et al., 1984). Cotinine levels may peak several hours after smoking a cigarette, with levels of 14 ng/mL typically indicating a smoking episode (Benowitz et al., 2002). Cotinine levels of 100 ng/mL roughly correspond to smoking consumption levels of 10 cigarettes per day (Benowitz, 1996), and regular smokers typically have cotinine levels of about 100–300 ng/mL, although individual variability may be substantial. In chronic smokers, cotinine levels may be measurable for up to 7 days following the last cigarette, thereby allowing greater measurement of nicotine use and long-term abstinence. Cotinine levels often require laboratory analysis, making it an expensive and slow means to verify smoking status. Dipstick semiquantitative measurement of salivary and urinary cotinine (e.g., NicAlert) has been found to be a sensitive and specific measurement that is well correlated with breath CO in predicting self-reported smoking status (Marrone et al., 2010; Schepis et al., 2008). Compared to laboratory analyzed blood and salivary cotinine measurement, semiquantitative dipstick measurement of salivary and urinary cotinine provides a more rapid and costly assessment of cotinine and therefore has greater utility in the clinical setting. The limitation of cotinine is that it measures nicotine levels specifically and does not differentiate between nicotine levels resulting from smoking and those from medicinal nicotine. Obtaining levels of urinary anabasine and anatabine, which are tobacco alkaloids, allows for longer-term measurement of tobacco use in individuals receiving nicotine replacement (Jacob et al., 2002). However, this is a laboratory measure not currently adapted for rapid and low-cost use in the clinic setting.

C. Neuroimaging

Neuroimaging studies suggest that over time in smokers compared to nonsmokers there is reduced density of gray matter and more nACH receptors in the brain (McClernon, 2009).

In addition, positron emission tomography (PET) scans show significantly lower levels of monoamine oxidase B (MAO B), a neurotransmitter involved in the breakdown of dopamine (Fowler et al., 1996). Dopamine has been implicated in appetitive behaviors (Salamone & Correa, 2002), which suggests a neurochemical mechanism responsible for the rewarding and reinforcing effects of smoking. In addition, cigarette smoking has been demonstrated to release dopamine in the left ventral basal ganglia (Scott et al., 2007) and specifically in the ventral striatum/nucleus accumbens (Brody et al., 2004).

When nonsmokers are administered nicotine, there is a reduction in cerebral metabolism in most brain regions. However, administration of nicotine to smokers causes increased activation in several brain areas, including the frontal lobes, amygdala, hypothalamus, limbic thalamus, insula, anterior and posterior cingulate cortex, and nucleus accumbens (Stein et al., 1998). Therefore, it appears that smoking history moderates brain activation when exposed to nicotine.

Abstinence—When a person tries to quit, α4β2 nACH receptors go unoccupied, and this lack of occupation appears to be responsible for the strong craving that the abstainer experiences. Of note, the binding potential of these receptors has been demonstrated to decrease to levels of nonsmokers after a period of 3 weeks (Mamede et al., 2007), at which point the physiological craving may be greatly reduced.

Smoking abstinence significantly alters brain functioning for a period of time following cessation. There is a reduction in cerebral blood flow (Wang et al., 2007) but increased responsiveness to smoking cues in the prefrontal and parietal cortex, as well as in dorsal brain structures involved in learning and reward (McClernon et al., 2007). Therefore, exposure to smoking-related cues (e.g., temporal cues, people, and objects associated with smoking) may significantly increase likelihood of lapse and relapse.

▶ Differential Diagnosis

Thirteen percent of smokers do not admit to their physician that they smoke cigarettes, with higher nondisclosure rates perhaps due to stigma, among pregnant women, estimated to be 23% in one study (Dietz et al., 2010; Legacy, 2012). Although this number is much lower than for alcohol and other substance use (National Center on Addiction and Substance Abuse, 2000), it still represents a substantial minority of patients who in most cases state that they do not want to be lectured to about their habit. In these cases, having an open and compassionate attitude while being aware of the signs and symptoms of nicotine use disorder and withdrawal may make patients more receptive to discussing their smoking.

In addition, signs of nicotine use disorder and withdrawal can often mimic other psychiatric or medical conditions and may therefore be prone to misinterpretation. As can be seen in Table 20–1 (signs and symptoms), the list of potential conditions or disorders that have overlapping signs and symptoms with nicotine poisoning, use disorder, and withdrawal is endless. However, it is important to be aware that certain psychiatric conditions increase risk for nicotine use disorder (e.g., panic disorder and generalized anxiety disorder; Moylan et al., 2012) and that the presentation of these conditions may be similar, as they all promote sympathetic nervous system arousal.

▶ Treatment

The 2018 American College of Cardiology consensus statement on tobacco cessation treatment transitioned the clinical approach to tobacco use disorder from a sometimes elusive "readiness for a quit attempt" negotiation to a "prescribe first" paradigm (ACC 2018). Previous clinical approaches tended to focus on motivating individuals to set a "quit date" prior to initiating pharmacotherapy. The 2018 ACC recommendations suggest that pharmacotherapy be initiated at the time of diagnosis with tobacco use disorder, increasing the proportion of patients receiving effective pharmacotherapy and assisting patients in reducing tobacco use, moving toward cessation.

The U.S. Public Health Service Clinical Practice Guideline "Treating Tobacco Use and Dependence, 2008 Update" (Fiore et al., 2009) reports on effective evidence-based tobacco treatments. This third edition of the guideline presents an update distilled from more than 8700 clinical research trials published between 1975 and 2007. The main findings include:

1. Tobacco dependence is seen as a chronic and recurring disorder with periods of relapse and remission. Multiple and repeated treatments are often needed. Effective treatments, such as those endorsed in the clinical practice guidelines, significantly increase the likelihood of long-term tobacco abstinence.

2. Every tobacco smoker seen in a health care setting should be screened for current tobacco use, and smoking status should be documented. At each session, every smoker should be assessed for motivation to quit smoking and advised to quit.

3. All smokers should be offered evidence-based smoking cessation medications to assist in quitting.

4. Brief interventions given by physicians and nonmedical clinicians are effective treatments, and all smokers should be offered at least brief interventions (≤3 minutes).

5. There is a dose–response relationship between intensity of behavioral counseling and treatment effectiveness. Effective behavioral interventions can be delivered in individual, group, and telephone formats.

6. Evidence-based medications and behavioral interventions are each effective for tobacco; however, a combination of medication and behavioral interventions is more effective than either type of treatment alone. Clinicians should encourage smokers to use both medication and counseling approaches to assist in quitting.

A. Pharmacological Interventions

U.S. Public Health Service (USPHS) clinical practice guidelines suggest that every smoker who is motivated to quit should be offered evidence-based smoking cessation medications, except in cases of contraindications, or for groups of smokers for which effectiveness has not been demonstrated (e.g., adolescent smokers, pregnant women). Guidelines recommend seven frontline FDA-approved smoking cessation medications, including five nicotine replacement therapies (nicotine patch, gum, lozenge, nasal spray, and inhaler), bupropion, and varenicline. Table 20–2 shows data from the 2008 USPHS clinical practice guidelines on the effectiveness and abstinence rates of FDA-approved tobacco cessation medications relative to placebo at 6 months (Fiore et al., 2009). Estimated odds ratios are presented with 95% confidence intervals, and estimated abstinence rates are shown in percent. These data suggest that, compared to placebo, most monotherapies are associated with a general doubling to tripling of quit rates at 6 months. All combination therapies listed were associated with at least a doubling of quit rates relative to placebo, with nicotine patch + long-term ad lib NRT (gum, lozenge, spray) associated with more than triple quit rates at 6 months. Therapies associated with significantly greater quit rates relative to nicotine patch alone are varenicline 2 mg and combination nicotine patch + long-term ad lib NRT (Fiore et al., 2009).

1. Nicotine replacement therapy—A regular smoker who abruptly stops tobacco use often experiences nicotine withdrawal symptoms, including restlessness, irritability, impatience, concentration impairment, increased appetite, mood and sleep disturbance, and craving. These symptoms are uncomfortable and may lead the smoker back to smoking to resolve withdrawal symptoms. Nicotine replacement therapy is an agonist therapy that serves to replace nicotine and attenuate nicotine withdrawal symptoms. Cigarette smoking delivers rapid and high peak plasma nicotine concentrations, making it an efficient nicotine delivery system. In comparison, NRT formulations generally deliver slower and lower peak plasma nicotine concentrations (30–75% of nicotine levels achieved by smoking cigarettes). Because of this different absorption pattern, NRT products are associated with lower nicotine neuroadaptation compared to inhaled tobacco products. Of the NRT formulations, absorption of nicotine is fastest with nicotine nasal spray, followed by comparable and moderate absorption rates in nicotine gum, lozenge, and inhaler, and is slowest with nicotine patch. Standard dosing regimens per clinical practice guidelines (Fiore et al., 2009) are described next. Given their demonstrated efficacy, safety, and availability, NRTs are considered a mainstay of smoking cessation treatments. NRT underutilization and early treatment discontinuation are common and can undermine treatment efficacy. Emerging data suggest that pretreatment

Table 20–2 Effectiveness and Abstinence Rates of Tobacco Use Monotherapies and Combination Therapies Versus Placebo at 6 Months ($N = 83$ Studies)

Medication	Estimated Odds Ratio	Estimated Abstinence Rates
Placebo	1.0	13.8
Nicotine patch (6–14 weeks)	1.9 (1.7–2.2)	23.4
Nicotine patch, long term (>14 weeks)	1.9 (1.7–2.3)	23.7
Nicotine patch, high dose (>25 mg)	2.3 (1.7–3.0)	26.5
Nicotine gum (6–14 weeks)	1.5 (1.2–1.7)	19.0
Nicotine gum, long term (>14 weeks)	2.2 (1.5–3.2)	26.1
Nicotine lozenge (2 mg)*	2.0 (1.4–2.8)	24.2
Nicotine inhaler	2.1 (1.5–2.9)	24.8
Nicotine nasal spray	2.3 (1.7–3.0)	26.7
Bupropion SR	2.0 (1.8–2.2)	24.2
Varenicline (1 mg)	2.1 (1.5–3.0)	25.4
Varenicline (2 mg)	3.1 (2.5–3.8)	33.2
Nicotine patch (18–24 weeks) + NRT PRN (gum, lozenge, spray 26–52 weeks)	3.6 (2.5–5.2)	36.5
Nicotine patch + nicotine inhaler	2.2 (1.3–3.6)	25.8
Nicotine patch + bupropion	2.5 (1.9–3.4)	28.9

*Data reflect one trial only.

use of NRT may improve a smoker's readiness to quit (Carpenter et al., 2011).

i. Nicotine patch—Transdermal nicotine patches deliver a steady state of nicotine for a 24-hour period and are available over the counter (OTC) in 21 mg, 14 mg, and 7 mg strengths. Standard dosing taper for individuals smoking 10 or more cigarettes per day is 21 mg per day for 4–6 weeks, 14 mg per day for 2 weeks, then 7 mg per day for 2 weeks. Standard dosing taper for individuals smoking less than 10 cigarettes daily is 14 mg per day for 6 weeks, then 7 mg per day for 2 weeks. As a monotherapy, longer-term patch dosing (>14 weeks) has not been found to be associated with significantly higher quit rates than standard patch dosing. Although clinical practice guidelines do not find higher dose (>25 mg) patches to be associated with higher abstinence rates than standard patches overall, some data suggest that higher dose patches may assist heavy smokers who have failed or have strong withdrawal symptoms because of being underdosed on a single patch (Dale et al., 1995; Hughes, 1995). High-dose nicotine patch has been shown to be well tolerated and safe for individuals who smoke more than 20 cigarettes per day and at dosing levels up to 63 mg per day (Dale et al., 1995; Frederickson et al., 1995; Zevin et al., 1998). To optimize nicotine patch dosing, baseline serum cotinine levels can be taken during ad lib smoking, and then again after the individual reaches steady state on nicotine patch (typically around 3 days after smoking cessation and use of nicotine patch). At that point, nicotine patch dosing can be readjusted to replace nicotine to baseline levels. Rough guidelines for initial patch dosing based on baseline cotinine levels are: 14–21 mg/day for cotinine level < 200 ng/mL, 21–42 mg day for cotinine level 200–300 ng/mL, and ≥42 mg/day for cotinine level >300.

Smokers were previously instructed to start nicotine patches on their quit day. However, initiating treatment regardless of quit date is now recommended by the 2018 ACC consensus statement. Patches should be applied between waist and neck on a non-hairy spot and worn for 24 hours. They may need to be discontinued during hours of sleep when used in psychiatric patients due to vivid dreams or nightmares (see below). One patch should be used per day for the duration of the scheduled course of treatment, and early discontinuation of patch should be discouraged.

Common side effects of nicotine patch include local skin irritation, which may occur in 30–50% of patch users. Most skin reactions are minor and respond to treatment with topical hydrocortisone cream (1%); however, some skin reactions are nonresponsive or severe and may require patch discontinuation. To reduce likelihood of skin irritation, patch users are instructed to apply the patch to a different site each day, not returning to a site for 7 days. Another side effect is vivid dreams, which may occur in about 10% of patch users. Often these dreams may diminish after several days' use; if they persist, the individual can remove the patch before sleep. However, this may diminish the impact of NRT, as nicotine patch

treatment formulated for 24-hour use (21 mg/24 hours) has been associated with greater relief of nicotine withdrawal and craving compared to patches formulated for 16-hour use (15 mg/16 hours) (Shiffman et al., 2000).

Based on review of scientific studies and safety reports, the FDA has recently updated labeling for OTC NRT reflecting decreased safety concerns (FDA, 2013). If unable to completely quit immediately or if they relapse to cigarettes, smokers should continue to use NRT and continue with their smoking cessation efforts. Patients are advised to complete NRT treatment and to consult with their providers if they need longer durations of NRT, acknowledging the need for some patients to have treatment for periods as long as 1 year.

The most recent ACOG committee opinion on tobacco cessation in pregnancy outlines the risk calculus to be reviewed with pregnant individuals experiencing ongoing tobacco use (ACOG, 2020). This opinion recommends individualized care that includes information about psychosocial, behavioral, and pharmacologic interventions, including nicotine replacement. The opinion discusses the mixed evidence for NRT in pregnancy and suggests that NRT should be "considered only after a detailed discussion with the patient of the known risks of continued smoking, the possible risks of nicotine replacement therapy, and need for close supervision" while on treatment. Pregnant smokers should be encouraged to stop smoking using behavioral strategies.

Despite initial concerns with smokers with cardiovascular disease, research has shown that treatment with 14- to 21-mg nicotine patches was not associated with increased adverse cardiovascular events for this population (e.g., Joseph et al., 1996). Although product information on nicotine patches includes a caution for use in smokers with cardiovascular disease, the USPHS clinical practice guideline summarizes that NRT is not a risk factor for acute cardiovascular effects. It recommends that NRT be used with caution in individuals who have had acute myocardial infarction within 2 weeks and in those with unstable angina and serious arrhythmias. Initiation of lower dosing (e.g., 14 mg per day) may be indicated with those smokers.

ii. Nicotine gum—Nicotine gum is an OTC preparation that is available in 2- and 4-mg strengths. It delivers nicotine through buccal absorption at peak levels well below that delivered by cigarette smoking. As a monotherapy, standard dosing is 4 mg for individuals smoking 25 or more cigarettes per day, and 2 mg for individuals smoking less than that amount. Smokers are encouraged to use at least 10 pieces per day and up to approximately 20 pieces per day, with scheduled use of 1 piece every 1–2 hours for 6 weeks, then 1 piece every 2–4 hours for 3 weeks, then 1 piece every 4–8 hours for 3 weeks, as well as ad lib smoking for breakthrough withdrawal and craving. Usual duration of nicotine gum treatment is 6–14 weeks; however, longer duration of gum treatment (>14 weeks) has been associated with higher quit rates. Combination therapy of nicotine patch + gum has been associated with higher quit rates than nicotine gum used as monotherapy. When used in combination with patch, nicotine gum is typically dosed at 2 mg, and individuals are encouraged to use gum as needed (up to 20 pieces per day) for withdrawal, craving, and in high-risk smoking situations. When used in combination, often nicotine patches and gum are administered for 8–12 weeks together, and gum continues to be used alone for additional periods of 12 weeks or longer according to the patient's need. Individuals using nicotine gum must be instructed in the "chew and park" method of use for proper release of nicotine. Gum is to be chewed until it releases a peppery taste or tingling sensation in the mouth, and then parked between gum and cheek until this sensation subsides. This process is then repeated many times for up to 30 minutes per piece of gum, or until taste and sensation no longer return. Absorption of nicotine is reduced by an acidic pH environment in the mouth, and therefore gum users should be instructed to not drink or eat for approximately 15 minutes before and after using gum. Underutilization of gum, in both amount and duration of treatment, is associated with lower quit rates and should be discouraged.

Common side effects of nicotine gum are soreness in mouth and teeth, jaw ache, hiccups and stomach upset. These may be temporary and improved by proper use of the "chew and park" method. Smokers with dentures or weak teeth may have difficulty using nicotine gum.

iii. Nicotine lozenge—Similar to nicotine gum, nicotine lozenge is an OTC agent available in 2- and 4-mg strengths, which delivers nicotine through buccal absorption. Standard dosing is based on time to first cigarette (a marker of nicotine dependence), with 4 mg lozenge used in individuals who smoke within 30 minutes of awakening and 2 mg lozenge used for those who smoke after 30 minutes. As a monotherapy, nicotine lozenge is used on a similar schedule to gum: 1 piece every 1–2 hours for 6 weeks, then 1 piece every 2–4 hours for 3 weeks, then 1 piece every 4–8 hours for 3 weeks. When initiating the first phase of monotherapy, it is recommended that at least 9 pieces be used per day, with a maximum of up to 20 pieces for up to 12 weeks' duration. When used as a combination therapy along with nicotine patch, it is recommended that 2 mg lozenge be used as needed for management of withdrawal, craving, and high-risk relapse situations. Individuals using nicotine lozenge should be instructed to allow the lozenge to dissolve slowly in the mouth, and to not chew it or swallow it whole. To not reduce transbuccal absorption, users should not drink or eat for about 15 minutes before or after use of nicotine lozenge. Because of its simpler method of use, compliance for nicotine lozenge may be better than for nicotine gum.

Common side effects of nicotine lozenge may be nausea, hiccups, indigestion and heartburn; 4 mg lozenge may be associated with experience of coughing and headaches.

Lozenge users should be advised in proper method of use, which may attenuate incidence of side effects.

iv. Nicotine nasal spray—Nicotine nasal spray is available by prescription only and delivers nicotine through the nasal mucosa at more rapid rates than other medicinal nicotine delivery systems. Each spray delivers 0.5 mg nicotine dose to each nostril for a total dose of 1.0 mg. When used as a monotherapy, initial dosing may be scheduled at 1–2 doses per hour, with recommended daily doses ranging from 8 (minimum) to 40 (maximum) doses per day. Guidelines recommend a treatment duration of 12–24 weeks of ad lib use, with taper of treatment near the end of its course to avoid potential of nicotine dependency. Nicotine nasal spray has been shown to be an effective ad lib agent when used in combination with nicotine patch. Nasal spray users should be instructed to tilt head back when using spray, to breathe through the mouth, and not to sniff nor inhale through the nose when administering spray.

The most common side effect listed in the package insert is nasal irritation, with 94% of users reporting moderate to severe irritation within the first few days of use and 81% of users reporting mild to moderate symptoms after 3 weeks of use. Other common side effects include runny nose, throat irritation, watery eyes, sneezing, coughing, and headaches. Side effects generally diminish over time and can be reduced by proper administration of spray. Despite being an effective smoking cessation agent, tolerability profiles and availability by prescription only may contribute to relatively lower use compared to OTC nicotine replacement products.

USPHS clinical practice guidelines recommend that nicotine nasal spray should not be used in individuals with severe reactive airway disease (Fiore et al., 2009).

v. Nicotine inhaler—Nicotine inhaler is a prescription-only agent that delivers nicotine vapor, which more accurately is absorbed through the oral mucosa. Cartridges are inserted into the plastic inhaler, which contain 10 mg but only delivers 4 mg nicotine (over 80 inhalations), as a small amount of the vapor actually reaches the lungs. As a monotherapy, the recommended dose is use of 6–16 cartridges per day for duration of up to 6 months. Tapering is recommended over the final 3 months of treatment. Nicotine inhaler ad lib use may be used in combination with steady-state nicotine patch. Although use of nicotine inhalers mimics hand-to-mouth behaviors of smoking, the recommended method of inhaler puffing is different from that of the deeper and longer inhalation on a cigarette. Inhaler users should be instructed to use short and frequent puffs for 15–20 minutes. The bioavailability of nicotine in inhalers is compromised when ambient temperatures are below 40°F; therefore, inhaler and cartridge products should be kept and used indoors in cold temperatures. To reduce interference with buccal absorption, food and drink should be avoided 15 minutes before and after inhaler use.

Common side effects noted in packet inserts are mouth and throat irritation, coughing, and runny nose, which were noted in 40%, 32%, and 23% respectively. These symptoms are generally rated as mild and diminish over time of use.

2. Bupropion—Bupropion is a nonnicotine prescription agent that is a dopaminergic antidepressant. Its mechanism of action is thought to block reuptake of dopamine and norepinephrine in primary reward centers, and it may also serve as a nicotine antagonist at the α4β2 receptor site (Slemmer et al., 2000). Studies have shown bupropion SR 150–300 mg per day to be effective for smoking cessation and associated with lower weight gain at 300 mg per day dosing (Hurt et al., 1997). An early randomized controlled trial found that bupropion alone was more effective than patch alone and as effective as patch + bupropion combined (Jorenby et al., 1999); however, subsequent research has led to clinical practice guidelines suggesting added benefit of combining bupropion SR and nicotine patch (Fiore et al., 2009). Bupropion SR has been shown to be an effective smoking treatment in smokers with cardiovascular disease and pulmonary disease (Tonstad et al., 2003; Tashkin et al., 2001), and as effective in smokers with and without a history of depression (Cox et al., 2004; Hayford et al., 1999). Standard dosing is to pretreat and titrate bupropion SR for 1–2 weeks before the targeted tobacco quit date, initiating with 150 mg/day for 3 days, then increasing to 150 mg twice per day. Duration of treatment is typically 7–12 weeks; however, longer duration of treatment (up to 6 months) of bupropion SR 150 mg/day dosing may be considered for maintenance of tobacco abstinence. Relevant to the treatment of smokers with history of depression, one study showed no drug-drug interaction when using bupropion SR for smoking cessation in individuals already receiving tricyclic antidepressants and selective serotonin reuptake inhibitors (SSRIs) (Chengappa et al., 2001); however, monitoring of side effects for those receiving more than one antidepressant would be advised.

Common side effects of bupropion SR are dry mouth (10%) and insomnia (35–40%), and users are recommended to take the last dosing several hours before bedtime to attenuate sleep disturbance effects. To minimize possibility of seizure, individuals are encouraged to moderate alcohol use while taking bupropion.

Bupropion is relatively contraindicated in individuals with history of seizures or eating disorders and is absolutely contraindicated in those taking MAO inhibitors or other forms of bupropion. Bupropion has no known risk of fetal anomalies or adverse pregnancy effects, though studies in pregnant patients are limited (ACOG 2020). An FDA black box warning was issued in February 2008 warning that changes in behavior, depressed mood, agitation, hostility, and suicidal thoughts and behavior had been reported in patients attempting to quit smoking while using bupropion. This black box warning was removed in 2016 after incorporating findings from a large multisite international trial demonstrating no significant increase in neuropsychiatric adverse events attributable to varenicline or bupropion relative to nicotine patch or placebo (Anthenelli et al., 2016).

3. Varenicline—Varenicline (Chantix), a prescription drug specifically developed for smoking cessation, is an α4β2 partial agonist. Varenicline stimulates release of dopamine (at levels lower and longer than for nicotine), thereby reducing nicotine craving and withdrawal, and blocks further nicotine binding at the α4β2 site, thereby reducing the rewarding effects of cigarette smoking. Studies have found 12 weeks of varenicline treatment to be associated with greater short-term tobacco abstinence than 12 weeks of placebo or bupropion SR (Gonzales et al., 2006; Jorenby et al., 2006). In a maintenance trial, individuals treated with varenicline for an additional 12 weeks (24 weeks total) had significantly higher tobacco abstinence rates at weeks 13–24 and at 1 year than did individuals treated with 12 weeks of varenicline (Tonstad et al., 2006). Varenicline has been associated with greater tobacco abstinence than placebo in a population of stable schizophrenic smokers (Williams et al., 2012). Further, the largest trial including all available pharmacotherapies for tobacco cessation demonstrated superiority for varenicline over bupropion, NRT monotherapy, and placebo (Anthenelli et al., 2016). The standard dosing regimen includes pretreatment and titration of varenicline 7 days before the targeted quit date, though it may be initiated without a specific quit date being set (that is, during continued tobacco use). Recommended dosing is varenicline 0.5 mg per day for days 1–3, then 0.5 mg twice per day for days 4–7, then 1.0 mg twice per day starting on day 8 (quit day) for a total of 12 weeks. Individuals who successfully quit with 12 weeks of treatment may be treated for another 12 weeks to better maintain tobacco abstinence.

A common side effect of varenicline is nausea (30%), which in early trials was found to be short term, mild to moderate in severity, and associated with a relatively small (>3%) medication discontinuation rate. Other common side effects include gastrointestinal distress, insomnia, and vivid dreams. Individuals taking varenicline should be encouraged to take their medication on a full stomach and with water to reduce nausea, and to take the evening dose at dinnertime rather than bedtime to reduce the chance of insomnia. Based on post marketing reports, FDA added a February 2008 warning of significant psychiatric symptoms and suicidal thoughts and behavior in individuals using varenicline and encouraged careful monitoring of psychiatric symptoms, particularly in individuals with psychiatric histories. Subsequent studies of smokers with a mental health diagnosis (Stapleton et al., 2008), in a large general-practice research data base (Gunnell et al., 2009), and with stable schizophrenia (Williams et al., 2012) have not found varenicline to be associated with significant increases in psychiatric risk. Retrospective review studies conducted in the Veterans Administration and Department of Defense health care systems compared large cohorts of smokers prescribed varenicline versus NRT and found no difference in psychiatric hospitalizations within 30 days of initiating medication (Meyer et al., 2013). Anthenelli and colleagues (2016) further investigated psychiatric safety and efficacy of varenicline, bupropion and nicotine patch in a recent large international multi-cite trial with more than 8000 participants. Using a randomized, double-blind, triple-dummy, placebo-controlled design, smoker with and without psychiatric disorders were randomized to 12 weeks of either varenicline, bupropion, nicotine patch or placebo and then were followed up for 12 weeks. Findings did not show a significant increase in a composite measure of moderate to severe psychiatric symptoms for varenicline or bupropion compared to nicotine patch or placebo. Varenicline was found to be associated with significantly higher tobacco quit rates compared to bupropion, nicotine patch and placebo. Based upon these recent safety trials, the black box warning for varenicline was removed by the FDA in December 2016.

There are limited data available regarding varenicline's safety and effectiveness as a smoking cessation treatment for pregnant smokers (ACOG, 2020). Precautions should be used in individuals with significant renal disease (i.e., creatinine clearance < 30 mL/min) or on dialysis, and dose reduction may be considered for these individuals. Individuals prescribed varenicline should be informed that it may impair ability to operate heavy machinery and drive. Based on data from a trial by Rigotti and colleagues (2010), FDA issued a June 2011 safety communication that varenicline may be associated with a small increase in risk of certain cardiovascular events, including angina, nonfatal myocardial infarction, need for coronary revascularization, and peripheral vascular disease in smokers with stable cardiovascular disease. However, this was updated in 2012 with additional meta-analytic data, and the 2018 ACC consensus statement continues to recommend varenicline as a first-line pharmacotherapy for individuals with coronary artery disease (ACC 2018).

4. Combination treatments—Combinations of certain frontline tobacco medications have been associated with higher quit rates than monotherapies (Fiore et al., 2009; see Table 20–2). The combination of long-term nicotine patches with ad lib nicotine gum, lozenge, or nasal spray has been associated with higher abstinence rates than nicotine patch alone. Nicotine patch provides a slow but steady nicotine delivery system for reduction of withdrawal and craving, whereas ad lib nicotine agents provide a faster delivery system that is used as a rescue medication to assist with breakthrough urges and high-risk circumstances. Clinical practice guidelines suggest that combination NRT in the form of patch + ad lib agents is associated with greater abstinence than combining more than one patch alone. Combination NRT regimens dose nicotine patch based on rate of cigarette consumption and prescribe for 8–12 weeks or longer based on need and response. Adjunct NRT using 2 mg gum or lozenge as needed is recommended for 12–52 weeks. Recent FDA update on NRT labeling indicates that there are no safety concerns in using more than one form of NRT (FDA, 2013). The combination of bupropion SR + NRT has been

associated with higher quit rates than either monotherapy alone and allows for the use of two different mechanisms of action. Bupropion SR may be combined with steady NRT (patch) or with ad lib NRT (patch, gum, etc.). Combination therapies involving varenicline have also been studied, including varenicline with single NRT and varenicline with bupropion; these may be considered as augmentation strategies if only a partial response to varenicline monotherapy is demonstrated (ACC 2018).

5. Second-line agents—Clonidine and nortriptyline have been identified as second-line medications. They have been shown to have some evidence of effectiveness in smoking cessation, however there are potential side effect concerns, and they are not FDA approved for tobacco treatment. These second-line treatments may be considered on a case-by-case basis if front line medications fail or are contraindicated.

6. Factors in selecting pharmacological treatments—Several factors influence selection of tobacco treatment medications, including history of response to treatment, heaviness of smoking and severity of nicotine use disorder, side effects and contraindications, ease of use, relative financial cost, and patient choice. For individuals with cardiovascular disease, the 2018 ACC consensus statements recommends either varenicline or dual NRT as first-line, given the superior efficacy of these two treatments (ACC 2018; Anthenelli et al., 2016). Generally, given the availability and ease of use, nicotine patches are often used as a front-line option for tobacco use disorder treatment. Smokers who have failed with prior standard patch treatment or have more severe nicotine use disorder may be treated with combination patch + ad lib NRT or trialed on heavy dose patch (more than one patch). Light smokers (<10 cigarettes per day) may respond well to bupropion SR or nicotine gum. Bupropion SR may also be a reasonable treatment choice for smokers with a history of depression. Recommended minimum durations for most tobacco treatment regimens is 6–12 weeks; however, longer duration may be helpful for smokers with vulnerabilities such as severe dependence, history of smoking relapse, co-morbid psychiatric conditions, etc. Selection of tobacco use disorder treatment medications should include careful consideration of side effects and risk; however this should be judged in light of the certain risk of continued smoking.

B. Behavioral Interventions

USPHS clinical practice guidelines (Fiore et al., 2009) suggest that counseling + medication combined are significantly more effective than medication treatment alone (odds ratio = 1.4), and that both counseling and medication should be offered to aid all smokers in quitting.

1. Brief interventions—Although more intensive and longer-duration behavioral treatments may be most efficacious, even brief interventions (≤3 minutes) can be effective in helping patients quit smoking. Brief advice offered by a physician is associated with a doubling of quit rates compared to no advice, suggesting that physician advice is a potent force in aiding patients to quit smoking. Treatment by nonphysician clinicians is also associated with increased abstinence rates, and guidelines suggest that treatment delivered by more than one type of clinician may increase quit rates.

USPHS clinical practice guidelines recommend the use of the "5A" model as a process for assessment and treatment of tobacco use disorder. An independent trial of the effectiveness of the 5A model across multiple treatment settings found that providers offered advice far more often than assistance. However, those smokers aided to stop smoking (e.g., smoking cessation medications and behavioral treatments) had significantly greater quit rates (Quinn et al., 2009), underscoring the importance of delivering assistance as part of brief tobacco treatment interventions. This is furthered by the "prescribe first" approach advocated by the 2018 ACC consensus statement, which recommends initiating pharmacotherapy regardless of an individual's readiness for cessation (ACC, 2018).

ASK about tobacco use. Tobacco use should be assessed at every visit (not just initial visit), and tobacco use status should be documented in the clinical record. Further questioning of smoking rate, history, patterns, cost, related health and function issues, history of quit attempts, and barriers to cessation may also be informative to treatment efforts.

ADVISE to quit. Providers should make clear, strong statements informing patients of the risks of their smoking, gains of their quitting, options for treatment, and recommendation to quit. Strong and effective messages should be personalized to the patient's specific medical, family, financial, or other needs and should include proximal as well as long-term benefits of smoking cessation for the patient.

ASSESS willingness to quit. Providers should assess a patient's proximal willingness to quit smoking (e.g., quitting within 2 weeks). Providers should normalize a patient's ambivalence to smoking cessation and seek to reassure patients that they can succeed and will be supported. For those smokers not willing to make a proximal quit attempt, motivational interventions are helpful (e.g., 5Rs; see later section).

ASSIST in quit attempt. For the patient willing to make a quit attempt, the provider should assist the patient in setting a specific targeted quit date (recommended within 2 weeks after advice to quit), offer effective smoking cessation medication, and provide or refer smokers to counseling. Effective brief interventions may include basic information about nicotine withdrawal symptoms and duration, and pragmatic tips in initiation and maintenance of quitting. Quitlines and interactive computer-based interventions have been associated with increased

quit rates (see later sections) and can be incorporated into brief interventions.

ARRANGE for follow-up. Follow-up sessions at 1 week and again at 1 month after targeted quit date should be provided by the clinician or trained associate. Smoking status, medication compliance and effectiveness, and behavioral coping strategies should be assessed. Patients who are smoke-free should be congratulated in their success and encouraged to continue using coping strategies and medications for the course of treatment. For patients who are still smoking, providers should help patients to recommit to abstinence, reset a proximal quit date, adjust tobacco medications for improved effectiveness, and offer new behavioral strategies to cope with challenges to quitting. Referrals to Quitlines or to intensive smoking cessation programs may be considered for additional support and treatment.

2. Motivating smokers unwilling to quit—Brief motivational interventions (MI) are effective in increasing future attempts to quit in smokers who are unwilling to stop smoking. MI is based on patient-centered principles developed by Miller and Rollnick (1991) to resolve ambivalence and promote movement toward change. MI is a teachable interpersonal style for clinicians that emphasizes a spirit of acceptance, partnership, evocation, and compassion in clinical interactions. MI-based interventions selectively evoke, attend to, and reflect back a patient's internal motivations for change, avoiding the common clinical "righting reflex" to focus on and correct the voiced reasons a person continues tobacco use.

3. Intensive smoking cessation treatments—For individuals who are motivated to quit but having difficulty obtaining abstinence, intensive smoking cessation treatments may be most helpful. There is a dose-dependent relationship between intensity of behavioral smoking cessation treatments and treatment outcome. Treatments are made more intensive by increasing amount of time per session, amount of total treatment time, and numbers of sessions. Intensive person-to-person treatments of at least 10 minutes per session, 90–300 minutes total duration and four to eight or more sessions, have been shown to be associated with the highest rates of positive smoking outcome. Intensive smoking cessation treatments may be offered individually or in groups, or a combination of modalities, and by a single or combination of trained providers (Fiore et al., 2009).

Clinical practice guidelines suggest that two broad behavioral treatment methods are associated with the best smoking outcomes. (1) **Pragmatic problem solving of challenges to smoking cessation** includes behavioral and cognitive behavioral strategies to identify urges and antecedents to smoking, and to use proactive coping skills such as avoidance of smoking cues and situations, altering habits associated with smoking, refusing smoking offers, use of substitutes to cigarettes, challenging smoking justification thoughts, and managing urges through cognitive distraction and delay techniques. (2) **Intra-treatment support for quitting** includes consistent provider communication of empathy for the smoker's quit experience, such as encouraging talk about quitting successes and barriers, encouraging the patient to continue with smoking cessation efforts, and expressing belief in a patient's ability to succeed in smoking cessation. As part of intensive treatment, effective and tailored pharmacotherapy should be selected and adjusted as needed and integrated as further tools within behavioral treatment sessions.

In addition, certain nonpharmacological interventions have shown notable promise in smoking cessation treatment. Contingency management (CM) for biochemically validated smoking abstinence has been associated with greater smoking outcomes across a range of groups of smokers, including adolescent smokers (Krishnan-Sarin et al., 2013), alcohol-dependent smokers (Cooney et al., 2010), pregnant and postpartum smokers (Higgins et al., 2004); and in work-site tobacco treatment (Volpp et al., 2009). Mindfulness-based training works to decouple urges to smoke from automatic smoking responses, allowing individuals to better cope with urges and to consider optimal coping strategies. In a randomized trial comparing mindfulness training (MT) to the American Lung Association's Freedom from Smoking (FFS) program, MT was associated with significantly lower smoking consumption, and greater quit rates at 17 weeks (Brewer et al., 2011). There is also emerging evidence for neuromodulation in tobacco cessation, with a recent large multisite, double-blind, randomized, sham-controlled trial demonstrating efficacy for rTMS (Zangen et al., 2021).

Certain behavioral interventions that have been used in smoking cessation have not been recommended by clinical practice guidelines (Fiore et al., 2009). Treatments such as acupuncture, hypnosis, tapering of cigarette consumption, and herbal medicine preparations are not recommended because of lack of evidence of effectiveness. Although recommended in past clinical practice guidelines, more recent analyses of aversive conditioning, or rapid smoking, and extra treatment support no longer find evidence of effectiveness, and these methods are no longer recommended.

4. Other interventions—New technologies offer effective treatments to be delivered in modalities other than face-to-face venues, therefore increasing access to care. **Quitlines** allow smokers to have rapid telephone access to trained smoking cessation counselors, and provide live, proactive telephone treatment with counselor-initiated sessions and call-back services. Data from a substantial growth in quitline research have been reviewed in several recent meta-analyses. Clinical practice guidelines (Fiore et al., 2009) found quitline counseling to be associated with significantly greater smoking quit rates compared to minimal counseling or self-help materials (OR = 1.6, 95% confidence index [CI] = 1.4–1.8), and combination of quitline + medication

to be more effective than medication alone (OR = 1.3, 95% CI = 1.1–1.6). Data from a recent Cochrane review (Stead et al., 2013) found highest quit rates for smokers randomized to multiple proactive quitline sessions (risk ratio [RR] = 1.37, 95% CI = 1.26–1.50) and suggest a dose-dependent relationship in which three or more sessions are associated with greater likelihood of smoking cessation than one or two sessions. A national network of quitlines is available by telephoning 1-800-QUIT-NOW, giving smokers broad access to a range of proactive smoking cessation counseling programs and in some states also providing a free course of nicotine replacement therapy.

Internet-based smoking cessation treatments allow for broad reach to easy-access and low-cost tobacco treatment and have particular appeal in a growing digital world (e.g., Brown et al., 2013). Web-based interventions may be used as stand-alone treatments or in conjunction with other brief or intensive smoking cessation protocols. Meta-analyses from a recent Cochrane review update on Internet-based tobacco interventions found mixed data; however, results show that interventions that were interactive and tailored treatments to individuals were associated with greater quit rates (Civljak et al., 2010).

Mobile phone–based smoking cessation treatments provide even greater access to treatment, as cell phones and smartphones are widely used and are nearly always in close proximity to their users. A recent Cochrane review of mobile phone–based treatment, mostly using text messaging interventions, found a significant increase in 6-month smoking outcome rates compared to control programs (RR = 1.71, 95% CI = 1.47–1.99; Whittaker et al., 2012). Smoking cessation mobile text messaging services have recently been launched by the National Cancer Institute (Smokefree TXT) and by the U.S. Department of Veterans Affairs (smokefreeVET) and can provide 24/7 text-based interventions with support, quit tips, and interactive options. The Cochrane review found no ongoing or published studies on the comparative effectiveness of smartphone apps for smoking cessation; however, a content analysis of 47 smoking cessation apps on iPhone suggest overall poor adherence to evidence-based clinical practice guideline recommendations (Abroms et al., 2011).

5. Factors in selecting behavioral treatment—Evidence-based behavioral treatments are effective for a broad range of smokers and should be part of any smoking cessation treatment. Brief interventions have broad reach and are useful in treating individuals self-motivated to quit smoking; however, intensive behavioral treatments should be considered for individuals who have difficulty in quitting or who have lower confidence in their ability to quit smoking. Certain groups of treatment-refractory smokers may benefit from adding specific treatments to the platform of evidence-based intensive tobacco treatments. Smokers with comorbid psychiatric disorders may benefit from additional stress and mood management treatments, tailored tobacco medications of longer duration, and the assurance that support for their smoking cessation efforts will be available for as long as it may take. Smokers with comorbid substance use disorders may benefit from integrative treatments that deliver intensive treatment for nicotine dependence concurrently or sequentially with addiction treatment. Smokers with weight concerns may benefit from adding weight management education and strategies to smoking cessation treatments. Hospitalized smokers who initiate tobacco abstinence while in the hospital may benefit from continued counseling following hospital discharge to maintain smoking abstinence.

▶ Electronic Nicotine Delivery Systems (ENDS), Electoronic Cigarettes (e-Cigs), or "Vapes"

These nicotine delivery systems are broadly marketed by their companies as a less harmful and more attractive cigarette alternative that can be used more discretely, and by implication, as a device that may be useful in smoking cessation. While cigarette use in youth has declined, e-cig use has increased, being the primary vehicle for introduction to nicotine use and developing nicotine use disorder for middle and high school students (National Youth Tobacco Survey, 2022). Given the proliferation of e-cig availability and sales, and growing concerns as to its risks and benefits—particularly among the rapidly increasing population of youth e-cig users—a discussion here is worthwhile.

E-cigs are battery-operated devices which use an atomizer to heat a refillable cartridge, releasing vapor containing nicotine and other substances (Kushner et al., 2011). E-cigs may have particular appeal to children and teenagers, as they have been available in a variety of desirable flavors (including vanilla, chocolate, strawberry, cotton candy, mint, piña colada), and have been widely sold online and in shopping mall kiosks—this targeted marketing toward youth has since been addressed by an FDA enforcement policy enacted in 2020 that bans the manufacture, distribution, and sale of flavored cartridge-based e-cigs that appeal to children. Cartridges generally contain approximately 20 mg nicotine (Cobb & Abrans, 2011); however, various levels of nicotine are claimed. Many cartridges are refillable, which may be dangerous as children and adult users may be exposed to unknown and potentially high concentrations of nicotine (Yamin et al., 2010).

The health consequences of e-cig use are not fully known, and there is limited scientific evidence establishing e-cig safety for direct or indirect users, particularly for the longer-term effects (Marques et al., 2021). In 2009, FDA analyzed ingredients from cartridges of two e-cig brands and found detectable levels of known carcinogens and toxins (diethylene glycol and nitrosamines), as well as low levels of nicotine in cartridges that were labeled as containing no nicotine (FDA, 2009). Of particular concern is the relatively rare cause of severe acute lung injury termed e-cigarette or vaping use-associated lung injury (EVALI), which was first identified in 2019 and is thought to be related to vitamin E acetate (among other possible contaminants) in the cartridge fluid (CDC, 2020). Due to high rate of e-cig use in youth, youth e-cig use associated with progression to nicotine use disorder, and documented health risks of e-cigs, FDA (2021) has described e-cig use in youths as "unsafe," and a public health concern.

E-cigs have been marketed for adult chronic smokers as a safer nicotine delivery system compared to combustible tobacco. Recent trials and analyses have begun to study if e-cigs can be helpful to help adult smokers quit. A recent large naturalistic study of tobacco users in the United States attempting to use e-cigs for smoking cessation did not demonstrate benefit, and actually suggested that e-cig use may be associated with greater relapse to tobacco smoking (Chen et al., 2022). This data is furthered by meta-analyses demonstrating e-cigs use to not be associated with significant increases in smoking cessation (Patil et al., 2020), as well as increased risk of relapse for former smokers using e-cigs (Barufaldi et al., 2021). In contrast, the most recent Cochrane review of randomized controlled trials comparing e-cig use to other NRT concluded that current evidence supports the efficacy of e-cigs for smoking cessation at 6 months' follow-up, although another meta-analysis clarified that prescribed e-cig use should be separated from consumer/commercial e-cig use, as only the former is associated with improved smoking cessation outcomes, while the consumer/commercial products were not associated with cessation (Hartmann-Boyce et al., 2022; Wang et al., 2021). This mixed evidence has led to widely divergent approaches to e-cig use for smoking cessation internationally, with some countries (e.g., the U.K.) more directly endorsing their use while others are exercising caution (e.g. Australia and the United States).

The FDA now regulates the manufacture, import, packaging, labeling, advertising, promotion, sale, and distribution of electronic nicotine delivery systems (ENDS). While the FDA has approved 23 tobacco-flavored e-cig devices and tobacco-flavored e-liquid cartridges, no e-cig has been approved as a smoking cessation device or reduced risk product and has indicated the need for further research on risks and benefits of these products on adult smokers. Controversy remains in the tobacco control field over the potential role of e-cigs. Although some experts argue that e-cigs have promised as a less lethal nicotine system for treatment-refractory smokers unable to quit (e.g., Etter & Bullen, 2011), others maintain that e-cigs serve to attract young people to nicotine use, may increase nicotine consumption in ongoing smokers through dual use of e-cig and combustible tobacco (Pearson et al., 2012), and work to undermine public indoor clean air regulation (World Health Organization, 2009). Further, nonbiased research on e-cig composition, safety in short-term and long-term use, and impact on public health is needed.

► Complications/Adverse Outcomes of Treatment

Information on common side effects, precautions, contraindications, and warnings for each smoking cessation medication was reviewed in the pharmacotherapy section. The potential risk of adverse events from treatment must be weighed against the certain risk of harm from ongoing smoking and tobacco use. Even when treated with smoking cessation medications, nicotine withdrawal symptoms may be difficult to tolerate, particularly for individuals with history of or sensitivity to mood, anxiety, and other psychiatric disorders. Even when using behavioral coping skills, individuals may experience strong urges to smoke in response to environmental and internal cigarette cues.

Early studies have found that for individuals with a history of major depressive disorder (MDD), long-term smoking cessation may be associated with an increased risk of MDD symptoms and depressed affect during the first 3 and 9 months, respectively, after quitting smoking (Covey et al., 1990, 1997). However, subsequent trials have found comparable rates of MDD episodes in smoking and tobacco-abstinent individuals with a history of MDD (Tsoh et al., 2000), and no increase in rates of depressive symptoms, psychiatric hospitalization, or suicidality after smoking cessation in individuals with current depressive disorder (Prochaska et al., 2008), making questionable the causative role of smoking cessation in MDD recurrence. Despite this, patients' concern about depressive symptoms following smoking cessation could undermine smoking cessation efforts and should be addressed clinically with education of normal mood symptoms that may be experienced with nicotine withdrawal, and monitoring of mood symptoms treatment if needed.

Smoking cessation is frequently associated with short-term, modest (<10 lb) weight gain; however, weight gain amounts may be substantially higher (e.g., 30 lb) in as many as 10% of former smokers (Fiore et al., 2009). Women, African Americans, heavy smokers, and individuals under age 55 are at higher risk for significant weight gain, and concerns over substantial weight gain may frequently undermine smoking cessation efforts. Weight gain after smoking cessation is linked to both an increase in caloric consumption and decreased metabolism following cigarette discontinuation. Smokers should be educated that most weight gain following smoking cessation presents a minor health risk compared to the certain and substantial health risks associated with smoking. Patients should be encouraged to use pragmatic weight management efforts to minimize high-calorie foods and increase exercise when they stop smoking. Clinical practice guidelines recommend that 4 mg nicotine gum and lozenge and bupropion may be effective smoking cessation treatments associated with less or delayed weight gain. A Cochrane database review found a lack of clear evidence that various behavioral weight loss treatments are effective at reducing short-term or long-term weight gain following smoking cessation (Farley et al., 2012); however, the review suggested that personalized weight management may show promise and that exercise may be related to longer-term weight reduction in smokers with weight concerns.

Contrary to common myth, smoking cessation treatment is not associated with an increased risk of relapse to alcohol (e.g., Cooney et al., 2003, 2007) in individuals with alcohol and nicotine dependence. Some trials have found that smoking cessation may be associated with improved alcohol treatment outcomes in smokers with alcohol use disorder (e.g., Cooney et al., 2010; Prochaska et al., 2004). Although one study has found that the sequencing of alcohol treatment prior to tobacco treatment may be associated with better maintenance of alcohol abstinence (Joseph et al., 2004), the USPHS clinical practice guidelines issued a consensus recommendation that smoking cessation does not interfere with substance use disorder recovery, and that smokers in addiction treatment programs should receive evidence-based treatments for tobacco use disorder (Fiore et al., 2009).

► Prognosis

Nicotine use disorder is a chronic and recurring condition, and smoking cessation is often marked by periods of remission and relapse. Although 70% of smokers report a wish to quit (CDC, 2002) and nearly 50% per year make a quit attempt (Shiffman, 2008), the majority of quit attempts are unassisted, without the benefit of treatment. Among untreated smokers, most relapse within 8 days of a quit attempt, and only 3–5% succeed in long-term abstinence (Hughes et al., 2004, 2008). Smokers frequently make as many as 10–14 quit attempts before they succeed in long-term abstinence (Hughes et al., 2008). Evidence-based treatments are effective and available but are not necessarily preferred as it is estimated that two-thirds of attempts to quit smoking are self-motivated and without treatment (Shiffman, 2008, 2010). Evidence-based smoking cessation medication and behavioral treatments as reported in this chapter are associated with a doubling to tripling of smoking abstinence at 6 months; however, smoking lapses may continue to occur. In a meta-analysis of prolonged abstinence in treated smokers, Hughes et al. (2008) found that following 1 year of established tobacco abstinence, abstinence rates tend to decline to levels of 10% or lower. Engaging smokers to accept, adhere to, and persist with smoking treatment enhances prognosis of long-term tobacco abstinence (Fiore et al., 2009, see Table 20-2). Shiffman et al. (2010) found that encouraging smokers to continue with use of high-dose patch during a lapse episode attenuated the rate of progression from lapse to continued relapse. In a shift from prior recommendations, FDA now recommends that individuals who lapse while using OTC NRT continue using NRT and continue with their attempt to quit (FDA, 2013). USPHS clinical practice guidelines recommend ongoing 5A care to combat the chronic nature of nicotine dependence and promote long-term smoking abstinence (Fiore et al., 2009).

Abroms L, Padmanabhan N, Thaweethai L, et al: iPhone apps for smoking cessation: a content analysis. *Am J Prev Med*. 2011;40: 279–285.

Allen M, Debanne M, Lazignac C, et al: Effect of nicotine replacement therapy on agitation in smokers with schizophrenia: a double-blind, randomized, placebo-controlled study. *Am J Psychiatry*. 2011;168:395–396.

American College of Obstetrics and Gynecology. Tobacco and nicotine cessation in pregnancy. Committee Opinion, Num 807. May 2020 (Reaffirmed 2023). https://www.acog.org/clinical/clinical-guidance/committee-opinion/articles/2020/05/tobacco-and-nicotine-cessation-during-pregnancy

American Psychiatric Association. *Diagnostic and Statistical Manual of Mental Health Disorders*. 5th ed. Washington, DC: American Psychiatric Publishing; 2013.

American Psychiatric Association. *Diagnostic and Statistical Manual of Mental Health Disorders*. 4th ed. Text revision. Washington, DC: American Psychiatric Publishing; 2000.

Anthenelli RM, Benowitz NL, West R, et al: Neuropsychiatric safety and efficacy of varenicline, bupropion, and nicotine patch in smokers with and without psychiatric disorders (EAGLES): a double-blind, randomised, placebo-controlled clinical trial. *Lancet*. 2016;387:2507–2520.

Barua RS, Rigotti NA, Benowitz NL, et al: 2018 ACC Expert Consensus Decision Pathway on Tobacco Cessation Treatment. *J Am Coll Cardiol*. 2018;72(25):3332–3365. doi:10.1016/j.jacc .2018.10.027

Barufaldi LA, Guerra RL, de Albuquerque RDCR, et al: Risk of smoking relapse with the use of electronic cigarettes: a systematic review with meta-analysis of longitudinal studies. *Tob Prevn Cessation* 29 (April 27, 2021):29. https://doi.org/10.18332/tpc/ 132964.

Benowitz N. Cotinine as a biomarker of environmental tobacco smoke exposure. *Epidemiol Rev*. 1996;18:188–204.

Benowitz N, Jacob P, Ahijevych K, et al: Biochemical verification of tobacco use and cessation. *Nicotine Tob Res*. 2002;4:149–159.

Biener L, Abrams D. Contemplation ladder: validation of a measure of readiness to consider smoking cessation. *Health Psychol*. 1991; 10:360–365.

Brewer J, Mallik S, Babuscio T, et al: Mindfulness training for smoking cessation: results from a randomized controlled trial. *Drug Alcohol Depend*. 2011;119:72–80.

Brody A, Olmstead R, London E, et al: Smoking-induced ventral striatum dopamine release. *Am J Psychiatry*. 2004;161:1211–1218.

Brown M, Michiee S, Raupach T. Prevalence and characteristics of smokers interested in internet-based smoking cessation interventions: cross-sectional findings from a national household survey. *J Med Internet Res*. 2013;15:e50.

Carpenter M, Hughes J, Gray K, et al: Nicotine therapy sampling to induce quit attempts among smokers unmotivated to quit. A randomized clinical trial. *Arch Intern Med*. 2011;171:1901–1907.

Centers for Disease Control and Prevention (CDC). Wide-ranging online data for epidemiologic research (WONDER). Atlanta, GA: CDC, National Center for Health Statistics; 2021. Available at http://wonder.cdc.gov.

Centers for Disease Control and Prevention. Outbreak of lung injury associated with the use of e-cigarette, or vaping, products. Updated February 25, 2020. https://www.cdc.gov/tobacco/basic_information/e-cigarettes/severe-lung-disease.html#epi-chart

Centers for Disease Control and Prevention. Cigarette smoking among adults—United States, 2000. *MMWR Morbid Mortal Wkly Rep*. 2002;51:642–645.

Centers for Disease Control and Prevention. Smoking-attributable mortality, years of potential life lost, and productivity losses—United States 2000–2004. *MMWR Morbid Mortal Wkly Rep*. 2009;57:1226–1228.

Centers for Disease Control and Prevention. Current cigarette smoking among adults—United States, 2011. *MMWR Morbid Mortal Wkly Rep*. 2012;61:889–894.

Chapman S, Ragg M, McGeechan K. Citation bias in reported smoking prevalence in people with schizophrenia. *Aust N Z J Psychiatry*. 2009;43:277–282.

Chen R, Pierce JP, Leas EC, et al: Effectiveness of e-cigarettes as aids for smoking cessation: evidence from the PATH study cohort, 2017–2019. *Tob Control*. January 11, 2022. https://doi .org/10.1136/tobaccocontrol-2021-056901.

Chengappa K, Kambhampati R, Perkins K, et al: Bupropion SR as a smoking cessation treatment in remitted depressed patients maintained on selective serotonin reuptake inhibitor antidepressants. *J Clin Psychiatry*. 2001;62:503–508.

Civljak M, Shikh A, Stead L, Car J. Internet-based interventions for smoking cessation, September 8, 2010. https://www.ncbi.nlm.nih .gov/pubmed/20824856.

Cobb H, Abrans D. E-cigarette or drug-delivery device? Regulating novel nicotine products. *N Engl J Med*. 2011;365:193–195.

Cooney N, Litt M, Cooney J. In vivo assessment of the effects of smoking cessation in alcoholic smokers. *Clin Exp Res*. 2003; 26:1952–1953.

Cooney N, Litt M, Cooney J. Alcohol and tobacco cessation in alcohol dependent smokers: analysis of real-time reports. *Psychol Addict Behav*. 2007;21:277–286.

Cooney J, Cooper S, Sevarino K, et al: *Frequent Brief Behavioral Intervention Plus Contingency Management vs. Cognitive Behavioral Treatment for Smoking Cessation for Alcoholic Smokers During Intensive Alcohol Treatment*. Baltimore, MD: Society for Research on Nicotine and Tobacco; 2010.

Covey L, Glassman A, Stetner F. Depression and depressive symptoms in smoking cessation. *Compr Psychiatry*. 1990;31: 350–354.

Covey L, Glassman A, Stetner F. Major depression following smoking cessation. *Am J Psychiatry*. 1997;154:263–265.

Cox L, Tiffany S, Christen A. Evaluation of the brief questionnaire of smoking urges (QSU-brief) in laboratory and clinical settings. *Nicotine Tob Res*. 2001;3:7–16.

Cox L, Patten C, Niaura N, et al: Efficacy of bupropion for relapse prevention in smokers with and without a past history of major depression. *J Gen Intern Med*. 2004;19:828–834.

Dale L, Hurt R, Offord K, et al: High-dose nicotine patch therapy. Percentage of replacement and smoking cessation. *JAMA*. 1995;274:1353–1358.

David S, Munafo M, Murphy M, et al: Genetic variation in the dopamine D4 receptor (DRD4) gene and smoking cessation: follow-up of a randomised clinical trial of transdermal nicotine patch. *Pharmacogenomics*. 2008;8:122–128.

Dietz PM, Homa D, England LJ, et al: Estimates of nondisclosure of cigarette smoking among pregnant and nonpregnant women of reproductive age in the United States. *Am J Epidemiol*. 2011; 173(3):355–359. doi:10.1093/aje/kwq381

Etter J, Bullen C. Electronic cigarette: user profile, utilization, satisfaction, and perceived efficacy. *Addiction*. 2011;106:2017–2028.

Farkas A, Pierce J, Zhu S, et al: Addiction versus stages of change models in predicting smoking cessation. *Addiction*. 1986;91:1271–1280.

Farley A, Hajek P, Lycett D, et al: Interventions for preventing weight gain after smoking cessation. January 18, 2012. https://www.ncbi.nlm.nih.gov/pubmed/22258966.

Fiore M, Jaén C, Baker T, et al: *Treating Tobacco Use and Dependence: 2008 Update. Quick Reference Guide for Clinicians*. Rockville, MD: Department of Health and Human Services; 2009.

Fowler J, Volkow N, Wang G, et al: Inhibition of monoamine oxidase B in the brains of smokers. *Nature*. 1996;379:733–736.

Frederickson P, Hurt R, Lee G. High dose transdermal nicotine therapy for heavy smokers: safety, tolerability and measurement of nicotine and cotinine levels *Psychopharmacology*. 1995;122: 215–222.

Gonzales D, Rennard S, Nides M, et al: Varenicline, an α4β2 nicotinic acetylcholine receptor partial agonist vs. placebo or sustained-release bupropion for smoking cessation. *JAMA*. 2006;296:47–55.

Gunnell D, Irvine D, Wise L, et al: Varenicline and suicidal behaviour: a cohort study based on data from the general practice research database. *BMJ*. 2009;339:3805.

Hartmann-Boycea J, Lindsona N, Butler AR, et al: Electronic cigarettes for smoking cessation. *Cochrane Database Syst Rev*. 2023;11. https://doi.org/10.1002/14651858.cd010216.pub7.

Hayford K, Patten C, Rummans R, et al: Efficacy of bupropion for smoking cessation in smokers with a former history of major depression or alcoholism. *Br J Psychiatry*. 1999;174:173–178.

Heatherton T, Kozlowski L, Frecker R, et al: Measuring the heaviness of smoking using self-reported time to the first cigarette of the day and number of cigarettes smoked per day. *Br J Addict*. 1989;84:791–800.

Heatherton T, Kozlowski L, Frecker R, Fagerström K. The Fagerström Test for Nicotine Dependence: a revision of the Fagerström Tolerance Questionnaire. *Br J Addict*. 1991;86:1119–1127.

Higgins S, Heil S, Solomon L, et al: A pilot study on voucher-based incentives to promote abstinence from cigarette smoking during pregnancy and postpartum. *Nicotine Tob Res*. 2004;6:1015–1020.

Hughes J. Treatment of nicotine dependence. Is more better? (editorial). *JAMA*. 1995;274:1390–1391.

Hughes J, Keely J, Naud S. Shape of the relapse curve and long-term abstinence among untreated smokers. *Addiction*. 2004;99:29–38.

Hughes J, Helzer J, S. Lindberg S. Prevalence of DSM/ICD-defined nicotine dependence. *Drug Alcohol Depend*. 2006;85:91–102.

Hughes J, Peters E, Naud S. Relapse to smoking after 1 year of abstinence: a meta-analysis. *Addict Behav*. 2008;33:1516–1520.

Hurt R, Sachs D, Glover E, et al: A comparison of sustained-release bupropion and placebo for smoking cessation. *N Engl J Med*. 1997;337:1195–1202.

Jacob P, Hatsukami D, Severson S, et al: Anabasine and anatabine as biomarkers for tobacco use during nicotine replacement therapy. *Cancer Epidemiol Biomarkers Prev*. 2002;11:1668–1673.

Jarvis M, Tunstall-Pedoe H, Feyerabend C, et al: Biochemical markers of smoke absorption and self reported exposure to passive smoking. *J Epidemiol Commun Health*. 1984;38:335–339.

Johnston LD, Miech RA, O'Malley PM, Bachman JG, Schulenberg JE, Patrick ME. (2020). Monitoring the future national survey results on drug use 1975–2019: 2019 overview, key findings on adolescent drug use. University of Michigan, Institute for Social Research. http://www.monitoringthefuture.org/pubs/monographs/mtf -overview2019.pdf

Jorenby D, Hays J, Rigotti N, et al: Efficacy of varenicline, an α4β2 nicotinic acetylcholine receptor partial agonist vs. placebo or sustained-release bupropion for smoking cessation. *JAMA*. 2006; 296:56–63.

Joseph A, Norma S, Ferry L. The safety of transdermal nicotine as an aid to smoking cessation in patients with cardiac disease. *N Engl J Med*. 1996;335:1792–1798.

Joseph A, Willenbring M, Nugent S, et al: A randomized trial of concurrent versus delayed smoking intervention for patients in alcohol dependence treatment. *J Stud Alcohol*. 2004;65: 681–691.

King DP, Paciga S, Pickering E, et al: Smoking cessation pharmacogenetics: analysis of varenicline and bupropion in placebo-controlled clinical trials. *Neuropsychopharmacology*. 2012;37(3):641–650. doi:10.1038/npp.2011.232

Krishnan-Sarin S, Cavallo D, Cooney J, et al: An exploratory randomized controlled trial of a novel high-school-based smoking cessation intervention for adolescent smokers using abstinence-contingent incentives and cognitive behavioral therapy. *Drug Alcohol Depend*. 2013;132:346–351.

Kushner W, Reddy S, Mehrotra N, et al: Electronic cigarettes and thirdhand tobacco smoke: two emerging healthcare challenges for the primary care provider. *Int J Gen Med*. 2011;4:115–120.

Lasser K, Boyd W, Woolhandler D, et al: Smoking and mental illness: a population-based prevalence study. *JAMA*. 2000; 284:2606–2610.

Legacy. National Survey: One-in-ten smokers reported they have concealed their smoking from health care providers. 2012. http://www.legacyforhealth.org/4973.aspx.

Levinson A, Camps S, Gascoigne J, et al: Smoking, but not smokers: Identity among college students who smoke cigarettes. *Nicotine Tob Res*. 2007;9:845–852.

Li M. The genetics of nicotine dependence. *Curr Psychiatry Rep*. 2006;8:158–164.

Lopez-Quintero C, Perez de los Cobos J, Hasin D, et al: Probability and predictors of transition from first use to dependence on nicotine, alcohol, cannabis, and cocaine: results of the National Epidemiologic Survey on Alcohol and Related Conditions (NESARC). *Drug Alcohol Depend*. 2011;115:120–130.

Lyon E. A review of the effects of nicotine on schizophrenia and antipsychotic medications. *Psychiatr Serv*. 1999;50:1346–1350.

Mamede M, Ishizu K, Ueda M, et al: Temporal changes in human nicotinic acetylcholine receptor after smoking cessation: 5IA SPECT study. *J Nuclear Med*. 2007;48:1829–1835.

Marrone G, Paulpillai M, Evan R, et al: Breath carbon monoxide and semiquantitative saliva cotinine as biomarkers for smoking. *Hum Psychopharmacol*. 2010;25:80–83.

Marques P, Piqueras L, Sanz MJ. An updated overview of e-cigarette impact on human health. *Resp Res*. May 18, 2021;22(1):151. https://doi.org/10.1186/s12931-021-01737-5.

McClernon F, Hiott F, Liu J, et al: Selectively reduced responses to smoking cues in amygdala following extinction-based smoking cessation: results of a preliminary functional magnetic resonance imaging study. *Addict Biol.* 2007;12:503–512.

McClernon FJ. Neuroimaging of nicotine dependence: key findings and application to the study of smoking-mental illness comorbidity. *J Dual Diagn.* 2009;5:168–178.

Meyer T, Taylor L, Xie S, et al: Neuropsychiatric events in varenicline and nicotine replacement patch users in the Military Health System. *Addiction.* 2013;108:203–210.

Miller W, Rollnick S. *Motivational Interviewing: Preparing People to Change Addictive Behavior.* New York: Guilford; 1991.

Moylan S, Jacka F, Pasco J, Berk M. Cigarette smoking, nicotine dependence and anxiety disorders: a systematic review of population-based, epidemiological studies. *BMC Med.* 2012;10.

National Center on Addiction and Substance Abuse. *Missed opportunity: National Survey of Primary Care Physicians and Patients on Substance Abuse.* New York: Columbia University; 2000.

Park-Lee E, Ren C, Cooper M, Cornelius M, Jamal A, Cullen KA. Tobacco product use among middle and high school students—United States, 2022. *MMWR Morb Mortal Wkly Rep.* 2022;71; 1429–1435. DOI: http://dx.doi.org/10.15585/mmwr.mm7145a1

Patil S, Arakeri G, Patil S, et al: Are electronic nicotine delivery systems (ENDs) helping cigarette smokers quit?—Current evidence. *J Oral Pathol Med.* 2020 Mar;49(3):181–189. doi: 10.1111/jop.12966. Epub 2019 Nov 8. PMID: 31642553.

Patkar A, Gopalakrishnan R, Lundy A, et al: Relationship between tobacco smoking and positive and negative symptoms in schizophrenia. *J Nerv Ment Dis.* 2002;190:604–610.

Pearson J, Richardson A, Niaura R, et al: E-cigarette awareness, use, and harm perceptions in U.S. adults. *Am J Public Health.* 2012;102:1758–1766.

Prochaska J, Delucchi K, Hall S. A meta-analysis of smoking cessation interventions in individuals in substance abuse treatment or recovery. *J Consult Clin Psychol.* 2004;72:1144–1156.

Prochaska J, Hall S, Tsoh J, et al: Treating tobacco dependence in clinically depressed smokers: effect of smoking cessation on mental health functioning. *Am J Public Health.* 2008;98:446–448.

Prom-Wormley EC, Ebejer J, Dick DM, Bowers MS. The genetic epidemiology of substance use disorder: a review. *Drug Alcohol Depend.* 2017;180:241–259. doi:10.1016/j.drugalcdep.2017.06.040

Quinn V, Hollis H, Smith K, et al: Effectiveness of the 5-As tobacco cessation treatments in nine HMOs. *J Gen Intern Med.* 2009;24:149–154.

Ray R, Loughead J, Wang Z, et al: Neuroimaging, genetics and the treatment of nicotine addiction. *Behav Brain Res.* 2008;193: 159–169.

Rigotti N, Pipe A, Benowitz N, et al: Efficacy and safety of varenicline for smoking cessation in patients with cardiovascular disease: a randomized trial. *Circulation.* 2010;121:221–229.

Salamone J, Correa M. Motivational views of reinforcement: implications for understanding the behavioral functions of nucleus accumbens dopamine. *Behav Brain Res.* 2002;137:3–25.

Schepis T, Duhig A, Liss T, et al: Contingency management for smoking cessation: enhancing feasibility through use of immunoassay test strips measuring cotinine. *Nicotine Tob Res.* 2008;10:1495–1501.

Scott D, Domino E, Heitzeg M, et al: Smoking modulation of mu-opioid and dopamine D2 receptor-mediated neurotransmission in humans. *Neuropsychopharmacology.* 2007;32:450–457.

Shiffman S. Individual differences in adoption of treatment for smoking cessation: demographic and smoking history characteristics. *Drug Alcohol Depend.* 2008;93:121–131.

Shiffman S. Smoking-cessation treatment utilization: the need for a consumer perspective. *Am J Prev Med.* 2010;38:S382–S384.

Shiffman S, Elash CA, Paton SM, et al: Comparative efficacy of 24-hour and 16-hour transdermal nicotine patches for relief of morning craving. *Addiction.* 2000;95:1185–1995.

Shiffman S, Scharf D, Shadel W. Analyzing milestones in smoking cessation: illustration in a nicotine patch trial in adult smokers. *J Consult Clin Psychol.* 2006;74:276–285.

Slemmer J, Norma S, Ferry L. Bupropion is a nicotinic antagonist. *J Pharmacol Exp Ther.* 2000;335:1792–1798.

Stapleton J, Watson L, Spirlin L, et al: Varenicline in the routine treatment of tobacco dependence: a pre-post comparison with nicotine replacement therapy and an evaluation in those with mental illness. *Addiction.* 2008;103:146–154.

Stead L, Hartmann-Boyce J, Perera R, et al: Telephone counseling for smoking cessation, 12 August 2013. https://www.ncbi.nlm.nih.gov/pubmed/23934971.

Stein E, Pankiewicz J, Harsch H, et al: Nicotine-induced limbic cortical activation in the human brain: a functional MRI study. *Am J Psychiatry.* 1998;155:1009–1015.

Substance Abuse and Mental Health Services Administration. (2022). Key substance use and mental health indicators in the United States: Results from the 2021 National Survey on Drug Use and Health (HHS Publication No. PEP22-07-01-005, NSDUH Series H-57). Center for Behavioral Health Statistics and Quality, Substance Abuse and Mental Health Services Administration. https://www.samhsa.gov/data/report/2021-nsduh-annual-national-report

Sullivan P, Kendler K. The genetic epidemiology of smoking, *Nicotine Tob Res.* 1999;1:S51–S57.

Tashkin D, Kanner R, Bailey W, et al: Smoking cessation in patients with chronic obstructive pulmonary disease: a double-blind placebo controlled, randomized trial. *Lancet.* 2001;357:1571–1575.

Tomaz PRX, Santos JR, Issa JS, et al: CYP2B6 rs2279343 polymorphism is associated with smoking cessation success in bupropion therapy. *Eur J Clin Pharmacol.* 2015;71(9):1067–1073. doi:10.1007/s00228-015-1896-x

Tonstad S, Frasang C, Klaene G, et al: Bupropion SR for smoking cessation in smokers with cardiovascular disease: a multicentre, randomized study. *Eur Heart J.* 2003;24:945–955.

Tonstadt S, Tonnesen P, Hajek P. Effect of maintenance therapy with varenicline on smoking cessation; a randomized controlled trial. *JAMA.* 2006;296:64–71.

Tsoh J, Humfleet G, Munoz R, et al: Development of major depression after treatment for smoking cessation. *Am J Psychiatry.* 2000;157:368–374.

U.S. Food and Drug Administration. (2020). 2019 National Youth Tobacco Survey shows youth e-cigarette use at alarming levels. https://www.fda.gov/media/132299/download

U.S. Food and Drug Administration. Summary of results: laboratory analysis of electronic cigarettes conducted by FDA. 2009, July 22. http://www.fda.gov/NewsEvents/PublicHealthFocus/ucm173146.htm.

U.S. Food and Drug Administration. Regulation of e-cigarettes and other tobacco products. 2011, April 25. http://www.fda.gov/NewsEvents/PublicHealthFocus/ucm252360.htm.

U.S. Food and Drug Administration. Federal Register, 2013, April 2. https://www.federalregister.gov/articles/2013/04/02/2013–07528/modifications-to-labeling-of-nicotine-replacement-therapy-products-for-over-the-counter-human-use.

U.S. Food and Drug Administration. Youth e-cigarette use remains serious public health concern amid COVID-19 pandemic. Updated September 30, 2021.

Volpp K, Troxel A, Paula M, et al: A randomized, controlled trial of financial incentives for smoking cessation. *N Engl J Med.* 2009;360:699–709.

Wang Z, Faith M, Patterson F, et al: Neural substrates of abstinence-induced cigarette cravings in chronic smokers. *J Neurosci.* 2007;27:14035–14040.

Wang RJ, Bhadriraju S, Glantz SA. E-cigarette use and adult cigarette smoking cessation: a meta-analysis. *American Journal of Public Health* 111, no. 2 (February 2021): 230–46. https://doi.org/10.2105/AJPH.2020.305999.

Whittaker R, McRobbie H, Bullen C. Mobile phone-based interventions for smoking cessation, November 14, 2012. https://www.ncbi.nlm.nih.gov/pubmed/23152238.

Williams J, Anthenelli R, Morris C, et al: A randomized, double-blinded, placebo-controlled study evaluating the safety and efficacy of varenicline for smoking cessation in patients with schizophrenia or schizoaffective disorder. *J Clin Psychiatry.* 2012;73:654–660.

World Health Organization, WHO Study Group on Tobacco Product Regulation. Report on the scientific basis of tobacco product regulation: Third report of a WHO study group. 2009. http://whqlibdoc.who.int/publications/2009/9789241209557_eng.pdf.

Yamin C, Bitton A, Bates D. E-cigarettes: a rapidly growing internet phenomenon. *Ann Intern Med.* 2010;153:607–609.

Zangen A, Moshe H, Martinez D, et al: Repetitive transcranial magnetic stimulation for smoking cessation: a pivotal multicenter double-blind randomized controlled trial. *World Psychiatry.* 2021;20(3):397–404. doi:10.1002/wps.20905

Zevin S, Jacob P, Benowitz L. Dose-related cardiovascular and endocrine effects of transdermal nicotine. *Clin Pharmacol Ther.* 1998;54:87–95.

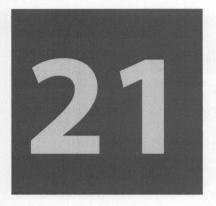

Cannabis Use Disorders

Ashley M. Schnakenberg Martin, PhD
Douglas L. Boggs, PharmD, MS
Halle Thurnauer, MA
Deepak Cyril D'Souza, MD

General Considerations

This chapter reviews the problems arising from the use and abuse of cannabis and related compounds. Cannabis refers to the herbal product prepared from cannabis plants, of which there are three species: *Cannabis indica*, *Cannabis sativa*, and *Cannabis ruderalis*. The principal constituents of cannabis are called cannabinoids. However, in addition to cannabinoids, cannabis contains several terpenoids and flavonoids. The principal psychoactive constituent of cannabis is delta-9-tetrahydrocannabinol (THC), which is present in the hair-like glandular trichomes located around the buds of the plants (Russo 2007). There is increasing recognition that other cannabinoids present in cannabis, such as cannabidiol (CBD), and possible complex interactions between the constituents of cannabis contribute to the overall effects (Potter et al. 2008). Cannabis or marijuana is referred to by several names including weed, pot, grass, ganja, and hash, some of which represent distinct forms of cannabis preparations. Cannabis is derived from the flowering tops and leaves of the cannabis plant. The THC content of cannabis varies according to the part of the plant: seeds > stems > leaves > flowers > bracts (Potter et al. 2008). The preparation from the buds and leaves of the pollinated female plants that have been grown outdoors is known as marijuana, whereas the preparation from the buds of female unfertilized plants is called sinsemilla (without seed). This form of cannabis is also known as skunk because of its pungent odor and because it contains higher levels of THC than most other forms. The resin secreted from the glandular trichomes is compressed to form hashish or subjected to solvent extraction to produce hash oil.

In addition to these plant-based cannabinoids or phytocannabinoids, a number of synthetic cannabinoids have been developed. The development of synthetic cannabinoids arose from scientific interest in the endogenous cannabinoid system. However, synthetic cannabinoids eventually started to be used by individuals for recreational purposes and became recognized substances of abuse in Europe in the early 2000s. Around 2009, synthetic cannabinoids started to appear in the United States under the name *Spice* and *K2* (Spaderna et al. 2013). These substances were marketed as potpourri and incense and labeled "not for human consumption" to circumvent regulatory restrictions. The chemical composition of the early synthetic cannabinoids included JWH-018, JWH-073, JWH-200, CP 47-497, and CP 47-497C8 homologue. In early 2011, the U.S. Drug Enforcement Agency classified these substances as schedule I substances to prevent their continued marketing. Several other synthetic cannabinoids have been developed and are found in products that are purchased for "herbal highs" (Zuba & Byrska 2013) (Table 21–1). The use of synthetic cannabinoids has declined considerably as enforcement has increased and as cannabis has been legalized in some states and has become more available.

A. Epidemiology

1. Prevalence of cannabis use—Globally, cannabis is the most widely used illicit substance according to the United Nations Office on Drugs and Crime (UNODC 2020). The prevalence of adult past-year cannabis use was estimated to be 7.8% in Western and Central Europe and 25% in Canada (UNODC 2020). The annual National Survey on Drug Use and Health (NSDUH) by the Substance Abuse and Mental Health Services Administration and surveys conducted by the National Institute on Alcohol Abuse and Alcoholism remain the important sources of cannabis use disorder (CUD) prevalence rate estimates in U.S. adults. The percentage of people aged 12 and older who used cannabis in the previous month according to the NSDUH has increased over the last two decades. In 2002, 6.2% of people reported cannabis use, and the percentage continued to decline until 2007, when it reached a low of 5.8%. The prevalence significantly increased from 2008 (6.1%) to 2009 (6.7 million) and has continued to climb. Data from 2011 found that 18.1 million people (7%) had used cannabis in the previous

Table 21–1 Some Synthetic Cannabinoids Found in Samples from Herbal Preparations

Compound	Type
Delta-9-THC	Classic cannabinoid
HU-210	Classic cannabinoid
AM-694	Benzoylindone
RCS-4*	Benzoylindone
WIN-48,098	Benzoylindone
CP-47,497	Cyclohexylphenol
JWH-018	Naphtoylindole
JWH-019	Naphtoylindole
JWH-073	Naphtoylindole
JWH-081	Naphtoylindole
JWH-122	Naphtoylindole
JWH-210	Naphtoylindole
AM-2201	Naphtoylindole
JWH-203	Phenylacetylindole
JWH-250	Phenylacetylindole
RCS-8**	Phenylacetylindole

month (NSDUH 2013), with most recent reports indicating that this number rose to 32.8 million people in 2020 (NSDUH 2021).

Adolescent use of cannabis is also tracked by the University of Michigan based Monitoring the Future program (MTF; Johnston et al. 2020). Similar to the data from the NSDUH, use of cannabis has increased among 8th, 10th, and 12th graders starting from around 2007; however, use remained stable from 2010, with the lifetime prevalence of adolescents who had used cannabis among 8th, 10th, and 12th graders 15.2, 34.0, 43.7%, respectively, as of 2019 (Miech et al. 2020). The most recent MTF reported lifetime cannabis use and annual prevalence of cannabis use declined in 2021 by 7.1 and 6.7%, respectively, for the three grades. Likewise, the 30-day prevalence of cannabis use also declined by 3.6%. Daily cannabis use in the prior 30 days also declined, with a relative decline across the three grades combined of 24%. The daily prevalence rates in 2021 across the three grades in 2021 were 0.6, 3.2, and 5.8%. In contrast, among young adults 19–30 years old, past-year cannabis use reached an all-time high in 2021 according to the MTF.

The annual prevalence of cannabis vaping has grown rapidly for the three grades combined, rising from 7% in 2017, when it was first measured, to 16% in 2020. But, in 2021 there was a decline in the three grades combined of 4.7 percentage points (which reflects a relative decline from 2020 of 29%, $p < .01$).

Lastly, synthetic cannabinoid use (e.g., spice, K2) appears to be relatively uncommon, with only 1.1% of young adults between the ages of 19 and 30 years, endorsing past-year use in 2019 (Schulenberg et al. 2020).

Perceived great risk in using cannabis regularly was lower in older than younger adolescents: 51.4% in 8th graders, 39.5% in 10th graders, and 30.5% in 12th graders (Johnston et al. 2020). The use of synthetic cannabis among this age group in 2012 was 4.4, 8.8, and 11.3%, respectively (Johnston et al. 2013); however, as of 2019 use has decreased in 8th, 10th, and 12th graders to 2.7, 2.6, and 3.3%, respectively (Miech et al. 2020).

Attitudes toward cannabis use among adults have also changed dramatically over the past 50 years. A 2013 Pew Research study found, for the first time since at least 1969, the majority of Americans (52%) favor legalization of cannabis versus the number that think it should be illegal (45%). As of 2023, 38 states, four territories, and the District of Columbia all have laws to decriminalize medical marijuana (Table 21–2). Further, 21 states have laws to legalize cannabis for recreational use. The increasing availability and acceptance of cannabis will likely lead to a growing prevalence rate of use and complications in the future.

2. Prevalence of cannabis use disorder—The rate of past-year DSM-5 CUD was 2.9% with higher rates in adults aged 18–29 years, in males and in individuals with the lowest incomes (Hasin et al. 2016). Among cannabis users, the rate of DSM-IV CUD was 30.6% with higher rates in younger males who had only high school education and belonged to

Table 21–2 US States and Territories with Laws for Medical Marijuana in 2023

Alabama	Louisiana	Ohio
Alaska	Maine	Oregon
Arizona	Maryland	Pennsylvania
Arkansas	Massachusetts	Puerto Rico
California	Michigan	Rhode Island
Colorado	Minnesota	South Carolina*
Connecticut	Mississippi	South Dakota
District of Columbia	Missouri	Tennessee*
Delaware	Montana	Texas*
Florida	Nevada	Utah
Georgia*	New Hampshire	Vermont
Guam	New Jersey	Virginia
Hawaii	New Mexico	Washington
Illinois	New York	West Virginia
Indiana*	North Carolina*	Wisconsin*
Iowa*	North Dakota	Wyoming*
Kentucky	Oklahoma	

Note: *While not considered a medical cannabis program, these states/territories have laws regarding the use of low THC, high CBD products for medical reasons in limited situations or as a legal defense.

the lowest income category (Hasin et al. 2015). The number of people aged 12 or older with disordered use (abuse/dependence/CUD) has increased over time. For example, the absolute values ranged from a low of 3.9 million in 2007, 4.5 million in 2004 and 2010, 4.2 million in 2011, to 14.2 million in the most recent estimate in 2020 (NSDUH 2013, 2021). Notably, disordered use was highest in young adults between the age of 18 and 25 years (NSDUH 2021).

The risk of CUD among adult cannabis users is now much higher than it was in the early 1990s. A commonly held view is that the prevalence of CUD among cannabis users is only 10%. Unfortunately, these estimates were based on studies conducted in the 1990s (Anthony et al. 1994), when cannabis was less potent, illegal, less available, and the definition of CUD has been redefined. In a recent meta-analysis, the prevalence of CUD among cannabis users in several countries was estimated to be 22% (Leung et al. 2020), while among frequent users, the risk of CUD was about 30%.

Critically, likely due to a decreasing perception of risk, the number of individuals receiving treatment of CUD has been decreasing. The Treatment Episode Data Set (TEDS) tracks the annual admissions to treatment centers that receive state funding. The number of admissions reported by TEDS in 2010, for cannabis as the primary substance of hospitalization, was 358,034 (18.6%), while by 2015 that number decreased to 242,386 (14.2% of all admissions), and just 139,481 (9.8%) by 2020 (TEDS 2021). Synthetic cannabinoid use (e.g., spice, K2) appears to be relatively uncommon, with only 1.1% of young adults between the ages of 19 and 30 years, endorsing past year use in 2019 (Schulenberg et al. 2020).

3. Prevalence of cannabis use adverse events—The Drug Abuse Warning Network (DAWN) is a national public surveillance system that monitors drug-related hospital admissions to hospital emergency departments (EDs). Cannabis-related ED visits have consistently increased over the past decade: a 70% increase has occurred since 2004 and a 27% increase since 2009. In 2021, cannabis was one of the top five drugs involved in drug-related ED visits (11.19%), following alcohol (41.70%), opioids (14.79%), and methamphetamine (11.29%; DAWN 2022). Further, there were 804,285 visits (11.19%) in 2021, nearly double the number of visits in 2011, which had 479,560 ED visits related to cannabis use, although in 2011 this constituted 38.3% of all ED visits (DAWN 2022, 2013).

Between 2012 and 2021, the American Association of Poison Control Centers reports 132,995 exposures to cannabinoid products, with annual increases since 2016 (Gummin et al. 2022). The first reports of synthetic cannabis exposure came in 2009 when 14 calls were received (Wood 2013), with a spike in synthetic cannabinoid exposure in 2015 (Gummin et al. 2022). Notably, despite its recent decline in exposure reports, synthetic cannabinoids remain associated with the highest rate of major adverse effects in clinical complications and hospital resource utilization (10.7% of 17,279 exposure

cases). There has been a significant increase (1804%) in ED visits by older adults for acute consequences of cannabis (Han et al. 2023) and cannabis legalization was associated with higher odds of cannabis-related problems in those ≥55 years (Imtiaz et al. 2023).

4. Risk of co-occurring psychiatric disorders—Because cannabis is the most commonly used substance of abuse in the general population, it is not surprising that CUD is common among people with other psychiatric illnesses, including affective disorders, anxiety disorders, and psychotic disorders (Hasin et al. 2016; Koskinen et al. 2010; Stinson et al. 2006). A representative sample of 36,309 American adults from the National Institute on Alcohol Abuse and Alcoholism 2012–2013 National Epidemiologic Survey on Alcohol and Related Conditions-III (NESARC-III) represents the best data about psychiatric comorbidity among CUDs (Hasin et al. 2016). According to the NESARC-III (Grant et al. 2014), individuals with a lifetime CUD were more likely to have other substance use disorders (OR = 6.6–14.5), mood disorders (OR = 2.6–3.8), anxiety disorders (OR = 2.1–3.2), PTSD (OR = 3.8), and personality disorders (OR = 4.0–4.7). Notably, with the exceptions of only a few disorders (bipolar II, agoraphobia and specific phobia), the associations between disorders increased with increasing severity of CUD (Hasin et al. 2016). Recent findings suggest that cannabis use or CUD is associated with worse prognosis for individuals with bipolar disorder (including increased suicidal behaviors) and depression (Kuhns et al. 2022). DSM-5 no longer lists post-traumatic stress disorder (PTSD) as an anxiety disorder, but as with other anxiety disorders, lifetime PTSD diagnosis is associated with a 2.5 times greater rate of lifetime cannabis use (Cougle et al. 2011).

A meta-analysis showed that approximately 25% of people with schizophrenia have lifetime cannabis use (Koskinen et al. 2010) and approximately one-third of individuals experiencing their first episode of psychosis endorse clinically significant cannabis use (Myles et al. 2016). Additionally, compared to the general population, individuals with psychosis are 3.5 times more likely to use cannabis heavily (Hartz et al. 2014). The rates of cannabis use are especially high during the first episode, with reported rates reaching 44.4%. Overall, the risk among people with schizophrenia is highest in younger males during their first episode.

B. Etiology

The risk factors for CUD are similar to those for other substances of abuse (Watson et al. 2000)—few factors specific to cannabis have been identified. A prospective study found that certain variables including living alone, having a CUD, using cannabis in the daytime, continual smoking, using cannabis to cope with situations, having motor and attentional impulsivity, and mean number of lifetime negative events all increase the likelihood of developing cannabis dependence (van der Pol et al. 2013). Social, psychological, environmental, and biological factors contribute to an individual's vulnerability to develop CUD. Social vulnerability factors are general and include family, neighborhood, peers, socioeconomic status, and delinquency. Biological vulnerability factors include hereditary (discussed later), brain developmental status (adolescence), biological sex, and other neuropsychiatric disorders (e.g., schizophrenia). Psychological factors include impulsivity and sensation seeking. Lastly, environmental factors including availability, price, potency of cannabis, THC:CBD ratio, and legal status, also play a role.

C. Genetics

Cannabis use and CUD are heritable (~50%) complex traits which are closely linked to several neuropsychiatric disorders. Similar to other substances of abuse, cannabis use has a strong genetic component. Results from eight twin studies suggest that heritability for CUDs is between 50 and 78% (Hines et al. 2018; Verweij et al. 2010). Heritable influences on cannabis use emerge during late adolescence and young adulthood and play a role in determining age at exposure, opportunity, and access to cannabis. For cannabis use, both non-shared and shared environmental factors explain ~25% of variance in the trait. In contrast, for CUD the role of non-shared environmental factors appears to be higher than shared environmental factors.

Several approaches have been used to find genetic variants that might underlie the above-mentioned heritability. Genes in regions known to be relevant to reward-related pathways and endocannabinoid signaling pathways have been studied. Linkage studies identified regions on seven chromosomes (1, 3, 4, 9, 14, 17, and 18) related to CUDs (Agrawal et al. 2008a, 2008b, 2008c; Hopfer et al. 2007). The gene coding for the cannabinoid 1 (CB1) receptor is found on chromosome 6q14–15, and this receptor is highly expressed in the brain, and is known to be responsible for the euphoric symptoms related to cannabis use. Two single-nucleotide polymorphisms (SNPs) of the CB1 receptor rs2023239 and rs806368 were linked to increased general substance-use dependence, and the SNP rs806380 was linked to cannabis dependence in some studies (Agrawal et al. 2009b; Hopfer et al. 2006) but not others (Herman et al. 2006). The gene that encodes for fatty acid amide hydrolase (FAAH), another enzyme responsible for breakdown of endogenous cannabinoids, has also been examined in several studies. Similar to the findings with CB1, SNPs of FAAH have been associated with general substance use disorders but not specifically cannabis use (Agrawal et al. 2009a). However, individuals with the A/A variant are less likely to be dependent on cannabis; the authors suggest this might be due to higher endogenous cannabinoid levels resulting from the less active variant (Tyndale et al. 2007). People with the A/A variant also report fewer withdrawal symptoms and do not experience the same degree of happiness after cannabis use (Schacht et al. 2009). Although monoglyceride lipase (MGL) has been implicated

in CUDs (Hopfer et al. 2006), no SNPs have been identified that correlate with cannabis dependence. The GABRA2 gene, which encodes the alpha$_2$ subunit of the gamma-aminobutyric acid (GABA) receptor, has the rs279858 polymorphism, which appears to be associated with cannabis dependence (Agrawal et al. 2006), but this was not replicated in another sample (Lind et al. 2008).

These candidate gene approaches have mixed results which do not offer conclusions. Furthermore, the candidate gene approach is fraught with a number of limitations including small sample sizes (Agrawal and Lynskey 2009). Many of these limitations of candidate gene approaches can be addressed by genome-wide association studies (GWASs) studies.

Several GWAS investigations have identified ANKFN1, NCAM1 CDAM2, SCOC, KCNT2, and *CHRNA2* (Agrawal et al. 2011; Demontis et al. 2019; Stringer 2016), as associated with lifetime cannabis use. The largest GWAS which included 185,000 individuals identified eight single nucleotide polymorphisms (SNPs) associated with lifetime cannabis use (Pasman et al. 2018); at the gene-wise level, 35 genes were found to be associated with cannabis use. The strongest link was to *CADM2* and *NCAM1* genes. Interestingly, the brain expressed CADM2 gene has been associated with alcohol use and risk-taking. The largest GWAS for CUD to date which included 21,000 individuals with CUD and >300,000 controls, identified significant association to *FOXP2* and *CHRNA2* genes (Johnson et al. 2020). The latter is implicated in tobacco smoking and schizophrenia, while the former has been implicated in the development of brain regions involved in reward processing. Furthermore, Johnson et al. showed partial genetic overlap between CUD and cannabis use ($r_g = 0.50$).

Despite the correlation between CUD and cannabis use, their genetic relationship with other traits and disorders varies. Both cannabis use and CUD are genetically correlated with other substance use disorders (e.g., tobacco and alcohol-use disorders), and other psychiatric disorders (e.g., major depression and schizophrenia).

▶ Clinical Findings

A. Signs & Symptoms

1. Cannabis intoxication and overdose—The acute effects of cannabis include euphoria, relaxation, increased appetite, cognitive impairment, and impaired motor coordination. In some instances, people report anxiety, paranoia, and, rarely, psychosis. The physiological effects of cannabis include dry mouth, conjunctival injection, tachycardia, and orthostatic hypotension. Generally, the symptoms of synthetic cannabis use are similar to those for cannabis, but there are important differences in the spectrum and intensity of the effects (Spaderna et al. 2013).

The risk of overdose from cannabis is extremely low. Animal studies suggest that cannabis is not lethal even at doses

5000 times greater than those needed to get high (Braude 1972; Chan et al. 1996).

2. Synthetic cannabinoid intoxication and overdose— Although many of the acute effects of synthetic cannabinoids are similar to those of cannabis, there are important differences in both the spectrum and intensity of effects. In general, the effects of spice include changes in mood, anxiety, perception, thinking, memory and attention, neurological function, cardiovascular function, and gastrointestinal function. The acute psychoactive effects of synthetic cannabinoids include euphoria, a feeling of well-being, calmness, relaxation, increased creativity, and mild perceptual alterations, as well as mild memory and attentional impairments. Effects at either end of the spectrum may occur, including anxiolysis or anxiety, stimulation or sedation, and euphoria or dysphoria. Panic attacks following the use of synthetic cannabinoids have been reported as including suicidal ideation and attempts (Gay 2010; Hurst et al. 2011; Shanks et al. 2012; Van der Veer & Fiday 2011). Given how little is known about the composition and pharmacology of the various synthetic cannabinoids, what constitutes an overdose remains unclear. Nevertheless, there are a number of reports of catastrophic effects of using synthetic cannabinoids, including myocardial infarction, seizures, and even death (Mir et al. 2011; St. James 2010; WYFF4.COM 2011).

One of the possible reasons why the rates of negative outcomes associated with the use of synthetic cannabinoids are higher than for cannabis is because the synthetic cannabinoids generally have higher affinity and potency.

3. Cannabis withdrawal—The DSM-5 is the first DSM to classify a cannabis withdrawal syndrome (CWS), although there has been increasing recognition of a withdrawal syndrome following the discontinuation of cannabis (Budney 1999). It was previously difficult to demonstrate a CWS in animals. The availability and application of CB1R antagonists to precipitate CWS has provided clear and robust support for a CWS. The CB1R antagonist SR141716A precipitates a withdrawal syndrome in rodents tolerant to THC that is characterized by the immediate emergence of ptosis, wet-dog shakes, "anxiety" reactions, and disorganized patterns of motor activity (Aceto et al. 1996, 2001; Lichtman & Martin 2002; Rodriguez de Fonseca et al. 1997; Tsou et al. 1995). A less dramatic syndrome occurs with discontinuation of chronic heavy exposure to cannabis, THC, or synthetic cannabinoids in both humans and animals. Observed withdrawal symptoms in CB1R agonist dependent animals following the abrupt discontinuation of CB1R agonist include hyper-irritability, tremors, and anorexia (Aceto et al. 1996, 2001; Beardsley et al. 1986; Lichtman et al. 2002).

In humans, a CWS has been reported from retrospective self-report studies (Wiesbeck et al. 1996), prospective outpatient studies (Budney et al. 2001, 2003), and human laboratory studies involving the administration and discontinuation of cannabinoids (Georgotas & Zeidenberg 1979; Haney et al.

1999a, 1999b; Jones et al. 1976). The typical withdrawal symptoms include anger, aggression, appetite change, weight loss, irritability, anxiety, restlessness, altered sleep, strange dreams, cannabis craving, and physical discomfort (Budney et al. 2002, 2004, 2007; Haney 2005; Haney et al. 1999a, 1999b; Jones et al. 1976; Kouri & Pope 2000; Kouri et al. 1999). Less common symptoms include chills, depressed mood, stomach pain, and sweating. Most symptoms appear within 1 day of abstinence, peak within 2–3 days, and resolve within 1–2 weeks. Two studies evaluated symptom time course for at least 4 weeks (45 days and 28 days, respectively). Both studies observed prominent withdrawal symptoms during the initial 2–3 weeks of abstinence, some of which persisted through the entire study period (Budney et al. 2003; Kouri et al. 2000). The findings of these studies suggest that withdrawal symptoms may persist longer than 4 weeks. Characteristic of a true withdrawal syndrome, abstinence symptoms occur with blind discontinuation and resolve with the administration of CB1R agonist readministration (Budney et al. 2007; Haney et al. 1999b, 2004; Jones et al. 1976, 1981).

Withdrawal reactions have also been reported with the use of synthetic cannabinoids. The symptoms include diaphoresis, internal restlessness, tremor, somatic pain, palpitations, insomnia, tachycardia, hypertension, hyperventilation, headache, diarrhea, nausea, vomiting, and depressed mood. Most severe withdrawal symptoms resolved within a week, although there were longer-lasting residual symptoms (Rominger et al. 2013; Zimmermann et al. 2009).

4. Cannabis addiction and sequelae—

i. Chronic cannabis use and cognitive function—The effects of chronic cannabis use are not as clear as acute effects and are difficult to study. Several studies suggest that chronic, heavy cannabis use may lead to memory impairments and attentional dysfunction (Bolla et al. 2002; Lundqvist 2005; Pope et al. 1995, 2001; Pope & Yurgelun-Todd 1996; Solowij & Battisti 2008). In a comprehensive review, Solowij and Battisti (2008) concluded that chronic heavy cannabis use is associated with impaired memory function. Impaired memory function persists beyond the period of acute intoxication and is related to the frequency, duration, dose, and age of onset of cannabis use. There is evidence for residual effects of cannabis on learning and memory in regular users (Broyd et al. 2016; Krzyzanowski and Purdon 2020; Lovell et al. 2020; Nader and Sanchez 2018; Schoeler et al. 2016). Heavy and prolonged use is associated with worse learning and memory (Broyd et al. 2016; Cuttler et al. 2012; Kroon et al. 2021; Solowij et al. 2011; Thames et al. 2014,). Lastly, greater cannabis use frequency during adolescence predicts poorer verbal memory (Duperrouzel et al. 2019). Whether these *persistent* cognitive deficits fully resolve with prolonged abstinence has not been conclusively determined. Pope et al (2003) demonstrated an absence of persistent neuropsychological deficits in frequent long-term cannabis users after 28 days of abstinence. However, others have found persistent cognitive impairments and other indices of alterations in brain function after 4 weeks of abstinence (Bolla et al. 2002, 2005; Eldreth et al. 2004; Pillay et al. 2008; Schweinsburg et al. 2008; Sneider et al. 2008). The findings are mixed whether there is complete recovery of verbal learning and memory deficits following months of abstinence from cannabis (Broyd et al. 2016; Kroon et al. 2021). Some studies found persistent deficits (Medina et al. 2007; Meier et al. 2012; Riba et al. 2015; Lorenzetti et al. 2021), while others found partial (Roten et al. 2015) or full recovery (Broyd et al. 2016; Pope et al. 2001; Tait et al. 2011; Thames et al. 2014). Although it is not clear whether complete recovery of function occurs following prolonged abstinence, it should not detract from the public health implications of millions of chronic cannabis users attempting to function with persistent cognitive deficits.

Solowij et al. (1995) showed that heavy, chronic use of cannabis may be associated with relatively subtle deficits in attentional processing as indexed by an electrophysiological indices of information processing. This evidence has been interpreted to indicate problems in the efficient selection of relevant stimulus information and in filtering out nonsalient information. Further work suggests that these deficits may endure over time. More recently, Ehrenreich et al. (1999) have reported that deficits in human visual scanning (which undergoes maturation between 12 and 15 years of age) are best predicted by earlier onset of cannabis use (before 16 years of age vs. after 16 years), suggesting that early use is associated with persistent deficits. Solowij and Michie (2007) suggested some similarities between the cognitive dysfunction associated with long-term, heavy cannabis use and the cognitive endophenotypes that have been proposed as vulnerability markers of schizophrenia (Solowij et al. 2007).

Previous cross-sectional experiments have reported inconsistent results with some suggesting that chronic cannabis use impairs performance on tests of intelligence (Stefanis et al. 1976; Wig & Varma 1977), while others find no impairment (Carlin & Trupin 1977; Culver & King 1974). More recently, it has also been observed that males, as opposed to females, may be more vulnerable to the neurocognitive deficits related to cannabis use in domains such as intelligence, psychomotor speed, and verbal learning (Hirst et al. 2021; Schnakenberg Martin et al. 2021). A longitudinal study examined 1037 subjects followed from birth to age 38 years (Meier et al. 2012). Subject cannabis use was evaluated at ages 18, 21, 26, 32, and 38 years; neuropsychological testing was conducted at ages 13 and 38 years. The experiment determined that those who persistently use cannabis are more likely than nonusers to experience a decline in IQ. The findings persisted even after controlling for level of education, and impaired IQ was found to be particularly true for the subjects who began to use cannabis during adolescence as opposed to during adulthood. Those who began to use cannabis during adolescence exhibited an 8-point decrease in IQ between childhood and adulthood. Another important finding of the study was that the decline in IQ did not appear

to reverse after cannabis use ceased (Meier et al. 2012). However, in a later study, more using data from the Environmental Risk Longitudinal Twin Study (E-Risk), Meier et al. (2018) did not find evidence that adolescent cannabis use or dependence was associated with IQ decline between the ages of 12 and 18 years. A more recent systematic review and metanalysis reported a significant effect for the association between frequent or dependent cannabis use in youth and IQ change; however, the magnitude of the effect was small.

It is noteworthy that the relationships between cognition and cannabis use as described above do not appear to translate to individuals with psychosis and regular cannabis use. For example, it has instead been observed that moderate, as opposed to heavy or no lifetime cannabis use is associated with fewer cognitive deficits in individuals with psychosis (Schnakenberg Martin et al. 2016; Yucel et al. 2012). Further, although many have suggested that greater executive cognition, and particularly social cognition, is required for the acquisition and use of cannabis, this notion has not been fully supported by the literature (Arnold et al. 2015; Helle et al. 2017; Sánchez-Torres et al. 2013). Given the cross-sectional nature of many of these studies, future research would benefit from considering the potential of baseline differences (pre-cannabis use) in cognition.

ii. Chronic cannabis use and amotivational syndrome— Chronic heavy cannabis use has also been associated with an "amotivational syndrome" (Halikas et al. 1982; Hall & Solowij 1998; Kolansky & Moore 1971; Millman & Sbriglio 1986; Tennant & Groesbeck 1972). This syndrome is characterized by apathy, amotivation, social withdrawal, narrowing of one's personal repertoire of interests, lethargy, impairment in memory and concentration, impaired judgment and decision making, and poor socio-occupational functioning. The existence of this syndrome is debated, and the confounding effects of concomitant polydrug abuse, poverty, low socio-economic status, or preexisting psychiatric disorders cannot be ruled out (Hollister 1988; Rubin & Comitas 1975). It has also been suggested that a decrease in dopamine brain reactivity due to disordered cannabis use is associated with negative emotionality and severity of cannabis use (Volkow et al. 2014). In the limited work in this area, one study demonstrated that individuals with schizophrenia spectrum disorders and regular cannabis use, compared to nonusing peers, expressed less ability to express emotion, were less likely to anticipate or expect pleasure, and had poorer social function (Schnakenberg Martin et al. 2020).

iii. Cannabis and psychosis—Several lines of evidence suggest an association between the use of cannabis and psychosis reviewed in D'Souza et al. (2022) and elsewhere (Radhakrishnan et al. 2012 and Sewell et al. 2010). The basis of this association remains unclear. Cannabinoids can produce a full range of acute, transient, schizophrenia-like positive, negative, and cognitive symptoms. Cannabinoids also produce some psychophysiological deficits that are known to be present in schizophrenia. It is also clear that in individuals with an established psychotic disorder, cannabinoids can acutely exacerbate symptoms, trigger relapse, and have negative consequences for the course of the illness. Furthermore, accumulating evidence suggests that early and heavy cannabis exposure may increase the risk of developing a persistent psychotic disorder such as schizophrenia. There appears to be a crucial role of age (with the period of adolescence being identified as a period of exquisite vulnerability), familial risk, degree of schizotypy, and the role of genetic factors in moderating this association between cannabis and schizophrenia.

iv. Cannabis and mood disorders—Converging lines of evidence from animal models and large epidemiological studies in humans suggest that cannabis consumption during adolescence is associated with an increased risk of developing mood disorders in adolescence or in young adulthood (Baggio et al. 2014; Fleming et al. 2008; Gobbi et al. 2019; Lev-Ran et al. 2014; Womack et al. 2016). The higher risk persists even after controlling for premorbid conditions, socio-economic status, and use of other drugs. The risk for depression is low-medium but given the high numbers of adolescents exposed to cannabis (20–30%), the increase in cases of depression remains high at a population level. Furthermore, cannabis consumption also increases the risk for both for suicidal behaviors and attempts (Gobbi et al. 2019).

v. Cannabis and anxiety disorders—The results of surveys suggest that individuals in the community are using cannabis to treat anxiety and report it to be efficacious. However, the results of surveys do not account for information about routes of administration, type of product used, frequency of use, dose, age of cannabis use onset, and expectancies (Mammen et al. 2018). In contrast, a recent systematic review spanning 11,959 individuals found that recent cannabis use over the past 6 months was associated with greater symptom severity, number of symptoms, and fewer instances of symptom remission and recovery for up to 5 years, compared to individuals without recent use (Mammen et al. 2018). Importantly, because investigators also observed that recent cannabis use was related to fewer treatment-related (e.g., psychotherapy, pharmacotherapy) gains, they further suggested that cannabis use may actually interfere with recovery and thus led to persistent long-term symptoms. The lack of evidence for cannabinoids as a treatment for anxiety has also been observed in follow-up systematic reviews and meta-analyses (Bilbao et al. 2022; Black et al. 2019).

B. Psychological Testing

There are no psychological tests that are specific to CUDs. Screening for cannabis is usually conducted using standardized rating scales for substance use disorders such as the Addiction Severity Index (Fureman et al. 1990). The prevalence and growing acceptance of cannabis necessitates screening of most individuals for CUD. DSM-5 now reports

specific symptoms associated with a CWS, but many other symptoms have been reported in cannabis-dependent individuals (Boggs et al. 2012; Budney & Hughes 2006a; Copersino et al. 2006a). At least three different scales have been published that measure CWS (Gorelick et al. 2012); however, none specifically meet DSM-5 criteria, although all capture the withdrawal symptoms reported in DSM-5.

C. Laboratory Findings

A standard urine toxicology screen is normally conducted for verification of cannabis intoxication. Urine tests generally analyze by immunoassay for a metabolite of THC, 11-nor-9-carboxy-tetrahydrocannabinol (Huestis 2007). Several factors are important when determining exposure to cannabis, such as route of administration and amount of prior exposure. Individuals with minimal cannabis exposure might not have traces of metabolites in their urine by immunoassay after a few hours. However, individuals with chronic exposure may have positive screens for weeks and in extreme cases, months. THC and other metabolites can also be detected in plasma, saliva, nails, and hair, but such tests are not done in routine clinical practice.

Synthetic cannabis will not be detected in the standard commercially available toxicological screens. A few specialized laboratories are now able to test for synthetic cannabinoids, using gas chromatography-mass spectrometry (GC/MS). As seen in Table 21–1, a large number of chemicals are sold as synthetic cannabis, and new compounds will probably continue to be developed. Therefore, detection of synthetic cannabis will likely continue to be difficult for the foreseeable future.

D. Neuroimaging

Many types of neuroimaging studies have been conducted addressing both the immediate and chronic effects of cannabis on the brain. THC administration generally shows marked enhancement in regional cerebral blood flow (rCBF) as measured by oxygen-15 labeled water. The greatest increases occur in the anterior cerebral cortex, frontal cortex, insula, and cerebellum (Mathew et al. 1997, 2002; O'Leary et al. 2000, 2007). Chronic cannabis users also have lower rCBF, especially in the cerebellum (Volkow et al. 1996). Structural imaging studies in chronic cannabis users have been inconsistent, likely due to variations in THC potency, other cannabinoid concentrations (and their unknown interaction with THC), routes of administration, and other use-related factors (e.g., age of cannabis initiation, recency of use, etc.). Global structural changes in the brain have not been detected, but specific changes in the hippocampus, orbitofrontal cortex, amygdala, and parahippocampus are seen in some but not all studies (Bloomfield et al. 2019; Chye et al. 2021; Lorenzetti et al. 2010, 2019). Unlike other substances of abuse, cannabis does not consistently increase striatal dopamine release, and chronic users do not have alterations of striatal dopamine release (Lorenzetti et al. 2010). However, many neuroimaging studies suggest that earlier and prolonged use of cannabis is correlated with more neurobiological changes. Magnetic resonance spectroscopy studies have shown glutamatergic and GABAergic abnormalities in chronic cannabis users that may also have sensitivity to biological sex and an association with taurine, a neuroprotective amino acid (Newman et al. 2019, 2020, 2022; Prescot et al. 2013). Recently, specific ligands have been developed that can bind to the CB1 receptor. Cannabis users seem to have globally lower availability of the CB1 receptor compared to controls but, return to normal levels with abstinence (D'Souza et al. 2016; Hirvonen et al. 2012). Although great strides are taking place in the area of neuroimaging, the increased availability and use of cannabis for medical conditions is going to require more research to determine how cannabis affects the brain.

E. Course of Illness

Cannabis use generally starts during adolescence, with CUD developing between 15 and 25 years (Perkonigg et al. 1998). Initiation of cannabis use before the age of 16 years increases the risk of developing CUD, other substance use disorders, and anxiety disorders (Connor et al. 2021). The short period of time since cannabis legalization in the United States makes it difficult to assess its full effect on the prevalence of disordered use. Historically, it has been estimated that approximately 10% of people who use cannabis develop dependence (Anthony et al. 1994). Newest estimates suggest that approximately 10% of those who endorse cannabis use over the past year identified as daily or near-daily users, with more than one-third considered to have CUD (UNODC 2020). The risk of cannabis dependence decreases over a 10-year period (Anthony et al. 1994). However, people who use cannabis at least five times a year are likely to continue the same level of use for at least 10 years (Perkonigg et al. 2008).

▶ Differential Diagnosis

Other substances may mimic cannabis intoxication, withdrawal, and use disorder.

▶ Treatment

A. Psychopharmacology Interventions

Although the number of people who seek out or have received formalized substance abuse treatment for cannabis has steadily increased over the past decade, the vast majority of individuals who use cannabis do not use medication to treat CUDs. This has led to a number of pharmacological trials to treat CUDs (Danovitch & Gorelick 2012). As reported, cannabis intoxication is usually well tolerated and self-limiting. Rarely, anxiolytics and/or antipsychotics are used to treat acute anxiety or psychotic symptoms.

Most pharmacological trials have focused on the initial and immediate goal of alleviating the unpleasant abstinence symptoms associated with CWS. Cannabis withdrawal has been found to be a significant negative reinforcement for relapse in people trying to abstain from cannabis use. Few studies have targeted the long-term goal of relapse prevention or reducing consumption.

The strategies tested include (1) drugs that directly target the CB-1R system, such as CB-1R agonists (e.g., THC, nabilone, and nabiximols) to substitute cannabis (Allsop et al. 2014; Budney et al. 2007; Haney et al. 2004; Hill et al. 2017; Levin & Kleber 2008; Levin et al. 2011; Lintzeris et al. 2019; Trigo et al. 2018), CB1R antagonists to block cannabis effects (Huestis et al. 2001, 2007), and inhibitors of the enzyme that breaks down the principal endocannabinoid, anandamide (D'Souza et al. 2019); (2) antidepressants including bupropion (Haney et al. 2001; McRae-Clark et al. 2009, 2015), nefazodone (Carpenter et al. 2009; Haney et al. 2003b), venlafaxine (Levin), escitalopram (Weinstein et al. 2014), fluoxetine (Findling et al. 2009), vilazodone (Mcrae-Clark et al. 2016), lofexidine (Haney et al. 2008), and baclofen and mirtazapine (Haney et al. 2010); (3) mood stabilizers such as lithium (Winstock et al. 2009) and divalproex (Haney et al. 2004; Levin et al. 2004); and (5) miscellaneous drugs including naltrexone (Cooper & Haney 2010; Greenwald & Stitzer 2000; Haney 2007; Haney et al. 2003a, 2015; Wachtel & de Wit 2000), topiramate (Miranda et al. 2017), N-acetylcysteine (Gray et al. 2010, 2012, 2017), atomoxetine (McRae-Clark et al. 2010; Tirado et al. 2008), buspirone (McRae-Clark et al. 2006, 2009), and entacapone (Shafa 2009).

The study designs were randomized, double-blind, placebo-controlled, and counterbalanced, with the exception of a few open-label studies (Weinstein & Gorelick 2011). The studies were generally small (mean 28.5 ± 33.7, range 6–156 subjects) and of varying duration (1–13 weeks). Subjects with DSM-IV cannabis dependence, a history of heavy cannabis use, or positive urine toxicology were included. Most of the subjects included in these studies were non–treatment seeking; this makes it difficult to generalize the findings to treatment-seeking populations.

Most of the approaches yielded negative results. The few that did yield promising results have not all been consistently replicated. Nefazodone decreased some withdrawal symptoms, but it had no effect on most other symptoms (Haney et al. 2003b). Baclofen dose-dependently decreased craving for cannabis (Haney et al. 2010). Mirtazapine improved sleep during abstinence and robustly increased food intake but had no effect on withdrawal symptoms and did not decrease relapse (Haney et al. 2010). Substitution with THC reduces cannabis withdrawal in a dose-dependent manner (Budney et al. 2007; Haney et al. 2004; Levin et al. 2011), although some studies have failed to observe the efficacy of cannabinoids like dronabinol, alone or in combination with lofexidine, an alpha-2 agonist (Levin et al. 2016). The reduction in cannabis withdrawal does not appear to translate into any reduction in relapse but may result in higher treatment retention (Levin et al. 2011). CB1R antagonism has also been studied to block the acute effects of cannabis (Huestis et al. 2001). However, the CB1R antagonist rimonabant was removed from the market because of concerns of anxiety, irritability, depression, and suicidal ideation (Despres et al. 2005; Gelfand & Cannon 2006). Thus, it is unlikely that an approach based on CB1R antagonism will be clinically feasible. A proof-of-concept study was conducted in treatment-seeking cannabis-dependent individuals with the antiepileptic gabapentin. The study found that 1200 mg/day of gabapentin over 12 weeks decreased both cannabis use and withdrawal in 50 people (Mason et al. 2012). A single-site, double-blind, randomized, placebo-controlled inpatient/outpatient study with a FAAH inhibitor showed a reduction in cannabis withdrawal, self-reported cannabis use, urinary THC-COOH levels and a normalization of stage 3 sleep deficits in CUD (D'Souza 2019). Lastly, neuromodulation techniques such as repetitive transcranial magnetic stimulation may be useful to treat comorbid CUD.

In summary, none of the medications that have been tested for cannabis withdrawal and/or use disorder have been shown to be consistently effective (Kondo et al. 2020; McRae-Clark et al. 2009; Nordstrom & Levin 2007; Vandrey & Haney 2009; Weinstein et al. 2011). The only treatment showing some promise in alleviating cannabinoid withdrawal is substitution therapy with CB1R agonists. The latter have potent psychoactive effects, and other side effects that limit tolerability and are not without risk. THC is unlikely to be a useful treatment for underage-21 patients with CUD because THC cannot be given to individuals who are under the age of 21—a group that has high rates of cannabis-related problems. Although low doses of oral THC might attenuate withdrawal symptoms, similar doses of THC have been shown to exhibit reinforcing properties in cannabis users, suggesting that abuse liability remains a concern with substitution therapy (Hart et al. 2005).

1. Drug interactions—Cannabis and its constituents do not have identified interactions related to the CYP450 system but a change in metabolism of medications or pharmacodynamic interactions can occur. According to the package insert for the oral THC medication dronabinol (Marinol), THC is highly protein bound and may displace other medications. Also, additive effects can be seen with sympathomimetic agents (hypertension, tachycardia, possible cardiotoxicity), anticholinergic agents (tachycardia, drowsiness), tricyclic antidepressants (tachycardia, hypertension, drowsiness), and central nervous system depressants (drowsiness and increased CNS depression). Hypomanic symptoms have been reported with fluoxetine and disulfiram. Cannabis combined with barbiturates can decrease the clearance of the barbiturate, possibly through competitive inhibition. Conversely, theophylline has increased metabolism with cannabis use which is similar to that seen with smoking tobacco.

B. Psychotherapeutic Interventions

A number of different psychotherapeutic interventions have been used in treating adults with CUDs including cognitive behavioral therapy (CBT), motivational enhancement therapy (MET), or contingency management (CM). Broadly, psychosocial interventions (vs. no treatment) have been observed to result in significant decreases in cannabis use (amount and frequency) and severity of disordered use, although many fail to maintain abstinence endorsing relapse within a month after treatment (Cooper et al. 2015; Gates et al. 2016; Winters et al. 2021). Also, it appears that treatment intensity is related to favorable outcomes, with inconsistent findings regarding to improvement in psychosocial outcomes like employment and mental health.

1. Cognitive behavioral therapy—CBT has emerged as the most widely used approach to psychotherapy in treating patients with substance use disorders. CBT has shown to have the largest treatment effect ($g = 0.5$) for CUD when compared to its efficacy in cocaine, opiate, or polysubstance-dependent populations (Magill & Ray 2009). CBT includes a large number of interventions and techniques that work in isolation as well as in tandem and can be applied in both an individual and group setting. These interventions target internal and external cues; enhance motivation for cessation, abstinence, and relapse prevention; address the cognitive distortions associated with cannabis use; provide enhanced problem-solving skills; and aid in the development of adaptive coping mechanisms and improved communication (McHugh et al. 2010). Randomized controlled trials have demonstrated that even a brief, 1-day intervention is more likely to elicit abstinence and decrease problems related to cannabis use than a delayed-treatment group (Copeland et al. 2001), and there are no substantial differences in improvement between a brief and extended CBT intervention (Stephens et al. 2000).

2. Motivational enhancement therapy—MET is a form of motivational interviewing stemming from Rogerian, client-centered therapy that empowers patients to become motivated to change beliefs and behaviors related to cannabis use. This is achieved through aiding patients in uncovering and resolving ambivalence related to making the changes necessary to cease and abstain from cannabis use (Hettema et al. 2005; Tevyaw & Monti 2004).

3. Contingency management—CM is based on the premise that substance use and addiction are forms of operant conditioning that are heavily influenced by consequences of maladaptive behaviors. One of the most widely used methods of contingency management is voucher-based reinforcement therapy, in which patients are awarded vouchers for small prizes or money in exchange for a cannabinoid-negative urine specimen (Prendergast et al. 2006). The abstinence-based incentive system has shown to enhance the effects of an adjunctive therapy or to be more effective than other treatment modalities. For example, MET has shown to be most efficacious when providing a voucher-based exchange program. Compared to MET with CBT interventions as well as MET alone, MET including the voucher-based incentives produced longer periods of abstinence during treatment (Budney et al. 2000). Furthermore, abstinence-based vouchers have been shown to be more effective than CBT alone in helping patients maintain abstinence. When used in combination, the addition of CBT increases the duration of the positive effects that vouchers have on abstinence from cannabis (Budney et al. 2006b). These findings suggest that incentive-based interventions provide an enhanced or even superior approach to other psychotherapeutic interventions in treating patients with cannabis dependence.

4. Combined psychosocial interventions (MET/CBT/CM)— Growing evidence suggest that the combination of psychosocial interventions (e.g., MET, CBT, CM) may offer increased effectiveness (Budney et al. 2018; Litt et al. 2013). Further, it has been suggested that a primary component may be the integration of abstinence-based CM with other treatment approaches (Winters et al. 2021).

5. Multidimensional family therapy (MDFT)—MDFT is a viable treatment option, particularly for adolescents with CUD. Because most cannabis users tend to be younger (NSDUH 2013), this presents a greater opportunity for family—particularly parents—to become involved with an adolescent's treatment for CUD. MDFT is typically delivered one to three times per week and can be performed in any setting (inpatient, outpatient, office-based, in-home) and for any duration of time (brief, day treatment, intensive outpatient), although it is typically completed over 4–6 months. MDFT structures the interventions into four domains: treating the adolescent, engaging parents in therapy, improving interaction between the parents and the adolescent, and enhancing familial competency of all of the systems in which the adolescent is involved (Liddle et al. 2008). It has been demonstrated that MDFT improves retention and outcomes, especially when conducted at home as well as in an outpatient clinic as a result of stronger family support and improved family relationships (Barrett et al. 1988; Brown et al. 1994; Diamond et al. 2002; Henggeler et al. 1991; Liddle et al. 2001).

6. Twelve-step programs—Historically, 12-step programs have been a standard approach to treatment for patients with substance use disorders. This form of treatment involves attending meetings such as Marijuana Anonymous (inspired by Alcoholics Anonymous). These programs rely on member-led groups, sponsorship, and adherence to the suggested 12 steps to recovery, which include acknowledgment of a problem and an improved relationship with a higher power (www.marijuana-anonymous.org/how-it-works/twelve-steps). There is virtually no research to support effectiveness of 12-step programs specifically for treating CUDs. Furthermore, 12-step programs

have been shown to be both effective and ineffective for other substance use disorders (i.e., alcohol dependence) when used in combination with other treatment modalities or alone (Ferri et al. 2006; Timko et al. 2006), so there is little empirical evidence to suggest that this approach would be effective for CUD.

C. Other Interventions

The vast majority of individuals who use cannabis are able to stop without formalized treatment (Stinson et al. 2006). Withdrawal symptoms are often a significant reason for relapse among individuals with CUD (Levin et al. 2010). Several individualized treatment strategies are used to deal with withdrawal symptoms, including increasing use of other substances such as nicotine, caffeine, alcohol, and prescription medications (Copersino et al. 2006b). A new model of behavioral intervention for CUD is the Individualized Assessment and Treatment Program (IATP; Litt et al. 2020). IATP provides highly individualized training on coping skills that are most relevant to each individual. Recent work has found that IATP leads to an increased use of coping skills compared to conventional MET-CBT treatment. Finally, to address the gap in care as many with disordered cannabis use do not seek treatment, there is an emerging interest in the development of technology-delivered interventions that may offer increased access to care, reduced cost of treatment delivery, and increased treatment fidelity (Marsch et al. 2014; Winters et al. 2021).

▶ Complications/Adverse Outcomes of Treatment

Currently, no standard pharmacotherapies or psychotherapies for CUD are available; therefore, no complications or adverse outcomes are associated with treatment.

▶ Prognosis

There are few empirical data supporting any trends in the outcome of CUD. It has been demonstrated that the rate of cannabis use is highest between the ages of 18 and 25 with approximately 18.7% of that population using at least once within the past month, with use tapering off to 7% after age 26. It can be inferred from these data that the rates of cannabis use and misuse tend to drop off in the late to mid-30s. However, recent surveys suggest that use of illicit drugs (particularly cannabis) among older adults (50 or older) has increased because of the progression of the baby boom cohort into this age demographic (Han et al. 2009). This suggests that the emergence of an older-adult subset of the population with CUD may not only alter the expected prognosis or remission of CUD but also have implications for treatment outcomes. It is important to note that the rates of cannabis use and misuse as well as prognosis of CUDs will likely change, given the trend toward the legalization of recreational cannabis use and "medical" marijuana.

Website
www.marijuana-anonymous.org/how-it-works/twelve-steps.

Aceto MD, Scates SM, Lowe JA, Martin BR. Dependence on delta 9-tetrahydrocannabinol: studies on precipitated and abrupt withdrawal. *J Pharmacol Exp Ther*. 1996;278(3):1290–1295.

Aceto MD, Scates SM, Martin BB. Spontaneous and precipitated withdrawal with a synthetic cannabinoid, WIN 55212-2. *Eur J Pharmacol*. 2001;416(1–2):75–81.

Agrawal A, Edenberg HJ, Foroud T, et al. Association of GABRA2 with drug dependence in the collaborative study of the genetics of alcoholism sample. *Behav Genet*. 2006;36(5):640–650.

Agrawal A, Hinrichs AL, Dunn G, et al. Linkage scan for quantitative traits identifies new regions of interest for substance dependence in the Collaborative Study on the Genetics of Alcoholism (COGA) sample. *Drug Alcohol Depend*. 2008a;93(1–2):12–20.

Agrawal A, Lynskey MT, Hinrichs A, et al. A genome-wide association study of DSM-IV cannabis dependence. *Addiction Biology*. 2011;16(3):514–518.

Agrawal A, 3 genes for cannabis use disorders: findings, challenges and directions. *Addiction*. 2009a; 104(4): 518–532.

Agrawal A, Morley KI, Hansell NK, et al. Autosomal linkage analysis for cannabis use behaviors in Australian adults. *Drug Alcohol Depend*. 2008b;98(3):185–190.

Agrawal A, Pergadia ML, Saccone SF, et al. An autosomal linkage scan for cannabis use disorders in the nicotine addiction genetics project. *Arch Gen Psychiatry*. 2008c;65(6):713–721.

Agrawal A, Wetherill L, Dick DM, et al. Evidence for association between polymorphisms in the cannabinoid receptor 1 (CNR1) gene and cannabis dependence. *Am J Med Genet*. 2009b;150B(5): 736–740.

Allsop DJ, Copeland J, Lintzeris N, et al. Nabiximols as an agonist replacement therapy during cannabis withdrawal: a randomized clinical trial. *JAMA Psychiatry*. 2014;71:281–291.

Anthony JC, Warner LA, Kessler RC. Comparative epidemiology of dependence on tobacco, alcohol, controlled substances, and inhalants: basic findings from the National Comorbidity Survey. *Exp Clin Psychopharmacol*. 1994;2(3):244.

Arnold C, Allot K, Farhall J, et al. Neurocognitive and social cognitive predictors of cannabis use in first-episode psychosis. *Schizophr Res*. 2015;168(1–2):231–237.

Baggio S, N'Goran AA, Deline S, et al. Patterns of cannabis use and prospective associations with health issues among young males. *Addiction*. 2014;109(6):937–945.

Barrett ME, Simpson DD, Lehman WE. Behavioral changes of adolescents in drug abuse intervention programs. *J Clin Psychol*. 1988;44(3):461–473.

Beardsley PM, Balster RL, Harris LS. Dependence on tetrahydrocannabinol in rhesus monkeys. *J Pharmacol Exp Ther*. 1986;239(2): 311–319.

Bilbao A, Spanagel R. Medical cannabinoids: a pharmacology-based systematic review and meta-analysis for all relevant medical indications. *BMC Med*. 2022;20:259.

Black N, Stockings E, Campbell G, et al. Cannabinoids for the treatment of mental disorders and symptoms of mental disorders: a systematic review and meta-analysis. *Lancet Psychiatry*. 2019; (6)12:995–1010.

Bloomfield MA, Hindocha C, Green SF, et al. The neuropsychopharmacology of cannabis: a review of human imaging studies. *Pharmacol Ther*. 2019;195:132–161.

Boggs DL, Kelly DL, Liu F, et al. Cannabis withdrawal in chronic cannabis users with schizophrenia. *J Psychiatr Res*. 2013;47(2):240–245.

Bolla KI, Brown K, Eldreth D, et al. Dose-related neurocognitive effects of marijuana use. *Neurology*. 2002;59(9):1337–1343.

Bolla KI, Eldreth DA, Matochik JA, Cadet JL. Neural substrates of faulty decision-making in abstinent marijuana users. *NeuroImage*. 2005;26(2):480–492.

Braude M. Toxicology of cannabinoids. In: Paton W, Crown J (eds). *Cannabis and Its Derivatives*. Oxford, UK: Oxford University Press, 1972, pp. 89–99.

Brown SA, Myers MG, Mott MA, Vik PW. Correlates of success following treatment for adolescent substance abuse. *Appl Prev Psychol*. 1994;3(2):61–73.

Broyd SJ, van Hell HH, Beale C, et al. Acute and chronic effects of cannabinoids on human cognition—a systematic review. *Biol Psychiatry*. 2016;79(7):557–567.

Budney AJ, Novy PL, Hughes JR. Marijuana withdrawal among adults seeking treatment for marijuana dependence. *Addiction*. 1999;94(9):1311–1322.

Budney AJ, Higgins ST, Radonovich KJ, Novy PL. Adding voucher-based incentives to coping skills and motivational enhancement improves outcomes during treatment for marijuana dependence. *J Consult Clin Psychol*. 2000;68(6):1051–1061.

Budney AJ, Hughes JR, Moore BA, Novy PL. Marijuana abstinence effects in marijuana smokers maintained in their home environment. *Arch Gen Psychiatry*. 2001;58(10):917–924.

Budney AJ, Hughes JR, Moore BA, Vandrey R. Review of the validity and significance of cannabis withdrawal syndrome. *Am J Psychiatry*. 2004;161(11):1967–1977.

Budney AJ, Hughes JR. The cannabis withdrawal syndrome. *Curr Opin Psychiatry*. 2006a;19(3):233–238.

Budney AJ, Moore BA, Rocha HL, Higgins ST. Clinical trial of abstinence-based vouchers and cognitive-behavioral therapy for cannabis dependence. *J Consult Clin Psychol*. 2006b;74(2): 307–316.

Budney AJ, Moore BA, Vandrey RG, Hughes JR. The time course and significance of cannabis withdrawal. *J Abnorm Psychol*. 2003;112(3):393–402.

Budney AJ, Moore BA. Development and consequences of cannabis dependence. *J Clin Pharmacol*. 2002;42(S1):28S–33S.

Budney AJ, Stranger C, Knapp AA, Walker DD. Status update on the treatment of cannabis use disorder. *Contemporary Health Issues on Marijuana*. New York: Oxford University Press, 2018, pp. 236–255.

Budney AJ, Vandrey RG, Hughes JR, et al. Oral delta-9-tetrahydrocannabinol suppresses cannabis withdrawal symptoms. *Drug Alcohol Depend*. 2007;86(1):22–29.

Carlin AS, Trupin EW (1977). The effect of long-term chronic marijuana use on neuropsychological functioning. *Int J Addict*. 1977;12(5):617–624.

Carpenter KM, McDowell D, Brooks DJ, et al. A preliminary trial: double-blind comparison of nefazodone, bupropion-SR, and placebo in the treatment of cannabis dependence. *Am J Addict*. 2009;18(1):53–64.

Chan PC, Sills RC, Braun AG, et al. Toxicity and carcinogenicity of delta 9-tetrahydrocannabinol in Fischer rats and B6C3F1 mice. *Fund Appl Toxicol.* 1996;30(1):109–117.

Chye Y, Kirkham R, Lorenzetti V, et al. Cannabis, cannabinoids, and brain morphology: a review of the evidence. *Biol Psychiatry Cogn Neurosci Neuroimaging,* 2021;6(6):627–635.

Connor JP, Stjepanović D, Le Foll B, et al. Cannabis use and cannabis use disorder. *Nat Rev Dis Primers.* 2021;7(1):16.

Cooper K, Chatters R, Kaltenthaler E, Wong R. Psychological and psychosocial interventions for cannabis cessation in adults: a systematic review short report. *Health Technol Assess.* 2015; 19(56):1–130.

Cooper ZD, Haney M. Opioid antagonism enhances marijuana's effects in heavy marijuana smokers. *Psychopharmacology. (Berl).* 2010;211(2):141–148.

Copeland J, Swift W, Roffman R, Stephens R. A randomized controlled trial of brief cognitive-behavioral interventions for cannabis use disorder. *J Subst Abuse Treat.* 2001;21(2):55–64; discussion 65–56.

Copersino ML, Boyd SJ, Tashkin DP, et al. Cannabis withdrawal among non-treatment-seeking adult cannabis users. *Am J Addict.* 2006a;15(1):8–14.

Copersino ML, Boyd SJ, Tashkin DP, et al. Quitting among non-treatment-seeking marijuana users: reasons and changes in other substance use. *Am J Addict.* 2006b;15(4):297–302.

Cougle JR, Bonn-Miller MO, Vujanovic AA, et al. Posttraumatic stress disorder and cannabis use in a nationally representative sample. *Psychol Addict Behav.* 2011;25(3):554–558.

Culver CM, King FW (1974). Neuropsychological assessment of undergraduate marihuana and LSD users. *Arch Gen Psychiatry.* 1974;31(5):707–711.

Cuttler C, McLaughlin RJ, Graf P. Mechanisms underlying the link between cannabis use and prospective memory. *PLoS One.* 2012;7(5), e36820.

D'Souza DC, Cortes-Briones J, Ranganathan M, et al. Rapid changes in cannabinoid 1 receptor availability in cannabis-dependent male subjects after abstinence from cannabis. *Biol Psychiatry Cog Neurosci Neuroimaging.* 2016;1(1)60–67.

D'Souza DC, DiForti M, Ganesh S, et al. Consensus paper of the WFSBP task force on cannabis, cannabinoids and psychosis. *World J Biol Psychiatry.* 2022;23(10):719–742.

Danovitch I, Gorelick DA. State of the art treatments for cannabis dependence. *Psychiatr Clin N Am.* 2012;35(2):309–326.

DAWN, 2013. Substance Abuse and Mental Health Services Administration, Drug Abuse Warning Network, 2011: national estimates of drug-related emergency department visits. HHS Publication No. (SMA) 13-4760 DSD. Rockville, MD: Substance Abuse and Mental Health Services Administration.

DAWN, 2022. Substance Abuse and Mental Health Services Administration, Drug Abuse Warning Network: Findings from Drug-Related Emergency Department Visits, 2021 (HHS Publication No. PEP22-07-03-002). Rochville, MD: Center for Behavioral Health Statistics and Quality.

Demontis D, Rajagopal VM, Thorgeirsson TE, et al. Genome-wide association study implicates CHRNA2 in cannabis use disorder. *Nat Neurosci.* 2019;22(7):846–850.

Despres JP, Golay A, Sjostrom L. Effects of rimonabant on metabolic risk factors in overweight patients with dyslipidemia. *N Engl J Med.* 2005;353(20):2121–2134.

Diamond G, Godley SH, Liddle HA, et al. Five outpatient treatment models for adolescent marijuana use: a description of the Cannabis Youth Treatment Interventions. *Addiction.* 2002;97 Suppl 1:70–83.

D'Souza DC, Cortes-Briones J, Creatura G, et al. Efficacy and safety of a fatty acid amide hydrolase inhibitor (PF-04457845) in the treatment of cannabis withdrawal and dependence in men: a double-blind, placebo-controlled, parallel group, phase 2a single-site randomised controlled trial. *Lancet Psychiatry;* 2019. 6(1):35–45.

Duperrouzel JC, Hawes SW, Lopez-Quintero C, et al. Adolescent cannabis use and its associations with decision-making and episodic memory: preliminary results from a longitudinal study. *Neuropsychology.* 2019;33(5):701.

Ehrenreich H, Rinn T, Kunert HJ, et al. Specific attentional dysfunction in adults following early start of cannabis use. *Psychopharmacology. (Berl).* 1999;142(3):295–301.

Eldreth DA, Matochik JA, Cadet JL, Bolla KI. Abnormal brain activity in prefrontal brain regions in abstinent marijuana users. *NeuroImage.* 2004;23(3):914–920.

Ferri M, Amato L, Davoli M. Alcoholics Anonymous and other 12-step programmes for alcohol dependence. *Cochrane Database Syst Rev.* 2006(3):CD005032.

Findling RL, Pagano ME, McNamara NK, et al. The short-term safety and efficacy of fluoxetine in depressed adolescents with alcohol and cannabis use disorders: a pilot randomized placebo-controlled trial. *Child Adolesc Psychiatry Ment Health.* 2009;3(1):11.

Fleming C B, Mason WA, Mazza JJ, et al. Latent growth modeling of the relationship between depressive symptoms and substance use during adolescence. *Psychol Addict Behav.* 2008;22(2):186.

Fureman B, Parikh G, Bragg A, McLellan AT. Addiction severity index. In: *A Guide to Training and Supervising ASI Interviews based on the past ten years.* 5th Edition. Philadelphia: University of Pennsylvania/Philadelphia VAMC Center for Studies of Addiction, 1990.

Gates PJ, Sabioni P, Copeland J, et al. Psychosocial interventions for cannabis use disorder. *Cochrane Database Syst Rev.* 2016;(5).

Gay M. Synthetic marijuana spurs state ban. *New York Times,* 2010. http://www.nytimes.com/2010/07/11/us/11k2.html?_r = 0.

Gelfand EV, Cannon CP. Rimonabant: a cannabinoid receptor type 1 blocker for management of multiple cardiometabolic risk factors. *J Am Coll Cardiol.* 2006;47(10):1919–1926.

Georgotas A, Zeidenberg P. Observations on the effects of four weeks of heavy marihuana smoking on group interaction and individual behavior. *Compr Psychiatry.* 1979;20(5):427–432.

Gobbi G, Atkin T, Zytynski T, et al. Association of cannabis use in adolescence and risk of depression, anxiety, and suicidality in young adulthood: a systematic review and meta-analysis. *JAMA Psychiatry.* 2019;76(4):426–434.

Gorelick DA, Levin KH, Copersino ML, et al. Diagnostic criteria for cannabis withdrawal syndrome. *Drug Alcohol Depend.* 2012; 123(1–3):141–147.

Grant BF, Chu A, Sigman R, et al. Source and accuracy statement: National Epidemiologic Survey on Alcohol and Related Conditions-III (NESARC-III). 2014; Available at: https://www.niaaa.nih.gov/sites/default/files/NESARC_Final_Report_FINAL_1_8_15.pdf (accessed 10 October 2021).

Gray KM, Carpenter MJ, Baker NL, et al. A double-blind randomized controlled trial of N-acetylcysteine in cannabis-dependent adolescents. *Am J Psychiatry.* 2012;169(8):805–812.

Gray KM, Sonne SC, McClure EA, et al. A randomized placebo controlled trial of N-acetylcysteine for cannabis use disorder in adults. *Drug Alcohol Depend.* 2017;177:249–257.

Gray KM, Watson NL, Carpenter MJ, Larowe SD. *N*-Acetylcysteine (NAC) in young marijuana users: an open-label pilot study. *Am J Addict.* 2010;19(2):187–189.

Greenwald MK, Stitzer ML. Antinociceptive, subjective and behavioral effects of smoked marijuana in humans. *Drug Alcohol Depend.* 2000;59(3):261–275.

Gummin, DD, Mowry JB, Beuhler MC, et al. Annual Report of the National Poison Data System (NPDS) from America's Poison Centers: 39th Annual Report, *Clinical Toxicology*, 2022. 60:12, 1381–1643.

Halikas J, Weller R, Morse C. Effects of regular marijuana use on sexual performance. *J Psychoact Drug.* 1982;14(1–2):59–70.

Hall W, Solowij N. Adverse effects of cannabis. *Lancet.* 1998;352(9140):1611–1616.

Han B, Gfroerer J, Colliver J. An examination of trends in illicit drug use among adults aged 50 to 59 in the United States: an OAS data review. Rockville, MD: Substance Abuse and Mental Health Services Administration Office of Applied Studies; 2009.

Han BH, Brennan JJ, Orozco MA, et al. Trends in emergency department visits associated with cannabis use among older adults in California, 2005–2019. *J Am Geriatr Soc.* 2023.

Haney M, Bisaga A, Foltin RW. Interaction between naltrexone and oral THC in heavy marijuana smokers. *Psychopharmacology.* 2003a;166(1):77–85.

Haney M, Hart CL, Vosburg SK, et al. Effects of baclofen and mirtazapine on a laboratory model of marijuana withdrawal and relapse. *Psychopharmacology. (Berl).* 2010;211(3):233–244.

Haney M, Hart CL, Vosburg SK, et al. Effects of THC and lofexidine in a human laboratory model of marijuana withdrawal and relapse. *Psychopharmacology. (Berl).* 2008;197(1):157–168.

Haney M, Hart CL, Vosburg SK, et al. Marijuana withdrawal in humans: effects of oral THC or divalproex. *Neuropsychopharmacology.* 2004;29(1):158–170.

Haney M, Hart CL, Ward AS, Foltin RW. Nefazodone decreases anxiety during marijuana withdrawal in humans. *Psychopharmacology. (Berl).* 2003b;165(2):157–165.

Haney M, Ramesh D, Glass A, et al. Naltrexone maintenance decreases cannabis self-administration and subjective effects in daily cannabis smokers. *Neuropsychopharmacology.* 2015;40(11):2489–2498.

Haney M, Ward AS, Comer SD, et al. Abstinence symptoms following oral THC administration to humans. *Psychopharmacology.* 1999a;141(4):385–394.

Haney M, Ward AS, Comer SD, et al. Abstinence symptoms following smoked marijuana in humans. *Psychopharmacology. (Berl).* 1999b;141(4):395–404.

Haney M, Ward AS, Comer SD, et al. Bupropion SR worsens mood during marijuana withdrawal in humans. *Psychopharmacology. (Berl).* 2001;155(2):171–179.

Haney M. Opioid antagonism of cannabinoid effects: differences between marijuana smokers and nonmarijuana smokers. *Neuropsychopharmacology.* 2007;32(6):1391–1403.

Haney M. The marijuana withdrawal syndrome: diagnosis and treatment. *Curr Psychiatry Rep.* 2005;7(5):360–366.

Hart CL, Haney M, Vosburg SK, et al. Reinforcing effects of oral Delta9-THC in male marijuana smokers in a laboratory choice procedure. *Psychopharmacology. (Berl).* 2005;181(2):237–243.

Hartz SM, Pato CN, Medeiros H, et al. Comorbidity of severe psychotic disorders with measures of substance use. *JAMA Psychiatry.* 2014;71(3):248–254.

Hasin DS, Kerridge BT, Saha TD, et al. Prevalence and correlates of DSM-5 cannabis use disorder, 2012–2013: findings from the National Epidemiologic Survey on Alcohol and Related Conditions-III. *Am J Psychiatry*, 2016;173(6):588–599.

Hasin DS, Saha TD, Kerridge BT, et al. Prevalence of marijuana use disorders in the United States between 2001-2002 and 2012-2013. *JAMA Psychiatry.* 2015;72(12):1235–1242.

Helle S, Løberg EM, Gjestad R, et al. The positive link between executive function and lifetime cannabis use in schizophrenia is not explained by current levels of superior social cognition. *Schizophr Res*; 2017;250:92–98.

Henggeler SW, Borduin CM, Melton GB, Mann BJ. Effects of multisystemic therapy on drug use and abuse in serious juvenile offenders: a progress report from two outcome studies. *Fam Dynam Addict Q.* 1991;1(3)40–51.

Herman AI, Kranzler HR, Cubells JF, et al. Association study of the CNR1 gene exon 3 alternative promoter region polymorphisms and substance dependence. *Am J Med Genet B Neuropsychiatr Genet.* 2006;141(5):499–503.

Hettema J, Steele J, Miller WR. Motivational interviewing. *Annu Rev Clin Psychol.* 2005;1:91–111.

Hill KP, Palastro MD, Gruber SA, et al. Nabilone pharmacotherapy for cannabis dependence: a randomized, controlled pilot study. *Am J Addict.* 2017;26:795–801.

Hines LA, Morley KI, Rijsdijk F, et al. Overlap of heritable influences between cannabis use disorder, frequency of use and opportunity to use cannabis: trivariate twin modelling and implications for genetic design. *Psychol Med.* 2018;48(16):2786–2793.

Hirst R, Vaughn D, Arastu S, et al. Female sex as a protective factor in the effects of chronic cannabis use on verbal learning and memory. *J Int Neuropsychol Soc.* 2021;27(6):570–580

Hirvonen J, Goodwin RS, Li CT, et al. Reversible and regionally selective downregulation of brain cannabinoid CB1 receptors in chronic daily cannabis smokers. *Mol Psychiatry.* 2012;17(6):642–649.

Hollister LE. Cannabis—1988. *Acta Psychiatr Scand Suppl.* 1988;345:108–118.

Hopfer CJ, Lessem JM, Hartman CA, et al. A genome-wide scan for loci influencing adolescent cannabis dependence symptoms: evidence for linkage on chromosomes 3 and 9. *Drug Alcohol Depend.* 2007;89(1):34–41.

Hopfer CJ, Young SE, Purcell S, et al. Cannabis receptor haplotype associated with fewer cannabis dependence symptoms in adolescents. *Am J Med Genet B Neuropsychiatr Genet.* 2006;141(8):895–901.

Huestis MA, Boyd SJ, Heishman SJ, et al. Single and multiple doses of rimonabant antagonize acute effects of smoked cannabis in male cannabis users. *Psychopharmacology. (Berl).* 2007;194(4):505–515.

Huestis MA, Gorelick DA, Heishman SJ, et al. Blockade of effects of smoked marijuana by the CB1-selective cannabinoid receptor antagonist SR141716. *Arch Gen Psychiatry.* 2001;58(4):322–328.

Huestis MA. Human cannabinoid pharmacokinetics. *Chem Biodivers.* 2007;4(8):1770–1804.

Hurst D, Loeffler G, McLay R. Psychosis associated with synthetic cannabinoid agonists: a case series. *Am J Psychiatry.* 2011;168(10):1119.

Imtiaz S, Nigatu YT, Ali F, et al. Cannabis legalization and cannabis use, daily cannabis use and cannabis-related problems among adults in Ontario, Canada (2001–2019). *Drug Alcohol Depend.* 2023;109765.

Johnson EC, Demontis D, Thorgeirsson TE, et al. A large-scale genome-wide association study meta-analysis of cannabis use disorder. *Lancet Psychiatry*; 2020;7(12):1032–1045.

Johnston LD, Miech RA, O'Malley PM, et al. *Demographic subgroup trends among adolescents in the use of various licit and illicit drugs, 1975–2019.* 2020; Available at: http://www.monitoringthefuture.org/pubs/occpapers/mtf-occ94.pdf (accessed October 17, 2021).

Johnston LD, O'Malley PM, Bachman JG, Schulenberg JE. *Monitoring the Future National Survey Results on Drug Use, 1975–2012. Volume I: Secondary School Students.* Ann Arbor: Institute for Social Research, The University of Michigan; 2013.

Jones RT, Benowitz N, Bachman J. Clinical studies of cannabis tolerance and dependence. *Ann N Y Acad Sci.* 1976;282:221–239.

Jones RT, Benowitz NL, Herning RI. Clinical relevance of cannabis tolerance and dependence. *J Clin Pharmacol.* 1981;21(8–9 Suppl):143S–152S.

Kolansky H, Moore WT. Effects of marihuana on adolescents and young adults. *J Psychiatr Nurs Ment Health Serv.* 1971;9(6):9–16.

Kondo KK, Morasco BJ, Nugent SM, et al. Pharmacotherapy for the treatment of cannabis use disorder: a systematic review. *Ann Intern Med.* 2020;172(6):398–412.

Koskinen J, Lohonen J, Koponen H, et al. Rate of cannabis use disorders in clinical samples of patients with schizophrenia: a meta-analysis. *Schizophr Bull.* 2010;36(6):1115–1130.

Kouri EM, Pope HG Jr, Lukas SE. Changes in aggressive behavior during withdrawal from long-term marijuana use. *Psychopharmacology. (Berl).* 1999;143(3):302–308.

Kouri EM, Pope HG Jr. Abstinence symptoms during withdrawal from chronic marijuana use. *Exp Clin Psychopharmacol.* 2000;8(4):483–492.

Kroon E, Kuhns, L, Cousijn J. The short-term and long-term effects of cannabis on cognition: recent advances in the field. *Curr Opin Psychol.* 2021;38:49–55.

Krzyzanowski DJ, Purdon SE. Duration of abstinence from cannabis is positively associated with verbal learning performance: a systematic review and meta-analysis. *Neuropsychology.* 2020;34(3):359.

Kuhns L, Kroon E, Colyer-Patel K, et al. Associations between cannabis use, cannabis use disorder, and mood disorders: longitudinal, genetic, and neurocognitive evidence. *Psychopharmacology.* 2022;239(5):1231–1249.

Leung J, Chan GCK, Hides L, et al. What is the prevalence and risk of cannabis use disorders among people who use cannabis? A systematic review and meta-analysis. *Addict Behav* 2020;109:106479.

Levin FR, Kleber HD. Use of dronabinol for cannabis dependence: two case reports and review. *Am J Addict.* 2008;17(2):161–164.

Levin FR, Mariani JJ, Brooks DJ, et al. Dronabinol for the treatment of cannabis dependence: a randomized, double-blind, placebo-controlled trial. *Drug Alcohol Depend.* 2011;116(1–3):142–150.

Levin FR, Mariani JJ, Pavlicova M et al. Dronabinol and lofexidine for cannabis use disorder: a randomized, double-blind, placebo-controlled trial. *Drug Alcohol Depend.*2016;159:53–60.

Levin FR, McDowell D, Evans SM, et al. Pharmacotherapy for marijuana dependence: a double-blind, placebo-controlled pilot study of divalproex sodium. *Am J Addict.* 2004;13(1):21–32.

Levin KH, Copersino ML, Heishman SJ, et al. Cannabis withdrawal symptoms in non-treatment-seeking adult cannabis smokers. *Drug Alcohol Depend.* 2010;111(1):120–127.

Lev-Ran S, Roerecke M, Le Foll B, et al. The association between cannabis use and depression: a systematic review and meta-analysis of longitudinal studies. *Psychol Med.* 2014;44(4):797–810.

Lichtman AH, Martin BR. Marijuana withdrawal syndrome in the animal model. *J Clin Pharmacol.* 2002;42(11 Suppl):20S–27S.

Liddle HA, Dakof GA, Parker K, et al. Multidimensional family therapy for adolescent drug abuse: results of a randomized clinical trial. *Am J Drug Alcohol Abuse.* 2001;27(4):651–688.

Liddle HA, Dakof GA, Turner RM, et al. Treating adolescent drug abuse: a randomized trial comparing multidimensional family therapy and cognitive behavior therapy. *Addiction.* 2008;103(10):1660–1670.

Lind PA, Macgregor S, Agrawal A, et al. The role of GABRA2 in alcohol dependence, smoking, and illicit drug use in an Australian population sample. *Alcohol Clin Exp Res.* 2008;32(10):1721–1731.

Lintzeris N, Bhardwaj A, Mills L, et al; Agonist Replacement for Cannabis Dependence (ARCD) study group. Nabiximols for the treatment of cannabis dependence: a randomized clinical trial. *JAMA Intern Med.* 2019;179(9):1242–1253.

Litt MD, Jadde RM, Tennen H, Petry NM. Individualized assessment and treatment program (IATP) for cannabis use disorder: randomized controlled trial with and without contingency management. *Psychol Addict Behav.* 2020;34(1):40.

Litt MD, Kadden RM, Petry NM. Behavioral treatment for marijuana dependence: randomized trial of contingency management and self-efficacy enhancement. *Addict* 2013;38(3):1764–1775.

Lorenzetti V, Chye Y, Silva P et al. Dose regular cannabis use affect neuroanatomy? An updated systematic review and meta-analysis of structural neuroimaging studies. *Eur Arch Psychiatry Clin Neurosci.* 2019;269:59–71.

Lorenzetti V, Lubman DI, Whittle S, et al. Structural MRI findings in long-term cannabis users: what do we know? *Subst Use Misuse.* 2010;45(11):1787–1808.

Lorenzetti V, Takagi M, van Dalen Y et al. Investigating the residual effects of chronic cannabis use and abstinence on verbal and visuospatial learning. *Front Psychiatry.* 2021;12663701.

Lovell ME, Akhurst J, Padgett C, et al. Cognitive outcomes associated with long-term, regular, recreational cannabis use in adults: a meta-analysis. *Exp Clin Psychopharmacol.* 2020;28(4):471.

Lundqvist T. Cognitive consequences of cannabis use: comparison with abuse of stimulants and heroin with regard to attention, memory and executive functions. *Pharmacol Biochem Behav.* 2005;81(2):319–330.

Magill M, Ray L. Cognitive-behavioral treatment with adult alcohol and illicit drug users: a meta-analysis of randomized controlled trials. *J Stud Alcohol Drug.* 2009;70(4):516.

Mammen G, Rueda S, Roerecke M, et al. Association of cannabis with long-term clinical symptoms in anxiety and mood disorders: a systematic review of prospective studies. *J Clin Psychol.*2018;79(4):2248.

Marsch LA, Carroll KM, Kiluk BD. Technology-based interventions for the treatment and recovery management of substance use disorders: a JSAT special issue. *J Subst Abuse Treat.* 2014;46(1):1–4.

Mason BJ, Crean R, Goodell V, et al. A proof-of-concept randomized controlled study of gabapentin: effects on cannabis use, withdrawal and executive function deficits in cannabis-dependent adults. *Neuropsychopharmacology.* 2012;37(7):1689–1698.

Mathew RJ, Wilson WH, Coleman RE, et al. Marijuana intoxication and brain activation in marijuana smokers. *Life Sci.* 1997;60(23):2075–2089.

Mathew RJ, Wilson WH, Turkington TG, et al. Time course of tetrahydrocannabinol-induced changes in regional cerebral blood flow measured with positron emission tomography. *Psychiatry Res Neuroimaging.* 2002;116(3):173–185.

McHugh RK, Hearon BA, Otto MW. Cognitive behavioral therapy for substance use disorders. *Psychiatr Clin N Am.* 2010;33(3):511–525.

McRae AL, Brady KT, Carter RE. Buspirone for treatment of marijuana dependence: a pilot study. *Am J Addict.* 2006;15(5):404.

McRae-Clark AL, Baker NL, Gray KM, et al. Buspirone treatment of cannabis dependence: a randomized, placebo-controlled trial. *Drug Alcohol Depend.* 2015;156:29–37.

McRae-Clark AL, Baker NL, Gray KM, et al. Vilazodone for cannabis dependence: a randomized, controlled pilot trial. *Am J Addict.* 2016;25:69–75.

McRae-Clark AL, Carter RE, Killeen TK, et al. A placebo-controlled trial of buspirone for the treatment of marijuana dependence. *Drug Alcohol Depend.* 2009;105(1–2):132–138.

McRae-Clark AL, Carter RE, Killeen TK, et al. A placebo-controlled trial of atomoxetine in marijuana-dependent individuals with attention deficit hyperactivity disorder. *Am J Addict.* 2010;19(6):481–489.

Medina KL, Hanson KL, Schweinsburg AD, et al. Neuropsychological functioning in adolescent marijuana users: subtle deficits detectable after a month of abstinence. *J Int Neuropsychol Soc.* 2007;13(5):807–820.

Meier MH, Caspi A, Ambler A, et al. Persistent cannabis users show neuropsychological decline from childhood to midlife. *Proc Natl Acad Sci U S A.* 2012;109(40):E2657–2664.

Meier MH, Caspi A, Danese A, et al. Associations between adolescent cannabis use and neuropsychological decline: a longitudinal co-twin control study. *Addiction.* 2018;113(2):257–265.

Miech RA, Johnston LD, O'Malley PM, et al. Monitoring the Future national survey results on drug use, 1975–2019: Volume I, Secondary school students. Ann Arbor: Institute for Social Research, The University of Michigan. 2020.

Millman RB, Sbriglio R. Patterns of use and psychopathology in chronic marijuana users. *Psychiatr Clin North Am.* 1986;9(3):533–545.

Mir A, Obafemi A, Young A, Kane C. Myocardial infarction associated with use of the synthetic cannabinoid K2. *Pediatrics.* 2011;128(6):e1622–1627.

Miranda R Jr, Treloar H, Blanchard A, et al. Topiramate and motivational enhancement therapy for cannabis use among youth: a randomized placebo-controlled pilot study. *Addict Biol.* 2017;22:779–790.

Myles H, Myles N, Large M. Cannabis use in first episode psychosis: meta-analysis of prevalence, and the time course of initiation and continued use. *Austr N Z J Psychiatry.* 2016;50(3):208–219.

Nader DA, Sanchez ZM. Effects of regular cannabis use on neurocognition, brain structure, and function: a systematic review of findings in adults. *Am J Drug Alcohol Abuse.* 2018;44(1):4–18.

Newman SD, Cheng H, Kim DJ, et al. An investigation of the relationship between glutamate and resting state connectivity in chronic cannabis users. *Brain Imaging Behav.* 2020;14:2062.

Newman SD, Cheng H, Schnakenberg Martin AM, et al. An investigation of neurochemical changes in chronic cannabis users. *Front Hum Neurosci.* 2019;13:318.

Newman SD, Schnakenberg Martin AM, Raymond D. et al. The relationship between cannabis use and taurine: a MRS and metabolomics study. *PLoS One.* 2022; 17(6):e0269280.

Nordstrom BR, Levin FR. Treatment of cannabis use disorders: a review of the literature. *Am J Addict.* 2007;16(5):331–342.

NSDUH, 2013. Substance Abuse and Mental Health Services Administration, Results from the 2012 National Survey on Drug Use and Health: summary of national findings. NSDUH Series H-46, HHS Publication No. (SMA) 13-4795. Rockville, MD: substance Abuse and Mental Health Services Administration

NSDUH, 2021. Substance Abuse and Mental Health Services Administration. Key substance use and mental health indicators in the United States: results from the 2020 National Survey on Drug Use and Health (HHS Publication No. PEP21-07-01-003, NSDUH Series H-56). Rockville, MD: Center for Behavioral Health Statistics and Quality, Substance Abuse and Mental Health Services Administration. Retrieved from https://www.samhsa.gov/data/

O'Leary DS, Block RI, Flaum M, et al. Acute marijuana effects on rCBF and cognition: a PET study. *Neuroreport.* 2000;11(17):3835–3840.

O'Leary DS, Block RI, Koeppel JA, et al. Effects of smoking marijuana on focal attention and brain blood flow. *Hum Psychopharmacol Clin Exp.* 2007;22(3):135–148.

Pasman JA, Verweij KJH, Gerring Z, et al. GWAS of lifetime cannabis use reveals new risk loci, genetic overlap with psychiatric traits, and a causal influence of schizophrenia. *Nat Neurosci* 2018;21(9):1161–1170.

Perkonigg A, Goodwin RD, Fiedler A, et al. The natural course of cannabis use, abuse and dependence during the first decades of life. *Addiction.* 2008;103(3):439–449.

Perkonigg A, Lieb R, Wittchen H-U. Prevalence of use, abuse and dependence of illicit drugs among adolescents and young adults in a community sample. *Eur Addict Res.* 1998;4(1–2):58–66.

Pillay SS, Rogowska J, Kanayama G, et al. Cannabis and motor function: fMRI changes following 28 days of discontinuation. *Exp Clin Psychopharmacol.* 2008;16(1):22–32.

Pope HG Jr, Gruber AJ, Hudson JI, et al. Early-onset cannabis use and cognitive deficits: what is the nature of the association? *Drug Alcohol Depend.* 2003;69(3):303–310.

Pope HG Jr, Gruber AJ, Hudson JI, et al. Neuropsychological performance in long-term cannabis users. *Arch Gen Psychiatry.* 2001;58(10):909–915.

Pope HG Jr, Gruber AJ, Yurgelun-Todd D. The residual neuropsychological effects of cannabis: the current status of research. *Drug Alcohol Depend.* 1995;38(1):25–34.

Pope HG Jr, Yurgelun-Todd D. The residual cognitive effects of heavy marijuana use in college students. *JAMA.* 1996;275(7):521–527.

Potter DJ, Clark P, Brown MB. Potency of delta 9-THC and other cannabinoids in cannabis in England in 2005: implications for psychoactivity and pharmacology. *J Forensic Sci.* 2008;53(1):90–94.

Prendergast M, Podus D, Finney J, et al. Contingency management for treatment of substance use disorders: a meta-analysis. *Addiction.* 2006;101(11):1546–1560.

Prescot AP, Renshaw PF, Yurgelun-Todd DA. γ-Amino butyric acid and glutamate abnormalities in adolescent chronic marijuana smokers. *Drug Alcohol Depend.* 2013;129(3):232–239.

Radhakrishnan R, Addy PH, Sewell RA, et al. Cannabis, cannabinoids, and the association with psychosis. In: Madras B, Kuhar MJ (eds). *The Effects of Drug Abuse on the Human Nervous System.* Neuroscience-Net; 2012.

Riba J, Valle M, Sampedro F, et al. Telling true from false: cannabis users show increased susceptibility to false memories. *Mol Psychiatry.* 2015;20(6):772–777.

Rodriguez de Fonseca F, Carrera MR, Navarro M, et al. Activation of corticotropin-releasing factor in the limbic system during cannabinoid withdrawal. *Science.* 1997;276(5321):2050–2054.

Rominger A, Cumming P, Xiong G, et al. Effects of acute detoxification of the herbal blend 'Spice Gold' on dopamine D receptor availability: a [18F]fallypride PET study. *Eur Neuropsychopharmacol.* 2013;23:1806–1810.

Roten A, Baker NL, Gray KM. Cognitive performance in a placebo-controlled pharmacotherapy trial for youth with marijuana dependence. *Addict Behav.* 2015;45:119–123.

Rubin V, Comitas L. *Ganja in Jamaica: A Medical Anthropological Study of Chronic Marihuana Use.* The Hague: Mouton; 1975.

Russo EB. History of cannabis and its preparations in saga, science, and sobriquet. *Chem Biodivers.* 2007;4(8):1614–1648.

Sánchez-Torres AM, Basterra V, Rosa A, et al. Lifetime cannabis use and cognition in patients with schizophrenia spectrum disorders and their unaffected siblings. *Eur Arch Psychiatry Clin Neurosci.* 2013;263:643–653.

Schacht JP, Selling RE, Hutchison KE. Intermediate cannabis dependence phenotypes and the FAAH C385A variant: an exploratory analysis. *Psychopharmacology. (Berl).* 2009;203(3):511–517.

Schnakenberg Martin AM, Bonfils KA, Davis BJ, et al. Compared to high and low cannabis use, moderate use is associated with fewer cognitive deficits in psychosis. *Schizophr Res Cogn.* 2016;6:15–21.

Schnakenberg Martin AM, D'Souza DC, Newman SD, et al. Differential cognitive performance in females and males with regular cannabis use. *J Int Neuropsychol Soc.* 2021;27(6):570–580.

Schnakenberg Martin AM, Lysaker PH. Individuals with psychosis and a lifetime history of cannabis use show greater deficits in emotional experience compared to non-using peers. *J Mental Health.* 2020;29(1):77–83.

Schoeler T, Petros N, Di Forti, M. et al. Association between continued cannabis use and risk of relapse in first-episode psychosis: a quasi-experimental investigation within an observational study. *JAMA Psychiatry.* 2016;73(11):1173–1179.

Schulenberg JE, Johnston LD, O'Malley PM, et al. Monitoring the Future national survey results on drug use, 1975-2019: Volume II, College Students and adults ages 19-60. 2020. Ann Arbor: Institute for Social Research, The University of Michigan.

Schweinsburg AD, Nagel BJ, Schweinsburg BC, et al. Abstinent adolescent marijuana users show altered fMRI response during spatial working memory. *Psychiatry Res.* 2008;163(1):40–51.

Sewell RA, Skosnik PD, Garcia-Sosa I, et al. [Behavioral, cognitive and psychophysiological effects of cannabinoids: relevance to psychosis and schizophrenia]. *Rev Bras Psiquiatr.* 2010;32 Suppl 1:S15–30.

Shafa R. COMT-inhibitors may be a promising tool in treatment of marijuana addiction Trials. *Am J Addict.* 2009;18:322.

Shanks KG, Dahn T, Terrell AR. Detection of JWH-018 and JWH-073 by UPLC-MS-MS in postmortem whole blood casework. *J Anal Toxicol.* 2012;36(3):145–152.

Sneider JT, Pope HG Jr, Silveri MM, et al. Differences in regional blood volume during a 28-day period of abstinence in chronic cannabis smokers. *Eur Neuropsychopharmacol.* 2008;18(8):612–619.

Solowij N, Battisti R. The chronic effects of cannabis on memory in humans: a review. *Curr Drug Abuse Rev.* 2008;1:81–98.

Solowij N, Jones KA, Rozman ME, et al. Verbal learning and memory in adolescent cannabis users, alcohol users and non-users. *Psychopharmacology.* 2011;216:131–144.

Solowij N, Michie PT, Fox AM. Differential impairments of selective attention due to frequency and duration of cannabis use. *Biol Psychiatry.* 1995;37(10):731–739.

Solowij N, Michie PT. Cannabis and cognitive dysfunction: parallels with endophenotypes of schizophrenia? *J Psychiatry Neurosci.* 2007;32(1):30–52.

Spaderna M, Addy PH, D'Souza DC. Spicing things up: synthetic cannabinoids. *Psychopharmacology.* 2013;228(4):525–540.

St. James J. Doctors concerned over possible link of K2, heart damage. 2010. http://www.wfaa.com/news/health/A-dangerous-link-100482134.html.

Stefanis C, Liakos A, Boulougouris J, et al. Chronic hashish use and mental disorder. *Am J Psychiatry.* 1976;133(2):225–227.

Stephens RS, Roffman RA, Curtin L. Comparison of extended versus brief treatments for marijuana use. *J Consult Clin Psychol.* 2000;68(5):898–908.

Stinson FS, Ruan WJ, Pickering R, Grant BF. Cannabis use disorders in the USA: prevalence, correlates and co-morbidity. *Psychol Med.* 2006;36(10):1447–1460.

Stringer S, Minică, CC, Verweij, KJ, et al. Genome-wide association study of lifetime cannabis use based on a large meta-analytic sample of 32 330 subjects from the International Cannabis Consortium. *Transl Psychiatry.* 2016;6(3):769.

Tait RJ, Mackinnon A, Christensen H. Cannabis use and cognitive function: 8-year trajectory in a young adult cohort. *Addiction.* 2011;106(12):2195–2203.

TEDS, 2021. Treatment Episode Data Set (TEDS). *Admissions to and Discharges from Publicly Funded Substance Use Treatment Facilities.* Rocville, MD: Substance Abuse and Mental Health Services Administration, Center for Behavioral Health Statistics and Quality.

Tennant FS Jr, Groesbeck CJ. Psychiatric effects of hashish. *Arch Gen Psychiatry.* 1972;27(1):133–136.

Tevyaw TO, Monti PM. Motivational enhancement and other brief interventions for adolescent substance abuse: foundations, applications and evaluations. *Addiction.* 2004;99(Suppl 2):63–75.

Thames AD, Arbid N, Sayegh P. Cannabis use and neurocognitive functioning in a non-clinical sample of users. *Addict Behav.* 2014;39(5):994–999.

Timko C, Debenedetti A, Billow R. Intensive referral to 12-Step self-help groups and 6-month substance use disorder outcomes. *Addiction.* 2006;101(5):678–688.

Tirado CF, Goldman M, Lynch K, et al. Atomoxetine for treatment of marijuana dependence: a report on the efficacy and high incidence of gastrointestinal adverse events in a pilot study. *Drug Alcohol Depend*. 2008;94(1–3):254–257.

Trigo JM, Soliman A, Quilty LC, et al. Nabiximols combined with motivational enhancement/cognitive behavioral therapy for the treatment of cannabis dependence: a pilot randomized clinical trial. *PLoS One*. 2018;13:e0190768.

Tsou K, Patrick SL, Walker JM. Physical withdrawal in rats tolerant to delta 9-tetrahydrocannabinol precipitated by a cannabinoid receptor antagonist. *Eur J Pharmacol*. 1995;280(3):R13–15.

Tyndale RF, Payne JI, Gerber AL, Sipe JC. The fatty acid amide hydrolase C385A (P129T) missense variant in cannabis users: studies of drug use and dependence in Caucasians. *Am J Med Genet B Neuropsychiatr Genet*. 2007;144(5):660–666.

UNODC, United Nationals Office on Drugs and Crime, *World Drug Report 2020: Global drug use rising; while COVID-19 has far reaching impact on global drug markets*. 2020.

van der Pol P, Liebregts N, de Graaf R, et al. Predicting the transition from frequent cannabis use to cannabis dependence: a three-year prospective study. *Drug Alcohol Depend*. 2013;133:352–359.

Van der Veer N, Fiday J. Persistent psychosis following the use of Spice. *Schizophrenia Res*. 2011;130:285–286.

Vandrey R, Haney M. Pharmacotherapy for cannabis dependence: how close are we? *CNS Drugs*. 2009;23(7):543–553.

Verweij KJ, Vinkhuyzen AA, Benyamin B, et al. The genetic aetiology of cannabis use initiation: a meta-analysis of genome-wide association studies and a SNP-based heritability estimation. *Addict Biol*. 2013;18(5):846–850.

Verweij KJ, Zietsch BP, Lynskey MT, et al. Genetic and environmental influences on cannabis use initiation and problematic use: a meta-analysis of twin studies. *Addiction*. 2010;105(3):417–430.

Volkow ND, Gillespie H, Mullani N, et al. Brain glucose metabolism in chronic marijuana users at baseline and during marijuana intoxication. *Psychiatry Res Neuroimaging*. 1996;67(1):29–38.

Volkow ND, Wang GJ, Telang F, et al. Decreased dopamine brain reactivity in marijuana abusers is associated with negative emotionality and addiction severity. *Proc Natl Acad Sci*. 2014; 111:3149–3156.

Wachtel SR, de Wit H. Naltrexone does not block the subjective effects of oral Delta(9)-tetrahydrocannabinol in humans. *Drug Alcohol Depend*. 2000;59(3):251–260.

Watson SJ, Benson Jr JA, Joy JE. Marijuana and medicine: assessing the science base: A summary of the 1999 Institute of Medicine report. *Arch Gen Psychiatry*. 2000;57(6):547.

Weinstein AM, Gorelick DA. Pharmacological treatment of cannabis dependence. *Curr Pharm Des*. 2011;17:1351–1358.

Weinstein AM, Miller H, Bluvstein I, et al. Treatment of cannabis dependence using escitalopram in combination with cognitivebehavior therapy: a double-blind placebo-controlled study. *Am J Drug Alcohol Abuse*. 2014;40:16–22.

Wiesbeck GA, Schuckit MA, Kalmijn JA, et al. An evaluation of the history of a marijuana withdrawal syndrome in a large population. *Addiction*. 1996;91(10):1469–1478.

Wig NN, Varma VK. Patterns of long-term heavy cannabis use in north India and its effects on cognitive functions: a preliminary report. *Drug Alcohol Depend*. 1977;2(3):211–219.

Winstock AR, Lea T, Copeland J. Lithium carbonate in the management of cannabis withdrawal in humans: an open-label study. *J Psychopharmacol*. 2009;23(1):84–93.

Winters KC, Mader J, Budney AJ, et al. Interventions for cannabis use disorder. *Curr Opin Psychol*. 2021;38:67–74.

Womack SR, Shaw DS, Weaver CM, Forbes EE. Bidirectional associations between cannabis use and depressive symptoms from adolescence through early adulthood among at-risk young men. *Journal of Studies on Alcohol and Drugs*. 2016;77(2):287–297.

Wood KE. Exposure to bath salts and synthetic tetrahydrocannabinol from 2009 to 2012 in the United States. *J Pediatr*. 2013;163(1):213–216.

WYFF4.COM. *Coroner: Synthetic pot killed college athlete; Anderson University basketball player collapsed on Oct. 4*. 2011. http://www.wyff4.com/Coroner-Synthetic-Pot-Killed-College-Athlete/-/9324882/6133626/-/10gxauh/-/index.html#ixzz1yHFVkCK7.

Yücel M, Bora E, Lubman DI, et al. The impact of cannabis use on cognitive functioning in patients with schizophrenia: a meta-analysis of existing findings and new data in a first-episode sample. *Schizophr Bull*. 2012;38(2):316–330.

Zimmermann US, Winkelmann PR, Pilhatsch M, et al. Withdrawal phenomena and dependence syndrome after the consumption of "spice gold". *Dtsch Arztebl Int*. 2009;106(27):464–467.

Zuba D, Byrska B. Analysis of the prevalence and coexistence of synthetic cannabinoids in "herbal high" products in Poland. *Forensic Toxicol*. 2013;31(1):21–30.

Hallucinogen Use Disorders

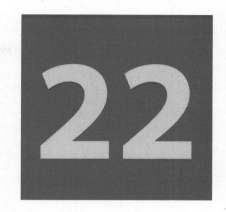

Anahita Bassir Nia, MD
Peter H. Addy, PhD
Deepak Cyril D'Souza, MD

22

▶ General Considerations

A. Classification of Hallucinogens and Hallucinogen-Related Disorders

It is difficult to narrowly define hallucinogens, given that drugs that can produce hallucinations are so diverse in chemical structure and mechanism/s of action. Many psychoactive drugs can induce hallucinations if given at high enough doses. For example, nicotine and even alcohol have been associated with hallucinations, even though these effects are not characteristic or desired. This chapter focuses on drugs that predominantly induce changes in thought, perception, and mood to a much greater extent than their other effects. In the past decade or so, the term hallucinogenic has been interchanged with psychedelic to refer to a class of drugs including psilocybin, N, N-dimethyltryptamine (DMT), and lysergic acid diethylamide (LSD), all of which share a mechanism that involves serotonin 2A receptors. In this chapter, hallucinogens are grouped into three categories: (1) serotonergic (tryptamine-like and phenethylamine-like), (2) N-methyl-D-aspartate (NMDA) antagonist, and (3) other.

B. Use of Hallucinogens

There is a long history of the use of hallucinogenic plants, commonly known as "psychedelics" (such as *Salvia divinorum*, psilocybin, mescaline, ibogaine, and the DMT-containing brew ayahuasca) by humans. Ceremonial hallucinogenic plant use can be found in cultures on most continents and in the histories of all the world's major religions (Schultes et al. 2001). As described later in further detail, hallucinogens are used to produce alterations in perception, as a means of reaching altered states of consciousness.

In addition to the naturally derived hallucinogens, several new hallucinogens have been synthesized over the past century, such as LSD and 3,4-methylenedioxyamphetamine (MDMA). These compounds have been characterized as extremely important to scientific research and clinical use. However, they have also been characterized as being dangerous addictive compounds with no accepted medical use.

C. Maladaptive Patterns of Hallucinogen Use

Hallucinogen-related disorders are classified into two categories: hallucinogen use disorders and hallucinogen-induced disorders. The *Diagnostic and Statistical Manual of Mental Disorders*, fifth edition (DSM-5) defines maladaptive patterns of drug use as involving tolerance and withdrawal. The U.S. National Institute of Drug Abuse (NIDA) does not consider LSD an "addictive drug since it does not produce compulsive drug-seeking behavior" (NIDA 2009). Tolerance develops rapidly to some effects of some hallucinogens but not to others. For example, tolerance develops in recreational users of LSD and "Ecstasy" but not in users of DMT. Discontinuation of most of these compounds does not appear to be associated with a withdrawal syndrome. Acute withdrawal is observed among regular users of "Ecstasy," but because of the varying and unknown purity and potency of "Ecstasy," it is difficult to draw conclusions about MDMA.

What does a maladaptive pattern of hallucinogen use look like? An analysis of the 1999 National Household Survey on Drug Abuse (NHSDA) (n = 1186) revealed that the most endorsed items indicative of hallucinogen *dependence* were emotional problems (11%), difficulty controlling use (7%), salience of use (7%), and tolerance (6%). Among adults who participated in the National Epidemiologic Survey on Alcohol and Related Conditions, the most and least commonly endorsed hallucinogen *dependence* items were "persistent desire or unsuccessful efforts to cut down or control use" (32%) and "important activities are given up or reduced" (5%), while the most and least commonly endorsed hallucinogen *abuse* items were "recent use in physically hazardous situations" (21%) and "legal problems related to use" (2%) (Kerridge et al. 2011). The most endorsed problems related to hallucinogen *use* among adult males in the Virginia Twin Registry were use in hazardous situations, physical and psychological consequences, and spending excessive time obtaining, using, or recovering from use (Gillespie et al. 2007).

Several demographic variables and subject characteristics have been correlated with hallucinogen use disorders. An Item Response Theory analysis of hallucinogen use disorders among adolescents revealed several effects of gender, race, and drug use patterns (Wu et al. 2010a). Adolescent males were more likely than females to endorse hazardous use of hallucinogens. Female adolescents were less likely than males to report use, but more likely to be diagnosed with a hallucinogen use disorder. Hispanic adolescents were more likely than Whites to endorse hazardous use and less likely to be diagnosed with a hallucinogen use disorder. The types of drugs people use were also correlated with the severity of hallucinogen use disorders they manifest. In adolescents, using "Ecstasy" and using hallucinogens more than 12 times were associated with increased odds of a hallucinogen use disorder (Wu et al. 2010a). In the 1999 NHSDA, adults were more likely to be diagnosed with hallucinogen dependence if they had recently begun using "Ecstasy" or mescaline (compared to LSD), or if they had ever used cocaine or other stimulants (compared to not having used) (Stone et al. 2006).

D. Epidemiology

1. Prevalence of hallucinogen use—One of the challenges in estimating the prevalence of hallucinogen use is the different definitions of hallucinogens and the drugs included in this category. The National Survey on Drug Use and Health (NSDUH) compiles annual data on drug use in the Unites States and defines LSD, PCP, ketamine, *S. divinorum*, peyote, mescaline, psilocybin mushrooms, and "Ecstasy" as "hallucinogens." According to the NSDUH, 2.2 million (0.8%) and 7.4 million (2.6%) persons aged 12 or older used hallucinogens over the past month and past year, respectively, in 2021 (Table 22–1). The rate of lifetime hallucinogen use was 16.4% among persons aged 12 or older and was higher for males (19.5%) than for females (13.4%). In 2021, 1.2 million (0.5%) persons aged 12 or older used hallucinogens for the first time within the past 12 months. Lifetime use of specific hallucinogens is reported in Table 22–2. LSD was the most often used hallucinogen (10.5%), followed by psilocybin (10.2%), "Ecstasy" (7.5%), mescaline (2.5%), PCP (2.3%), and peyote (1.9%). However, in the past decade, interest in the use of hallucinogens for recreational and "therapeutic" purposes has surged and therefore, current attempts to accurately estimate the prevalence of use may be challenging.

2. Prevalence of hallucinogen use disorders—An estimated 493,000 people (0.2%) met criteria for hallucinogen use disorder over the past year in 2021 (Table 22–3). Of all people surveyed in 2021 who had received substance-use treatment in the past year, 4.8% received treatment for hallucinogen use.

Table 22–1 Hallucinogen Use in Lifetime, Past Year, and Past Month Among Persons Aged 12 or Older, by Demographic Characteristics: Percentages, 2011 and 2012

Demographic Characteristic	Lifetime (2011)	Lifetime (2012)	Past Year (2011)	Past Year (2012)	Past Month (2011)	Past Month (2012)
Total	14.1	14.6	1.6	1.7	0.4	0.4
Age						
12–17	3.7	3.3	2.6	2.2	0.9	0.6
18–25	17.6	17.6	6.8	6.5	1.6	1.7
26 or older	14.8	15.4	0.6**	0.8	0.1**	0.2
Gender						
Male	17.6	18.2	2	2.2	0.5	0.6
Female	10.8	11.2	1.1	1.1	0.3	0.3
Hispanic Origin and Race						
Not Hispanic or Latino	15	15.3	1.5	1.7	0.4**	0.4
White	16.9	17.2	1.6	1.7	0.4**	0.5
Black or African American	6.6	7.8	0.9**	1.3	0.3	0.4
American Indian or Alaska Native	28.7	31.9	4.1	4.2	0.6	1.3
Native Hawaiian or other Pacific Islander	11.4	11	3.2	1.1	0.3	*
Asian	4.7	6	1.1	1.3	0.2	0.1
Two or more races	25.5	20.2	2.6	3.1	0.7	0.7
Hispanic or Latino	9.3	10.4	1.8	1.6	0.5	0.4

*Low precision; no estimate reported.

**Difference between estimate and 2012 estimate is statistically significant at the 0.05 level.

Adapted from SAMHSA, Center for Behavioral Health Statistics and Quality, National Survey on Drug Use and Health, 2011 and 2012.

Table 22–2 Specific Hallucinogen Use in Lifetime, by Age Group: Percentages, 2011 and 2012

Drug or Method of Administration	Total (2011)	Total (2012)	Aged 12–17 (2011)	Aged 12–17 (2012)	Aged 18–25 (2011)	Aged 18–25 (2012)	Aged 26+ (2011)	Aged 26+ (2012)
Hallucinogens	14.1	14.6	3.7	3.3	17.6	17.6	14.8	15.4
PCP (angel dust, phencyclidine)	2.4	2.5	0.3	0.4	1	1	2.9	3
LSD (acid)	8.9	9.1	0.9	1	6	5.9	10.4	10.7
Peyote	2	2.3	0.2	0.2	0.8	0.9	2.5	2.8
Mescaline	3	3	0.1	0.1	1.1	1	3.8	3.8
Psilocybin (mushrooms)	8.1	8.1	1.4	1.3	10.1*	9.3	8.6	8.7
Ecstasy (MDMA)	5.7**	6.2	2.4*	2	12.3	12.9	4.9**	5.6

*Difference between estimate and 2012 estimate is statistically significant at the 0.05 level.
**Difference between estimate and 2012 estimate is statistically significant at the 0.01 level.
Adapted from SAMHSA, Center for Behavioral Health Statistics and Quality, National Survey on Drug Use and Health, 2011 and 2012.

Studies using national data comparing the trends of hallucinogen use in the United States from 2002 to 2019 reported that hallucinogen use increased in adults aged 26 or older and decreased in adolescents aged 12–17 years in this period (Livne et al. 2022). Though the use of hallucinogens generally has similar trends, some differences exist. Lifetime use of some hallucinogens such as peyote has remained stable from 2002 to 2019. However, the lifetime use of mescaline has significantly decreased, and the lifetime use of ketamine and psilocybin has significantly increased over this time (Walsh et al. 2022). The overall past-year use of hallucinogens has increased in 2019 compared to 2015. Looking at different age groups, hallucinogen use has increased in adults aged 26 or older and decreased in adolescents aged 12–17 years in 2019 compared to 2002. Over this time period, the use of Ecstasy has decreased in adolescents, adults aged 18–25 years and 26 or older (Livne et al. 2022) and the use of LSD has increased overall and in all age groups (Livne et al. 2022).

3. Risk of co-occurring psychiatric diagnoses—In 2021, among adults aged 18 or older, 6.4% of those who had mental illness and 1.7% of those who did not have mental illness had used hallucinogens in the past year. Of adults with a major depressive episode, 8.4% had used hallucinogens in the past

year compared to 2.3% of adults without a major depressive episode. Among youth aged 12–17, 2.8% with and 1% without a major depressive episode had used hallucinogens in the past year.

Data drawn from 2001 to 2004, NSDUH suggested no significant associations between lifetime use of serotonergic hallucinogens (LSD, psilocybin, and mescaline) and past-year mental health outcomes or symptoms (Krebs & Johansen 2013). But in young adults (age 18–25), past-year LSD users had greater risk of suicidal ideation, serious psychological distress, major depressive disorder, and any/serious mental illness than those who never used illicit LSD (Han et al. 2022). However, use of serotonergic hallucinogens was reported in several observational studies to be associated with lower rates of mental health disorders, including substance use disorders (Jones & Nock 2022). Whether these associations reflect the effects of serotonergic hallucinogens or not is still unclear.

4. Prevalence of hallucinogen-related adverse events—National Inpatient Sample data show that the rate of hospitalizations with hallucinogen use disorder as the primary or secondary diagnosis has increased from 22.8 to 40.4 (1.8-fold), from 1998 to 2014. In addition, the rate of

Table 22–3 Substance Dependence or Abuse for Specific Substances in the Past Year, by Age Group: Percentages, 2011

Past Year Dependence or Abuse	Total (2011)	Total (2012)	Aged 12–17 (2011)	Aged 12–17 (2012)	Aged 18–25 (2011)	Aged 18–25 (2012)	Aged 26+ (2011)	Aged 26+ (2012)
Hallucinogens	0.1	0.1	0.3	0.3	0.5	0.4	0.1	0.1

Note: Dependence or abuse is based on definitions found in the 4th edition of the *Diagnostic and Statistical Manual of Mental Disorders* (DSM-IV).
Adapted from SAMHSA, Center for Behavioral Health Statistics and Quality, National Survey on Drug Use and Health, 2011 and 2012.

in-hospital mortality rate has increased from 0.3 to 0.6 (2.3-fold); and the rate of non-home discharge has increased from 4.2 to 6.3 (1.5-fold) (Singh 2021).

E. Etiology

There is little information on the etiology of maladaptive hallucinogen use. Given that hallucinogen use tends to be sporadic, the rates of maladaptive use are low, and there is little evidence to support physical dependence to these drugs, it is difficult to study the basis of vulnerability to hallucinogen use. In contrast, much research has been conducted to explain the high inter- and intra-variability of the psychoactive effects of hallucinogens. The net effect of any psychoactive drug is a complex interaction between the individual's current mood, expectations, and personality structure ("set"); environmental factors including immediate cultural, physical, and social variables in which the drug is used ("setting"); and the pharmacological effects of the drug (Johnson et al. 2008; Studerus et al. 2012).

1. Set (individual factors)—Performance anxiety and emotional excitability can have strong influences on the acute subjective response to hallucinogens. Being in a relaxed state of mind and being willing to let go control tends to decrease the likelihood of unpleasant experiences ("bad trips"). Previous experience with hallucinogens may be correlated with an overall less intense experience. Age has been correlated with outcomes in research studies, with older subjects reporting less impaired control and more blissful states (Studerus et al. 2012). Preparation for the experience also tends to make the experience more tolerable.

2. Setting (environmental factors)—The physical location and sociocultural environment may have strong influences on the acute subjective response to hallucinogens. For example, whether psilocybin is administered in a laboratory setting or as part of a positron emission tomography scan significantly predicts subjective anxiety (Studerus et al. 2012). However, there remains some debate about how critical the setting is for the "therapeutic" effects of psychedelic drugs used in treating psychiatric disorders. "Ecstasy" is often used in a dance club environment, which can consist of extreme heat and decreased water intake, leading to negative physical effects not seen in a laboratory setting (Parrott 2012a).

F. Genetics

Studies of large cohorts of twins suggest that hallucinogens show the least relative risk of addiction and furthermore, hallucinogen use disorders show the least heritability of all studied addictive agents (weighted mean 0.39) (Goldman et al. 2005). A population-based survey of female twins examining hallucinogen use disorders reported a lifetime prevalence of these disorders at less than 1%, and no cases of current abuse or dependence in dizygotic twins (Kendler et al. 1999). In this sample, it was suggested that hallucinogen use was the result of genetic and familial-environmental factors acting together.

Several gene × "Ecstasy" interaction effects have been demonstrated. COMT val/val and SERT s/s genotypes are associated with worse performance on visuospatial and perceptual attention tasks, the Tyr polymorphism of 5-HT2a receptor is associated with worse delayed recall, and extra-high CYP2D6 metabolizers show lower verbal fluency among polydrug "Ecstasy" users (Cuyas et al. 2011). The LPR polymorphism of 5-HTT and the rs165599 polymorphism of COMT were independently associated with reduced verbal fluency in polydrug "Ecstasy" users (Fagundo et al. 2011). MDMA reinforcing effects are much higher in the presence of a genetic deletion of the serotonin transporter in rats (Oakly et al. 2014). In summary, the genetic basis of vulnerability to hallucinogen use is still inconclusive.

G. Environmental Factors

Early life adversity is one of the major environmental factors known to increase the risk of substance use disorders in general. The underlying biological mechanism of this association is still poorly understood. But it is observed that early life adversity induces alterations in the endocannabinoid (Bassir Nia et al. 2019) and serotonergic systems (Llorente-Berzal et al. 2013), which play a critical role in the rewarding effects of several drugs, including MDMA (Llorente-Berzal et al. 2013). Animal models of maternal deprivation in early childhood have shown development of conditioned place preference (CPP) in male rodents with maternal deprivation, but not females or control males and females (Llorente-Berzal et al. 2013).

▶ Clinical Findings

A. Signs & Symptoms

The acute effects of various hallucinogens differ most likely based on their mechanism of action. NMDA receptor antagonists, 5-HT_{2A} agonists, and κ-opioid receptor (KOR) agonists have distinct profiles of effects. Furthermore, the time course of acute effect of hallucinogens varies considerably according to the route of administration. The KOR Salvinorin A, when smoked, produces effects lasting around 10 minutes, while ibogaine, when orally ingested, can last up to 28 hours. Perceptual effects most often include a lucid awareness of the drug-induced nature of the perceptions—that is, hallucinations are not accompanied by loss of insight into the drug-induced nature of the phenomena. DMT and Salvinorin A reportedly produce complex visual imagery and immersive "waking dream" like experiences. Even though these drugs are characterized as hallucinogens, they rarely produce true hallucinations—as defined as perceptions in the absence of external stimuli. These drugs more likely induce misperceptions of existing stimuli by removing the top-down influences that help us perceive our world the way that we do. Drug effects may change over time. For example, LSD, one of the most potent hallucinogens (psychoactive effects may begin at 50 mcg), initially produces somatic symptoms including paresthesia (tingling of the extremities), dizziness, weakness, and tremor. Later, individuals commonly see abstract geometric patterns with closed eyes.

1. Acute intoxication—Although these drugs differ in the onset, duration, and intensity of effects, their acute subjective effects are quite similar (Table 22–4). Hallucinogens produce a range of perceptual alterations and distortions. Sensory inputs are heightened or diminished (colors, textures, sounds, tastes, and touch become more intense or less intense). Sensations may assume compelling significance to the point that an individual becomes completely immersed in the experience and disregards more salient stimuli. Individuals may experience illusions (distortions in the perceived nature or meaning of real objects), such as seeing a grotesque distortion of a familiar face. Frank hallucinations (perceptions in the absence of any obvious stimuli) are rare but may occur. Typically, the hallucinations produced by serotonergic hallucinogenic drugs tend to be in the visual domain, and individuals generally realize that the perceptions are false. Synesthesia may also occur wherein individual perceptions cross sensory modalities (e.g., "seeing" sounds, or "hearing" colors).

Often the body or its parts may appear larger, smaller, heavier, or lighter than it normally feels. Time perception may be distorted, with time seeming to pass slower or faster. Concentration and attention can also be impaired, and subjects may sometimes focus on seemingly trivial details instead of more salient parts of an experience. Similarly, individuals may have difficulty "filtering" out irrelevant or trivial external or internal stimuli from more salient ones, resulting in the feeling of being overwhelmed by sensations. Individuals may experience feeling detached from themselves or the immediate environment (depersonalization). This may be described as watching oneself as a spectator or observer. Similarly, individuals may experience their surroundings as unreal or dreamlike (derealization). Depersonalization and derealization are more common for NDMA-antagonists and

KOR agonists than for 5-HT_{2A} agonists. Individuals may describe their experience as having "greater understanding" or enlightenment of events, their existence or the motivation of others, while under the influence of hallucinogens. These experiences have been described as "transformative" or "life changing." Rarely, individuals may develop false fixed beliefs or inferences that are not consistent with reality (delusions, e.g., ideas that people in the environment are trying to harm or kill the individual).

These effects on perceptions and thinking are invariably accompanied by changes in the individual's mood. Thus, individuals may experience intense and often rapidly shifting mood states ranging from mild apprehension to panic, severe depression, or elation or by concurrent emotions (e.g., sadness and joy) that are not ordinarily experienced simultaneously.

NMDA antagonists are likely to produce feelings of dissociation from the body and external world and can lead to a dreamlike disconnected state. Users of ketamine describe higher doses leading to a "k-hole" consisting of intense dissociation, out-of-body experiences, and delusions, usually associated with decreased volition and motor skills.

Salvinorin A inhalation can lead to very short (5–10 minutes) and intense hallucinatory-like experiences during which subjects become incapacitated and without volition. The intensity and suddenness of these experiences may lead to anxiety, fear, and panic. Inhalation can also lead to spontaneous, uncontrollable laughter and disorganized speech and movements (Addy 2012; Ranganathan et al. 2012).

A state of consciousness known to be facilitated by psilocybin, DMT, and salvinorin A under supportive conditions in research settings has been termed "mystical-type experience" (Griffiths et al. 2006; Johnson et al. 2011; Reissig et al. 2012). Subjects who undergo mystical-type experiences describe the experience as having substantial personal meaning. These are some of the reported effects associated with a mystical-type experience (Griffiths et al. 2006):

- internal unity (pure awareness, a merging with ultimate reality)
- external unity (unity of all things, all things are alive, all is one)
- transcendence of time and space
- ineffability and paradoxicality (claim of difficulty in describing the experience in words)
- sense of sacredness (awe)
- noetic quality (claim of intuitive knowledge of ultimate reality)
- deeply felt positive mood (joy, peace, and love) (Griffiths et al.

Table 22–4 Signs and Symptoms of Hallucinogen Intoxication

Autonomic arousal
Depersonalization
Derealization
Impaired judgment
Marked anxiety or depression
Mystical-type experiences
Perceptual changes
Synesthesia
Thought disorders

2. Neuroadaptation—Not much is known about neuroadaptation to hallucinogens. Serotonergic hallucinogens and KOR agonists produce little to no dependence and do not cause conditioned place aversion in animals, except for MDMA, which causes conditioned place preference. NMDA antagonists produce robust (CPP. Frequent users of serotonergic hallucinogens rarely report craving. Acute MDMA use leads to depleted neuronal serotonin levels for 24–48 hours after use, which can lead to depressive symptoms, restlessness, fatigue, and muscle ache (Benningfield & Cowan 2013).

Tolerance refers to a gradual decrease in responsiveness to a drug after repeated administration. Tolerance to the behavioral effects has been observed in humans and animals for some but not other of serotonergic hallucinogens. Strassman et al. (2000) did not observe physiological tolerance with repeated administration of DMT. In humans, acute tolerance to the behavioral and subjective effects of LSD emerges quickly (24 hours after its first exposure) and peaks 4 days later (Belleville et al. 1956; Buchborn et al. 2016). Interestingly, tolerance to the psychoactive effects of LSD generalizes to some other classic serotonergic hallucinogens including psilocybin and mescaline but not to tetrahydrocannabinol or amphetamine. Once tolerance develops, it cannot be overcome with doses higher than the initial dose. Tolerance abates within about 5 days of abstinence. Importantly, abstinence is not associated with symptoms of withdrawal. When tolerance occurs rapidly, it is referred to as tachyphylaxis. In animals, there is tachyphylaxis to LSD-induced behaviors. Mechanistically, pharmacodynamic adaptations of serotonin 5-HT$_{2A}$ and/or (downstream) glutamate receptors are likely to account for tolerance; a learning-related precipitation, however, has also been described. Adaptive changes in LSD-stimulated serotonin receptor signaling and/or (downstream) glutamate receptor signaling may mediate tolerance to the discriminative stimulus effects of LSD. The rapid onset of tolerance to the psychoactive effects of LSD is probably the main reason why LSD is not used daily. Tolerance is more often reported among "Ecstasy" users than users of other types of hallucinogens (Wu et al. 2010a).

Withdrawal symptoms are extremely uncommon (Gillespie et al. 2007) and are not considered necessary to diagnose hallucinogen use disorder according to DSM-5. There is little evidence to suggest that the use of serotonergic or KOR hallucinogens is associated with a withdrawal syndrome. Physical dependence has not been shown in animals or humans (Ross 2012). NMDA antagonists, including the over-the-counter antitussive dextromethorphan, have documented abuse potential including tolerance, withdrawal, and craving.

3. Long-term effects—There are differences in the long-term sequelae of different hallucinogens.

i. Serotonergic hallucinogens—Serotonergic hallucinogens have a long history of safe single dose administration in controlled research settings (Strassman 1994), and several attempts to quantitatively analyze and rank drug harms score hallucinogens as among the less harmful known psychoactive substances, in terms of both harm to the user and harm to others (Nutt et al. 2010; van Amsterdam et al. 2010).

Hallucinogen-Induced Psychotic Disorder includes labile affect; delusions, often of a religious nature; and hallucinations. During early research in the 1950s, the incidence of LSD-related psychosis in experimental subjects was estimated at 0.8 per 1000 (Cohen 1960).

Hallucinogen Persisting Perception Disorder (HPPD) ("flashbacks") is an uncommon condition characterized by the spontaneous recurrence of perceptual distortions (usually visual) first encountered under the influence of a hallucinogen. Evidence suggests that HPPD may be more common with recreational LSD use than with research or therapeutic use, and there is no known proven treatment (Halpern & Pope 2003). Analysis of 2001–2004 NSDUH data (Krebs & Johansen 2013) showed that past-year use of LSD was *not* associated with past-year symptoms of visual phenomena, panic attacks, or psychosis. Subjects in randomized controlled trials with psilocybin do not report "flashbacks" or HPPD symptoms (Griffiths et al. 2008 2011; Studerus et al. 2011). Regular members of the Native American Church, who use mescaline-containing peyote in its rituals, similarly do not report "flashbacks" or persistent visual symptoms (Halpern et al. 2005).

The use of psychedelics has historically involved the infrequent or sporadic consumption of moderate to high doses in a single or otherwise limited number of exposures. In recent and current clinical research with LSD and other hallucinogens, participants are carefully selected for a lack of significant medical or serious psychiatric conditions (e.g., psychosis) and undergo careful screening and preparation. The studies are conducted in a controlled setting with careful preparation, medical and psychiatric oversight, access to emergency care during dosing sessions, and extensive post-dosing follow-up. Such historical and research practices support the safety and a lack of socioeconomic consequences or addictive potential of psychedelics (van Amsterdam et al. 2011). However, the safety of multiple, repeated dosing, and dosing without careful preparation and medical/psychiatric supervision may have a different safety profile. Some serotonergic hallucinogens are now legal in some U.S. states. The availability of these compounds has increased, as also interest in using them outside controlled medical/psychiatric supervision.

Furthermore, one increasingly popular use of serotonergic hallucinogens involved the practice of "microdosing." This practice involves taking low or subpsychedelic doses repeatedly (daily or weekly) over a prolonged period. Given that the safety profile is derived from typical use of these compounds, which is sporadic and often with medical/psychiatric supervision, the safety of repeated use even with microdoses has not been established and is a cause for concern. A clear warning exists in the LSD derivative, methysergide, a highly effective migraine and cluster headache preventive (taken daily) that was removed from the market after cases of cardiac valve and other tissue fibrosis emerged.

Individuals with underlying cardiovascular or cerebrovascular disease or with a history of serious mental illnesses are at higher risk for serious adverse events with psychedelics. Even in those without such underlying health conditions, there is a potential for unpleasant or dangerous outcomes, particularly if taking an unknown dose, combining drugs, and/or not being informed on the range of acute effects. Thus, given the rapidly changing landscape of serotonergic hallucinogens, the safety of these compounds needs to be reexamined.

ii. NMDA antagonists—The safety of ketamine is derived from two sources. The recreational use of ketamine and the use of ketamine/esketamine for therapeutic purposes (Nikayin et al. 2022). Long-term recreational ketamine users may develop cognitive impairments (Liang et al. 2013; Zhang et al. 2020) and brain lesions after 2–4 years of use (Hung, Zhang, et al. 2020; Wang et al. 2013). A review (Morgan et al. 2012) lists the several effects of chronic ketamine use, including ulcerative cystitis, kidney dysfunction, depression, and cognitive impairments. A recent articles reported the increased risk of cholestatic liver injury in COVID-19-associated acute respiratory distress syndrome (Wendel-Garcia et al. 2022), and other hepatobiliary adverse events (Cotter et al. 2021).

Beyond the acute transient, generally mild and self-limited side effects of ketamine and esketamine observed in ketamine administration studies, treatment with esketamine has been associated with an increased risk of dysuria and urinary urgency (Nikayin et al. 2022). However, severe bladder pathology, which has been observed in chronic recreational ketamine users, has not been reported among patients receiving doses of esketamine/ketamine for depression. Likewise, in contrast to long-term impairments in cognition observed in chronic recreational ketamine users, the esketamine clinical trials did not find evidence for increased risk of cognitive impairment. More studies are needed to conclusively assess the potential long-term side negative effects of repetitive use of ketamine on health.

B. Psychological Testing

There are no known psychological tests available that are specific to hallucinogen use disorders. Screening for hallucinogen use is usually conducted using standardized rating scales such as the Addiction Severity Index (McLellan et al. 1980) or standardized interviews such as the Structured Clinical Interview for DSM-IV-TR Diagnoses (Lobbestael et al. 2011).

C. Laboratory Findings

Although LSD and psilocin can be detected in urine, standard urine tests do not typically include them. The detection window for LSD and psilocin is rather small: 8 hours for LSD and up to 24 hours for psilocin. Furthermore, samples are photosensitive and must be kept away from light. MDMA use can be assessed through hair samples. Commercial urine toxicology tests exist to capture recent use of PCP and ketamine. There are no current commercially available urine tests for salvinorin A.

D. Neuroimaging

This section is focused on imaging findings associated with long-term and/or repeated use of hallucinogens. Chronic use of "Ecstasy" is associated with reduced serotonin transporter (SERT) in the midbrain, thalamus, and cortical regions (Benningfield & Cowan 2013; Martinez et al. 2007; Parrott 2013a). This reduction in SERT is more pronounced in women and appears to be reversible, as ex-users did not differ from healthy controls. A meta-analysis of 16 studies with a total of 356 MDMA users and 311 controls reported decreased SERT density in most of the investigated brain regions, which may be reversible to some extent after abstinence (Müller et al. 2019). Interestingly, while animal studies demonstrated MDMA-induced axonal degradation, it was not shown in humans with chronic MDMA use (Zimmermann et al. 2022).

Structural magnetic resonance imaging scans of ketamine-dependent subjects have revealed decreased frontal cortex gray matter volume and white matter abnormalities in frontal and left temporoparietal cortices (Liao et al. 2010, 2011); cortical atrophy in the frontal, parietal, or occipital cortices (Wang et al. 2013); right insula, left inferior parietal lobule, left dorsolateral prefrontal cortex/superior frontal gyrus, and left medial orbitofrontal cortex (Hung, Liu, et al. 2020) and decreased white matter microstructural integrity in the right hemisphere, which was associated with increased dissociative experiences in chronic ketamine users. Furthermore, the decreased gray matter volume has negative associations with amount, frequency, and duration of ketamine use (Zhong et al. 2021).

There is also increasing evidence of functional connectivity alterations in chronic hallucinogen users. Compared to controls, Hung et al. (2020) reported that ketamine users showed higher connectivity between caudate and dorsal anterior cingulate cortex and between pallidum and bilateral cerebellum. Furthermore, putamen showed higher connectivity with the left orbitofrontal cortex in ketamine users, in association with higher scores of impulsivity and longer ketamine use.

E. Course of Hallucinogen Use

It is difficult to ascertain whether long-term use of any one drug or class of drugs causes impairment or neurotoxicity. Preclinical studies do not allow exact prediction of adverse events in humans (Green et al. 2012a) for several reasons. For example, users rarely stick to one substance or substance class exclusively, and in the case of "Ecstasy" one cannot assume it to be equivalent to MDMA (Green et al. 2012b). Furthermore, the rates of hallucinogen use are quite low. Given these limitations, it seems that physical toxicity from hallucinogens is rare (Nutt et al. 2010; van Amsterdam et al. 2010) but may occur. Recreational use of "Ecstasy" can lead to cardiovascular emergencies, liver failure, and potentially fatal dehydration. The association between LSD and HPPD may suggest neurotoxic changes in the perceptual system, but there is no clear evidence at present. A recent systematic review of 48 studies of serotonergic psychedelics (LSD, psilocybin, DMT, 5-MeO-DMT, mescaline, or ayahuasca) that included 1774 participants reported adverse effects for up to 1 month after use. The adverse events included a wide range of complaints, including headaches, sleep disturbances, and individual cases of increased psychological distress (Evens et al. 2023). Another meta-analysis of 44 articles, describing the therapeutic use of serotonergic psychedelics (psilocybin, LSD, and ayahuasca) and MDMA in 598 unique patients, reported that the main acute side effects are nausea, headaches, and anxiety (Breeksema et al. 2022). One serious adverse event was reported during MDMA administration, which was an increase in premature ventricular contractions and needed brief hospitalization.

The use of serotonergic hallucinogens is typically sporadic. In a survey of the population-based Virginia Twin Registry (n = 4234 adult males), 91% of people who had ever used hallucinogens reported using them fewer than six times in their life (in this survey hallucinogen was defined as LSD, mescaline, and PCP). Although most users take hallucinogens sporadically and infrequently, there are two notable exceptions. Members of the Native American Church use mescaline-containing peyote in regular ceremonies (Halpern et al. 2005; Kulis et al. 2012), and members of the União do Vegetal church use ayahuasca as part of their ceremonies. In both groups, the use of other drugs and alcohol is forbidden. These religious groups are sanctioned by the U.S. government to use these hallucinogens under the aegis of religious freedom (Ross 2012). Longitudinal and cross-sectional studies using control groups suggest no long-term ill-effects of ceremonial use of these substances and reduced use of alcohol and cocaine among group members (Barbosa et al. 2012).

More recently however, as discussed earlier, microdosing has become increasingly popular. This practice involves taking low or sub-psychedelic doses repeatedly (daily or weekly) over a prolonged period. The safety of this practice has not been fully determined.

Differential Diagnosis

Clinicians are most likely to encounter patients presenting either with acute hallucinogen intoxication or for complications related to use. Acute hallucinogen intoxication may present with symptoms that overlap to some extent with endogenous psychotic states. A history of recent consumption of a hallucinogenic drug and the typically transient nature of symptoms should help determine the diagnosis. It is important to consider other conditions that may cause hallucinations, delusions, and cognitive impairment, such as

traumatic brain injury, delirium, and acute psychosis. Severe adverse effects and fatalities associated with psilocybin are usually due to the coingestion of other drugs such as alcohol (van Amsterdam et al. 2011), and this is likely true for other serotonergic hallucinogens as well.

Co-occurring Disorders

There is no clear pattern of co-occurring disorders in those who use hallucinogens. See also the earlier discussion of co-occurring psychiatric disorders assessed by the NSDUH. According to the self-medication hypothesis, people who use substances of all kinds often take them to self-medicate underlying psychiatric conditions, but this has not been supported by compelling evidence.

However, in the last few decades, the increasing interest in the use of serotonergic psychedelic drugs and ketamine as treatments for neuropsychiatric disorders would be expected to be associated with an increase in individuals with comorbid neuropsychiatric disorders using these compounds. Patients who use hallucinogens should be investigated for self-medication of co-occurring psychiatric disorders since certain diagnostic groups (e.g., those with psychotic disorders) may be more vulnerable to the negative consequences of psychedelics. Users of MDMA and classic serotonergic hallucinogens are likely to use other types of drugs as well, particularly alcohol and cannabis (Licht et al. 2012). Therefore, patients who use hallucinogens may initially present with other substance use disorders.

Treatment

A. Psychotherapeutic Interventions

People acutely under the influence of hallucinogens may require supportive engagement: being nondirective and nonconfrontational while waiting for the effects of the drug to wear off. Acute intoxication leading to emergency intervention may include confusion, disordered self-control, fear of death or permanent psychosis, and paranoia. Such symptoms generally resolve within 6 hours, but some substances last longer than others, as mentioned earlier. Hallucinogen use disorder is not common, and treatment follows that of substance use disorder in general: psychoeducation, cognitive–behavioral therapy, mindfulness-based relapse prevention, 12-step groups, and other psycho-social-spiritual support (Table 22–5).

B. Psychopharmacologic Interventions

In general, psychopharmacological interventions are not necessary to manage the acute effects of hallucinogen use. However, benzodiazepines may be used to relieve distress if the individual is experiencing a "bad trip." If psychotic symptoms during a bad trip are distressing, antipsychotic drugs particularly ones that have a serotonergic mechanism, e.g., risperidone, may reduce psychotic symptoms.

Table 22–5 Nonpharmacologic Modalities of Hallucinogen-Abuse Treatment

12-Step support program facilitation
Aftercare
Enhancement of coping strategies
Family therapy
Health and nutritional counseling
Lifestyle change
Psychotherapy
Recreational therapy
Relaxation training
Sexual education
Spiritual growth
Vocational and physical rehabilitation

▶ Complications

A. Cognition

Though some animal studies showed that MDMA induces impairment of long-term memory in rodents (Ros-Simó et al. 2013), a recent systematic review of 25 years of animal studies on MDMA reported that they did not find any evidence that doses of less than 3 mg/kg MDMA (which is in the range of recreational use of MDMA) produce cognitive deficits in animals. This study reported that even much higher doses of MDMA (up to 20 times) did not produce cognitive impairment in most studies (Pantoni & Anagnostaras 2019).

The evidence on the effects of MDMA on cognition in humans has several limitations such as co-occurring use of other drugs. Some studies reported that recreational users of "Ecstasy" demonstrate deficits in retrospective memory, prospective memory, cognition, attentional shifting, problem solving, social intelligence, and sleep architecture (Parrot 2013a, 2013b; Roberts et al. 2013) and long-term ecstasy users demonstrate impairment in visual perception processes (White et al. 2013). Moreover, lower serotonin transporter (SERT) binding in abstinent Ecstasy/MDMA users have been shown in neuroimaging studies (Parrott 2013). However, a recent review article on the cognitive effects of MDMA summarized the evidence from human studies and concluded that repeated use of ecstasy produces mild short to medium term neurocognitive impairments that are potentially reversible with abstinence (Montgomery & Roberts 2022).

The acute and long-term effects of ketamine use on health have been the subject of considerable research. Animal models demonstrated that ketamine impairs visual perception (Ward et al. 2013). Clinical studies demonstrated that frequent daily ketamine use is associated with neurocognitive impairments including working and episodic memory deficits (Morgan et al. 2006, 2012). More recently, verbal/visual memory and executive function dysfunction have been reported in heavy, chronic recreational users of ketamine

(Zhang et al. 2020). Most of these studies have been cross-sectional and unable to determine causation.

However, it is important to note that both preclinical and clinical studies on the use of ketamine in the treatment of depression and other psychiatric disorders not only failed to show any negative effects of therapeutic use of ketamine but also reported potential positive effects of ketamine on cognition (Nikayin et al. 2022; Shiroma et al. 2022; Xu et al. 2022).

B. Drug Interactions

Classic hallucinogens increase serotonin levels in the brain, thus, in theory, they may increase the risk of serotonin syndrome, particularly if coadministered with medications such as selective serotonin reuptake inhibitors (SSRIs). However, several small clinical trials reported very low risk. In fact, SSRIs may reduce the effects of hallucinogens such as MDMA, if taken in advance. However, recent studies have shown that treatment with SSRIs does not reduce the positive mood effects of psychedelic psilocybin in healthy subjects (Becker et al. 2022). SSRIs taken along with ayahuasca (which contains MAOIs) can, in theory, lead to serotonin syndrome, and many psychedelic phenethylamines like MDMA are generally considered contraindicated in combination with MAOIs (Malcolm & Thomas 2022). Lastly, MDMA inhibits CYP2D6 and affects the metabolism of medications when coadministered with MDMA (Papaseit et al. 2020).

C. Other

The main physical harm associated with chronic frequent ketamine use is ulcerative cystitis. The etiology has not been sufficiently described, but symptoms include frequent and urgent need to urinate, dysuria, incontinence, and painful hematuria. Symptoms usually resolve on cessation of ketamine use, but not always (Morgan et al. 2012).

▶ Prognosis

Hallucinogen use disorder is typically sporadic and experimental in nature. Long-term hallucinogen use can lead to HPPD, mood lability, cognitive deterioration, and personality alterations. It is important to treat co-occurring medical and psychiatric disorders to maximize abstinence.

▶ Sex differences

There is increasing evidence of sex differences in various aspects of substance use disorders, including subjective effects, abuse liability, prevalence, course of substance use disorders, and prognosis. Though the evidence is limited for hallucinogen substances, similar patterns have been reported.

Observational studies reported that among ecstasy users, men reported taking larger amounts of ecstasy, but the frequency of use was similar between men and women (Ogeil et al. 2013).

▶ Potential therapeutic effects

Though the focus of this chapter is on the development of hallucinogen use disorder and harmful effects of these drugs, there is emerging research suggesting beneficial effects of hallucinogenic drugs. The U.S. Food and Drug Administration (FDA) approved esketamine, s-enantiomer of ketamine, for the treatment of treatment-resistant depression in 2019 (Young et al. 2023), and MDMA will most likely receive FDA approval for the treatment of posttraumatic stress disorder. Furthermore, increasing evidence supports the potential effects of psilocybin in the treatment of depression (Goodwin et al. 2022, 2023; Sloshower et al. 2023) and substance use disorders (van der Meer et al. 2023), particularly alcohol use disorder (Bogenschutz et al. 2022). Though the underlying mechanism of action of these effects is still poorly understood, increased neuroplasticity is one of the leading theories (Calder & Hasler 2023; Vargas et al. 2023). Positive personality changes such as increased openness up to 14 months after a single dose of psilocybin (MacLean et al. 2011) and MDMA-induced enhancement of emotional empathy and prosocial behaviors have been demonstrated in experimental studies (Hysek et al. 2014). More studies are needed to confirm these reported effects, and the required dose, set, setting, and potential correlators.

Addy P, Radhakrishnan R, Cortes J, D'Souza D. Comorbid alcohol, cannabis, and cocaine use disorders in schizophrenia: epidemiology, consequences, mechanisms and treatment. *Focus.* 2012;2(10):140–153.

Addy PH. Acute and post-acute behavioral and psychological effects of salvinorin A in humans. *Psychopharmacology (Berl).* 2012;220(1):195–204.

Barbosa PC, Mizumoto S, Bogenschutz MP, Strassman RJ. Health status of ayahuasca users. *Drug Test Anal.* 2012;4(7–8):601–609.

Bassir Nia A, Bender R, Harpaz-Rotem I. Endocannabinoid system alterations in posttraumatic stress disorder: a review of developmental and accumulative effects of trauma. *Chronic Stress (Thousand Oaks).* 2019;3. https://doi.org/10.1177/2470547019864096

Becker AM, Holze F, Grandinetti T, et al. Acute effects of psilocybin after escitalopram or placebo pretreatment in a randomized, double-blind, placebo-controlled, crossover study in healthy subjects. *Clin Pharmacol Ther.* 2022;111(4):886–895. https://doi.org/10.1002/cpt.2487

Belleville RE, Fraser HF, Isbell H, et al. Studies on lysergic acid diethylamide (LSD-25). I. Effects in former morphine addicts and development of tolerance during chronic intoxication. *AMA Arch Neurol Psychiatry.* 1956;76(5):468–478.

Benningfield MM, Cowan RL. Brain serotonin function in MDMA (ecstasy) users: evidence for persisting neurotoxicity. *Neuropsychopharmacology.* 2013;38(1):253–255.

Bogenschutz MP, Ross S, Bhatt S, et al. Percentage of heavy drinking days following psilocybin-assisted psychotherapy vs placebo in the treatment of adult patients with alcohol use disorder: a randomized clinical trial. *JAMA Psychiatry.* 2022;79(10):953–962. https://doi.org/10.1001/jamapsychiatry.2022.2096

Breeksema JJ, Kuin BW, Kamphuis J, et al. Adverse events in clinical treatments with serotonergic psychedelics and MDMA: a mixed-methods systematic review. *J Psychopharmacol.* 2022;36(10):1100–1117. https://doi.org/10.1177/02698811221116926

Calder AE, Hasler G. Towards an understanding of psychedelic-induced neuroplasticity. *Neuropsychopharmacology.* 2023;48(1):104–112. https://doi.org/10.1038/s41386-022-01389-z

Cohen S. LSD: Side effects and complications. *J Nerv Ment Dis.* 1960;130:20–40.

Cotter S, Wong J, Gada N, et al. Repeated or continuous medically supervised ketamine administration associated with hepatobiliary adverse events: a retrospective case series. *Drug Saf.* 2021;44(12):1365–1374. https://doi.org/10.1007/s40264-021-01120-9

Cuyas E, Verdejo-Garcia A, Fagundo AB, et al. The influence of genetic and environmental factors among MDMA users in cognitive performance. *PLoS One.* 2011;6(11):e27206.

Drug Abuse Warning Network (DAWN). *Selected Tables of National Estimates of Drug-Related Emergency Department Visits.* Rockville, MD: Center for Behavioral Health Statistics and Quality, 2011.

Elie MP, Elie LE, Baron MG. Keeping pace with NPS releases: fast GC-MS screening of legal high products. *Drug Test Anal.* 2013;5:281–290.

Evens R, Schmidt ME, Majić T, Schmidt TT. The psychedelic afterglow phenomenon: a systematic review of subacute effects of classic serotonergic psychedelics. *Ther Adv Psychopharmacol.* 2023;13, 20451253231172254. https://doi.org/10.1177/20451253231172254

Fagundo AB, Cuyas E, Verdejo-Garcia A, et al. The influence of 5-HTT and COMT genotypes on verbal fluency in ecstasy users. *J Psychopharmacol.* 2010;24(9):1381–1393.

Gillespie NA, Neale MC, Prescott CA, et al. Factor and item-response analysis DSM-IV criteria for abuse of and dependence on cannabis, cocaine, hallucinogens, sedatives, stimulants and opioids. *Addiction.* 2007;102(6):920–930.

Goldman D, Oroszi G, Ducci F. The genetics of addictions: uncovering the genes. *Nat Rev Genet.* 2005;6(7):521–532.

Goodwin GM, Aaronson ST, Alvarez O, et al. Single-dose psilocybin for a treatment-resistant episode of major depression. *N Engl J Med.* 2022;387(18):1637–1648. https://doi.org/10.1056/NEJMoa2206443

Goodwin GM, Aaronson ST, Alvarez O, et al. Single-dose psilocybin for a treatment-resistant episode of major depression: impact on patient-reported depression severity, anxiety, function, and quality of life. *J Affect Disord.* 2023;327:120–127. https://doi.org/10.1016/j.jad.2023.01.108

Green AR, King MV, Shortall SE, Fone KC. Lost in translation: preclinical studies on 3,4-methylenedioxymethamphetamine provide information on mechanisms of action, but do not allow accurate prediction of adverse events in humans. *Br J Pharmacol.* 2012a;166(5):1523–1536.

Green A, King M, Shortall S, Fone K. Ecstasy cannot be assumed to be 3,4-methylenedioxyamphetamine (MDMA). *Br J Pharmacol.* 2012b;166(5):1521–1522.

Griffiths R, Richards W, Johnson M, et al. Mystical-type experiences occasioned by psilocybin mediate the attribution of personal meaning and spiritual significance 14 months later. *J Psychopharmacol.* 2008;22(6):621–632.

Griffiths RR, Richards WA, McCann U, Jesse R. Psilocybin can occasion mystical-type experiences having substantial and sustained personal meaning and spiritual significance. *Psychopharmacology (Berl)*. 2006;187(3):268–283; discussion 84–92.

Griffiths RR, Johnson MW, Richards WA, et al. Psilocybin occasioned mystical-type experiences: immediate and persisting dose-related effects. *Psychopharmacology (Berl)*. 2011;218(4):649–665.

Halpern JH, Pope HG Jr. Hallucinogen persisting perception disorder: what do we know after 50 years? *Drug Alcohol Depend*. 2003;69(2):109–19.

Halpern JH, Sherwood AR, Hudson JI, et al. Psychological and cognitive effects of long-term peyote use among Native Americans. *Biol Psychiatry*. 2005;58(8):624–631.

Han B, Blanco C, Einstein EB, Compton WM. Mental health conditions and receipt of mental health care by illicit lysergic acid diethylamide (LSD) use status among young adults in the United States. *Addiction*. 2022;117(6):1794–1800. https://doi.org/10.1111/add.15789

Hung CC, Liu YH, Huang CC, et al. Effects of early ketamine exposure on cerebral gray matter volume and functional connectivity. *Sci Rep*. 2020;10(1):15488. https://doi.org/10.1038/s41598-020-72320-z

Hung CC, Zhang S, Chen CM, et al. Striatal functional connectivity in chronic ketamine users: a pilot study. *Am J Drug Alcohol Abuse*. 2020;46(1):31–43. https://doi.org/10.1080/00952990.2019.1624764

Hysek CM, Schmid Y, Simmler LD, et al. MDMA enhances emotional empathy and prosocial behavior. *Soc Cogn Affect Neurosci*. 2014;9(11):1645–1652. https://doi.org/10.1093/scan/nst161

Jones GM, Nock MK. Exploring protective associations between the use of classic psychedelics and cocaine use disorder: a population-based survey study. *Sci Rep*. 2022;12(1):2574. https://doi.org/10.1038/s41598-022-06580-2

Johnson M, Richards W, Griffiths R. Human hallucinogen research: guidelines for safety. *J Psychopharmacol*. 2008;22(6):603–620.

Johnson MW, MacLean KA, Reissig CJ, et al. Human psychopharmacology and dose-effects of salvinorin A, a kappa opioid agonist hallucinogen present in the plant *Salvia divinorum*. *Drug Alcohol Depend*. 2011;115(1–2):150–155.

Kendler KS, Karkowski L, Prescott CA. Hallucinogen, opiate, sedative and stimulant use and abuse in a population-based sample of female twins. *Acta Psychiatr Scand*. 1999;99(5):368–376.

Kerridge BT, Saha TD, Smith S, et al. Dimensionality of hallucinogen and inhalant/solvent abuse and dependence criteria: implications for the *Diagnostic and Statistical Manual of Mental Disorders*—Fifth Edition. *Addict Behav*. 2011;36(9):912–918.

Kobayashi H, Ujike H, Iwata N, et al. The adenosine A2A receptor is associated with methamphetamine dependence/psychosis in the Japanese population. *Behav Brain Funct*. 2010;6:50.

Krebs TS, Johansen PO. Psychedelics and mental health: a population study. *PLoS One*. 2013;8(8):e63972.

Kulis S, Hodge DR, Ayers SL, et al. Spirituality and religion: intertwined protective factors for substance use among urban American Indian youth. *Am J Drug Alcohol Abuse*. 2012;38(5):444–449.

Liang HJ, Lau CG, Tang A, et al. Cognitive impairments in poly-drug ketamine users. *Addict Behav*. 2013;38(11):2661–2666.

Liao Y, Tang J, Ma M, et al. Frontal white matter abnormalities following chronic ketamine use: a diffusion tensor imaging study. *Brain*. 2010;133(Pt 7):2115–2122.

Liao Y, Tang J, Corlett PR, et al. Reduced dorsal prefrontal gray matter after chronic ketamine use. *Biol Psychiatry*. 2011;69(1):42–48.

Licht CL, Christoffersen M, Okholm M, et al. Simultaneous polysubstance use among Danish 3,4-methylenedioxymethamphetamine and hallucinogen users: combination patterns and proposed biological bases. *Hum Psychopharmacol*. 2012;27(4):352–363.

Livne O, Shmulewitz D, Walsh C, Hasin DS. Adolescent and adult time trends in US hallucinogen use, 2002-19: any use, and use of ecstasy, LSD and PCP. *Addiction*. 2022;117(12):3099–3109. https://doi.org/10.1111/add.15987

Llorente-Berzal A, Manzanedo C, Daza-Losada M, et al. Sex-dependent effects of early maternal deprivation on MDMA-induced conditioned place preference in adolescent rats: possible neurochemical correlates. *Toxicology*. 2013;311(1–2):78–86. https://doi.org/10.1016/j.tox.2012.12.003

Lobbestael J, Leurgans M, Arntz A. Inter-rater reliability of the Structured Clinical Interview for DSM-IV Axis I Disorders (SCID I) and Axis II Disorders (SCID II). *Clin Psychol Psychother*. 2011;18(1):75–79.

MacLean KA, Johnson MW, Griffiths RR. Mystical experiences occasioned by the hallucinogen psilocybin lead to increases in the personality domain of openness. *J Psychopharmacol*. 2011;25(11):1453–1461.

Malcolm B, Thomas K. Serotonin toxicity of serotonergic psychedelics. *Psychopharmacology (Berl)*. 2022;239(6):1881–1891. https://doi.org/10.1007/s00213-021-05876-x

Martinez D, Kim JH, Krystal J, Abi-Dargham A. Imaging the neurochemistry of alcohol and substance abuse. *Neuroimaging Clin North Am*. 2007;17(4):539–555, x.

McLellan AT, Luborsky L, Woody GE, O'Brien CP. An improved diagnostic evaluation instrument for substance abuse patients. The Addiction Severity Index. *J Nerv Ment Dis*. 1980;168(1):26–33.

Montgomery C, Roberts CA. Neurological and cognitive alterations induced by MDMA in humans. *Exp Neurol*. 2022;347:113888. https://doi.org/10.1016/j.expneurol.2021.113888

Morefield KM, Keane M, Felgate P, et al. Pill content, dose and resulting plasma concentrations of 3,4-methylendioxymethamphetamine (MDMA) in recreational "ecstasy" users. *Addiction*. 2011;106(7):1293–1300.

Morgan CJ, Perry EB, Cho HS, et al. Greater vulnerability to the amnestic effects of ketamine in males. *Psychopharmacology (Berl)*. 2006;187(4):405–414.

Morgan CJ, Curran HV; Independent Scientific Committee on D. Ketamine use: a review. *Addiction*. 2012;107(1):27–38.

Müller F, Brändle R, Liechti ME, Borgwardt S. Neuroimaging of chronic MDMA ("ecstasy") effects: a meta-analysis. *Neurosci Biobehav Rev*. 2019;96:10–20. https://doi.org/10.1016/j.neubiorev.2018.11.004

NIDA https://nida.nih.gov/research-topics/publications/drugfacts Nutt DJ, King LA, Phillips LD; Independent Scientific Committee on D. Drug harms in the UK: a multicriteria decision analysis. *Lancet*. 2010;376(9752):1558–1565.

Nikayin S, Murphy E, Krystal JH, Wilkinson ST. Long-term safety of ketamine and esketamine in treatment of depression. *Exp Opin Drug Saf.* 2022;21(6):777–787.

Oakly AC, Brox BW, Schenk S, Ellenbroek BA. A genetic deletion of the serotonin transporter greatly enhances the reinforcing properties of MDMA in rats. *Mol Psychiatry.* 2014;19(5): 534–535. https://doi.org/10.1038/mp.2013.75

Ogeil RP, Rajaratnam SM, Broadbear JH. Male and female ecstasy users: differences in patterns of use, sleep quality and mental health outcomes. *Drug Alcohol Depend.* 2013;132(1–2): 223–230. https://doi.org/10.1016/j.drugalcdep.2013.02.002

Pantoni MM, Anagnostaras SG. Cognitive effects of MDMA in laboratory animals: a systematic review focusing on dose. *Pharmacol Rev.* 2019;71(3):413–449. https://doi.org/10.1124/pr.118.017087

Papaseit E, Pérez-Mañá C, Torrens M, et al. MDMA interactions with pharmaceuticals and drugs of abuse. *Expert Opin Drug Metab Toxicol.* 2020;16(5):357–369. https://doi.org/10.1080/17425255.2020.1749262

Parrott AC. MDMA and 5-HT neurotoxicity: the empirical evidence for its adverse effects in humans—no need for translation. *Br J Pharmacol.* 2012a;166(5):1518–1520; discussion 1521–1522.

Parrott AC. MDMA and temperature: a review of the thermal effects of "Ecstasy" in humans. *Drug Alcohol Depend.* 2012b;121(1–2):1–9.

Parrott AC. MDMA, serotonergic neurotoxicity, and the diverse functional deficits of recreational 'Ecstasy' users. *Neurosci Biobehav Rev.* 2013;37(8):1466–1484. https://doi.org/10.1016/j.neubiorev.2013.04.016

Parrott AC. Human psychobiology of MDMA or "Ecstasy": an overview of 25 years of empirical research. *Hum Psychopharmacol.* 2013b;28(4):289–307.

Ranganathan M, Schnakenberg A, Skosnik PD, et al. Dose-related behavioral, subjective, endocrine, and psychophysiological effects of the kappa opioid agonist salvinorin A in humans. *Biol Psychiatry.* 2012;72:871–879.

Reissig CJ, Carter LP, Johnson MW, et al. High doses of dextromethorphan, an NMDA antagonist, produce effects similar to classic hallucinogens. *Psychopharmacology (Berl).* 2012;223(1):1–15.

Roberts CA, Fairclough SH, McGlone FP, et al. Electrophysiological evidence of atypical processing underlying mental set shifting in ecstasy polydrug and polydrug users. *Exp Clin Psychopharmacol.* 2013;21(6):507–515. https://doi.org/10.1037/a0034002

Ros-Simó C, Moscoso-Castro M, Ruiz-Medina J, et al. Memory impairment and hippocampus specific protein oxidation induced by ethanol intake and 3, 4-methylenedioxymethamphetamine (MDMA) in mice. *J Neurochem.* 2013;125(5):736–746. https://doi.org/10.1111/jnc.12247

Ross S. Serotonergic hallucinogens and emerging targets for addiction pharmacotherapies. *Psychiatr Clin North Am.* 2012;35(2):357–374.

Schultes RE, Hofmann A, Rätsch C. *Plants of the Gods: Their Sacred, Healing and Hallucinogenic Powers.* 2nd ed. Rochester, VT: Inner Traditions; 2001.

Shiroma PR, Velit-Salazar MR, Vorobyov Y. A systematic review of neurocognitive effects of subanesthetic doses of intravenous ketamine in major depressive disorder, post-traumatic stress disorder, and healthy population. *Clin Drug Investig.* 2022;42(7):549–566. https://doi.org/10.1007/s40261-022-01169-z

Singh JA. Epidemiology of hospitalizations with hallucinogen use disorder: a 17-year U.S. National study. *J Addict Dis.* 2021; 39(4):545–549. https://doi.org/10.1080/10550887.2021.1907503

Sloshower J, Skosnik PD, Safi-Aghdam H, et al. Psilocybin-assisted therapy for major depressive disorder: an exploratory placebo-controlled, fixed-order trial. *J Psychopharmacol.* 2023; 2698811231154852. https://doi.org/10.1177/02698811231154852

Stone AL, Storr CL, Anthony JC. Evidence for a hallucinogen dependence syndrome developing soon after onset of hallucinogen use during adolescence. *Int J Methods Psychiatr Res.* 2006;15(3):116–130.

Strassman R. *DMT: The Spirit Molecule.* Rochester, VT: Park Street Press; 2000.

Strassman RJ. *Human Hallucinogenic Drug Research: Regulatory, Clinical, and Scientific Issues.* NIDA research monograph. 1994; 146:92–123.

Studerus E, Kometer M, Hasler F, Vollenweider FX. Acute, subacute and long-term subjective effects of psilocybin in healthy humans: a pooled analysis of experimental studies. *J Psychopharmacol.* 2011;25(11):1434–1452.

Studerus E, Gamma A, Kometer M, Vollenweider FX. Prediction of psilocybin response in healthy volunteers. *PLoS One.* 2012; 7(2):e30800.

van Amsterdam J, Opperhuizen A, Koeter M, van den Brink W. Ranking the harm of alcohol, tobacco and illicit drugs for the individual and the population. *Eur Addict Res.* 2010;16(4):202–207.

van Amsterdam J, Opperhuizen A, van den Brink W. Harm potential of magic mushroom use: a review [Research Support, Non-U.S. Gov't, Review]. *Regul Toxicol Pharmacol.* 2011;59(3):423–429. https://doi.org/10.1016/j.yrtph.2011.01.006

van der Meer PB, Fuentes JJ, Kaptein AA, et al. Therapeutic effect of psilocybin in addiction: a systematic review. *Front Psychiatry.* 2023;14:1134454. https://doi.org/10.3389/fpsyt.2023.1134454

Vargas MV, Dunlap LE, Dong C, et al. Psychedelics promote neuroplasticity through the activation of intracellular 5-HT2A receptors. *Science.* 2023;379(6633):700–706. https://doi.org/10.1126/science.adf0435

Vogels N, Brunt TM, Rigter S, et al. Content of ecstasy in the Netherlands: 1993-2008. *Addiction.* 2009;104(12):2057–2066.

Walsh CA, Livne O, Shmulewitz D, et al. Use of plant-based hallucinogens and dissociative agents: U.S. Time Trends, 2002-2019. *Addict Behav Rep.* 2022;16:100454. https://doi.org/10.1016/j.abrep.2022.100454

Wang C, Zheng D, Xu J, et al. Brain damages in ketamine addicts as revealed by magnetic resonance imaging. *Front Neuroanat.* 2013;7:23.

Ward KC, Khattak HZ, Richardson L, et al. NMDA receptor antagonists distort visual grouping in rats performing a modified two-choice visual discrimination task. *Psychopharmacology (Berl).* 2013;229(4):627–637. https://doi.org/10.1007/s00213-013-3123-8

Wendel-Garcia PD, Erlebach R, Hofmaenner DA, et al. Long-term ketamine infusion-induced cholestatic liver injury in COVID-19-associated acute respiratory distress syndrome. *Crit Care.* 2022;26(1):148. https://doi.org/10.1186/s13054-022-04019-8

White C, Brown J, Edwards M. Altered visual perception in long-term ecstasy (MDMA) users. *Psychopharmacology (Berl).* 2013;229(1):155–165. https://doi.org/10.1007/s00213-013-3094-9

Wu LT, Pan JJ, Yang C, et al. An item response theory analysis of DSM-IV criteria for hallucinogen abuse and dependence in adolescents. *Addict Behav.* 2010a;35(3):273–277.

Wu LT, Pan JJ, Blazer DG, et al. Using a latent variable approach to inform gender and racial/ethnic differences in cocaine dependence: a National Drug Abuse Treatment Clinical Trials Network study. *J Subst Abuse Treat*. 2010b;38 Suppl 1:S70–S79.

Xu G, Wang Y, Chen Z, et al. Esketamine improves propofol-induced brain injury and cognitive impairment in rats. *Transl Neurosci*. 2022;13(1):430–439. https://doi.org/10.1515/tnsci-2022-0251

Young AH, Abdelghani M, Juruena MF, et al. Early clinical experiences of esketamine nasal spray in the UK in adults with treatment-resistant major depressive disorder: advisory panel recommendations. *Neuropsychiatr Dis Treat*. 2023;19:433–441. https://doi.org/10.2147/ndt.S388392

Zhang C, Xu Y, Zhang B, et al. Cognitive impairment in chronic ketamine abusers. *Psychiatry Res*. 2020;291:113206. https://doi.org/10.1016/j.psychres.2020.113206

Zhong J, Wu H, Wu F, et al. Cortical thickness changes in chronic ketamine users. *Front Psychiatry*. 2021;12:645471. https://doi.org/10.3389/fpsyt.2021.645471

Zimmermann J, Friedli N, Bavato F, et al. White matter alterations in chronic MDMA use: evidence from diffusion tensor imaging and neurofilament light chain blood levels. *Neuroimage Clin*. 2022;36:103191. https://doi.org/10.1016/j.nicl.2022.103191

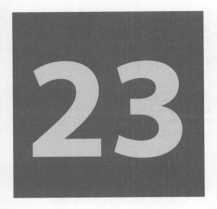

23 Gambling and Behavioral Addictions

Yvonne H. C. Yau, MSc
James W. B. Elsey, BSc
Marc N. Potenza, PhD, MD

The term "addiction" is derived from the Latin word *addicere*, meaning "bound to" or "enslaved by" (Potenza 2006). In its original formulation, addiction was not linked exclusively to substance-use behaviors. Several behaviors, besides psychoactive substance ingestion, may produce short-term reward that may engender persistent behavior despite knowledge of adverse consequences and may result in diminished control over the behaviors. Potential endophenotypes or underlying constructs such as aspects of motivation, reward processing, and decision making (Chambers et al. 2007; Redish et al. 2008; Goldstein et al. 2007) may be shared across a spectrum of substance- and non–substance-related addictive disorders. Aided by data from neurobiological studies, addiction professionals and the public are recognizing that certain nondrug behaviors warrant consideration as non-substance or "behavioral" addiction (Frascella et al. 2010; Karim & Chaudhri 2012). Behaviors such as gambling, Internet use, video-game play, sex, shopping, and eating may be addictive in nature (Holden 2010), with a minority of individuals thought to display habitual or compulsive engagement in these behaviors (Chambers et al. 2007; Karim & Chaudhri 2012).

Some of these potentially addictive behaviors were considered as "Impulse Control Disorders Not Elsewhere Classified" in the *Diagnostic and Statistical Manual of Mental Disorders*, 4th ed., Text Revision (DSM-IV-TR), and this category was distinct from that containing substance-use disorders (SUDs). Although the conceptualization of impulse-control disorders (ICDs) as addictions or obsessive–compulsive spectrum disorders are not mutually exclusive and data exist to support both conceptualizations, these frameworks have important clinical implications with respect to prevention and treatment strategies. An important departure from past diagnostic manuals is the renaming of the "Substance-Related Disorders" diagnostic category to "Substance-Related and Addictive Disorders" in the DSM-5. Pathological gambling (now termed gambling disorder [GD]) has been included in this category by the American Psychiatric Association in the DSM-5. This change reflects the increasing evidence that certain disorders resemble SUDs both behaviorally (e.g., involving diminished control, salience of behaviorally related cues) and neurobiologically (e.g., involving alterations in brain function, structure, and neurochemistry). Several other behavioral addictions were considered for inclusion; however, it was concluded that there is presently insufficient research to warrant their inclusion in the main section, although criteria for Internet gaming disorder (focusing on multiplayer online gaming) were included in Section III. This section, unlike the appendix of DSM-IV, contains diagnostic categories that require further research and ultimately aims to enhance our capacity to recognize and define the presence of these maladaptive behaviors as well as to promote further research.

More recently, the 11th revision of the International Classification of Diseases (ICD-11) included both GD and gaming disorder as "disorders due to addictive behaviors," formally designating both gambling as gaming as the focus of clinically diagnosable addictive disorders. However, other behaviors (e.g., shopping/buying, social media use) are not specifically identified as the focus of disorders in either the ICD-11 or DSM-5, despite high-level engagement in such behaviors being clinically concerning at times. As such, it has been proposed that the designation of "other specified disorders due to addictive behaviors" be considered as a diagnostic entity in such circumstances (Brand et al. 2022). Furthermore, compulsive sexual behavior disorder has been included as an ICD in the ICD-11 (Kraus et al. 2018), although hypersexual disorder was considered but excluded from DSM-5.

GD represents the most thoroughly investigated behavioral addiction; consequently, this chapter largely focuses on GD, the relationships of GD and SUDs, and the current treatment and prevention strategies for GD. We also review and discuss other behavioral addictions including "Internet addiction," problematic video-game playing, hypersexual disorder/compulsive sexual behavior disorder, compulsive shopping behavior, and food addiction that, despite having been less well studied, have been receiving attention from clinicians and researchers.

American Psychiatric Association. *Diagnostic and Statistical Manual of Mental Disorders*. 5th ed. Washington, DC: American Psychiatric Press; 2013.

Brand M, Rumpf HJ, Demetrovics Z, et al. Which conditions should be considered as disorders in the ICD-11 designation of "other specified disorders due to addictive behaviors"? *J Behav Addict*. 2022;11(2):150–159.

Brewer JA, Potenza MN. The neurobiology and genetics of impulse control disorders: relationships to drug addictions. *Biochem Pharmacol*. 2008;75(1):63–75.

Chambers RA, Bickel WK, Potenza MN. A scale-free systems theory of motivation and addiction. *Neurosci Biobehav Rev*. 2007;31(7):1017–1045.

Frascella J, Potenza MN, Brown LL, Childress AR. Shared brain vulnerabilities open the way for nonsubstance addictions: carving addiction at a new joint? *Ann N Y Acad Sci*. 2010;1187(1):294–315.

Goldstein RZ, Alia-Klein N, Tomasi D, et al. Is decreased prefrontal cortical sensitivity to monetary reward associated with impaired motivation and self-control in cocaine addiction? *Am J Psychiatry*. 2007;164(1):43–51.

Holden C. Behavioral addictions debut in proposed DSM-V. *Science*. 2010;327(5968):935.

Karim R, Chaudhri P. Behavioral addictions: an overview. *J Psychoactive Drugs*. 2012;44(1):5–17.

Kraus SW, Krueger RB, Briken P, et al. Compulsive sexual behaviour disorder in the ICD-11. *World Psychiatry*. 2018;17(1):109–110.

Potenza MN. Should addictive disorders include non-substance-related conditions? *Addiction*. 2006;101(1):142–151.

Redish AD, Jensen S, Johnson A. A unified framework for addiction: vulnerabilities in the decision process. *Behav Brain Sci*. 2008;31(4):415–437.

► General Considerations

A. Epidemiology

Gambling is a common recreational pastime, and community surveys from several countries indicate that most people have gambled in their lifetime and engage in at least occasional gambling. The U.S. National Comorbidity Survey Replication reported that 78.4% of adults reported lifetime gambling (Kessler et al. 2008). Lifetime at-risk/problem gambling (meeting at least one DSM-IV inclusionary criterion for GD) (2.3%) and GD (0.6%) were significant but much less common. Prevalence of GD is estimated to be as high as 1–3% in the United States as well as in other countries such as Australia, Canada, China, Norway, Sweden, Switzerland, Spain, and the United Kingdom (Sussman et al. 2011).

These prevalence estimates are elevated in certain demographic sectors. With respect to age, meta-analyses have consistently shown higher rates of GD among adolescents (0.8–13%) (Volberg et al. 2010) and college students (7.9–10.2%) (Blinn-Pike et al. 2007; Nowak & Aloe 2014).

The typical age for the development of problem gambling is thought to be in the 20s, with researchers estimating that approximately 75% of college students have gambled legally or illegally during the past year (Barnes et al. 2010). Moreover, individuals with GD typically report initiation of recreational gambling at a younger age than individuals with nonproblem gambling (Kessler et al. 2008)—a trend that is also evident in SUDs (Grant & Dawson 1998).

With respect to gender, much of the gambling literature suggests that males are more likely to gamble and have gambling problems (Wardle et al. 2011). For example, data from the U.S. National Comorbidity Survey Replication suggest that men were four times more likely than women to meet criteria for DSM-IV GD (Kessler et al. 2008). Males also account for a greater proportion of treatment-seeking cases (Petry 2002), although "telescoping"—the phenomenon whereby the time between initiation and problematic engagement in the addictive behavior is shorter in females than in males—has been observed in GD (as well as for SUDs) and is important to consider (Potenza et al. 2001). Prevalence surveys have shown that greater proportions of women are now gambling (Wardle et al. 2011). The recent British Gambling Prevalence Survey in 2010 found that although there had been a general increase in gambling engagement since the 2007 survey (from 68 to 73%), this increase was greater among women (from 65 to 71%) than men (from 71 to 75%) (British Gambling Commission 2010).

Although prevalence estimates of other behavioral addictions are less well studied, high preliminary prevalence estimates for Internet addiction (adolescents, 4.0–19.1%; adults, 0.7–18.3%) (Yau et al. 2012), problematic video-game playing (adolescents, 4.2–20.0%; adults 1.1–11.9%) (Yau et al. 2012), and hypersexual disorder (adult 5–6%) (Coleman et al. 2000; Schaffer & Zimmerman 1990) have been reported. However, given that these prevalence findings may be influenced by the lack of a common definition coupled with differences in assessment measures, estimates of prevalence are best considered preliminary.

Comorbidity—GD is a serious public and mental health concern, with implications for individual families and communities. GD is associated with impaired psychological functioning, reduced quality of life, legal problems, and high rates of bankruptcy, divorce, and incarceration (Grant & Kim 2005). Gambling problems are also associated with various mental health problems and disorders. Data from the U.S. National Comorbidity Survey Replication, a U.S.-based community survey, reported that 0.6% of respondents met criteria for lifetime GD (2.3% reported at least one core symptom), but of these, 96% met criteria for at least one other lifetime diagnosis and 49% had been treated for another mental illness (Kessler et al. 2008).

Existing epidemiology data support a relationship between GD and SUDs, with a recent meta-analysis suggesting a mean co-occurrence of 57.5% (Lorains et al. 2011). In particular, the highest rates of co-occurrence are typically observed between gambling and alcohol use (Cunningham-Williams et al. 1998). Among individuals with SUDs, the risk of moderate- to high-severity gambling was roughly threefold higher (El-Guebaly et al. 2006). A Canadian epidemiological survey estimated that the relative risk for alcohol-use problems increased roughly fourfold when disordered gambling (a term used to describe the full range of gambling problems, which includes disordered and subclinical gambling) was present (Bland et al. 1993). Moreover, data from the National Epidemiological Survey on Alcohol and Related Conditions (NESARC) suggest that rates of alcohol- and nicotine-use disorders are positively associated with problem-gambling severity (Morasco et al. 2006). Clinical samples of other behavioral addictions suggest that co-occurrence with SUDs is common (Yau et al. 2014). For example, in a study of 2453 college students, individuals meeting the criteria for Internet addiction were roughly twice as likely to report harmful alcohol use, after controlling for gender, age, and depression (Yen et al. 2009). Taken together, these findings suggest that behavioral addictions may share a common pathophysiology with SUDs.

Behavioral addictions frequently co-occur not only with SUDS but also with various psychiatric conditions including impulse-control, mood, and personality disorders (Brewer & Potenza 2008; Dowling & Brown 2010; Mazhari 2012). The linkage between GD and obsessive–compulsive disorder (OCD) has been debated following the proposal that GD and other behavioral addictions may lie on an impulsive–compulsive spectrum (McElroy et al. 1994). At the present time, comorbidity data do not clearly support a close relationship. The St. Louis Epidemiological Catchment Area study, which assessed many co-occurring conditions, found no significant relationship between GD and OCD (Cunningham-Williams et al. 1998). In contrast, other disorders (e.g., SUDs, affective and psychotic disorders) were found to be elevated among individuals with GD. In a separate study, attention-deficit/hyperactivity disorder (ADHD) was elevated in people with gambling problems, and longitudinal work has shown that persistent ADHD symptoms in childhood and adolescence statistically predicted gambling problems later in life (Breyer et al. 2009). Together, these data suggest that GD shares substantial co-occurrence with other mental health problems, particularly those characterized by impulsivity.

B. Etiology

GD may be a more complex and unstable disorder (LaPlante et al. 2008) than originally and traditionally thought (DSM-IV-TR; National Gambling Impact Study Commission 2010). As with most addictive disorders, the majority of those who experience disordered gambling do not develop addiction after their initial gambling experience. Contrary to predictions derived from the traditional exposure model

(i.e., exposure to gambling opportunities is sufficient to stimulate the development of GD) (Kindt 1993), gambling escalates—sometimes rapidly and other times slowly—as individuals may develop neuroadaptations (e.g., withdrawal and tolerance) (LaPlante et al. 2008). In addition to physical signs and symptoms, individuals with GD typically experience negative psychosocial consequences (e.g., debt, guilt, or depression). Recreational gambling may transition to disordered gambling when individuals persist in gambling behaviors despite adverse consequences, exhibit diminished control over gambling behaviors, and crave and desire opportunities to gamble.

Barnes GM, Welte JW, Hoffman JH, Tidwell MC. Comparisons of gambling and alcohol use among college students and noncollege young people in the United States. *J Am Coll Health*. 2010;58(5):443–452.

Bland RC, Newman SC, Orn H, Stebelsky G. Epidemiology of pathological gambling in Edmonton. *Can J Psychiatry*. 1993; 38(2):108–112.

Blinn-Pike L, Worthy SL, Jonkman JN. Disordered gambling among college students: a meta-analytic synthesis. *J Gambl Stud*. 2007;23(2):175–83.

Brewer JA, Potenza MN. The neurobiology and genetics of impulse control disorders: relationships to drug addictions. *Biochem Pharmacol*. 2008;75(1):63–75.

Breyer JL, Botzet AM, Winters KC, et al. Young adult gambling behaviors and their relationship with the persistence of ADHD. *J Gambl Stud*. 2009;25(2):227–238.

British Gambling Commission. British Gambling Prevalence Survey 2010. http://www.gamblingcommission.gov.uk/PDF/British%20 Gambling%20Prevalence%20Survey%202010.pdf;2010

Coleman E, Gratzer T, Nesvacil L, Raymond NC. Nefazodone and the treatment of nonparaphilic compulsive sexual behavior: a retrospective study. *J Clin Psychiatry*. 2000;61(4):282–284

Cunningham-Williams RM, Cottler LB, Compton WM 3rd, Spitznagel EL. Taking chances: problem gamblers and mental health disorders—results from the St. Louis Epidemiologic Catchment Area Study. *Am J Public Health*. 1998;88(7):1093–1096.

Dowling NA, Brown M. Commonalities in the psychological factors associated with problem gambling and Internet dependence. *Cyberpsychol Behav Soc Netw*. 2010;13(4):437–441.

El-Guebaly N, Patten SB, Currie S, et al. Epidemiological associations between gambling behavior, substance use & mood and anxiety disorders. *J Gambl Stud*. 2006;22(3):275–287.

Grant BF, Dawson DA. Age of onset of drug use and its association with DSM-IV drug abuse and dependence: results from the National Longitudinal Alcohol Epidemiologic Survey. *J Subst Abuse*. 1998;10(2):163–173.

Grant JE, Kim SW. Quality of life in kleptomania and pathological gambling. *Compr Psychiatry*. 2005;46(1):34–37.

Kessler RC, Hwang I, LaBrie R, et al. DSM-IV pathological gambling in the National Comorbidity Survey Replication. *Psychol Med*. 2008;38(9):1351–1360.

Kindt JW. The economic impacts of legalized gambling activities. *Drake L Rev*. 1993;43:51.

LaPlante DA, Nelson SE, LaBrie R, Shaffer HJ. Stability and progression of disordered gambling: lessons from longitudinal studies. *Can J Psychiatry*. 2008;53:52–60.

Lorains FK, Cowlishaw S, Thomas SA. Prevalence of comorbid disorders in problem and pathological gambling: systematic review and meta-analysis of population surveys. *Addiction*. 2011; 106(3):490–498.

Mazhari S. Association between problematic Internet use and impulse control disorders among Iranian university students. *Cyberpsychol Behav Soc Netw*. 2012;15(5):270–273.

McElroy SL, Phillips KA, Keck PE Jr. Obsessive compulsive spectrum disorder. *J Clin Psychiatry*. 1994;55 Suppl:33–51; discussion 2–3.

Morasco BJ, Pietrzak RH, Blanco C, et al. Health problems and medical utilization associated with gambling disorders: results from the National Epidemiological Survey on Alcohol and Related Conditions. *Psychosom Med*. 2006;68:976–984.

National Gambling Impact Study Commission. What is problem gambling? 2010. http://www.ncpgambling.org/i4a/pages/index.cfm?pageid=1.

Nowak DE, Aloe AM. The prevalence of pathological gambling among college students: a meta-analytic synthesis, 2005–2013. *J Gambl Stud*. 2014;30:819–843.

Petry NM. A comparison of young, middle-aged, and older adult treatment-seeking pathological gamblers. *Gerontologist*. 2002;42(1):92–99.

Potenza MN, Steinberg MA, McLaughlin SD, et al. Gender-related differences in the characteristics of problem gamblers using a gambling helpline. *Am J Psychiatry*. 2001;158(9):1500–1505.

Schaffer SD, Zimmerman ML. The sexual addict: a challenge for the primary care provider. *Nurse Pract*. 1990;15(6):25–26, 28, 33.

Sussman S, Lisha N, Griffiths M. Prevalence of the addictions: a problem of the majority or the minority? *Eval Health Prof*. 2011;34(1):3–56.

Volberg RA, Gupta R, Griffiths MD. An international perspective on youth gambling prevalence studies. *Int J Adolesc Med Health*. 2010;22(1):3–38.

Wardle H, Moody A, Griffiths M, et al. Defining the online gambler and patterns of behaviour integration: evidence from the British Gambling Prevalence Survey 2010. *Int Gambl Stud*. 2011;11(3):339–356.

Yau Y, Yip S, Potenza MN. Understanding "behavioral addictions": insights from research. In: Fiellin DA, Miller SC, Saitz R, eds. *Principles of Addiction Medicine*. 5th ed. Philadelphia: Lippincott Williams & Wilkins; 2014:55–83.

Yau YHC, Crowley MJ, Mayes LC, Potenza MN. Are Internet use and video-game-playing addictive behaviors? Biological, clinical and public health implications for youths and adults. *Minerva Psichiatr*. 2012;53:153–170.

Yen J-Y, Ko C-H, Yen C-F, et al. The association between harmful alcohol use and Internet addiction among college students: comparison of personality. *Psychiatry Clin Neurosci*. 2009;63(2):218–224.

▶ Clinical Findings

A. Signs and Symptoms

A core feature of behavioral addictions is a failure to resist an impulse, drive, or craving to perform an act that is harmful to oneself or to others (DSM-5). Each behavioral addiction is characterized by a recurrent pattern of a certain behavior; extended and repetitive engagement in this behavior ultimately interferes with functioning. Symptoms typically include an increasing sense of tension or arousal before committing the act and subsequent experiences of pleasure, gratification, or relief at the time of committing the act (DSM-5). In this respect, the ego-syntonic nature of these behaviors is similar to the experience of substance-use behaviors. This contrasts with the ego-dystonic nature of OCD. However, both behavioral and substance addictions may become less ego-syntonic and more ego-dystonic over time, as the behavior itself becomes less pleasurable, more of a habit or compulsion, and motivated less by positive reinforcement (e.g., rewarding effects of the behavior) and more by negative reinforcement (e.g., relief of dysphoria or withdrawal).

B. Personality

Individuals with behavioral addictions may share similar personality profiles to those with SUDs. Individuals with behavioral and substance addictions both score high on self-report measures of impulsivity and sensation-seeking and generally low on measures of harm avoidance (Leeman & Potenza 2012; Verdejo-Garcia et al. 2008). As with SUDs, it has been hypothesized that a shift from impulsive (often entailing rash action in pursuit of reward) to compulsive (i.e., action taken with diminished regard for reward) behavior may take place with GD and SUDs (Brewer & Potenza 2008). However, there also exist data that individuals with Internet addiction, gaming disorder, or GD may exhibit high levels of harm avoidance (Tavares et al. 2005; Yau et al. 2014). The extent to which behavioral tendencies such as harm avoidance may shift (e.g., over time) or differ (e.g., according to geographic region or other factors) warrants additional research.

C. Neurocognition

Behavioral and substance addictions may share common cognitive features. For example, both individuals with GD and individuals with histories of alcohol-use disorder had impaired performance on neurocognitive tasks involving inhibition, time estimation, cognitive estimation, and planning tasks in comparison to healthy comparison subjects and to individuals with Tourette syndrome, who only had an impaired performance on inhibition tasks (Goudriaan et al. 2006). Neurocognitive measures of disinhibition and decision making are also positively associated with problem-gambling severity (Odlaug et al. 2011) and may predict the relapse of GD (Goudriaan et al. 2008). Both individuals with GD and those with alcohol-use disorder display alterations in risky decision making and reflection impulsivity in comparison to matched comparison subjects (Lawrence et al. 2009). Individuals with GD display impaired performance on the Iowa Gambling Task (IGT), a task involving risk/reward decision making (Bechara 2003; Goudriaan et al. 2005). In contrast, a study of individuals with Internet addiction demonstrated no such deficits in decision making on the IGT (Ko et al. 2010).

D. Neurochemistry

Multiple neurotransmitter systems (e.g., serotonergic, dopaminergic, opioidergic, noradrenergic) have been implicated in the pathophysiology of behavioral addictions and SUDs (Koob & Volkow 2010; Yau et al. 2014). Dysregulated dopamine systems, which are involved with learning, motivation, and salience of stimuli and rewards, have been frequently implicated in studies of addiction (Heinz et al. 2004), although dopaminergic findings for behavioral addictions have presented a complicated picture. Using positron emission tomography (PET) with the tracer [^{11}C]raclopride, a study reported that not only did people with GD perform worse on the IGT than controls, but among those with GD, dopamine release in the ventral striatum (a key component of the "reward pathway") was positively associated with excitement levels (Linnet et al. 2011a). Although there were no differences in the magnitude of dopamine release between individuals with GD and controls during a slot machine gambling task, among those with GD, dopamine release correlated positively with problem-gambling severity (Joutsa et al. 2012). Increased dopamine levels may serve a "double deficit" function by reinforcing GD behavior through increasing excitement levels while simultaneously reducing inhibition of risky decisions. D_2/D_3 receptor availability has also been shown to negatively correlate with mood-related impulsivity ("urgency") within the striatum (Clark et al. 2012) and positively correlate with problem-gambling severity within the dorsal striatum (Boileau et al. 2013) among individuals with GD. Similar to findings in substance addiction literature (Volkow et al. 2001), studies using [^{11}C]raclopride (PET) scanning have reported reductions in dopamine D_2-like receptor availability in the striatum among individuals with Internet addiction (Kim et al. 2011), and obese individuals (Wang et al. 2009) and mice (Geiger et al. 2008; Huang et al. 2006). Alsiö, Olszewski, and Norbäck (2010) found that rats fed a high-fat (vs. unrestricted) diet showed decreased expression of D_1 and D_2 receptors in the ventral tegmental area (VTA), nucleus accumbens (NAc), and prefrontal cortex (PFC) following an 18-day withdrawal. However, in contrast to results from SUDs (Dalley et al. 2007), no significant difference in D_2/D_3 receptor availability at resting state was observed between GD and control subjects (Boileu et al. 2013; Clark et al. 2012; Linnet et al. 2011a). Taken together, these data (which should be considered preliminary given the small samples involved in each study) suggest a possible role for dopamine in GD, although the nature of the relationship remains unclear.

Studies have also implicated serotonin systems—thought to be involved in behavioral control and inhibition of behavior—in behavioral addictions. Serotonin neurons project from the raphe nucleus of the brainstem to multiple brain regions including the hippocampus, amygdala, and PFC that together support a variety of functions including emotion, motivation, and decision making. It has been hypothesized that dysregulated serotonin functioning may mediate behavioral inhibition and impulsivity in GD (Brewer & Potenza 2008; Linnet et al. 2011a, 2011b). Low cerebral spinal fluid (CSF) levels of the 5-HT metabolite 5-hydroxyindoleacetic acid (5-HIAA) have been reported in individuals with GD (Norden & Eklundh 1999). Evidence from preclinical research suggests a correlation between risk-taking behaviors and lowered CSF levels of 5-HIAA in monkeys (Cardinal 2006) and rats (Ettenberg et al. 2011). Moreover, low levels of platelet monoamine oxidase (MAO) activity, considered a peripheral marker of serotonin activity, have been reported among males with GD (Ibanez et al. 2000; Pérez de Castro et al. 2002). Like that observed among individuals with alcohol or cocaine-use disorders (Moss et al. 2007; Patkar et al. 2006), acute administration of sumatriptan (a selective serotonin 1B receptor agonist) to individuals with GD resulted in blunted growth hormone response, suggesting downregulation of these receptors (Pallanti et al. 2010a).

Other neurotransmitter systems may also contribute to GD, although less is known about their integrity. Dysregulated hypothalamic–pituitary–adrenal axis and increased levels of noradrenergic metabolites have been observed in GD (Meyer et al. 2004). Adrenergic drugs influence specific aspects of impulse control in animal and human studies (Chamberlain & Sahakian 2007), suggesting an avenue of intervention. Noradrenaline may be involved in peripheral arousal associated with gambling, although the direction of effect is currently unclear (Elman et al. 2012; Pallanti et al. 2010b). Opioidergic systems have also been implicated in GD. Opioid antagonists (e.g., naltrexone and nalmefene) have demonstrated superiority over placebo in multiple randomized clinical trials (Bullock & Potenza 2012; Grant et al. 2010a; Kim et al. 2001).

E. Neuroimaging

Neuroimaging studies suggest shared neurocircuitry (particularly involving frontal and striatal regions) between behavioral and substance addictions. Functional magnetic resonance imaging (fMRI) studies during cognitive tasks have implicated frontal areas; investigations have observed differences in ventromedial prefrontal cortex (vmPFC) function in GD (Potenza et al. 2003a). Diminished activity of the vmPFC has been associated with reward processing, simulated gambling, and decision making in GD (Balodis et al. 2012; Choi et al. 2012; Reuter et al. 2005; Tanabe et al. 2007). Seemingly contradictory findings have also been reported. A recent fMRI study reported greater frontal lobe and basal ganglia activation, particularly in the vmPFC, caudate, and amygdala, during high-risk gambling decisions during the IGT (Power et al. 2012). Differences in findings across studies may relate to the specific tasks used, populations studied, or other factors. Cue-induction studies have also reported both relatively decreased (Potenza et al. 2003b) and increased (Crockford et al. 2005; Goudriaan et al. 2010) vmPFC activity has been reported for

GD (vs. control) in response to gambling stimuli. Similarly, game cue–associated brain activation in individuals with online gaming problems occurs in the same brain regions (orbitofrontal, dorsolateral prefrontal, anterior cingulate, NAc) as with drug cue–associated brain activation in individuals with substance dependence (Ko et al. 2009). In response to anticipated receipt of food, activation in the medial orbitofrontal cortex, anterior cingulate, and amygdala was positively correlated with food addiction scores (Gearhardt et al. 2011). Taken together, dysfunction in frontal areas appears to contribute to behavioral addictions, although the precise nature of the dysfunction warrants additional study.

Brain imaging research also implicates the dopaminergic mesolimbic pathway (commonly known as the "reward pathway") from the VTA to the NAc in behavioral and substance addiction. Decreased ventral striatal activation to impulsive decision making in risk–reward assessment (Balodis et al. 2012) and during simulated gambling (Reuter et al. 2005) has been reported in GD. In gambling cue-exposure tasks, subjects with GD exhibited decreased activation in the ventral (Potenza 2008) and dorsal (de Greck et al. 2010) striatum compared to non-GD subjects. A recent fMRI study found stronger NAc activity among people with compulsive shopping (vs. controls) during the initial product presentation phase of a multiphase purchasing task (Raab et al. 2011). These findings implicating ventral striatal function (either increased or decreased) during reward anticipation in behavioral addictions are reminiscent of findings from substance addictions (Hommer et al. 2011; Wrase et al. 2007). Moreover, both ventral striatal and vmPFC activity were inversely correlated with severity of problem-gambling severity in GD subjects, such that greater severity was associated with lower ventral striatal and vmPFC activity during simulated gambling (Reuter et al. 2005).

Neuroanatomical alterations may also exist in behavioral addictions. Diffusion tensor imaging findings suggest reduced fractional anisotropy (FA) values—indicating reduced white-matter integrity—in regions including the corpus callosum in GD compared to control subjects (Joutsa et al. 2011; Yip et al. 2013). Research regarding widespread reduction of FA in major white-matter pathways and abnormal white-matter structure has yielded both positive (Lin et al. 2012) and negative results (Yuan et al. 2011) for Internet addiction. Despite hypothesized inferior frontal white-matter disorganization (i.e., low FA and high mean diffusivity), no difference between individuals with and without hypersexual disorder was noted (Miner et al. 2009). Taken together, these data suggest involvement of white-matter microstructures in the pathophysiology of some behavioral addictions, although the precise relationship warrants further research.

F. Family History and Genetics

Small family studies of probands with GD (Black et al. 2006), hypersexual disorder (Schneider & Schneider 1996), and compulsive-shopping behavior (McElroy et al. 1994) have found that first-degree relatives of the probands had significantly higher lifetime rates of SUDs, depression, and other psychiatric disorders. These findings support the view that behavioral addictions may have a genetic relationship to SUDs and other disorders.

Like those from substance addictions (Kreek et al. 2005), data from the Vietnam Era Twin Registry estimate the heritability of GD to be 50–60% (Lobo & Kennedy 2009; Shah et al. 2005). Twin studies suggest that genetic factors may contribute more than environmental factors to the overall variance of risk for developing of GD (Blanco et al. 2012; Slutske et al. 2010).

There are currently few molecular genetic studies of behavioral addictions. Genetic polymorphisms putatively related to dopamine transmission (e.g., *DRD2* Taq1A1, which is in linkage with *Ankk1*, which appears to relate more closely to SUDs than does TaqA1 in some studies) have been associated with GD (Comings et al. 1996; Lobo et al. 2010) as well as problematic video-game playing (Han et al. 2007). Genetic polymorphisms related to serotonin transmission (e.g., *5HTTLPR* and *MAO-A*) have also been associated with GD (Ibanez et al. 2000; Pérez de Castro et al. 1999) and Internet addiction disorder (Lee et al. 2008). These genes may have addictive effects (Comings et al. 2001). However, genetic studies are best considered preliminary given the small sample sizes and lack of consideration of potential influences related to race/ethnicity in multiple studies; replication of candidate gene studies using alternate designs is needed. Small genome-wide association studies for GD have been performed, but no single-nucleotide polymorphism reached genome-wide significance (Lang et al. 2016; Lind et al. 2013).

G. Course of Illness

Repeated failed attempts to control gambling are a diagnostic feature of GD and suggest that it may be a chronic, relapsing disorder. However, more recent data are challenging this notion and indicate more variability in the trajectories of gambling problems (LaPlante et al. 2008; Potenza 2006; Slutske 2006). Data from the NESARC indicate that among individuals with a lifetime history of GD, 36–39% did not experience any gambling-related problems in the past year despite only 7–12% having received treatment for gambling problems (Slutske 2006). Results from a longitudinal study suggest that young adults frequently move in and out of gambling problems (Slutske et al. 2003). Vitaro and colleagues (2001) have found that gambling participation at age 16 was a better predictor of gambling problems 1 year later than disordered gambling itself at age 16; moreover, only in individuals with high levels of disinhibition did stability of gambling problems resemble the moderate stabilities of other problem behaviors, suggesting that other risk factors may explain observed lagged links between gambling participation and gambling problems (Wanner et al. 2009).

A meta-analysis of five longitudinal studies did not find evidence for the persistence of several gambling problems or that mild disordered gamblers were more at risk of progression to GD than people with nonproblem gambling (LaPlante et al. 2008). More prospective studies are needed to fully understand the natural course of GD and other behavioral addictions.

▶ Differential Diagnosis

Gambling and GD represent heterogeneous entities. Psychological processes may relate differently to specific forms of gambling, and specific forms of gambling may appeal more to certain individuals than to others. One important distinction within the varieties of gambling is between nonstrategic (e.g., lottery, slot machines) and strategic (e.g., blackjack, poker, and sports betting) forms of gambling. Other parameters that vary between forms of gambling and may relate to addictive potential include wager size (e.g., often relatively small in slot machines, potentially very large in poker), the jackpot/winning size (e.g., often modest in slot machine, large in lottery), the delay between wager and outcome (e.g., short for many forms of casino gambling and instant [scratch] lotteries, typically longer for sport betting and traditional lotteries), and the potential for continuous play (e.g., "double or nothing" in poker, one-off for lotteries). Short delays between wager and outcome and the potential for continuous play may relate to greater problem-gambling severity and a more rapid onset of gambling problems (Breen & Zimmerman 2002; Morgan et al. 1996). However, other studies have failed to support these findings, suggesting that the highest risks of disordered gambling may be associated with casino gambling, card gambling, and sports betting (LaPlante et al. 2011; Welte et al. 2009).

Other behavioral addictions also represent heterogeneous constructs. For example, individuals with problematic video-game playing may be addicted to certain genres of game play (e.g., massive multiplayer online role playing, puzzle and strategy, action) that may differ on a range of dimensions and engage different cognitive, behavioral, and affective systems.

As previously discussed, individuals with versus without GD are more likely to exhibit non-GD psychiatric disorders (e.g., mood, anxiety, substance-use, and personality disorders) (Kessler et al. 2008; Petry et al. 2005). Individuals with a diagnosis of GD may experience distinctive subclinical symptom patterns that are associated with symptom clusters often related to other diagnostic categories. For example, individuals with GD and co-occurring depression may be predisposed to emotional vulnerability, whereas individuals with co-occurring ADHD may be predisposed to impulsive tendencies. However, clinicians may fail to attend to behavioral addictions when in the presence of treating these psychiatric disorders. For example, none of the participants from a nation-wide study, U.S. National Comorbidity Survey Replication (Kessler & Merikangas 2004), with a GD diagnosis

received treatment for gambling problems; however, 49% were treated for other mental disorders (Kessler et al. 2008). By identifying and addressing behavioral addictions as well as associated clinical and subclinical syndromes, clinicians and health professionals might be better able to treat the needs of their patients and, in turn, improve clinical outcomes.

Alsiö J, Olszewski PK, Norbäck AH, et al. Dopamine D1 receptor gene expression decreases in the nucleus accumbens upon long-term exposure to palatable food and differs depending on diet-induced obesity phenotype in rats. *Neuroscience*. 2010; 171(3):779–787.

Balodis IM, Kober H, Worhunsky PD, et al. Diminished frontostriatal activity during processing of monetary rewards and losses in pathological gambling. *Biol Psychiatry*. 2012;71: 749–757.

Bechara A. Risky business: emotion, decision-making, and addiction. *J Gambl Stud*. 2003;19(1):23–51.

Black DW, Monahan PO, Temkit MH, Shaw M. A family study of pathological gambling. *Psychiatry Res*. 2006;141(3):295–303.

Blanco C, Myers J, Kendler KS. Gambling, disordered gambling and their association with major depression and substance use: a web-based cohort and twin-sibling study. *Psychol Med*. 2012; 42(3):497–508.

Boileau I, Payer D, Chugani B, et al. The D2/3 dopamine receptor in pathological gambling: a positron emission tomography study with [^{11}C]-(+)-propyl-hexahydro-naphtho-oxazin and [^{11}C] raclopride. *Addiction*. 2013;108:953–963.

Breen RB, Zimmerman M. Rapid onset of pathological gambling in machine gamblers. *J Gambl Stud*. 2002;18(1):31–43.

Brewer JA, Potenza MN. The neurobiology and genetics of impulse control disorders: relationships to drug addictions. *Biochem Pharmacol*. 2008;75(1):63–75.

Bullock SA, Potenza MN. Pathological gambling: neuropsychopharmacology and treatment. *Curr Psychopharmacol*. 2012;1(1):67–85.

Cardinal RN. Neural systems implicated in delayed and probabilistic reinforcement. *Neural Netw*. 2006;19(8):1277–1301.

Chamberlain SR, Sahakian BJ. The neuropsychiatry of impulsivity. *Curr Opin Psychiatry*. 2007;20(3):255–261.

Choi J-S, Shin Y-C, Jung WH, et al. Altered brain activity during reward anticipation in pathological gambling and obsessive-compulsive disorder. *PLoS One*. 2012;7(9):e45938.

Clark L, Stokes PR, Wu K, et al. Striatal dopamine D2/D3 receptor binding in pathological gambling is correlated with mood-related impulsivity. *NeuroImage*. 2012;63(1):40–46.

Comings DE, Gade-Andavolu R, Gonzalez N, et al. The additive effect of neurotransmitter genes in pathological gambling. *Clin Genet*. 2001;60(2):107–116.

Comings DE, Rosenthal RJ, Lesieur HR, et al. A study of the dopamine D2 receptor gene in pathological gambling. *Pharmacogenetics*. 1996;6(3):223–234.

Crockford DN, Goodyear B, Edwards J, et al. Cue-induced brain activity in pathological gamblers. *Biol Psychiatry*. 2005;58(10): 787–795.

Dalley JW, Fryer TD, Brichard L, et al. Nucleus accumbens D2/3 receptors predict trait impulsivity and cocaine reinforcement. *Science*. 2007;315(5816):1267–1270.

de Greck M, Enzi B, Prösch U, et al. Decreased neuronal activity in reward circuitry of pathological gamblers during processing of personal relevant stimuli. *Hum Brain Mapp.* 2010;31(11):1802–1812.

Elman I, Becerra L, Tschibelu E, et al. Yohimbine-induced amygdala activation in pathological gamblers: a pilot study. *PLoS One.* 2012;7(2):e31118.

Ettenberg A, Ofer OA, Mueller CL, et al. Inactivation of the dorsal raphé nucleus reduces the anxiogenic response of rats running an alley for intravenous cocaine. *Pharmacol Biochem Behav.* 2011;97(4):632–639.

Gearhardt AN, Yokum S, Orr PT, et al. Neural correlates of food addiction. *Arch Gen Psychiatry.* 2011;68(8):808–816.

Geiger BM, Behr GG, Frank LE, et al. Evidence for defective mesolimbic dopamine exocytosis in obesity-prone rats. *FASEB J.* 2008;22(8):2740–2746.

Goudriaan AE, De Ruiter MB, Van Den Brink W, et al. Brain activation patterns associated with cue reactivity and craving in abstinent problem gamblers, heavy smokers and healthy controls: an fMRI study. *Addict Biol.* 2010;15(4):491–503.

Goudriaan AE, Oosterlaan J, de Beurs E, van den Brink W. Decision making in pathological gambling: a comparison between pathological gamblers, alcohol dependents, persons with Tourette syndrome, and normal controls. *Cogn Brain Res.* 2005;23(1):137–151.

Goudriaan AE, Oosterlaan J, De Beurs E, Van Den Brink W. Neurocognitive functions in pathological gambling: a comparison with alcohol dependence, Tourette syndrome and normal controls. *Addiction.* 2006;101(4):534–547.

Goudriaan AE, Oosterlaan J, De Beurs E, Van den Brink W. The role of self-reported impulsivity and reward sensitivity versus neurocognitive measures of disinhibition and decision-making in the prediction of relapse in pathological gamblers. *Psychol Med.* 2008;38:41–50.

Grant JE, Odlaug BL, Potenza MN, et al. Nalmefene in the treatment of pathological gambling: multicentre, double-blind, placebo-controlled study. *Br J Psychiatry.* 2010a;197(4):330–331.

Han DH, Lee YS, Yang KC, et al. Dopamine genes and reward dependence in adolescents with excessive Internet video game play. *J Addict Med.* 2007;1(3):133–138.

Heinz A, Siessmeier T, Wrase J, et al. Correlation between dopamine D2 receptors in the ventral striatum and central processing of alcohol cues and craving. *Am J Psychiatry.* 2004;161(10):1783–1789.

Hommer DW, Bjork JM, Gilman JM. Imaging brain response to reward in addictive disorders. *Ann N Y Acad Sci.* 2011;1216(1):50–61.

Huang XF, Zavitsanou K, Huang X, et al. Dopamine transporter and D2 receptor binding densities in mice prone or resistant to chronic high fat diet-induced obesity. *Behav Brain Res.* 2006;175(2):415–419.

Ibanez A, Pérez de Castro I, Fernandez-Piqueras J, et al. Pathological gambling and DNA polymorphic markers at MAO-A and MAO-B genes. *Mol Psychiatry.* 2000;5(1):105–109.

Joutsa J, Johansson J, Niemelä S, et al. Mesolimbic dopamine release is linked to symptom severity in pathological gambling. *NeuroImage.* 2012;60(4):1992–1999.

Joutsa J, Saunavaara J, Parkkola R, et al. Extensive abnormality of brain white matter integrity in pathological gambling. *Psychiatry Res Neuroimaging.* 2011;194(3):340–346.

Kessler RC, Hwang I, LaBrie R, et al. DSM-IV pathological gambling in the National Comorbidity Survey Replication. *Psychol Med.* 2008;38(9):1351–1360.

Kessler RC, Merikangas KR. The National Comorbidity Survey Replication (NCS-R): background and aims. *Int J Methods Psychiatr Res.* 2004;13(2):60–68.

Kim SH, Baik S-H, Park CS, et al. Reduced striatal dopamine D2 receptors in people with Internet addiction. *NeuroReport.* 2011;22(8):407–411.

Kim SW, Grant JE, Adson DE, Shin YC. Double-blind naltrexone and placebo comparison study in the treatment of pathological gambling. *Biol Psychiatry.* 2001;49(11):914–921.

Ko CH, Hsiao S, Liu GC, et al. The characteristics of decision making, potential to take risks, and personality of college students with Internet addiction. *Psychiatry Res.* 2010;175(1–2):121–125.

Ko C-H, Liu G-C, Hsiao S, et al. Brain activities associated with gaming urge of online gaming addiction. *J Psychiatr Res.* 2009;43(7):739–747.

Koob GF, Volkow ND. Neurocircuitry of addiction. *Neuropsychopharmacology.* 2010;35(1):217–238.

Kreek MJ, Nielsen DA, Butelman ER, LaForge KS. Genetic influences on impulsivity, risk taking, stress responsivity and vulnerability to drug abuse and addiction. *Nat Neurosci.* 2005;8(11):1450–1457.

Lang M, Leménager T, Streit F, et al. Genome-wide association study of pathological gambling. 2016;36:38–46.

LaPlante DA, Nelson SE, LaBrie R, Shaffer HJ. Stability and progression of disordered gambling: lessons from longitudinal studies. *Can J Psychiatry.* 2008;53:52–60.

LaPlante DA, Nelson SE, LaBrie RA, Shaffer HJ. Disordered gambling, type of gambling and gambling involvement in the British Gambling Prevalence Survey 2007. *Eur J Public Health.* 2011;21(4):532–537.

Lawrence A, Luty J, Bogdan N, et al. Problem gamblers share deficits in impulsive decision-making with alcohol-dependent individuals. *Addiction.* 2009;104(6):1006–1015.

Lee YS, Han D, Yang KC, et al. Depression like characteristics of 5HTTLPR polymorphism and temperament in excessive Internet users. *J Affect Disord.* 2008;109:165–169.

Leeman RF, Potenza MN. Similarities and differences between pathological gambling and substance use disorders: a focus on impulsivity and compulsivity. *Psychopharmacology.* 2012;219(2):469–490.

Lin F, Zhou Y, Du Y, et al. Abnormal white matter integrity in adolescents with Internet addiction disorder: a tract-based spatial statistics study. *PLoS One.* 2012;7(1):e30253.

Lind PA, Zhu G, Montgomery GW, et al. Genome-wide association study of a quantitative disordered gambling trait. *Addict Biol.* 2013;18:511–522.

Linnet J, Møller A, Peterson E, et al. Dopamine release in ventral striatum during Iowa Gambling Task performance is associated with increased excitement levels in pathological gambling. *Addiction.* 2011a;106(2):383–390.

Linnet J, Moller A, Peterson E, et al. Inverse association between dopaminergic neurotransmission and Iowa Gambling Task performance in pathological gamblers and healthy controls. *Scand J Psychol.* 2011b;52(1):28–34.

Lobo DS, Kennedy JL. Genetic aspects of pathological gambling: a complex disorder with shared genetic vulnerabilities. *Addiction.* 2009;104(9):1454–1465.

Lobo DSS, Souza RP, Tong RP, et al. Association of functional variants in the dopamine D2-like receptors with risk for gambling behaviour in healthy Caucasian subjects. *Biol Psychol.* 2010;85(1):33–37.

McElroy SL, Keck PE Jr, Pope HG Jr, et al. Compulsive buying: a report of 20 cases. *J Clin Psychiatry.* 1994;55(6):242–248.

Meyer G, Schwertfeger J, Exton MS, et al. Neuroendocrine response to casino gambling in problem gamblers. *Psychoneuroendocrinology.* 2004;29(10):1272–1280.

Miner MH, Raymond N, Mueller BA, et al. Preliminary investigation of the impulsive and neuroanatomical characteristics of compulsive sexual behavior. *Psychiatry Res Neuroimaging.* 2009; 174(2):146–151.

Morgan T, Kofoed L, Buchkoski J, Carr RD. Video lottery gambling: effects on pathological gamblers seeking treatment in South Dakota. *J Gambl Stud.* 1996;12(4):451–460.

Moss HB, Hardie TL, Dahl JP, et al. Diplotypes of the human serotonin 1B receptor promoter predict growth hormone responses to sumatriptan in abstinent alcohol-dependent men. *Biol Psychiatry.* 2007;61(8):974–978.

Nordin C, Eklundh T. Altered CSF 5-HIAA disposition in pathologic male gamblers. *CNS Spectr.* 1999;4:25–33.

Odlaug BL, Chamberlain SR, Kim SW, et al. A neurocognitive comparison of cognitive flexibility and response inhibition in gamblers with varying degrees of clinical severity. *Psychol Med.* 2011;41:2111–2119.

Pallanti S, Bernardi S, Allen A, et al. Noradrenergic function in pathological gambling: blunted growth hormone response to clonidine. *J Psychopharmacol.* 2010b;24(6):847–853.

Pallanti S, Bernardi S, Allen A, Hollander E. Serotonin function in pathological gambling: Blunted growth hormone response to sumatriptan. *J Psychopharmacol.* 2010a;24(12):1802–1809.

Patkar AA, Mannelli P, Hill KP, et al. Relationship of prolactin response to meta-chlorophenylpiperazine with severity of drug use in cocaine dependence. *Hum Psychopharmacol Clin Exp.* 2006;21(6):367–375.

Pérez de Castro I, Ibanez A, Saiz-Ruiz J, Fernandez-Piqueras J. Concurrent positive association between pathological gambling and functional DNA polymorphisms at the MAO-A and the 5-HT transporter genes. *Mol Psychiatry.* 2002;7:927–928.

Pérez de Castro I, Ibáñez A, Saiz-Ruiz J, Fernández-Piqueras J. Genetic contribution to pathological gambling: possible association between a functional DNA polymorphism at the serotonin transporter gene (5-HTT) and affected men. *Pharmacogenetics.* 1999;9(3):397–400.

Petry NM, Stinson FS, Grant BF. Comorbidity of DSM-IV pathological gambling and other psychiatric disorders: results from the National Epidemiologic Survey on Alcohol and Related Conditions. *J Clin Psychiatry.* 2005;66(5):564–574.

Potenza MN, Leung HC, Blumberg HP, et al. An FMRI Stroop task study of ventromedial prefrontal cortical function in pathological gamblers. *Am J Psychiatry.* 2003a;160(11):1990–1994.

Potenza MN, Steinberg MA, Skudlarski P, et al. Gambling urges in pathological gambling: a functional magnetic resonance imaging study. *Arch Gen Psychiatry.* 2003b;60(8): 828–836.

Potenza MN. Should addictive disorders include non-substance-related conditions? *Addiction.* 2006;101(1):142–151.

Potenza MN. The neurobiology of pathological gambling and drug addiction: an overview and new findings. *Phil Trans R Soc B.* 2008;363(1507):3181–3189.

Power Y, Goodyear B, Crockford D. Neural correlates of pathological gamblers preference for immediate rewards during the Iowa Gambling Task: an fMRI study. *J Gambl Stud.* 2012;28:623–636.

Raab G, Elger C, Neuner M, Weber B. A neurological study of compulsive buying behaviour. *J Consum Pol.* 2011;34(4):401–413.

Reuter J, Raedler T, Rose M, et al. Pathological gambling is linked to reduced activation of the mesolimbic reward system. *Nat Neurosci.* 2005;8:147–148.

Schneider JP, Schneider BH. Couple recovery from sexual addiction: research findings of a survey of 88 marriages. *Sex Addict Compulsivity.* 1996;3:111–126.

Shah KR, Eisen SA, Xian H, Potenza MN. Genetic studies of pathological gambling: a review of methodology and analyses of data from the Vietnam Era Twin Registry. *J Gambl Stud.* 2005;21(2):179–203.

Slutske WS, Jackson KM, Sher KJ. The natural history of problem gambling from age 18 to 29. *J Abnorm Psychol.* 2003;112(2):263.

Slutske WS, Zhu G, Meier MH, Martin NG. Genetic and environmental influences on disordered gambling in men and women. *Arch Gen Psychiatry.* 2010;67(6):624–630.

Slutske WS. Natural recovery and treatment-seeking in pathological gambling: results of two national surveys. *Am J Psychiatry.* 2006;163:297–302.

Tanabe J, Thompson L, Claus E, et al. Prefrontal cortex activity is reduced in gambling and nongambling substance users during decision-making. *Hum Brain Mapp.* 2007;28(12):1276–1286.

Tavares H, Zilberman ML, Hodgins DC, El-Guebaly N. Comparison of craving between pathological gamblers and alcoholics. *Alcohol Clin Exp Res.* 2005;29(8):1427–1431.

Verdejo-Garcia A, Lawrence AJ, Clark L. Impulsivity as a vulnerability marker for substance-use disorders: review of findings from high-risk research, problem gamblers and genetic association studies. *Neurosci Biobehav Rev.* 2008;32(4):777–810.

Vitaro F, Brendgen M, Ladouceur R, Tremblay RE. Gambling, delinquency, and drug use during adolescence: mutual influences and common risk factors. *J Gambl Stud.* 2001;17(3):171–190.

Volkow ND, Chang L, Wang GJ, et al. Low level of brain dopamine D2 receptors in methamphetamine abusers: association with metabolism in the orbitofrontal cortex. *Am J Psychiatry.* 2001; 158(12):2015–2021.

Wang GJ, Volkow ND, Thanos PK, Fowler JS. Imaging of brain dopamine pathways: implications for understanding obesity. *J Addict Med.* 2009;3(1):8–18.

Wanner B, Vitaro F, Carbonneau R, Tremblay RE. Cross-lagged links among gambling, substance use, and delinquency from midadolescence to young adulthood: additive and moderating effects of common risk factors. *Psychol Addict Behav.* 2009;23(1):91.

Welte JW, Barnes GM, Tidwell M-CO, Hoffman JH. The association of form of gambling with problem gambling among American youth. *Psychol Addict Behav.* 2009;23(1):105.

Wrase J, Schlagenhauf F, Kienast T, et al. Dysfunction of reward processing correlates with alcohol craving in detoxified alcoholics. *NeuroImage.* 2007;35(2):787–794.

Yau Y, Yip S, Potenza MN. Understanding "behavioral addictions": insights from research. In: Fiellin DA, Miller SC, Saitz R, eds. *Principles of Addiction Medicine*. 5th ed. Philadelphia, PA: Lippincott Williams & Wilkins; 2014:55–83.

Yau YHC, Crowley MJ, Mayes LC, Potenza MN. Are Internet use and video-game-playing addictive behaviors? Biological, clinical and public health implications for youths and adults. *Minerva Psichiatr*. 2012;53:153–170.

Yip SW, Lacadie CM, Xu J, et al. Reduced genual corpus callosal white matter integrity in pathological gambling and its relationship to alcohol abuse or dependence. *World J Biol Psychiatry*. 2013;14(2):129–138.

Yuan K, Qin W, Wang G, et al. Microstructure abnormalities in adolescents with Internet addiction disorder. *PLoS One*. 2011;6(6):e20708.

▶ Treatment

A. Psychopharmacologic Interventions

Despite the personal and societal impact of GD, no medication has yet received regulatory approval in the United States as a treatment for GD. There have been, however, multiple double-blind, placebo-controlled trials of various pharmacological agents for the treatment of GD and other behavioral addictions, and these have been recently reviewed with a treatment algorithm proposed based on patient willingness to take medication (vs. dietary supplement) and presence (vs. absence) of specific co-occurring disorders or familial tendencies (Bullock & Potenza 2012). A treatment algorithm that considers both behavioral and pharmacological interventions has also been proposed (Potenza et al. 2019). Although placebo-controlled randomized clinical trials provide the strongest support for valid therapies, open-label trials and case reports may provide insight into new approaches for treating conditions, and these have also been reviewed for GD (Bullock & Potenza 2013; Kraus et al. 2020). Overall, data suggest that psychopharmacological therapies (as well as behavioral therapies) may be beneficial in treating GD.

1. Serotonin reuptake inhibitors and other antidepressants—Antidepressants were one of the first medications used to treat GD; however, controlled clinical trials have demonstrated mixed results for both behavioral and substance addictions (Potenza et al. 2009). Several randomized control trials have found selective serotonin reuptake inhibitors (SSRIs) such as fluvoxamine and paroxetine to be superior to placebo in treatment of GD (Hollander et al. 2000; Kim et al. 2002), whereas others have reported negative findings (Blanco et al. 2002; Grant et al. 2003). Citalopram, another SSRI, was found effective in reducing hypersexual disorder symptoms in homosexual and bisexual men without lessening sexual satisfaction (Wainberg et al. 2006). In contrast, among individuals with Internet addiction disorder, citalopram did not significantly differ from placebo groups in terms of reduction of hours spent online and global functioning improvements (Dell'Osso et al. 2008). Heterogeneity

in treatment response may result from individual differences. For example, individuals with GD and co-occurring anxiety disorders may respond well to SSRIs (Bullock & Potenza 2012). A case report using fMRI demonstrated differential effects before and after fluvoxamine treatment including decreased self-reported desire to gamble and increased activation in frontal and parietal areas during a card-game task—these effects were maintained at 6 and 9 months (Chung et al. 2009). SSRI treatments remain an active area of investigation (Brewer & Potenza 2008; Bullock & Potenza 2012); further research is needed to assess the potential clinical utilization of SSRIs for GD and other behavioral addictions.

2. Opioid antagonists—Opioids have been implicated in pleasurable and rewarding processes, and opioid function can influence neurotransmission in mesolimbic pathways (Spanagel et al. 1992). Based on these findings and similarities between behavioral and substance addictions, opioid antagonists have been evaluated in the treatment of GD and other behavioral addictions. An initial double-blind study suggested the efficacy of naltrexone—a treatment approved by the U.S. Food and Drug Administration (FDA) for alcohol use disorder—in reducing the intensity of urges to gamble, gambling thoughts, and gambling behavior (Kim et al. 2001). Individuals reporting higher intensity of gambling urges responded preferentially to treatment (Kim et al. 2001). Findings from this initial study have been replicated in a larger, longer study of 77 subjects randomized to either naltrexone or placebo over an 18-week period (Grant et al. 2008). A separate study found positive effects to be maintained after naltrexone discontinuation (Dannon et al. 2007). Naltrexone has also appeared effective in treating hypersexual disorder, with high doses (100–200 mg/day) reported to successfully reduce hypersexual disorder symptoms, sexual urges, sexual fantasies, and masturbation in two case report studies (Grant & Kim 2001; Raymond et al. 2002); these features, however, recurred following naltrexone discontinuation (Grant & Kim 2001). Another opioid antagonist, nalmefene, has also shown promise in the treatment of GD. In two large, multi-center trials using double-blind, placebo-controlled, designs, nalmefene was superior to placebo, although in one study only higher doses of nalmefene (40 mg/day) showed statistically significant differences from placebo in treatment outcome (Grant et al. 2006, 2010a). These findings suggest that medication dosing may be an important consideration in achieving improvement or remission.

3. Glutamate antagonists—Glutamatergic tone in the NAc has been implicated in reducing the reward-seeking behavior in substance addictions (Chambers & Potenza 2003; Kalivas et al. 2006;). The glutamatergic nutraceutical N-acetylcysteine has shown promise in small, controlled trials (Bullock & Potenza 2012). Memantine, an N-methyl-D-aspartate-type glutamate receptor antagonist, reduced both the number of hours spent gambling per week and money spent gambling in GD after 10 weeks of medication in an open-label trial. In addition, GD subjects reported improved cognitive flexibility posttreatment, suggesting that glutamate may contribute to impulsive and compulsive behaviors (Grant et al. 2010b). These preliminary data indicate a need for additional investigations into glutamatergic contributions to GD and glutamatergic therapies for its treatment.

4. Other psychopharmacological treatments—Dopamine receptor antagonists have not shown promise in the treatment of GD. Oral administration of a D_2-like receptor antagonist, haloperidol, increased gambling motivations among GD (but not control) subjects (Zack & Poulos 2007), although individual differences appear to be important (Tremblay et al. 2011). D_2-like antagonist drugs (e.g., olanzapine) have also not shown superiority to placebo in the treatment of GD (Fong et al. 2008; Grant & Potenza 2004; McElroy et al. 2008).

Preliminary studies investigating mood stabilizers such as lithium have shown some positive effects. Although sustained-release lithium carbonate did not have any significant effects on the number of episodes of gambling per week or time spent per gambling episode in individuals with GD (Hollander et al. 2005), lithium demonstrated efficacy in reducing gambling thoughts and urges, as well as GD severity in individuals with co-occurring GD and bipolar-spectrum disorder (Hollander et al. 2005). These findings suggest that co-occurring disorders may have important treatment implications for GD.

B. Psychotherapeutic Interventions

Multiple psychotherapeutic interventions have been proposed and investigated for the treatment of GD. Meta-analyses of psychotherapeutic approaches to the treatment of GD suggest they can result in significant improvements, with these positive effects retained, though to a lesser degree, over follow-ups of up to 2 years (Pallesen et al. 2005). However, these findings should be interpreted with caution, as the typical "no-treatment" or "wait-list" controls for psychological interventions promote greater differences between treatment and control than do pharmacological "placebo" controls.

1. Cognitive–behavioral therapy (CBT)—CBT is a semi-structured and problem-oriented approach that focuses in part on challenging the irrational thought processes and beliefs thought to maintain compulsive behaviors (such as ideas regarding lucky streaks, or the anticipated reversal of losing streaks in the case of GD). Learned behavioral tendencies, such as engaging in gambling after exposure to gambling-related cues, can also be tackled through exposure and desensitization techniques. Imaginal desensitization appears to be a successful approach (McConaghy et al. 1991), perhaps because once it is learned from a therapist, it can be practiced independently in any location, without immediate risk of gambling engagement as in in vivo exposure to a gambling environment. Therapists work to replace dysfunctional emotions, maladaptive behaviors, and cognitive processes

through goal-oriented, explicit systematic procedures and by facilitating engagement in non-gambling activities. The therapeutic technique varies according to the patient or issue but typically involves keeping a diary of significant events and associated feelings, thoughts, and behaviors; recording cognitions, assumptions, evaluations, and beliefs that may be maladaptive; and trying new ways of behaving and reacting. Management of finances is also an important factor that is addressed in CBT for GD. Such factors are important not only for initial abstinence but also for relapse prevention.

CBT approaches have arguably the strongest evidence base of any of the psychotherapeutic approaches, with a meta-analysis of randomized controlled trials demonstrating improvement in gambling-related variables after treatment and at follow-ups in people with GD (Pallesen et al. 2005). CBT also benefits from having multiple manualized treatment protocols for GD (Grant et al. 2011; Ladouceur & Lachance 2007; Petry 2005).

2. Gamblers Anonymous (GA)—GA is based on the 12-step model of Alcoholics Anonymous, with a focus on acceptance of powerlessness over the behavior (gambling) and a commitment to abstinence, facilitated by the development of a support network with more experienced members ("sponsors") in the group. The process involves admitting loss of control over gambling behavior; recognizing a higher power that can give strength; examining past errors (with the help of a sponsor or experienced member) and making amends; learning to live a new life with a new code of behavior; and helping and carrying the message to other people with gambling problems (Gamblers Anonymous 2013). Although studies have shown a beneficial effect in those attending GA vs. those who do not, attrition rates are often high, which may limit the efficacy of GA alone (Brewer et al. 2008). However, enrollment in a GA group may be a beneficial adjunct to more personalized therapy, with studies showing that those who attended GA in addition to individual therapy attended more individual therapy sessions (Grant & Odlaug 2012).

3. Motivational interviewing/enhancement (MI)—Motivational approaches are person-centered and revolve around exploring and resolving a patient's ambivalence toward change, with the aim of facilitating their intrinsic motivation and self-efficacy about dealing with their problem behavior. Such interventions are typically brief, even as little as a 15-minute telephone consultation. Research suggests that even such a brief intervention can prove efficacious in reducing GD symptoms and promoting duration of abstinence (Hodgins et al. 2004). Hence, such interventions could provide a cost-effective and resource-conserving treatment, especially for people with mild to moderate problems. Moreover, such brief interventions are not necessarily experienced as "treatments" by those receiving them. As such, MI techniques might be particularly useful with individuals reluctant to engage in prolonged therapy on account of stigma, shame, or financial concerns.

4. Mindfulness-based approaches—Mindfulness-based approaches incorporate Eastern meditation principles into more traditionally cognitive treatments. Key features of mindfulness are the cultivation of curiosity toward and acceptance of present-moment internal and external experiences, as well as an increasing capacity to control one's attention. It has been shown that low dispositional mindfulness is associated with gambling problems, leading to the suggestion that enhancing mindfulness may benefit problem gamblers. However, the evidence base is limited including several successful, open-label case studies (Toneatto et al. 2007). These patients had failed to benefit from traditional CBT but were aided by mindfulness-based meditation, suggesting that mindfulness-based therapies may be useful in helping people who did not respond to other forms of treatments. Mindfulness-based therapies may hold promise as an adjunctive intervention to help people with gambling problems learn to cope with gambling-related cognitive distortions by making patients more aware of their moment-to-moment experience and may be beneficial in relapse prevention, as patients could become aware of, but detached from, addictive urges. However, controlled trials are needed to examine these possibilities.

5. Psychodynamic psychotherapy (PDPT)—Psychodynamic approaches share an emphasis on assuming underlying meanings behind addictive behaviors, with treatment focused on unearthing these meanings. Emphasis is also placed on the interpersonal therapist–patient dynamic, or "transference," which may prove informative in revealing unconsciously repeated behaviors that could underpin a patient's difficulties. Long-term PDPT could last as long as several years, with multiple sessions per week. More directive and problem focused short-term PDPT can last from 16 to 30 sessions. However, psychodynamic approaches are limited by a lack of randomized controlled trials to evaluate their efficacy, especially about behavioral addictions. Moreover, because psychodynamic approaches can be prolonged and expensive, treatment may be complicated by commitment and financial difficulties.

6. Self-help interventions—In addition to GA, other self-help options exist. Individuals seeking treatment for gambling-related problems often display variations in types and frequencies of gambling and compositions of symptoms. Many patients may not meet diagnostic criteria for GD, and it is common for patients to migrate between GD and subsyndromal gambling. Although psychotherapy may be beneficial, this type of intervention is costly and may be unnecessarily intensive for some individuals. Self-help interventions may facilitate the dissemination of treatment to a wider population of individuals and can be distributed through various media such as textual, audio and audiovisual, and multimedia formats. One study suggested that Internet-based programs can have beneficial effects in GD, including at 3-year follow-up (Carlbring et al. 2012).

Meta-analyses indicate that self-help approaches have yielded significantly better results than no treatment or placebo for GD, although these positive effects are typically not as strong as other empirically tested psychotherapeutic approaches (Pallesen et al. 2005).

C. Other Interventions

In addition to treatment interventions, prevention interventions are also important in curbing addictive behaviors. Introduction and implementation of effective educational campaigns that promote community awareness about the potentially deleterious health effects of these behaviors and campaigns that alert the medical community to the importance of evaluating and treating behavioral addictions could help reduce the cost of these disorders to society. Increased awareness can facilitate early detection of behavioral addictions and may help in reducing the costs of treatment. Policies, programs, or strategies with the purpose of identifying risk factors and promoting resilience may further this endeavor. Given the high prevalence rates of behavioral addictions among youth, school-based prevention programs could be particularly beneficial. Furthermore, government and the industry should adopt policies and practices that promote responsible engagement in behaviors and access to treatment interventions for those with problems.

Blanco C, Petkova E, Ibanez A, Saiz-Ruiz J. A pilot placebo-controlled study of fluvoxamine for pathological gambling. *Ann Clin Psychiatry*. 2002;14(1):9–15.

Brewer JA, Potenza MN. The neurobiology and genetics of impulse control disorders: relationships to drug addictions. *Biochem Pharmacol*. 2008;75(1):63–75.

Brewer JA, Grant JE, Potenza MN. The treatment of pathologic gambling. *Addict Disord Treat*. 2008;7(1):1–13.

Bullock SA, Potenza MN. Pathological gambling: neuropsychopharmacology and treatment. *Curr Psychopharmacol*. 2012;1(1):67–85.

Bullock SA, Potenza MN. Update on the pharmacological treatment of pathological gambling. *Curr Psychopharmacol*. 2013;2:204–211.

Carlbring P, Degerman N, Jonsson J, Andersson G. Internet-based treatment of pathological gambling with a three-year follow-up. *Cogn Behav Ther*. 2012;41(4):321–334.

Chambers RA, Potenza MN. Neurodevelopment, impulsivity, and adolescent gambling. *J Gambl Stud*. 2003;19(1):53–84.

Chung SK, You IH, Cho GH, et al. Changes of functional MRI findings in a patient whose pathological gambling improved with fluvoxamine. *Yonsei Med J*. 2009;50(3):441–444.

Dannon PN, Lowengrub K, Musin E, et al. 12-month follow-up study of drug treatment in pathological gamblers: a primary outcome study. *J Clin Psychopharmacol*. 2007;27(6):620–624.

Dell'Osso B, Hadley S, Allen A, et al. Escitalopram in the treatment of impulsive-compulsive Internet usage disorder: an open-label trial followed by a double-blind discontinuation phase. *J Clin Psychiatry*. 2008;69(3):452–456.

Fong T, Kalechstein A, Bernhard B, et al. A double-blind, placebo-controlled trial of olanzapine for the treatment of video poker pathological gamblers. *Pharmacol Biochem Behav.* 2008;89(3):298–303.

Gamblers Anonymous. Gamblers Anonymous: Recovery Program. http://www.gamblersanonymous.org/ga/content/recovery-program; 2013.

Grant J, Kim SW. A case of kleptomania and compulsive sexual behavior treated with naltrexone. *Ann Clin Psychiatry.* 2001; 13(4):229–231.

Grant JE, Odlaug BL. Psychosocial interventions for gambling disorders. In: *Increasing the Odds. Vol 7: What Clinicians Need to Know About Gambling Disorders.* National Center for Responsible Gaming; 2012:38–52.

Grant JE, Potenza MN. Impulse control disorders: clinical characteristics and pharmacological management. *Ann Clin Psychiatry.* 2004;16(1):27–34.

Grant JE, Kim SW, Potenza MN, et al. Paroxetine treatment of pathological gambling: a multi-centre randomized controlled trial. *Int Clin Psychopharmacol.* 2003;18(4):243–249.

Grant JE, Potenza MN, Hollander E, et al. Multicenter investigation of the opioid antagonist nalmefene in the treatment of pathological gambling. *Am J Psychiatry.* 2006;163(2):303–312.

Grant JE, Kim SW, Hartman BK. A double-blind, placebo-controlled study of the opiate antagonist naltrexone in the treatment of pathological gambling urges. *J Clin Psychiatry.* 2008;69(5):783–789.

Grant JE, Odlaug BL, Potenza MN, et al. Nalmefene in the treatment of pathological gambling: multicentre, double-blind, placebo-controlled study. *Br J Psychiatry.* 2010a;197(4):330–331.

Grant JE, Chamberlain SR, Odlaug BL, et al. Memantine shows promise in reducing gambling severity and cognitive inflexibility in pathological gambling: a pilot study. *Psychopharmacology.* 2010b;212(4):603–612.

Grant JE, Donahue CB, Odlaug BL. *Treating Impulse Control Disorders: A Cognitive-Behavioral Therapy Program (Treatments That Work).* New York: Oxford University Press; 2011.

Hodgins DC, Currie S, el-Guebaly N, Peden N. Brief motivational treatment for problem gambling: a 24-month follow-up. *Psychol Addict Behav.* 2004;18(3):293.

Hollander E, DeCaria CM, Finkell JN, et al. A randomized double-blind fluvoxamine/placebo crossover trial in pathologic gambling. *Biol Psychiatry.* 2000;47(9):813–817.

Hollander E, Pallanti S, Allen A, et al. Does sustained-release lithium reduce impulsive gambling and affective instability versus placebo in pathological gamblers with bipolar spectrum disorders? *Am J Psychiatry.* 2005;162(1):137–145.

Kalivas PW, Peters J, Knackstedt L. Animal models and brain circuits in drug addiction. *Mol Interv.* 2006;6(6):339–344.

Kim SW, Grant JE, Adson DE, Shin YC. Double-blind naltrexone and placebo comparison study in the treatment of pathological gambling. *Biol Psychiatry.* 2001;49(11):914–921.

Kim SW, Grant JE, Adson DE, et al. A double-blind placebo-controlled study of the efficacy and safety of paroxetine in the treatment of pathological gambling. *J Clin Psychiatry.* 2002;63(6):501–507.

Kraus SW, Etuk R, Potenza MN. Current pharmacotherapy for gambling disorder: a systematic review. *Expert Opin Pharmacother.* 2020;21(3):287–296.

Ladouceur R, Lachance S. *Overcoming Pathological Gambling: Therapist Guide (Treatments That Work).* New York: Oxford University Press; 2007.

McConaghy N, Blaszczynski A, Frankova A. Comparison of imaginal desensitisation with other behavioural treatments of pathological gambling. A two-to nine-year follow-up. *Br J Psychiatry.* 1991;159(3):390–393.

McElroy SL, Nelson EB, Welge JA, et al. Olanzapine in the treatment of pathological gambling: a negative randomized placebo-controlled trial. *J Clin Psychiatry.* 2008;69(3):433–440.

Pallesen S, Mitsem M, Kvale G, et al. Outcome of psychological treatments of pathological gambling: a review and meta-analysis. *Addiction.* 2005;100(10):1412–1422.

Petry NM. *Pathological Gambling: Etiology, Comorbidity, and Treatment.* Washington, DC: American Psychological Association; 2005.

Potenza MN, Balodis IM, Derevensky J, et al. Gambling disorder. *Nat Rev Dis Primers* 2019;5:51.

Potenza MN, Koran LM, Pallanti S. The relationship between impulse-control disorders and obsessive–compulsive disorder: a current understanding and future research directions. *Psychiatry Res.* 2009;170(1):22–31.

Raymond NC, Grant JE, Kim SW, Coleman E. Treatment of compulsive sexual behaviour with naltrexone and serotonin reuptake inhibitors: two case studies. *Int Clin Psychopharmacol.* 2002;17(4):201–205.

Spanagel R, Herz A, Shippenberg TS. Opposing tonically active endogenous opioid systems modulate the mesolimbic dopaminergic pathway. *Proc Natl Acad Sci U S A.* 1992;89(6): 2046–2050.

Toneatto T, Vettese L, Nguyen L. The role of mindfulness in the cognitive-behavioural treatment of problem gambling. *J Gambl Issues.* 2007:91–100

Tremblay A-M, Desmond RC, Poulos CX, Zack M. Haloperidol modifies instrumental aspects of slot machine gambling in pathological gamblers and healthy controls. *Addict Biol.* 2011; 16(3):467–484.

Wainberg ML, Muench F, Morgenstern J, et al. A double-blind study of citalopram versus placebo in the treatment of compulsive sexual behaviors in gay and bisexual men. *J Clin Psychiatry.* 2006;67(12):1968–1973.

Zack M, Poulos CX. A D2 antagonist enhances the rewarding and priming effects of a gambling episode in pathological gamblers. *Neuropsychopharmacology.* 2007;32(8):1678–1686.

▶ Complications/Adverse Outcomes of Treatment

People with gambling problems are often hesitant to enter treatment, and many factors may contribute to this hesitancy. For example, individuals with gambling problems may be ashamed, unaware that help is available, uninsured or without financial resources to enter treatment, of the opinion that they can change on their own, or repelled by the treatments that are available (Pulford et al. 2009). Moreover, the wide varieties of symptoms that accompany behavioral addictions and the lack of formal diagnostic criteria for some of these disorders, as well as potential inaccuracies in patients' reports, may make the diagnosis of these disorders difficult. It is important that clinicians and other health professionals learn about behavioral addictions and be prepared to identify them to attend to them in an appropriate manner. A first step in this process is to provide clinical tools (e.g., development of formal diagnostic tools and health screens based on these criteria) and public policies that will help guide clinicians.

Treatment outcome is also complicated by high rates of treatment discontinuation (e.g., 40–60% among individuals with GD; Grant et al. 2006). Before engaging in any treatment, clinicians should carefully consider the applicability of different approaches to the specific patient. For example, in cases of GD, patients may be severely limited financially. Such practical factors could effectively preclude certain types of treatment, such as long-term psychodynamic psychotherapy, that can be very costly. If treatment is initiated but financial difficulties persist or worsen, it could be detrimental to a patient's condition to curtail such long-term therapies without proper closure.

Another factor that may contribute to high treatment-discontinuation rates is that patients with GD and other behavioral addictions are often assigned to treatment facilities lacking the clinical expertise needed to manage these disorders and their associated complications. Clinicians and health professionals should develop the expertise to recognize and diagnose behavioral addictions. In addition, clinicians should be aware of potential co-occurring psychiatric disorders that can worsen prognosis if not addressed. The presence of co-occurring disorders in GD has been associated with increased gambling problems and severity of associated consequences (Ladd & Petry 2003). Co-occurring disorders may also partly determine compliance to gambling treatment (Milton et al. 2002) and may influence the efficacy of pharmacological (Dell'Osso et al. 2005) and psychological (Winters & Kushner 2003) interventions. Treatment plans that appropriately address co-occurring illnesses may improve efficacy and treatment compliance. Retrospective studies suggest that simultaneous treatment of GD and alcohol-use disorder improves the outcome of GD treatment (Lesieur & Blume 1991). Complete psychiatric evaluations are therefore important in patients with behavioral addictions. These points are discussed in greater detail in the earlier section "Differential Diagnosis."

Potentially negative effects of cognitive strategies should also be considered, particularly with respect to challenging patients' cognitions and beliefs. Challenging deeply held cognitions could significantly threaten a patient's self-esteem and sense of self and thus should be done sensitively and with respect. The rate of attrition is also noteworthy in treatments for addiction. In the event of noncompletion of a program of treatment, especially self-help interventions, patients should be provided with a means of noncompletion that does not elicit concomitant feelings of failure and guilt.

No medication has yet been approved by the FDA for treating GD or other behavioral addictions. There are questions regarding adequate drug dosing for the treatment of GD, and relatively scant data exist on the optimal durations of treatments, rates of relapse associated with discontinuation, and associated adverse effects of pharmacological treatments. Despite the relatively early stage of investigations into efficacious and well-tolerated drug treatments for behavioral addictions, it is important to consider whether distinct groups of individuals with GD may respond better or worse to specific pharmacotherapies and whether distinct groups might represent treatment-resistant populations. In clinical settings, it is not unusual to encounter patients who have had no response or only a partial response to treatment and thus require further treatment. Among individuals with alcohol-use disorder, combinations of different treatments such as SSRIs and opioid antagonists have produced higher alcohol abstinence rates and longer delays before relapse to heavy drinking than administration of either treatment alone (Pettinati et al. 2010). The extent to which these combinations may be effective and well tolerated in the treatment of behavioral addictions requires additional investigation.

Multiple options are available for the treatment of behavioral addictions, and clinicians should be aware that treatments are not mutually exclusive. For example, brief motivational interviewing may supplement a patient's self-help efforts if full treatment is not an option. Further research should investigate combinations of pharmacological and psychotherapeutic treatments to determine whether they may prove more effective than either alone. Future research should also address whether individual differences may indicate that a particular intervention might be more appropriate and whether treatment should start with medication or therapy or both.

With addictions, relapse prevention may be of equal importance to problem behavior reduction or abstinence. Clinicians and health professionals should anticipate that people with GD may struggle with gambling problems and co-occurring disorders and therefore may require intermittent treatment over an extended duration.

Finally, it should be noted that research into behavioral addictions is at a relatively early stage; treatment options discussed in the present chapter should be considered as informative but preliminary. Work is ongoing about which specific elements of different therapies should be considered active ingredients of treatment, and clinicians should expect innovations in the future that might necessitate significant changes in their therapeutic approach. Moreover, many of the randomized controlled trials that demonstrate the efficacy of different treatments have excluded individuals with co-occurring disorders. As this group may reflect the bulk of patients encountered in practice by clinicians, clinicians should use their judgment in deciding which issues are of primary importance and consider flexibility in how they approach treatment.

Dell'Osso B, Allen A, Hollander E. Comorbidity issues in the pharmacological treatment of pathological gambling: a critical review. *Clin Pract Epidemiol Ment Health.* 2005;1:21.

Grant JE, Potenza MN, Hollander E, et al. Multicenter investigation of the opioid antagonist nalmefene in the treatment of pathological gambling. *Am J Psychiatry.* 2006;163(2):303–312.

Hall GW, Carriero NJ, Takushi RY, et al. Pathological gambling among cocaine-dependent outpatients. *Am J Psychiatry.* 2000; 157(7):1127–1133.

Ladd GT, Petry NM. A comparison of pathological gamblers with and without substance abuse treatment histories. *Exp Clin Psychopharmacol.* 2003;11(3):202–209.

Lesieur HR, Blume SB. Evaluation of patients treated for pathological gambling in a combined alcohol, substance abuse and pathological gambling treatment unit using the Addiction Severity Index. *Br J Addict.* 1991;86(8):1017–1028.

Milton S, Crino R, Hunt C, Prosser E. The effect of compliance-improving interventions on the cognitive-behavioural treatment of pathological gambling. *J Gambl Stud.* 2002;18(2):207–229.

Pettinati HM, Oslin DW, Kampman KM, et al. A double blind, placebo-controlled trial that combines sertraline and naltrexone for treating co-occurring depression and alcohol dependence. *Am J Psychiatry.* 2010;167(6):668.

Pulford J, Bellringer M, Abbott M, et al. Barriers to help-seeking for a gambling problem: the experiences of gamblers who have sought specialist assistance and the perceptions of those who have not. *J Gambl Stud.* 2009;25(1):33–48.

Winters KC, Kushner MG. Treatment issues pertaining to pathological gamblers with a comorbid disorder. *J Gambl Stud.* 2003;19(3):261–277.

▶ Prognosis

Development of problem gambling is frequently in the third decade of life (in the 20s), with those initiating recreational gambling at a younger age more likely to develop GD (Kessler et al. 2008). Biological, psychological, and environmental factors contribute to GD. Co-occurring psychiatric and medical disorders, abilities to cope in high-risk situations, developmental histories, socioeconomic status, peer support, genetic predispositions, willingness to engage in treatment, treatment choices, and other aspects may all influence treatment outcome. Consequently, the gambling behavior of patients seeking treatment for gambling problems may vary over the course of treatment—as might the intensities and influences of co-occurring clinical disorders.

Few direct examinations of gambling relapse exist. Generally, factors that may contribute to relapse are varied.

Optimism about winning, a perceived need to make money, lack of structured time or boredom, "giving in" to craving, difficulties coping with negative emotions, a perceived need to socialize or fit in, and excitement seeking were among the top reasons respondents cited for their gambling relapses (Hodgins & el-Guebaly 2004).

Hodgins DC, el-Guebaly N. Retrospective and prospective reports of precipitants to relapse in pathological gambling. *J Consult Clin Psychol.* 2004;72(1):72.

Kessler RC, Hwang I, LaBrie R, et al. DSM-IV pathological gambling in the National Comorbidity Survey Replication. *Psychol Med.* 2008;38(9):1351–1360.

CONCLUSION

Behavioral addictions have received little attention from clinicians and researchers, with few empirical studies of treatment strategies for these disorders. Consequently, our understanding of efficacious and well-tolerated psychopharmacological and psychotherapeutic strategies for behavioral addictions lags significantly behind our understanding of treatment for other major neuropsychiatric disorders. Data, however, suggest that individuals with behavioral addictions frequently respond positively to pharmacological and psychotherapeutic interventions for SUDs, with the best data existing for GD.

An important first step in treating behavioral addictions involves proper diagnoses. Many people with behavioral addictions may not recognize or acknowledge their maladaptive engagement in these behaviors or may be ashamed to report that they might have a problem. For these reasons, clinicians should screen for GD and other behavioral addictions if these disorders are to be identified and treated properly. Although behavioral addictions share some characteristics with ICDs, OCD, and SUDs, there also exist important differences that may necessitate different treatment strategies. As with SUDs, co-occurring disorders may complicate treatment, and such conditions should be addressed to provide the most comprehensive and complete treatment.

Approaches and data from this chapter represent significant advances compared to what was available several years ago. Continued advances in our understanding of these disorders hold the potential for significantly improving the lives of individuals with behavioral addictions as well as those who are affected by their conditions.

Schizophrenia

Rajiv Radhakrishnan, MD
Suhas Ganesh, MD
Herbert Y. Meltzer, MD
William V. Bobo, MD
Stephan H. Heckers, MD
S. Hossein Fatemi, MD, PhD
Deepak Cyril D'Souza, MD

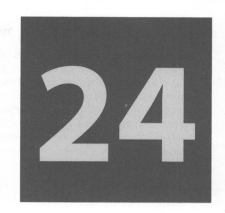

Schizophrenia is one of the most complex of psychiatric disorders which is ranked among the top 10 illnesses contributing to the global burden of disease, per the World Health Organization (WHO).

- **Diagnosis is based on a standardized psychiatric interview and the use of diagnostic criteria**, as specified below. Note that these criteria allow the diagnosis in the absence of prominent hallucinations or delusions (e.g., there is instead some combination of negative symptoms, disorganized speech, and/or disorganized or catatonic behavior).

- **Duration of active psychotic symptoms** for at least 1 month, or for a shorter duration if successfully treated.

- **Total duration of illness for at least 6 months**, including prodrome, acute phase, and residual symptoms.

- **Cognitive impairment and disorganization** characterized by disorganized, illogical, loosely associated or bizarre **speech**, or by inappropriate or bizarre **behaviors**.

- **The above symptoms are idiopathic in nature**—that is, they are not attributable to the physiological effects of a substance (e.g., a drug of abuse, a medication) or another medical condition.

- **Dysfunction in one or more life domains** as a result of the above signs or symptoms.

Other common features:

- **Lack of insight** that symptoms and difficulties that stem from them are products of a mental illness that requires treatment.

- **Deterioration in personal appearance and hygiene.**

- **Depression and anxiety symptoms**, including **suicidal thinking**.

- **Abnormal motor activity**, including rocking, pacing, grimacing, maintaining uncomfortable postures, stereotypies, and odd mannerisms.

- **Poor adherence** with treatment.

- Comorbid **drug** (including nicotine) **and alcohol use-disorders**, and chronic **physical health problems**.

▶ DSM-5 Diagnostic Criteria for Schizophrenia

A. Two (or more) of the following, each present for a significant portion of time during a 1-month period (or less if successfully treated). At least one of these must be delusions, hallucinations, or disorganized speech:

1. Delusions

2. Hallucinations

3. Disorganized speech (e.g., frequent derailment or incoherence)

4. Grossly disorganized or catatonic behavior

5. Negative symptoms (i.e., diminished emotional expression or avolition)

B. Continuous signs of the disturbance persist for at least 6 months. This 6-month period must include at least 1 month of symptoms (or less if successfully treated) that meet the above criteria (i.e., active phase symptoms) and may include periods of prodromal or residual symptoms. During these prodromal or residual periods, the signs of the disturbance may be manifested only by negative symptoms or by two or more symptoms listed above present in an attenuated form.

C. For a significant portion of time since the onset of the disturbance, the level of functioning in one or more major areas, such as work, interpersonal relations, or self-care, is markedly below the level achieved prior to the onset (or when the onset is in childhood or adolescence, there is a failure to achieve expected level of interpersonal, academic, or occupational functioning).

D. Schizoaffective disorder and depressive or bipolar disorder (BD) with psychotic features have been ruled out.

E. The disturbance is not attributable to the physiological effects of a substance (e.g., a drug of abuse, a medication) or another medical condition. If there is a history of autism spectrum disorder or a communication disorder of childhood onset, the additional diagnosis of schizophrenia is made only if prominent delusions or hallucinations, in addition to the other required symptoms of schizophrenia, are also present for at least 1 month (or less if successfully treated).

▶ General Considerations

Schizophrenia is a heterogenous clinical syndrome characterized by a constellation of symptoms that have been broadly classified into three domains: positive, negative, and cognitive dysfunction. It typically has a chronic, relapsing course with incomplete remissions and is associated with significant impairment in most domains of functioning. Schizophrenia is one of the top 10 leading causes of disability worldwide. In the United States, the estimated excess economic burden of schizophrenia in 2019 was $343.2 billion, including $251.9 billion in indirect costs (73.4%), $62.3 billion in direct health care costs (18.2%), and $35.0 billion in direct non–health care costs (10.2%). Disability accounted for approximately 80% of total costs with the largest drivers of indirect costs being caregiving ($112.3 billion), premature mortality ($77.9 billion), and unemployment ($54.2 billion). The economic burden of schizophrenia was estimated to be 1.6% of the gross domestic product.

The positive symptoms of schizophrenia include hallucinations and other perceptual alterations, delusions, disorganized thinking and speech, and disorganized behavior (including catatonia). The negative symptoms of schizophrenia include amotivation, blunted affect, social withdrawal, avolition (diminished interests, sense of purpose, and social drive), diminished emotional expression, alogia (diminished quantity of speech and amount of spontaneous elaboration), and anhedonia (diminished capacity to experience pleasure or interest). The cognitive symptoms of schizophrenia include deficits in memory, attention, reasoning and problem solving, processing speed, social cognition, and intelligence quotient (IQ). Together, these positive, negative, and cognitive symptoms have an adverse impact on work and/or interpersonal functioning and self-care. This in turn results in a failure to reach the expected level of academic, interpersonal, or work functioning. The clinical diagnosis of schizophrenia is currently made on the basis of these characteristic signs and symptoms, their time course, their adverse impact on functional capacity, and their idiopathic nature (e.g., they are not the psychiatric manifestations of general medical conditions or effects of substances, and they are not better accounted for by other diagnoses that feature psychotic symptoms or severe

functional or cognitive incapacity). The negative symptoms and cognitive deficits are more enduring and chronic, whereas the positive symptoms (psychosis) have an episodic pattern. The exacerbation of psychotic symptoms is often a cause for hospitalization. Of note, none of the signs or symptoms described earlier are pathognomonic of schizophrenia, although historically certain symptoms (called first-rank symptoms) were thought to be pathognomonic, as described later. Rather, it is the constellation of signs and symptoms, and the chronic course of illness that typify schizophrenia. Finally, there is a high degree of variability in the expression of these symptoms.

Even after excluding the secondary causes of psychotic symptoms, the diagnosis of schizophrenia and related disorders remains challenging. For one, the etiology and the pathophysiology of schizophrenia is unknown. It is likely that within the current nosology several disorders are lumped under schizophrenia. As Eugen Bleuler first noted, schizophrenia could be more accurately referred to as "the group of schizophrenias." This is analogous to pneumonias, which at one time were viewed as one condition and that were diagnosed based on a constellation of clinical symptoms (e.g., cough) and signs (e.g., fever). Following the discovery of bacteria, viruses, and fungi, and the differentiation of bacteria into gram-positive and -negative subtypes, pneumonias were differentiated into specific types. Similarly, "dropsy" was at one time considered a single entity that presented with common signs and symptoms including edema. However, over time it was differentiated based on pathophysiology into congestive heart failure, hepatic failure, primary and secondary nephrotic syndrome, and eventually classified histologically. For schizophrenia, there is no clinically reliable biological marker, including functional or structural neuroimaging or pattern of genetic heritability. Thus, it is conceivable that schizophrenia will in due course be subtyped as distinct pathophysiologies underlying chronic psychoses are discovered. Second, no single sign or symptom is pathognomonic of schizophrenia.

Although schizophrenia has been described in one form or another since ancient times, the twentieth-century observations of Emil Kraepelin, Eugen Bleuler, and Kurt Schneider have influenced the conceptualization of the disorder. Their descriptions of the phenomenology of the disorder have influenced the development of diagnostic criteria for the *Diagnostic and Statistical Manual of Mental Disorders* (DSM) and *International Classification of Disease* (ICD). Emil Kraepelin was credited for distinguishing manic–depressive illness (now called BD) from **dementia praecox** (the forerunner of schizophrenia) based on relative age of onset (younger in the case of manic–depressive illness), symptom course (episodic for manic–depressive illness, chronic for dementia praecox), vocational/social outcome (better for manic–depressive illness), and level of cognitive impairment (more severe in dementia praecox). Eugen Bleuler coined the term "schizophrenia" based on his observation that long-term outcome was quite variable among patients with dementia praecox and on the hypothesis that a split between thought and affect was the central feature of the illness. Bleuler specifically identified four components (also known as Bleuler's "four A's") as the essence of the syndrome: **Autism** (i.e., a withdrawal from reality), **Ambivalence** (of affect and will), **Affectivity** (in Bleuler's words: an "indifference to everything"), and **Association** (in Bleuler's words: "the associations lose their continuity"). Kurt Schneider introduced the concept of **first-rank symptoms** (e.g., thought insertion, thought withdrawal, thought broadcast, voices arguing or discussing, delusions of control), which he believed were pathognomonic of schizophrenia and became the forerunner of the notion of positive symptoms. Schneider's first-rank symptoms are now known not to be specific for schizophrenia, for they may also occur in mania, drug-induced states, and other disorders. Nonetheless, these and other signs and symptoms together have undergone extensive empirical testing to be criteria with sufficient diagnostic specificity, reliability, and validity for use in clinical practice. The concept of schizophrenia as a diagnostic entity continues to evolve as evidenced by changes to the diagnostic criteria in the latest version of the *Diagnostic and Statistical Manual of Mental Disorders, Fifth Edition* (DSM-5) and the *International Classification of Diseases (ICD)-10.*

In recent years, there has also been a call for abandonment of the concept of schizophrenia as a discrete diagnostic entity and preference for a more general concept of "psychosis spectrum disorder" since individual symptoms of schizophrenia may also be seen in otherwise healthy individuals in the general population (e.g., "voice-hearers") and as part of personality constructs such as paranoid, schizoid, or schizotypal personality disorder.

Owen MJ, Sawa A, Mortensen PB. Schizophrenia. *Lancet.* 2016; 388:86–97.

Kadakia A, Catillon M, Fan Q, et al. The economic burden of schizophrenia in the United States. *J Clin Psychiatry.* 2022; 83(6):22m14458. doi: 10.4088/JCP.22m14458.

A. Epidemiology

1. Incidence & prevalence—The **incidence** of schizophrenia ranges from 8 to 43 new cases per 100,000 population, whereas the age-corrected median **point prevalence** and **lifetime prevalence** estimates of the disorder are 4.6 and 4.0 cases per 1000 population, respectively. Of note, for a long time, schizophrenia was believed to have a uniform lifetime morbid risk of 1% worldwide. More recent studies, however, suggest that there may be considerable variability (more than five times) in the lifetime risk for schizophrenia reported in studies that cannot be explained away by methodological differences but is likely real and related to differences in the rate and exposure to a variety of factors. While the yearly incidence of schizophrenia spectrum disorders (per 10,000 individuals) in the Danish registry in 2018 was

1.6 for schizophrenia, 0.1 for schizoaffective disorder, and 1.3 for schizotypal disorder, in a review of studies between 1974 and 2022, the incidence rate in low-middle income countries varied around 4.2 times, from 10.0 per 100,000 person-years in Brazil to 42.0 in India. The numbers for lifetime prevalence estimate are lower than the often reported range of 0.5–1.0%, which is believed to be an overestimate. However, the estimated prevalence is higher by two to three times when broader diagnostic criteria are applied.

2. Life expectancy, drug use, & physical health problems—Life expectancy in schizophrenia is lower by about 20% (i.e., 15–25 years lower) relative to the general population. The majority of deaths are due to preventable physical diseases, especially cardiovascular disease, respiratory disease, and infections. Up to 75% of persons with schizophrenia (compared to 33% of the general population) die of coronary heart disease. The rates of respiratory diseases are two to six times higher than the rate in the general population (even after controlling for tobacco smoking and substance abuse), and individuals with this condition die of infectious diseases at about two to four times the rate of the general population. Patients with schizophrenia are also more likely to die of diabetes mellitus. The cancer fatality rate in this population is also higher, although the incidence of cancer is comparable to the general population.

Increased early mortality among patients with schizophrenia is attributed to increased rates of **suicide** (10–13% lifetime risk of completed suicide, 18–55% risk for attempted suicide), accidents, and poor physical health. Factors associated with suicidality include age (younger), stage of illness (earlier), gender (male), family socioeconomic status (higher), intelligence (higher), expectations (higher), marital status (single), (lack of) social supports, awareness of symptoms, and being recently discharged from the hospital. Other factors that may contribute include low self-esteem, stigma, recent loss or stress, hopelessness, isolation, treatment nonadherence, and substance abuse. Both depression and the severity of psychosis contribute to the risk for suicide in schizophrenia.

At baseline, patients with schizophrenia appear to be at higher risk for a host of metabolic and cardiovascular disorders, including obesity, diabetes, dyslipidemia, and coronary artery and cerebrovascular disease. Other contributors to the medical morbidity of schizophrenia include sedentary lifestyle, alcohol and drug abuse, and high rates (60–80%) of chronic heavy smoking. High rates of substance abuse alone contribute to poor physical health, infrequent medical and psychiatric follow-up, and poor adherence with medical and psychiatric treatment. In addition, most available antipsychotic treatments elevate cardiovascular risk as a result of weight gain, dyslipidemia, and glucose elevation.

In spite of the health concerns that accompany schizophrenia, there is a disproportionately low rate of health service utilization among this population. Cognitive dysfunction, paranoid symptoms, apathy, comorbid disorders, poverty, and illness-associated stigma may all impede utilization of necessary medical services. Collectively these factors contribute to a reduction in life expectancy of 10–25 years in schizophrenia. There appears to be a widening gap in longevity between persons with schizophrenia and the general population. Concrete recommendations for health screening and monitoring for individuals with schizophrenia are provided later (see section "Treatment").

B. Demographics

1. Gender—Schizophrenia is slightly more common in males than in females (male:female risk ratio is 1.4); however, as noted earlier, the average age of onset of schizophrenia for women is at least 5 years later than for men. Others have found no statistically significant differences in prevalence estimates between males and females. In contrast to the preponderance of males among those diagnosed with schizophrenia in adolescence and early adulthood, after the age of 45 there appears to be a 2:1 gender ratio in favor of women. The age of onset distribution for women is bimodal with two peaks: one in the 20s and the second after the age of 45. Compared with men, women with schizophrenia tend to have better premorbid functioning, fewer negative symptoms, more prominent mood symptoms, more complete recovery from episodes, better clinical response to antipsychotic medication, milder long-term course, better social functioning, less comorbid substance abuse, and less potential for suicide. Symptoms in women may worsen after menopause.

2. Age—The age of onset for men appears to be earlier (age 18–25 years) than for women (age 25–35 years). Onset prior to the age of 10 is considered rare, though when it does occur, symptoms are typically very severe. Onset after the age of 45 (**late onset**) is also uncommon, and very uncommon after the age of 65 (**very late onset**). An early age of onset is associated with a worse outcome—conversely, later age of onset is associated with a better outcome.

3. Socioeconomic status—The prevalence of schizophrenia is thought to be lower in developing countries compared with developed nations. This finding is limited by a relative lack of data from low- vs. higher-income nations and the use of a single economic variable to classify countries. Patients in developing countries are also thought to have a more benign illness course than those in developed countries. In Western societies, individuals with schizophrenia are at higher risk for poverty, unemployment, homelessness or inadequate housing, ill health, and poor access to health care. It has been theorized that the limitations posed by the symptoms of schizophrenia result in a **downward social drift** in socioeconomic status, or prevent upward social mobility, or both.

Some evidence suggests an association between neighborhood-level socioeconomic deprivation and increased incidence of schizophrenia. In contrast, other evidence suggests that the prevalence of schizophrenia is lower in developing countries and that the course of the illness is more benign. However, recent evidence for the "better prognosis of schizophrenia" hypothesis has been inconclusive.

Individuals in lower socioeconomic classes have higher rates of schizophrenia. Additionally, individuals with ultrahigh-risk mental states (attenuated, brief, or limited intermittent psychotic symptoms) have higher rates of unemployment. Recent studies using genetic data to address the **social causation** vs. **social selection** hypothesis for the noted inverse correlation between schizophrenia and socioeconomic status suggest some support for the latter theory. Preliminary emerging evidence suggests that the genetic risk for schizophrenia also predicts residence in deprived neighborhoods.

4. Social support—Individuals with schizophrenia are more likely to be single (never married), divorced, or separated relative to age-matched controls. Individuals with schizophrenia who are unmarried are more likely to have had an earlier onset of psychosis, poorer premorbid functioning, and more severe illness, relative to those who are married. Conversely, adequate social support in any form and avoidance of high "**expressed emotion**" environments (overcritical or overprotective) both predict better long-term course. A high degree of expressed emotion (e.g., hostility, emotional over-involvement, and criticism) has been associated with increased psychotic relapse.

5. Ethnicity—Schizophrenia affects individuals from all racial and ethnic groups. Schizophrenia has been reported to be more prevalent among immigrant minority groups in the United Kingdom and the Netherlands. Studies done in the United Kingdom and the Netherlands have observed a higher incidence of psychotic disorders in ethnic minority groups in areas with low ethnic density than in areas with high ethnic density, suggestive of a "**social defeat**" hypothesis. Studies from several countries and a recent meta-analysis have shown an increased prevalence of schizophrenia in migrants when compared with native-born populations. However, the disproportionately high prevalence of schizophrenia observed among first-generation immigrants in Western countries appears to normalize in subsequent generations.

6. Other factors—Epidemiologic data consistently show that patients with schizophrenia have an increased likelihood of having been born in the **late winter and spring months**. The seasonal effect has been linked to epidemics of influenza or viral infections that occur more frequently during winter months. A number of epidemiologic studies have attributed the increased rate of schizophrenia births to maternal influenza or other viral infections during the second trimester. Maternal influenza during the second trimester may impair fetal growth and predispose to obstetric complications and lower birth weight in about 2% of individuals destined to develop schizophrenia. Other complicating factors such as maternal malnutrition and Rh incompatibility during gestation have been associated with increased vulnerability to schizophrenia. The rates of schizophrenia have been noted to be greater in people living in higher latitudes compared to lower latitudes. This finding has led to interesting hypotheses about exposure to sunlight and the role of vitamin D in the pathophysiology of schizophrenia.

C. Etiopathophysiology

Kraepelin conjectured that schizophrenia was caused by a biological abnormality, even though the attempts to identify an abnormality (including neuropathological studies by Alois Alzheimer) were unsuccessful. In the middle of the twentieth century, the view that schizophrenia was the result of specific disturbances in childrearing received considerable attention. In particular, communication deviance between parents and the child who was diagnosed with schizophrenia was considered by some clinicians to be a sufficient cause of schizophrenia. Although communication deviance in families with a child with schizophrenia has been demonstrated in a number of studies, evidence that this feature was specific for schizophrenia or causative was unconvincing. Nevertheless, this line of research led to a continual interest in how family (and other caregiver) interactions can contribute to or diminish the stress and coping skills of patients with schizophrenia and, thus, modulate the course of the illness.

The current view is that schizophrenia is a brain disease. However, as discussed earlier, schizophrenia is likely a collection of disorders, and therefore it is highly unlikely that one etiology will explain the disorder. A number of factors contributing to an increased risk of schizophrenia have been identified, as shown in Table 24–1.

▶ Pathophysiology of Schizophrenia

A. Dopamine Hypothesis

The most widely accepted original hypothesis of the etiology of schizophrenia and of the action of antipsychotic drugs implicates the neurotransmitter dopamine (DA). Dopaminergic neurons arise from two midbrain nuclei: (1) the **nigrostriatal tract** originates in the substantia nigra, terminates in the striatum, and is involved in modulation of motoric behavior, cognition, and sensory gating; and (2) the **mesolimbic** and **mesocortical tracts** originate in the ventral tegmental area and terminate in limbic and cortical structures, respectively, affecting cognitive, motivational, and reward systems. The dopamine 1 (D_1) receptor family, which includes D_1 and D_5 receptors, is present in high concentration in the cortex and striatum. The dopamine 2 (D_2) receptor family consists of D_2, D_3, and D_4 receptors and is concentrated in the limbic and striatal regions. Presynaptic DA receptors (i.e., D_2 and D_3) can consist of either somatodendritic autoreceptors localized to cell bodies in the substantia nigra and ventral tegmental area or terminal autoreceptors limited to axons of these DA cells. The somatodendritic and terminal autoreceptors affect the firing of DA cells and the synthesis and release of DA, respectively.

1. Positive symptoms—The DA hypothesis is one of the oldest biological explanations for schizophrenia and has evolved considerably since its inception. When originally postulated, it was proposed that schizophrenia is due to an excess of DA activity in limbic brain areas, especially the nucleus accumbens, as well as the stria terminalis, lateral septum, and olfactory tubercle (e.g., **mesolimbic dopamine hyperactivity**). This hypothesis was based on evidence that chronic administration of the stimulant D-amphetamine produced a psychosis that resembles paranoid schizophrenia. D-Amphetamine increases the release of DA and norepinephrine (NE) and inhibits their reuptake. Isomers of D-amphetamine with differential effects on the availability of NE and DA in rodents demonstrated increased locomotor activity, an animal model correlate of psychosis in humans. This evidence led to the attribution of an increased release of DA rather than NE as the cause of psychosis.

The second line of evidence relating DA to schizophrenia is that antipsychotic drugs decrease DA activity by receptor depletion (reserpine) and blockade (D_2 antagonists). The most compelling evidence that linked DA to the positive symptoms of schizophrenia was the finding that chlorpromazine was an effective antipsychotic drug and that it blocked DA receptors in vivo, inhibiting the effect of D-amphetamine on locomotor activity. The discovery that several different chemical classes of DA-receptor antagonists are effective as antipsychotic drugs and that there is a high correlation between the drug's average daily dosage and its affinity for the D_2-receptor family led to the view that increased stimulation of these receptors caused schizophrenia. More recently, studies using positron emission tomography (PET) have consistently demonstrated increased availability of presynaptic DA in patients who were acutely ill with psychotic symptoms of schizophrenia.

Table 24–1 Risk Factors for Schizophrenia

Prenatal	Paternal age >50 years at birth Maternal malnutrition Maternal infection: influenza Maternal stress
Perinatal	Obstetric complications
Postnatal	Low birth weight
Childhood	Trauma CNS infections
Adolescence	Cannabis use Stimulant use

2. Negative symptoms and cognitive dysfunction—

The concept of increased DA activity as the core deficit in schizophrenia was developed at the time when delusions and hallucinations were central to the diagnosis of schizophrenia. Emerging evidence from early PET studies demonstrating reduced cerebral blood flow to the frontal cortex and inconsistencies in the cerebrospinal fluid (CSF) levels of DA metabolites in persons with schizophrenia suggested possible region-specific disruptions in DA function. A reduced DA transmission in the prefrontal cortex populated by D_1 receptors (prefrontal hypodopaminergia) emerged as a potential explanation for negative and cognitive symptoms. An increased DA activity in the striatum populated by D_2/D_3 receptors (striatal hyperdopaminergia) found further support as an explanation for the psychotic symptoms of schizophrenia.

3. Limitations of the dopamine hypotheses—One of

the factors that challenges the primacy of DA imbalance at the expense of other transmitter systems stems from a clinical observation. Drugs that act on other transmitter systems, such as hallucinogens (e.g., lysergic acid, psilocybin) and dissociative anesthetics (e.g., phencyclidine, ketamine), also cause psychotic symptoms. Phencyclidine exposure results in a psychotic syndrome that models the psychosis seen in schizophrenia more accurately than amphetamine does.

Furthermore, postmortem studies of patients with schizophrenia have not found consistent abnormalities in the density of any of the five DA receptors or changes in their affinities for DA, with the possible exception of the D_3 receptor, which may have an abnormal form. Several research groups have also reported a link between D_3 polymorphisms and schizophrenia. There is no reliable evidence, from either postmortem studies or PET studies, for an increase in the density of D_2 receptors in schizophrenia. Recent PET studies of the release of DA in the striatum of patients with schizophrenia suggest that the extracellular concentration of DA in this region is increased compared to that in normal subjects. Plasma and CSF levels of homovanillic acid, the major metabolite of DA, are not elevated in patients who have schizophrenia. Some researchers have suggested that DA-receptor sensitization occurs in schizophrenia, but only indirect evidence supports this hypothesis. Taken together, dopaminergic dysfunction as a standalone hypothesis may be insufficient to explain the complete spectrum of schizophrenia pathology, but it does play a significant role potentially through its interaction with the other neurotransmitter systems in the brain.

Abi-Dargham A, Gil R, Krystal J, et al. Increased striatal dopamine transmission in schizophrenia: confirmation in a second cohort. *Am J Psychiatry*. 1998;155:761–767.

Capuano B, Crosby IT, Lloyd EJ. Schizophrenia: genesis, receptorology and current therapeutics. *Curr Med Chem*. 2002;9:521.

Charney DS, Nestler EJ, eds. *Neurobiology of Mental Illness*. 2nd ed. New York: Oxford; 2004.

Heinz A, Romero B, Gallinat J, et al. Molecular brain imaging and the neurobiology and genetics of schizophrenia. *Pharmacopsychiatry*. 2003;36(suppl 3):S152.

Howes OD, Kapur S. The dopamine hypothesis of schizophrenia: version III—the final common pathway. *Schizophr Bull*. 2009; 35(3):549.

Jaskiw GE, Weinberger DR. Dopamine and schizophrenia: a cortically correct perspective. *Semin Neurosci*. 1992;4:179.

Laruelle M. Imaging dopamine transmission in schizophrenia. A review and meta analysis. *Q J Nucl Med*. 1998;42:211–221.

Weinstein JJ, Chohan MO, Slifstein M, et al. Pathway-specific dopamine abnormalities in schizophrenia. *Biol Psychiatry*. 2017; 81(1):31.

B. Serotoninergic Hypothesis

Serotonin (5-HT) neurons originate in the midbrain dorsal and median raphe nuclei, which project to the cortex, striatum, hippocampus, and other limbic regions. There are at least 15 types of 5-HT receptors; of these, the most relevant to schizophrenia are the 5-HT_1, 5-HT_{1D}, 5-HT_2, 5-HT_3, 5-HT_6, and 5-HT_7 receptors. Somatodendritic autoreceptors (of the 5-HT_{1A} type) are present on the cell bodies of 5-HT raphe neurons and inhibit firing of serotonergic neurons. Terminal autoreceptors (5-HT_{1D} in humans) regulate the synthesis and release of 5-HT. 5-HT_3 receptors stimulate DA release. Postsynaptic 5-HT_{2A} receptors are localized on pyramidal neurons in mesocortical areas. The complex interaction between 5-HT and DA varies by brain region and by types of 5-HT and DA receptor.

An early theory of the etiology of schizophrenia was that it is due to an abnormality of brain serotonergic activity. This theory was based on the belief that the psychotomimetic properties of lysergic acid diethyl amide (LSD), an indole compound, are due to its 5-HT blocking properties. This led to a search for endogenous indole hallucinogens in the brain, blood, and urine of patients with schizophrenia. However, the studies that followed did not note an increase in the activity of the enzyme required for the synthesis of these compounds or their metabolites in patients with schizophrenia.

The notion that the effects of LSD and other indole hallucinogens, such as psilocybin and N,N-dimethyltryptamine, provide an adequate model of schizophrenia was also rejected because the primary effect of these drugs is to cause visual hallucinations. The potency of these agents as hallucinogens is highly correlated with their 5-HT_{2A}-receptor affinity. The thought disorder, auditory hallucinations, and bizarre behavior usually present in schizophrenia are generally absent in normal individuals given these agents. However, ingestion of these agents can cause an exacerbation of positive symptoms in patients with schizophrenia.

More selective DA D_2 antagonist drugs are not particularly useful in decreasing the effects of the indole hallucinogens. Antipsychotic drugs such as clozapine, olanzapine, risperidone, quetiapine, sertindole, and lurasidone are potent antagonists of the 5-HT$_{2A}$ receptor. Some of the advantages of these drugs may result from their greater potency as 5-HT$_{2A}$-receptor antagonists, relative to D$_2$-receptor blockade. The most likely advantages of these drugs, related to their higher affinity to 5-HT$_{2A}$ versus DA receptors, are their low D$_2$-induced extrapyramidal symptoms (EPS) profile and their ability to improve negative and cognitive symptoms. However, this explanation has been challenged by several other lines of evidence and partly by the complex interaction of serotonergic network with itself other neurotransmitter systems including DA and acetylcholine. In addition to 5HT$_{2A}$-mediated activity, 5HT$_{2C}$ and 5HT$_{1A}$ receptors also seem to play an important role in the biology of schizophrenia, and many atypical antipsychotics have variable affinities for these receptors. Broadly, antagonism of 5HT$_{2A}$ and 5HT$_{2C}$ receptors and agonism of 5HT$_{1A}$ seem to define the favorable properties of a drug in the treatment of schizophrenia.

Abi-Dargham A, Laruelle M, Aghajanian GK, et al. The role of serotonin in the pathophysiology and treatment of schizophrenia. *J Neuropsychiatry Clin Neurosci.* 1997;9:1.

Capuano B, Crosby IT, Lloyd EJ. Schizophrenia: genesis, receptorology and current therapeutics. *Curr Med Chem.* 2002; 9:521.

Eggers AE. A serotonin hypothesis of schizophrenia. *Med Hypotheses.* 2013;80:79.

Meltzer HY, Fatemi SH. The role of serotonin in schizophrenia and the mechanisms of action of antipsychotic drugs. In: Kane JM, Möller HJ, Awouters F, eds. *Serotonin in Antipsychotic Treatment: Mechanisms and Clinical Practice.* New York: Marcel Dekker; 1996:77–107.

Selvaraj S, Arnone D, Cappai A, Howes O. Alterations in the serotonin system in schizophrenia: a systematic review and meta-analysis of postmortem and molecular imaging studies. *Neurosci Biobehav Rev.* 2014;45:233.

C. Glutamatergic Hypothesis

Clinical and experimental evidence has supported a complex role for glutamate in the etiology of schizophrenia. The original evidence for an abnormality of the glutamatergic system was a decreased level of glutamate in the CSF of patients with schizophrenia. Subsequent studies have revealed decreased expression of glutamatergic receptors, such as the *N*-methyl-D-aspartate (NMDA) and AMPA/kainate receptors. Evidence indicates that decreased glutamatergic activity is the result of decreased levels of glutamate receptors of the NMDA subtype. Consistent with the role of glutamate in schizophrenia, three noncompetitive antagonists of NMDA receptors (phencyclidine [PCP], ketamine, and MK-801) and three competitive antagonists (CPP, CPP-ene, and CGS 19,755) have been shown to induce a range of positive and negative symptoms and cognitive dysfunction in normal control subjects closely mimicking the clinical signs and symptoms of schizophrenia. In contrast to DA agonists that generally only induced positive symptoms of psychosis in healthy individuals, NMDAR antagonists induce positive, negative, and cognitive symptoms resembling those seen in schizophrenia. Furthermore, the administration of NMDAR antagonists has been shown to exacerbate symptoms in patients with schizophrenia.

NMDA receptor function may be central to the pathophysiology of schizophrenia. While early studies revealed decreased expression of glutamatergic receptors, such as the NMDA and AMPA/kainate receptors, the evidence has largely been inconsistent. More recent studies suggest that the primary abnormality in schizophrenia is in NMDA and AMPA receptor trafficking and downstream signaling, rather than the level of global receptor expression. This is reflected in decreased expression of postsynaptic density 95 (PSD95) and of proteins involved in receptor trafficking.

Antipsychotics have been shown to block some of the clinical effects of PCP. In addition, the preclinical effects of PCP, such as disruption of sensory gating, can be blocked by selective 5-HT$_{2A}$-receptor antagonists, such as MDL100,907, and by clozapine. Preliminary studies have shown that compounds that enhance NMDA receptor function (e.g., glycine, D-serine, D-cycloserine, glycine transporter inhibitors) reduce negative and positive symptoms of schizophrenia to some degree when administered in conjunction with typical antipsychotic drugs.

Coyle JT. Glutamate and schizophrenia: beyond the dopamine hypothesis. *Cell Mol Neurobiol.* 2006;26:365–384.

Goff DC, Coyle JT. The emerging role of glutamate in the pathophysiology and treatment of schizophrenia. *Am J Psychiatry.* 2001;158:1367.

Hammond J, Shan D, Meador-Woodruff J, McCullumsmith R. Evidence of glutamatergic dysfunction in the pathophysiology of schizophrenia. In: Popoli M, Diamond D, Sanacora G, eds. *Synaptic Stress and Pathogenesis of Neuropsychiatric Disorders.* New York: Springer; 2014:265–294.

Olney JW, Farber NB. Glutamate receptor dysfunction and schizophrenia. *Arch Gen Psychiatry.* 1995;52:998.

D. GABAergic (Gamma-Aminobutyric Acid) Hypothesis

The major inhibitory neurotransmitter gamma-aminobutyric acid (GABA) has been implicated in the pathophysiology of schizophrenia. Converging lines of evidence indicate that alterations in both presynaptic and postsynaptic components of GABA neurotransmission may contribute to the pathophysiology of schizophrenia. Reduced levels of GAD67 mRNA or a reduced density of neurons positive for GAD67 mRNA in the dorsolateral prefrontal cortex (DLPFC) are one of the most consistent neuropathological findings in schizophrenia. This decrease is likely a consequence of a reduction of GAD67 mRNA in subsets of GABA neurons, including primarily the parvalbumin-containing GABAergic neurons, but also other subclasses of GABAergic neurons. Experiments in mouse models where NMDA receptors were selectively deleted on cortical and hippocampal GABAergic interneurons resulted in phenotypes that correlated with human schizophrenia, suggesting that the NMDA receptor antagonist-mediated psychotic symptoms in otherwise healthy individuals could be mediated by GABA interneurons. These GABA deficits may play a crucial role in the modulation of pyramidal cell firing and the synchronization of cortical activity. Electrophysiologically, this translates to an abnormality in the gamma band oscillation that has been observed in schizophrenia. Experimental evidence suggests that an aberration in the number and/or function of a subtype of parvalbumin-positive GABA interneurons (basket cells) underlies this defect.

Benes FM, Berretta S. Gabaergic interneurons: implications for understanding schizophrenia and bipolar disorder. *Neuropsychopharmacology*. 2001;25:1–27.

Gonzalez-Burgos G, Cho RY, Lewis DA. Alterations in cortical network oscillations and parvalbumin neurons in schizophrenia. *Biol Psychiatry*. 2015;77(12):1031.

Lewis DA, Hashimoto T, Volk DW. Cortical inhibitory neurons and schizophrenia. *Nat Rev Neurosci*. 2005;6:312–324.

Nakazawa K, Zsiros V, Jiang Z, et al. GABAergic interneuron origin of schizophrenia pathophysiology. *Neuropharmacology*. 2012;62:1574–1583.

E. Cannabinoid Hypothesis

The cannabinoid hypothesis of schizophrenia includes exogenous and endogenous components. According to the *exogenous* hypothesis of cannabinoids, exposure to natural (cannabis) and synthetic cannabinoids ("Spice," "K-2") is associated with psychotic states and psychotic disorders. For example, experimental and nonexperimental studies have shown that exposure to natural (cannabis) and synthetic cannabinoids ("Spice," "K-2") can induce a full range of schizophrenia-like transient positive, negative, and cognitive deficits in healthy individuals. In addition, cannabinoids can also transiently induce several psychophysiological effects that are relevant to schizophrenia. Cannabinoids are also known to exacerbate psychotic symptoms, trigger relapse, and negatively impact the course of illness in patients with schizophrenia. Finally, several epidemiological studies suggest that exposure to cannabinoids in adolescence may contribute to the risk (between two- and fourfold) of later developing schizophrenia. Animal studies suggest that exposure to cannabinoids during critical phases of adolescent brain development can have long-lasting effects that persist even after cannabinoids are withdrawn. These studies suggest a mechanism by which exposure to cannabinoids during adolescence can results in a very different path.

Emerging evidence also suggests the presence of abnormalities in the brain endocannabinoid (eCB) system in schizophrenia (i.e., the endogenous hypothesis). Several groups have reported elevated levels of the eCB anandamide in the blood or CSF of patients with schizophrenia. Furthermore, anandamide levels are inversely correlated with psychotic

symptoms and normalize following treatment with antipsychotics and with clinical remission. Reductions in synthesizing enzymes and increased degrading enzymes of eCBs have been reported in the peripheral mononuclear cells of first-episode psychosis patients. The results of postmortem studies of cannabinoid receptors (CB1Rs) have been mixed with studies reporting increases, decreases, or no changes in either CB1R protein or mRNA levels in schizophrenia. Relevant to interpreting eCB abnormalities in schizophrenia, reports on the effects of antipsychotics on CB1R availability are mixed. The results of in vivo brain imaging studies of CB1R availability have also been mixed. These mixed results could be due to differences in methodologies, the regions studied, or the presence of comorbidities in the patient groups.

D'Souza DC, Deepak C, Radhakrishnan R, et al. Cannabinoids and psychosis. *Curr Pharm Des*. 2016;22(42):6380–6391.

Gage SH, Hickman M, Zammit S. Association between cannabis and psychosis: epidemiologic evidence. *Biol Psychiatry*. 2016;79(7): 549–556.

Leweke FM, Rohleder C. Putative role of endocannabinoids in schizophrenia. In: Murillo-Rodríguez E, ed. *The Endocannabinoid System: Genetics, Biochemistry, Brain Disorders, and Therapy*. New York: Academic Press; 2017:83.

Sherif M, Radhakrishnan R, D'Souza DC, Ranganathan M. Human laboratory studies on cannabinoids and psychosis. *Biol Psychiatry*. 2016:79(7):526–538.

F. Immune Dysregulation

Multiple lines of evidence suggest the role of abnormal immune processes in schizophrenia. Ecological studies relying on historical and serological evidence for gestational viral infection exposure during influenza pandemics showed evidence for an association between second-trimester influenza exposure and psychotic outcome in the offspring. However, recent meta-analysis of eight ecological studies concluded that the evidence was insufficient. Studies have also shown an association of schizophrenia with higher rates of antibodies to *Toxoplasma gondii*, herpes simplex virus, type 1 (HSV-1), anti-NMDA antibodies, and antineuronal antibodies. Postmortem studies have been variable, demonstrating an increase, decrease, or no change in inflammatory markers such as glial, astrocytic, microglial markers, and cytokines. Patients with schizophrenia have also been shown to have elevated cytokine levels in peripheral blood samples, both as a state and a trait marker. Some markers such as interleukin 6 (IL-6), tumor necrosis factor α (TNFα), soluble IL-2 receptor (sIL-2R), and IL-1 receptor antagonist (IL-1RA) have been shown to be elevated not just in schizophrenia, but also in BD and major depressive disorder.

Genome-wide association studies (GWAS) of schizophrenia revealed a strong signal at a locus on chromosome 6 that covers the major histocompatibility complex (MHC) region. Subsequent studies indicated that this signal was likely to reflect abnormalities in the complement C4 gene.

Because complement C4 is known to play a role in synaptic pruning and plasticity, this has renewed interest in an inflammatory hypothesis of schizophrenia and implicated the role of glial cells such as microglia, astrocytes and oligodendrocytes.

In-vivo positron imaging tomography imaging studies of microglia, using radioligands that bind to translocator protein, a protein expressed on activated microglia, have been mixed. Whereas the early studies demonstrated evidence for an increased microglial activation in schizophrenia, subsequent studies failed to find any difference. Nevertheless, research into the contribution of immune processes to the pathophysiology of schizophrenia remains an area of active interest.

Kenk M, Selvanathan T, Rao N, et al. Imaging neuroinflammation in gray and white matter in schizophrenia: an in-vivo PET study with [18F]-FEPPA. *Schizophr Bull.* 2015;41(1):85–93.

Radhakrishnan R, Kaser M, Guloksuz S. The link between the immune system, environment, and psychosis. *Schizophr Bull.* 2017;43(4):693–697.

Sekar A, Bialas AR, de Rivera H, et al. Schizophrenia risk from complex variation of complement component 4. *Nature.* 2016; 530(7589):177–183.

Selten JP, Termorshuizen F. The serological evidence for maternal influenza as risk factor for psychosis in offspring is insufficient: critical review and meta-analysis. *Schizophr Res.* 2017:183:2–9.

G. Synaptic Loss and Altered Excitatory/Inhibitory Balance as a Final Common Pathway:

It is now possible to image synaptic vesicles in-vivo using PET ligands specific for synaptic vesicle protein 2A (SV2A). Loss of synaptic spines is the most consistent finding in postmortem studies of schizophrenia. Studies in patients with chronic schizophrenia using [11C]UCB-J, a SV2A PET ligand, have shown reductions in synaptic density across brain regions, including the hippocampus and cortical regions. This reduction was also found to correlate with symptom severity and cognitive performance. Recent genetic studies including GWAS from the Psychiatric Genomics Consortium (PGC-SSZ) and exome sequencing from SCHEMA consortium show a convergence on synaptic function. The highest peak of the Manhattan plot of GWAS at the MHC region of chromosome 6 has been mapped to structural variation of the complement C4A gene. Importantly, C4A has been shown to play a key role in synaptic pruning during adolescence and consistent with this, animal studies with C4A over-expressing mice show a reduction in synaptic spines. It is likely that altered excitatory/inhibitory balance resulting from the loss of synaptic spines contribute to the pathophysiology of schizophrenia. Evidence points to the existence of synaptic pruning during adolescence followed by an age-related decline in synaptic density, with some evidence to suggest that the decline in brain volumes due to aging begins after age 40–50 years. Synaptic loss is also a point of convergence for environmental risks factors such as childhood trauma, stress, cannabis use, and inflammatory processes. The interactive effects of genetic risk, pathological processes, and environmental risk factors on synaptic loss could thus tip the balance below a "synaptic threshold" (or a critical level of excitatory/inhibitory balance) resulting in psychosis-like experiences and schizophrenia.

Howes OD, Onwordi EC. The synaptic hypothesis of schizophrenia version III: a master mechanism. *Mol Psychiatry.* 2023. doi: 10.1038/s41380-023-02043-w. Online ahead of print.

Radhakrishnan R, Skosnik PD, Ranganathan M. In vivo evidence of lower synaptic vesicle density in schizophrenia. *Mol Psychiatry.* 2021;26(12):7690–7698.

Onwordi EC, Halff EF, Whitehurst T. Synaptic density marker SV2A is reduced in schizophrenia patients and unaffected by antipsychotics in rats. *Nat Commun.* 2020;11(1):246.

▶ Structural Brain Abnormalities

A. Gray Matter Abnormalities

Schizophrenia had for long been considered the "graveyard of neuropathologists" because no distinct pathological finding was evident in postmortem brain studies. With advances in neuroimaging technology coupled with newer methods of data analysis and interpretation, this notion has undergone a revision. Structural brain imaging studies have noted enlarged lateral and third ventricles and decreased volume in medial temporal lobe structures in schizophrenia. A recent meta-analysis of 37 studies examining gray matter volume using voxel-based morphometry noted extensive volume reductions in reductions in the bilateral insula/inferior frontal cortex, superior temporal gyrus, anterior cingulate gyrus/medial frontal cortex, thalamus, and left amygdala in patients with schizophrenia when compared to healthy controls. Whereas initial reports indicated a significant decrease of mediodorsal thalamic nucleus volume, subsequent rigorous, larger studies have not replicated the finding of thalamic neuronal loss. The basal ganglia have been studied extensively in schizophrenia, as they constitute one of the projection sites of dopaminergic fibers from the substantia nigra. Although several studies have demonstrated increased striatal DA release (especially during periods of acute psychosis), there is little consistent evidence of a volume abnormality in basal ganglia, cell number, or protein and gene expression.

At the cellular level of cortical organization, abnormalities of cell number, protein expression, and gene expression have been reported. The well-established finding of decreased cortical volume in schizophrenia is not mirrored, as in most neurological disorders, by reports of marked neuronal loss. On the contrary, there is evidence for increased neural cell density in schizophrenia. The volume reduction on the macroscale is attributed to reduction in the neuronal size as well as dendritic and axonal arborization (neuropil density), which is in turn attributed to excessive synaptic pruning during neurodevelopment.

The application of sophisticated methods of protein and gene expression in postmortem brain tissue has provided researchers with the opportunity to study subtle abnormalities of cellular architecture that are not detected by the standard neuropathological examination of brain tissue. Such studies have demonstrated deficits in cortical and hippocampal neurons, such as subtypes of GABAergic neurons in the prefrontal cortex. More recently, studies in animal models of schizophrenia and postmortem studies in humans have demonstrated a disruption in perineuronal nets. These microstructures, composed of components of the extracellular matrix that coats a variety of cells, seem to play a vital role in neuronal migration, formation of neural circuits, and synaptic plasticity.

Longitudinal neuroimaging studies have shown convincingly that the changes in cortical structure are visible at the time of the first episode of schizophrenia, and not simply the effect of longstanding illness or treatment. Furthermore, some studies provide evidence that abnormalities of brain structure can be found in individuals who are at high risk of developing schizophrenia but have not yet become symptomatic. Finally, neuroimaging studies reveal that some of the abnormalities found in schizophrenia are also present in unaffected first-degree relatives.

B. White Matter Abnormalities

Recent studies reveal abnormalities of glial cells and myelinated fiber pathways in schizophrenia. The cellular abnormalities include fewer oligodendroglia and a decreased expression of myelin-related genes. Either abnormality could lead to a disturbance of myelinated fiber pathways in the brain. Neuroimaging studies of fractional anisotropy, a measure of the alignment and organization of fiber bundles in the brain, have indeed revealed such patterns of cortical disconnection. They appear to affect regions in the prefrontal cortex as well as several large-scale networks of brain regions, such as the frontal and tempo-ro-parietal brain regions subserving language function.

The past two decades have seen a surge in neuroimaging studies that examine structural and functional connectivity between the brain regions rather than isolated volumetric abnormality in a localized brain region. Structural connectivity alludes to anatomical connections between defined brain regions, whereas functional connectivity refers to statistically determined functional relations between brain regions. Emerging evidence points to a definite reduction in structural connectivity and aberrant functional connectivity in patients with schizophrenia.

▶ Functional Brain Abnormalities

There is little doubt that the core features of schizophrenia (i.e., the positive and negative symptoms and the significant decline in social functioning) are caused by abnormalities of brain function. The extensive literature on neuropsychological deficits in schizophrenia is supported by more recent reports of the neural basis of such deficits.

A. Neuropsychological Studies

Most patients with schizophrenia show significant deficits on standard neuropsychological tests. Although some investigators have proposed a selective pattern in such deficits (e.g., verbal memory or attention), meta-analyses reveal abnormalities in most aspects of cognition (including neurocognition and social cognition) in schizophrenia. The deficits of cognition are present in the early stages of the illness. Cohort studies of subjects who later develop schizophrenia reveal significant cognitive deficits even before the onset of clinically defined illness. Although cognitive deficits are conceptualized as the core of schizophrenia symptomatology, there is notable heterogeneity in their severity and their influence on functional outcomes.

B. Prefrontal Cortex Function

Behavioral, neuroimaging, and electrophysiological studies have shown convincingly that several functions of the prefrontal cortex are impaired in schizophrenia. These include DLPFC function during the storage as well as the retrieval of information from working memory. Abnormal anterior cingulate cortex function is found when inhibiting responses to sensory stimuli. Decreased activation of the inferior prefrontal cortex has been noted in the learning phase of the verbal learning tasks.

Functional neuroimaging studies using PET and functional magnetic resonance imaging reveal a complex pattern of abnormal DLPFC activation in schizophrenia. Whereas patients show a decreased activation of the DLPFC compared to healthy control subjects (referred to as hypo-frontality) during some cognitive tasks, they show normal or increased DLPFC activation on other tasks. Task performance, which is typically lower in schizophrenia, explains some of these variable patterns. When the performance on tasks of DLPFC function is equilibrated between subjects, subjects with schizophrenia typically show an increased pattern activation. This has been interpreted as a sign of decreased cortical efficiency, because greater DLPFC activation (i.e., more activity in the same number of cortical neurons or the same degree of activity in a larger number of neurons) is required for the same level of task performance. Some have speculated that such patterns could be the result of abnormal dopaminergic modulation of cortical neurons, whereas others have proposed decreased cortical inhibition and impaired cortical synchronization as the cause.

C. Hippocampal Function

Some aspects of hippocampal function during the encoding and retrieval of memory are abnormal in schizophrenia.

There are patterns of increased hippocampal activity at baseline and during passive viewing of stimuli, and a decreased ability to modulate hippocampal responses during the retrieval of previously stored information. The impairment of hippocampal function appears to be particularly pronounced when the relationship between previously learned items must be recalled.

D. Sensory Functions

The reception and integration of sensory information is abnormal in schizophrenia. Extensive electrophysiological literature has documented abnormalities in early sensory processing. These abnormalities involve the thalamic nuclei, the primary sensory cortices, and the multimodal cortices.

E. Other Functions

Several other brain regions, including thalamus, basal ganglia, and cerebellum, have been shown to be impaired during the performance of cognitive tasks in schizophrenia. Recent functional imaging studies have examined the deficits in specific aspects of social cognition in patients with schizophrenia. Notably, abnormal activation patterns in amygdala and other limbic circuits have been demonstrated, especially in the context of negatively valent stimuli.

Bakhshi K, Chance SA. The neuropathology of schizophrenia: aelective review of past studies and emerging themes in brain structure and cytoarchitecture. *Neuroscience* 2015;303:82–102.

Bora E, Fornito A, Radua J, et al. Neuroanatomical abnormalities in schizophrenia: a multimodal voxelwise meta-analysis and meta-regression analysis. *Schizophr Res.* 2011;127:46–57.

Davis KL, Stewart DG, Friedman JI, et al. White matter changes in schizophrenia: evidence for myelin-related dysfunction. *Arch Gen Psychiatry.* 2003;60:443–456.

Gur RE, Gur RC. Functional magnetic resonance imaging in schizophrenia. *Dialogues Clin Neurosci.* 2010;12(3):333–343.

Lewis DA, Lieberman JA. Catching up on schizophrenia: natural history and neurobiology. *Neuron.* 2000;28:325–334.

Sim K, Cullen T, Ongur D, Heckers S. Testing models of thalamic dysfunction in schizophrenia using neuroimaging. *J Neural Transm.* 2006;113:907–928.

Wright IC, Rabe-Hesketh S, Woodruff PW, et al. Meta-analysis of regional brain volumes in schizophrenia. *Am J Psychiatry.* 2000;157:16–25.

► Genetic Hypothesis

Family history of schizophrenia is one of the consistently observed risk factors and is known to increase the lifetime morbid risk for schizophrenia with an inverse relationship to the degree of relatedness (Table 24–2). Family, twin, and adoption studies have successfully demonstrated the significant role of genetic disposition in the occurrence of schizophrenia with an estimated heritability as high as 80%. Heritability is the proportion of phenotypic variance

Table 24–2 Lifetime Expectancy (Morbid Risk) Estimates of Schizophrenia

	Lifetime Expectancy (%)
If no relative has schizophrenia	1
If the following relative has schizophrenia:	
One parent	10
Both parents	46
Sibling	10
Child	6
For twin if cotwin has schizophrenia:	Proband-wise concordance (%)
Dizygotic twin	14
Monozygotic twin	46

accounted for by genetic variation. It refers to variance in the population and does not translate into a straightforward risk assessment for an individual. Furthermore, high heritability does not exclude a role for nongenetic factors and accounts only for an additive etiological model. Despite the high heritability of schizophrenia, the concordance rate in monozygotic twins is only 50%, suggesting the importance of environmental factors. Taken together, there is convincing evidence that a combination of risk genes contributes to the development of schizophrenia.

The exact genetic mechanism underlying the risk for schizophrenia remains elusive to date. Early linkage studies in large loaded families identified several potential candidate regions under the assumption of an "oligogenic" model, i.e., that a limited number of genes contribute to the manifestation of the disorder. The replication of the results in subsequent studies was modest at the best. However, the adoption of fine mapping of the linkage regions has resulted in several intriguing leads. Neuregulin coded by *NRG1* gene on the short arm of chromosome 8 (8p) exemplifies such a discovery. The other linkage hits that have found support in replication studies with positional cloning include dysbindin (*DTNBP1*) gene on 6p22, proline dehydrogenase (*PRODH2*), and catechol-*O*-methyltransferase (*COMT*) on 22q11 and G72/ᴅ-amino acid-oxidase (*DAAO*) on 13q34 (Table 24–3). The proteins coded by these genes play critical roles in important neural pathways such as dopaminergic and glutamatergic transmission and could further serve as potential targets for drug development.

The relatively common occurrence of severe mental illnesses such schizophrenia in the population posits a challenge to the "rare variant oligogenic hypothesis" of genetic etiology, in the absence of evidence for natural selection. Hence, disorders such as schizophrenia, diabetes, and hypertension, which are relatively common, are presumed to be caused by common variants prevalent in the population that, when they come together above a threshold, result in disease expression

Table 24–3 Resources for Schizophrenia Genomics

Study Type	Genetic Risk Targeted and Technology	Selected Resources
Genome-wide association studies	Common variants (MAF > 5%)—representative genome wide microarrays	https://pgc.unc.edu/for-researchers/download-results/
Whole-exome sequencing studies (population scale)	Rare coding variations (MAF < 1% or 0.1%)—whole-exome sequencing	https://schema.broadinstitute.org/
Targeted genetic studies	Targeted sequencing of selected genes, linkage and fine mapping	https://www.omim.org/entry/181500

(the "polygenic threshold model"). GWAS paved the way for exploring the "common disease, common variant" hypothesis. Notably, the results of the most recent publication of the schizophrenia working group of the Psychiatric Genomics Consortium involving 76,755 individuals with schizophrenia and 243,649 controls identified 287 distinct genomic loci and about 120 genes likely to be implicated in disease. This and earlier GWAS have reported significant associations spanning several genes critical not only to neuronal processes such as dopaminergic and glutamatergic transmission but also to several ion-channel- and immune-related functions, neurodevelopment, and synaptic biology.

Despite the apparent success of large-scale GWAS in identifying common variants, they are estimated to explain only a part of the estimated heritability. Recent advances in our ability to sequence entire genomes coupled with falling costs have renewed the interest in decoding the "missing heritability" of schizophrenia. The application of whole-exome (WES) and whole-genome sequencing in schizophrenia is still in its early stages, but the emerging results have renewed interest in the "oligogenic model" of its genetic basis, i.e., limited number of rare variants of large effect-size. One such population scale WES study in 24,248 cases and 97,322 controls identified ultra-rare coding variants in 10 genes that conferred substantial risk for schizophrenia. Majority of the genes identified to carry such variation in cases had important role to play in synaptic function. In summary, individuals with schizophrenia tend to carry a higher burden of rare protein altering variations in evolutionarily conserved genes relevant to brain development and synaptic functioning and this pattern has been observed across ancestries.

The **stress–diathesis model** posits that a biological predisposition toward developing schizophrenia is inherited genetically and that this vulnerability interacts with environmental challenges, which together lead to development of the full syndrome. Several nongenetic factors have been explored, including obstetric, birth, and early childhood complications; season of birth (e.g., during spring and early winter months); exposure to infection; drug use; stressful life events; and societal modernization. The precise contribution of these and other factors to the overall risk of developing schizophrenia is difficult to assess, given the heterogeneity of the disorder, its course, and the wide variety of exposures that individuals with the disorder encounter. It is also possible that these environmental factors exert epigenetic effects that influence gene expression. This is also an area of ongoing research.

Bromet EJ, Fennig S. Epidemiology and natural history of schizophrenia. *Biol Psychiatry*. 1999;46:871.

Brown S, Inskip H, Barraclough B. Causes of excess mortality of schizophrenia. *Br J Psychiatry*. 2000;177:212.

Gulsuner S, Stein DJ, Susser ES, et al. Genetics of schizophrenia in the South African Xhosa. *Science*. 2020;367(6477):569–573.

Haefner H, An der Heiden W. Epidemiology of schizophrenia. *Can J Psychiatry*. 1997;42:139.

Jablensky A. Epidemiology of schizophrenia: aglobal burden of disease and disability. *Eur Arch Psychiatry Clin Neurosci*. 2000;250:274.

Jones P, Cannon M. The new epidemiology of schizophrenia. *Psychiatr Clin North Am*. 1998;21:1.

Kato T. Whole genome/exome sequencing in mood and psychotic disorders: whole genome/exome in mental disorders. *Psychiatry Clin Neurosci*. 2015;69(2):65–76.

Liu D, Meyer D, Fennessy B, et al. Schizophrenia risk conferred by rare protein-truncating variants is conserved across diverse human populations. *Nat Genet*. 2023;55(3):369–376.

McGrath JJ. Myths and plain truths about schizophrenia epidemiology: the NAPE lecture 2004. *Acta Psychiatr Scand*. 2005;111:4–11.

Mortensen PB, et al. Effects of family history and place and season of birth on the risk of schizophrenia. *N Engl J Med*. 1999;340:603.

Owen MJ, Craddock N, O'Donovan MC. Schizophrenia: genes at last? *Trends Genet*. 2005;21:518–525.

Saha S, Chant D, Welham J, McGrath J. A systematic review of the prevalence of schizophrenia. *PLoS Med*. 2005;2:413.

Singh T, Poterba T, Curtis D, et al. Rare coding variants in ten genes confer substantial risk for schizophrenia. *Nature*. 2022;604(7906):509–516.

Stefansson H, Sigurdsson E, Steinthorsdottir V, et al. Neuregulin 1 and susceptibility to schizophrenia. *Am J Hum Genet*. 2002;71(4):877–892.

Trubetskoy V, Pardinas AF, Qi T, et al. Mapping genomic loci implicates genes and synaptic biology in schizophrenia. *Nature*. 2022;604(7906):502–508.

Tsuang MT, Tohen M, eds. *Textbook in Psychiatric Epidemiology*. 2nd ed. New York: Wiley-Liss, 2002.

▶ Clinical Findings

The *Diagnostic and Statistical Manual of Mental Disorders, Fifth Edition* requires at least two of five types of symptoms

(Criterion A) to make a diagnosis of schizophrenia. The four positive symptoms (Criteria A1–A4)—delusions, hallucinations, disorganized speech, and grossly disorganized or catatonic behavior—are considered psychotic symptoms, in that these behaviors, beliefs, and percepts are not considered consistent with normal human experience. The fifth criterion, A5, is negative symptoms characterized by diminished emotional expression or avolition. DSM-5, unlike its previous version DSM IV-TR, does not recognize the subtypes of schizophrenia. However, it allows a specifier "with catatonia" when catatonic symptoms are noted in a patient. The other specifiers that are delineated in DSM-5 include eight course specifiers to be used after 1-year duration of illness.

A. Signs & Symptoms

1. Delusions—Delusions are defined by the DSM-5 as "fixed beliefs that are not amenable to change in light of conflicting evidence" and "false belief based on incorrect inference about external reality that is firmly held despite what almost everyone else believes and despite what constitutes incontrovertible and obvious proof or evidence to the contrary." Most often, delusions have the form of distorted and highly illogical misinterpretations of actual events or experiences (**errors of inference**). In the clinical setting, it can sometimes be difficult to determine if a patient's conviction is so distorted, illogical, and impermeable as to be considered delusional. It is helpful to garner as much detail as possible from the patient about his or her belief(s) in order to uncover errors of inference. Suggesting rational explanations for a patient's belief may elicit a willingness to consider alternatives (less consistent with delusional thought). On the other hand, it may demonstrate that the patient is unwilling or incapable of doing so (more consistent with delusional thought, especially if the belief clearly leads to dysfunctional behavior). Common delusional themes are exemplified in Table 24–4.

2. Hallucinations—Hallucinations are typically prominent, occurring several times a day. They usually appear in the form of one or more voices that keep a running commentary on the patient's everyday activities. They occasionally are unfriendly, insulting, or accusatory. Hallucinations are usually associated with delusions and are consistent with delusional themes. On occasion, voices command patients to perform acts that could result in harm to themselves or others (**command auditory hallucinations**). Only rarely do patients carry out the commands; however, command auditory hallucinations increase risk of suicidal and violent behaviors. Although patients with schizophrenia can experience visual, olfactory, gustatory, somatosensory, viscerosensory, or tactile hallucinations, these types of hallucinatory activity should raise the suspicion of a general medical cause (Table 24–5). The same may generally be said for single auditory hallucinations that occur in the context of cognitive dysfunction and altered sensorium, or in the absence of delusion.

Table 24–4 Common Types of Delusions

Delusions of control: Belief that one's thoughts, feelings, or actions are being controlled or actively manipulated by outside forces or agencies.

Delusions of grandiosity: Belief that one has extraordinary powers, gifts, or abilities that are clearly exaggerated and often bizarre.

Delusions of guilt: Belief that one has committed a terrible act or crime. Often, there is also the belief that transgressions will lead to impossibly terrible outcomes, and that they are deserving of punishment.

Delusions of reference: Belief that actions or remarks of others, or external events, have a significant personal and often private meaning for the patient.

Persecutory delusions: Belief that one is being conspired against or threatened by others, including but not limited to individuals, organizations (such as the FBI), religious figures, or extraterrestrials.

Somatic delusions: Belief that one is carrying a severe disease or other malfunction not supported by medical evidence; often bizarre and attributed to outside forces.

Thought insertion, withdrawal, or broadcasting: Belief that one's own thoughts have been implanted by an outside agency (insertion), that one's thoughts have been taken out of their mind (withdrawal), or that one's thoughts can be read or heard by others via telepathy or other passive means (broadcasting).

3. Disorganized speech, grossly disorganized or abnormal motor behavior, and catatonia—Examples of **disorganized speech** (Criterion A3) **and grossly disorganized or abnormal motor behavior** (Criterion A4) are many,

Table 24–5 Characteristics of Psychiatric Presentations That Raise Suspicion of Medical Etiology*

Atypical age at first symptom onset

Atypical symptom presentation (e.g., does not conform to descriptive diagnostic criteria)

Fluctuations in sensorium

Rapid-onset cognitive impairment

Abnormal vital signs

History of chronic general medical problems or use of substances that cause psychotic symptoms

Recent deterioration or change in physical health status coincident with onset of psychotic symptoms

History of significant polypharmacy, including use of over-the-counter preparations

Abnormal body habitus, neurological examination

Absence of personal or family history of psychiatric illness

Atypical or absence of response to established treatment(s)

*No single factor alone can establish an organic cause for psychiatric symptoms. A thorough evaluation taking into account history from the patient and collateral informants, available medical records, physical and neurological examination, appropriate laboratory and neurodiagnostics, and clinical observation is required.

Table 24–6 Disorganized/Catatonic Speech and Behavior

Speech

Circumstantiality: Speech that is goal directed but excessive in unneeded detail. Questions are eventually answered; however, direct answers are difficult to come by.

Tangentiality: Speech that begins in a goal-directed manner but deviates gradually and consistently such that answers to questions are not reached. New topics arise from the topic previously under discussion, so an association between thoughts can be appreciated.

Derailment: Speech that begins in a goal-directed manner, but topics shift rapidly between sentences with no logical connection to the topic previously under discussion.

Illogicality: Speech that is goal directed but gives illogical responses to logical questions, or bases assertions on premises that have no logical or coherent basis.

Concrete speech: Speech that reflects an inability to use abstract thinking, which may bring about literal interpretations of proverbs during mental status examination, or a pattern of speech that conveys little to no information due to use of excessively vague or meaningless phrases (**verbigeration**).

Incoherence: Incomprehensible speech due to loss of logical connections between words, phrases, and sentences, the extreme form of which is termed **word salad**.

Clanging: Words are used based on how they sound rather than what they mean.

Neologism: Use of nonsensical words, often as a combination of parts of two or more different words.

Thought blocking: Sudden and involuntary interruption in the progress of speech or thought.

Behavior

Unprovoked outbursts of laughter or other emotions

Unprovoked outbursts of hyperactive, agitated, or violent behavior

Inappropriate social behaviors

Severe neglect of hygiene or bizarreness of choice in clothing and general appearance

Table 24–7 Selected Catatonic Signs

Psychomotor Signs

Excitement: Extreme but purposeless hyperactivity

Stupor: Extreme hypoactivity or immobility with little if any responsiveness to external stimuli

Staring

    Maintaining postures for long periods without reacting

    Maintaining odd facial expressions (several seconds to several minutes)

Echopraxia

    Stereotypies: Repetitive but purposeless (non–goal-directed) activity

Rigidity

    Mannerisms: Purposeful movements executed in an odd or exaggerated manner

    Negativism: Purposeless resistance to instructions or efforts at being moved

Waxy flexibility

    Refusal to eat, drink, and/or make eye contact

    Sudden and inappropriate behaviors, with no apparent provocation (including combativeness)

    Perseveration: Repeatedly returns to same movement or motor activity

Speech

Mutism: Absent or minimal verbal responses

Echolalia

    Verbigeration: Aimless repetition of phrases or sentences

    Perseveration: Repeatedly returns to same topic

Other

Primitive reflexes

Autonomic hyperactivity

as summarized in Table 24–6. In general, disorganized speech is believed to reflect an underlying impairment in thought processes—that is, the inability to process stimuli accurately and link thoughts or ideas in a coherent and logical manner. Alternatively referred to as **thought disorder**, these clinical signs are believed by many to be the cardinal feature of schizophrenia and to be more closely associated with functional disability than positive symptoms are. **Grossly disorganized or abnormal motor behavior** may manifest itself in a variety of ways, ranging from difficulty performing goal-directed behaviors and activities of daily living to child-like "silliness" and unpredictable agitation. As is the case with speech, for a behavior to be considered disorganized, it must result in significant impairment and be obvious to casual observers. Organized behaviors that occur in response to delusions are not considered to be "disorganized." **Catatonia**

refers to a marked decrease in reactivity to the environment. **Catatonic behaviors** (Table 24–7) are found in other mental disorders, medical conditions, and drug toxicity. They warrant immediate medical evaluation if of new onset.

4. Negative symptoms—The fifth group of symptoms (Criterion A5) is referred to as **negative symptoms** because they represent deficits of normal function and are not psychotic, per se (Table 24–8). It is generally accepted that there are **primary and secondary negative symptoms**, the former of which represent longstanding illness features that persist between psychotic episodes and may even predate the onset of psychotic symptoms. Primary negative symptoms tend to respond less well to drug treatment and cause more dysfunction than positive symptoms. Secondary negative symptoms are believed to stem from side effects of medication, from depression or demoralization associated with the illness, or as a reaction to psychotic symptoms. Secondary negative symptoms may not persist and can respond to treatment of the underlying cause.

5. Diagnostic threshold—The diagnostic threshold put forth by the DSM-5 calls for two or more symptoms from Criteria A1–A5. DSM-5 does not recognize the importance

Table 24–8 Negative Symptoms of Schizophrenia

Affective flattening: Absence of outward emotional reaction to stimuli. There is a decrease in or absence of spontaneous movement, expressive gestures, eye contact, shifts in vocal inflections

Avolition: Lack of motivation for initiating or completing tasks, reflective of a loss of drive and of interest in one's surroundings

Alogia: Decrease in the production and fluency of spontaneous speech (but not refusal to speak), which is believed to reflect poverty of thought. Abnormalities may also include prolonged pauses before answering questions

Anhedonia: Diminished or absent capacity to experience pleasure

Attention deficits: Inability to maintain engagement in a goal-directed activity or task

Social withdrawal, diminished capacity to feel close to others

of **bizarre delusions** (i.e., completely implausible beliefs), or the auditory hallucinations of a voice keeping a **running commentary** on the subject's daily activities, or **two or more voices conversing** with each other, as standalone criteria for the diagnosis of schizophrenia.

Even though the foregoing symptoms are not necessarily present in all patients with schizophrenia, many patients express these symptoms at one time or another. The clinical manifestations of the illness as described above can vary greatly in intensity over time in a particular patient. The DSM-5 requires that the symptoms result in significant **functional impairment** in work, relationships, self-care, or other life domains. The symptoms must be present in one form or another (e.g., prodromal or residual symptoms) for a period of 6 months or greater, but with at least 1 month of fully expressed, active symptoms as described in Criterion A. The signs and symptoms should not be better accounted for by another psychiatric disorder, general medical illnesses, or the effects of substances (see section "Differential Diagnosis" later).

6. Other clinical features—Mild neurologic deficits are often present in schizophrenia: abnormal body movements, gait, mannerisms, or reflexes; increased or decreased muscle tone; abnormal rapid eye movements (saccades); frequent blinking; dysdiadochokinesis; astereognosis; and poor right–left discrimination.

Cognitive dysfunction is a cardinal feature of schizophrenia. On average, the intelligence quotient (IQ) of patients with schizophrenia, when first diagnosed with the disorder, is 10 points lower than comparison groups, including unaffected siblings or co-twins. Children at risk of schizophrenia have lower IQs than do control subjects with abnormalities in attention and concentration. Patients in their first episode of schizophrenia exhibit impairments in attention, working memory, visual–spatial memory, semantic memory, recall memory, and executive function.

The diverse nature of the cognitive disturbance in schizophrenia suggests that the disturbance is based on diffuse rather than localized brain disease. With treatment, that impairment might improve slightly, but there is little evidence that antipsychotic drugs, with the exception of clozapine, have a significant effect on the cognitive disturbance in schizophrenia. Cognitive impairment is often independent of positive and negative symptoms and even of disorganization. Over the course of the illness, a small percentage of patients with schizophrenia experience a great deterioration in cognition and reach the levels of impairment of patients with senile psychosis, such as Alzheimer disease. The majority of patients with schizophrenia do not exhibit such marked dilapidation of cognitive function. Cognitive disturbance plays a major role in limiting the social life and occupational performance of patients with schizophrenia. For this reason, therapies that reverse cognitive disturbance in schizophrenia will be of immense value.

American Psychiatric Association. *Diagnostic and Statistical Manual of Mental Disorders.* 5th ed. Arlington, VA: American Psychiatric Association; 2013.

B. Psychological Testing

The usefulness of **projective** and **personality tests** in the diagnosis of schizophrenia may be limited because, although these tests identify bizarre ideations and abnormal personality traits, respectively, they are prone to unreliable, subjective interpretation. **Neuropsychological testing** may be useful in establishing a cognitive pretreatment baseline but not for diagnosis. Furthermore, neuropsychological testing may help guide targeted cognitive remediation.

Lesak MD, Howieson DB, Loring DW, eds. *Neuropsychological Assessment.* Oxford, UK: Oxford University Press; 2004.

C. Laboratory & Neuroimaging Findings

No laboratory or neuroimaging findings are considered pathognomonic for schizophrenia. The utility of these investigations is therefore limited to the ruling out of nonpsychiatric etiologies for psychotic presentations (discussed later). Some findings have been replicated and have shed light on neuropathological processes that may eventually be found to characterize schizophrenia.

1. Cerebral ventricular enlargement—Despite the large body of supportive imaging studies, ventricular enlargement is not present in all patients with schizophrenia and is not specific for schizophrenia. For example, ventricular enlargement and increased sulcal prominence can also be observed in patients with mood disorders.

2. Structural and functional brain abnormalities—A number of brain abnormalities have been identified with neuroimaging (reviewed earlier). However, none of the findings reported so far have achieved the status of a diagnostic test. There is an emerging literature on the longitudinal aspects of brain changes in schizophrenia. Such studies will be helpful in gaining a better understanding of the differences in disease outcome and treatment response.

▶ Course of Illness

A. Onset & Natural Course

1. Onset—The **onset** of the disorder is quite variable. The peak age at onset for the first psychotic episode is in the early to mid-20s for males and in the late 20s for females. Although onset can be abrupt, classically, it is insidious, with a **prodromal** phase of varying duration that predates the first psychotic break. The prodromal phase is generally considered the first of **three phases** of schizophrenia (prodromal, active, and residual phases). During this time, patients may evidence gradually increasing social withdrawal, poor motivation, restricted affective range, cognitive difficulties, and increasingly odd behavior. These changes are subthreshold for a diagnosis of schizophrenia. For others, the onset can be quite rapid, evolving over a period of weeks.

2. Course—**Active-phase** symptoms emerge following the prodrome (referred to as a "first psychotic break" or "first-episode schizophrenia") often in the context of significant life stress or substance use. Treatment may begin after a variable period of time, referred to as the **duration of untreated psychosis**. There is considerable evidence that the longer the duration of untreated psychosis, the poorer the response to treatment, though not all studies are in agreement. After initiation of treatment, pooled data analysis suggests that about one-third of patients with first-episode schizophrenia have a benign **illness course** (i.e., they fully or nearly fully recover, with minimal or no impairment), while the remainder have either an intermediate or poor outcome.

The **residual phase** is characterized by persisting schizophrenia symptoms. Of the two-thirds of patients who do not achieve full or nearly full recovery during active-phase treatment, approximately half experience a stable course without further deterioration, but significant residual deficits remain. The remaining group of patients with poor treatment outcome often exhibit progressive deterioration. Thus, the level of psychopathology and impairment during the residual phase can vary considerably. In general, the more incomplete the symptom recovery, the more likely the patient is to function poorly and relapse in the future. Relative to positive symptoms, negative symptoms and cognitive deficits are less responsive to medication.

3. Early-onset, very-early-onset, late-onset, and very-late-onset disease—Most older patients with schizophrenia have had an onset of illness during early adulthood, that is, adult-onset schizophrenia (AOS). A small proportion of cases manifest as early-onset schizophrenia (EOS) (onset before age 18 years but after the age of 13 years), or very-early-onset schizophrenia (VEOS; also called "childhood-onset schizophrenia"; onset before the age of 13 years). EOS and VEOS differ from AOS in the following: insidious onset; more severe premorbid neurodevelopmental abnormalities; more frequent visual hallucinations; higher rate of inappropriate or blunted affects; higher rate of familial psychopathology; poorer response to treatment; and poorer outcome. About 20% of patients manifest psychotic symptoms for the first time during middle (**late-onset**, after age 45 years) or old age (**very-late-onset**, after age 65 years). In general, the clinical symptoms of AOS and late-onset schizophrenia are similar, though some important differences characterize late-onset illness. These include higher prevalence among women, less severe negative symptoms and cognitive impairment, the predominance of paranoid delusions, and lower dose requirement for antipsychotic medication.

Driver DI, Gogtay N, Rapoport JL. Childhood onset schizophrenia and early onset schizophrenia spectrum disorders. *Child Adolesc Psychiatr Clin N Am.* 2013;22(4):539–555.

Hafner H, an der Heiden W. Epidemiology of schizophrenia. *Can J Psychiatry.* 1997;42:139.

Harrison G, Hopper K, Craig T, et al. Recovery from psychotic illness: a 15- and 25-year international follow-up study. *Br J Psychiatry.* 2001;178:506.

Howard R, Rabins PV, Seeman MV, et al. Late-onset schizophrenia and very-late-onset schizophrenia-like psychosis: an international consensus. *Am J Psychiatry.* 2000;157:172.

Margari F, Presicci A, Petruzzelli MG, et al. Very early onset and greater vulnerability in schizophrenia: a clinical and neuroimaging study. *Neuropsychiatr Dis Treat.* 2008;4(4):825–830.

McGrath J, Saha S, Chant D, Welham J. Schizophrenia: a concise overview of incidence, prevalence, and mortality. *Epidemiol Rev.* 2008;30:67–76.

Perkins DO, Gu H, Boteva K, Lieberman JA. Relationship between duration of untreated psychosis and outcome in first-episode schizophrenia: a critical review and meta-analysis. *Am J Psychiatry.* 2005;162:1785.

▶ Differential Diagnosis

A detailed workup, often in the context of the safety and structure afforded by psychiatric hospitalization, is necessary, especially at the first onset of psychotic symptoms. Serial patient interviews and additional history from collateral sources (e.g., prior medical records, collateral informants) are required.

A. Secondary Etiologies of Psychotic Symptoms

Most reversible secondary causes of psychosis (Table 24–9) can be ruled out on the basis of a meticulous history, mental status examination, physical and neurological examination, and appropriate laboratory and neurodiagnostic

Table 24–9 Selected Secondary Causes of Psychotic Symptoms

CNS infections
  Viral
    Herpes, Mumps, Mononucleosis
  Bacteria
    Syphilis
  Parasitic
    Schistosomiasis, trypanosomiasis
Substance related
  Medications
    Anticholinergic drugs
    Prodopaminergic agents
    Antimalarials
    Antiparkinson drugs
    Antihypertensives
    Antituberculous agents
    Over-the-counter stimulants (ephedrine, phenylephrine, pseudoephedrine)
    Methylphenidate, psychostimulants
    Corticosteroids
    Certain antiarrhythmics (digitalis, procainamide)
  Agents of abuse
    Hallucinogens
    Cannabis
    Psychostimulants
    Dissociative anesthetics (phencyclidine, ketamine, dextromethorphan)
Withdrawal states (alcohol, sedative–hypnotic, psychostimulant)
Acute cardiovascular
  Anoxia, any cause
Metabolic
  Hypoglycemia, hyponatremia, hypercalcemia
  Hepatic or uremic encephalopathy, postdialysis state
  Porphyria
  Postoperative state
Traumatic brain injury
Other CNS pathology
  Demyelinating (e.g., multiple sclerosis)
Primary dementing disorders
  Alzheimer disease, Pick disease
  Dementia with Lewy bodies
Epilepsy
Cerebrovascular disease
Space occupying lesions
  Malignancy, abscesses
Endocrine
  Hypo- or hyperthyroidism
  Hypo- or hyperadrenalism
  Hypo- or hyperparathyroidism
  Postpartum psychosis
Connective tissue disorders
  Systemic lupus erythematosus, temporal arteritis Sarcoidosis
Toxicological (drug overdose, heavy metal poisoning)
Nutritional
  Deficiency in thiamine, vitamin B_{12}, folate, niacin

Table 24–10 Suggested Diagnostic Workup for First-Break Psychotic Symptoms

Serial (repeated) histories from patient and collateral informants
Thorough review of all available medical records
Complete physical and neurological examinations
Routine laboratory tests
  Electrolytes, blood urea nitrogen, creatinine
  Glucose
  Complete blood count, with differential
  Thyroid panel
  Liver function tests
  Syphilis screening (VDRL, etc.)
  Vitamin B_{12}, folate levels
  HIV screen (if indicated)
  Urine drug/toxicology screen, blood alcohol level
  Routine urinalysis
Other laboratory tests to consider
  Pregnancy test
  Serum drug levels
  Lumbar puncture for CSF analysis
  Coagulation studies
Radiographic tests to consider
  Indications for cranial CT or MRI
    Previously unevaluated psychotic symptoms
    New onset cognitive deficits
    Atypical psychotic presentation
      Nonauditory hallucinations
      Rapid onset
      Onset age > 50 years
      Altered/fluctuating sensorium
      Focal neurological deficits or soft signs
      History of recent head injury
    Electroconvulsive therapy being considered
  Chest X-ray (geriatric patients)
Electroencephalogram (as clinical situation warrants)

testing (Table 24–10). Some general clinical guidelines can be applied to the raising of suspicion of an organic etiology for psychotic symptoms. They must always be followed by adequate clinical assessment.

Secondary etiologies of altered mental status presenting with psychotic symptoms include temporal lobe epilepsy, anti-NMDA receptor encephalitis, Hashimoto encephalopathy, Graves disease, steroid-responsive encephalopathy associated with autoimmune thyroiditis, hypothyroidism, Wilson disease, neurosyphilis, adrenocortical insufficiency (Addison disease), hypercortisolism (Cushing syndrome), acute intermittent porphyria, Huntington chorea, dementia with Lewy bodies, Creutzfeldt–Jakob disease, HIV, and vitamin B_{12} deficiency. Other disorders associated with high rates of psychosis include Down syndrome, 22q11.2 deletion syndrome or velocardiofacial syndrome, and autism spectrum disorders.

B. Psychiatric Disorders That Present with Psychotic (or Psychotic-Like) Symptoms

1. Other psychotic disorders—In differentiating schizophrenia from other psychotic disorders, the duration of symptoms must be accurately assessed. **Schizophreniform disorder** involves prodromal, active-phase, and residual symptoms identical to those of schizophrenia, but the total duration of illness is less than 6 months before full recovery. It should be noted, however, that whereas about one-third of patients fully recover within 6 months and retain a diagnosis of schizophreniform disorder, two-thirds eventually progress to schizophrenia or schizoaffective disorder. With **brief psychotic disorder**, psychotic symptoms endure for less than 1 month before full recovery. **Delusional disorder** is distinguished by its later age of onset (35–50 years) and the persistence of nonbizarre delusions in the absence of hallucinations, disorganized thoughts or behaviors, and negative symptoms. Patients with delusional disorder do not typically manifest the degree of functional incapacity observed among patients with schizophrenia and do not experience significant changes in cognition. Therefore, delusional disorder is a very difficult diagnosis to recognize in the clinical setting.

2. Substance/medication-induced psychotic disorder—History of recent use of drugs of abuse, such as alcohol, marijuana, synthetic cannabinoids, amphetamine, methamphetamine, cocaine, hallucinogens, opioids, Ecstasy (MDMA), LSD, PCP, "bath salts" (cathinones), other synthetic psychoactive "designer" drugs, or prescription medications such as steroids, amphetamine, digoxin, disulfiram, or varenicline should raise the possibility of a substance/medication-induced psychotic disorder. A negative urine drug screen may not be sufficient to rule out the diagnosis, because many of the newer "designer" drugs of abuse are not detectable on standard drug screens. Substance/medication-induced psychotic disorders usually resolve following 4 weeks of abstinence from the offending substance/medication, although in rare cases a prolonged psychotic disorder indistinguishable from schizophrenia may emerge.

3. Mood disorders with psychotic features—In distinguishing between **mood disorders (bipolar I disorder and major depression)** with psychotic features, **schizoaffective disorders (bipolar or depressed subtype)** and schizophrenia, it is helpful to determine whether the mood and psychotic symptoms occurred simultaneously, whether the psychotic symptoms persisted at any point independent of mood symptoms, and whether the mood symptoms were brief relative to the total period of the disturbance. In mood disorder with psychotic features and schizoaffective disorder, psychotic symptoms occur at the same time as mood symptoms; however, in schizoaffective disorder, psychotic symptoms exist independently of mood changes for at least 2 weeks (and often longer). For mood disorders with psychotic features, psychotic symptoms do not persist apart from mood dysfunction. Another important distinction between mood disorder and schizophrenia is that, after resolution of acute mood and psychotic symptoms, there is a return to normal functioning. Patients with schizophrenia rarely return to baseline functioning, and each subsequent psychotic relapse may result in progressive deficits.

4. Personality disorders—Individuals with personality disorders may be suspicious and hypervigilant (**paranoid personality disorder**), with marked eccentricities of appearance and behavior, perceptual distortions, and diminished capacity for close relationships (**schizotypal personality disorder**). They may evidence an incapacity for relationships of any kind and extreme isolation (**schizoid personality disorder**). Individuals with cluster B personality disorders and those with **borderline personality disorder** are prone to severe stress-induced paranoia and hallucinations, which may be difficult to distinguish from a primary psychotic disturbance on the basis of only one clinical encounter. However, personality disorders have mild relative symptoms compared to those observed among patients with schizophrenia, and the symptoms have been present throughout the patient's lifetime. Rarely do those with personality disorder present with prominent hallucinations or frank delusions. They also lack chronic negative symptoms or disorganization.

5. Anxiety disorders—Patients with **posttraumatic stress disorder (PTSD)** are prone to severe hallucination-like symptoms and fearful (paranoid) behavior; however, patients with PTSD usually retain insight in to the nature of their disturbances, which are inextricably linked to exposure to past traumatic event(s). Insight is typically preserved in **obsessive–compulsive disorder (OCD)**, even though uncontrollable intrusive thoughts and compulsive mental or physical rituals can mimic psychosis. A rare subtype of OCD is characterized by poor insight; however, these disorders do not feature negative or disorganization symptoms and are not associated with the same degree of functional incapacity as the typical patient with schizophrenia.

6. Other disorders—Patients with **hypochondriasis** or **body dysmorphic disorder** are convinced of the presence of an occult disease or bodily defect in the absence of objective evidence to support their belief(s). The absence of hallucinations and disorganization symptoms, and exclusively somatically circumscribed preoccupations, quickly distinguish these disorders from schizophrenia.

C. Differential Diagnosis of Negative Symptoms

The workup of a patient who presents with prominent negative symptoms must be especially thorough. Many conditions, some very serious, can mimic the negative symptoms of schizophrenia. These include malignant catatonia, delirium, frontal lobe injury, intracranial space-occupying lesions (e.g., tumors), substance abuse, hypothyroidism, severe depression, bipolar mania (catatonic presentation), parkinsonism (idiopathic or antipsychotic-induced), and antipsychotic-induced akinesia.

American Psychiatric Association. *Diagnostic and statistical manual of mental disorders*, 5th ed. (DSM-5). Washington, DC: American Psychiatric Association, 2013.

Fiorentini A, Volonteri LS, Dragogna F, et al. Substance-induced psychoses: a critical review of the literature. *Curr Drug Abuse Rev*. 2011;4(4):228–240.

Fraser S, Hides L, Philips L, et al. Differentiating first episode substance induced and primary psychotic disorders with concurrent substance use in young people. *Schizophr Res*. 2012; 136(1–3):110–115.

Goff DC, Freudenreich O, Henderson DC. Psychotic patients. In: Stern TA, Fricchione GL, Cassem NH, et al., eds. *Handbook of General Hospital Psychiatry*. Philadelphia: Mosby; 2004:37–48.

Marsh CM. Psychiatric presentations of medical illness. *Psychiatr Clin North Am*. 1997;20:181.

Schooler NR. Deficit symptoms in schizophrenia: negative symptoms versus neuroleptic-induced deficits. *Acta Psychiatr Scand Suppl*. 1994;380:21.

Siris SG. Depression in schizophrenia: perspective in the era of "Atypical" antipsychotic agents. *Am J Psychiatry*. 2000;157:1379.

Whiteford HA, Peabody CA. The differential diagnosis of negative symptoms in chronic schizophrenia. *Aust N Z J Psychiatry*. 1989;23:491.

▶ Treatment

The modern treatment of schizophrenia has as its broad **goals** the reduction of symptoms and the maximization of functioning. To achieve this, several **treatment targets** have been identified, including (1) positive symptoms, (2) negative symptoms, (3) conceptual disorganization, (4) neurocognitive deficits, and (5) anxious/depressive symptoms and suicidality. The situation is more complicated in cases of comorbid substance abuse or severe physical morbidity, both of which are common among patients with schizophrenia. In addition, improvements in positive symptoms do not always result in improved functioning in relationships, work capacity, and other important life domains. Therefore, a number of treatment modalities—both pharmacological and nonpharmacological—must be utilized.

Generally, **positive symptoms** such as hallucinations and delusions, as well as **disorganized speech and behavior** and psychotic **agitation**, respond well to antipsychotic drug treatment. Though dramatic in appearance and potentially dangerous to the patient and others, the severity of positive symptoms does not appear to correlate significantly with long-term functioning.

By contrast, **negative symptoms** such as anhedonia, affective flattening, alogia, avolition, and social withdrawal are far more difficult to treat pharmacologically and are robust predictors of long-term functional incapacity. Both first-generation ("typical") antipsychotic medications, such as haloperidol and perphenazine, and second-generation ("atypical") antipsychotic drugs have limited efficacy in treating negative symptoms.

Cognitive function is severely impaired for most patients with schizophrenia. Patients demonstrate neuropsychological deficits in a broad array of domains; however, impairments in executive skills, working memory, verbal skills, and learning and memory are especially severe. Cognitive impairment has important consequences for everyday functioning and is a critical determinant of capacity for work, social functioning, and independent living. Not surprisingly, cognitive impairment is an important therapeutic target, based on the rationale that improvements in cognitive function will lead to subsequent improvement in functional status.

An underappreciated phenomenon is the severity and pervasiveness of **depression and anxiety** symptoms associated with schizophrenia. Depression in schizophrenia is very common and is often observed during acute psychotic episodes or shortly after their resolution (i.e., **post-psychotic depression**). Over time, they tend to re-occur and persist independently of positive symptoms and may occur at any stage of the illness. By the same token, **suicidal behavior**, also common among patients with schizophrenia, has become an independent treatment target.

A. Psychopharmacologic Interventions

Antipsychotic drugs are the treatment of choice for patients with schizophrenia. There are two broad classes of antipsychotic drugs: the **first-generation** (a.k.a., "typical") antipsychotic drugs (first-generation antipsychotics [FGAs]) that were available on the market before 1990, and the second-generation (a.k.a., "atypical") antipsychotics (second-generation antipsychotics [SGAs]) (Table 24–11) that were generally available on the market after 1990. What follows is a description of each of these broad classes, followed by guidelines for choosing antipsychotic medications and for their clinical use in treating schizophrenia during the acute phase and long-term treatment.

1. Second-generation antipsychotics (SGAs)—The SGAs are also known as "atypical" antipsychotic drugs because they have antipsychotic effects at doses that produce less acute EPS and have a lower but not absent risk of tardive dyskinesia. The prototypical atypical antipsychotic drug is clozapine, a dibenzodiazepine, which was first identified in 1959. After the hypothesis was advanced that its atypicality was due to a weak D_2-receptor blockade coupled to potent serotonin (5-HT_{2A}) antagonism (**mechanism of action**) several other atypical antipsychotic drugs were developed that shared this mechanism, including risperidone, olanzapine, quetiapine, ziprasidone, paliperidone, lurasidone, asenapine, iloperidone, and lumateperone. Some SGAs have additional mechanisms of action in addition to 5-HT_{2A} and D_2 antagonism such as 5-HT_{1A} agonism (lurasidone, asenapine), 5-HT_{2A} antagonism combined with D_2 and D_3 partial agonism (cariprazine), and 5-HT_{2A} receptor antagonism combined with

Table 24–11 Drugs Used in the Treatment of Schizophrenia

	Potency	Oral Starting Dose (mg)	Oral Target Dose Range (mg/day)	Motor Side Effects	Endocrine (Prolactinemia)	Hypotension	Anticholinergic	Sedation	Weight	Metabolic Dysfunction	Miscellaneous	Dosage Strengths	Other Formulations
First Generation Antipsychotics (FGAs)													
Chlorpromazine (Thorazine)	Lo	50 BID	400–1000	Lo	+++	+++	+++	Hi	+++	+		10, 25, 50, 100, 200 mg tablets	25 mg/mL inj.
Loxapine (Loxitane)		20 BID	60–100	+	++	++	+		±↓	±		5, 10, 25, 50 mg capsules	10 mg inhal. powder
Perphenazine (Trilafon)		4–8 BID	24–48		++	+	+		++	±		2, 4, 8, 16 mg tablets	—
Thiothixene (Navane)		5–10 QD	10–60		++	+	+		±	±	Rare lens pigmentation, long ½ life	1, 2, 5, 10 mg capsules	—
Trifluoperazine (Stelazine)		2–5 BID	10–30		++	+	+		±	±		1, 2, 5, 10 mg tablets	—
Fluphenazine (Prolixin)		2–5 BID	5–20		+++	+	+		+	±	Depot: 25–75 mg q 2 weeks	1, 2.5, 5, 10 mg tablets	5 mg/mL oral sol, 2.5 mg/mL inj. & 25 mg/mL depot
Haloperidol (Haldol)		2–5 BID	5–20		+++	+	+		+	±	Depot: 100–200 mg q 4 weeks	0.5, 1, 2, 5, 10, 20 mg tablets	2 mg/mL oral sol, 5 mg/mL inj. & 50, 100 mg/mL depot
Pimozide (Orap)		1–2 QD	2–8	Hi	+++	+	+	Lo	+	±	↑QTc—monitor EKG and K$^+$, CYP3A & 1A2, long ½ life	1, 2 mg tablets	—
Second-Generation Antipsychotics (SGAs)													
Quetiapine (Seroquel)	Lo	50–100 BID	400–1000	↕	↕	++	+	+++	++	++	SE: activation, insomnia, Should be taken WITH food	25, 50, 100, 200, 300, 400 mg tablets	50, 150, 200, 300, 400 mg extended release tablets
Ziprasidone (Geodon)		20 BID	160–320	+	↕	+	↕	↕	↕	↕	Dose dependent increase in SE, should be taken WITH food. CYP3A4 interaction	20, 40, 60, 80 mg capsules	20 mg inj.
Lurasidone (Latuda)		40 QD	40–80	↕	↕	+	↕	++	±	↕	On Formulary only for Bipolar Depression	20, 40, 60, 80, 120 mg tablets	—
Olanzapine (Zyprexa)		5–10 QD	10–40	±	↕	+	+	++	+++	+++	LAI: 210 or 300 mg q 2 weeks, 405 mg q 4 weeks	2.5, 5, 7.5, 10, 15, 20 mg tablets	10 mg inj., 210, 300, 405 mg LAI, 5, 10, 15, 20 mg ODT
Lumateperone (Caplyta)		42 QD	42	↕	↕	+	↕	+	↕	↕	SE: sedation, dry mouth, headache, EPS	10.5, 21, 42 mg capsules	—
Aripiprazole (Abilify)		10–15 QD	10–45	+	↕	+	↕	↕	+	↕	SE: activation, insomnia, nausea, vomiting LAI (once-monthly): 400 mg q 4 weeks LAI (lauroxil): maintenance doses = 441–882 mg q 4 weeks, 882 mg q 6 weeks, or 1064 mg q 8 weeks	2, 5, 10, 15, 20, 30 mg tablets	300, 400 mg LAI (once-monthly), 441, 662, 882 mg LAI (lauroxil), 9.75 mg/1.3 mL inj., & 10, 15 mg ODT, 1mg/mL oral sol
Brexpiprazole (Rexulti)		0.5–1 QD	2–3	+	↕	↕	↕	+	↕	↕	SE: dizziness, akathisia, headache, constipation, fatigue. Titrate dose in 7-day intervals until initial target dose of 2 mg is reached.	0.25, 0.5, 1, 2, 3, 4 mg tablets	Titration pack available
Iloperidone (Fanapt)		1 BID titrated slowly	6–12 BID	↕	↕	+++	↕	++	+	↕	SE: dizziness, somnolence, dyspepsia, dry mouth. Gradually titrate over 1 week and dose BID to avoid orthostatic hypotension. Kit available to determine CYP2D6 genotype.	1, 2, 4, 6, 8, 10, 12 mg tablets	Titration pack available

Drug								SE	Oral forms	LAI / other
Cariprazine (Vraylar)	1.5 QD	3-6	+	↔	+	↔	+	↔	SE: EPS, dizziness, blurred vision, balance problems	1.5, 3, 4.5, 6 mg capsules	
Paliperidone (Invega)	3-6 QD	12	+	+++	+	↔	+	++	SE: headache, tachycardia Renal metabolism Sustenna q 4 weeks IM injection, start with 234 mg and then 156 mg 1 week later; dosing options 39 mg, 78mg 117 mg, 156 mg, 234mg. Trinza q 3 months IM injection following treatment with Sustenna for atleast 4 months, depending on last dose of Sustenna dosing options: 273mg, 410mg, 546mg, 819mg Hafyera q 6 months IM injection following treatment with Sustenna for atleast 4 months (with last 2 doses being 156 mg or 234 mg or Trinza (at doses of 546 mg or 819 mg) for atleast one 3-month cycle; dosing options: 1,092 mg or 1560 mg	1.5, 3, 6, 9 mg tablets	39, 78, 117, 156, 234 mg LAI
Asenapine (Saphris)	5 BID	5-10	+	↔	+	↔	+	↔	SE: oral hypoesthesia, constipation, nausea and vomiting, insomnia	5, 10 mg SL tablets	—
Risperidone (Risperdal)	1-2 QD	4-8	+	+++	+	↔	+	++	ᵃConsta: 25–50 mg q 2 weeks	0.25, 0.5, 1, 2, 3, 4 mg tablets	1 mg/mL oral sol & 12.5, 25, 37.5, 50 mg inj,. ODT
Clozapine (Clozaril)	Lo	25 QD	300–600	↔	+++	↔	+++	+++	+++	SE: agranulocytosis, seizures, myocarditis, cardiomyopathy Weekly CBC x 6 months → q 2 weeks x 6 months → q month	25, 50, 100, 200 mg tablets	12.5, 25, 100 mg ODT, 50 mg/mL oral susp

1. SIDE EFFECTS PROFILE

Relative risk of EPS: High-potency FGAs > mid-potency FGAs = risperidone = paliperidone > low-potency FGA > aripiprazole = brexpiprazole ≥ ziprasidone = asenapine = olanzapine = cariprazine > lurasidone > iloperidone = lumateperone > quetiapine > clozapine

Relative risk of TD: FGA > SGA > clozapine

Relative risk of weight gain: clozapine = olanzapine > low-potency FGA > risperidone = paliperidone = quetiapine > iloperidone > asenapine > mid- potency FGA > high-potency FGA = aripiprazole = brexpiprazole = ziprasidone = lurasidone = cariprazine = lumateperone

Relative risk of prolactin elevation and sexual side effects: risperidone = paliperidone > FGA > olanzapine > ziprasidone > quetiapine = clozapine > aripiprazole = brexpiprazole > asenapine > lurasidone > iloperidone = cariprazine = lumateperone

2. EFFICACY: No significant differences in efficacy—except clozapine

3. FIRST EPISODE: Any FGA or SGA—choice driven by side effects. Use lower dose of FGA (half†) to reduce the risk of EPS.

Quicker response to positive symptoms, more motor side effects and poor adherence is usually seen, so closer monitoring is recommended.

4. CLOZAPINE USE: After failure of 2 antipsychotic trials. Can be the initial choice in patients with suicidality, violence, and substance use. In patients with 2 years of positive symptoms on medication treatment and 5 years of inadequate response, clozapine should be considered.

Table 24-11 Drugs Used in the Treatment of Schizophrenia (Continued)

Metabolic Screening and Monitoring Guidelines		Recommended intervals*
Definitions: Adult treatment panel III (ATPIII)—presence of 3 or more of the following, International Diabetes Federation (IDF)-central obesity plus 2 of the following:		
Waist circumference	Male ≥102 cm, Female ≥88 cm (ATPIII) Male ≥94 cm, Female ≥80 cm (IDF)	Baseline and then annually
BP	SBP ≥130 mmHg or DBP ≥85 mmHg **or** on drug treatment for elevated blood pressure	Baseline, at 12 weeks, and then annually
HDL-C	Male <40 mg/dL, Female <50 mg/dL **or** on drug treatment for reduced HDL-C	Fasting lipid profile at baseline, then at 12 weeks and then annually
TGL	≥150 mg/dL (1.7 mmol/L) **or** on drug treatment for raised triglycerides	Fasting lipid profile at baseline, then at 12 weeks and then annually
Glucose	Fasting plasma glucose ≥100 mg/dL (5.6 mmol/L) **or** on drug treatment for elevated glucose	Baseline, at 12 weeks and then annually

QD = daily, BID = twice daily, SE = side effects, ODT = orally disintegrating tablets, LAI = long-acting injection, SL = sublingual.

*More frequent assessments of BMI (every 4 weeks for 12 weeks and then quarterly); also monitoring for family history of diabetes, dyslipidemia, and hypertension or cardiovascular diseases is recommended. Adverse effect monitoring can occur more frequently, as clinically indicated.

Some Side Effects Common to Many of the Drugs:

Blockade of D_2 dopamine receptors:
  Motor side effects: dystonia, akathisia, tremor, rigidity, bradykinesia, akinesia, tardive dyskinesia
  Endocrinopathy: gynecomastia, galactorrhea, amenorrhea, sexual dysfunction, decreased libido
  Neuroleptic malignant syndrome
Blockade of H_1 histaminic receptors: sedation, weight gain
Blockade of muscarinic receptors: dry mouth, constipation, blurred vision, urinary retention, sinus tachycardia, amnesia
Blockade of α_1 adrenergic receptors: hypotension, dizziness, syncope, reflex tachycardia, priapism
Most drugs can be administered once per day.

Adapted from:

TMAP = The Texas Medication Algorithm Project (Moore TA, et al. The Texas Medication Algorithm Project antipsychotic algorithm for schizophrenia. *J Clin Psychiatry*. 2007;68(11)1751–1762).
PORT = The Schizophrenia Patient Outcomes Research Team (Kreyenbuhl J et al. The Schizophrenia Patient Outcomes Research Team [PORT]: Updated Treatment Recommendations 2009. *Schizophr Bull*. 2010;36(1):94–103). © Copyright 2004–2006 International Psychopharmacology Algorithm Project (IPAP) www.ipap.org

D_2 receptor presynaptic partial agonist and postsynaptic antagonist effects plus D1 receptor-dependent modulation of glutamate neurotransmission (lumateperone). Beyond their effects on D_2 and 5-HT_{2A} receptors, the role of additional mechanisms to the net antipsychotic effects of atypical antipsychotic drugs is not clear. Two SGAs demonstrate 5-HT2A antagonism combined with D2 partial agonism (aripiprazole, brexpiprazole). Finally, pimavanserin, a drug that does not block D_2 receptors but is instead a $5HT_{2A}$ antagonist/inverse agonist, is approved for the treatment of hallucinations and delusions associated with Parkinson disease psychosis.

i. Clozapine—Clozapine was the first antipsychotic drug shown in controlled clinical trials to alleviate both positive and negative symptoms in patients who had failed to respond to adequate trials of typical antipsychotic drugs. In this treatment-resistant group, clozapine treatment results in a clinical response in 30–60% of cases. It produces almost no EPS, akathisia, tardive dyskinesia, or hyperprolactinemia. The onset of a significant response to clozapine in treatment-resistant patients may be delayed for up to 6 months. Primary negative symptoms tend to improve more slowly than do other types of symptoms such as hallucinations and delusions. The response to clozapine is usually only partial, but for patients whose symptoms have been virtually nonresponsive to all other therapies, the change can be highly significant.

The remarkable advantages of clozapine (described later in this section) must be balanced against its ability to cause **agranulocytosis** in 0.8% of patients. As a result, clozapine is reserved for patients with schizophrenia who have failed to respond adequately to two or more adequate therapeutic trials of other antipsychotic drugs (**treatment-resistant schizophrenia**), or who are intolerant of typical antipsychotic drugs because of EPS or tardive dyskinesia, or who are at high risk for **suicide** or manifest persistent self-injury. Poor work function or moderate-to-severe residual negative symptoms are considered a poor response, even if only mild positive symptoms are present. Due to the risk of agranulocytosis, clozapine prescribing requires periodic monitoring of absolute neutrophil count (ANC) in treated patients. In the United States, ANC monitoring is regulated by a specific Risk Evaluation and Mitigation Strategy program.

Clozapine has been shown to reduce depression and suicidality. The latter effect leads to a major decrease in the overall mortality rate associated with schizophrenia, despite the slight increase due to agranulocytosis. Numerous studies have reported that clozapine can improve some aspects of cognitive function, especially verbal fluency, attention, and recall memory. This effect appears to be unrelated to the drug's lack of adverse effect on motor function.

About 40% of patients have positive symptoms that fail to respond adequately to clozapine monotherapy. As previously mentioned, it often takes 6 months and sometimes longer for positive symptoms to be controlled in very treatment-resistant patients. Patience is required. Polypharmacy with other antipsychotic drugs should be avoided, if possible. For patients who respond poorly to clozapine, electroconvulsive therapy (ECT) has sometimes been found to be effective as an adjunctive treatment. The effectiveness of adding other (nonclozapine) antipsychotic drugs, mood stabilizers, and antidepressants for managing residual psychotic symptoms, mood instability or depression to ongoing treatment with clozapine is not supported by strong clinical evidence. However, on clinical grounds, trials with various antipsychotic drugs such as aripiprazole or mood stabilizers such as lamotrigine may be attempted.

Most cases of clozapine-induced **agranulocytosis** (CIA) occur within 4–18 weeks after treatment begins, but it can occur rarely at later times. In the United States, ANC must be monitored weekly for 6 months, then every 2 weeks for months 7–12, followed by monthly monitoring on an indefinite basis. In cases of mild treatment-emergent neutropenia (ANC 1000–1499/μL), clozapine can be continued but ANS monitoring must increase in frequence to three times per week until counts normalize. For moderate neutropenia (ANC 500–999/μL), clozapine treatment must be interrupted. The ANC must be monitored daily until counts increase to 1000/μL or higher, at which time clozapine treatment can be reinitiated. For severe neutropenia/agranulocytosis (ANC drops below 500/μL), clozapine should be stopped. In such cases, rechallenging with clozapine can be considered only if benefits clearly outweigh risks, generally in consultation with a hematology specialist. If agranulocytosis has developed, filgrastim, a granulocyte colony stimulating factor (G-CSF) analog, can be used to hasten the recovery process. Recovery generally takes 7–14 days. Hospitalization to prevent or treat sepsis is essential. To date, the death rate from clozapine due to agranulocytosis is about 1 per 10,000. CIA may be a heritable trait, with GWAS implicating the involvement of human leukocyte antigen locus. Furthermore, most likely CIA is a complex, polygenic trait; this in turn may make it challenging to develop genetic predictors.

Some healthy individuals may have a lower baseline ANC than normal. This condition, now referred to as Duffy-null associated neutrophil count (DANC), is considered a normal variant associated with the null form of the Duffy phenotype (an antigen on RBCs). DANC, now the preferred term, was once referred to as "benign ethnic neutropenia" because it is thought to be more common among members of certain ethnic groups. Because DANC is not considered a pathological trait (another reason for preferring the term, DANC, over "benign ethnic neutropenia), it is not associated with higher risk of clozapine-induced agranulocytosis and should not be considered a contraindication to treatment with clozapine. However, ANC-based guidelines for continuation vs. discontinuation of clozapine are different for persons with DANC in the United States.

Other life-threatening side effects of clozapine include **myocarditis, paralytic ileus or megacolon (Ogilvie syndrome), and pulmonary embolism.** Clozapine can also cause **leukocytosis** and **eosinophilia**. The development of these disorders does not predict later development of agranulocytosis. However, clozapine must be discontinued in patients who develop these severe adverse effects (along with urgent evaluation and management), and such patients should not be rechallenged unless there is a greater risk of harm from avoiding clozapine. Other side effects of clozapine include sedation, postural hypotension (orthostatic hypotension), QT interval prolongation, metabolic syndrome, weight gain, type 2 diabetes, hyperlipidemia and atherosclerotic heart disease, major motor **seizures**, obsessive–compulsive symptoms or treatment-emergent obsessive–compulsive disorder, hypersalivation, tachycardia, neuroleptic malignant syndrome, urinary incontinence, and constipation. Many of these side effects diminish over time or are responsive to pharmacologic agents and decreased dosage. Neuroleptic malignant syndrome (NMS) classically presents with mental status changes, hyperthermia, muscular rigidity, and unstable vital signs. A high index of suspicion is important, as NMS can be fatal and rapid diagnosis and management can be life-saving. The management of NMS includes, at minimum, discontinuation of the causative medication (including antipsychotic and any other dopamine D_2-blocking medications) and supportive measures (cardiovascular support, management of hyperthermia, correction of fluid, and electrolyte disturbances).

The dosage of clozapine ranges from 100 to 900 mg/d for most patients. It must be titrated slowly because of tachycardia and hypotensive side effects, with a starting dosage of 25 mg/d. The average dosage is 400–500 mg/d, usually given twice daily. Plasma levels of 250–350 ng/mL are more likely to be associated with clinical response than are lower levels. The risk of treatment-emergent seizures with clozapine is thought to be higher as the dose is increased, especially at a daily dose of 600 mg or higher. Many clinicians will indicate treatment with an anticonvulsant medication such as divalproex for patients who are treated with clozapine at daily doses of 600 mg or more.

Clozapine has a very complex pharmacologic profile. It has a high affinity for serotonergic (5-$HT_{2A,2C,6,7}$), adrenergic ($\alpha_{1,2}$), muscarinic, and histaminergic receptors. Clozapine and related drugs are inverse agonists at 5-HT_{2A} and 5-HT_{2C} receptors, meaning they can block the constitutive activity of these receptors (i.e., activation of the receptor that is independent of 5-HT stimulation). The major metabolite of clozapine, N-desmethylclozapine, is an M1 muscarinic agonist. This mechanism may improve cognitive function and reduce psychosis. No other atypical or metabolite thereof has M1 muscarinic properties.

ii. Other D_2 and 5-HT_{2A} antagonists—This group of drugs includes **quetiapine, olanzapine, risperidone, ziprasidone, paliperidone, iloperidone, and lumateperone.** Most of these agents are as effective as the FGA drugs with regard to the control of positive symptoms as evidenced by the CATIE and CUtLASS studies. The newer agents within this group are not thought to be more efficacious than FGA drugs for controlling positive symptoms, though head-to-head studies are lacking. In a 2013 network meta-analysis comparing the efficacy of 15 antipsychotics in treating schizophrenia symptoms as measured by Positive and Negative Syndrome Scale or Brief Psychiatric Rating Scale, the effect size of change was large for clozapine; intermediate for olanzapine, risperidone, and paliperidone; and small for haloperidol, quetiapine, aripiprazole, ziprasidone, chlorpromazine, asenapine, lurasidone, and iloperidone. In an updated network meta-analysis that compared the clinical effects of 32 antipsychotic drugs for symptoms of schizophrenia, the same general conclusions about clinical efficacy were reached. Therefore, at clinically equivalent doses, there is no reliable evidence that any of the nonclozapine atypical antipsychotic drugs are significantly more efficacious than the other antipsychotics.

Similar to how FGAs were differentiated, SGAs are differentiated based on their side-effect profiles (Table 24–12). Olanzapine, like clozapine, has the greatest likelihood of causing metabolic side effects. Both drugs show relatively high-affinity binding to H1, α-1, and M1 receptors and thus are associated with corresponding adverse effects. Metabolic effects include weight gain and abnormalities in indices of insulin resistance, including increased fasting blood sugar and an atherogenic lipid profile. Some patients develop type 2 diabetes or diabetic ketoacidosis. In rank order, the other drugs likely to produce these effects are quetiapine and risperidone (moderate risk), and ziprasidone and aripiprazole (lowest risk). Lurasidone is thought to also be relatively lower in terms of risk for treatment-emergent weight gain, dysglycemia, and atherogenic lipidoses. Nevertheless, some

Table 24–12 Common Causes of Suboptimal Response to Antipsychotic Treatment in Schizophrenia

Misdiagnosis of schizophrenia
Diagnosis of schizophrenia should be reconfirmed in every instance of suboptimal treatment response
Undiagnosed psychiatric comorbidity
Comorbid substance use disorder(s)
Poor compliance with treatment
Can confirm using plasma levels for haloperidol and clozapine
Inadequate drug dose (see Table 24–10)
400–600 mg/d chlorpromazine equivalents for all typical agents
Target serum level of 250–350 ng/mL for clozapine
Inadequate trial length
≥4–6 weeks is usually necessary
Possibly longer for clozapine treatment or history of refractory disease
Possibly longer for any agent where negative symptoms are prominent
Intolerable side effects, especially:
EPS, including akathisia and parkinsonism
Sedation
Cognitive dulling (with traditional neuroleptics)
Worsening affective symptoms (with traditional neuroleptics)
Intolerable drug–drug interactions
Poor social support

patients treated with any of these drugs will gain weight or have glucose and lipid changes. Despite the fact that many patients who develop insulin resistance also experience significant weight gain, these two factors are not highly correlated in many patients. Patients who do not gain weight may therefore show other facets of the insulin resistance syndrome and vice versa. When initiating treatment with antipsychotic drugs, inquiring about a personal and family history of cardiovascular disease, diabetes, hypertension, lifestyle factors (e.g., diet, exercise, smoking status, etc.) and assessing baseline blood pressure, body weight, fasting glucose or glycosylated hemoglobin (HgbA1c), and lipid profile is recommended. During subsequent phases of treatment, periodic assessments of body weight, blood pressure, fasting glucose (or HgbA1c), and lipid profile are recommended, generally at 6 weeks, 3 months, 12 months, and quarterly to annually afterward depending on clinical status. Although the risk of weight gain and metabolic adverse effects appears to vary between individual antipsychotic drugs, screening and monitoring recommendations apply to all patients who are treated with SGAs, regardless of diagnosis or specific agent.

Most atypical antipsychotic drugs have less treatment-emergent antidopaminergic side effects than typical antipsychotics. Dose-dependent EPS and hyperprolactinemia can be observed with risperidone and paliperidone, however.

The dose of these drugs should be kept as low as possible in non–treatment-resistant patients. First-episode patients and those within the first 5 years of illness can often be successfully treated with antipsychotic doses at or near the lower end of their approved dose ranges. Most atypical antipsychotic drugs can be given once a day, generally before sleep (for agents with a relatively higher propensity for sedating side effects) to minimize daytime sedation: for example, olanzapine, 10–20 mg/d; quetiapine, 200–1000 mg/d; and risperidone, 2–8 mg/d. Polypharmacy with two antipsychotic drugs should be avoided for the great majority of patients. If control of positive symptoms is inadequate at these dosages after 6 weeks, it might be useful to increase the dose. However, a switch to clozapine, where the dose can be relatively high with minimal EPS, is often a better strategy, especially after the failure of two adequate antipsychotic trials (e.g., 6 or more weeks at an adequate dose). As with clozapine, augmentation with mood stabilizers, antidepressant drugs, or ECT may be attempted on clinical grounds, but only after a careful risk-benefit assessment.

Currently, risperidone, paliperidone, aripiprazole, and olanzapine are available in a long-acting form. Long-acting injectable risperidone must be given intramuscularly (IM) in the deltoid or gluteal muscles every 2 weeks and takes 6 weeks before steady-state plasma levels are achieved. Therefore, oral risperidone must be continued for at least 3 weeks after the first long-acting risperidone injection, or even longer in some cases. The typical dose of long-acting injectable risperidone is between 25 and 50 mg every 2 weeks. Risperidone is also available in a subcutaneously (SQ)-injected (into the back of the upper arm or abdominal area) biodegradable polymer form that is dosed according to the patient's average daily dose of oral risperidone. The equivalent dose of long-acting SQ injectable risperidone is 90 mg every 4 weeks for patients taking oral risperidone 3 mg/day (120 mg of risperidone long-acting SQ injectable every 4 weeks for patients taking 4 mg/day of oral risperidone). Patients who are taking less than 3 mg/day of oral risperidone may not be eligible for long-acting SQ injectable risperidone. Unlike risperidone long-acting intramuscular injection, patients who are converted from oral risperidone to long-acting SQ injectable risperidone do not need to continue to supplement with oral risperidone. Paliperidone, which is the active metabolite of risperidone, is available in once-monthly (Sustenna: 39, 78, 117, 156 mg, 234 mg IM in deltoid or gluteal muscles), trimonthly (Trinza: 273, 410, 546, 819 mg IM), and semi-annual (Hafyera: generally 1092 or 1560 mg IM) depot formulations. Deltoid injection is associated with higher serum concentrations and is hence preferred. Continuation of oral paliperidone is not required when converting from oral to once-monthly IM paliperidone; however, loading doses of once-monthly IM paliperidone must be given. For patients with no evidence of renal impairment, loading doses are injected in the deltoid muscle on treatment days 1 (234 mg) and 8 (156 mg). Maintenance doses are then given every 4 weeks following the week 8 injection, generally at a dose of 117 mg, although the dose range is 39–234 mg IM every 4 weeks. Loading and maintenance doses have to be adjusted downward in patients with mild renal impairment (Cl_{cr} 50–80 mL/min). Paliperidone long-acting IM injection therapy should generally not be offered to patients with Cl_{cr} <50 mL/min. The trimonthly formulation is to be used only after the patient has been on 4 months of the once-monthly IM paliperidone. The semi-annual formulation can only be used in patients who are stable on 4 months of once-monthly IM paliperidone (with last two doses being 156 or 234 mg) or at least one cycle (3 months) of trimonthly IM paliperidone (at doses of 546 or 819 mg).

Olanzapine is available as a long-acting IM (gluteal) injection that is recommended for use every 2 weeks in 150, 210, or 300-mg doses; or every 4 weeks in 300 or 405-mg doses. The dose of long-acting IM (depot) olanzapine is based on the oral daily dose of olanzapine; however, supplementation with oral olanzapine is not required after converting to depot olanzapine. Olanzapine depot injection has been associated with post-injection delirium sedation syndrome and sudden death. For this reason, patients should be observed for at least 3 hours post-injection by appropriately qualified personnel in a health care facility with ready access to emergency response services, and concomitant administration of intravenous benzodiazepines is not recommended.

iii. **Partial D_2 agonists**—**Aripiprazole** was the first partial DA agonist approved for the treatment of schizophrenia. The basis of partial DA agonism as a mechanism for antipsychotic effect is that aripiprazole occupies the receptor but causes significantly less activation of the receptor than the full agonist, DA. That aripiprazole can reduce prolactin levels and produce nausea is evidence of its partial D_2 receptor agonist effects. Aripiprazole is also a 5-HT$_{2A}$ antagonist and a 5-HT$_{1A}$-partial agonist, both of their effects would be expected to minimize EPS. Aripiprazole is generally given once daily, at a dose of 15 mg/d. Sometimes, doses of 20–30 mg are required. Combination with a typical antipsychotic should be avoided, as that may interfere with the partial DA agonist properties. Aripiprazole produces milder metabolic side effects than many SGAs. It may also be associated with activation when first administered, and it can cause nausea.

Aripiprazole is available as long-acting IM (depot) formulations that can be given once-monthly (400 mg initially in the deltoid or gluteal muscle and as a once-monthly maintenance dose) or once every 4–8 weeks (referred to as aripiprazole lauroxil). Following the first aripiprazole once-monthly depot injection of 400 mg, oral aripiprazole should be continued for 2 weeks. The typical maintenance dose of 400 mg once-monthly can be reduced to 300 mg IM monthly in case of side effects. Unlike the aripiprazole once-monthly depot injection form, aripiprazole lauroxil long-acting injection can be initiated in one of two ways, both of which require the concurrent use of oral aripiprazole—either by starting aripiprazole lauroxil and supplementing with oral aripiprazole for 21 days following the initial injection or by providing a 675 mg injection with a one-time oral 30 mg dose of aripiprazole. Maintenance doses of aripiprazole lauroxil range are generally 441–882 mg once-monthly, 882 mg every 6 weeks, or 1064 mg every 8 weeks.

Brexpiprazole, a medication chemically similar to aripiprazole, is a partial agonist of the 5-HT1A, D2, and D3 receptors and antagonist of the 5-HT2A, 5-HT2B, 5-HT7, α1A-, α1B-, α1D-, and α2C-adrenergic and H1 receptors. Brexpiprazole and aripiprazole both appear to have relatively low risk for body weight gain compared with many other antipsychotic drugs. The comparative risk of clinically significant body weight gain in patients with schizophrenia appears to be similar between brexpiprazole and aripiprazole.

iv. D_2, 5HT$_{2A}$ antagonism combined with 5-HT$_{1A}$ agonism— **Lurasidone and asenapine** are relatively newer SGAs designed to have partial agonist effects on 5-HT$_{1A}$ receptor. Theoretically this is thought to improve negative symptoms and depression, improve EPS profile, have a more favorable metabolic profile, and improve cognitive functioning. While clinical trials have not been able to demonstrate robust effects on negative symptoms and cognitive functioning, these compounds do have a favorable metabolic profile. Of note, lurasidone (like ziprasidone) must be taken with food and asenapine has to be taken sublingually.

v. D_2 and D_3 partial agonism—**Cariprazine** is a novel SGA with a proposed unique mechanism of action, namely dopamine D_3 and D_2 receptor partial agonism with preferential binding to D_3 receptors and does not involve 5-HT$_{2A}$ antagonism. Cariprazine has been shown to be safe, well tolerated, and efficacious in the treatment of acute schizophrenia. The risk of body weight gain with cariprazine appears to be low during short-term treatment.

1. FGA—The discovery of chlorpromazine in 1950 revolutionized the treatment of schizophrenia. The **mechanism of action** responsible for its antipsychotic property is dopamine D_2-receptor antagonism. Thus, chlorpromazine and other FGAs block D_2 receptors in each of the relevant DA pathways, including the mesolimbic tract (where excessive DA transmission is believed to underlie positive symptoms), mesocortical tract (where deficits in DA transmission are thought to cause cognitive dysfunction and negative symptoms), nigrostriatal tract (where D_2 blockade results in extrapyramidal adverse effects, as will be discussed shortly), and tuberoinfundibular tract (where activation of D_2 receptors controls pituitary prolactin release). By this one mechanism, typical antipsychotics remedy positive symptoms but coincidentally result in troublesome antidopaminergic adverse effects (EPS, hyperprolactinemia).

i. Clinical use—In terms of **treatment response**, about 70% of patients with schizophrenia who experience delusions or hallucinations will have a good response of those symptoms to FGAs. For many, an antipsychotic response will be observed sooner, sometimes within the first week of treatment. The remaining 30% will have moderate to severe positive symptoms despite adequate doses of FGAs for at least 6 weeks, which is considered the minimum adequate **therapeutic trial length**. Relative to practice in the past, lower **dosages** of FGAs have been shown to be as effective as higher doses but with fewer side effects. For instance, daily dosages of 5–10 mg of haloperidol, or its equivalent (see Table 24–11), may be adequate for many, if not most, patients with acute psychosis. First-episode and recent-onset patients almost always respond to lower dosages. Ordinarily, the dose may be titrated up if there is no or poor response after 1–2 weeks of confirmed adherence to treatment. Switching medications can be considered in case of no or poor response after 4–6 weeks of treatment for most antipsychotics. Plasma levels of antipsychotics and their metabolites vary greatly between patients. The only FGA with a possible therapeutic window is haloperidol. For haloperidol, a steady-state plasma range of 12–17 ng/L has been associated with optimal antipsychotic action.

ii. Adverse effects—The old term for FGA, **neuroleptic**, refers to the neurologic side effects of the FGAs, such as catalepsy in rodents and **EPS** in humans. These effects occur in the same dose range as is associated with an antipsychotic effect; therefore, for typical antipsychotics, treatment-emergent EPS is a common and significant treatment-limiting factor. The EPS may be divided into acute and delayed effects. The predominant acute effects are **parkinsonism** (coarse resting tremor, bradykinesia, hypertonia, unstable gait), **akathisia** (subjective restlessness and psychomotor agitation), and **dystonic reactions** (sudden, sustained, intense, and often painful muscular contraction). The late-occurring side effects are **tardive dyskinesia** and **tardive dystonia**. The late-occurring effects are sometimes irreversible and, rarely, life threatening.

As mentioned earlier, the antipsychotic action and motor side effects of antipsychotics are secondary to their ability to block D_2 receptors in the mesolimbic and nigrostriatal pathways of the brain, respectively. The affinities that antipsychotic agents have for D_2, $5\text{-}HT_{2A}$, and muscarinic receptors are key determinants of their liability to cause EPS. These drugs also have variable affinities for other neurotransmitter receptors that have predictable effects on antipsychotic profile (see Table 24–12). These receptors include histamine 1 (H1, antagonism of which may result in sedation and weight gain), alpha-1 (α-1) adrenergic (antagonism of which may result in sedation, orthostatic hypotension, and reflex tachycardia), muscarinic-1 (M1) cholinergic (antagonism of which may result in blurring of vision, dry mouth, urinary retention, constipation, and cognitive dulling) receptors. Hematologic effects, jaundice, cardiac effects (e.g., electrocardiographic changes such as QTc interval prolongation, especially for thioridazine, pimozide, and droperidol), photosensitivity, and retinitis pigmentosa (associated especially with the use of higher doses of thioridazine, which may result in blindness) result from toxic effects on specific target tissues.

iii. Choice of agent—The choice of typical antipsychotic drug is based on a variety of initial considerations, which include the following:

- Side-effect profile.
- Past response(s) to antipsychotic drugs.
- The availability of long-acting preparations (e.g., fluphenazine and haloperidol decanoate) required for patients who frequently relapse due to poor medication adherence. In chronically noncompliant patients who are unwilling to take oral medication, long-acting injectables may decrease relapse rates.
- The availability of short-acting injectable or intravenous formulations for use in acute situations (to control agitation and combative behavior) where oral dosing is not feasible, or when the oral route is not available. Of note, the use of intravenous haloperidol requires cardiac monitoring due to increased risk of QTc interval prolongation.

Other considerations are based on the side-effect profile. Differences in side-effect profile between low- and high-potency typical antipsychotics are predicted to a great degree by their receptor-binding profiles. For instance, low-potency drugs (e.g., chlorpromazine, thioridazine, mesoridazine), so named because of their relatively lower affinity for D_2 receptors and therefore higher dose requirement for antipsychotic potency (300 mg/d or greater), may result in lower EPS or hyperprolactinemic liability compared to high-potency agents (e.g., haloperidol, fluphenazine). However, low-potency drugs result in more sedation, weight gain, orthostasis, and antimuscarinic effects than high-potency agents do because of their higher affinities for H1, α-1, and M1 receptors. The latter agents produce more EPS than do the low-potency agents (see Table 24–12). Individuals with a history of congenital long QT syndrome or those who are at risk of acquired prolongation of the QT interval (e.g., patients who are taking antiarrhythmic agents or other QT interval-prolonging drugs; those with a history of cardiac arrythmias, recent myocardial infarction, electrolyte imbalances [particularly hypokalemia or hypomagnesemia]; and persons with a family history of sudden cardiac death owing to cardiac arrhythmias, etc.) should generally be channeled away from antipsychotic drugs that are more strongly associated with QT interval lengthening. These medications include, but are not limited to, IV haloperidol and certain oral antipsychotic medications such as chlorpromazine, pimozide, thioridazine, quetiapine, and ziprasidone. Antipsychotic drugs with strong anticholinergic side effects should be avoided when possible in older persons and in patients who are cognitively impaired or have certain general medical conditions such as acute angle closure glaucoma, chronic constipation, and benign prostatic hypertrophy.

If the patient's history of drug response does not indicate an unusual sensitivity to EPS, high-potency agents such as haloperidol and fluphenazine are preferred to low-potency agents. Thioridazine is believed to have more risk of causing a ventricular arrhythmia than other typical antipsychotic drugs. If EPS develop, anticholinergic agents such as benztropine, diphenhydramine, biperiden, or trihexyphenidyl can be used as a pharmacological adjunct, or the patient can be switched from a high-potency agent to a medium-potency drug (e.g., trifluoperazine) or to a low-potency drug (e.g., thioridazine). A more important strategy for the minimization of EPS is to keep the dose as low as possible (e.g., no more than 5–10 mg/d of haloperidol equivalents), assuming there is a reason why an atypical antipsychotic drug could not be substituted. Persistent EPS, especially akathisia, can contribute to nonadherence or lead to increased agitation or even suicide risk. Thus, in cases of apparently increased agitation and disorganized behavior in the face of ongoing treatment, especially with typical antipsychotics, screening for akathisia should always be considered.

Regardless of the type of antipsychotic drug chosen, monitoring for tardive dyskinesia should occur periodically. Tardive dyskinesia can be assessed clinically at each visit and every 3–6 months (in high-risk patients) or every 12 months (most patients) using the Abnormal Involuntary Movement Scale. When tardive dyskinesia is detected, discontinuation of the offending agent—most typically an antipsychotic drug (though occasionally DA receptor-blocking antiemetics such as metoclopramide)—should be attempted or considered. For antipsychotic drugs, this should occur slowly, over several weeks, as sudden cessation of antipsychotic medication can worsen tardive dyskinesia symptoms (withdrawal dyskinesia). Most cases of withdrawal dyskinesia will resolve spontaneously; however, several weeks may be needed for that to occur. In cases of severe withdrawal dyskinesia (e.g., to the point of impairing speaking or swallowing), reintroducing the antipsychotic drug will often result in improvement of dyskinetic movements. At that point, a slower tapering can be attempted. For the great majority of patients with schizophrenia, ongoing antipsychotic treatment will be needed to prevent acute psychotic relapses. In such cases, switching to medication with a lower risk of tardive dyskinesia can be considered. This may include switching from an FGA to an SGA. Of all potential options for switching antipsychotics in patients with tardive dyskinesia, clozapine is the most-preferred due to low affinity for D_2 receptors, low risk of tardive dyskinesia, and the possibility of improvement in tardive dyskinesia symptoms. However, the potential benefits of switching to clozapine must be weighed against the risks of agranulocytosis, treatment-emergent weight gain and dysmetabolic side effects, and other clozapine-associated adverse effects. Quetiapine and iloperidone both have low affinities for D2 receptors and may be potential alternatives to clozapine, although their respective roles as switch options for patients with schizophrenia and antipsychotic-associated tardive dyskinesia have not been extensively investigated. For cases of severe tardive dyskinesia that persists despite switching to lower-risk agents (or if switching antipsychotic medication is infeasible), oral vesicular monoamine transporter type 2 (VMAT2) inhibitors (such as deutetrabenazine, valbenazine, or tetrabenazine) or botulinum toxin injections may be helpful, often in consultation with a movement disorder specialist. The management of common side effects is listed in Table 24–13.

Table 24–13 Management of Medication Side Effects in Schizophrenia

Side Effects	Better Outcome
Extrapyramidal side effects (tremor, stiffness)	Antiholinergics (Benztropine, Trihexyphenidyl)
Acute dystonia	Diphenhydramine
Akathisia	Propranolol. Mirtazepine
Tardive dyskinesia	Valbenazine, deutetrabenazine, botulinum toxin
Weight-gain, metabolic syndrome	Metformin, Topiramate, Glucagon-like peptide-1 receptor agonists (GLP-1 agonists) (e.g., semaglutide, trizepatide, liraglutide), sodium-glucose cotransporter-2 (SGLT-2) inhibitors (canagliflozin, dapagliflozin, and empagliflozin)
Clozapine-induced agranulocytosis	Lithium, Fligastim
Clozapine-induced sialorrhea	Atropine, Glycopyrrolate
Clozapine-induced constipation	Senna, polyethylene glycol, lactulose

Principles of treatment:

The management of schizophrenia is often conceived of as occurring in three phases of treatment (acute, continuation, and maintenance).

1. Acute-phase treatment—The acute phase of schizophrenia is characterized by fully expressed psychotic symptoms. The acuity of symptoms is often such that hospitalization is necessary for control of acute, life-threatening agitation and combativeness. To avoid use of physical restraints, oral antipsychotic medication may be offered; however, oral medication is often refused or, more commonly, cannot be safely administered in an acute situation. For patients who are acutely agitated or likely to harm themselves or others, short-acting injectable antipsychotics may be considered. Currently, ziprasidone, aripiprazole, and olanzapine are the atypical antipsychotics available in an acute injectable form. Several FGAs are available in this form (e.g., haloperidol, 5 mg IM) and are often administered alone or in combination with an injectable benzodiazepine (e.g., lorazepam) and/or an anticholinergic drug (e.g., benztropine or diphenhydramine). It is necessary to isolate such patients in a quiet room, with as much supervision as possible. Parenteral haloperidol may be repeated, as needed, every 2–4 hours. An important caveat is that, whenever possible, antipsychotic medications should be held or delayed in patients with schizophrenia who present acutely with catatonia, including agitated catatonia. The use of antipsychotic medications in patients with catatonia can lead to a worsening of catatonic symptoms and unstable vital signs (malignant catatonia).

Once agitation has been controlled or if injectable medication is not indicated, treatment with an orally administered antipsychotic may be initiated. Ordinarily, the first antipsychotic administered should be chosen from the SGAs in a treatment-naïve patient or in a medication-free patient who has a prior history of response to antipsychotic drug treatment (Figure 24–1). The choice may be based on several factors including past response, family history of response, history of side effects, and current metabolic profile. Thus, in individuals with a high body mass index, SGAs with the greatest likelihood of metabolic syndrome should be avoided. For patients on one of these drugs for whom a switch is indicated to another of the same class, there is no accepted preferred way to do this. Stopping the current drug as the new drug is introduced may be as safe and effective as rapid or slow cross-titration.

In choosing among the various first-line options, no convincing data suggest superior efficacy in target symptom domains for a particular agent. The clinical decision about which agent to use is based on other factors: side-effect profile, past therapeutic response to agent(s), and patient/caregiver preference. For patients with a history of frequent psychotic relapses due to nonadherence to otherwise effective oral antipsychotic treatment, acute treatment with an oral medication that can be converted to a long-acting

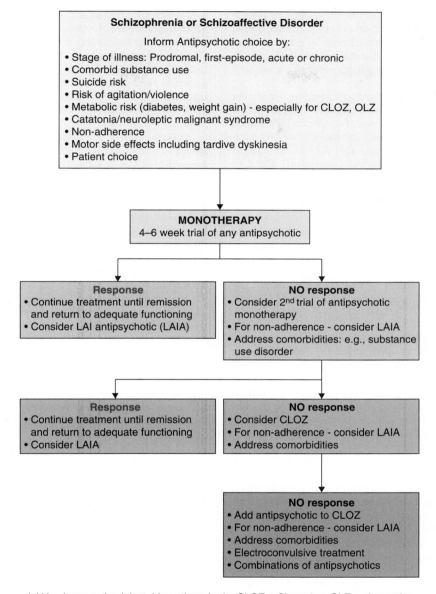

LAIA = Long-acting injectable antipsychotic, CLOZ = Clozapine, OLZ = olanzapine

▲ **Figure 24–1** Algorithm for the pharmacological treatment of patients with schizophrenia or schizoaffective disorder. First-line options include amisulpride (AMI, not available in the United States), aripiprazole (ARIP), olanzapine (OLZ), quetiapine (QTP), risperidone (RISP), paliperidone (PALI), or ziprasidone (ZIP). An adequate trial of medication is 4–6 weeks at an adequate dosage before trying a different agent. Clozapine should be considered if a patient does not respond to two or more adequate medication trials. Patients should receive 6 months of clozapine treatment before adequacy of treatment response is judged. If response is inadequate, a number of less well-studied options may be considered. At first assessment and at each initial visits, there are a number of clinical considerations and other important areas that should be assessed.

injectable form in the future may be preferred. The adverse effect burden of acute phase antipsychotic medication must also be considered because relapse into acute-phase illness is often preceded by unilateral discontinuation of medication due to side effects, even if the patient achieves a good antipsychotic response.

If circumstances are such that a patient requires treatment with a FGA (i.e., prior treatment response to typical rather than atypical drugs in the absence of significant EPS, limited formularies, cost considerations, or patient/caregiver preference), treatment is best commenced with an oral drug at low dosage (i.e., 10 mg/d haloperidol equivalent). The dose should not be increased for 4–6 weeks unless psychotic or aggressive symptoms or sleeplessness are severe. Rapid dose increases the risk of EPS and secondary negative symptoms without added antipsychotic benefit.

Long-acting injectable antipsychotic medications should not be given initially except to those patients noncompliant with other forms of treatment. On the other hand, and as discussed previously, acute-phase symptoms due to illness relapse in the setting of poor adherence call specifically for consideration of long-acting injectable antipsychotic medication.

2. Continuation-phase treatment—Psychotic symptoms respond, usually partially, within the first several days of treatment. However, most patients do not achieve a full antipsychotic response at a given dose for 2–6 weeks and remain vulnerable to early relapse if treatment is interrupted. The purpose of continuation-phase treatment is to monitor patient adherence, therapeutic response, and treatment tolerance. In addition, because a significant lag time may be required to full therapeutic effect at a given dose of drug, it is inadvisable to discontinue a drug prematurely and substitute a different class of antipsychotic agent before the optimal 4–6 weeks of therapy has passed, unless significant side effects develop that are not amenable to treatment. After initial stabilization, continuation treatment ranges in duration up to 6–8 weeks, depending upon treatment response.

In general, the same medication dosage that resulted in control of acute-phase symptoms is appropriate for the continuation phase, though the dose may be "fine-tuned" during this time to minimize adverse effects or bring about a more adequate clinical response. Although some evidence supports intermittent dosing of antipsychotic medication, this strategy has been associated with increased rates of relapse. Continuous dosing is therefore preferred.

The use of more than one antipsychotic at the same time should be avoided. There is no justification for the concomitant use of two classes of typical antipsychotic drugs (e.g., a parenteral and an oral antipsychotic) unless the patient's route of treatment is being converted from intramuscular to oral or the patient is being converted from an oral to long-acting injectable antipsychotic medication that requires continuing oral therapy for a specific period of time.

3. Maintenance treatment—The primary goals of maintenance treatment are prevention of relapse and optimization of psychosocial functioning. Long-term illness management also calls for monitoring and treating medical comorbidities (including the effects of antipsychotic treatment), addressing comorbid psychiatric and substance-use disorders, monitoring for long-term adverse effects (and working to minimize them when possible), and addressing the important issue of medication adherence.

As is the case with continuation-phase treatment, the dosage used to achieve clinical response in the acute phase is often continued but may be subject to "fine tuning" for the reasons specified above. Continuous dosing is preferred. Ongoing monitoring of medication adherence must be paramount, as this is still the most common reason for relapse. Nonadherence stems from several factors: denial of illness (poor insight); intolerable side effects; suboptimal management of clinical symptoms; cognitive deficits; and other reasons. Side effects such as weight gain, EPS (especially akathisia), sexual dysfunction, and sedation can also be distressing to patients. Because many of the adverse effects of medication are dose dependent, problems with adherence may be managed by lowering the dosage or switching to agents that result in fewer side effects. Pharmacological adjuncts may be required to counter certain adverse effects if dosage adjustment or switching are not clinically feasible. For most patients, treatment with antipsychotic medications will be of indefinite duration.

Despite recent advances in antipsychotic treatment, a significant proportion of patients are left with persisting symptoms, especially negative and neurocognitive symptoms. Even under the best of circumstances, however, positive symptoms also frequently persist, though in a less acute form. Incompletely treated symptoms are associated with significant psychiatric and physical health-related morbidity, and with an increased risk of relapse and rehospitalization. Thus, management during maintenance phase must endeavor to achieve as optimal a treatment response as possible. If at least a partial response to a well-executed antipsychotic trial has been achieved, remaining options include watchful waiting (because some treatment effects may take longer to appear), increasing the drug dosage, using adjunctive medication, or switching to another medication if other factors that contribute to suboptimal treatment response have been ruled out (see Table 24–12). For FGAs, clinical evidence indicates that either the dose–response profiles eventually plateau or the side-effect liability begins to outweigh therapeutic benefit as doses are increased. For SGAs, the dose–response interactions have been less well studied, though there is some evidence in favor of high-dose strategies for olanzapine and other atypicals.

The evidence for augmenting nonclozapine atypical antipsychotics is generally lacking. In an analysis comprising 42 medication combinations for augmenting antipsychotic monotherapy, evidence was favorable for 14 such combinations, although the quality of the meta-analyses limited specific recommendations. Serial trials of antipsychotic monotherapy are preferred. For treatment-refractory patients, a trial of clozapine monotherapy is clearly indicated (discussed later). However, when dosages of antipsychotic medication cannot be raised, when the risk of losing the partial response already achieved outweighs the potential benefit of switching medication, or when no other options are feasible, augmentation may be considered for specific target symptoms or psychiatric comorbidities that antipsychotic monotherapy cannot address. When an adjunct is being considered, great care must be taken to review all medications, in order to anticipate unwanted drug interactions and other risks of combining medications. Specific clinical subgroups for whom adjuncts have at least some support include patients with aggressive behavior (valproate, benzodiazepines), anxiety (benzodiazepines, antidepressants), tobacco-use disorders (nicotine replacement), other substance-use problems (naltrexone), prominent affective symptoms (valproate, lithium, antidepressants), positive symptoms (benzodiazepines), negative symptoms (antidepressants), and cognitive difficulties (antidepressants, buspirone). These strategies, again, are based on anecdotal reporting and, in cases where the evidence is stronger, clinical responses can be highly variable or even worse, especially in the case of benzodiazepines.

An important consideration for treating the symptoms of schizophrenia with antipsythoic drugs is the potential effect of restrictions against smoking tobacco that are part of most modern hospital settings. As mentioned earlier, many patients with schizophrenia are especially heavy smokers and the inhaled polycyclic aromatic hydrocarbons in cigarette smoke act as inducers of several cytochrome P450 isoenzymes including 1A1, 1A2, and 2E1. In such cases, the doses of certain antipsychotic drugs that are metabolized by these enzymes may be higher (in some cases, much higher) while actively smoking than if smoking is suddenly stopped. The latter can occur when patients require psychiatric hospitalization, as an example, where smoking cigarettes is often disallowed. When smoking stops, the induction of the aforementioned CYP450 enzymes also stops. Therefore, if medications such as clozapine, olanzapine, haloperidol, perphenazine, fluphenazine, and chlorpromazine are reinitiated at the patient's "usual" outpatient dose while in a no-smoking environment, the dose of drug may actually be excessive in absence of concurrent smoking, leading to higher side effect burden or excessively high drug levels in the case of clozapine. The opposite may occur if any of these medications are initiated in a smoke-free environment, as the dose may need to be upwardly adjusted to maintain efficacy, especially if heavy cigarette smoking is subsequently resumed by the patient.

4. Treatment-resistant schizophrenia—Treatment-resistant schizophrenia is variously defined. Failure of two well-carried-out therapeutic trials of antipsychotics from any pharmacological class is a generally accepted definition.

The atypical antipsychotic, clozapine, is the only drug with proven efficacy for treatment-resistant patients. It remains the gold standard in this subgroup. Approximately 30–60% of all patients with schizophrenia who fail to respond to typical antipsychotics respond to clozapine. Data concerning the usefulness of other atypical antipsychotics at conventional doses are not convincing, though higher-than-usual doses of other atypical antipsychotics may occasionally be of benefit. As was previously discussed, there are several potentially useful adjuncts for addressing a partial antipsychotic response to clozapine, though none have a particularly strong empirical basis. To date, the most evidence is for ECT. Although the rationale for the use of augmenting therapies would be the strongest for clozapine, given its status as a treatment of last resort, the potential for dangerous adverse effects with certain drug combinations is considerable. Thus, the need for caution may be even greater when augmenting clozapine partial response than for other agents. Numerous psychosocial stressors can precipitate a worsening of symptoms of schizophrenia and a range of psychosocial interventions are needed for most patients for optimal outcomes of treatment. Therefore, although absent from most definitions of treatment-resistant schizophrenia, the adequacy of nonpharmacological treatments and psychosocial supports should be considered carefully when assessing any patient with schizophrenia who is not responding adequately to treatment.

Artukoglu BB, Li F, Szejko N, Bloch MH Pharmacologic treatment of tardive dyskinesia: a meta-analysis and systematic review. *J Clin Psychiatry* 2020;81(4):19r12798. doi: 10.4088/JCP.19r12798.

Barton BB, Segger F, Fischer K, et al Update on weight-gain caused by antipsychotics: a systematic review and meta-analysis. *Expert Opin Drug Saf.* 2020;19:295–314.

Bobo WV. Asenapine, iloperidone and lurasidone: critical appraisal of the most recently approved pharmacotherapies for schizophrenia in adults. *Exp Rev Clin Pharmacol.* 2013;6:61–91.

Caroff SN, Hurford I, Lybrand J, Campbell EC. Movement disorders induced by antipsychotic drugs: implications of the CATIE schizophrenia trial. *Neurol Clin.* 2011;29:127–48, viii.

Casey DE. Neuroleptic drug-induced extrapyramidal syndromes and tardive dyskinesia. *Schizophr Res.* 1991;4:109–120.

Christison GW, Kirch DG, Wyatt RJ. When symptoms persist: choosing among alternative somatic treatments for schizophrenia. *Schizophr Bull.* 1991;17:217–245.

Citrome L. A review of the pharmacology, efficacy and tolerability of recently approved and upcoming oral antipsychotics: an evidence-based medicine approach. *CNS Drugs.* 2013;27(11):879–911.

Conley RR, Buchanan RW. Evaluation of treatment-resistant schizophrenia. *Schizophr Bull.* 1997;23:663–674.

Correll CU, Kim E, Sliwa JK, et al. Pharmacokinetic characteristics of long-acting injectable antipsychotic drugs for schizophrenia: an overview. *CNS Drugs.* 2021;35:39–59.

Correll CU, Rubio JM, Inczedy-Farkas G, et al. Efficacy of 42 pharmacologic cotreatment strategies added to antipsychotic monotherapy in schizophrenia: systematic overview and quality appraisal of the meta-analytic evidence. *JAMA Psychiatry.* 2017;74(7):675–684.

De Hert M, Detraux J, van Winkel R, Correll CU. Metabolic and cardiovascular adverse effects associated with antipsychotic drugs. *Nat Rev Endocrinol.* 2012;8:114–126.

Desai HD, Seabolt J, Mann MW. Smoking in patients receiving psychotropic medications: a pharmacokinetic perspective. *CNS Drugs.* 2001;15:469–494.

Goldman LS. Medical illness in patients with schizophrenia. *J Clin Psychiatry.* 1999;60:10–15.

Gurrera RJ, Gearin PF, Love J, et al. Recognition and management of clozapine adverse effects: a systematic review and qualitative synthesis. *Acta Psychiatr Scand.* 2022;145:423–441.

Howes OD, McCutcheon R, Agid O, et al. Treatment-Resistant Schizophrenia: Treatment Response and Resistance in Psychosis (TRRIP) Working Group Consensus Guidelines on Diagnosis and Terminology. *Am J Psychiatry.* 2017;174:216–229.

Huhn M, Nikolakopoulou A, Schneider-Thoma J, et al. Comparative efficacy and tolerability of 32 oral antipsychotics for the acute treatment of adults with multi-episode schizophrenia: a systematic review and network meta-analysis. *Lancet.* 2019;10202:939–951.

Keepers GA, Frochtmann LJ, Anzia JM, et al. The American Psychiatric Association Practice Guideline for the treatment of patients with schizophrenia. 2020;177:868–872.

Keith SJ, Kane JM. Partial compliance and patient consequences in schizophrenia: our patients can do better. *J Clin Psychiatry.* 2003;64:1308–1315.

Kreyenbuhl J, Buchanan RW, Dickerson FB, Dixon LB. The Schizophrenia Patient Outcomes Research Team (PORT): updated treatment recommendations 2009. *Schizophr Bull.* 2010;36:94–103.

Lally J, Tully J, Robertson D, et al. Augmentation of clozapine with electroconvulsive therapy in treatment resistant schizophrenia: a systematic review and meta-analysis. *Schizophr Res.* 2016;171:215–224.

Leucht S, Cipriani A, Spineli L, et al. Comparative efficacy and tolerability of 15 antipsychotic drugs in schizophrenia: a multiple-treatments meta-analysis. *Lancet.* 2013;382(9896):951–962.

Leucht S, Crippa A, Siafis S, et al. Dose-response meta-analysis of antipsychotic drugs for acute schizophrenia. *Am J Psychiatry.* 2020;177:342–353.

Lobo MC, Whitehurst TS, Kaar SJ, et al. New and emerging treatments for schizophrenia: a narrative review of their pharmacology, efficacy and side effect profile relative to established antipsychotics. *Neurosci Biobehav Rev.* 2022;132:324–361.

Lybrand J, Caroff S. Management of schizophrenia with substance use disorders. *Psychiatr Clin North Am.* 2009;32:821–833.

Manu P, Sarvaiya N, Rogozea NM, et al. Benign ethnic neutropenia and clozapine use: a systematic review of the evidence and treatment recommendations. *J Clin Psychiatry* 2016;77:e909–e916.

Meltzer HY, Bobo WV, Nuamah IF, et al. Efficacy and tolerability of oral paliperidone extended-release tablets in the treatment of acute schizophrenia: pooled data from three 6-week, placebo-controlled studies. *J Clin Psychiatry.* 2008;69:817–829.

Norman R, Lecomte T, Addington D, Anderson E. Canadian Treatment Guidelines on psychosocial treatment of schizophrenia in adults. *Can J Psychiatry.* 2017;62:617–623.

Remington G, Foussias G, Fervaha G, et al. Treating negative symptoms in schizophrenia: an update. *Curr Treat Options Psychiatry.* 2016;3:133–150.

Weiss C, Weiller E, Baker RA, et al. The effects of brexpiprazole and aripiprazole on body weight as monotherapy in patients with schizophrenia and as adjunctive treatment in patients with major depressive disorder: an analysis of short-term and long-term studies. *Int Clin Psychopharmacol.* 2018;33:255–260.

Wicinski M, Weclewicz M. Clozapine-induced agranulocytosis/granulocytopenia: mechanisms and monitoring. *Curr Opin Hematol.* 2018;25:22–28.

B. Psychotherapeutic Interventions

Although antipsychotic drugs are the mainstay of treatment of schizophrenia, significant residual symptoms often remain, even with optimal management. Furthermore, the rate of nonadherence to pharmacological treatment is high and even marked improvement in psychotic symptoms does not necessarily translate to improved occupational and social functioning. These facts make it imperative for every clinician to explore nonpharmacological modalities of treatment. Such treatments are aimed at improving adherence with drug therapy, supporting the patient, fostering independent living skills, improving psychosocial and work functioning, and reducing caretaker burden.

Psychosocial interventions are crucial for optimizing therapeutic outcomes in patients with schizophrenia and are, therefore, considered important adjuncts to pharmacotherapy. The major forms of psychotherapeutic interventions for schizophrenia are cognitive–behavioral therapy (CBT) (including social skills training and cognitive therapy), cognitive remediation, psychoeducation, acceptance and commitment therapy, family-based interventions, and supportive psychotherapy. Although the specific approaches to treatment differ between modalities, most of these psychosocial treatments include education about the nature and treatment of schizophrenia, the need for adherence to treatment, identification of early warning signs of relapse, management of behavioral crises, and improvements in certain types of skills needed for everyday functioning. The goals of CBT in the treatment of schizophrenia include belief modification, reattribution, and reframing of psychotic experiences so that the intensity of hallucinations and delusions, and the levels of distress associated with each, are reduced. Meta-analyses of CBT trials in schizophrenia reported a small to modest effect size for the reduction of positive symptoms. Social skills training focuses on bolstering basic skills involved in everyday social interactions (such as basic conversational skills and engaging in leisure activities) and independent living (including self-care and management of medications). Social skills training has been found to lead to improvements in interpersonal communication, social interaction and independent living skills despite mixed evidence regarding symptom reduction and relapse. A variation of CBT is acceptance and commitment therapy, which does not aim to change thoughts and feelings, but to "just notice" and accept them. Cognitive remediation is focused on improving relative weaknesses in cognitive functioning and is often coupled with activities meant to extend these improvements into real-world situations and activities. The utility of cognitive remediation in improving aspects of cognitive and global functioning is supported by meta-analyses. The effectiveness of cognitive remediation for improving the symptoms of schizophrenia is less clear. Psychoeducation includes proving information about the illness and its treatment and uses motivational interviewing to improve medication adherence in the acute stage of the illness (often at the time of hospitalization).

Providing education and support to family members is a crucial component of comprehensive treatment. Family treatment that reduces high expressed emotion reduces the likelihood of relapse, especially if the patient's response to antipsychotic medication is less than optimal. Other components of family-based interventions will often include strategies for resolving disputes and related interpersonal difficulties among family members that can arise during the course of treatments and for collaborating with clinicians and interacting within the broader health care system.

In most mental health systems, case management has been developed to provide low-cost support for patients living in the community, many of whom were formerly institutionalized. Case managers help patients find housing; manage financial resources; get access to psychiatric clinics, rehabilitation services, and crisis intervention; and comply with medication regimens. Such assistance enables patients to live in settings with no or minimal mental health-worker–provided supervision. Some mental health systems assign patients at especially high risk of rehospitalization to a multidisciplinary team that is available around the clock, an approach termed "assertive community treatment."

Finally, many communities offer additional services including supported employment programs, whereby patients are assessed for skills and are matched with an appropriate job with on-site support and training from a work coach familiar with the special needs of patients with schizophrenia. The goal of supported employment is similar to that of sheltered work programs—assisting patients to obtain employment. For patients with schizophrenia who are homeless and are prone to psychotic relapses due to gaps in treatment and other challenges, many communities also offer assertive community treatment programs in which small but mobile teams of health care professionals, including a psychiatrist or other clinicians, a nurse, and a social worker will provide evaluation and treatment to patients in the field, rather than in clinics or hospitals. For patients with co-occurring substance-use disorders, integrated treatment programs that combine pharmacotherapy with substance-focused psychosocial treatments and broader wrap-around services such as case management may provide the best chances of achieving sustained sobriety, enduring symptom control, and enhanced functioning.

Addington D, Anderson E, Kelly M, et al. Canadian Practice Guidelines for Comprehensive Community Treatment for Schizophrenia and Schizophrenia Spectrum Disorders. *Can J Psychiatry.* 2017;62:662–672.

Cella M, Preti A, Edwards C, et al. Cognitive remediation for negative symptoms of schizophrenia: a network meta-analysis. *Clin Psychol Rev.* 2017;52:43–51.

Garety PA, Fowler D, Kuipers E. Cognitive–behavioral therapy for medication-resistant symptoms. *Schizophr Bull.* 2000;26:73–86.

Heinssen RK, Libwerman RP, Kopelowicz A. Psychosocial skills training for schizophrenia: lessons from the laboratory. *Schizophr Bull.* 2000;26:21–46.

Jauhar S, McKenna PJ, Radua J, et al. Cognitive-behavioural therapy for the symptoms of schizophrenia: systematic review and meta-analysis with examination of potential bias. *Br J Psychiatry.* 2014;204(1):20–29.

Kern RS, Glynn SM, Horan WP, Marder SR. Psychosocial treatments to promote functional recovery in schizophrenia. *Schizophr Bull.* 2009;35:347–361.

Lenroot R, Bustillo JR, Lauriello J, Keith SJ. Integrated treatment of schizophrenia. *Psychiatr Serv.* 2003;54:1499–1507.

McGurk SR, Twamley EW, Sitzer DI, et al. A meta-analysis of cognitive remediation in schizophrenia. *Am J Psychiatry.* 2007;164(12):1791–1802.

Morin L, Franck N. Rehabilitation interventions to promote recovery from schizophrenia: a systematic review. *Front Psychiatry.* 2017;8:100.

Penn DL, Mueser KT, Tarrier N, et al. Supportive therapy for schizophrenia: possible mechanisms and implications for adjunctive psychosocial treatments. *Schizophr Bull.* 2004;30:101–112.

Wykes T, Huddy V, Cellard C, et al. A meta-analysis of cognitive remediation for schizophrenia: methodology and effect sizes. *Am J Psychiatry.* 2011;168(5):472–485.

Prognosis

As indicated earlier, the course of schizophrenia is highly variable; however, the typical pattern is of relative remissions with residual symptoms and dysfunction, punctuated by periodic symptom exacerbation. About 10% of patients eventually recover, and an additional 20% have a good outcome. One-third of treated patients have a stable but only intermediate outcome; the remaining one-third have a deteriorating course.

Thus, a significant proportion of treated patients (about 40%) continue to manifest psychotic symptoms. Even low-grade residual symptoms can be enough to impede functional capacity (e.g., to work, sustain meaningful relationships, maintain adequate self-care, and live independently). Therefore, despite advances in the treatment of the disorder, more is needed before patients with schizophrenia can enjoy a quality of life comparable to that of the general population.

A. Predictors of Better Long-Term Course

Predictors of better long-term course are summarized in Table 24–14. Even under these circumstances, return to a full

Table 24–14 Predictors of Course and Outcome in Schizophrenia

Factor	Better Outcome	Poorer Outcome
Age at onset*	About 20–25	Below 20
CT/MRI studies*	Normal morphology	Dilated ventricles, brain atrophy
Initial clinical symptoms*,†	Catatonia, paranoia, depression, schizoaffective diagnosis, atypical symptoms, confusion	Negative symptoms (e.g., flat affect, poverty of thought, apathy, asociality); obsessive–compulsive symptoms
Occupational record*	Stable	Irregular
Onset*	Acute, late	Insidious
Rate of progression*	Rapid	Slow
Sex*	Possibly females	Possibly males
Length of episode prior to assessment†	Months or less	Years
Being in a developing country‡	Present	Absent
Cannabis use‡	Absent	Present
Optimal prenatal care‡	Present	Absent
Precipitating factors‡	Present	Absent
Socioeconomic status‡	Middle, high	Low
Substance abuse‡	Absent	Present
Stressful life‡	Absent	Present
Early treatment with medications§	Present	Absent
Long-term drug maintenance§	Present	Absent
Response to medications initially§	Present	Absent
Family history of mental illness¶	Affective	Schizophrenia
Other adverse social factors¶	Absent	Present
Prenatal adverse events¶	None	Present
Presence of certain gene polymorphism, e.g., COMT. NMDA2A¶	Absent	Present

*Clinical; †diagnosis; ‡environment; §treatment; ¶genetic.

premorbid level of functioning is rarely observed, and milder residual deficits persist as indicated earlier. Early treatment, shorter duration of untreated psychosis and fewer relapses are associated with better outcomes.

B. Predictors of Poorer Long-Term Course

Predictors of poorer long-term course are summarized in Table 24–14. Taking into account the different syndromal domains of schizophrenia, negative symptoms and cognitive dysfunction are more closely tied than positive symptoms to functional disability and problems with independent living. This is probably due to the combination of illness-specific factors and the limitations of available treatment, the latter of which may successfully address combativeness, agitation, neurovegetative problems, and positive symptoms such

as hallucinations and delusions but provide less benefit for negative symptoms, social dysfunction, impaired cognition, and poor insight.

More than half of patients with schizophrenia have poor insight. Many are unaware that their symptoms are attributable to mental illness. Even if appropriate treatment is initiated, the rates of relapse are high, especially in the context of poor treatment adherence, the most common form of which is "partial" nonadherence rather than outright treatment refusal or discontinuation.

C. Early Mortality

Early mortality is frequently encountered among patients with schizophrenia, roughly 1.5–2.0 times more often than in the general population, corresponding to a 10–25-year reduction in life expectancy. Excess mortality is attributed not only to illness-related psychopathological symptoms and cognitive dysfunction but also to medical comorbidity, accidents, and suicide. The standardized mortality ratios for "natural causes," accidents, and suicide among patients with schizophrenia are approximately 1.1, 2.2, and 8.4, respectively. The lifetime risk for suicide among patients with schizophrenia is 10–13%. At some point during their lifetime, 18–55% of patients attempt suicide. Other contributors to the increased mortality include lifestyle factors such as unhealthy diets, excessive smoking, alcohol and other substance use, lack of exercise, delayed diagnosis, inadequate treatment of physical disorders, and the metabolic and cardiovascular side effects of antipsychotic medications.

Successful treatment of the disorder, therefore, requires attention not only to psychopathological domains such as positive and negative symptoms but also to cognition, functional capacity, treatment adherence, affective/anxiety symptoms, psychosocial support, comorbid conditions (psychiatric and substance related), and general medical care. Advances in pharmacological and psychosocial treatment, and increased attention to medical problems and the other special needs of patients with schizophrenia, offer hope to many.

Davidson L, McGlashan TH. The varied outcomes of schizophrenia. *Can J Psychiatry*. 1997;42:34.

Jobe TH, Harrow M. Long-term outcome of patients with schizophrenia: a review. *Can J Psychiatry*. 2005;50:892.

Laursen TM, Munk-Olsen T, Vestergaard M. Life expectancy and cardiovascular mortality in persons with schizophrenia. *Curr Opin Psychiatry*. 2012;25(2):83–88.

Tsuang MT, Tohen M, eds. *Textbook in Psychiatric Epidemiology*. 2nd ed. New York: Wiley-Liss; 2002.

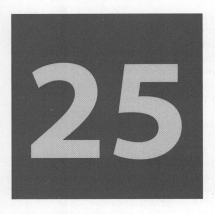

Other Psychotic Disorders

Richard C. Shelton, MD

SCHIZOPHRENIFORM DISORDER

▶ General Considerations

A. Epidemiology

Diagnostically, schizophreniform disorder is "positioned" in time between brief psychotic disorder (discussed later in this chapter), which lasts 1 month or less, and schizophrenia (see Chapter 24), which by definition continues beyond 6 months. Although many patients will eventually develop schizophrenia, a small but significant number of patients with persisting psychotic disorders will show complete recovery of their illness. The proportion that recover is likely small, although the exact percentage is unknown. Those who do show recovery typically exhibit characteristics known to predict better outcome in other diagnostic categories (e.g., acute onset, brief prodrome, lack of psychosocial deterioration, and prominent mood symptoms).

B. Etiology

Schizophreniform disorder is a heterogeneous category; therefore, in all likelihood, it has several distinct etiologies. Because most patients will go on to meet diagnostic criteria for schizophrenia, the etiologies will be the same as for that condition, discussed in detail in Chapter 24. Some patients with this disorder appear to recover significantly and thus represent a manifestation that is distinct from typical schizophrenia.

C. Genetics

Because schizophreniform disorder is likely to be an etiologically heterogeneous disorder, genetic relationships are unclear. Those persons who proceed on to manifest typical schizophrenia show genetic predispositions that are similar to this condition. Those who recover completely may have increased family histories of both psychotic and affective disorders, especially bipolar disorder.

▶ Clinical Findings

A. Signs & Symptoms

Patients with schizophreniform disorder exhibit symptoms consistent with Criterion A of schizophrenia (i.e., hallucinations; delusions; negative symptoms; disorganization of thought, speech, and behavior) that last between 1 and 6 months. Patients with these symptoms may proceed on to a typical pattern of schizophrenia and should be diagnosed as such if the symptoms are present for more than 6 months. However, others may proceed to complete or near-complete resolution of their symptoms. These patients generally have good premorbid function, acute onset (often after a stressor), and complete resolution without residual deficits in psychosocial function. In addition, mood symptoms tend to be more prominent, and a family history of mood disorder is common in these patients.

B. Psychological Testing

Psychological testing will reveal a pattern of symptoms more typical of schizophrenia (see Chapter 24). These findings will include the common symptoms of thought disorganization, hallucinations, and delusions. However, overt cognitive impairment (including memory problems) is uncommon, and prominent mood symptoms may occur. Persons with schizophreniform disorder may demonstrate frontal-cortical regional deficits such as impaired performance on the Wisconsin Card Sorting Test.

C. Laboratory Findings & Neuroimaging

Brain imaging studies may show the same results as those reported for schizophrenia. However, the differences often are less prominent, owing to the shorter duration of the condition. Alternatively, many patients do not show differences from normal controls, which may be associated with recovery. However, diagnostic imaging studies are not routinely indicated.

A relative activation deficit in the inferior prefrontal region while performing the Wisconsin Card Sorting Test has been reported in both patients with schizophrenia and schizophreniform disorder.

Course of Illness

Schizophreniform disorder often follows a course typical of schizophrenia. If symptoms are present for more than 6 months, psychological and social deterioration typically associated with schizophrenia may occur. First-generation antipsychotics such as haloperidol reduce the symptoms of the illness but will not prevent deterioration if the symptoms are present for more than 6 months. The potential beneficial effects of newer, atypical antipsychotics (e.g., clozapine, risperidone, olanzapine, quetiapine) in preventing psychosocial deterioration or cognitive impairment have been hypothesized but not conclusively established.

Differential Diagnosis (Including Comorbid Conditions)

Although the major differential diagnoses are brief psychotic disorder and schizophrenia, the rapid onset of acute psychosis may be the most important diagnostic point. Attention should focus on the prior 6 months, the pattern of onset, and the presence of mood changes, substance abuse, and other medical illness and medications.

Treatment

The treatment of schizophreniform disorder is similar to that of schizophrenia (see Chapter 24).

Hospitalization is usually required in the acute stages of overt psychotic symptoms.

A. Psychopharmacologic Interventions

Antipsychotic drugs represent the mainstay of symptomatic management, and resolution of psychosis often is fairly rapid. It has been shown that patients with schizophreniform disorder respond to antipsychotic treatment more rapidly than do patients with schizophrenia. Sedative agents, especially benzodiazepines, may be needed to manage acute agitation. Electroconvulsive therapy may also be indicated for some refractory patients.

B. Psychotherapeutic Interventions

Psychotherapy is usually needed to help patients integrate the psychotic experience. Psychosocial support and rehabilitation is critical with these patients to help reduce the deterioration in function more typical of schizophrenia. Therefore, rapid treatment of symptoms and social reintegration of the patient are important.

C. Other Interventions

After acute symptoms resolve, psychological, social, occupational, and educational interventions become the main focus of treatment. An acute schizophreniform psychotic episode represents a catastrophic event in the life of the patient, and psychotherapy is needed to help the patient understand the event and gain a sense of control over future episodes. A variety of issues should be discussed with the patient and his or her support system: (1) the fundamental biological nature of the disorder; (2) the role of medication in controlling current and future symptoms, particularly the possible effect of symptom management on the evolution of the disorder; (3) the early warning signs that indicate a return of psychosis; (4) the impact of the disturbance on the person's life and that of the family; (5) the need for gradual reintegration into work or school; and (6) the importance of future psychosocial management, including intensive case management or occupational or educational rehabilitation.

Prognosis

Most individuals with schizophreniform disorder are simply in the early stages of the development of more typical schizophrenia. The 6-month cutoff for the diagnosis of schizophreniform disorder acknowledges that although patients with typical schizophrenia symptoms sometimes show complete resolution, this seldom occurs when the symptoms have been present for 6 months or more. Almost all patients will then proceed to a course more consistent with schizophrenia, with persistent deterioration and impairment in psychosocial functioning. Exceptions to this rule are very rare.

Benazzi F. Outcome of schizophreniform disorder. *Curr Psychiatry Rep.* 2003;5(3):192–196.

Fusar-Poli P, Cappucciati M, Rutigliano G, et al. Diagnostic stability of ICD/DSM first episode psychoses diagnoses: meta-analysis. *Schizophr. Bull.* 2016;42(6):1395–1406.

Strakowski SM. Diagnostic validity of schizophreniform disorder. *Am j psychiatry.* 1994;151:815.

SCHIZOAFFECTIVE DISORDER

General Considerations

A. Epidemiology

The lifetime prevalence of schizoaffective disorder is less than 1%. Schizoaffective disorder is characterized by prominent mood symptoms (mania or depression) occurring during the course of a chronic psychotic disorder. Phenomenologically, schizoaffective disorder holds the middle ground between mood disorders (especially psychotic mood disorders) and chronic psychotic conditions such as schizophrenia. The debate continues over whether schizoaffective disorder "belongs" to the spectrum of either schizophrenia or affective disorders or represents a distinct category. Schizoaffective disorder likely represents a heterogeneous disorder with multiple distinct etiologies.

B. Etiology

Recent research indicates that there appear to be distinct etiologies and outcomes depending on whether the course of schizoaffective disorder is typified by episodes of bipolar-type cycling or simple depressive episodes in the absence of mania.

C. Genetics

In the bipolar variant, there is an increased proportion of family history of bipolar disorder (but not schizophrenia) and a better overall outcome. Although a family history of affective disorder is observed in the depressive variant, a history of psychotic disorder seems to be more common and outcome is poorer than in the bipolar form. Both variants usually have a better prognosis than does schizophrenia without prominent mood symptoms.

▶ Clinical Findings

A. Signs & Symptoms

Patients with schizoaffective disorder exhibit symptoms consistent with DSM-5-TR diagnostic Criterion A for schizophrenia. However, during the course of illness, there are superimposed episodes of depressive or manic symptoms. These patients would be diagnosed as having schizoaffective disorder, depressed or manic types, respectively. However, psychotic symptoms consistent with schizophrenia must be present for at least 2 weeks independently of the mania or depression syndromes.

Schizoaffective disorder, bipolar type, usually involves cycling of mania, depression, or mixed states in a way that is consistent with bipolar disorder. Similarly, patients with schizoaffective disorder, depressive type, may have repeated episodes of major depression, as in major depressive disorder. However, unlike depressive or bipolar disorders, there are consistent symptoms of schizophrenia in the absence of overt mood disorder. In schizoaffective disorder, depressive type, depressive episodes in which the patient meets full diagnostic criteria for major depression must be distinguished from the mood and negative symptoms associated with schizophrenia. Similarly, care should be taken to avoid misdiagnosing as mania agitation, hostility, insomnia, and other symptoms of an acute exacerbation of schizophrenia.

B. Psychological Testing

The results of psychological tests depend on the state of illness of a given patient. That is, although the typical results of schizophrenia usually are present (see Chapter 24), characteristics of mood disorders also may be present. For example,

psychological testing results will be consistent with depression or mania during corresponding episodes of illness. However, schizoaffective disorder, bipolar type, may be associated with less psychosocial and cognitive impairments than are schizophrenia or schizoaffective disorder, depressive type.

▶ Course of Illness

Generally, persons with schizoaffective disorder have a course of illness that is intermediate between the mood disorders (with a relatively better prognosis) and schizophrenia (with marked residual psychosocial deterioration). However, distinctions also can be made for patients within the schizoaffective spectrum. Patients with schizoaffective disorder, bipolar type have a course of illness that is more similar to bipolar disorder. These patients often have better functioning between acute episodes of illness than patients with either schizophrenia or schizoaffective disorder, depressive type. Patients with schizoaffective disorder, depressive type, tend to exhibit more typical schizophrenic symptoms and course, although when the disorder is managed properly, the prognosis may be better than typical schizophrenia without comorbid depression.

▶ Differential Diagnosis (Including Comorbid Conditions)

Persons with schizophrenia are not immune to the occurrence of mood symptoms. When these features meet the diagnostic criteria for a mood disorder concurrently with features of schizophrenia, the diagnosis of schizoaffective disorder may be made. However, great care must be exercised in the evaluation in order to provide appropriate management of the disorder. For example, depressive symptoms not meeting full diagnostic criteria for a major depressive episode are common in schizophrenia and do not warrant a diagnosis of schizoaffective disorder per se. In fact, treatment of schizophrenia, especially management with atypical antipsychotics, may reduce these symptoms in many patients without reliance on antidepressants. Alternatively, the negative symptoms of schizophrenia (e.g., apathy, withdrawal, avolition, blunted affect) may be confused with the symptoms of depression. Again, these symptoms generally are treated more effectively with atypical antipsychotics. Finally, the agitation, insomnia, and grandiose delusions of an acutely psychotic patient with schizophrenia sometimes can be confused with mania. However, a careful examination of the course of illness, prodromal symptoms, and acute presentation can be helpful in making the correct diagnosis. For example, the acutely agitated patient who presents for treatment after a period of progressive withdrawal, isolation, and bizarre behavior is unlikely to have mania. A good diagnostic rule of thumb is to evaluate the patient for the presence of current or past mood disorder by excluding the symptoms of schizophrenia, prior to confirming the diagnosis of schizoaffective disorder.

Psychotic mood disorders also may present with a confusing picture. DSM-5-TR diagnostic criteria are written to aid the clinician in making this distinction. The presence of mood symptoms concurrent with psychosis, even symptoms that otherwise appear to be more like typical schizophrenia (i.e., bizarre behavior or disorganized speech) are not adequate to make the diagnosis of schizoaffective disorder. This condition is understood as representing a mood disorder superimposed on a course of schizophrenia. Therefore, the criteria require the symptoms of schizophrenia to be present for at least 2 weeks in the absence of prominent mood symptoms meeting diagnostic criteria for major depression, mania, or mixed state. A course consistent with dysthymia concurrent with schizophrenia does not constitute a diagnosis of schizoaffective disorder.

Treatment

A. Psychopharmacologic Interventions

Once a definite diagnosis of schizoaffective disorder is made, treatment must take into consideration the necessity of managing both mood symptoms and psychotic symptoms (Table 25–1). Antipsychotics are required for the management of the psychotic features (see Chapter 26) and are typically used in these patients in acute manic states. Atypical antipsychotics are the first treatments of choice for several reasons. They can reduce both psychotic and more purely manic symptoms. They also exhibit mood-stabilizing effects, which are needed if cycling is present. Antidepressant drugs should be used as required in a manner similar to that discussed in Chapter 26 for the treatment of major depression. Alternatively, mood-stabilizing agents such as lithium, carbamazepine, or divalproex may be required adjunctively for the treatment of mood cycling. The effectiveness of lamotrigine as an adjunctive antidepressant or mood stabilizer in this population is not as well-studied. Finally, psychosocial management often is needed in much the same fashion as with

Table 25–1 Principles of Management of Schizoaffective Disorder

- Acute and chronic antipsychotic drug therapies usually are required.
- Atypical antipsychotics may be more effective in managing psychotic and mood symptoms.
- Additional mood stabilizers may be needed for patients with a history of mania.
- Antidepressants will sometimes be required for both depressive and bipolar types; however, exposure to antidepressant medications should be minimized for patients with a history of mania.
- Psychological, social, educational, and occupational support and rehabilitation usually are needed as with schizophrenia.

schizophrenia or schizophreniform disorder to aid in social reintegration.

B. Psychotherapeutic Interventions

No single specific psychotherapeutic intervention has been recommended for schizoaffective disorder. However, patients may benefit from a combination of family therapy, social skills training, and cognitive rehabilitation.

Prognosis

Regardless of the diagnostic category (i.e., bipolar or depressive type), certain factors are associated with a poor outcome. They include insidious onset prior to the first psychotic episode; early onset of illness; poor or deteriorating premorbid functioning; the absence of a clear precipitating stressor; prominent negative symptoms in the prodromal, acute, or residual phases of illness; and a family history of schizophrenia. These factors are also associated with a poorer outcome in persons with schizophrenia without prominent mood symptoms.

Kantrowitz JT, Citrome L. Schizoaffective disorder: a review of current research themes and pharmacological management. *CNS Drugs.* 2011;25(4):317–331.

Marneros A. The schizoaffective phenomenon: the state of the art. *Acta Psychiatr Scand Suppl.* 2003;418:29–33.

Miller JN, Black DW. Schizoaffective disorder: a review. *Ann Clin Psychiatry.* 2019;31(1):47–53.

DELUSIONAL DISORDER

General Considerations

A. Epidemiology

The cause of delusional disorder is unknown. A very small proportion of the population (roughly 0.03%) experience persistent, relatively fixed delusions in the absence of the characteristic features of other psychotic disorders such as schizophrenia.

B. Etiology

Etiologic theories about the development of delusional disorder abound, but systematic study is sparse. Early concepts of etiology focused on the denial and projection of unacceptable impulses. Hence, as examples, homosexual attraction would be reformulated unconsciously to homosexual delusions or a belief in a love relationship with a famous person. Other theories focus on projection of unacceptable sexual and aggressive drives, leading to paranoid fears of others. These and other psychodynamic theories have certain heuristic appeal, but little systematic study has been done to support these conjectures.

C. Genetics

Little is known about the genetics of delusional disorder. Family studies have suggested a decided lack of increased family history of psychotic or mood disorder.

▶ **Clinical Findings**

A. Signs & Symptoms

Delusional disorder is characterized by delusions lasting greater than 1 month. Most often the delusional content appears possible, albeit far-fetched. For example, people with this condition may have fixed delusions that they are being watched by the CIA. More traditionally, delusional disorder excluded bizarre or non-plausible delusions (such as their movements are being controlled by an external force), but this is no longer a core diagnostic feature. Persons with this condition may appear otherwise quite normal. They often hold jobs and may be married. The oddness and eccentricity of their beliefs and behavior may manifest itself only around the topic of the delusion.

The diagnosis of delusional disorder depends on the presence of delusions for more than 1 month in the absence of meeting Criterion A for schizophrenia (see Chapter 24). Specifically, there should not be significant hallucinatory experiences, marked thought disorder, prominent negative symptoms, or psychosocial deterioration. Except for the behaviors associated with the delusions (e.g., delusional accusations of unfaithfulness in the spouse), the actions of the individual are not otherwise impaired. Although people with delusional disorder may have comorbid major depression or bipolar disorder, the delusions should be present at times when a mood disorder is not present and not just concurrently with an episode of depression or mania. Under these circumstances, however, care must be taken to distinguish this condition from schizoaffective disorder. Specifically, the symptoms must not meet Criterion A of the schizophrenia diagnostic criteria.

Specific types of delusional disorder have distinguishing features. The most familiar is the so-called **persecutory type**, in which patients experience fixed (and often focal) paranoid delusions that other persons are intending to harm them in some way. These patients may believe that they are being watched or followed or that malevolent parties are engaging in other persecutory or threatening behavior. The affected person will act in a way that is consistent with the content of the persecutory delusion but will otherwise be normal.

Another common variant is the **jealous type**. These patients exhibit delusional beliefs that their significant other is being unfaithful. As with the persecutory type, the plausible nature of the belief system may make it difficult to distinguish delusional beliefs from normal fears or real experiences. Patients with delusional disorder, jealous type, either have beliefs that cross the threshold of credibility or refuse to accept reasonable reassurances. For example, a 90-year-old man who believes that his 88-year-old wife is having sex regularly with young men may be more suspicious for delusional disorder.

In delusional disorder, **erotomanic type** (also referred to as de Clerambault syndrome), the delusion is that another person (usually someone who is famous or of higher social status) is in love with the affected individual. These beliefs may be highly elaborate, although plausibility is maintained. For example, a young woman with delusional disorder, erotomanic type, may travel around the country to attend the concerts of a famous performer. She may believe that the performer gives her secret signals during his concert that indicate his love. However, she also may believe that there is some external reason that he cannot express his love more directly, for example, because he is married. Persons with this condition seldom make direct contact with their paramour, although they may, occasionally, engage in more aggressive stalking behavior. Whenever the disorder occurs, it typically becomes the central focus of the person's life.

In the **grandiose type** of the disorder, the person experiences fixed, false beliefs of power (e.g., being the owner of a major corporation), money, identity (e.g., being the Prince of Wales), a special relationship with God (e.g., being Jesus Christ) or famous people, or some other distinguishing characteristic. These patients may be quietly psychotic but may come to treatment as a result of a contact with a government agency or other organization. For example, a person who believes that he is the President of the United States may be picked up trying to enter the grounds of the White House.

The **somatic type** of delusional disorder involves a fixed belief of some physical abnormality or characteristic. Distinguishing this disorder from illness anxiety disorder may be difficult and generally depends on the content of the belief and the degree to which the belief is held in spite of evidence to the contrary. People with somatoform disorders such as illness anxiety disorder or body dysmorphic disorder may have a fixed belief regarding a specific, serious, but plausible physical illness, such as cancer or acquired immunodeficiency syndrome (AIDS). In illness anxiety disorder, these beliefs often relate to specific symptoms, such as pain, stiffness, or swelling. Patients with delusional disorder, somatic type, may have beliefs about other, more unusual conditions. These delusions may involve beliefs about contamination with toxic substances, infestations of insects (parasitosis) or other vermin, foul body odors, malfunctions of specific body parts such as the liver or intestines, or other unusual content.

Finally, the **mixed type** of delusional disorder involves more than one of the types just described, without one taking prominence, and the **unspecified type** involves delusions that do not fall into one of the other categories. For example, the delusion of Capgras syndrome is the belief that a familiar person has been replaced by an imposter.

B. Psychological Testing

Psychological testing will reveal the presence of the delusional psychotic material in these patients but, most often, little else. The cognitive impairments or social deterioration seen in schizophrenia are absent; if such impairments are present, the diagnosis of schizophrenia should be considered. Similarly, prominent mood symptoms might suggest a diagnosis of a psychotic mood disorder.

C. Laboratory Findings & Imaging

Neuroimaging data on delusional disorder are rare. Limited evidence indicates that persons with delusional disorder show reduced cortical gray matter and increased ventricular and sulcal size similar to that seen in schizophrenia. However, there has been little systemic study of this condition.

▶ Course of Illness

Occasionally, patients with delusional disorder will go on to develop schizophrenia. This is an exception, though; most patients maintain the delusional diagnosis. About half of patients recover fully and about one-third improve significantly. Only about 20% maintain the delusion indefinitely.

▶ Differential Diagnosis (Including Comorbid Conditions)

The differential diagnosis of delusional disorder encompasses broad categories of disorders. For example, delusional thinking may occur in patients with other psychotic disorders such as schizophrenia, schizoaffective disorder, mood disorders (bipolar disorder, manic or depressed type, or major depression) with psychotic features, psychotic disorders due to a general medical condition, or substance-induced psychotic disorder. In delusional disorder, however, important features of those conditions will be absent. For example, the prominent hallucinations, negative symptoms, thought disorder, or social deterioration consistent with schizophrenia are not present. Similarly, mood symptoms, if present, are not prominent. The delusional thinking should not be accounted for by the presence of a medical condition or substance, including substances of abuse. For example, a young patient with a history of stimulant abuse who exhibits paranoid ideation after a recent cocaine binge would not necessarily have delusional disorder.

A delusional diagnosis also may be easily confused with the obsessions of obsessive–compulsive disorder (OCD; see Chapter 30); however, in OCD the patient almost always has at least some insight into the exaggerated nature of the thoughts. Further, obsessions associated with OCD most often involve an inappropriate or exaggerated appraisal of a real threat. This could include a fear of contamination, loss of control of impulses, loss of important documents, and similar threats. When delusional disorder involves a fear of a specific threat, the fears are more typically paranoid or persecutory in nature.

Somatoform disorders such as illness anxiety disorder or somatization disorder are easily confused with delusional disorder, somatic type (see Chapter 16). As noted earlier, delusional disorder, somatic type, generally differs in both degree and type of belief. That is, in delusional disorder the beliefs are held tenaciously and often will involve implausible content. Alternatively, people with body dysmorphic disorder often hold tenaciously to their preoccupation with a specific body part and are not easily dissuaded from the belief. In this case, the belief may seem like a delusion. The distinction is that the problem is perceptual—that is, it is fixed on the appearance of a body part and does not extend to other types of delusional beliefs.

Paranoid personality disorder also may be confused with delusional disorder (see Chapter 21). Two significant characteristics distinguish these disorders. In paranoid personality disorder, the hostility and paranoid thinking most often are generalized and affect multiple areas of the person's life. For example, the patient may be jealous of the spouse but also will exhibit hypersensitivity at work and in other areas. By contrast, the psychotic thoughts of delusional disorder usually are focused in a single area with remarkable preservation of other areas of thinking and functioning. Another feature distinguishing the disorders is the tenacity of the delusional belief. Persons with delusional disorder most often will maintain a stable but false belief system for long periods. Alternatively, the threatening beliefs of the person with paranoid personality disorder do not reach delusional proportions and often wax and wane in intensity.

▶ Treatment

A. Psychopharmacologic Interventions

The treatment of delusional disorder relies heavily on the use of antipsychotic drugs, particularly the atypical antipsychotics; however, little systematic study has examined the effectiveness of this approach. Pharmacotherapy should be undertaken with caution: patients with delusional disorder are convinced of the delusional beliefs and will usually resist medication management. Drug treatment should only be undertaken in the context of an ongoing therapeutic relationship in which there has been an effort to establish rapport, collaboration, and shared goals. For example, it is of little use to try to convince patients who have persecutory delusions that medicine will help them by changing how they think about the feared situation. Patients may be willing to take a drug that will calm the anxiety that has resulted from the persecution. Pimozide has historically been recommended for this condition; however, systematic study showing particular superiority is lacking.

B. Psychotherapeutic Interventions

Individual supportive psychotherapy as well as family therapy may also be required.

Complications/Adverse Outcomes of Treatment

The main complication of delusional disorder has to do with whether the affected person acts on the delusion in some way. Most people with this disorder lead quiet, uneventful lives otherwise. However, a sudden, unexpected event may intervene, such as the stalking of a famous person. These events may lead to incarceration or involuntary hospitalization, which may surprise friends and coworkers. These actions are consistent with the content of the delusion. Unfortunately, treatment, at least in the short term, often is ineffective, leading to a repetition of the behaviors related to the false beliefs.

Prognosis

The prognosis of delusional disorder is good in most cases. About two-third of patients recover or improve significantly; however, in about 20% of patients delusional symptoms persist and are usually treatment-resistant.

Manschreck TC, Khan NL. Recent advances in the treatment of delusional disorder. *Can J Psychiatry*. 2006;51:114.

Muñoz-Negro JE, Cervilla JA. A systematic review on the pharmacological treatment of delusional disorder. *J Clin Psychopharmacol*. 2016;36(6):684–690.

Skelton M, Khokhar WA, Thacker SP. Treatments for delusional disorder. *Cochrane Database Syst Rev*. 2015;2015(5):CD009785. Published 2015 May 22.

BRIEF PSYCHOTIC DISORDER

General Considerations

The emergence of transient psychotic symptoms, particularly after a severe psychological or social stressor such as a move or loss of a loved one, is not rare. Brief psychotic symptoms in the absence of a clear stressor are less common but also may occur. This disorder is generally associated with very acute onset and florid symptoms that decline rapidly even in the absence of the use of antipsychotic drugs. A diagnosis of brief psychotic disorder should be considered if a psychotic patient has a history of good premorbid functioning and an acute onset that resolves rapidly and completely in response to antipsychotic therapy.

A. Epidemiology

Reliable estimates of the frequency of this disorder are not available; however, an increased frequency is observed in populations that have experienced significant life stresses (e.g., immigrants, refugees, military recruits, and persons who have experienced a disaster such as an earthquake or hurricane). Therefore, the frequency is going to depend on the population under study. Predisposing variables include comorbidity of personality disorder, substance-use disorder, or dementia, or low socioeconomic status. Socioeconomic status may be associated with brief psychotic disorder in part because persons of lower social class may be at increased risk for major life stresses.

B. Etiology

A variety of stressors may occur prior to the onset of brief psychotic disorder. For example, the disorder may occur after the death of a loved one, after a move to a new country (culture shock), during a natural disaster, or during combat or other military activity. A variety of factors are associated with the occurrence of brief psychotic disorder. They can be associated with either an increased likelihood of experiencing a stressor (e.g., lower socioeconomic status, refugee or immigrant status, presence in a war zone) or limitations in coping skills (e.g., persons with personality disorders, children or adolescents). However, the problem may also occur in people experiencing mild or no stressor and without predisposing characteristics.

C. Genetics

Family history relationships are unclear; however, there may be an increased risk of psychotic disorder (including brief psychotic episodes) or affective disorder in relatives of persons with this condition.

Clinical Findings

A. Signs & Symptoms

Psychotic symptoms occurring for 1 month or less with complete resolution constitute brief psychotic disorder. This condition occurs most often after a significant external stressor, although DSM-V-TR allows the diagnosis without an obvious stress. The presentation is usually particularly florid. Patients can exhibit confusion, marked agitation or catatonia, emotional lability, and psychotic symptoms such as hallucinations or delusions. The symptoms may be so severe as to mimic the appearance of delirium.

B. Psychological Testing

Psychological testing has not been shown to be useful in adding to the diagnosis of brief psychotic disorder.

C. Laboratory Findings

There are no laboratory findings suggestive or supportive of brief psychotic disorder.

Course of Illness

Though by definition symptoms are brief and time limited, recurrence of psychotic events often occurs, especially in the face of ongoing stressors or comorbid conditions such as personality disorder. When recurrence is frequent, long-term management with an antipsychotic (usually an atypical antipsychotic agent) may be indicated.

Differential Diagnosis (Including Comorbid Conditions)

The diagnosis of brief psychotic disorder is often difficult to make, and corroborative information from a family member or friend may be required to distinguish this problem from another psychotic disorder or cognitive disorder such as delirium.

A variety of disorders should be considered in the differential, including schizophrenia spectrum disorders (i.e., schizophreniform disorder, schizophrenia, or schizoaffective disorder), psychotic affective disorders, delusional disorder, personality disorder, substance-use disorder (including withdrawal), substance-induced psychosis, delirium, or psychotic disorder due to medical condition. Schizophrenia and related disorders (including delusional disorder) are distinguished by the duration of psychotic symptoms and impairments. Persons with brief psychotic disorder show complete resolution of their psychotic symptoms and impairments within the 30 days allotted for the diagnosis. The symptoms of persons with delusional disorder are more confined to the delusional content and are not as pervasive as that usually seen in brief psychotic disorder.

A diagnosis of psychotic affective disorder should be made in the presence of prominent mood symptoms meeting diagnostic criteria for mania or depression. This distinction may be difficult to make, especially in highly agitated or otherwise distressed patients. The mood, psychotic, and behavioral symptoms of affective psychosis rarely resolve completely within 30 days of initiation of treatment; therefore, if patients show complete return of baseline function within this time frame, a diagnosis of brief psychotic disorder should be considered, especially in the absence of a history of mood disorder.

Patients with personality disorder may present transient episodes of psychosis. This is particularly true of borderline personality disorder but may be seen in other disorders, including histrionic, schizotypal, or obsessive–compulsive personality. These events almost always follow a significant stressor, especially an interpersonal stressful event. These occurrences may be very brief (i.e., less than 1 day) and would be included in the category of psychotic disorder not otherwise classified. However, if they occur for more than 1 day but less than 1 month, the patient should be given a diagnosis of brief psychotic disorder along with the personality disorder diagnosis. Finally, if the psychotic symptoms seem related to substance use or withdrawal or to a medical condition, the alternatives of substance-use disorder (including substance-induced psychotic disorder) or psychotic disorder due to medical condition should be given diagnostic primacy.

Table 25–2 Principles of Management of Brief Psychotic Disorder

- Hospitalization usually is indicated.
- Undertake a thorough psychiatric and medical evaluation and laboratory testing to rule out other major psychiatric, medical, or substance-use disorders.
- Attempt to identify and eliminate or modify significant stressors.
- Antipsychotic and sedative drugs (such as benzodiazepines) often are indicated in acute management; however, long-term treatment with these medicines should be avoided when the diagnosis of brief psychotic disorder is clear and the patient experiences complete resolution of symptoms.
- Long-term treatment should focus on several major elements:
  Improving coping skills
  Eliminating or stabilizing ongoing psychological or social stressors
  Establishing a network of social support
  Managing comorbid conditions, including personality disorders
  Reintegrating the patient into the social, educational, or occupational milieu
  Helping the patient and social network to understand the condition and to recognize early prodromal symptoms of impending psychosis, especially sleeplessness
  Facilitating sleep, nutrition, and hygiene

Treatment

Treatment proceeds as with any other form of psychosis (Table 25–2). Hospitalization is usually required, and a reduction in sensory stimulation is helpful.

A. Psychopharmacologic Interventions

Antipsychotics and sedatives help to ameliorate the symptoms, especially by inducing sleep. Response to antipsychotic drug treatment is often rapid and complete. If complete resolution of psychotic symptoms occurs, the duration of treatment can be relatively brief—1 to 3 months. If brief psychotic disorder is recurrent, then longer-term treatment with an atypical antipsychotic should be considered.

B. Psychotherapeutic Interventions

Subsequent psychotherapeutic management should be aimed at three goals. The first goal of treatment is to help the person understand the nature of the problem, especially as it relates to the reaction to a specific stressor (if any). An acute onset of a major psychotic episode is a highly disruptive and disturbing event. Any person so affected needs to make sense of the experience. The second goal is rapid reintegration into the environment.

C. Other Interventions

Third, longer-term goals include the development of coping skills to help prevent subsequent episodes of illness. Because the problem may recur, it is important to help the patient and family recognize early prodromal signs (e.g., sleeplessness) of an impending episode.

Complications/Adverse Outcomes of Treatment

The principal complications of brief psychotic disorder have to do with the disruptions of social function, including employment, that may occur. As a result, rapid but stepwise reintegration is indicated in most patients. Careful attention should be paid to predisposing variables, including ongoing stressors (e.g., relationship stress, especially abuse) and comorbid disorders (e.g., comorbid personality or substance use disorders or medical conditions). Longer-term adverse outcomes may be more related to the outcome of these predisposing variables (especially personality disorder) than to the brief psychotic disorder per se. Some patients will never experience another psychotic event, whereas others will experience recurrences.

Prognosis

By definition, the short-term outcome of this disorder is good, though recurrence of symptoms is common, especially in the face of stressors or comorbid conditions. Long-term antipsychotic management may be indicated in some cases. Table 25–3 summarizes the favorable prognostic indicators of brief psychotic disorder.

Fusar-Poli P, Cappucciati M, Rutigliano G, et al. Diagnostic stability of ICD/DSM first episode psychosis diagnoses: meta-analysis. *Schizophr Bull.* 2016;42(6):1395–1406.

Fusar-Poli P, Cappucciati M, Bonoldi I, et al. Prognosis of brief psychotic episodes: a meta-analysis. *JAMA Psychiatry.* 2016;73(3):211–220. doi:10.1001/jamapsychiatry.2015.2313

Provenzani U, Salazar de Pablo G, Arribas M, et al. Clinical outcomes in brief psychotic episodes: a systematic review and meta-analysis. *Epidemiol Psychiatr Sci.* 2021;30:e71. Published 2021 Nov 4. doi:10.1017/S2045796021000548

Table 25–3 Favorable Prognostic Indicators of Brief Psychotic Disorder

Good premorbid adjustment
Few premorbid schizoid traits
Severe precipitating stressors
Sudden onset of symptoms
Affective symptoms
Confusion and perplexity during psychosis
Little affective blunting
Short duration of symptoms
Lack of schizophrenic relatives

SHARED PSYCHOTIC DISORDER

General Considerations

A. Epidemiology

The exact frequency of shared psychotic disorder is not known. It may occur with greater frequency in certain groups or situations, especially with social isolation of the involved parties.

B. Etiology

The etiology of shared psychotic disorder is generally thought to be psychological. The dominant, psychotic person simply imposes the delusional belief on the submissive party.

C. Genetics

A genetic predisposition to idiopathic psychoses has been suggested as a possible risk factor for shared psychotic disorder.

Clinical Findings

A. Signs & Symptoms

Shared psychotic disorder, commonly referred to as *folie à deux,* occurs when a delusion develops in a person who has a close relationship with another person who already has a fixed delusion in the context of another psychotic illness such as schizophrenia or delusional disorder. Most often the person experiencing shared psychotic disorder is in a dependent or submissive position. This would include, as examples, the position of a dependent spouse or child of a psychotic person. Most cases involve members of a family, although it may occur in other situations (e.g., religious cults). Moreover, other factors such as old age, social isolation, low intelligence, sensory deprivation, cerebrovascular disease, and alcohol abuse are associated with shared psychotic disorder.

Course of Illness

In shared psychotic disorder, the patients must be separated for treatment purposes. In general, the healthier of the two will give up the delusional belief. The sicker of the two will maintain the false fixed belief.

Differential Diagnosis (Including Comorbid Conditions)

Differential diagnosis should consider the following: delirium and dementia; alcohol-induced psychotic disorder; intoxications with sympathomimetics (including MDMA, amphetamine, marijuana, L-dopa); mood disorders; schizophrenia; and malingering and factitious disorders.

Table 25–4 Principles of Management of Shared Psychotic Disorder

Separate the involved persons. Make an effort to maintain separation if possible.
Hospitalization or alternative community residence (such as respite care) may be needed.
Avoid the use of medications if possible.
Provide ongoing psychological and social support after acute treatment.
Ongoing psychological treatment should focus on the development of coping skills and social independence.
Social monitoring and intervention (including family therapy) are indicated if the patient is going to return to the same environment.

▶ Treatment

A. Psychotherapeutic Interventions

In the most common situation, simple separation results in resolution of the delusional belief in the submissive member (folie imposée). Less commonly, the delusion fails to remit in either of the parties at separation (folie simultanée). In the rarest form, the dominant person induces a delusion in a second person, but that person goes on to develop his or her own additional delusional ideation (folie communiquée).

In the latter two conditions, antipsychotic drug therapy may be required to help reduce the psychosis of the submissive person. Table 25–4 summarizes the treatment options.

Mentjox R, van Houten CA, Kooiman CG. Induced psychotic disorder: clinical aspects, theoretical considerations, and some guidelines for treatment. *Compr Psychiatry.* 1993;34:120.

Silveira JM, Seeman MV. Shared psychotic disorder: a critical review of the literature. *Can J Psychiatry.* 1995;40:389.

PSYCHOTIC DISORDER DUE TO A GENERAL MEDICAL CONDITION & SUBSTANCE-INDUCED PSYCHOTIC DISORDER

▶ General Considerations

Many medical illnesses (Table 25–5) and drugs (Table 25–6) can induce psychotic symptoms. Other medical conditions, toxins, and drugs should be considered with any patient presenting with psychosis or with an exacerbation of a pre-existing psychotic disorder. Psychotic conditions related to medical conditions are very common, especially in the hospital setting. Clinicians should be prepared to treat these conditions vigorously.

Table 25–5 Medical Conditions Associated with Psychotic Symptoms

Brain neoplasm
Cerebrovascular accident
Creutzfeldt–Jakob disease
Encephalitis
Deficiency states (vitamin B_{12}, folate, thiamin, niacin)
Dementias (e.g., Alzheimer disease, Pick disease)
Fabry disease
Fahr disease
Hallervorden–Spatz disease
Heavy metal poisoning
Herpes encephalitis
HIV/AIDS
Huntington disease
Lewy body disease
Metachromatic leukodystrophy
Neurosyphilis
Parkinson disease
Porphyria
Seizure disorder (complex partial seizures)
Systemic lupus erythematosus
Wilson disease

▶ Clinical Findings

Signs & Symptoms

Hallucinations and delusions are common; however, the hallucinations of illness-related psychosis tend to be fairly specific to the underlying illness. For example, olfactory (smell) and gustatory (taste) hallucinations are associated with basal lesions of the brain or seizure disorders involving the temporal lobe or hippocampus. Alcohol or other sedative withdrawal may result in tactile (touch) hallucinations. Visual hallucinations may be reported in psychotic states induced by dopamine agonists, sympathomimetics, anticholinergics, or hallucinogenic drugs.

Table 25–6 Drugs Associated with the Induction of Psychosis

Anticholinergics (atropine)
Antidepressants
Dopamine agonists (L-dopa, bromocriptine, pramipexole)
Hallucinogens (D-lysergic acid diethylamide, phencyclidine, cannabis, mescaline)
Histamine-2 antagonists (cimetidine)
Inhalants (toluene)
Psychostimulants (cocaine, amphetamine, sympathomimetics)
Sedative-hypnotic, alcohol, or anxiolytic withdrawal
Sympathomimetics (pseudoephedrine)

Table 25–7 Management of Psychotic Disorder Due to Medical Condition and Substance-Induced Psychotic Disorder

Evaluate all acutely psychotic patients for medical or substance-induced causes, even those with chronic psychotic conditions.
Identify and vigorously treat the underlying medical or substance use disorder (including withdrawal).
Minimize exposure to all drugs.
Judiciously use antipsychotics or sedatives (including benzodiazepines).
Drug management may include low-dose typical (e.g., haloperidol 0.5–2 mg/d) or atypical (e.g., risperidone 0.5–2 mg/d, olanzapine 2.5–5 mg/d) antipsychotics or low-dose, short-acting benzodiazepines (e.g., alprazolam, lorazepam 0.25–1 mg/d).
Lower the dose or discontinue psychotropic medications as soon as possible.
Longer-term management should focus on the vigorous treatment of the underlying condition. In addition, special attention should be paid to sleep hygiene.

▶ Treatment

A. Psychotherapeutic Interventions

The management of these disorders requires identification and aggressive management of the underlying illness or drug that has induced the psychosis (Table 25–7).

B. Psychopharmacologic Interventions

In addition, antipsychotics may be required to treat the psychotic symptoms acutely. Generally, elimination of the offending illness or drug will resolve the psychotic state. Drug treatment should be conservative and targeted to the offending symptoms, such as psychosis, insomnia, or agitation.

▶ Prognosis

The long-term prognosis of these conditions relates to the course of the underlying illness. Psychosis in the face of medical conditions does not portend a favorable outcome in many patients and may be seen in parallel with delirium, a poor prognostic feature. In addition, psychosis may recur if the fundamental medical disorder recurs.

Fricchione GL, Carbone L, Bennett WI. Psychotic disorder caused by a general medical condition, with delusions. Secondary "organic" delusional syndromes. *Psychiatr Clin North Am.* 1995;18:363.
Keshavan MS, Kaneko Y: Secondary psychoses: an update. *World Psychiatry.* 2013;12(1):4–15.

PSYCHOTIC DISORDER NOT OTHERWISE SPECIFIED (NOS)

Certain psychotic states cannot be classified into one of the foregoing categories of psychoses and are referred to as psychotic disorder NOS.

Kendler KS, Walsh D. Schizophreniform disorder, delusional disorder and psychotic disorder not otherwise specified: clinical features, outcome and familial psychopathology. *Acta Psychiatr Scand.* 1995;91:370.

OTHER SPECIFIED OR CULTURE-BOUND PSYCHOTIC DISORDERS

Several psychotic disorders have specific presentations or are contained within certain demographic groups (although DSM-V-TR has created a separate diagnostic section for "Culture and Psychiatric Diagnosis"). These disorders are widely recognized but are not accorded formal diagnostic status in DSM-5-TR.

1. Capgras syndrome (delusion of doubles)—This disorder represents a fixed belief that familiar persons have been replaced by identical imposters who behave identically to the original person.

2. Lycanthropy—This is a delusion that the person is a werewolf or other animal.

3. Frégoli phenomenon—In this delusion, a persecutor (who usually is following the person) changes faces or makeup to avoid detection.

4. Cotard syndrome (délire de négation)—A false perception of having lost everything, including money, status, strength, health, but also internal organs. This may be seen in schizophrenia or psychotic depression and responds to treatment of the underlying condition.

5. Autoscopic psychosis—The main symptom is a visual hallucination of a transparent phantom of one's own body.

6. Koro—This disorder in males is characterized by a sudden belief that the penis is shrinking and may disappear into the abdomen. An associated feature may be the belief that when this occurs the person will die. A similar condition may be seen in women with fears of the loss of the genitals or breasts. Although this problem is seen more commonly in Asia, presentations in Western countries occur occasionally.

7. Amok—The amok syndrome consists of an abrupt onset of unprovoked and uncontrolled rage in which the affected person may run about savagely attacking and even killing people and animals in his or her way. It is seen most often in Malayan native peoples but has been reported in other cultures. In some circumstances, this problem is observed in individuals with preexisting psychotic disorders.

8. Piblokto (Arctic hysteria)—This disorder occurs among the Eskimos and is characterized by a sudden onset of screaming, crying, and tearing off of clothes. The affected person may then run or roll about in the snow. It usually resolves rapidly, and the person will usually have no memory of the event.

9. Windigo (witigo)—Specific North American Indian tribes, including the Cree and Ojibwa, manifest this rare psychotic state. People affected may believe that they are possessed by a demon or monster that murders humans and eats their flesh. Trivial symptoms including hunger or nausea may induce intense agitation because of a fear of transformation into the demon.

Bernstein RL, Gaw AC. Koro: proposed classification for DSM-IV. *Am J Psychiatry.* 1990;147:1670.

Berrios GE, Luque R. Cotard's syndrome: analysis of 100 cases. *Acta Psychiatr Scand.* 1995;91:185.

Koehler K, Ebel H, Vartzopoulos D. Lycanthropy and demonomania: some psychopathological issues. *Psychol Med.* 1990;20:629.

Kon Y. Amok. *Br J Psychiatry.* 1994;165:685.

Mojtabai R. Fregoli syndrome. *Aust N Z J Psychiatry.* 1994;28:458.

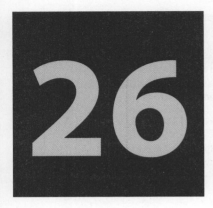

Mood Disorders

Keming Gao, MD, PhD

The depressive disorders (DDs) and bipolar and related disorders (BRDs) have their own chapter in the DSM-5-TR (*Diagnostic and Statistical Manual of Mental Disorder, 5th Edition, Text Revision*). Both DDs and BRDs have significant impact on patients' life and society. In 2019, globally, DDs were ranked #13 of all ages in disability adjusted life years (DALYs) and #2 in years lived with disability (YLDs) among the 369 diseases. BRDs were ranked #67 in DALYs and #28 in YLD. Clinical studies have shown that correct diagnosis and adequate treatment of mood disorders can improve functioning and prevent disability. The focus of this chapter is to discuss the diagnosis of DDs and BRDs based on the DSM-5-TR and the differential diagnosis between major depressive disorder (MDD) also known as unipolar depression (UPD) and bipolar depression (BPD). For treatment, commonly used pharmacological and nonpharmacological treatments will be discussed.

MAJOR DEPRESSIVE DISORDER

▶ Essentials of Diagnosis

The etiology and neuropathophysiology of MDD remain unclear, although studies have shown that genetic vulnerability, social environment, and personality play an important role in the development of MDD and response to treatment. Still, no diagnostic test is available for MDD, although some studies have shown that functional imaging with network analysis and protein markers in blood cells or serum/plasma are promising. Currently, the diagnosis of MDD is based on the criteria of the DSM-5 provided by the American Psychiatric Association, ICD (*International Classification of Diseases Tenth Revision-10 or 11* provided by the World Health Organization, or local professional societies.

▶ General Considerations

A. Epidemiology

MDD is a highly prevalent psychiatric disorder. Twelve-month prevalence in the United State is about 7%. The prevalence of individuals in the 18–29 year old group is threefold higher than in individuals of age 60 years or older. Females have 1.5–3 time higher rates than males beginning from early adolescence. Globally, the prevalence of DDs varied widely with higher rates in developed countries. Worldwide, there is an increase of 50% in cases of MDD from 1990 to 2017, although the prevalence of DDs remains stable.

GBD 2019 Mental Disorders Collaborators. Global, regional, and national burden of 12 mental disorders in 204 countries and territories, 1990-2019: a systematic analysis for the Global Burden of Disease Study 2019. *Lancet Psychiatry.* 2022;9(2):137–150.

Liu Q, He H, Yang J, et al. Changes in the global burden of depression from 1990 to 2017: findings from the Global Burden of Disease study. *J Psychiatr Res.* 2020;126:134–140.

B. Etiology

Despite intensive attempts to establish its etiologic or pathophysiologic basis, the precise cause of MDD remains unknown. There is consensus that multiple etiologic factors—genetic, biochemical, psychodynamic, and socioenvironmental—may interact in complex ways and that the modern-day understanding of DDs requires an understanding of the interrelationships among these factors.

1. Life events—Recent evidence confirms that crucial life events, particularly the death or loss of a loved one, can precede the onset of depression. However, such losses precede only a small (though substantial) number of cases of depression. Fewer than 20% of individuals experiencing losses become clinically depressed. Although other major life events may occur prior to the onset of depression, many patients become depressed with little or no apparent provocation. These observations argue strongly for a predisposing factor, probably genetic, developmental, or temperamental in nature.

2. Biological theories

i. Neurotransmitters—Associations between mood and monoamines (i.e., norepinephrine, serotonin, and dopamine) were first indicated serendipitously by the mood-altering effects of isoniazid (used initially for the treatment of tuberculosis) and later by reports that isoniazid (a monoamine oxidase inhibitor [MAOI]) affects monoamine concentrations in the brains of laboratory animals. We now know that all traditional antidepressants affect postsynaptic signaling of serotonin, norepinephrine, or both at the postsynaptic membrane. This action has led to the hypothesis that depression is caused by a neurotransmitter deficiency and that antidepressants exert their clinical effect by treating this imbalance.

However, new antidepressants targeting glutamatergic (ketamine) and GABAergic (neurosteroid) systems have demonstrated efficacy in the treatment of MDD. Other neurotransmitters (e.g., acetylcholine, melatonin, glycine, histamine), hormones (e.g., thyroid and adrenal hormones), and neuropeptides (e.g., corticotrophin-releasing hormone, endorphins, enkephalins, vasopressin, cholecystokinin, substance P) may play a significant role in the modulation of mood.

ii. Neuroendocrine factors—Emotional trauma sometimes immediately precedes the onset of depression. Emotional trauma can also precede the onset of endocrine disorders such as hyperthyroidism and Cushing disease, both of which are commonly associated with psychological disturbance, most commonly in mood and cognition. When endocrine changes are associated with psychological disturbance, it is often unclear whether such changes are precipitants, perpetuating influences, or secondary effects.

The hypothalamic–pituitary–adrenal (HPA) axis and the hypothalamic–pituitary–thyroid (HPT) axis are extensively studied. About half of patients with MDD exhibit cortisol hypersecretion that returns to normal once the depression is cured. However, medications targeting this system have not been successful. In contrast, depression and cognitive decline are the most frequently observed psychiatric symptoms in patients who have adult hypothyroidism. A small dose of thyroid hormone, preferably triiodothyronine (T_3), will accelerate the therapeutic effect of various antidepressants. Administration of thyrotropin-releasing hormone (TRH) may induce an increased sense of well-being and relaxation in normal subjects and in patients with neurologic and psychiatric disease, especially depression. Overt thyroid disease is rare in MDD, although subtle forms of thyroid dysfunction are common, suggesting that role of HPT axis remains unclear.

iii. Early life stress—In recent years, an increasing number of studies have evaluated both the immediate and long-term neurobiological effects of early childhood trauma. Studies of traumatized persons or animal models of early life stress suggest long-lasting effects on neuroendocrine, psychophysiological, neurochemical, and inflammatory systems. Together, these effects may present the biological basis of an enhanced risk for psychopathology, including depression.

C. Genetics

DDs are familial to some extent although the genetic determination is not as strong as for bipolar disorder (BD), schizophrenia, or alcoholism. In addition, the exact mode of transmission remains unclear (see Chapter 3).

▶ Clinical Findings

A. Signs & Symptoms

1. Major depressive episode—The prerequisite symptom of a major depressive episode (MDE) is depressive mood or the loss of interest or pleasure that predominates for at least 2 weeks, nearly every day, and most of the time. During the same period, the individual must also have at least three or four other symptoms (Table 26–1) to a total of five symptoms. Meanwhile, the symptoms cause significant distress or impairment in the individual's social, occupational, or other important areas of functioning and are not because of a substance or a medical condition.

i. Depressed mood—Depressed mood is the most characteristic symptom, occurring in over 90% of patients. The patient usually describes himself or herself as feeling sad, low, empty, hopeless, gloomy, or down in the dumps. The quality of mood is often described as different from a normal sense of sadness or grief. Changes in the patient's posture, speech, face, dress, and grooming are observable by others, which are consistent with the patient's self-report. Some depressed patients state that they are unable to cry, but others report frequent weeping spells that occur without significant precipitants. A small percentage of patients do not report feeling depressed, sometimes referred to as masked depression. Family members, friends, or coworkers who have noticed the patients' social withdrawal or decreased activity commonly bring these patients to their physicians. Patients may associate depression with feelings of sadness. However, depression as often involves emotional numbness or lack of positive reactivity. Similarly, some children and adolescents do not exhibit a sad demeanor but report feeling irritable instead.

ii. Anhedonia—An inability to enjoy usual activities is almost universal among depressed patients. However, it is relatively rare that patients only have anhedonia without having depressed mood. The patients or their families may report

Table 26–1 Symptom Presentations for Diagnosis of a Major Depressive Episode According to the DSM-5

Core Symptoms	Symptom Presentations	Frequency
Depressed mood	Subjective report feeling depressed, sad, empty, hopeless, discouraged, "down in the dumps," "blah," "have no feeling," or "anxious"; or observed by others, such as tearful and sad affect.	Most of the day Nearly every day
Loss of interest or pleasure	Subjective report or observed by others: marked diminished in interest or pleasure in all or almost all activities or hobbies, "not caring anymore."	Most of the day Nearly every day
Weight or appetite changes	>5% body weight loss unintentionally or weight gain. Decrease or increase appetite, force to eat or carving sweets or other carbohydrates.	A month Nearly every day
Sleep disturbances	Initial insomnia: problem of falling asleep. Middle insomnia: problem with staying asleep (wake up in the middle of night and then being unable to return to sleep). Terminal insomnia: waking up too early and being unable to return to sleep. Hypersomnia: oversleeping, prolonged sleep episodes at night, or increased daytime sleep.	Nearly every day Nearly every day
Psychomotor changes	Agitation: inability to sit still, pacing, handwringing; pulling or rubbing of the skin, clothing or other objects; severe enough to be observable by others. May express as irritability, hostility, poor impulsive control, uncooperative, or violent behavior. Retardation: slowed speech, thinking, and body movements; increased pause before answering; speech with decrease in volume, infection, amount or variety of content, or muteness; severe enough to be observable by others.	Nearly every day Nearly every day
Decreased energy	Sustained fatigue without physical exertion, less efficiency on tasks, tired or exhausted easily, taking much longer time for the same task.	Nearly every day
Worthless or guilt	Feeling worthless (unrealistic negative self-evaluation); excessive or inappropriate guilt (guilty preoccupation or rumination over minor past failings); misinterpretation of natural or trivial day-to-day events as evidence of personal defects; exaggerated sense of responsibility for untoward events; convinced of being responsible for natural disasters and world fairs (delusional thinking); blaming oneself for being sick and for failing to meet occupational responsibilities.	Nearly every day
Concentration and decision making	Unable to think or concentrate or even make minor decisions by subjective report or observed by others; complaint of easily distracted and poor memory, poor school performance of students or "pseudodementia" for elderly.	Nearly every day
Suicidality	Passive suicidal ideation: wish not waking up the morning or a belief that others would be better off if the individual was dead. Active suicidal ideation: recurrent thoughts of committing suicides with or without a plan (hanging, shooting, or overdosing) or intent (updated wills, settle debts, giving away personal belongs, or suicide note). A suicide attempt.	Not specified

Note: A major depressive episode requires that depressed mood or loss of interest or pleasure must be present for at least 2 weeks most of the day and nearly every day along with four of the other seven symptoms to a total of five symptoms. The symptoms cause significant distress or impairment in the individual's social, occupational, or other important areas of functioning.

markedly diminished interest in all, or almost all, activities previously enjoyed such as sex, hobbies, and daily routines.

iii. **Change in appetite**—About 70% of patients observe a reduction in appetite with accompanying weight loss. It is important to differentiate intentional weight loss from unintentional loss. Only a minority of patients experience an increase in appetite and gain weight, which is also known as a presentation of MDD with "atypical features." Some are often associated with cravings for particular foods such as sweets and other carbohydrates.

iv. **Change in sleep**—About 80% of depressed patients complain of some type of sleep disturbance, the most common being insomnia including initial, middle, or late insomnia. The most common and unpleasant form of sleep disturbance is late insomnia, with awakenings in the early morning (usually around 4–5 AM) and unable to return to sleep. Subsequently, depressive symptoms significantly worsen in the first part of the day. In contrast, initial insomnia is especially common in those with significant comorbid anxiety. On the other hand, some patients complain of hypersomnia that is another presentation of MDD with "atypical features," and/or MDD with seasonal patterns. Some patients with hypersomnia may have hyperphagia and weight gain.

v. Psychomotor retardation/agitation—About one-half of depressed patients develop slowness or retardation of their normal level of activity. About 75% of depressed women and 50% of depressed men, anxiety or restless is expressed in the form of psychomotor agitation. Both signs of psychomotor agitation and retardation must be observable by others, not merely feeling slowed down for psychomotor retardation or feeling inner restless for psychomotor agitation.

vi. Loss of energy—Almost all depressed patients report a significant loss of energy, unusual fatigue, tiredness, or exhaustion. Some may feel inefficient in accomplishing usualtasks. Others may need more time to complete the same tasks compared to before.

vii. Worthlessness and guilt—Feeling excessive worthlessness, decreased self-esteem, or inappropriate guilt is common in depressed patients. Some patients may be preoccupied with excessive and inappropriate guilt over trivial day-to-day events or feel responsible for untoward events including natural disasters and world events, evento the level of delusion. In European cultures, depressed patients may exhibit some guilt, ranging from a vague feeling that their current conditions are the result of something they have done previously to frank delusions and hallucinations of having committed an unpardonable sin. In other cultures, excessive shame or humiliation may be dominant.

viii. Indecisiveness or decreased concentration—About half of depressed patients complain that they are not able to think as well as before, cannot concentrate, or are easily distracted. Frequently, they doubt their ability to make good judgments and find themselves unable to make even small decisions. On formal psychological testing, accuracy is usually retained, but speed and performance are low. In severe forms, particularly among the elderly, memory deficits may be mistaken for early signs of dementia (pseudodementia). In contrast to dementia, pseudodementia usually reverses after treatment of the underlying depression. However, when cognitive symptoms are comorbid with depression, they may represent an emerging dementia that can persistafter the depression has resolved.

ix. Suicidal ideation—Many depressed individuals experience recurrent thoughts of death, ranging from transient feelings that others would be better off without them to the actual planning and implementing of suicide (Table 26–1).

2. Subtype of MDD

i. Subtypes of MDD—Subtypes of MDD are listed as specifiers in the DSM-5, DSM-5-TR, and DSM-IV. In DSM-5, specifiers of "with anxious distress," "with mixed feature," were added to the DSM-IV specifiers that include melancholic, atypical, psychotic, and catatonic features, seasonal pattern" for recurrent episode, and postpartum onset that was changed to peripartum onset in DSM-5. The "Chronic" specifier in the DSM-IV was deleted in the DSM-5 and -5-TR since MDD with chronic course (i.e., not meeting the remission criteria for 2 months in a row in a 2 year period) was re-classified as "persistent depressive disorder" in DSM-5. In addition, premenstrual dysphoric disorder (PMDD) was listed in the DSM-IV as a "depressive disorder not otherwise specified" in the diagnostic class of conditions for further study and is included in the DDs in the DSM-5. Disruptive mood dysregulation disorder (DMDD) is a new subtype of DD in the DSM-5.

ii. MDD with anxious distress—To diagnose MDD with anxious distress, at least two of the following symptoms have to be present during the majority of days of the current or most recent MDE: (1) feeling keyed up or tense; (2) feeling unusually restless; (3) difficulty concentrating because of worry; (4) fear that something awful may happen; (5) feeling that individual might lose control of himself or herself. The severity of anxiety can be defined as mild (two symptoms), moderate (three symptoms), moderate-severe (four or five symptoms), or severe (four or five symptoms with motor agitation). High anxiety has been associated with an increased risk for suicide, longer duration to reach remission, and greater risk for treatment-resistance. Specific monitoring and treatment planning may be necessary for those with high anxiety. Selecting an antidepressant without or with minimal activating effect and/or adding an anxiolytic early may be necessary to control depressive and anxious symptoms.

iii. MDD with mixed features—To diagnose MDD with mixed features, at least three of the following manic/hypomanic symptoms have to be present during the majority of days of the current or most recent MDE: (1) elevated, expansive mood; (2) inflated self-esteem or grandiosity; (3) more talkative than usual or pressure to keep talking; (4) flight of ideas or subjective experience that thoughts are racing; (5) increase in energy or goal-directed activities, either socially, at work or school, or sexually; (6) increased or excessive involvement in activities that carry a high potential for painful consequences, such as engaging in unrestrained buying sprees, sexual indiscretions, unnecessary legal activities, or foolish business investments; (7) decreased need for sleep such as feeling rested despite sleeping less than usual. Meanwhile, the mixed symptoms are observable by others and present a change from the person's usual behavior and are not due to the physiological effects of a substance such as a substance of abuse or a medication or a nonpharmacological treatment. For patients whose symptoms meet full episode criteria for both mania/hypomania and MDE simultaneously, the diagnosis should be mania/hypomania with mixed features. This subtype is likely a byproduct of the elimination of DSM-IV's mixed episode category in DSM-5. Lurasidone and lumateperone monotherapy have shown efficacy in treating this subtype of MDD.

iv. MDD with peripartum onset—The specifier of MDD with postpartum onset in DMS-IV was changed to MDD with peripartum onset in DSM-5. This change reflects the fact that about 50% of postpartum MDEs begin prior to delivery. To diagnose MDD with peripartum onset, the onset of depressive symptoms of the current MDE or the most recent MDEs in partial or full remission occurs during the pregnancy or within 4 weeks after delivery. About 9% of pregnant women will have a MDE from their baby's conception to birth. By the best estimate, about 7% will have a MDE between birth and 12 months after delivery. Postpartum depression (PPD) can present with or without psychotic features. Infanticide is often associated with postpartum psychotic episodes characterized by command hallucinations to kill the infant or delusions that the infant is possessed as compared to severe PPD with psychotic features that do not have specific delusions or hallucinations. The risk of recurrence for PPD with psychotic features in each subsequent delivery is about 30–50%. Postpartum DDs must be differentiated from the much common mood disturbance "maternity blues" or "baby blues" which is characterized by sudden mood changes such as sudden onset of tearfulness without feeling depressed. Maternity blues is not a mental disorder and does not cause functional impairment. It is temporary and self-limited and improves quickly (within a week) without the need of treatment.

3. Other depressive disorders

i. Persistent depressive disorder—There is no diagnosis of persistent DD in the DSM-IV, although it is included in ICD-10. In the DMS-5, persistent DD includes dysthymia and chronic MDD. In order to diagnose persistent DD, the following criteria must be met: (1) depressed mood (can be irritable mood for children and adolescents) for most the day, for more day than not, either subjectively feels or observed by others for at least 2 years in adults (1 year for children and adolescents) and never being without significant symptoms for 2 months at a time; (2) the presence of two or more of poor appetite or overeating, insomnia or hypersomnia, low energy or fatigue, low self-esteem, poor concentration or difficulty making decisions, or feelings of hopelessness while depressed; (3) a MDE continuously lasting 2 years or more; (4) has never been manic or hypomanic episode; (5) the disturbances are not due to psychotic disorders, a substance or another medical condition; (6) the symptoms cause clinically significant distress and impairment in any domains of patient's life. The 12-month prevalence of chronic MDD is about 1.5% and dysthymia is about 0.5%. The prevalence in women is approximately 1.5–2 times higher than in men.

ii. Premenstrual dysphoric disorder—In order to diagnose PMDD, the following criteria must be met in most menstrual cycles that occurred the preceding year: (1) in the majority of menstrual cycles, at least five symptoms as listed below must be present in the final week before the onset of menses, start to improve with a few days after the onset of menses, and become minimal or no symptoms in a week post menses; (2) one or more of the following symptoms must be present: (a) marked affective lability (mood swings, increased sensitivity to rejection, or feeling suddenly sad or tearful), (b) marked irritability or anger or increased personal conflicted, (c) marked depressed mood, feeling hopeless, or self-deprecating thoughts, (d) marked anxiety, tension and/or feeling being keyed up or on edge; (3) one or more of the following must be present to a total of five symptoms: (a) anhedonia (no interest in usual activities), (b) difficult concentrating, (c) lack of energy or fatigued easily, (d) marked change in appetite, overeating or craving for certain foods, (e) insomnia or hypersomnia, (f) feeling overwhelmed or out of control, (g) physical symptoms including breast tenderness or swelling, joint or muscle pain, bloating or weight gain. As other DDs, these symptoms must cause clinically significant impairment in any domains of patient's life, and the symptoms were not due to an exacerbation of another psychiatric disorder, a substance or another medical condition.

The prevalence of PMDD acrosstwo menstrual cycles is 1.3% in the United States. In a large study from Germany, the 12-month prevalence of PMDD is estimated at 5.8%. Premenstrual syndrome (PMS) does not require a minimum of five symptoms nor mood-related symptomatology as does PMDD, and it is generally considered less severe than PMDD. The prevalence of PMS is estimated at about 20%. For menstrual women with somatic or behavioral symptoms but without affective symptoms during the premenstrual phase of the menstrual cycles, PMS is likely the diagnosis instead of PMDD.

iii. Disruptive mood dysregulation disorder—The addition of DMDD in the DSM-5 is to emphasize the difference between severe, nonepisodic irritability and distinct episodes of mania or hypomania thatqualify for the diagnosis of a BD in both children and adults and to reduce the risk of children with severe, nonepisodic irritability from being diagnosed with BD (Chapter 57).

iv. Substance/medication-induced depressive disorder—Any substance that directly and/or indirectly affects the central nervous system (CNS) has the potential to cause DDs. The substances can be illicit street drugs, prescribed medications, over-the-counter medications or nutritional/metabolic supplements. The risk and rate of substance-induced DD from each substance is difficult to determine, but the impact of a substance-induced DD should not be ignored. In addition, substances/medications can worsen and trigger relapse for those who have preexisting DDs. In order to diagnose a substance-induced DD, the history, physical exam, and/or laboratory results must support that the DD develops during or within a month of substance intoxication or withdrawal or taking a medication, and that the substance is capable of producing the DDs. The DD is not due to another psychiatric disorder. If the disorder preceded the onset of intoxication, withdrawal, or exposure to a substance, and/or persisted for more than a month after the cessation of acute intoxication, withdrawal, or exposure, a diagnosis of substance-induced DD should not be given.

v. Depressive disorder due to another medical condition— Any medical condition that directly orindirectly affects the CNS can cause or worsen DDs. The requirement of "direct" pathophysiological effect of another medical condition on a DD makes this diagnosis more challenging. Strictly speaking, DD purely due to direct pathophysiological effect of another medical condition is relatively rare. According to DMS-5, the cause–effect relationship between DD and another medical condition should be based on the best clinical evidence, which is the key variable in diagnosing DD due to another medical condition (Table 26–2). The association of depression with some neurological conditions such as stroke, Huntington disease, Parkinson disease, traumatic brain injury, and some neuroendocrine conditions like hypothyroidism or Cushing disease were used for this justification. Without a complete list of medical conditions that can induce depression, "the clinician's best judgment is essence of this diagnosis."

vi. Other specified depressive disorder—Other specified DDs include recurrent brief depression, short-duration depressive episode (4–13 days), depressive episode with insufficient symptoms, and MDE superimposed on psychotic disorders with the exception of schizoaffective disorder. These disorders cause clinically significant distress and impairment in an individual who has never met the criteria any other DDs or BD. For recurrent brief depression, concurrence of depressive mood and four other symptoms of depression lasts for 2–13 days at least once a month (not associated with menstrual cycles) for at least 12 consecutive months in an individual who has never met the criteria any other DDs or BD, and does not currently meet active or residual criteria for any psychotic disorder.

Gaebel W, Stricker J, Kerst A. Changes from ICD-10 to ICD-11 and future directions in psychiatric classification. *Dialogues Clin Neurosci.* 2020;22(1):7–15.

Uher R, Payne JL, Pavlova B, Perlis RH. Major depressive disorder in DSM-5: implications for clinical practice and research of changes from DSM-IV. *Depress Anxiety.* 2014;31(6):459–71.

American Psychiatric Association. *Diagnostic and Statistical Manual of Mental Disorders,* 5th ed. Arlington VA: American Psychiatric Association; 2013.

American Psychiatric Association. *Diagnostic and Statistical Manual of Mental Disorders,* 5th ed, Text revision. Washington, DC: American Psychiatric Association; 2022.

3. Treatment-resistant depression—It is well known that a significant number of patients with DDs fail to achieve remission with antidepressants and nonpharmacological treatments. However, the prevalence of treatment-resistant depression (TRD) varies widely depending on the models of TRD is used. The Thase and Rush model defines levels of treatment-resistance by using the failure of responses to

Table 26–2 Depressive Disorders Due to Another Medical Condition

- Cardiovascular diseases
  Outpatients with coronary artery disease:
    12–23% with major depressive disorder
  Survivors of acute myocardial infarction
    16–20% with major depressive disorder
    Up to 45% having significant depressive symptoms
    ≈ 55% of episodes have onset prior to the cardiac event
- Central nerve system
  Cerebrovascular disease:
    ≈ 20% with major depressive disorder
    20% with minor depression
  Epilepsy:
    29% with depression based on Patient Health Questionnaire -9 (PHQ-9) score
  Headache:
    34% with lifetime major depressive disorder among migraine patients
  Movement disorders:
    ≈ 40–50% of patients with Parkinson's disease have depression
  Multiple sclerosis:
    > 50% with depressive symptoms,
    50% with lifetime major depressive disorder
  Traumatic brain injury:
    77% with depression among those with more severe injuries.
- Endocrine diseases
  Diabetes ellitus:
    ≈ 30% with depressive symptoms
    12–18% with major depressive disorder
  Thyroid dysfunction:
    64% with depressive symptoms in subclinical hypothyroidism
- Infectious diseases
  HIV (human immunodeficiency *virus*)–AIDS (acquired immunodeficiency syndrome):
    ≈ 20–36% patients have depression
  Hepatitis C:
    Up to 25% with serious mental illness
- Oncology
    18% having significant depressive symptoms among cancer patients

Data from Rivelli SK, Shirey KG. Prevalence of psychiatric symptoms/syndromes in medical settings. In: *Integrated Care in Psychiatry: Redefining the Role of Mental Health Professionals in the Medical Setting.* Summergrad P, Kathol RG (eds). New York, NY: Springer, 2014, pp. 5–27.

different classes of antidepressants in a sequential manner and ECT (electroconvulsive therapy) and was used in the Sequential Treatment Alternatives to Relieve Depression (STAR*D) project sponsored by the National Institute of Mental Health (NIMH). Based on the STAR*D, the overall remission rate was 67% after four levels of treatments with different classes of antidepressants. The remission rates after level one (citalopram) or level two (venlafaxine, bupropion, or sertraline monotherapy, or buspirone or bupropion adjunctive to citalopram) treatment were similar, 36.8 versus

30.6%. The remission rates after level three (augmentation with lithium or T3, nortriptyline monotherapy, or mirtazapine monotherapy) and level four (venlafaxine and mirtazapine combination or tranylcypromine monotherapy) were also similar, 13.7 versus 13%.

Sackeim HA, Aaronson ST, Bunker MT, et al. The assessment of resistance to antidepressant treatment: rationale for the Antidepressant Treatment History Form: Short Form (ATHF-SF). *J Psychiatr Res.* 2019;113:125–136.

Pitsillou E, Bresnehan SM, Kagarakis EA, et al. The cellular and molecular basis of major depressive disorder: towards a unified model for understanding clinical depression. *Mol Biol Rep.* 2020; 47(1):753–770.

B. Psychological testing

Psychological testing has not been found useful in aiding the diagnosis of MDD. However, psychological testing may identify personality traits or disorders that may help in understanding the psychopathology of patients, especially for those who are treatment-resistant to both pharmacological and nonpharmacological treatments.

C. Laboratory findings

There is no objective laboratory test to diagnose MDD, but some tests may help clinicians to rule out DDs due to another medical condition or substance-induced DDs. Commonly used tests include urine drug screening, thyroid-stimulating hormone (TSH), complete blood count (CBC), and comprehensive metabolic panel (CMP). In addition, several laboratory findings are abnormal in some patients with MDD as compared to the general population. Most laboratory abnormalities appear state dependent (i.e., they occur while patients are depressed) or precede the onset of an episode or persist after its remission. However, only TSH level monitoring in patients with hypothyroidism has been used in routine clinical practice.

1. HPA axis

i. Dexamethasone suppression test—The dexamethasone suppression test (DST) has limited use as a clinical marker for depression. Within the depression spectrum, the rates of DST nonsuppression increased strikingly from grief reactions (10%) and dysthymic disorders (23%) to MDD (44%), MDD with melancholia (50%), psychotic affective disorders (69%), and depression with serious suicidality (78%). DST-positive patients appeared to respond more favorably to biological interventions such as antidepressants or ECT. Among depressed patients, abnormal DST results correlated mostly with initial insomnia, weight loss, loss of sexual interest, ruminative thinking, and psychomotor retardation or agitation. HPA axis dysregulation contributed to cognitive dysfunction, although it is not known whether hypercortisolemia and cognitive impairment in depression are related indirectly or causally.

ii. Corticotrophin-releasing hormone test—A blunted adrenocorticotropic hormone response after corticotrophin-releasing hormone administration is another HPA axis abnormality commonly observed in major depression.

2. HPT axis

i. T_4 concentrations—Most depressed patients appear to be euthyroid; however, longitudinal studies consistently found significant serum T_4 reductions during a wide range of somatic treatments, including various antidepressants, lithium, sleep deprivation, or ECT. Evidence indicates that the T_4 reduction was greater in treatment responders than in nonresponders. It is not known whether the initial T_4 increase in depression is part of the pathophysiology of the illness, or it is a compensatory mechanism for the low thyroid hormone to the brain.

ii. Subclinical hypothyroidism—Subtle thyroid dysfunctions are common in depression. Between 1% and 4% of patients show evidence of overt hypothyroidism, and between 4% and 40% show evidence of subclinical hypothyroidism. Comorbid subclinical hypothyroidism can be associated with cognitive dysfunction or with a diminished response to standard psychiatric treatments. Some depressed patients with subclinical hypothyroidism may respond to thyroid hormone treatment.

iii. TRH test—The TRH test (i.e., measurement of serum TSH following TRH administration) has been used widely in psychiatry. More than 3000 patients have been studied, the majority of whom had MDD. Approximately 30% of patients had a blunted TSH response during depression, and a smaller number showed TSH blunting during remission; however, definitions of TSH blunting have varied among studies, different assays have been used, and a standard amount of TRH has not always been injected. The TRH test does not aid in the distinction between primary and secondary depression or between unipolar and bipolar subgroups. Preliminary evidence suggests that TSH blunting may be associated with a more prolonged course of depression and with a history of violent suicidal behavior.

3. Sleep electroencephalogram—Sleep electroencephalogram (EEG) recordings reveal the following: (1) a shortened rapid eye movement (REM) latency, more commonly in elderly depressed patients and often associated with UPD; (2) a shift of slow-wave sleep (i.e., sleep stages 3 and 4), normally occurring during the first non-REM period, into the second non-REM period; and (3) an increased REM density (i.e., more frequent REM episodes) during the first few hours of sleep. Because most of these sleep EEG abnormalities can be found in other illnesses, and some accompany normal aging, there is no agreement as to whether these abnormalities constitute diagnostic markers of depression. There is evidence that EEG sleep variables are normal in depressed patients 6 months after an acute episode. A recent review suggested that gamma rhythms on EEG might provide objective information on MDD and differentiate MDD from BD and healthy controls.

D. Neuroimaging

There is no neuroimaging test to diagnose MDD, but for patients with neurological symptoms, a computerized tomography scan and a structural MRI (magnetic resonance imaging) scan may provide useful information to help in the diagnosis of DDs due to another medical condition. With the rapidly increasing sophistication of neuroimaging techniques, neuroimaging studies have been provided useful characterization of the circuitry underlying emotional disorders and mood regulations. Global cerebral blood flow and glucose metabolism appear normal in most patients but may be decreased in late life depression. Decreased prefrontal cortex (PFC) blood flow and metabolism, especially in the left PFC of MDD patients are the most consistently replicated findings. The finding of hypofunction of the PFC has helped in the development of rTMS (repetitive transcranial magnetic stimulation) for the treatment of MDD. Subcortical areas including amygdala, hippocampus, cingulate, striatum, insula, and thalamus are also involved in MDD. The finding of decreased activity in anterior cingulate in MDD provides a basis for deep brain stimulation (DBS) and imaging-guided rTMS such as SAINT (the Stanford Accelerated Intelligent Neuromodulation Therapy) for the treatment of MDD.

E. Couse of illness

According to the number of episodes at the time of assessment, MDD is coded as a single or recurrent episode. Based on the number, severity and length of depressive symptoms and the impact at the follow-up assessments, the episode is coded as partial remission, full remission or unspecified. This information is not only essential for selecting acute treatment option(s) but also important for future planning or preventing relapse. The onset of MDD is common in early 20s for females and late 20s for males. Symptoms typically develop over days to weeks, and prodromal symptoms and preexisting comorbid conditions such social anxiety disorder, generalized anxiety disorder (GAD), and/or panic disorders are common. A MDE often follows acute psychosocial stressors, such as death, loss of a loved one, divorce, or acute medical illness.

The course of recurrent depression is variable. Some patients have a few isolated episodes separated by stable intervals (years) of normal functioning. Others have clusters of episodes, and still others have increasingly frequent episodes with shortening of the interepisode interval and generally increasing disease severity. Some patients experience a MDE without full remission before the next during a 2-year period. About 50% of patients with one depressive episode will have a recurrence, and about 90% of patients who have had three episodes can be expected to have a fourth. Thus, the number of past episodes can serve as a predictor of the future relapses. The average number of lifetime episodes is around five. About 5–10% of patients with an initial diagnosis of MDD subsequently develop a manic/hypomanic episode, and then are diagnosed with BD.

Depressive episodes may remit completely with or without treatment, partially or fully. The patient's functioning usually returns to the premorbid level between episodes, but 20–35% of patients show persistent residual symptoms and social or occupational impairment. Data from the pre-psychopharmacology era (i.e., before 1960) suggest that, if untreated, a MDE may last about 12 months. Relapse is common. The risk of relapse during early remission can be reduced significantly by maintaining patients on antidepressants for at least 6 months—a regimen now generally viewed as important in managing the recurring nature of the illness.

▶ Differential Diagnosis

1. Bipolar depression—Since a MDE can be present exactly same in both UPD and BPD, the differential diagnosis of UPD and BPD is critical because the treatment for the two disorders are quite different. For UPD, antidepressants are the first-line treatment. For BPD, mood stabilizers (MSs) are the first-line treatment. Most MS have more side effects than antidepressants. A careful evaluation of manic/hypomanic symptoms is the only way to separate BPD from UPD.

2. Psychotic disorders—In MDD, 12–20% patients may have psychotic symptoms. A differential diagnosis between MDD and a psychotic disorder, especially one with depressive symptoms is essential for proper treatment planning. MDD with psychotic features and a psychotic disorder with depressive symptoms need both antidepressant and antipsychotic treatments, but the course of using these two groups of medications is different. For patients with MDD with psychotic features, antipsychotic can be discontinued in 3–6 months after psychotic symptoms are under control or 12 months for patients with a history of relapse after stopping antipsychotics. By contrast, antipsychotics should be continued for psychotic disorders with depressive symptom even after the psychotic symptom(s) resolves.

3. Psychiatric comorbidities—Psychiatric comorbidity in DDs is the rule rather than exception. An epidemiological study based on DSM-5 found that the 12-month prevalence of MDD comorbid with an anxiety disorder (AD) was about 36%, with PTSD (posttraumatic stress disorder) 16%, and with any SUD (substance use disorder) about 45%. Clinical samples have shown that more than 80% of MDD are associated lifetime comorbid ADs and 40–50% with a lifetime comorbidity of any SUD and that 80% of patients have one or more comorbidities (Figure 26–1). Ten percent of patients have four or more other psychiatric disorders.

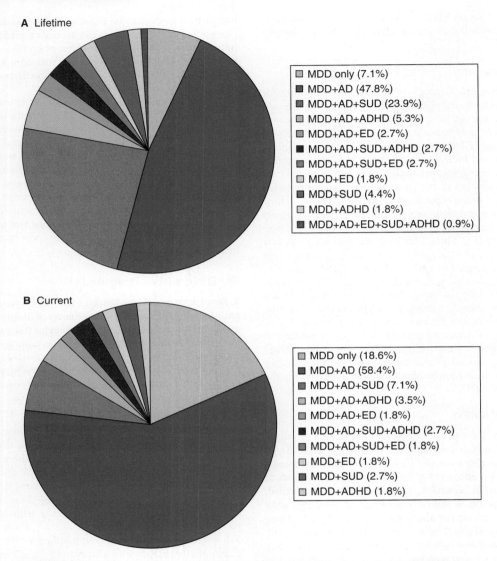

A Lifetime

☐ MDD only (7.1%)
■ MDD+AD (47.8%)
■ MDD+AD+SUD (23.9%)
☐ MDD+AD+ADHD (5.3%)
☐ MDD+AD+ED (2.7%)
■ MDD+AD+SUD+ADHD (2.7%)
■ MDD+AD+SUD+ED (2.7%)
☐ MDD+ED (1.8%)
■ MDD+SUD (4.4%)
■ MDD+ADHD (1.8%)
■ MDD+AD+ED+SUD+ADHD (0.9%)

B Current

☐ MDD only (18.6%)
■ MDD+AD (58.4%)
■ MDD+AD+SUD (7.1%)
☐ MDD+AD+ADHD (3.5%)
☐ MDD+AD+ED (1.8%)
■ MDD+AD+SUD+ADHD (2.7%)
■ MDD+AD+SUD+ED (1.8%)
☐ MDD+ED (1.8%)
■ MDD+SUD (2.7%)
☐ MDD+ADHD (1.8%)

Note: The diagnoses were according to DSM-IV diagnostic criteria. Anxiety disorder includes generalized anxiety disorder, panic disorder, social phobia, posttraumatic stress disorder, and obsessive-compulsive disorder. Eating disorder includes anorexia nervosa and bulimia nervosa. Substance use disorder including alcohol use disorder, cannabis use disorder, cocaine/stimulant use disorder, opiate use disorder and benzodiazepine/hypnotic use disorder.

Abbreviations: AD, anxiety disorder; ADHD, attention deficit hyperactivity disorder; ED, eating disorder; MDD, major depressive disorder; SUD, substance disorder.

▲ **Figure 26–1** Lifetime and current comorbid patterns of MDD with other psychiatric disorder in a clinical sample (*n*=113)

Arnaud AM, Brister TS, Duckworth K, et al. Impact of major depressive disorder on comorbidities: a systematic literature review. *J Clin Psychiatry.* 2022;83(6):21r14328.

Gao K, Wang Z, Chen J, et al. Should an assessment of Axis I comorbidity be included in the initial diagnostic assessment of mood disorders? Role of QIDS-16-SR total score in predicting number of Axis I comorbidity. *J Affect Disord.* 2013; 148(2–3):256–264.

Hasin DS, Sarvet AL, Meyers JL, et al. Epidemiology of adult DSM-5 major depressive disorder and its specifiers in the United States. *JAMA Psychiatry.* 2018;75(4):336–346.

4. Medical comorbidities—Co-occurrence of MDD and medical conditions are also common, although the sequence of most comorbidities is difficult to determine. MDD can not only significantly exacerbate preexisting medical conditions but also precipitate the onset of new medical conditions. Conversely, a medical condition may directly and/or indirectly cause depression or worsen pre-existing MDD. The interaction between depression and its comorbidities is still not fully understood. However, 63% of total MDD-related to costs in the United States in 2018 were due to the cost of treating medical and psychiatric comorbidities instead of MDD itself.

Thom R, Silbersweig DA, Boland RJ. Major depressive disorder in medical illness: a review of assessment, prevalence, and treatment options. *Psychosom Med.* 2019;81(3):246–255.

▶ Treatment

A. Psychopharmacologic Interventions

One important aspect for successful treatment after diagnosis is to discuss with patients and their families the symptoms of depression, the course of illness, and treatment options. At the beginning, educating patients and their families on the presentations of depressive symptoms and impact of each symptom is necessary to ease the concern of patients and their families and to increase insight of patients on their illness. At each follow-up visit, discussing the changes in each depressive symptom and understanding the patient's concerns is helpful in deciding whether to continue or modify the treatment plan. Using a self-reported depression rating scale such as PHQ-9 (Patient Health Questionnaire- 9) to monitor depressive symptom severity should be a routine clinical practice. Discussing the importance of self-monitoring emergent depressive symptoms after remission is key to preventing depression relapses.

All options including pharmacological and nonpharmacological treatments should be discussed with patients before forming a personalized treatment plan. A treatment plan should depend on clinical factors, demographics, and preferences of patients. Previous studies have shown that patients who received a treatment they preferred had a higher completion rate than those who received a treatment they did not prefer, suggesting that following a patient's preference is likely to increase treatment compliance. Currently available pharmacological treatments include selective serotonin reuptake inhibitors (SSRIs), serotonin–norepinephrine reuptake inhibitors (SNRIs), dopamine reuptake inhibitors, tricyclic antidepressants (TCAs), MAOIs, atypical antidepressants, NMDA (N-methyl-D-aspartate) receptor antagonists, and neurosteroids. Nonpharmacological treatments include psychotherapies, ECT, rTMS, transcranial direct current stimulation (tDCS), DBS, and vagus nerve stimulation (VNS).

Overall, a treatment plan should include acute, continuation, and maintenance phases. The goal in the acute phase is to achieve remission. The continuation phase and maintenance phase are to prevent early and late relapse. Managing subtle changes such as insomnia and/or newly emergent anxiety symptoms during the continuation and maintenance phases is essential to preventing relapse. In addition, it is important to understand the designs and conduct of clinical trials: Phase III trials are required by regulatory agencies for approving an indication for a mediation. Commonly, the FDA requires two positive studies for an indication approval regardless of how many studies are conducted. It is only about one-third of patients with MDD who may be eligible for a phase III study; therefore, the results from phase III studies are not generalizable. In contrast, results from "real world" studies like the STAR*D project with broad inclusion and limited exclusion criteria are more generalizable.

1. Acute treatments of MDD

i. SSRI and related antidepressants—SSRIs are the most prescribed antidepressants for the treatment of DDs and anxiety disorders. This group includes fluoxetine, paroxetine, sertraline, citalopram, escitalopram, and fluvoxamine. As a group, they potently and selectively block the reuptake of serotonin by presynaptic serotonergic neurons. However, their potency and selectivity to serotonin transporters are not uniform, especially at higher doses of these medications. In addition to these "standard" SSRIs, there are a number of medications developed targeting serotonin reuptake blockade and 5-HT receptors. One early example is trazodone, which not only blocks serotonin reuptake but also antagonizes 5-HT2 receptors.A example is vortioxetine, which blocks serotonin reuptake, antagonizes 5-HT3, and agonizes 5-HT1A (Table 26–3). These additional effects on 5-HT receptors do not appear to improve efficacy in reducing depressive symptoms, but lower rates of sexual side effects;and significant cognitive improvements with some of newer medications are reported.

The side effects from SSRIs and serotonin-related antidepressants depend on the locations of serotonin receptors that are distributed in the CNS and peripheral organs, but their distributions are not homogenous. Most common side effects such as nausea, dry mouth, weight change, agitation, anxiety, tremor, and headache are short-term, but sexual dysfunction and sweating can be persistent. Unless a side effect(s) is severe

Table 26–3 Selective Serotonin Reuptake Inhibitors and Related Medications

Citalopram	10–40	33	5-TH↑ via inhibition of SERT
Escitalopram	5–20	27–32	5-TH↑ via inhibition of SERT
Fluoxetine	10–80	Parent: 4–6 days, Metabolite 4–16 days	5-TH↑ via inhibition of SERT, NE↑? DA↓?
Fluvoxamine	25–300	15–26	5-TH↑ via inhibition of SERT
Paroxetine	20–50	24–31	5-TH↑ via inhibition of SERT, NE↑ via inhibition of NET
Sertraline	25–200	27	5-TH↑ via inhibition of SERT, DA↑ via inhibition of DAT
Vilazodone	10–40	25	5-TH↑ via inhibition of SERT, 5HT$_{1A}$ partial agonist
Vortioxetine	5–20	66	5-TH↑ via inhibition of SERT, 5-HT$_{1A}$ partial agonist, 5-HT$_3$ antagonist
Serotonin–norepinephrine reuptake inhibitors			
Desvenlafaxine	50–100	10–11	5-TH↑ and NE↑ via inhibition of SERT and NET (SERT:NET=14:1)
Duloxetine	30–120	12	5-TH↑ and NE↑ via inhibition of SERT and NET (SERT:NET=10:1)
Levominacipran	40–120	8–12	5-TH↑ and NE↑ via inhibition of SERT and NET (SERT:NET=1:2)
Venlafaxine	37.5–225	4–5	5-TH↑ and NE↑ via SERT and NET (SERT:NET=30:1)
Dopamine Reuptake Inhibitor			
Bupropion	150–450	21	DA↑ via inhibition of DAT NE↑ via inhibition of NET Antagonist of nicotinic acetylcholinergic receptor (nAChR)
Atypical antidepressants			
Mirtazapine	15–60	20–40	5-TH↑ and NE↑ via presynaptic inhibition of α$_2$ receptor 5-TH$_{1A}$ transmission↑ via antagonism of 5-HT$_2$ and 5-HT$_3$ Hypnotic: H$_1$ receptor antagonism
Nefazodone	200–600	Parent: 2–4 mCPP 4–8 Triazole dione 18	5-TH↑ and NE↑ via weak SERT and NET 5-HT$_2$ antagonist a weak α$_1$ adrenergic receptor antagonist
Trazodone	300–600 50–100 for sleep	10–12 hours	Simultaneous inhibition of serotonin transporters, 5-HT$_{2A}$, and 5-HT2C receptors Hypnotic: antagonism of 5-HT$_{2A}$ receptor, H$_1$ receptor, and α-adrenergic receptors

Abbreviations: DA, dopamine, DAT, dopamine transporter; 5-HT, 5-hydroxytryptamine (serotonin); 5-TH$_{1A}$, 5-hydroxytryptamine 1A receptor; 5-HT$_2$, 5-hydroxytryptamine 2 receptor; 5-HT$_3$, 5-hydroxytryptamine 3 receptor; H$_1$, histamine 1 receptor; mCPP, *meta-chlorophenylpiperazine*, an active metabolite of nefazodone; NE, norepinephrine; NET, norepinephrine transporter; SERT, serotonin transporter.

or intolerable, staying on the medication for several weeks is reasonable before discontinuing the medication. For sexual side effects, reducing the dosage is worthy of trying as the first step, although the sexual side effects are not dose-dependent for some medications. Waiting for developing tolerance may work for some patients. Switching to bupropion, mirtazapine or nefazodone may be appropriate for some patients. However, nefazodone can cause idiopathic hepatic failure and mirtazapine can cause severe sedation and weight gain. Adding cyproheptadine, yohimbine, or methylphenidate may be useful in some patients. Finally, sildenafil may be beneficial for SSRI-induced anorgasmia, delayed ejaculation, or impotence in men and anorgasmia or delayed orgasm in women.

Severe side effects from antidepressants including SSRIs can occur (Table 26–4). Serotonin syndrome is considered a severe, but low prevalence condition. The syndrome is usually mild in nature and resolves within 24 hours after drug discontinuation. Delayed diagnosis and treatment of serotonin syndrome can be life threatening. Early identification and proper treatment is the key to prevent severe consequences of serotonin syndrome. Another uncomfortable but not life-threatening condition from antidepressants including SSRIs is antidepressant withdrawal syndrome. After a long-term therapy with a SSRI, about 10–15% of patients may experience a withdrawal syndrome, especially after suddenly stopping the medication either intentionally or

Table 26–4 Risks for Potential Severe Side Effects from Commonly Used Antidepressants in Major Depressive Disorder

- Risk of suicidality—younger than 24 years old.
- Risk of hypertension—venlafaxine and desvenlafaxine.
- Risk for serotonin syndrome—selective serotonin reuptake inhibitors, serotonin norepinephrine reuptake inhibitors.
- Risk of hepatoxicity—duloxetine, nefazodone (250,000 to 300,000 patient-years).
- Risk of seizures—bupropion, clomipramine.
- Risk of neuropsychiatric events with bupropion when used for smoking cessation—behavioral changes, agitation, depression, hostility, suicidality.
- Risk of cardiac arrhythmias with fluoxetine and citalopram—not recommended in patients with underlying heart conditions (bradycardia, QTc prolongation, heart failure, recent myocardial infarction), hypokalemia, or hypomagnesemia.
- Risk of hyponatremia—selective serotonin reuptake inhibitors, serotonin norepinephrine reuptake inhibitors.
- Risk of angle-closure glaucoma—antidepressants with anticholinergic effect.

https://www.cms.gov/Medicare-Medicaid-Coordination/Fraud-Prevention/Medicaid-Integrity-Education/Pharmacy-Education-Materials

unintentionally. Withdrawal symptoms should start within 5 days after discontinuing the medication for the most of antidepressants. Common symptoms include paresthesia, dizziness, irritable and anxious mood, nausea, insomnia, tremors, and vivid dreams. The symptoms can last up to 3 weeks. The severity and duration of withdrawal symptoms are related to the half-life of a medication. Among all commonly used antidepressants, venlafaxine has the shortest half-life. A small number of patients on venlafaxine are unable to discontinue it because of intolerable withdrawal symptoms. Tapering off instead of sudden discontinuation can minimize or avoid the withdrawal syndrome.

ii. SNRI antidepressants—SNRI antidepressants include venlafaxine, desvenlafaxine (a metabolite of venlafaxine), duloxetine, and levomilnacipran. Although all these antidepressants target serotonin and norepinephrine, their potency to serotonin and norepinephrine presynaptic transporters is different (Table 26–3). Because of the weak blockade of norepinephrine transporters by venlafaxine, it has to be dosed toat least 150 mg per day in order to work as an SNRI antidepressant. Doses of lower than 150 mg per day are more likely functioning as SSRIs. In addition to MDD, duloxetine is also used to treat anxiety and relieve nerve pain due to diabetic peripheral neuropathy or ongoing pain due to medical conditions such as arthritis, chronic back pain or fibromyalgia. Levomilnacipran are not indicated for fibromyalgia or chronic pain, although a similar medication milnacipran, manufactured by a different company, is used to treat fibromyalgia.

Patients taking an SNRI may experience the same side effects related to serotonin with additional side effects related to norepinephrine such as tachycardia and increase in blood pressure. For duloxetine, anticholinergic effects may cause dry mouth, constipation, urinary retention, and/or blurred vision. Duloxetine also potentially causes liver damage and severe skin reactions.

iii. Dopamine reuptake inhibitor—Bupropion is the only medication in the class and may be able to block norepinephrine reuptake at high doses, but the potency of bupropion to dopamine transporters is about four time stronger than its potency to norepinephrine transporters. It remains unclear at doses of 150–450 mg per day how much norepinephrine is involved in the total antidepressant effect of bupropion. In the STAR*D, bupropion monotherapy had a similar remission rate as venlafaxine and sertraline monotherapy in patients who failed citalopram monotherapy, suggesting that bupropion can be the first medication for those who present with severe anhedonia, lack of energy, poor concentration, and/or hypersomnia without much anxiety. For patients who have sexual side effects from SSRIs and/or SNRIs in previous episodes, bupropion can be the first medication prescribed for a recurrent episode.

The common side effects from bupropion include headache, insomnia, dizziness, agitation, decreased appetite and weight loss, dry mouth, nausea, constipation, tachycardia, tremor, excessive sweating, rhinitis, and pharyngitis. Bupropion can lower the seizure threshold. Therefore, bupropion is contraindicated for patients with seizure disorders and any other factors predisposing to seizures, such as withdrawal from alcohol or benzodiazepines, eating disorders (anorexia nervosa or bulimia nervosa), brain tumors, traumatic brain injury, arteriovenous malformations, and severe stroke. Bupropion can also cause false-positive results for amphetamine and methamphetamine on a urine drug test.

iv. Tricyclic antidepressants—TCAs including tertiary (amitriptyline, clomipramine, doxepin, imipramine, trimipramine), secondary (desipramine, nortriptyline, protriptyline) and tetracyclic (amoxapine, maprotiline) antidepressants started being available from 1950s. Their efficacy is believed through the blocking of reuptake of serotonin and norepinephrine, but their potency is different. For blocking serotonin reuptake, clomipramine is the stongest, followed by imipramine and amitriptyline. For blocking norepiphrine reuptake, desipramine is the strongest, followed by protriptyline and nortriptyline. Their potency of blocking dopamine reuptake is negligible. Some evidence also supports the 5-TH2 antagonism involvement in their antidepressant efficacy. For blockade of 5-HT2 receptors, amoxapine is the strongest, followed by amitriptyline, clomipramine and doxpin.

In the STAR*D, nortriptyline, an active metabolite of amitriptyline, had a remission rate of 20% for patients who failed an SSRI, SNRI, and/or bupropion. This remission rate is lower than that of rTMS and ketamine treatment. With other new medications and newer adjunctive therapies to antidepressants becoming available, the role of tricyclics in the treatment of DDs likely continues declining although tricyclics may be more effective than SSRIs in MDD melancholic type. For those who are indicated for a tricyclic for MDD, monitoring the blood level may be necessary. The effective blood levels of amitriptyline, nortriptyline, imipramine, desipramine, and doxepin are established, however, nortriptyline level is in a bell shape with a narrow window of efficacy.

Side effects from TCAs are through anticholinergic, antihistaminergic, and α_1 adrenergic blocking mechanism in addition to inhibiting the reuptake of serotonin and norepinephrine. Their anticholinergic effect can cause blurred vision, dry mouth, urinary retention, constipation, and acute organic brain syndrome (delirium), especially on multiple anticholinergic drugs. The affinity to muscarinic 1 receptor is the strongest for amitriptyline, followed by protritypline and clomipramine. Blocking α_1 adrenergic receptors relates to hypotension and orthostasis. The affinity to α_1 adrenergic receptors is the strongest for doxpin and trimipramine, followed by amitriptyline. Antihistaminic effect relates sedation and weight gain. The affinity to histaminic 1 receptors is the strongest for doxpine and trimipramine, followed by amitriptyline, maprotiline, impipriane and nortriptyline. Tremor, nocturnal myoclonus, photosensitivity, heat intolerance, atrioventricular (AV) block, quinidine-like antiarrhythmic effects are also common. Increases risk for seizure with maprotiline, clomipramine, amoxapine was reported. Suddenly stopping tricyclics can cause withdrawal symptoms (cholinergic rebound) including excessive salivation, diarrhea, headache, and vivid dreams. The frequency and severity of aforementioned side effects depend on their pharmacological profiles with each of those neurotransmitters. Before SSRIs were available, tricyclics were the number one medication causing death by overdose.

v. Monoamine oxidase inhibitor antidepressants—MAOIs werethe first group of antidepressants developed in 1950s. Due to theirstrict dietary restrictions, side effects and safety concerns, MAOIs have fallen out of favor in the treatment of MDD, although newer MAOIs with reversibility and transdermal delivery have beendeveloped (Table 26–5). Before rTMS and ketamine treatment became available, MAOIs were considered as fourth-line antidepressants for those who failed trials of a first- and second-line antidepressant (SSRIs and SNRIs) and a TCA. In the STAR*D, only about 7% of patients who failed nortriptyline achieved remission with treatment ontranylcypromine (an MAOI). In addition, only less than 5% of patients who achieved remission with nortriptyline or tranylcypromine remained in remission in 12 months. With these low remission rates and high relapse rates, some researchers have questioned the value of including TCAs and MAOIs in stage II or III TRD.

The most common side effects from MAOIs include dry mouth, nausea, diarrhea, constipation, drowsiness, insomnia or sedation, dizziness, lightheadedness, weight gain, orthostatic hypotension, and sexual dysfunction (dose-related impotence or anorgasmia). Less common side effects include hepatitis, ataxia, and color blindness. The main concern from taking an MAOI is the potential forhypertensive crisis that includes headache, diaphoresis, anxiety/nervousness, increased BP, and neck stiffness. Without immediate intervention, cerebral hemorrhage or even death can occur. A hypertensive crisis is a medical emergency and should be treated with slow intravenous

Table 26–5 Summary of Commonly Used Monoamine Oxidase Inhibitors in the Treatment of Depressive Disorders

Medication	Selectivity	Reversibility	Dose (mg/day)	Half-life (hours)	Common Side Effects
Phenelzine	No	No	30–90	11.6	Blurred vision, constipation, dry mouth, headache, insomnia, liver enzyme elevation, myoclonus, nausea, orthostatic hypotension, paresthesia, peripheral edema, sedation, sexual dysfunction, urinary hesitancy, weight gain.
Tranylcypromine	No	No	10–60	2-2.5	
Isocarboxazid	No	No	10–60	1.5–4	
Selegiline oral	Yes*	No	1.25–10	1.5–3.5	Constipation, dizziness, headaches, insomnia, nausea, xerostomia.
Selegiline transdermal	Yes*	No	6–16	18–25	Dizziness, drowsiness, dry mouth, headache, insomnia, irritation at application site, nausea.
Moclobemide	Yes**	Yes	300–600	1–4	Dizziness, headache, gastrointestinal discomfort, nausea, insomnia.

Note: *Selective for monoamine oxidase inhibitors B subtype (MAO-B) at lower doses and nonselective at higher doses; **selective for monoamine oxidase inhibitors A subtype (MAO-A). Moclobemide is not available in the United States and has negligible risk to induce hypertensive crisis after ingestion of tyramine-rich food/drinks when it is used in the recommended doses.

administration of phentolamine, 5 mg (repeated hourly as needed), or with sublingual or oral 10–20 mg of nifedipine. Early diagnosis and intervention are the key to preventing severe consequences. To avoid these possibly severe side effects, educating patients to the risks of drug–food and drug–drug interactions is essential before considering an MAIO (Table 26–6).

As tyramine is mainly derived from fermented food and drinks, those who are taking an MAOI should be advised to eat fresh foods instead of leftovers or food prepared hours earlier. When switching from MAOIs to another antidepressant or switching from an SSRI, SNRI, or TCA to an MAOI, patients should wait for at least 14 days after discontinuation before initiating the new treatment. Those who take fluoxetine should wait for 5 weeks before starting an MAOI. For patients anticipatingelective surgery that requires general anesthesia, MAOIs should be stopped for at least 10 days before surgery to minimizedrug interactions with general anesthetics, barbiturates and other sedatives, antihistamines, or narcotics (particularly meperidine). Over-the-counter medications such as anticholinergic agents and sympathomimetic amines (e.g., pseudoephedrine used commonly in decongestants) should be avoided.

vi. Atypical antidepressants—There is no standard definition for an atypical antidepressant, although mirtazapine along with nefazodone, trazodone, and a few other medications are considered as atypical antidepressants.

Mirtazapine increases serotonin and norepinephrine in the synaptic cleft through increased release of these two neurotransmitters rather than blockade of reuptake. It also acts as a potent antagonist of H1 histamine receptors (producing a sedating, calming effect) as well as 5-HT2A, 5-HT2C, and 5-HT3 serotonin receptors (Table 26–3).

Common side effects include drowsiness, weight gain, xerostomia, increased serum cholesterol, constipation, increase in appetite, and sedation. Rare, but potential life-threatening side effects include thrombocytopenia, bone marrow suppression and neutropenia, and acute pancreatitis. Mirtazapine is less likely to cause tremors and sexual dysfunction compared to other antidepressants. Mirtazapine can antagonize clonidine's hypotensive effect; therefore, patients with cardiovascular disease should be cautious when using mirtazapine. Low dose mirtazapine is associated with anti-histamine H1 effects such as excessive sedation and weight gain. Drowsiness can paradoxically be diminished ata higher doses. Mirtazapine is associated with weight gain in

Table 26–6 Dietary and Drug Restrictions Associated with Monoamine Oxidase Inhibitor Antidepressants

Danger Level	Foods	Drugs
Very dangerous (must be avoided under all circumstances)	All cheese (cottage cheese, cream cheese) Sauerkraut yogurt are safe	Amphetamines, asthma inhalants (*pure* steroid inhalants are safe), cyclopentamine, decongestants, cold, and sinus medications, ephedrine, meperidine, metaraminol, methylphenidate, phenylephrine, phenylpropanolamine, pseudoephedrine, serotonin-active antidepressants (clomipramine, fluoxetine, sertraline, paroxetine, fluvoxamine)
Moderately dangerous (should be avoided)	All fermented or aged foods (aged corned beef, salami, fermented sausage, pepperoni, summer sausage, pickled herring) Broad bean pods (English broad beans, Chinese pea pods) Fermented alcohol beverages (red wine, sherry, vermouth, cognac, beer, and ale) Liver (chicken, beef or pork) or liverwurst Meat or yeast extracts Spoiled fruit (spoiled bananas, pineapples, avocados, figs, raisins)	Antihistamines, buspirone, carbamazepine, detromethorphan high doses, Dopamine, fenfluramine, L-Dopa Local anesthetics with epinephrine (safe without epinephrine—e.g., carbocaine) L-tryptophan Narcotics (codeine is safe) Tricyclic antidepressants (e.g., imipramine, amitriptyline, nortriptyline, desipramine, doxepin)
Minimal danger (rarely causing hypertensive episodes and can be used in moderation)	Anchovies, beets, caviar, chocolate, clear alcoholic drinks coffee, colas, curry powder, figs, junket, licorice, mushrooms, rhubarb, snails, soy sauce, tea, worcestershire sauce	

Note: Diabetics taking insulin may have increased hypoglycemia, requiring adjustment in dose of insulin (otherwise safe); patients taking hypotensive agents for high blood pressure may have more hypotension, also requiring adjustment (but also otherwise safe).

short- and long-term but appears less likely to cause weight gain than TCAs.

Nefazodone is a serotoninergic modulating antidepressant through the inhibition of serotonin and norepinephrine reuptake, and weak serotonin and α₁ adrenergic antagonism. Its rare risk of fatal idiopathic hepatic failure limits its usein practice. Trazodone simultaneously inhibits serotonin transporters 5-HT2A and 5-HT2C receptors, allowingtrazodone to largely avoid the issue of sexual dysfunction (Table 26-3). Low-dose trazodone exerts a sedative effect for sleep through antagonism of 5-HT-2A receptor, H1 receptor, and α₁ adrenergic receptors. Priapism has been reported in men taking Trazodone and is considered a medical emergency.

vii. NMDA receptors-related medications

a. Ketamine—Ketamine, a noncompetitive NMDA antagonist, became available in1962 and was approved as an anesthetic agent in 1970. The fast onset of antidepressant effects in TRD after intravenous ketamine infusion at 0.5 mg/kg over 40 minutes was first reported by researchers at Yale University School of Medicine and subsequently confirmed by other researchers after single or repeated infusions. However, the magnitude of efficacy of Ketamine was much smaller in patients who had more advanced TRD and failed trials of two antidepressant monotherapies and two adjunctive therapies. In more advanced TRD, only 27% of patients achieved a response as defined by ≥ 50% reduction in MADRS (Montgomery–Asberg Depression Rating Scale) total score and only 5% met remission criteria (MADRS total score ≤ 10) after a single ketamine infusion. After six repeated infusions in 2 weeks, a total of 59% of patients achieved response and 23% patients achieved remission.

Ketamine infusion at a fixed dose of 0.5 mg/kg over 40 minutes was not as effective as right unilateral ECT in hospitalized patients who had at least moderate severity of UPD. After 12 ECT or ketamine infusion treatments in 4 weeks, the remission rate was 46% for ketamine infusion and 63% of ECT. Both ketamine and ECT required a median of six treatment sessions to achieve remission. However, a more recent study of ketamine infusion versus ECT in outpatients with TRD did not find significant difference between the two treatments.

The most common side effects associated with ketamine infusion were dissociation (feeling of floating), sleepiness/drowsiness/sedation, numbness or tingling, dizziness andvisual disturbances (blurry vision or diplopia). Long-term side effects from ketamine infusion remain unknown. However, cystitis and hepatic toxicity have occurred in ketamine abusers, who typically use much higher doses of ketamine.

b. Esketamine—Esketamine is more potent than the racemic ketamine. Intranasal esketamine doses of 56 mg and 84 mg per session produce similar clinical outcomes as i.v. ketamine infusion at 0.5 mg/kg. The FDA approved intranasal esketamine plus an antidepressant for the treatment of TRD in

2019. Three acute studies and two long-terms studies supported its approval, but only one of the three phase III studies demonstrated intranasal esketamine plus an antidepressant was superior to placebo plus an antidepressant in reducing depression. The other two studies did not show superiority of intranasal esketamine over placebo in the primary outcome, but some secondary outcomes were significantly in favor of the active treatment over placebo. One of the long-term studies also favored active treatment over placebo.

The effect size of intranasal esketamine relative to placebo in the MADRS score change from baseline to the end of study was 0.30 (small), even in the positive study. However, the significant difference occurred from the day 2. A post-hoc analysis of all RCTs (randomized, controlled trials) found that response rates were 63.4% for active treatment versus 49.5% for placebo with an NNT (number needed to treat to benefit) of eight. The remission rates were 48.2% for active treatment versus 30.3% for placebo with an NNT of six. In evidence-based medicine, an NNT < 10 indicates clinical relevance. The significant difference in common side effects with an NNH (the NNT to harm) of <10 included dissociation, vertigo, nausea, dizziness, and dysgeusia. The discontinuation rate due to adverse events (DAEs) was also significantly different, with an NNH of 17. Other side effects (>10%) included headache, somnolence, hypoesthesia, paresthesia, and oral hypoesthesia. Most side effects peak at 20–30 minutes after administering the third dose of intranasal esketamine.

Because ketamine has pro-cardiovascular and sedation effects, barbiturates, benzodiazepines, narcotics, stimulants, modafinil/armodafinil, and MAOIs should be decreased or withheld for 4–24 hours depending on their half-life on the day of treatment. Patients may be precluded from receiving ketamine if they have unstable cardiovascular disease, elevated intracranial or intraocular pressure, hyperthyroidism, pheochromocytoma, severe liver disease, full stomach (due to aspiration risk), pregnancy, intoxication by a substance, active SUD, delirium, acute psychosis or limited exercise tolerance/physical activity.

c. Dextromethorphan + bupropion—Dextromethorphan, an uncompetitive NMDA receptor antagonist, an agonist at the sigma-1 receptor, and an inhibitor of serotonin and norepinephrine transporters, plus bupropion was approved by the US FDA for acute treatment of MDD in adults in 2022. Dextromethorphan is an active ingredient of cough medicine for decades, but its rapid and extensive metabolism through cytochrome P450 (CYP 2D6) makes it difficult to maintain at therapeutic levels. The combination of dextromethorphan and bupropion (105 mg/day), itself a moderate inhibitor of CYP2D6, has demonstrated superiority over placebo in MDD.

The combination of dextromethorphan and bupropion has more adverse events than placebo, but serious adverse events are rareSide effects at least two time higher than placebo were dizziness, nausea, headache, diarrhea, somnolence, dry mouth, hyperhidrosis, anxiety, constipation decreased appetite, and insomnia. Because dextromethorphan also increases serotonin levels, taking this combination with SSRIs, SNRIs, MAOIs, and other serotonin-increasing agents should be undertaken with caution. Dextromethorphan–bupropion was not associated with psychotomimetic effects, weight gain, or sexual dysfunction.

Anand A, Mathew SJ, Sanacora G, et al. *N Engl J Med.* 2023 May 24. doi: 10.1056/NEJMoa2302399. Online ahead of print.

Citrome L, DiBernardo A, Singh J. Appraising esketamine nasal spray for the management of treatment-resistant depression in adults: number needed to treat, number needed to harm, and likelihood to be helped or harmed. *J Affect Disord.* 2020; 271:228–238.

Ekstrand J, Fattah C, Persson M, et al. Racemic ketamine as an alternative to electroconvulsive therapy for unipolar depression: a randomized, open-label, non-inferiority trial (KetECT). *Int J Neuropsychopharmacol.* 2022;25(5):339–349.

Iosifescu DV, Jones A, O'Gorman C, et al. Efficacy and safety of AXS-05 (dextromethorphan-bupropion) in patients with major depressive disorder: a phase 3 randomized clinical trial (GEMINI). *J Clin Psychiatry.* 2022;83(4):21m14345.

Nelson JC. Tricyclic and tetracyclic drugs. In Schatzberg AF, Nemeroff CB, eds. The Textbook of Psychopharmacology, 5th ed. Arlington: American Psychiatric Association Publishing; 2017:305–333.

Phillips JL, Norris S, Talbot J, et al. Single, Repeated, and maintenance ketamine infusions for treatment-resistant depression: a randomized controlled trial. *Am J Psychiatry.* 2019; 176(5):401–409.

Rhee TG, Shim SR, Forester BP, et al. Efficacy and safety of ketamine vs electroconvulsive therapy among patients with major depressive episode: a systematic review and meta-analysis. *JAMA Psychiatry.* 2022;79(12):1162–1172.

Tabuteau H, Jones A, Anderson A, et al. Effect of AXS-05 (dextromethorphan-bupropion) in major depressive disorder: a randomized double-blind controlled trial. *Am J Psychiatry.* 2022;179(7):490–499.

vii. Neurosteroids—Neurosteroids are steroid-derived molecules synthesized from cholesterol in the CNS and alter neuronal excitability through modulating gamma-aminobutyric acid (GABA) receptors, especially $GABA_A$ receptors. Dysregulation of neurosteroidogenesis has been observed in neuropsychiatric disorders including PPD and MDD. Lower levels allopregnanolone in the cerebral spinal fluid of depressed patients than healthy control, and its normalization after administeringSSRIs, supports the involvement of neurosteroids in MDD.

a. Brexanolone for PPD—Brexanolone is the first neurosteroid that was approved by the FDA for the treatment of PPD in 2019. Brexanolone was superior to placebo in reducing depressive symptoms of PPD. However, continuous i.v. infusion of brexanolone is under a Risk Evaluation and Mitigation Strategy (REMS) program in which health care facilities and pharmacies are certified and patients are required to enroll beforeinfusion in order to mitigate the potential risk for excessive sedation and sudden loss of consciousness during the infusion. Because of the REMS requirement and its 60 hour continuous infusion protocol, currently brexanolone has very limited use in clinical practice. However, brexanolone infusion was generally well tolerated. The most common treatment-emergent adverse events in the brexanolone groups were headache, dizziness, and somnolence.

b. Zuranolone for postpartum depression—Zuranolone is a synthetic and oral neuroactive steroid and acts as a positive allosteric modulator on $GABA_A$ receptors. It has been evaluated as a rapid acting, once daily, 14-day oral short course therapy for adult patients with MDD and PPD. There are two positive studies of zuranolone versus placebo in the treatment of PPD. Zuranolone demonstrated significant difference in changes of HAMD-17 (Hamilton Depression Rating Scale-17) total scores from baseline to day 15 compared to placebo. Sustained differences in HAMD-17 scores favoring zuranolone were observed from day 3 through day 45. The response rate was significantly higher with zuranolone than with placebo from day 15 to day 45. The remission rate (HAMD-17 ≤ 7) was significantly higher with zuranolone at day 3, and at day 15. Zuranolone was well tolerated. The common side effects with a higher rate in zuranolone group were somnolence, dizziness, upper respiratory tract infection, diarrhea, and sedation.

c. Zuranolone for MDD—There are four phase III and two phase II studies of zuranolone in the treatment of MDD, but all excluded patients with TRD. The first phase II trial also known as SAGE-217 or MDD-201B showed that zuranolone 30 mg/day for 2 weeks was significantly superior to placebo in reducing depression symptoms starting for from day 2 to day 28. At the day 15, the NNT for response and remission was both of three. However, the phase III studies did not produce robust results. In the MOUNTAIN study, zuranolone 20 mg/day or 30 mg/d was not superior to placebo in primary outcomes. In the WATERFALL, zuranolone 50 mg/d was significantly superior to placebo in reducing depressive symptoms at day 15, but the difference in HAMD-17 scores was small (−1.8 points). Similarly, in the CORAL study, zuranolone 50 mg plus one of the five antidepressants (sertraline, escitalopram, citalopram, duloxetine, or desvenlafaxine) was significantly superior to placebo in reducing HAMD-17 total scores at day 3, but again, small (−1.9 points). In addition to the side effects reported in the PPD studies, chromaturia, decreased appetite, pruritus, dry mouth, insomnia, irritability, fatigue, headache, and nausea were reported.

Clayton AH, Lasser R, Nandy I, et al. Zuranolone in major depressive disorder: results From MOUNTAIN-A phase 3, multicenter, double-blind, randomized, placebo-controlled Trial. *J Clin Psychiatry.* 2023;84(2):22m14445.

Deligiannidis KM, Meltzer-Brody S, Gunduz-Bruce H, et al. Effect of zuranolone vs placebo in postpartum depression: a randomized clinical trial. *JAMA Psychiatry.* 2021;78(9):951–959.

Gunduz-Bruce H, Silber C, Kaul I, et al. Trial of SAGE-217 in patients with major depressive disorder. *N Engl J Med.* 2019; 381(10):903–911.

Gunduz-Bruce H, Takahashi K, Huang MY. Development of neuroactive steroids for the treatment of postpartum depression. *J Neuroendocrinol.* 2022;34(2):e13019

Kanes S, Colquhoun H, Gunduz-Bruce H, et al. Brexanolone (SAGE-547 injection) in post-partum depression: a randomised controlled trial. *Lancet.* 2017;390(10093):480–489.

viii. Psilocybin—Psychedelics, also known as serotonergic hallucinogens, are agonists or partial agonists of serotonin 5-hydroxytryptamine 2A receptors in the brain. The activation of serotonin 5-hydroxytryptamine 2A receptors in the brain is necessary for the therapeutic effects in psychiatric disorders from psychedelics. Psilocybin is the most studied psychedelic and is able to "destabilize" the default mode network (DMN) that is critical for integrating information for complex cognitive functions. DMN is believed being hyperactive in different psychiatric disorders including depression. Reduction in the hyperactive DMN by psilocybin can dramatically increase global brain connectivity including synchronization of sensory networks and disintegration in associative ones that change or retune of negative thoughts and behaviors of depression.

Several small studies have demonstrated efficacy of psilocybin in the treatment of depression. One phase II study in patients with long-standing MDD with moderate-to-severe symptoms found oral psilocybin 25 mg plus placebo twice, 3 weeks apart, in 6 weeks was superior to escitalopram plus psilocybin 1 mg in remission rate. In another phase II study with double-blind design, a single dose of a proprietary, synthetic formulation of psilocybin at a dose of 25, 10, or 1 mg (control) were given along with psychological support adults with TRD. The mean changes from baseline to week 3 in MADRS total score were significantly different between 25 mg group and the 1 mg group, but no significant difference between the 10 mg group and 1 mg group. The incidences of response and remission at 3 weeks were generally supportive of the primary results. A single, moderate dose of psilocybin (0.215 mg/kg body weight) in conjunction with psychological support versus placebo found that at 14 days after the intervention, the psilocybin condition was significantly superior to placebo in reducing MADRS scores with large effect size (Cohens' $d = 0.97$). Headache, nausea, dizziness, suicidal ideation or behavior, or self-injury were reported.

Carhart-Harris R, Giribaldi B, Watts R, et al. Trial of psilocybin versus escitalopram for depression. *N Engl J Med.* 2021;384(15): 1402–1411.

Goodwin GM, Aaronson ST, Alvarez O, et al. Single-dose psilocybin for a treatment-resistant episode of major depression. *N Engl J Med.* 2022;387(18):1637–1648

von Rotz R, Schindowski EM, Jungwirth J, et al. Single-dose psilocybin-assisted therapy in major depressive disorder: a placebo-controlled, double-blind, randomised clinical trial. *EClinicalMedicine.* 2022;56:101809.

ix. Atypical antipsychotics—Aripiprazole, brexpiprazole, cariprazine, olanzapine, quetiapine-extended release (XR), risperidone, and ziprasidone have been studied with RCTs as adjunctive therapy to an antidepressant for the treatment of TRD, but only aripiprazole, brexpiprazole, cariprazine, olanzapine, and quetiapine-XR have been approved by the FDA for this indication. Amisulpride, sulpride, quetiapine-XR, ziprasidone, olanzapine, lurasidone, and lumateperone monotherapy showed efficacy in MDD in RCTs. There are no head-to-head comparisons of atypical antipsychotics in the acute treatment of TRD, although the efficacy of each antipsychotics relative to its placebo varies (Table 26–7). The challenge of comparing the efficacy of these antipsychotics in the treatment of TRD or non-TRD MDD is that the definitions of TRD were different in different studies, and inclusion and exclusion criteria for each study were also different. For TRD, most studies used a historical failure of an antidepressant and a prospective failure of another antidepressant to define TRD, but others just used retrospective reviews to determine treatment failure (Table 26–7). Without head-to-head comparison data, multiple network meta-analyses have been used to indirectly compare differences among the treatments in MDD and other psychiatric disorders. For clinicians, it is important to understand that meta-analysis is not hypothesis testing although results from a meta-analysis are commonly considered as the best evidence for clinical practice. However, misinterpretation of the results can occur if attention is not paid to which studies are included in the meta-analysis.

Among the FDA-approved antipsychotics for TRD, the side effects from antipsychotics are quite different (Table 26–7). Weight gain is a common side effect from olanzapine; and somnolence is a common side effect from olanzapine, quetiapine-XR, and ziprasidone. In contrast, akathisia is common from aripiprazole, brexpiprazole, and cariprazine. Like efficacy data, head-to-head comparison studies are important for safety and tolerability comparisons. A large 12-week study from the Veteran Health Admission comparing the efficacy and safety of switching to bupropion, augmentation with bupropion, or augmentation with aripiprazole in patients with MDD who failed an SSRI or SNRI is a good example for this argument. In the study, there was no significant difference between augmentation with bupropion and augmentation with aripiprazole, but the augmentation with aripiprazole had significantly more side effects compared to augmentation with bupropion, including somnolence, akathisia, extrapyramidal side effect (EPS), lab abnormality, increased appetite, weight gain, ≥ 7% weight again, and muscle spasm. Atypical antipsychotic adjunctive therapies to an antidepressant have been widely

Table 26–7 Summary of Treatment Response and Common Side Effects of Second-Generation Antipsychotics as Adjunctive Therapy to Antidepressant in Major Depressive Disorder

Drugs	Patient Population	Duration (weeks)	Dose	Response** NNT Mean (95% CI)	Somnolence NNH Mean (95% CI)	≥ 7% or Self-Reported Weight Gain NNH Mean (95% CI)	Akathisia NNH Mean (95% CI)
Aripiprazole	Historical failure of 1–3 antidepressants during current depressive episode, with subsequent prospective treatment failure with another antidepressant for 8 weeks.	6	Aripiprazole 2–20 mg/day	7 (5, 11)	24 (14, 87)	24 (16, 44)	5 (4, 7)
Brexpiprazole	Historical failure of 1–3 antidepressants during current depressive episode, with subsequent prospective treatment failure with another antidepressant for 8 weeks.	6	Brexpiprazole 1 mg/day Brexpiprazole 2 mg/day Brexpiprazole 3 mg/day	13 (7, 83) 13 (6, 98) 13 (7, 98)	29 (14, 81) 27 (13, 75) 19 (11, 39)	32 (14, 257) 32 (14, 431) 2538 (35, ∞, -49)	37 (16, 2090) 17 (10, 44) 8 (6, 13)
Cariprazine	Failed an ongoing medication for 6–8 weeks.	6	Cariprazine 1–2 mg/day Cariprazine 2–4.5 mg/day	11 (7, 29) 13 (7, 52)	31 (17, 248) 30 (16, 174)	76(31, -217) 30 (37, -127	28 (15, 48) 7 (6, 9)
Cariprazine	Failed 1 or 2 previous antidepressants for the current episode, and then failed a prospective 8-week open-label treatment with a new antidepressant.	8	Cariprazine 1–4.5 mg/day	32 (10, −27)	34 (18, 162)	43 (18, 118)	9 (6. 16)
Olanzapine-fluoxetine combination (OFC)*	History of treatment failure (lifetime) with two antidepressants of different classes, with subsequent prospective treatment failure with fluoxetine.	8	OFC 5–20/ 20–60 mg/day Fluoxetine 20–60 mg/day	15 (7, ∞ -6533)	8 (5, 17)	13 (8, 29) $^{\pi}$ 4 (3, 5) $^{\Omega}$	n/a
Quetiapine extended release	History of an inadequate response during the current episode to an adequate trial of an antidepressant during current depressive episode. No prospective treatment.	6	Quetiapine-XR 150 mg/day Quetiapine XR 300 mg/day	14 (7, ∞, -250) 8 (5, 24)	6 (5, 9) 4 (4, 6)	81 (26, ∞ -79) 22 (13, 69)	148 (24, ∞, -40) 51 (17, ∞ -68)
Risperidone	Insufficient response to an antidepressant monotherapy in prospective treatment for 4–5 weeks.	6	Risperidone 0.5–3 mg/day	5 (3, 12)	28 (11, ∞, -92)	46 (17, ∞, -56) $^{\Omega}$	137 (25, ∞, -46)

(Continued)

Table 26–7 Summary of Treatment Response and Common Side Effects of Second-Generation Antipsychotics as Adjunctive Therapy to Antidepressant in Major Depressive Disorder (*Continued*)

Drugs	Patient Population	Duration (weeks)	Dose	Response** NNT Mean (95% CI)	Somnolence NNH Mean (95% CI)	≥ 7% or Self-Reported Weight Gain NNH Mean (95% CI)	Akathisia NNH Mean (95% CI)
Ziprasidone	Insufficient response to escitalopram monotherapy in prospective treatment for 8 weeks.	8	Ziprasidone 40–160 mg/day	7 (3, ∞, -292)	5 (3, 12)	-22 (- 38, ∞, 8) $^{\Omega}$	12 (5, ∞, -36)

Note: *Olanzapine-fluoxetine combination versus fluoxetine 20–60 mg/day; **Response rates are defined as ≥ 50% reduction (improvement) from baseline values in MADRS (Montgomery–Asberg Depression Rating Scale) or HRSD-17 (Hamilton Depression Rating Scale-17 items) total scores in all studies. $^{\pi}$ ≥ 10% weight gain; $^{\Omega}$ Self-reported weight gain.

NNT and NNH = 1 ÷ (active response rate – placebo response rate). A positive number of NNT indicates that the response rate in active treatment is higher than that in placebo. A positive number of NNH indicates that the rate of a side effect in the active treatment is higher than that of placebo. The 95% of CI does not cross zero is indicative of significant difference between the groups. A small NNT is indicative of a medication having a larger effect relative to placebo in response compared to a medication for response with a large NNT relative to placebo. A small NNH is indicative of a medication having a higher risk for a side effect relative to place than a medication for the same side effect with a large NNH relative to placebo.

Abbreviations: CI, confidence interval; n/a, not available; NNT, number needed to treat to benefit; NNH, number needed to treat to harm.

marketed and used in the treatment of early stage of TRD. However, clinicians should consider the risk and benefit from an atypical antipsychotic compared to other options because most atypical antipsychotics can cause long-term side effects such as obesity, metabolic syndrome, diabetes, and tardive dyskinesia.

Aftab A, Gao K. The preclinical discovery and development of brexpiprazole for the treatment of major depressive disorder. *Expert Opin Drug Discov*. 2017;12(10):1067–1081.

Jha MK, Mathew SJ. Pharmacotherapies for treatment-resistant depression: how antipsychotics fit in the rapidly evolving therapeutic landscape. *Am J Psychiatry*. 2023;180(3):190–199.

Kishimoto T, Hagi K, Kurokawa S, et al. Efficacy and safety/tolerability of antipsychotics in the treatment of adult patients with major depressive disorder: a systematic review and meta-analysis. *Psychol Med*. 2022 May 5:1–19. Online ahead of print

Mohamed S, Johnson GR, Chen P, et al. Effect of antidepressant switching vs augmentation on remission among patients with major depressive disorder unresponsive to antidepressant treatment: the VAST-D randomized clinical trial. *JAMA*. 2017; 318(2):132–145.

x. Mood stabilizers—Commonly used non-antipsychotic MSs for TRD include lithium, valproate (VPA)/divalproex (DIV), and lamotrigine (LTG). However, RCTs of lithium as an adjunctive therapy to antidepressant have been small, with short duration, and mainly focusing on tricyclics. A network meta-analysis of 48 trials at different stages of TRD found the efficacy of adjunctive therapies with quetiapine, aripiprazole, thyroid hormone, and lithium to besuperior to placebo with an odds ratio for response of 1.92 for quetiapine, 1.85 for aripiprazole, 1.84 for thyroid hormone, and 1.56 for lithium, respectively. There were no significant differences between active treatments and placebo in acceptability. Lithium was better tolerated compared to quetiapine, olanzapine, aripiprazole. However, a remission rate of 15.9% with lithium augmentation in patients with stage II TRD of a STAR*D study suggests that the benefit with lithium augmentation is relatively small. Some evidence suggested that adjunctive VPA and LTG had beneficial effects for MDD. An RCT in TRD found that VPA augmentation to paroxetine was as effective as risperidone, buspirone, trazodone, or thyroid hormone augmentation with the highest remission rate of 48.7%. For LTG, three large RCTs in non-TRD did not find significant difference from placebo. LTG adjunctive therapy to antidepressant in MDD also did not significantly differ from placebo in an early meta-analysis. A more recent meta-analysis including all studies of LTG in MDD and BPD found that LTG was significantly superior to placebo as a whole, but less robust in subgroups.

Gao K, Bai Y, Calabrese JR. Lithium and mood stabilizers. In: Nemeroff CB, Rasgon N, Schatzberg AF, Strakowski SM, eds. *The American Psychiatric Association Publishing Textbook of Mood Disorders*, 2nd ed, Washington DC; 2022:271–284.

Zhou X, Ravindran AV, Qin B, et al. Comparative efficacy, acceptability, and tolerability of augmentation agents in treatment-resistant depression: systematic review and network meta-analysis. *J Clin Psychiatry*. 2015;76(4):e487–498.

xi. Psychostimulants—A systematic review of psychostimulants in treatment of TRD including 12 RCT and 19 retrospective chart reviews or open studies (14 in MDD and 7 in BD) suggested that adjunctive therapies with stimulants are effective in reducing depressive symptoms, but atomoxetine did not show benefit for improving depressive symptoms. Side effects from stimulants such as psychosis, anorexia, anxiety, insomnia, mood changes (irritability or anger), misuse, addiction, mania, and cardiovascular problems may occur. Lisdexamfetamine, as a prodrug, has less abuse potential compared with dextroamphetamine and methylphenidate. A retrospective cohort study did not find significant increase in the number of cardiac events in patients receiving dextroamphetamine or methylphenidate. Physical examination including vital signs, height, weight, and an electrocardiogram as indicated may be considered before starting a stimulant. Throughout treatment, monitoring the changes in blood pressure, pulse, weight or mood, as well as dependence or misuse may be necessary. Regular urine drug screening should be a part of treatment plan for those are taking a psychostimulant.

Pary R, Scarff JR, Jijakli A, et al. A review of psychostimulants for adults with depression. *Fed Pract*. 2015;32(Suppl 3):30S–37S.

xii. Other pharmacological agents—Buspirone is indicated for the treatment of anxiety disorder and commonly used an adjunctive therapy to an antidepressant for patients who do not fully respond to the antidepressant monotherapy. In the STAR*D, adjunctive buspirone to citalopram was as effective as adjunctive bupropion to citalopram in patients who failed citalopram monotherapy. Dizziness is a common side effect that occurs in over 10% of patients.

Triiodothyronine (T3) or levothyroxine (T4) has been used as an adjunct therapy to an antidepressant for TRD. In the STAR*D, about 25% of patients with Thase and Rush Stage II TRD achieved remission compared to 16% of patients received lithium. Checking thyroid function including TSH, free T3, and free T4 and a thorough medical history are necessary before starting thyroid hormone. Rechecking TSH at 3 months, then every 6 months, or at least once a year should follow. The goal of the treatment is the TSH level is at the lower limit of the normal range or below in the absence of hyperthyroid symptoms. The T3 levels can be maintained at the upper limit of the normal range based the severity of depression and response to T3. Monitor bone density with densitometry every 2 years in postmenopausal women and referring for evaluation of osteoporosis if bone density is declining. Cardiovascular monitoring may be necessary for patients with preexisting cardiovascular diseases.

Nuñez NA, Joseph B, Pahwa M, et al. Augmentation strategies for treatment resistant major depression: a systematic review and network meta-analysis. *J Affect Disord*. 2022;302:385–400.

2. Maintenance treatment of MDD—The goal for the acute treatment of MDE in patients with MDD is to achieve full remission, not simply response or partial remission. The STAR*D study found that patients who did not achieve full remission relapsed much earlier than those who achieved remission during a 12-month follow-up period. In a clinical sample, patients in remission had a similar level of quality of life, enjoyment, and satisfaction as general population, and depression severity was the only independent factor significantly associated with poor quality of life. Currently, the field agrees that for patients who have three or more MDEs, a life-long maintenance treatment is necessary to prevent future relapses. In terms of how to maintain the treatment after achieving remission, there is no standard protocol, although continuing the medication(s) and/or non-pharmacological treatment(s) that helps patients achieve remission is a common practice. For those who relapse with ongoing treatments, the next-step treatment options are more challenging, especially for patients who are in the late stage of TRD.

A meta-analysis of 40 studies with 8890 patients on antidepressants for preventing depressive relapse found that the relapse rate within 6 months was significantly lower in patients who continued the same antidepressant that achieved remission than those switched to placebo, 20.9 versus 39.7%. The difference in relapse rate was similar from a maintenance period of 6 months to over 1 year. To prevent relapse and treatment failure, maintenance therapy and careful attention for at least 6 months after remission is recommended. Overall, the acceptability is greater for SSRIs than for other antidepressants. SSRIs are well-balanced agents, and flexible dose adjustments are more effective for relapse prevention. In a more recent systematic review and network meta-analysis of 34 RCTs with 9384 patients in the efficacy, acceptability, tolerability, and safety on 20 antidepressants also found similar results. However, the results from studies with relapse prevention (enrichment) designs are not generalizable (see maintenance treatment of BD).

As for nonpharmacological treatments, early studies indicated that ECT monotherapy was as effective as lithium plus nortriptyline in preventing depression relapse in 6 months in patients who achieve remission with ECT. Combination of right unilateral ECT and an antidepressant was effective as compared to an antidepressant alone in geriatric depression. A recent systematic review of psychotherapy combination with pharmacology after remission found the combination is superior over medication alone in preventing depressive relapse/recurrence. Ketamine infusion and intranasal esketamine have demonstrated efficacy in preventing relapse. Continuation of TMS after remission to preventing depressive relapse has been reported, but currently, maintenance treatment with TMS is not allowed in the United States.

In addition to those aforementioned continuation treatments, managing residual symptoms such as insomnia and lack of motivation, and comorbidities such as ADs, PSTD, obsessive-compulsive disorder (OCD), ADHD, and SUD are also critical to prevent depressive relapse. Medications such as hypnotics for insomnia, benzodiazepines for ADs, and simulants for ADHD and specific psychosocial interventions of PTSD, OCD, and SUD may be necessary to control residual symptoms and prevent relapse (see below).

Culpepper L, Muskin PR, Stahl SM. Major depressive disorder: understanding the significance of residual symptoms and balancing efficacy with tolerability. *Am J Med*. 2015;128(9 Suppl): S1–S15.

Gao K, Su M, Sweet J, et al. Correlation between depression/anxiety symptom severity and quality of life in patients with major depressive disorder or bipolar disorder. *J Affect Disorders*. 2019;244:9–15.

Kellner CH, Knapp RG, Petrides G, et al. Continuation electroconvulsive therapy vs pharmacotherapy for relapse prevention in major depression: a multisite study from the Consortium for Research in Electroconvulsive Therapy (CORE). *Arch Gen Psychiatry*. 2006;63(12):1337–1344.

Kellner CH, Husain MM, Knapp RG, et al. A novel strategy for continuation ECT in geriatric depression: phase 2 of the PRIDE study. *Am J Psychiatry*. 2016;173(11):1110–1118.

Kato M, Hori H, Inoue T, et al. Discontinuation of antidepressants after remission with antidepressant medication in major depressive disorder: a systematic review and meta-analysis. *Mol Psychiatry*. 2021;26(1):118–133.

Kishi T, Ikuta T, Sakuma K, et al. Antidepressants for the treatment of adults with major depressive disorder in the maintenance phase: a systematic review and network meta-analysis. *Mol Psychiatry*. 2023;28(1):402–409.

Rush AJ, Trivedi MH, Wisniewski SR, et al. Acute and longer-term outcomes in depressed outpatients requiring one or several treatment steps: a STAR*D report. *Am J Psychiatry*. 2006;163(11):1905–1917.

B. Psychotherapeutic Interventions

During an acute depressive phase, supportive therapy may be the first-step to build a therapeutic relationship and to prevent deteriorating of depressive symptoms. Afterwards, therapies targeting different areas related to depression such as cognition, behavior, interpersonal relationship, and coping mechanisms may follow. Psychoeducation on the nature of illnesses, treatment options, side effects from medications,

importance of treatment compliance, harm from using drugs and alcohol, regular sleep-wake cycles, and other strategies should be an ongoing intervention at each visit. Each type of psychotherapy can be used alone or combination with antidepressant(s) and/or other somatic treatments, mainly depending on the depression severity and the preference of patients. Each patient can have different therapies at different times during the course of treatment. For patients with mild depression, psychotherapy alone is appropriate. For patients with moderate depressive severity, psychotherapy alone is as effective as an antidepressant alone, but the combination of both therapies is more effective than either one alone. For patients with severe depression, medication(s) or other somatic treatments should be the priority.

1. Cognitive–behavioral therapy (CBT)—CBT is based on the premise that helping patients recognize and correct erroneous beliefs and maladaptive behaviors can relieve their affective distress (Chapter 9). CBT can be effective in the acute treatment of MDD and may have an enduring effect that protects the patient against subsequent relapse following treatment termination. In a meta-analysis of five trials of CBT versus SGA (second-generation antidepressants) in patients with moderate to severe MDD, response and remission rates after 8–16 weeks were similar in the two groups. However, adding CBT to SGA did not show any benefit in remission or response compared to antidepressant monotherapy after 12–52 weeks of treatment. The efficacy of behavioral activation compared with an SGA was mixed with regard to response and remission.

In a large systematic review and meta-analysis of 11,374 participants, CBT and interpersonal therapy (IPT) were equally effective across all, but for psychotherapy delivered without concomitant antidepressant treatment, CBT was superior to IPT. Within-CBT moderator analyses showed that increased CBT efficacy was associated with younger age, high initial depression severity, individual format and no adjunctive antidepressants. For IPT, all moderators had comparable efficacy. Some studies have shown that in very severe depressed outpatients, neither IPT nor CBT is quite as effective as antidepressant drugs. A study of patients with chronic depression who received nefazodone or CBT indicated that a history of early childhood trauma or abuse mediated the efficacy of CBT.

2. Interpersonal psychotherapy—IPT is to identify precipitants and triggers that involve in four areas of interpersonal relationships: (1) interpersonal losses; (2) role disputes and transitions; (3) social isolation; or (4) deficits in social skills. IPT focuses on here and now interpersonal problems and try to avoid childhood antecedents or transference in the therapeutic relationship. IPT can be effective in reducing depressive symptoms in the acute phase of DDs. Four trials (872 participants) that compared SGA monotherapy with IPT alone found that SGAs and IPT had similar response or remission rates, and the combination of SGA and IPT had 25% higher remission rates than SGA alone.

3. Brief psychodynamic therapy (BPT)—BPT is derived from traditional psychoanalytic theory that focuses on unconscious processes as they are manifested in patients' present behavior (Chapter 7). The number of sessions BPT is typically considered no more than 25 sessions, but some allow up to 40 sessions. BPT has been used in different psychiatric disorders including DDs and commonly studied as an adjunctive therapy instead of monotherapy. SGA monotherapy and BPT monotherapy did not significantly differ in remission rates or improvements in functional capacity. SGAs and BPT had similar rates of overall discontinuation over 8–16 weeks, 48 weeks, and 96 weeks of follow-up. Suicidal ideas or behaviors also did not differ statistically for patients on SGAs, long-term psychodynamic therapy, or a combination of the two. Adding long-term (96 weeks) of psychodynamic therapy to SGA treatment led to lower rates of overall discontinuation compared with SGA monotherapy. Studies that are more recent have shown that BPT is comparable to CBT, but patients with feeling of chronic emptiness, lack of self-esteem, childhood trauma or loss, chronic conflict of interpersonal relationships, and rigid belief and behaviors may benefit more from BPT than from other psychotherapies.

4. Dialectical behavior therapy (DBT)—DBT was developed for the treatment for borderline personality disorder (BPD). DBT has many similarities with other cognitive-behavioral approaches but focuses on skills training including mindfulness, emotion regulation, interpersonal effectiveness, and distress tolerance. In a pilot study of a 16-week DBT-based skills training group for TRD as an adjunctive treatment to pharmacotherapy, patients who were randomized to the DBT-based skill training showed increases in emotional processing that were associated with decreases in depression symptoms compared those on the waiting list. In contrast, the waiting list group showed increases in emotional processing that were associated with increases in depression, suggesting that DBT-based skills training may help individuals with TRD to reduce depressive symptoms through developing skills that facilitate processing emotions in a way that helps to reduce rather than exacerbate depression symptoms.

5. Family therapy/couple therapy—Overall evidence supports that family therapy is more effective than no treatment or waiting list condition in decreasing depression and increasing family functioning. A more recent review on the evidence of couple and family interventions for depressive and BDs published from 2010 to 2019 found that the study designs including interventional approaches, settings, comparison groups, study duration, and outcome measure are heterogeneous. Attachment-based couple and family interventions for depression are probably efficacious as well as

family psychoeducation. Couple and family interventions can improve relationship dynamics that may improve treatment response and reduce relapse and recurrence associated with poor relationships. However, integrative couple interventions and family play-based interventions for depression are regarded as experimental.

Di Salvo G, Bianco M, Teobaldi E, et al. A psychoanalytic-derived brief psychotherapeutic approach in the treatment of major depression: monotherapy studies. *Medicina (Kaunas)*. 2022;58(10):1335.

Feldman G, Harley R, Kerrigan M, et al. Change in emotional processing during a dialectical behavior therapy-based skills group for major depressive disorder. *Behav Res Ther*. 2009; 47(4):316–321.)

Guidi J, Fava GA. Sequential combination of pharmacotherapy and psychotherapy in major depressive disorder: a systematic review and meta-analysis. *JAMA Psychiatry*. 2021;78(3):261–269.

Gartlehner G, Gaynes BN, Amick HR, et al. Comparative benefits and harms of antidepressant, psychological, complementary, and exercise treatments for major depression: an evidence report for a clinical practice guideline from the American College of Physicians. *Ann Intern Med*. 2016;164(5):331–341.

Whiston A, Bockting CLH, Semkovska M. Towards personalising treatment: a systematic review and meta-analysis of face-to-face efficacy moderators of cognitive-behavioral therapy and interpersonal psychotherapy for major depressive disorder. *Psychol Med*. 2019;49(16):2657–2668.

Whiston A, Lennon A, Brown C, et al. A systematic review and individual patient data network analysis of the residual symptom structure following cognitive-behavioral therapy and escitalopram, mirtazapine and venlafaxine for depression. *Front Psychiatry*. 2022;13:746678.

Wittenborn AK, Woods SB, Priest JB, et al. Couple and family interventions for depressive and bipolar disorders: evidence base update (2010-2019). *J Marital Fam Ther*. 2022;48(1):129–153.

6. Psychotherapy for maintenance treatment of MDD—In a naturalistic study of comparing CBT and BPT to the treatment as usual (TAU) for 3 years, 50-minute sessions CBT or BPT once a week therapy for 14–16 weeks were superior over TAU in reducing depressive symptoms and improving functioning. However, the functional capacity during long-term maintenance depended on the education level, the work situation, and the severity of depressive symptoms at the beginning of the treatment. One early study of mindfulness-based cognitive therapy (MBCT) found that the maintenance benefit from the MBCT with weekly 8 sessions depended on the remission status before the initiation of the therapy, i.e., patients with unstable remission, but not those with stable remission, had significant benefit from MBCT during 18-month follow-up period. In contrast, a large multicenter trial in child and adolescent (aged 11–17 years) did not find significant differences among CBT, short-term psychoanalytical therapy, and brief psychological intervention in reducing depressive symptoms at weeks 36, 52, or 86.

Dos Santos ÉN, Molina ML, Mondin T, et al. Long-term effectiveness of two models of brief psychotherapy for depression: a three-year follow-up randomized clinical trial. *Psychiatry Res.* 2020;286:112804.

Goodyer IM, Reynolds S, Barrett B, et al. Cognitive behavioral therapy and short-term psychoanalytical psychotherapy versus a brief psychosocial intervention in adolescents with unipolar major depressive disorder (IMPACT): a multicenter, pragmatic, observer-blind, randomized controlled superiority trial. *Lancet Psychiatry.* 2017;4(2):109–119.

Segal ZV, Bieling P, Young T, et al. Antidepressant monotherapy vs sequential pharmacotherapy and mindfulness-based cognitive therapy, or placebo, for relapse prophylaxis in recurrent depression. *Arch Gen Psychiatry.* 2010;67(12):1256–1264.

C. Other Interventions

1. Neuromodulation therapies for acute depression

i. Electroconvulsive therapy

a. ECT and FDA—There is a long history between ECT and the FDA, although prior to 1976, the FDA did not regulate medical devices including ECT (Chapter 10). During a final ruling in 2018, the FDA reclassified the use of ECT devices into Class II, limited to the treatment of catatonia or a severe MDE associated with MDD or BD in patients age 13 years and older who are treatment-resistant or who require a rapid response treatment due to the severity of their psychiatric or medical condition. This final ruling made ECT an indication for MDD, BPD, and catatonia. The use of ECT for other disorders is "off-label" and manufactures of ECT devices cannot market their devices for other disorders other than depression and catatonia.

b. Indication of ECT—ECT is indicated for UPD and BPD with MDEs accounting 80–90% of all ECT treatments. ECT can also be used for acute mania as monotherapy or adjunctive therapy to MSs. Studies have also shown that ECT are effective and safe in treating treatment-resistant schizophrenia and schizoaffective disorders. However, there is no compelling evidence of ECT in treatment of dysthymia, ADs, SUDs, eating disorders, or personality disorders. In contrast, some general medical conditions such as neuroleptic malignant syndrome and refractory Parkinson disease may benefit from ECT treatment.

c. Contraindication to ECT—There is no absolute contraindication to ECT. However, some medical conditions may potentially increase the risk for complication related ECT. These conditions include, but not limit to the following: (1) recent Intracranial hemorrhage; (2) recent thromboembolic stroke; (3) intracranial lesion (tumor or infection) causing mass effect; (4) unruptured cerebral aneurysm or peripheral vascular aneurysm; (5) recent myocardial infarction, particularly sequelae are present; (6) unstable angina or decompensating heart failure; and (7) unstable vertebral fracture. For patients with any of these contraindications or other unstable medical conditions such as unstable hypertension or severe chronic obstructive pulmonary disease, a consultation from related specialties should be sought before considering ECT. For patients with a recent heart attack or stroke in 6 months, ECT should not be considered unless it is an emergency, in which the risk and benefit should be carefully balanced.

d. Types of ECT—The ECT can be classified based on the electrode placement such as right unilateral ECT (RUL ECT), bilateral (bitemporal) ECT (BL ECT), or bifrontal ECT (BF ECT); the time of treatment such as acute and continuation/maintenance; and the pulse width such as brief pulse versus ultrabrief pulse.

e. Efficacy of ECT—The most studies in ECT are in adult population. Overall remission rate was about 65%, similar for UPD and BPD. As mentioned earlies, ECT may be more effective than ketamine infusion, especially in severe cases. In terms of the efficacy with different electrode placements, one relative large study supported by the NIMH did not find significant differences among the three electrode placements. Other studies also found that BL and BF ECT have similar efficacy, and high dose of RUL ECT had similar efficacy as BL ECT. In terms of ECT in special populations, here is more data on the elderly than on children/adolescents and pregnant women. Overall evidence suggests that ECT is effective and safe in geriatric and pediatric population.

f. Safety of ECT—The fatality from ECT is extremely low (around 2.1 per 100,000), which is roughly the same ratio as for the induction of brief general anesthesia (3.4 per 100,000). The most common side effects are headache and nausea. Both can be managed with appropriate pre-ECT medications. Post-ictal delirium/agitation also occurs in a small number of patients and commonly responds to a low dose of midazolam. Memory impairment, cognitive change, and/or executive function impairment are the most notable and distressing side effects. The memory impairment can be present as retrograde amnesia and/or anterograde amnesia. Most memory loss will recover after stopping ECT or finishing the acute series of ECT, but some patients may claim they have "permanent" memory loss, especially for the memory before the initiation of ECT treatment. There is not good evidence that supports a relationship between ECT and brain damage. In contrast, some studies have shown that ECT may increase neuronal sprouting and synaptic strength.

g. Predictors of acute treatments—Because of potential side effects from ECT, predictors for ECT treatment response are important to minimize unnecessary ECT exposures or decrease the number of ECT treatment. However, only personality disorders have been consistently shown to predict less response to ECT. Psychiatric comorbidities also predict less response to ECT. In contrast, the relationship between MDD with melancholic features, psychotic depression, resistant to antidepressants, age, baseline severity, episode duration, chronic course, or sex and response to ECT has been inconsistent.

h. Continuation and maintenance ECT—After an acute ECT series, most patients may benefit from continuation and maintenance treatment to prevent quick relapse. Patients who have an increased risk factors for relapse should consider continuation and maintenance ECT. The risk factors for relapse include: (1) MDD with melancholic features; (2) delusional depression; (3) medication-resistance pre-ECT; (4) comorbid SUD; (5) treatment of benzos and/or antipsychotics; and (6) personality disorders, especially cluster B personality disorder. However, logistic requirements for outpatient ECT may prevent a number of patients from having continuation and maintenance ECT.

The options to consider for continuation/maintenance treatment after an acute ECT series may includemedication alone, or medication and ECT with or without psychotherapy. A small number of patients need medication(s) with ECT for months or even years to maintain mood stability.

i. Concurrent medication during ECT—ECT providers and other prescribers commonly manage concurrent medication(s) during ECT treatment. Some medications need stop, some need hold, and some need continue. The decision on concurrent medications depends on their potential interactions with medications associated with ECT treatment, their interferences on seizure threshold, and their roles in managing comorbid medical and psychiatric conditions.

Martin DM, Tor PC, Waite S, et al. The utility of the brief ECT cognitive screen (BECS) for early prediction of cognitive adverse effects from ECT: a CARE network study. *J Psychiatr Res.* 2021;145:250–255.

McDonald WM, Weiner RD, Fochtmann LJ, et al. The FDA and ECT. *J ECT.* 2016;32(2):75–77.

Rasmussen KG. Principles and Practice of Electroconvulsive Therapy, 1st ed. Washington, DC, American Psychiatric Association Publishing; 2019.

Ross EL, Zivin K, Maixner DF. Cost-effectiveness of electroconvulsive therapy vs pharmacotherapy/psychotherapy for treatment-resistant depression in the United States. *JAMA Psychiatry.* 2018;75(7):713–722.

Sigström R, Nordenskjöld A, Juréus A, et al. Long-term subjective memory after electroconvulsive therapy. *BJPsych Open.* 2020; 6(2):e26.

Slade EP, Jahn DR, Regenold WT, et al. Association of electroconvulsive therapy with psychiatric readmissions in US hospitals. *JAMA Psychiatry.* 2017;74(8):798–804.

Zhang J, Wang G, Yang X, et al. Efficacy and safety of electroconvulsive therapy plus medication versus medication alone in acute mania: a meta-analysis of randomized controlled trials. *Psychiatry Res.* 2021;302:114019.

ii. **Vagus nerve stimulation**—In 2005, FDA approved VNS for treatment-refractory MDD and BPD in patients who failed ≥ 4 treatments including ECT (Chapter 10). After the rejection for coverage by the CMS (Center of Medicare and Medicaid Service) in 2007, the company conducted a 5-year study of VNS versus TAU and found that VNS was superior to TAU in response and remission rates and time to reach response and remission. Although the 5-year observation confirmed the previous findings, CMS, again, rejected the coverage application of VNS for treatment-refractory MDD and BPD in 2013.

LivaNova (a reorganized company from Cyberonic) initiated a RCT to study the safety and effectiveness of VNS as an adjunctive therapy versus sham in subjects with TRD in 2019. The inclusion and exclusion criteria for this study are the same as previous studies. The study was designed in accordance with the CMS coverage. If the results demonstrate that active VNS is superior to sham VNS in reducing depressive symptoms, the VNS will likely be a part of the routine clinical practice.

Aaronson ST, Sears P, Ruvuna F, et al. A 5-year observational study of patients with treatment-resistant depression treated with vagus nerve stimulation or treatment as usual: comparison of response, remission, and suicidality. *Am J Psychiatry.* 2017; 174(7):640–648.

https://www.livanova.com/depression/en-us/insurance-and-clinical-trial

iii. **Repetitive transcranial magnetic stimulation**

a. Current TMS system—The first rTMS device approved by the FDA for depression in 2008 was Neuronetics' Neuro-Star system that uses figure 8 coil for patients who failed one antidepressant. In 2014, the indication was changed to intend use of a NeuroStar TMS device for patients who had failed at least one antidepressant medication after the company provided new evidence. Currently, companies using the figure 8 coils include Magstim Rapid, Magventure, MagVista system, NeuroSoft TSM system and all were approved for the treatment of TRD. Brainsway and its partners use H coils that are patented by the company. Brainsway system with H1coil was approved by for the treatment of TRD in 2013, and H7 coil system was approved for treatment-resistant OCD.

Other forms of TMS include intermittent theta-burst stimulation (iTBS) and accelerated TMS. Several TMS systems with iTBS have been approved for the treatment of TRD. One of the accelerated TMS treatments is the Stanford Accelerated Intelligent Neuromodulation Therapy (SAINT) that uses functional MRI to map out an individual's brain connectivity to identify the optimal anatomic region for the condensed course of magnetic stimulation. The accelerated stimulation regimen of the SAINT involves multiple short TMS sessions daily for 5 days instead of 4–6 week regular TMS. After 5 days of treatment, patients with active treatment had an average a 62% reduction in their MADRS scores compared with a 14% decrease in those receiving sham stimulation. At the 4-week follow-up, the reduction was 53% versus 11%.

b. TMS in special population—There is no large study of rTMS in special populations. Systematic reviews and meta-analyses suggest that rTMS is safe and effective in MDD for adolescents, elderly, and pregnant women.

c. rTMS versus ECT in MDD—An early meta-analysis with 294 patients with an average of 15.2 high frequency rTMS or 8.2 ECT sessions found that the remission rate of ECT (52%) was significantly higher than rTMS (33.6%) with an NNT for remission of six favoring ECT. An umbrella review of neurostimulation and other nonpharmacological treatments in psychiatric disorders found that ECT has a large effect size, but TMS has a moderate effect size for DDs. Similarly, a systematic review and network meta-analysis of 113 nonsurgical brain stimulation trials (262 treatment arms) with 6750 patients with MDD or BPD found that BL ECT and high dose RUL ECT are more effective than any form of rTMS in reducing depressive symptoms.

Perera T, George MS, Grammer G, et al. The clinical TMS society consensus review and treatment recommendations for TMS therapy for major depressive disorder. *Brain Stimul.* 2016;9(3):336–346.

Blumberger DM, Vila-Rodriguez F, Thorpe KE, et al. Effectiveness of theta burst versus high-frequency repetitive transcranial magnetic stimulation in patients with depression (THREE-D): a randomised non-inferiority trial. *Lancet.* 2018; 391(10131):1683–1692.

Berlim MT, Van den Eynde F, Daskalakis ZJ. Efficacy and acceptability of high frequency repetitive transcranial magnetic stimulation (rTMS) versus electroconvulsive therapy (ECT) for major depression: a systematic review and meta-analysis of randomized trials. *Depress Anxiety.* 2013;30(7):614–623.

Rosson S, de Filippis R, Croatto G, et al. Brain stimulation and other biological non-pharmacological interventions in mental disorders: an umbrella review. *Neurosci Biobehav Rev.* 2022;139:104743.

Qiu H, Liang K, Lu L, et al. Efficacy and safety of repetitive transcranial magnetic stimulation in children and adolescents with depression: a systematic review and preliminary meta-analysis. *J Affect Disord.* 2023;320:305–312.

Kaster TS, Daskalakis ZJ, Noda Y, et al. Efficacy, tolerability, and cognitive effects of deep transcranial magnetic stimulation for late-life depression: a prospective randomized controlled trial. *Neuropsychopharmacology.* 2018;43(11):2231–2238.

Kim DR, Wang E, McGeehan B, et al. Randomized controlled trial of transcranial magnetic stimulation in pregnant women with major depressive disorder. *Brain Stimul.* 2019;12(1):96–102.

Cole EJ, Phillips AL, Bentzley BS, et al. Stanford neuromodulation therapy (SNT): a double-blind randomized controlled trial. *Am J Psychiatry.* 2022;179(2):132–141.

Mutz J, Vipulananthan V, Carter B, et al. Comparative efficacy and acceptability of non-surgical brain stimulation for the acute treatment of major depressive episodes in adults: systematic review and network meta-analysis. *BMJ.* 2019;364:l1079.

iv. Deep brain stimulation—DBS in the treatment of TRD remains uncertain. A recent systematic review and meta-analysis of 17 studies (3 RCTs and 14 open) involving seven DBS targets found that DBS treatment significantly reduced depressive symptoms in TRD compared to before DBS, with the response, remission, and recurrence rates of 56, 35, and 14%, respectively. However, two RCTs did not find significant difference in response rates between active and control groups. One study reported that a number of patients attempted suicide during the study period.

Wu Y, Mo J, Sui L, et al. Deep brain stimulation in treatment-resistant depression: a systematic review and meta-analysis on efficacy and safety. *Front Neurosci.* 2021;15:655412.

v. Transcranial current stimulation or transcranial electrical stimulation—Transcranial alternating current stimulation (tACS), transcranial random noise stimulation, cranial electrotherapy stimulation, and tDCS have been studied in the treatment of depression and anxiety. The FDA grandfathered some devices for the treatment of insomnia, depression, and anxiety in 1970s. No new device using transcranial current stimulation is approved for any psychiatric disorder. In a systematic review of 12 RCTs of tDCS in the treatment of depression, active treatment with tDCS, especially along with medication, was superior to sham in reducing depressive symptoms, but the combination of tDCS and psychotherapy did not have significant benefit. The current intensity was the only predictor for treatment response. A recent relatively large study of tACS at 77.5 Hz, 15 mA for 40 minutes 5 days a week for 4 weeks found the active treatment was superior over sham in reducing depressive symptoms of patients with MDD and the efficacy lasted beyond the time of active treatment.

Wang J, Luo H, Schülke R, et al. Is transcranial direct current stimulation, alone or in combination with antidepressant medications or psychotherapies, effective in treating major depressive disorder? A systematic review and meta-analysis. *BMC Med.* 2021;19(1):319.

Wang H, Wang K, Xue Q, et al. Transcranial alternating current stimulation for treating depression: a randomized controlled trial. *Brain.* 2022;145(1):83–91.

2. Nonpharmacological maintenance treatments of MDD—There is no good evidence for most nonpharmacological treatments in the maintenance treatment of MDD. Some small studies suggested that subjects with MDD who had remitted with acute ECT or TMS might benefit from continuation of ECT or TMS.

3. Medicinal agents and other treatments

i. S-adenosyl-ʟ-methionine—ʟ-methylfolate and S-adenosyl-methionine (SAMe) monotherapy or adjunctive therapy to an antidepressant have been studied in the treatment of non-resistant MDD and TRD. ʟ-methylfolate is approved by the FDA as a medicinal supplement for augmentation antidepressant for TRD. The efficacy and safety of SAMe in the treatment of MDD were compared with placebo or other antidepressants as monotherapy or adjunctive therapy. A recent systematic review of eight trials with a total of 11 arms and 1011 subjects found that the results of the difference between SAMe and placebo had been inconsistent. Studies comparing the differences between SAMe and other antidepressants (imipramine or escitalopram) did not find significant difference. One study showed that SAMe combined with an SSRI was better than an SSRI alone.

ii. St. John's Wort—The results of individual studies comparing St. John's Wort with an antidepressant or placebo for depression have been mixed. Different studies used different doses and different formulations. A meta-analysis of nine trials with 1513 patients found similar response rates between SGAs and St. John's Wort, 52 versus 54%. However, all trials compared St. John's Wort and SGAs were confounded by using moderate- or low-dose SGA regimen as a comparator. The overall risk of adverse events was higher among patients receiving SGAs than those receiving St. John's Wort, but the risk of serious adverse events did not differ significantly.

iii. Omega-3 fatty acids—Most studies of Omega-3 fatty acids (Omega-3) were compared with placebo. A Cochrane Database Systematic Review of 34 studies with 1924 patients comparing Omega-3 with placebo found that Omega-3 supplementation results in a small to modest benefit for reducing depressive symptoms, with a between group difference in HAMD-17 scores of about 2.5 points. Commonly, a minimal change score on this scale of 3.0 points is considered clinically meaningful. However, in a small study comparing Omega-3 with an antidepressant, there was no significant differences between Omega-3 and the antidepressant. Overall, the quality of the evidence for all outcomes was as low to very low. Likely, Omega-3 supplementation has some, but limited relevance in clinical practice.

Appleton KM, Voyias PD, Sallis HM, et al. Omega-3 fatty acids for depression in adults. *Cochrane Database Syst Rev.* 2021;11(11):CD004692.

Cuomo A, Beccarini Crescenzi B, Bolognesi S, et al. S-Adenosylmethionine (SAMe) in major depressive disorder (MDD): a clinician-oriented systematic review. *Ann Gen Psychiatry.* 2020;19:50.

Gartlehner G, Gaynes BN, Amick HR, et al. Comparative benefits and harms of antidepressant, psychological, complementary, and exercise treatments for major depression: an evidence report for a clinical practice guideline from the American College of Physicians. *Ann Intern Med.* 2016;164(5):331–341.

Halaris A, Sohl E, Whitham EA. Treatment-resistant depression revisited: a glimmer of hope. *J Pers Med.* 2021;11(2):155.

iv. Light therapy—The efficacy of light therapy was initially assessed in patients with MDD or BPD with season patterns, in which 10,000-lux cool-white florescent light 30 minutes each morning for 6 weeks was as effective as 12 sessions of 90 minutes twice a week CBT in a group format. The efficacy of light therapy was further investigated in a mixed group of patient with BPD (n = 50) and MDD (n = 45) without a seasonal pattern. After 14 days of treatment, the light therapy did not significantly differ in the improvement in depression symptom scores compared to the sham, but response and remission rates were significantly higher in the active treatment group than in the sham group. The efficacy of light therapy with 10,000-lux fluorescent white light for 30 min/d in the early morning was further observed in MDD without season pattern in a 4-arm study. The combination of fluoxetine 20 mg/day with light therapy was significantly superior to placebo in reducing depression, but fluoxetine monotherapy was not superior to placebo. Light therapy alone had numerically higher response and remission rates than placebo.

Chojnacka M, Antosik-Wójcińska AZ, Dominiak M, et al. A sham-controlled randomized trial of adjunctive light therapy for non-seasonal depression. *J Affect Disord.* 2016;203:1–8.

Lam RW, Levitt AJ, Levitan RD, et al. Efficacy of bright light treatment, fluoxetine, and the combination in patients with nonseasonal major depressive disorder: a randomized clinical trial. *JAMA Psychiatry.* 2016;73(1):56–63.

v. Exercise—There is a long history of using exercise to treat acute MDD in different age groups.

A recent meta-analysis of 41 studies with 2264 participants found large effects favoring exercise interventions, and the effect sizes of supervised exercise interventions were even larger. A meta-analysis of 15 studies with 1331 adolescents also found that physical exercise significantly reduced depressive symptoms with a moderate effect size. For adolescents with depression, exercise interventions lasting 6 weeks, 30 minutes a time, and four times a week had optimal results. For adolescents with depressive symptoms, aerobic exercise and resistance + aerobic exercise had significant effect, and aerobic exercise lasting 8 weeks, 75–120 minutes a time, and three times a week had optimal results. However, physical and mental exercise (yoga) did not have significant antidepressant effects in this subgroup. Overall, physical exercise with moderate intensity is a better choice for adolescents with depression and depressive symptoms. Two trials comparing sertraline and aerobic exercise in MDD did not find significant difference in remission rates after 16 weeks. However, combination therapy with antidepressant and exercise yielded mixed results.

Heissel A, Heinen D, Brokmeier LL, et al. Exercise as medicine for depressive symptoms? A systematic review and meta-analysis with meta-regression. *Br J Sports Med.* 2023: bjsports-2022-106282. Online ahead of print.

Wang X, Cai ZD, Jiang WT, et al. Systematic review and meta-analysis of the effects of exercise on depression in adolescents. *Child Adolesc Psychiatry Ment Health.* 2022;16(1):16.

vi. Acupuncture—A systematic review and meta-analysis of 22 trials from China and 7 outside China found that acupuncture significantly reduced depression severity compared to usual care or sham acupuncture. There was a significant correlation between an increase in the number of acupuncture treatments and the reduction in depression severity. However, the majority of the included trials were at a high risk of blind bias and poor quality. In three trials (263 participants) comparing an SGA with acupuncture that were all conducted in China, pooled results did not show significant differences between SGA and acupuncture. Adding acupuncture to the SGA appeared more effective than SGA alone.

D. Treatment of Psychiatric Comorbidity

1. Anxiety disorders—There is no large study to assess the efficacy and safety of a medication in the treatment of this comorbid condition. Most antidepressants including SSRIs, SNRIs, and atypical antidepressants have been used as the first-line medication for ADs, PTSD and OCD (Table 26–8). For patients who continue having anxiety symptoms with an antidepressant, other options approved for an AD such as buspirone and benzodiazepines, and agents showing anxiolytic effect such as some antipsychotics, antihistamines (e.g., hydroxyzine), alpha- and beta-adrenergic medications (e.g., propranolol, clonidine), and GABAergic medications (benzodiazepines, pregabalin, and gabapentin) can be considered (Chapter 27).

2. Posttraumatic stress disorder—For MDD with comorbid PTSD, current guidelines for the treatment of PTSD recommend initiation of an SSRI or SNRI. Prazosin may be added as adjunctive therapy for PTSD-related nightmares.

Table 26–8 Current Pharmacotherapies Approved by the Food and Drug Administration of the United States and/or the European Commission for Anxiety Disorders, Obsessive-Compulsive Disorder and/or Posttraumatic Stress Disorder

Disorder	Medications
Generalized anxiety disorder	Escitalopram, duloxetine, paroxetine, pregabalin*, venlafaxine-XR.
Obsessive-compulsive disorder	Clomipramine, fluoxetine, fluvoxamine, paroxetine, sertraline.
Panic disorder	Alprazolam, clonazepam fluoxetine, citalopram paroxetine, sertraline, venlafaxine.
Posttraumatic stress disorder	Paroxetine, sertraline.
Social anxiety disorder	Fluvoxamine-CR, paroxetine, sertraline, venlafaxine-XR.
Anxiety disorders or anxiety symptoms	Alprazolam, buspirone, chlordiazepoxide, hydroxyzine, lorazepam, oxazepam, trifluoperazine.

Note: *Approved by the European Commission. Based on Garakani A, et al., *Front Psychiatry.* 2020;11:59558; Sheehan DV, Sheehan KH. *Psychopharmacol Bull.* 2007;40(1):98–109.

If the first SSRI or SNRI is not effective after 4–8 weeks, a second SSRI/SNRI, mirtazapine or amitriptyline may be considered. A recent meta-analysis showed that the effect sizes for pharmacological treatments for PTSD are small (comparable to effect sizes for MDD) and may be smaller relative to effect sizes from psychotherapies. Some evidence support that people with PTSD and comorbid depression respond more poorly to antidepressants than people with PTSD alone. The poor response may be associated with childhood trauma.

There is no conniving evidence of benefit from treatment with the antipsychotic compared to placebo. Other treatments such as ketamine infusion and intranasal esketamine may reduce depression and PTSD symptoms. One study of TMS has shown efficacy reducing depressive and PTSD symptoms. The most promising medication for PTSD and MDD is MDMA (3, 4-methylenedioxymethamphetamine) as used in assisted psychotherapy. So far, two large RCTs of MDMA-assisted psychotherapy have demonstrated efficacy in PTSD and depressive symptom with large effect sizes. Psychotherapies specific for PTSD such as Eye Movement Desensitization and Reprocessing (EMDR) may be considered for MDD and comorbid PTSD (Chapter 28).

3. Obsessive-compulsive disorder—For comorbid OCD in MDD, prolonged administration of SSRIs is effective. Combination of a SSRI with CBT or exposure and response prevention (ERP) therapy is the most effective. Refractory OCD may be treated with different strategies, including a switch to another SSRI or clomipramine, or augmentation with an atypical antipsychotic. Deep rTMS and DBS have been approved for treatment-resistant OCD. Other options for "pure" OCD can also be considered (Chapter 30).

4. Attention deficit hyperactivity disorder—In patients with DDs, ADHD (attention deficit hyperactivity disorder) is best to diagnose when typical symptoms of ADHD are persistently present during periods of euthymia. In patients with MDD + ADHD and moderate to severe depression, MDD should be treated first. In contrast, mild cases or euthymic patients ADHD may be treated first even without an ongoing antidepressant. Bupropion, an SSRI/SNRI plus a long-acting stimulant, or an antidepressant plus CBT are first-line treatments for MDD+ADHD. Desipramine, nortriptyline, and venlafaxine are second-line antidepressant options. For MDD patients with comorbid ADHD and AD, the ADHD should be treated after the depression and anxiety symptoms are under control. Controlling depression and anxiety likely reduces the dosages of stimulants or non-stimulants to address ADHD—related symptoms. For patents with comorbid ADHD and SUD, non-stimulant or less addictive stimulant medications for ADHD should be tried first after controlling depressive symptoms.

5. Substance use disorders—Most studies in MDD and SUD are conducted in patients with MDD and an alcohol use disorder (AUD). Overall, the effects of antidepressants on drinking outcomes are modest, and depression may mediate the effect of antidepressants on drinking outcomes. Medications such as naltrexone for AUD are safe and effective for reducing drinking and depression symptoms in patients with DDs and AUD. A meta-analysis of studies using acamprosate to treat AUD found similar effects among people with and without depression, and alcohol abstinence has a strong effect on remission of depression. Combination of an antidepressant and AUD medication such as sertraline with naltrexone or acamprosate with escitalopram has shown positive outcomes for both AUD and depressive symptoms. In addition to pharmacotherapy, patients with a current comorbid SUD should receive specialized treatments (Chapters 16–23).

Bond DJ, Hadjipavlou G, Lam RW, et al. The Canadian Network for Mood and Anxiety Treatments (CANMAT) task force recommendations for the management of patients with mood disorders and comorbid attention-deficit/hyperactivity disorder. *Ann Clin Psychiatry*. 2012;24(1):23–37.

Del Casale A, Sorice S, Padovano A, Simmaco M, et al. psychopharmacological treatment of obsessive-compulsive disorder (OCD). *Curr Neuropharmacol*. 2019;17(8):710–736.

Gao K, Sheehan DV, Calabrese JR. Atypical antipsychotics in primary generalized anxiety disorder or comorbid with mood disorders. *Expert Rev Neurother*. 2009;9(8):1147–58.

Garakani A, Murrough JW, Freire RC, et al. Pharmacotherapy of anxiety disorders: current and emerging treatment options. *Front Psychiatry*. 2020;11:595584.

Li R, Wu R, Chen J, et al. A randomized, placebo-controlled pilot study of quetiapine-XR monotherapy or adjunctive therapy to antidepressant in acute major depressive disorder with current generalized anxiety disorder. *Psychopharmacol Bull*. 2016;46(1):8–23.

McHugh RK, Weiss RD. Alcohol use disorder and depressive disorders. *Alcohol Res*. 2019;40(1):arcr.v40.1.01.

Mitchell JM, Bogenschutz M, Lilienstein A, et al. MDMA-assisted therapy for severe PTSD: a randomized, double-blind, placebo-controlled phase 3 study. *Nat Med*. 2021;27(6):1025–1033.

Williams T, Phillips NJ, Stein DJ, et al. Pharmacotherapy for post traumatic stress disorder (PTSD). *Cochrane Database Syst Rev*. 2022;3(3):CD002795.

E. Treatment of suicidality

Suicidality is a diagnostic criterion for a MDE. Death by suicide is the leading cause of death in the United States, especially in young adults. It accounts for more than 30,000 deaths each year. The risk for suicide attempt (SA) likely decrease in the middle and late life, but the death by suicide does not. Among patients with MDD who are older than 55 years, the death rate is increased fourfold. The rates of suicide in the United States have increased from 10.5 to 14.0 per 100,000 over the past two decades. Mental illness is the number one cause of suicide in the United States. MDD accounts for the highest number of suicides, although patients with BD have the highest risk for suicide. An earlier review indicated that patients with a DD have a 17-fold increased risk for

suicide over the age- and gender-adjusted general population rate. Thirty-one percent of patients with MDD had SA and 10–15% completed suicide during their lifetime.

The severity of suicidality is commonly associated with depression severity and psychiatric comorbidity such as aggression-impulsivity, BPD, SUD, anxiety disorders, comorbid medical conditions, and/or functional impairment. Anhedonia is strongly associated with suicidal ideation. Other factors associated with an increased risk for suicide include being single, living alone, social disconnection, early childhood trauma, availability of lethal methods, sleep disturbance, cognitive and decision-making deficits, and profound feeling of hopelessness. Approximately 25–30% of persons who attempted suicide will go on to make more attempts. However, there is significant variability in terms of frequency, method, and lethality. A history of previous SA is a reliable predictor for future SA.

Intranasal esketamine is approved for the acute treatment of MDD with suicidal ideation or behavior. Since the severity of suicidality is associated with depressive symptom severity, rapid reduction of depression severity is the key to prevent SA and completed suicide. Aggressively treating comorbidity can also reduce the severity of suicidality. Lithium has anti-suicidal effect, although it may be not safe for patients with acute suicide risk. Traditional antidepressants may increase risk for suicidality in patients who are younger than 24 years old. Careful monitoring for this group after starting a new antidepressant is necessary to minimize the risk for suicide.

Canuso CM, Singh JB, Fedgchin M, et al. Efficacy and safety of intranasal esketamine for the rapid reduction of symptoms of depression and suicidality in patients at imminent risk for suicide: results of a double-blind, randomized, placebo-controlled study. *Am J Psychiatry*. 2018;175(7):620–630.

Gao K, Ming R, Wang Z, et al. Differential association of the number of comorbid conditions and the severity of depression and anxiety with self-reported suicidal ideation and attempt in major depressive disorder and bipolar disorder. *J Depress Anxiety*. 2015;4:173.

Fu DJ, Ionescu DF, Li X, et al. Esketamine nasal spray for rapid reduction of major depressive disorder symptoms in patients who have active suicidal ideation with intent: double-blind, randomized study (ASPIRE I). *J Clin Psychiatry*. 2020;81(3):19m13191.

Ionescu DF, Fu DJ, Qiu X, et al. Esketamine nasal spray for rapid reduction of depressive symptoms in patients with major depressive disorder who have active suicide ideation with intent: results of a phase 3, double-blind, randomized study (ASPIRE II). *Int J Neuropsychopharmacol*. 2021;24(1):22–31.

▶ Complications/Adverse Outcomes of Treatment

MDD exacts a large toll on patients, family members, and society because of its high level of morbidity, disability, and mortality. Compared to nondepressive subjects, patients with MDD admitted to a nursing home are more likely to die within the first 5 years. Among patients in general medical settings, physically ill patients with depression have increased pain and physical illness and decreased social and role functioning as compared to those who are not depressed. It may account for more bed days than any other physical disorder except cardiovascular disease, and it may be more costly to the economy than chronic respiratory illness, diabetes, arthritis, or hypertension. The incremental economic burden of individuals with MDD increased by 21.5% between 2005 and 2010 (from $173.2 billion to $210.5 billion, inflation-adjusted dollars). The costs are approximately 45% attributable to direct costs, 5% to suicide-related costs, and 50% to workplace costs. It was estimated that only 38% of the total costs were due to MDD per se and the rest were likely due to comorbid conditions.

However, MDD and depressive symptoms are often underdiagnosed and undertreated. In patients with cardiovascular disease, stroke, cancer and other chronic medications, treatment of depression may stabilize mood, improve quality of life, and perhaps positively affect such outcome measures as longevity. Although current commonly used antidepressants are relatively safe in patients with depression and medical conditions, their safety and tolerability and interactions with medications for medical conditions have never been systematically studied. With the exception of rare cases of death from ECT, hypertensive crisis from MAOIs, or neuroleptic malignant syndrome from antipsychotics, severe acute adverse outcomes from currently commonly used treatments for depression are relatively rare. However, some treatments may cause long-term complications such as metabolic syndrome, diabetes mellitus, and tardive dyskinesia from antipsychotics, renal deficiency from lithium, and liver damage from anticonvulsants and antidepressants. Clinicians should be thoughtful when forming a treatment plan to avoid or minimize the risk of these potential adverse outcomes.

Rivelli SK, Shirey KG. Prevalence of psychiatric symptoms/syndromes in medical settings. *Integr Care Psychiatry*. 2014. https://www.wjgnet.com/2220-3206/CitedArticlesInF6?id=10.4088%2Fpcc.v09n0401.

Greenberg PE, Fournier AA, Sisitsky T, et al. The economic burden of adults with major depressive disorder in the United States (2005 and 2010). *J Clin Psychiatry*. 2015;76(2):155–162.

▶ Prognosis

MDD is not a benign condition, but an early correct diagnosis and proper therapeutic intervention can largely improve depressive symptoms, restore function, prevent morbidity, and reduce mortality. Euthymic patients with MDD have similar quality of life as general population. The prognosis of MDD depends on the response to treatment(s). Studies on the long-term outcome of MDD have produced variable results because of different study designs and different case definitions. A longitudinal study lasted for up to 6 years found that patients with MDD had a very low full recovery (including recovery from other psychiatric disorders) of less than 20% during the 6-year follow-up. Compared to well-matched patients with minor surgery or schizophrenia, the depressed patients' outcome was intermediate.

Positive prognostic indicators include an absence of psychotic symptoms, a short hospitalization or duration of depression, none or a few psychiatric and/or medical comorbidities, and good family functioning. Poor prognostic indicators include negative affectivity, adverse childhood experience, a comorbid psychiatric disorder, chronic or disabling medical conditions, early age at onset, long duration of the index episode, and inpatient hospitalization. A patient who has MDD with comorbid addiction is more likely to require hospitalization, more likely to attempt suicide, and less likely to comply with treatment than is a patient with depression of similar severity but not complicated by comorbid addiction. The most significant factor contributing to mortality is suicide, although other factors such as malnutrition and comorbid medical illness are also likely to contribute.

Verduijn J, Verhoeven JE, Milaneschi Y, et al. Reconsidering the prognosis of major depressive disorder across diagnostic boundaries: full recovery is the exception rather than the rule. *BMC Med*. 2017;15(1):215.

BIPOLAR DISORDER

▶ Diagnosis

The diagnosis of BD has been evolved in the development of different versions of the DSM. In order to diagnose a BD, manic or hypomanic symptoms must be present, and the manic/hypomanic symptoms are not due to a medical condition or a substance. The main difference between the DSM-IV and the DSM-5 for diagnosis of a manic/hypomanic episode is that "abnormally and persistently increased energy and/or activity" becomes a prerequisite in the DSM-5 in addition to the requirement of "abnormally and persistently elevated or irritable mood" as in the DSM-IV. The DSM-5 adds other specified BDs such as MDEs with 3 days of hypomania in addition to bipolar I disorder, bipolar II disorder, cyclothymic disorder, BD not otherwise specified as in the DMS-IV. In addition, the DSM-5 does not have mania in mixed state anymore so that patients with the DSM-IV mixed state are likely to be reclassified as manic or as MDD with mixed features.

Since the existence of manic/hypomanic symptoms is a pre-requisite for diagnosis of BD, uncovering manic/hypomanic symptoms is key to the correct diagnosis of BD. A good rapport with patients is essential to collecting reliable information regarding manic/hypomanic symptoms. Collateral information from patients' family and friends may be necessary to obtain the information to make a final diagnosis. Structured diagnostic interview and screening tools such an MDQ (mood disorder questionnaire) and HCL-32 (hypomania checklist 32 item) can elicit manic/hypomanic symptoms.

▶ General Considerations

A. Epidemiology

Twelve-month prevalence in the United States for the DSM-IV-defined bipolar I disorder (BPI) is about 0.6% and lifetime prevalence is about 1%. The prevalence of male and female for BPI is similar. The 12-month prevalence for the DSM-IV-defined bipolar II disorder (BPII) is about 0.8% and lifetime prevalence is about 1.1%. BPII is more prevalent in female than male. The 12-month prevalence of subthreshold BD is 1.4% and lifetime is 2.4%. Lumping different types of BDs together, 2.8% in 12-months and 4.4% in lifetime. Overall, the prevalence of BDs is higher in North American and European counties than the rest parts of the world.

The prerequisite of "persistently increased energy/activities" in the diagnosis of mania/hypomania in the DSM-5 might be expected to reduce the apparent prevalence of BD. However, the results of these changes have been inconsistent. About a half of patients with BD present with the first mood episode as a depressive episode. A small number of adult patients with MDD will have their first manic/hypomanic episode/symptom cluster each year, and subsequently, their diagnoses are changed from DDs/MDD to BD. In contrast, approximately 10–15% of adolescents with the diagnosis of recurrent MDD will later develop BD. The key risk factors for BD are being female (BPII), having a family history of BD, and coming from an upper socioeconomic class. Data also suggest that people under age 50 years are at higher risk of a first episode of mania/hypomania, whereas someone who already has the disorder faces an increasing risk of a recurrent manic or depressive episode as he or she grows older. In contrast, when the first manic/hypomanic episode occurs after the age of 50 years one should consider organic origins or a substance-induced disorder. Patients with early-onset BD are more likely to display psychotic symptoms and to have a poorer lifetime prognosis. BDs often have seasonal patterns. Acute episodes of depression are common in spring and fall, whereas mania appears to cluster in the summer months. Corresponding data on suicides also show a peak in the spring and a (smaller) peak in the late fall.

Blanco C, Compton WM, Saha TD, et al. Epidemiology of DSM-5 bipolar I disorder: results from the National Epidemiologic Survey on Alcohol and Related Conditions - III. *J Psychiatr Res.* 2017;84:310–317.

Calabrese JR, Gao K, Sachs G. Diagnosing mania in the age of DSM-5. *Am J Psychiatry.* 2017;174(1):8–10.

Fassassi S, Vandeleur C, Aubry JM, et al. Prevalence and correlates of DSM-5 bipolar and related disorders and hyperthymic personality in the community. *J Affect Disord.* 2014;167:198–205.

Kessing LV, González-Pinto A, Fagiolini A, et al. DSM-5 and ICD-11 criteria for bipolar disorder: implications for the prevalence of bipolar disorder and validity of the diagnosis - a narrative review from the ECNP bipolar disorders network. *Eur Neuropsychopharmacol.* 2021;47:54–61.

Merikangas KR, Akiskal HS, Angst J, et al. Lifetime and 12-month prevalence of bipolar spectrum disorder in the National Comorbidity Survey replication. *Arch Gen Psychiatry.* 2007;64(5):543–552.

B. Etiology

Despite intensive attempts to establish its etiologic or pathophysiologic basis, the precise cause of BD remains unknown. As in MDD, there is consensus that multiple etiologic factors—genetic, biochemical, and socioenvironmental—may interact in complex ways. BD has a strong genetic association with two-thirds or more of patients showing evidence for a family history.

1. Life events—Although psychosocial stressors can occasionally precede the onset of BD, there is no clear association between life events and the onset of manic or hypomanic episodes. In fact, given the disruptive nature of mood cycling, BD may be more likely to induce negative life events. For example, poor judgment during a manic episode may expose people to greater risk for trauma, sexual abuse, or debt.

2. Biological theories

i. **Neurotransmitters**—Neurotransmitter theories initially conceptualized that depression and mania are on the opposite ends of the same continuum. For example, the norepinephrine hypothesis of affective illness centered on the availability of norepinephrine at synaptic sites, with less norepinephrine being available in depression and more in mania. This theory and its later modifications have been largely dismissed as overly simplistic, especially as they pertain to the separation DDs and BDs. The role of dopamine in acute mania is not only supported by the efficacy of antipsychotic in reducing manic/hypomanic symptoms but also confirmed by amphetamine-included mania-like symptoms in animal models. Simple models of variable transmitter levels have given way to more complex conceptualizations of the illness.

ii. **Neuroendocrine factors**—Abnormalities in the HPA axis and, more so in the HPT axis are common in BD. They are discussed later in the Laboratory Findings section.

iii. **Systematic toxicity**—The data from last several decades support the hypothesis of systematic toxicity in the pathogenesis of BD. This hypothesis is believed that the interaction between genetic factors (susceptibility) and predisposing, precipitating, and perpetuating environmental factors (stress and traumatic events) could cause dysfunctions in intracellular biochemical cascades, oxidative stress, and mitochondrial dysfunction that impair the processes linked to neuroplasticity. The impairment of neuroplasticity can lead to cell damage and neuronal loss that are present in postmortem and neuroimaging studies. This hypothesis is supported by peripheral biomarkers related to hormones, inflammation, oxidative stress, and neurotrophins that are altered in BDs, especially during acute mood episodes.

3. Psychosocial theories—Psychosocial theories pertaining to the etiology of BDs are the same as those described for MDD. Environmental conditions contribute more to the timing of a bipolar episode than to the patient's inherent underlying vulnerability. In other words, more stressful life events appear to precede early episodes than later ones, and there is a pattern of increased frequency over time. It is possible that early precipitating events merely activate preexisting vulnerability, thereby making an individual more vulnerable for future episodes.

This clinical observation is conceptualized with a **kindling model** that provides a better understanding of several phenomena inherent in the illness, including the just-mentioned effects of repeated episodes on disease severity and outcome (e.g., rapid-cycling BD usually develops late in the course of the illness) and the acute and prophylactic treatment effects of ECT and anticonvulsants such as carbamazepine and valproic acid. Because these therapies inhibit kindling in laboratory animals, their therapeutic effect in BD may involve interruption of kindling. However, the kindling model is not fully supported by other anticonvulsants that are lack of antimanic effect. Regardless, preventing or treating early episodes will favorably affect outcome. This pertains particularly to younger patients who are likely to have more episode during adolescence and early adulthood.

Young AH, Juruena MF. The neurobiology of bipolar disorder. *Curr Top Behav Neurosci.* 2021;48:1–20.

C. Genetics

Twin and family studies provide strong evidence for a genetic component in BD, but the precise mechanisms of inheritance are not known. In monozygotic twins, the concordance rate is higher for BDs (80%) than for DDs (54%). In dizygotic twins, concordance rates are 24% for BDs and 19% for DDs. Adoption studies have shown that the biological children of affected parents have an increased risk for developing a mood disorder, even when reared by unaffected parents, although the data are not uniform. Finally, first-degree biological relatives of BPI patients have elevated rates of BPI (4–20%), BPII (1–5%), and MDD (4–24%).

Genome-wide association studies have been the most successful strategy for identifying specific genetic variants associated with BD but have not yield a gene or a panel of genes for the diagnosis or treatment of BD. Polygenic risk score analysis found that BD has significant genetic overlap with schizophrenia, and other psychiatric disorders. Extensive genetic overlaps are also identified between all personality traits and BD, most notably that > 90% of the genetic variants estimated to influence BD are also estimated to influence educational attainment. Certain copy number variants (CNVs) known to be associated with elevated risk for developing neurodevelopmental such as autistic spectrum disorder and mental disorders like schizophrenia as well as somatic conditions like diabetes and hypertension are also found in BD, but the frequency of CNVs in BD is less than that observed for neurodevelopmental disorders or schizophrenia.

Harrison PJ, Geddes JR, Tunbridge EM. The emerging neurobiology of bipolar disorder. *Trends Neurosci.* 2018;41(1):18–30

O'Connell KS, Coombes BJ. Genetic contributions to bipolar disorder: current status and future directions. *Psychol Med.* 2021; 51(13):2156–2167.

▶ Clinical Findings

A. Signs & Symptoms

Although mania/hypomania is a required symptom for BD, patients with BD spend more time in depression than in mania/hypomania when they are symptomatic regardless of diagnostic subtypes. For this reason, patients with BPD are commonly misdiagnosed as UPD and receive antidepressant treatments. It is also common that patients with a diagnosis of BD are subsequently misdiagnosed as MDD or other disorders by different clinicians during the course of treatment. Adolescents with BD are often misdiagnosed as ADHD or other behavior disorders. For BD, the standard treatments are MSs instead of antidepressants. The misdiagnosis and mistreatment can worsen the course of illness, increasing burden to patients and society. To avoid impropr treatment, to improve quality of life and functioning, and to reduce mortality, the correct diagnosis of BD is critical.

1. Manic episode—Manic or hypomanic symptoms must be present for diagnosing a BD, and the manic/hypomanic symptoms are not due to a medical condition or a substance. According to the severity and length of manic/hypomanic symptoms, a manic episode, a hypomanic episode, or other hypomanic episodes can be established. To diagnose a manic episode, a distinct period of "abnormally and persistently elevated mood (euphoria) or irritable mood (dysphoria)" with "abnormally and persistently increased goal-directed activity or energy," lasting at least a week and present most of day, nearly every day must be present. Additional symptoms are needed to meet full criteria for a manic episode (Table 26–9). If the manic symptoms are so severe that hospitalization is needed or psychotic features are present, the duration of manic symptoms and other additional symptoms is not required for diagnosing a manic episode.

For patients who do not need hospitalization or do not have psychosis, in addition to mood disturbance and increased activity/energy at least 3 of 7 symptoms (Table 26–9) have to be present to a significant degree and represent a noticeable change from usual behavior during the same periodfor euphoric mania, and at least 4 of 7 symptoms have to be

Table 26–9 Symptom Presentations for Diagnosis of a Manic Episode According to the DSM-5

Core Symptoms	Symptom Presentations
Abnormally and persistently elevated, expansive, or irritable mood, and abnormally and persistently increased goal-directed activity and energy	Euphoric mania is often described as euphoric, excessive cheerful, high, or "on top of the world," more sociable and outgoing"; and happiness, silliness, and goofiness, especially in children. Dysphoric mania is often with predominant irritability, especially when individual's wishes are denied or the individual have been using substances.
Increase self-esteem or grandiosity	Ranging from uncritical self-confidence to grandiose delusions.
Decreased need for sleep (feel rested after only 3 hours of sleep)	Sleep little, if at all or may waken up several hours earlier than usual, feeling rested and full of energy; some may go for days without sleep, yet not feel tired. Often decreased need for sleep is an indication of the onset of a manic episode.
More talkative than usual or pressure to keep talking	Can be rapid, pressured, loud, and difficult to interrupted; sometimes characterized by jokes, puns, amusing irrelevancies, and theatricality with dramatic mannerisms, singing, and excessive gesturing. If mood is dysphoric, complaints, hostile comments, or angry tirades may be the main presentation.
Flight of ideas or subjective experience that thoughts are racing	Flight of ideas can be evidenced by a nearly continuous flow of accelerated speech, with abrupt shifts from one topic of another; severe cases may present as disorganized, incoherent, or unable to speak because thoughts are so crowded.
Distractibility	Evidenced by inability to censor immaterial external stimuli such as interviewer's attire, background noises or conversations, or furnishings in the room, and often prevents individuals from holding a rational conversation or following instructions.
Increased in goal-directed activity or psychomotor agitation	Often consists of excessive planning and participating in multiple activities including sexual, occupational, political, or religious activities. Increased sexual drive, fantasies, and behavior are often present. Some may renew old acquaintances, call, or contact friends or even strangers. Some may display purposeless activity by pacing around or holding multiple conversations simultaneously. Some write excessive letters, emails, and test messages on different topics to friends, public figures, or the media.
Excessive involvement in activities that have a high potential for pain consequences	Poor judgement often lead to reckless involvement in activities such as spending sprees, giving away possessions, reckless driving, foolish business investments, sexual promiscuity, and legal complications. Some may purchase many unneeded items without the money to pay for them. Sexual behavior may including infidelity or indiscriminate sexual encounters with strangers, often disregarding the risk for sexual transmitted disease or interpersonal consequences.

Note: The abnormally and persistently elevated, expansive, or irritable mood and abnormally and persistently increased goal-directed activity or energy must last for at least 1 week and present most of the day and nearly every day along with three of the other seven symptoms for euphoric mania and four of the seven symptoms for dysphoric mania. The symptoms cause significant distress or impairment in the individual's social, occupational, or other important areas of functioning.

present for dysphoric mania,. Meanwhile, the severity of the mood disturbance and other symptoms must be sufficiently severe to cause marked impairment in social or occupational functioning.

2. Hypomanic episode—As compared to a manic episode, a hypomanic episode is shorter (≥ 4 days) and not sufficiently severe to cause marked impairment in social or occupational functioning, require hospitalization, or demonstrate psychosis. The episode is associated with an unequivocal change in functioning that is uncharacteristic of the individual when not symptomatic, and the mood disturbance and change in functioning are observable by others. The main differences between a manic and a hypomanic episode are duration and severity (Table 26–10).

Table 26–10 Difference Between a Manic and a Hypomanic Episode

Presentations	Mania	Hypomania
Duration	≥ 7 days	≥ 4 days
Marked impairment	Yes	No
Hospitalization	Yes	No
Psychosis	Yes	No
Unequivocal change in function	Yes, but not required	Yes
Observable by others	Yes, but not required	Yes

3. Bipolar I disorder—At least one manic episode is required for the diagnosis of BPI. Although a MDE is not required, more than 90% of patients with BPI also have MDEs. In 50–60% of cases, a depressive episode immediately precedes or follows a manic episode.

4. Bipolar II disorders—At least one hypomanic episode and a MDE is required for the diagnosis of BPII. A bipolar II diagnosis should never be made in the presence or history of a manic episode. Clinically significant distress or impairment in social, occupational, or other important areas of functioning due to the symptoms of depression or hypomania is also required for the diagnosis of bipolar II disorder. The presentations of MDE in BDs are the same as those in MDD, although some atypical features such as hypersomnia and weight gain are present more often in MDEs of BPD than the MDEs of UPD. As mentioned before, as the treatments of BPD and UPD are different it is important to differentiate BPD from UPD (see differential diagnosis). However, some symptomatic patients with hypomania do not perceive themselves as being ill and are likely to minimize their symptoms and to resist treatment or acceptance of the diagnosis of BD.

5. Specifiers/subtypes of bipolar I or II disorder—Subtypes of BPI are listed as specifiers in the DSM-5 and the DMS-IV. In the DSM-5, specifiers of "with anxious distress" and "with mixed features" were added to the DSM-IV specifiers that include melancholic, atypical, psychotic, and catatonic features, seasonal pattern for recurrent episodes, and postpartum onset (that is changed to peripartum onset in the DSM-5). In the DSM-5, the psychotic features are divided "mood-congruent psychotic features" and "mood-incongruent psychotic features." The "Chronic" specifier in the DSM-IV was deleted in the DSM-5. Most of these specifiers can be applied to a manic, hypomanic, or depressive episode, but some can only be applied to a specific episode. For instance, melancholic or atypical features are specifiers for a MDE. In contrast, peripartum onset can be used for a manic, hypomanic, or depressive episode. As in MDD, these specifiers are not for coding purposes.

i. Rapid cycling—Rapid cycling is defined as the presence of at least four mood episodes in the previous 12 months. The episodes need meet the criteria of manic, hypomanic or MDE in BPI or hypomanic or MDE in BPII. The episodes are demarcated by either partial or full remission for at least 2 months or directly switch to an episode of opposite bipolarity of the index episode. Approximately 10–15% of bipolar patients experience rapid cycling and tend to have a longer duration and a more refractory course of the illness. Women represent up to 80–95% of rapid-cycling cases. A variety of factors may predispose bipolar illness to a rapid-cycling course, including treatment with antidepressants. The development of clinical or subclinical hypothyroidism (spontaneously or during lithium treatment) in a manic patient predisposes to a more rapid cycling course.

ii. Manic/hypomanic with mixed features—In order to diagnose mania/hypomania with mixed features, the full criteria of a manic/hypomanic episode must be met along with the presence of at least three of following six symptoms during the majority of days of the current or most recent episode of mania/hypomania: (1) persistent dysphoria or depressed mood either with subjective report or observed by others; (2) diminished interest or pleasure in all or almost all activities either subjective account or observed by others; (3) psychomotor retardation nearly every day; (4) fatigue or loss of energy; (5) feeling worthless and excessive inappropriate guilt; (6) recurrent thoughts if death, suicidal ideation with or without a plan or intent, or a suicide attempt. Mixed features are observable by others and represent a change from the individual's usual behaviors. If the symptoms meet the full criteria for both mania and MDE simultaneously, the diagnosis should be manic with mixed feature.

Cegla-Schvartzman F, Ovejero S, López-Castroma J, et al. Diagnostic stability in bipolar disorder: a follow-up study in 130,000 patient-years. *J Clin Psychiatry*. 2021;82(6):20m13764.

Gao K, Ayati M, Kaye NM, et al. Differences in intracellular protein levels in monocytes and CD4+ lymphocytes between bipolar depressed patients and healthy controls: a pilot study with tyramine-based signal-amplified flow cytometry. *J Affect Disord*. 2023;328:116–127.

iii. Treatment-resistant bipolar disorder—A significant number of patients with BRD fail to achieve remission with pharmacologic and non-pharmacological treatments. However, the prevalence of treatment-resistant bipolar disorder (TRBD), mainly treatment-resistant BPD varies widely depending on the models/definitions of TRBD are used. Compared to the models used to define treatment-resistant MDD, there is no widely accepted model to define TRBD.

Fountoulakis KN, Yatham LN, Grunze H, et al. The CINP guidelines on the definition and evidence-based interventions for treatment-resistant bipolar disorder. *Int J Neuropsychopharmacol*. 2020;23(4):230–256.

Hidalgo-Mazzei D, Berk M, Cipriani A, et al. Treatment-resistant and multi-therapy-resistant criteria for bipolar depression: consensus definition. *Br J Psychiatry*. 2019;214(1):27–35.

6. Cyclothymic disorder—To diagnose cyclothymic disorder, patients musthave numerous periods with hypomanic symptoms that do not meet criteria for a hypomanic episode and numerous periods with depressive symptoms that do not meet the criteria for an MDE for at least 2 years for adults and at least 1 year for children and adolescents. During the 2-year (1-year for children and adolescents), the hypomanic and depressive periods must be present for at least half of the time, and the patient has not been without the symptoms for more than 2 months at a time.

7. Other specified bipolar and related disorders— DSM-5 adds four other BRD including short-duration hypomanic episodes (2–3 days) and MDEs, hypomanic episodes with insufficient symptoms and MDEs, hypomanic episodes without prior MDEs, and short-duration cyclothymia (less than 24 months). In the DSM-IV, these disorders are lumped into the BD not otherwise specified category.

B. Psychological Testing

Psychological testing for BD has also not been found useful in aiding the diagnosis or managing BD. High rates of personality disorder, especially BPD, with BD have been reported. As in MDD, psychological testing may identify personality trait or disorders and coping skills to help clinicians understand the psychopathology of patients.

C. Laboratory Findings

There is no objective test to diagnose BRD, but some tests may help clinicians to rule out BRD due to another medical condition or a substance. Commonly used tests include urine drug screening, TSH, CBC, and CMP. Compared to MDD, research in laboratory findings in BD is in general scarce and inconclusive. For one thing, BD is not as common as MDD. Beyond that, patients in acute manic states are not as likely to collaborate in laboratory research studies.

1. HPA axis—A few available cross-sectional and longitudinal studies reveal increased plasma cortisol levels in some depressed bipolar patients. Abnormalities in the DST have also been noted. DST nonsuppression occurs more frequently in the mixed phase of the illness (78%) but also occurs in BPD (38%) and mania (49%). Both hypercortisolemia and DST results normalize after the acute episode subsides, suggesting that these abnormalities are state, but not trait dependent. Although these abnormalities are not specific for BD or even MDD, their pathophysiology is suggestive of central (i.e., hypothalamic) rather than peripheral dysregulation of cortisol.

2. HPT axis—HPT axis abnormalities are rather common in BD, especially in rapid-cycling BD, but the precise relationship of these abnormalities with the illness and its various clinical presentations is not known. Among these abnormalities are an attenuated nocturnal TSH peak, a blunted TSH response to TRH administration, and a high prevalence of various degrees of hypothyroidism. The associations among thyroid function, BD, and gender are complex. Hypothyroidism is very common in patients with BD, especially in female patients who present with a rapid-cycling course. Treatment with hypermetabolic doses of T_4 has shown some promise that it may reduce acute symptoms, number of relapses, and duration of hospitalizations. Overall impression has been that comorbid hypothyroidism seems to negatively affect disease outcome by predisposing the individual patient to a rapid-cycling course; and

substitution with T_4 has proven useful in some patients, but often, high doses are necessary to induce clinical response. Conceptually these findings support the hypothesis that a relative central thyroid hormone deficit may predispose to the marked and frequent mood swings that characterize rapid-cycling BD.

3. Sleep EEG—Sleep EEG recordings have revealed normal results in acutely ill bipolar patients, including normal REM latencies, but not all studies agree. Bipolar patients in remission can exhibit an increased density and percentage of REM and a sleep architecture more sensitive to arecoline (an acetylcholine agonist known to produce a shortened REM latency). Under certain conditions, gamma rhythms on EEG can distinguish subjects with BPD from UPD.

D. Neuroimaging

Brain imaging: The most consistent neuroimaging findings in depressed (unipolar and bipolar) patients are decreased blood flow and metabolism in PFC. It remains unclear if decreased activity of the PFC in depressed bipolar patients are state- or trait-dependent. Basal ganglia abnormalities including decreased blood flow and metabolism have also been found in depressed bipolar patients. In BDs, structural imaging studies suggest an increased number of white matter hyperintensities, which may be unique to BD and its treatment, or related to cardiovascular factors.

Numerous studies have reported distinct functional and structural alterations in emotion- or reward-processing neural circuits between BPD depression and UPD. During emotion-, reward-, or cognition-related tasks, different activation patterns in neural networks including the amygdala, anterior cingulate cortex (ACC), PFC, and striatum have been observed between BPD and UPD. A stronger functional connectivity pattern in BPD compared to UPD was observed in default mode, frontoparietal networks, and brain regions including the PFC, ACC, parietal and temporal regions, and thalamus. Gray matter volume differences between BPD and UPD in the ACC, hippocampus, amygdala, and dorsolateral prefrontal cortex have also been reported. BPD showed reduced integrity in the anterior part of the corpus callosum and posterior cingulum compared to UPD. A review of nine studies with six comparing bipolar versus unipolar found that differentiation are most common in the ACC, insula, and dorsal striatum (putamen and caudate) brain areas.

Han KM, De Berardis D, Fornaro M, et al. Differentiating between bipolar and unipolar depression in functional and structural MRI studies. *Prog Neuropsychopharmacol Biol Psychiatry.* 2019;91:20–27.

Kelberman C, Biederman J, Green A, et al. Differentiating bipolar disorder from unipolar depression in youth: a systematic literature review of neuroimaging research studies. *Psychiatry Res Neuroimaging.* 2021;307:111201.

E. Course of Illness

The natural course of BD is variable. Patients usually experience their first manic episode in their late teens or early 20s, but BDs sometimes start in adolescence or after age 40 years. Psychosocial stressors often trigger manic episodes and typically begin suddenly with a rapid escalation of symptoms over a few days. In about 50% of patients, an MDE immediately precedes a manic episode. Some patients have multiple depressive episodes before having the first manic/hypomanic episode.

Although medications are effective in treating acute episodes and maintaining patients in remission, they are not completely effective in preventing future episodes. Effectively preventing relapse is not only important for minimizing interruption of normal life but also essential for preventing memory and cognition decline, morbidity and mortality. Studies have shown that the number of mood episodes is associated with the decline in memory and cognition. A review of 8942 patients found that psychological and pharmacological treatments in the early stages of illness are more effective than in the later stages of BD across multiple domains, suggesting that an early intervention in BD can improve patient outcomes.

Joyce K, Thompson A, Marwaha S. Is treatment for bipolar disorder more effective earlier in illness course? A comprehensive literature review. *Int J Bipolar Disord*. 2016;4(1):19.

Vieta E, Salagre E, Grande I, et al. Early intervention in bipolar disorder. *Am J Psychiatry*. 2018;175(5):411–426.

▶ Differential Diagnosis

A. MDD

As mentioned earlier, the presentations of a MDE in UPD and BPD are the same, but the treatments of UPD and BPD are quite different. Therefore, the differential diagnosis between UPD and BPD is critical to avoid inappropriate treatments and minimize treatment-emergent side effect(s). There is no test or biomarkers to differentiate these two conditions. A careful evaluation of manic/hypomanic symptoms and a thorough history collection are the key to differentiate BPD from UPD. Some variables may suggest BD instead of MDD (Table 26–11). A longitudinal approach is essential for a correct diagnosis of BD.

B. Psychotic Disorders

Rates of psychosis are highest during acute episodes of mania, with between 50 and 80% of patients showing evidence of psychotic symptoms. Delusions are the most frequent psychotic symptoms experienced in mania, occurring in approximately 50% of patients. Hallucinations are present in only 15% of patients, with auditory and olfactory hallucinations occurring with equal frequency. Visual

Table 26–11 Cues and Presentations that "Unipolar" Depression May Be Bipolar Depression

- Early age of onset
- Postpartum onset
- Seasonal mood changes and diurnal preference
- Atypical features (hypersomnia, psychomotor slowing and/or weight gain/increased appetite during depression)
- Severe depression and severe anhedonia during depressive episodes
- Depression with catatonia and/or psychotic features
- Bipolar family history
- Pharmacological-induced mania or hypomania
- History of recurrent but brief depressive episodes and many previous depressive episodes
- Circadian rhythmic disturbance, day/night reversal
- A higher frequency of childhood traumatic experiences
- Severe substance disorders
- Multiple treatment failures, nonresponse or erratic response to antidepressants
- Unevenness in intimate relationships and marital problem
- Frequent career changes
- Legal problems

hallucinations occur with less frequency, at approximately half the frequency of auditory and olfactory hallucinations. A longitudinal study showed that 10% of previously hospitalized psychotic patients with BD were still delusional 2 years after hospitalization.

During BPD, 25% of the individuals with BPI and 6–20% of the individuals with BPII reported having psychosis. In a Bipolar CHOICE study, psychosis was present in 10.6% of the depressed outpatient BPI or II participants. Although antipsychotics are commonly used for the treatment of BD with or without psychotic features and psychotic disorders, the prognosis of these two group disorders is different. For BD, in addition to antipsychotics, lithium and some anticonvulsants are also first-line medications for treatments of mania or BPD. Differentiation of BD with psychotic features from psychotic disorders is important for planning short-term and long-term treatment. The sporadic nature of manic and depressive episodes of BD is helpful to differentiate bipolar with psychosis from psychotic disorders.

Caldieraro MA, Sylvia LG, Dufour S, et al. Clinical correlates of acute bipolar depressive episode with psychosis. *J Affect Disord*. 2017;217:29–33.

Frankland A, Cerrillo E, Hadzi-Pavlovic D, et al. Comparing the phenomenology of depressive episodes in bipolar I and II disorder and major depressive disorder within bipolar disorder pedigrees. *J Clin Psychiatry*. 2015;76(1):32–38.

Goes FS, Sadler B, Toolan J, et al. Psychotic features in bipolar and unipolar depression. *Bipolar Disord*. 2007;9(8):901–906.

C. Substance/Medication-Induced Bipolar and Related Disorder

As in MDD, a large number of substances have the potential of causing manic/hypomanic symptoms. The substance can be illicit street drugs, prescribed medications, over-the-counter medications or nutritional/metabolic supplements. Several substances/medications have considerable evidence that support their ability to cause BRD during intoxication or withdrawal or regular use. They include, but not limit, alcohol, phencyclidine, other hallucinogens, sedatives, hypnotics, anxiolytics, amphetamine and other stimulants, cocaine, and other substances/medications such as steroids. As diagnosing a substance-induced DD, history, physical exam, and/or laboratory results support the BRD develops during or within a month of substance intoxication or withdrawal or taking a medication. If the symptoms preceded the onset of intoxication, withdrawal, or exposure to a substance, and/or persisted for more than a month after the cessation of acute intoxication, withdrawal, or exposure, a diagnosis of substance-induced BRD should not be given.

Mania/hypomania that occurs after starting antidepressant or other treatments such electroconvulsive therapy or light therapy and persists beyond the physiological effect of the medication or treatment is considered as an indicator of true BD instead of substance/medication-induced BRD. However, side effects from some antidepressants and other psychotropic drugs can cause agitation, irritability, and edginess that may resemble a primary symptom of dysphoria mania, but they are distinct from bipolar symptoms. Unless the symptoms meet the criteria of mania/hypomania, a single symptom of agitation cannot make a bipolar diagnosis.

D. Bipolar and Related Disorder Due to Another Medical Condition

As with DD due to another medical condition, any medical condition that directly and indirectly affects the CNS can cause or worsen BRD. Similarly, the cause–effect relationship between BRD and another medical condition should be based on the best clinical evidence including history, physical exam, and/or laboratory findings, and "the clinician's best judgment…."

E. Psychiatric Comorbidities

Psychiatric comorbidity in BPI or II disorder is the role rather than the exception. In epidemiological studies, BD has the highest comorbidity among all psychiatric disorders. More than 80% patients with BPI or II disorder have an AD and more than half of them have a lifetime SUD (Table 26–12).

Clinical patients with BD also have high rates of comorbidity with AD and SUD. The most common comorbid patterns were BD with an AD, BD with an AD and a SUD, and BD with an AD, a SUD and ADHD (Figure 26–2).

Table 26–12 Lifetime Prevalence of Comorbid Psychiatric Disorders in Bipolar Disorders

Disorders	Any Bipolar Disorder (n=408) %	Bipolar I Disorder (n=93) %	Bipolar II Disorder (n=102) %	Subthreshold Bipolar Disorder (n=223) %
Any anxiety disorder	**74.9**	**86.7**	**89.2**	**63.1**
Agoraphobia w/o panic disorder	5.7	5.6	8.1	4.6
Panic disorder	20.1	29.1	27.2	13.1
Posttraumatic disorder	24.2	30.9	34.3	16.5
Generalized anxiety disorder	29.6	38.7	37.0	22.3
Specific phobia	35.5	47.1	51.1	23.3
Social phobia	37.8	51.6	54.6	24.1
Obsessive compulsive disorder	13.6	25.2	20.8	4.3
Any substance disorder	**42.3**	**60.3**	**40.4**	**35.5**
Alcohol abuse	39.1	56.3	36.0	33.2
Alcohol dependence	23.2	38.0	19.0	18.9
Drug abuse	28.8	48.3	23.7	22.9
Drug dependence	14.0	30.4	8.7	9.5
Any impulse control disorder	**62.8**	**71.2**	**70.6**	**56.1**
Intermittent explosive disorder	28.9	38.1	22.9	27.9
Attention deficit hyperactive disorder	31.4	40.6	42.3	23.0
Oppositional defiance disorder	36.8	44.4	38.2	32.8
Conduct disorder	30.3	43.8	18.6	28.9

Note: The diagnoses were based on DSM-IV.

Adapted from Merikangas KR, et al. *Arch Gen Psychiatry.* 2007;64(10):1180–1188.

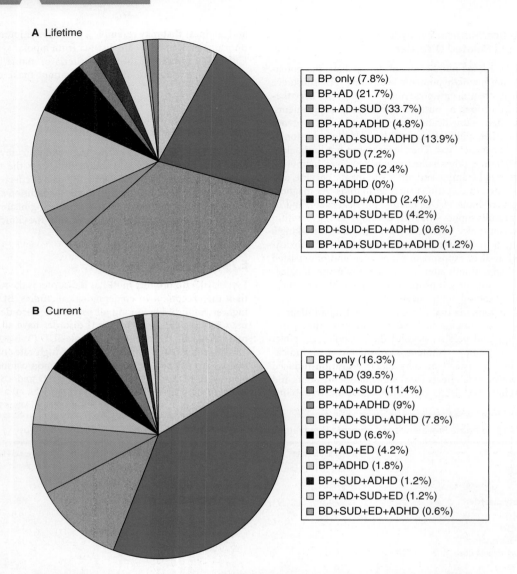

A Lifetime

☐ BP only (7.8%)
■ BP+AD (21.7%)
■ BP+AD+SUD (33.7%)
■ BP+AD+ADHD (4.8%)
■ BP+AD+SUD+ADHD (13.9%)
■ BP+SUD (7.2%)
■ BP+AD+ED (2.4%)
☐ BP+ADHD (0%)
■ BP+SUD+ADHD (2.4%)
☐ BP+AD+SUD+ED (4.2%)
■ BD+SUD+ED+ADHD (0.6%)
■ BP+AD+SUD+ED+ADHD (1.2%)

B Current

☐ BP only (16.3%)
■ BP+AD (39.5%)
■ BP+AD+SUD (11.4%)
■ BP+AD+ADHD (9%)
■ BP+AD+SUD+ADHD (7.8%)
■ BP+SUD (6.6%)
■ BP+AD+ED (4.2%)
☐ BP+ADHD (1.8%)
■ BP+SUD+ADHD (1.2%)
☐ BP+AD+SUD+ED (1.2%)
■ BD+SUD+ED+ADHD (0.6%)

Note: The diagnoses were according to DSM-IV diagnostic criteria. Anxiety disorder includes generalized anxiety disorder, panic disorder, social phobia, posttraumatic stress disorder, and obsessive-compulsive disorder. Eating disorder includes anorexia nervosa and bulimia nervosa. Substance use disorder including alcohol use disorder, cannabis use disorder, cocaine/stimulant use disorder, opiate use disorder and benzodiazepine/hypnotic use disorder.

Abbreviations: AD, anxiety disorder; ADHD, attention deficit hyperactivity disorder; BP, bipolar disorder; ED, eating disorder; SUD, substance disorder.

▲ **Figure 26–2** Lifetime and current comorbid patterns of bipolar disorder with other psychiatric disorders in a clinical sample (*n*=166)

Gao K, Wang Z, Chen J, et al. Should an assessment of Axis I comorbidity be included in the initial diagnostic assessment of mood disorders? Role of QIDS-16-SR total score in predicting number of Axis I comorbidity. *J Affect Disord.* 2013;148(2–3):256–264.

Merikangas KR, Akiskal HS, Angst J, et al. Lifetime and 12-month prevalence of bipolar spectrum disorder in the National Comorbidity Survey replication. *Arch Gen Psychiatry.* 2007;64(5):543–552.

Passos IC, Jansen K, Cardoso Tde A, et al. Clinical outcomes associated with comorbid posttraumatic stress disorder among patients with bipolar disorder. *J Clin Psychiatry.* 2016;77(5): e555–e560.

F. Medical Comorbidities

Medical comorbidities in BD are also common. Arthritis, hypertension, angina, tachycardia, gastritis, metabolic syndrome, and migraine headache are among the common ones (Table 26–13). In patients with rapid cycling BD and a SUD, about 60% of patients have at least one medical comorbidity with an average of five medical conditions. The leading cause of premature death among patients with seriously mental illnesses including BD is heart disease. The risk for metabolic syndrome in BD is the second highest after schizophrenia. The number of medical comorbidities and metabolic syndrome affect treatment response to MSs.

Table 26–13 Medical Comorbidities in Patients with Bipolar I or II Disorder (*N*=264)

Medical conditions	%
Obesity	36.9
Migraines	24.5
Head trauma with loss of consciousness	18.5
Hypertension	17.0
Hyperlipidemia	16.0
Asthma	14.4
Polycystic ovarian syndrome	9.4
Thyroid Disease	6.5
Diabetes	5.7
Hepatitis	4.2
Seizures	3.1
Cancer	2.7
Previous myocardial infarction	1.9
Coronary artery disease	1.1
Kidney disease	1.1

Reproduced with permission from Kemp DE, et al. *Acta Psychiatr Scand.* 2014;129(1):24–34.

Kemp DE, Gao K, Ganocy SJ, et al. Medical and substance use comorbidity in bipolar disorder. *J Affect Disord.* 2009; 116(1–2):64–69.

Kemp DE, Gao K, Chan PK, et al. Medical comorbidity in bipolar disorder: relationship between illnesses of the endocrine/metabolic system and treatment outcome. *Bipolar Disord.* 2010; 12(4):404–413.

Miller BJ, Paschall CB 3rd, Svendsen DP. Mortality and medical comorbidity among patients with serious mental illness. *Psychiatr Serv.* 2006;57(10):1482–1487.

▶ Treatments

The unique clinical challenges of bipolar treatment posed by this chronic illness include various acute phases of mood instability: depressive, hypomanic, and manic episodes. BD mandates prescription of lifelong maintenance treatment in an effort to minimize relapse, recurrence, and functional impairment. These wide affective presentations require thoughtful psychopharmacologic and non-pharmacological strategies that often must be individually adjusted over time. Lithium is the first medication approved by the FDA in 1970 for acute mania. The first approved medication for treatment of acute BPD was the combination of olanzapine and fluoxetine (OFC) in 2003. The core principles of medication management for BD revolve around the use of "mood stabilizers." However, most approved medications for BD are antipsychotics (Table 26–14). MSs are developed through regulatory approval with phase III studies. Similar to MDD phase III trials, it is only about one-third of patients with BD may be eligible for a phase III study. Therefore, the results from phase III studies in BD are also not generalizable. The effectiveness studies in BD are scarce.

A. Psychopharmacologic Interventions

1. Acute treatment of mania—The available evidence suggests that lithium, certain anticonvulsants, and most atypical antipsychotic drugs are effective for acute mania and may possess other therapeutic properties that could support calling them "mood stabilizers." Among approved medications, all with efficacy are clinically relevant with NNTs for response less than 10 (Table 26–15). Hospitalization is most often necessary when attempting to control acute manic symptoms. The first step in choosing initial MS therapy for mania should involve assessment of the severity of symptoms, which may guide need for monotherapy versus combination therapy. Patients with hypomanic to mild manic presentations may be candidates for monotherapy, whereas patients with more severe mania should usually be treated urgently with combinations of antimanic agents or ECT for treatment-resistant cases. Other considerations, such as first episode versus break-through episode, rapid cycling or refractory illness, and patient preference and tolerability issues also affect decisions for initial management choices.

Table 26–14 Approved Medications in the United States for Bipolar Disorder

Drug	Mania	Mixed	Maintenance	Depression
Aripiprazole	X	X	X	
Aripiprazole-LAI			X	
Asenapine	X	X		
Carbamazepine ER	X	X		
Cariprazine	X			X
Chlorpromazine	X			
Divalproex DR	X			
Divalproex ER	X	X		
Lamotrigine			X	
Lithium	X		X	
Lumateperone				X*
Lurasidone				X*
Olanzapine	X*	X	X	
Olanzapine-fluoxetine				X
Olanzapine-samidorphan¥	X		X	
Quetiapine	X*		X**	X
Risperidone	X*	X		
Risperidone-LAI			X	
Ziprasidone	X	X	X**	

*Adjunctive therapy with lithium or valproate, or monotherapy.

**Adjunctive therapy with lithium or valproate only.

¥Approval based on the data from schizophrenia.

Abbreviations: DR, delayed release; ER, extended release; LAI, long-acting injection.

i. Lithium—The efficacy of lithium in the treatment of acute mania is supported by numerous RCTs. With a few exceptions, overall evidence supports that lithium monotherapy is as effective as other antimanic agents, and combining lithium with an anticonvulsant MS or an antipsychotic is more effective than lithium alone. However, lithium has not been shown to be superior to placebo or DIV in reducing manic symptoms in children and adolescents. While lithium is effective for mania, clinical improvement is relatively slow, with an initial onset of therapeutic response generally occurring no sooner than 7–14 days after it is started. Additionally, lithium has a significant adverse effect profile that complicates long-term management (Table 26–16). These effects may be less apparent during acute treatment with lithium than during maintenance treatment.

For the acute treatment of mania, lithium should be dosed to achieve therapeutic serum concentrations (sampled 12 hours after the last dose) between 0.8 and 1.2 mEq/L. For healthy patients with severe mania, lithium carbonate 300 mg can be started three or four times daily with trough plasma level determination on Day 4 or Day 5 of the treatment. A lower starting dose and slower titration are recommended in older patients and those with impaired renal function. When used to treat milder mania or hypomania, lower starting doses (300 mg bid) and lower blood levels (0.6–0.8 mEq/L) may sufficiently stabilize mood over a period of several weeks to months. For patients with BPD, lithium may start with 300 mg at bedtime for 3 nights, and then 600 mg at bedtime with trough plasma level determination on Day 4 or Day 5 of 600 mg/day treatment. The final dose is adjusted according to the serum level of lithium and the goal of treatment. Lower doses and levels of lithium may be sufficient when combination pharmacotherapy strategies, such as lithium plus an anticonvulsant or antipsychotic, are used. These lower doses may greatly reduce the frequency of troublesome side effects during early treatment and thus enhance adherence.

The side effects of lithium are involved in many organ systems (Table 26–16). Some are short-term and some are long-term. Most side effects typically subside within 1–2 weeks, but they can persist. Lithium toxicity may be heralded by emergence or aggravation of any of the common side effects, progressing to include one or more other symptoms such as coarsening tremor, sluggishness, slurred speech, Parkinsonism, hyperreflexia, myoclonic twitches, and mental status changes. Early recognition of toxicity is critical, as is investigation of cause (Table 26–16). The possibility of drug–drug interactions with lithium must always be considered, particularly with thiazide (and possibly loop) diuretics, angiotensin converting enzyme inhibitors, nonsteroidal anti-inflammatory drugs, and other psychotropics.

Lithium is absorbed completely within 8 hours of oral intake with peak plasma levels reached between 1 and 3 hours after ingestion. Absorption is not affected by the presence of food, making it preferable for some patients experiencing gastric irritation to take lithium right after meals. Distribution of lithium after absorption into the bloodstream is rapid with the majority entering the intracellular space. Its final concentration in blood and tissue is determined by complicated transport mechanisms. On an average, the brain concentration of lithium is lower than the plasma concentration, while the half-life of lithium in the brain is longer than in blood. Renal clearance is the primary route of lithium elimination. Age-related changes necessitate more careful use of lithium in the elderly as elimination may be significantly decreased, lending to greater risk of elevated or toxic levels. It is reabsorbed from the glomerular filtrate in the proximal tubule so clinicians must know that lithium elimination may be substantially increased by certain medications, while certain diuretics that act at the distal tubule may lead to unwanted lithium retention. Pretreatment procedures and testing are recommended before beginning therapy with lithium: general medical history, physical

Table 26–15 Number Needed to Treat to Benefit for Response from Psychotropics Relative to Placebo in Acute Treatment of Mania

Drug	Dose or Serum Level	NNT Mean (95% CI)
Monotherapy		
Aripiprazole	15 or 30 mg/day	6 (5, 10)
Asenapine	10–20 mg/day	8 (5, 21)
Carbamazepine-ER	up to 1600 mg/day	4 (3, 6)
Cariprazine	3–12 mg/day	5 (4, 8)
Divalproex-DR	up to 150 µg/mL	4 (3, 13)
Divalproex-ER	75–125 µg/mL	9 (5, 27)
Haloperidol*	2–30 mg/day	6 (5, 10)
Lithium	0.6–1.5 mEq/L	6 (4, 10)
Olanzapine	5–20 mg/day	4 (3, 4)
Paliperidone*	3–12 mg/day	11 (8, 65)
Quetiapine-IR	up to 800 mg/day	6 (4, 11)
Quetaipine-XR	400–800 mg/day	5 (3, 9)
Risperidone	1–6 mg/day	4 (3, 5)
Ziprasidone	80–160 mg/day	6 (4, 12)
Adjunctive therapy to lithium or valproate		
Aripiprazole + Li or Val	15 or 30 mg/day + Li (0.6–1.0 mEq/L) or Val (50–125 µg/mL)	7 (4, 27)
Asenapine + Li or Val	10-20 mg/day + Li (0.6–1.2 mEq/L) or Val 5(0–125 µg/ml)	8 (4, 41)
Olanzapine + Li or Val	5–20 mg/day + lithium or valproate	4 (3, 8)
Olanzapine + DIV	5–20 mg/day + divalproex	8 (4, 648)
Paliperidone-ER + Li or Val	3–12 mg/day + Li (0.6–1.2 mEq/L) or Val (50–125 µg/mL)	13 (5, ∞, -29)
Quetiapine-IR + Li or Val	up to 800 mg/d day + Li (0.7–1.0 mEq/L) or Val (50–100 µg/mL)	8 (5, 17)
Quetiapine-XR + Li	400 to 800 mg/day + Li (600 to 1,800 mg/d).	9 (5, 57)
Risperidone + Li, Val,or Car	1–6 mg/day + ongoing Li, Val, or Car for at least 2 weeks	6 (3, 162)
Neuroleptic + Val	Basic antipsychotics, preferably haloperidol and/or perazine. + Val 20 mg/kg/day	4 (3, 16)
Ziprasidone low dose + Li or valproate	40–80 mg/day + Li (0.6–1.2 mEq/L) or Val (50–125 µg/mL)	ns
Ziprasidone high dose + Li or Val	120–160 mg/day + Li (0.6–1.2 mEq/L) or Val (50–125 µg/mL)	ns

Note: Ziprasidone study does not have responder data to calculate. NNT = 1 ÷ (active response rate–placebo response rate). A positive number of NNT indicates that the response rate in active treatment is higher than that in placebo. The 95% of CI does not cross zero is indicative of significant difference between the groups. A small NNT is indicative of a medication having a larger effect relative to placebo in response compared to a medication for response with a large NNT relative to placebo.

Abbreviation: Car, carbamazepine; CI, confidence interval; DR, delayed release; ER, extended release, IR; immediate release; L, litter; Li, lithium; mL, milliliter; ns, not significant different from placebo; Val, valproate.

exam and weight, BUN and creatinine determination, thyroid function studies, and pregnancy testing for women of childbearing age. Lithium carries a teratogenicity category D warning. Electrocardiography and CBC measurement should be obtained if necessary, especially for patients over the age of 40 years old.

ii. **Anticonvulsants**—The kindling theory of BD has helped the development of anticonvulsants in the treatment of BD. However, despite assumed primary modes of action for any individual anticonvulsant, each has a different profile in terms of the mechanisms that may confer anticonvulsant properties. The differences in mechanisms among anticonvulsants may explain why not all anticonvulsant can effectively treat mania. Based on RTCs with adequate sample size, other than DIV and carbamazepine, other anticonvulsants

including LTG, topiramate, and gabapentin have not demonstrated strong enough evidence for treatment of acute mania.

a. *Divalproex/valproate*—DIV sodium became the first anticonvulsant approved for bipolar mania by the FDA in 1995. Its antimanic effect was further verified during the development of olanzapine. As lithium, VPA/DIV was commonly used as adjunctive therapies to antipsychotics or other medications for mania. VPA monotherapy was not found to be significantly superior to placebo in 10–17 years old children and adolescents with manic or mixed symptoms but was superior to placebo in 3–7 years old. Like lithium, VPA appeared to be less effective than antipsychotics in children and adolescents with acute mania.

DIV/VPA is recommended as a first-line acute treatment option for mania in most evidence-based practice guidelines,

Table 26–16 Adverse Effects of Lithium and Their Managements

System Affected	Adverse Effect(s)	Treatment/Comments
Cardiovascular	Bradycardia, syncope, AV block, EKG changes, sick-sinus syndrome	Infrequent or rare events; EKG monitoring; do not use lithium with sick sinus syndrome; discontinuation of lithium may be needed.
Central Nervous System	Mental dullness, headache, memory troubles, muscle weakness, poor concentration	Commonly seen, especially at start of therapy; dose reduction may help.
Dermatologic	Acne, hair loss, psoriasis, skin reactions	Standard dermatologic treatments; avoid or discontinue lithium if severe.
Endocrine	Goiter, elevated TSH (5%), hypothyroidism (3%), hyperparathyroidism with hypocalcemia	Thyroid problems common with long-term therapy; can be treated with exogenous L-thyroxine.
Gastrointestinal	Nausea, GI pain/distress, vomiting, diarrhea, frequent loose stools	More common at start of therapy but may indicate toxicity, check lithium levels to rule out toxicity; take lithium with food or change preparation; lower/slower dosing may help.
Hematological	Leukocytosis	Common, reversible.
Metabolic	Weight gain	Avoid caloric beverages, eat healthy diet, and increase physical activity.
Neurologic	Postural tremor, confusion, ataxia	Fine tremor is a frequent side effect (up to 50%) and worsened by caffeine use, anxiety, and muscle tension; dosage reduction and/or β-blockers may help. Other presentations should prompt lithium level check.
Ophthalmic	Blurry vision, nystagmus, eye pain, tearing, itching.	Rare. May occur during the first week of treatment. Reduce dose or discontinue lithium if necessary.
Renal	Polydipsia, polyuria, diabetes insipidus, structural kidney damage	Polydipsia and polyuria usually occur in the early of treatment (up to 60%) and persist for up to more than 20%. Diuretics should be used with caution. Lower dosage with once daily at bedtime may help. Decrease dietary protein intake may reduce polyuria. Diabetes insipidus is reversible and may need treatment in a small number of patients. Structural damage may occur after long-term use. Early identification is the key to prevent renal failure.
Pregnancy	Congenital abnormalities (Ebstein anomaly)	Avoid lithium in the first trimester if possible or use low dose if necessary. Monitor fetal development with ultrasound as recommended.
Toxicity*	1.0–1.5 Fine tremor, nausea 1.5–2.0 Cogwheeling tremor, nausea, vomiting, somnolence 2.0–2.5 Ataxia, confusion 2.5–3.0 Dysarthria, gross tremor >3.0 Delirium, seizures, coma, death	Avoid dehydration or increase in lithium level unintentionally (perspiration, diarrhea, vomiting, thiazide diuretics, and salt-free diets). Early identification is the key to prevent severe consequences. Dialysis may be necessary for a small number of patients.

Note: *The representations of lithium toxicity depends on the serum level of lithium.

either as monotherapy or in combination with antipsychotics for more severe manic episodes. Its absolute bioavailability quickly approaches 100% after oral administration. The DIV ER (extended release) preparation bioavailability is closer to 90%, suggesting a slightly higher dose (8–20%) of the DIV ER form is needed in order to reach bioequivalence with the immediate release preparation. Peak plasma concentrations are achieved within 3–5 hours although up to 17 hours may be needed to reach peak concentration for the ER form. Mean terminal half-life is about 12–16 hours for either preparation, with steady state conditions usually being achieved within 3–4 days.

For acute management of severely ill manic patients, DIV oral loading with a therapeutic starting dose of 20–30 mg/kg per day is suggested over standard, gradual titration schedules.

Oral-loading typically achieves serum concentrations of valproic acid greater than 50 mg/L by Day 2, which represents the low end of the therapeutic range of serum concentrations for this agent of 50–125 mg/L. Similar results can be obtained by using the ER preparation. This oral-loading strategy for DIV has been demonstrated to lead to a more rapid antimanic effect when compared with standard-titration DIV, lithium, or placebo; it is also better tolerated than olanzapine and as well tolerated as lithium or standard-titration DIV. Divided doses are recommended (250 mg three times a day or 500 mg twice a day) for patients with less severe mania or in elderly patients.

Before initiating acute treatment of mania with DIV/VPA, a general medical history with special attention to any past problems of hepatic or hematological nature should be obtained, as well as baseline liver profile, and complete blood cell count. Pregnancy screening should be conducted before starting DIV/VPA, particularly given its FDA black-box warning of teratogenicity category D.

DIV/VPA is metabolized almost entirely by liver via the cytochrome P450 2D6 system. It does not induce its own metabolism. It inhibits drug oxidation and may increase serum levels of other oxidatively metabolized drugs, such as phenytoin, phenobarbital, LTG, and TCAs. It inhibits LTG metabolism by 50% resulting in the critical need to initiate LTG at 50% lower doses when coadministered with DIV/VPA. Coadministration with other microsomal enzyme-inducing drugs, such as carbamazepine, will decrease plasma valproic acid levels. Inhibitors of the P450 system, such as SSRIs, can increase levels of valproic acid in the plasma. Toxicity can also be induced when DIV/VPA is given along with other drugs that may be highly protein bound.

Adverse effects seen during initial therapy with DIV/VPA are usually mild, transient, and easily managed. Gastrointestinal distress and sedation are the most commonly seen side effects during acute treatment, although other dose-related effects including tremor and benign hepatic transaminase elevations are occasionally encountered. Reduced dosage or slower upwards titration can be helpful. In addition, using DIV or DIV ER instead of valproic acid may also lessen these side effects. Tremor may be minimized through dose reduction or concomitant beta-blocker medication. During acute treatment with DIV, clinicians should consider the possibility of rare but potentially serious adverse effects such as irreversible hepatic failure (especially in patients younger than 12 year old), hemorrhagic pancreatitis, or hyperammonemic encephalopathy when patients experience severe abdominal distress, confusion, or delirium.

b. *Carbamazepine and oxcarbazepine*—Two large well-designed RCTs of carbamazepine, a beaded, extended-release formulation, monotherapy in acute mania confirmed its efficacy in reducing manic symptoms from early small sample studies. A Cochrane Database Systematic Review found the quality of studies of oxcarbazepine in BD was poor. Oxcarbazepine was not significantly superior to placebo in reducing manic symptoms in children and adolescents with BD. There is no clear target serum level of carbamazepine for acute mania although a range of 6–16 µg/mL is recommended. Immediate release carbamazepine therapy may be started at a total divided daily dose of 200–600 mg, with incremental increase to 200–1000 mg/day followed by careful monitoring of blood levels, side effects, and clinical efficacy. The beaded, ER form may be started at 400 mg/day and increased as tolerated up to 1600 mg/day. Many factors can affect carbamazepine blood levels beyond direct dosing, including auto-induction of metabolism and significant drug–drug interactions.

During acute treatment with carbamazepine, the most commonly observed side effects are nausea, fatigue, blurred vision, and ataxia. More gradual initial titration of the dose may minimize these effects. Infrequently, liver transaminase elevations, rash, hyponatremia, and blood dyscrasias may complicate acute treatment with carbamazepine. Before treatment with carbamazepine, a general history and physical exam should be performed, including screening for any history of liver disease or blood dyscrasias. Routine laboratories including CBC, liver profile, and electrolytes with creatinine should be obtained. More frequent monitoring is indicated in the elderly or in any individual on carbamazepine who develops fever, easy bruising or bleeding, weakness, or infection.

Carbamazepine is 80% bioavailable after oral administration, with immediate and beaded release formulations bioequivalent. Nearly 80% is protein bound with the primary route of hepatic metabolism via the cytochrome 3A4 system to its active epoxide form. With initial administration of the ER form, half-life averages between 35 and 40 hours, but with repeated administration this falls to 12–17 hours due to auto-induction. Inhibitors of the P450 system will increase carbamazepine levels, while inducers can decrease the levels.

iii. Antipsychotics—With the exception of lurasidone and lumateperone without investigation in mania, all other atypical antipsychotics along with chlorpromazine and haloperidol have been studied with RTCs in the treatment of acute mania with or without psychotic features (Table 26–15). The antipsychotics approved for acute mania are chlorpromazine, olanzapine, risperidone, quetiapine, ziprasidone, aripiprazole, asenapine, cariprazine. Almost all approved agents are also for mixed states in BD, but DSM-5 does not have this mood state anymore. Overall, there are no significant differences in efficacy among the FDA approved antipsychotics in acute mania (Table 26–15), and the combination of atypicals and lithium or VPA was more effective than lithium or VPA alone. Most head-to-head comparisons did not find significant differences between antipsychotics and lithium or VPA, although some meta-analyses suggested some antipsychotics may be more effective than other antipsychotics, lithium or VPA. In addition to FDA-approved antimanic agents, haloperidol, tamoxifen, are paliperidone are also superior to placebo in reducing manic symptoms. However, brexpiprazole, endoxifen, eslicarbazepine, LTG, licarbazepine, topiramate, and verapamil are not superior to placebo. Olanzapine/samidorphan is also approved for the acute mania and long-term treatment of BD, but the approval was based on the evidence of safety and tolerability in the treatment of schizophrenia.

Although the efficacy of FDA-approved antipsychotics is similar, there are significant differences in safety and tolerability among them. Atypical antipsychotics generally have superior tolerability when compared with typical antipsychotics in BD. Side-effect profiles vary among the atypical agents, while monitoring need remain the same. The risk for metabolic derangements, weight gain, type-2 diabetes, and lipid elevations is a major concern. Prior to initiating therapy for mania with any atypical antipsychotic, baseline determination of fasting glucose, weight, waist circumference, and lipid profile is recommended. More importantly, patients with mania are more sensitive to antipsychotics than patients with schizophrenia. Even though all atypical antipsychotics were as well as tolerated as placebo, side effects like EPS should be closely monitored.

Bai YH, Yang HC, Chen GJ, et al. Acceptability of acute and maintenance pharmacotherapy of bipolar disorder: a systematic review of randomized, double-blind, placebo-controlled clinical trials. *J Clin Psychopharmacol.* 2020;40:167–179.

Citrome L, Graham C, Simmons A, et al. An evidence-based review of OLZ/SAM for treatment of adults with schizophrenia or bipolar I disorder. *Neuropsychiatr Dis Treat.* 2021;17:2885–2904.

Gao K, Bai Y, Calabrese JR. Lithium and mood stabilizers. In: Nemeroff CB, Rasgon N, Schatzberg AF, Strakowski SM, eds. *The American Psychiatric Association Publishing Textbook of Mood Disorders*, 2nd ed. Washington DC; 2022:271–284.

Gao K, Kemp D E, Wu R, et al. Mood stabilizers. In: Tasman A, Kay J, Lieberman, JA, First MB, Riba MB, eds. *Psychiatry*, 4th ed. Chichester, UK: John Wiley & Sons, Ltd; 2015:2129–2153.

Vieta E, Durgam S, Lu K, et al. Effect of cariprazine across the symptoms of mania in bipolar I disorder: analyses of pooled data from phase II/III trials. *Eur Neuropsychopharmacol.* 2015;25(11):1882–1891.

Kishi T, Ikuta T, Matsuda Y, et al. Pharmacological treatment for bipolar mania: a systematic review and network meta-analysis of double-blind randomized controlled trials. *Mol Psychiatry.* 2022;27(2):1136–1144.

2. Acute treatment of bipolar depression

i. Lithium—Early studies of lithium in BPD were confounded by study designs and small sample sizes. In a quetiapine BPD study, lithium monotherapy was not significantly superior to placebo in reducing depressive symptoms regardless of lithium levels. However, lithium plus adjunctive personalized treatment (APT) was as effective as quetiapine plus APT in BD. Lithium reduced depression and anxiety symptoms as effective as quetiapine in patients with BPD and different comorbidities. Lithium or DIV plus lurasidone or lumateperone are indicated for BPD. Lithium and LTG alone were not very effective in reducing depressive symptoms, but lithium and LTG were significantly superior to lithium alone (Table 26–17). Lithium plus modafinil was also more efficacious than lithium alone in patients who failed lithium monotherapy, but the results of adjunctive armodafinil or antidepressant(s) to lithium or other MS were inconsistent. One possible reason is that different studies used different inclusion and exclusion criteria. In bipolar II depression, lithium monotherapy appeared significantly less effective than antidepressants for acute and long-term treatments in some studies.

ii. Anticonvulsant mood stabilizers

a. Divalproex/valproate—There is no large study of the efficacy and safety of DIV/VPA in the treatment of acute BPD. A meta-analysis with 142 patients found that response (39.3% vs. 17.5%) and remission (40.6% vs. 24.3%) rates are significantly greater for DIV/VPA than placebo. The efficacy for response is comparable to other FDA-approved medications for BPD (Table 26–17). The most common side effects include gastrointestinal distress, fatigue, and weight gain.

b. Lamotrigine—The results from the first RCT of LTG in the acute treatment of BPD have contributed to its common off-label use even though the results from this study were not replicated with four additional trials of LTG in acute BPD. In a meta-analysis of five RCTs with 1072 participants, more patients treated with LTG than placebo responded to treatment as measured with two different depression-rating scales. Moreover, the significant difference between LTG and placebo was related to baseline depression severity, i.e., LTG was significantly superior to placebo in severely depressed patients, but not in moderately depressed patients. A head-to-head 7-week comparison of OFC and LTG in the acute treatment of BPD showed similar response rates: 68.8% for OFC and 59.7% for LTG, and remission rates: 56.4% for OFC and 49.2% for LTG (Table 26–17). The efficacy of LTG as an adjunctive therapy to lithium, DIV, or quetiapine was more effective than these three medications alone. In contrast, LTG adjunctive therapy to lithium and VPA in rapid cycling BD with or without a current SUD was not significantly superior to placebo. There is limited evidence of LTG in pediatric and geriatric patients with BD. However, DIV/VPA and LTG may have potential benefit for comorbid SUD in BD.

Steven–Johnson syndrome or toxic epidermal necrolysis from LTG is a major concern. A recent systematic review of LTG in 122 RCTs found that 8.6% of patients with BD developed skin reactions and only 0.02% developed Steven–Johnson syndrome or toxic epidermal necrolysis. In early epilepsy trials, rash lead to hospitalization and treatment discontinuation or Stevens–Johnson syndrome in 0.3% of adults treated with LTG. As of 2013, the starting dose and the rate of titration were widely recognized as two factors for an increased risk of LTG-induced rash. The risk is also greater in children younger than 12 years old. To minimize the risk of rash, LTG should be prescribed as described in the prescribing information of LTG to avoid life-threatening rash. Clinicians should not deviate from the recommended guidance, especially when coadministering with DIV/VPA. Rare cases of aseptic meningitis and emophagocytic lymphohistiocytosis have occurred with LTG.

iii. Atypical antipsychotics for acute bipolar depression—Over the years, the use of typical antipsychotics to treat affective disorders gradually faded because of concerns on the acute and long-term neurological side effects such as tardive dyskinesia. The emergence of atypical antipsychotics with less neurological complications has placed these drugs on the frontline in treating BPD. So far, OFC, quetiapine, lurasidone, cariprazine, and lumateperone have been approved by

Table 26–17 Number Needed to Treat to Benefit for Response from Psychotropics Relative to Placebo or Active Control in Bipolar Depression

Drugs	Dosage	Patients	NNT Mean (95% CI)
Monotherapy			
Aripiprazole	5–30 mg/day	Bipolar I	44 (10, ∞, −20)
Cariprazine	0.75 mg/day	Bipolar I	15 (6, ∞, −22)
Cariprazine	1.5 mg/day	Bipolar I	10 (6, 27)
Cariprazine	3 mg/day	Bipolar I	9 (6, 23)
Divalproex-ER*	62–82 µg/mL	Bipolar I or II	5 (3, 15)
Lamotrigne	100–400 mg/day	Bipolar I or II	12 (7, 39)
Lithium	600–1800 mg/day	Bipolar I or II	15 (5, ∞, −20)
Lumateperone	42 mg/day	Bipolar I or II	8 (4. 33)
Lurasidone	20–60 mg/day	Bipolar I or II	4 (3, 8)
Lurasidone	80–120 mg/day	Bipolar I or II	5 (3,10)
Olanzapine+fluoxetine	6/25, 6/50, or 12/50 mg/day	Bipolar I	4 (3, 7)
Olanzapine	5-20 mg/d	Bipolar I	9 (6, 18)
Olanzapine+fluoxetine versus Lamotrigine	6/25, 6/50, or 12/50 mg/d versus 150–200 mg/day	Bipolar I	16 (7, ∞, −62)
Quetiapine-IR	300 mg/day	Bipolar I or II	6(3, 4)
Quetiapine-IR	600 mg/day	Bipolar I or II	6 (4, 8)
Quetiapine-XR	300 mg/day	Bipolar I or II	4 (3, 10)
Paroxetine	20 mg/day	Bipolar I or II	46 (7, ∞, −10)
Ziprasidone	40–80 mg/day	Bipolar I	23 (7, 15)
Ziprasidone	120–160 mg/day	Bipolar I	-34 (13, ∞, −7)
Adjunctive therapy			
MS + armodafinil	150 mg/day	Bipolar I	-90 (9, ∞,−8)
MS + armodafinil	150 mg/day	Bipolar I	8 (5, 43)
MS+ armodafinil	150 mg/day	Bipolar I	12 (6, ∞,−71)
Lithium + lamotrigine	0.6–1.2 mEq/L+200 mg/d	Bipolar I or II	5 (3, 39)
MS + lurasidone	20–120 mg/day	Bipolar I or II	7 (4, 24)
MS + lumateperone	28 mg/day	Bipolar I or II	9 (5, 663)
MS + lumateperone	42 mg/day	Bipolar I or II	17 (6, ∞, −22)

Note: Cariprazine, lumateperone monotherapy or adjunctive therapy, lurasidone monotherapy or adjunctive therapy, olanzapine-fluoxetine combination, quetiapine-IR, and quetiapine-XR were approved for bipolar depression.* The result is from a meta-analysis. MS in lurasidone and lumateperone studies were lithium or valproate, but in armodafinil studies, MS included lithium, valproate, and/or antipsychotics.

NNT= 1 ÷ (active response rate–placebo response rate). A positive number of NNT indicates that the response rate in active treatment is higher than that in placebo. The 95% of CI does not cross zero is indicative of significant difference between the groups. A small NNT is indicative of a medication having a larger effect relative to placebo in response compared to a medication for response with a large NNT relative to placebo.

Abbreviation: ER, extended release; IR, immediate release; MS, mood stabilizer; NNT, number needed to treat to benefit; XR, extended release.

the FDA for the acute treatment of BPD with a similar efficacy as reflected by similar NNTs for response (Table 26–17). Similar to mania, the safety and tolerability of among the antipsychotics are different (Table 26–18). Two large RTCs of aripiprazole did not show its superiority over placebo in reducing depressive symptoms. The efficacy of ziprasidone as monotherapy or adjunctive therapy to a MS in BPD did not show superiority over placebo in RCTs.

Bai YH, Yang HC, Chen GJ, et al. Acceptability of acute and maintenance pharmacotherapy of bipolar disorder: a systematic review of randomized, double-blind, placebo-controlled clinical trials. *J Clin Psychopharmacol.* 2020;40:167–179.

Calabrese JR, Durgam S, Satlin A, et al. Efficacy and safety of lumateperone for major depressive episodes associated with bipolar I or bipolar II disorder: a phase 3 randomized placebo-controlled trial. *Am J Psychiatry.* 2021;178(12):1098–1106.

Gao K, Bai Y, Calabrese JR. Lithium and mood stabilizers. In: Nemeroff CB, Rasgon N, Schatzberg AF, Strakowski SM, eds. *The American Psychiatric Association Publishing Textbook of Mood Disorders,* 2nd ed. Washington DC; 2022:271–284.

Gao K, Kemp D E, Wu R, et al. Mood stabilizers. In: Tasman A, Kay J, Lieberman, JA, First MB, Riba MB, eds. *Psychiatry,* 4th ed. Chichester, UK: John Wiley & Sons, Ltd; 2015:2129–2153.

Gao K, Calabrese JR. 'Lamotrigine'. In: Schatzberg AF, Nemeroff CB, eds. *The American Psychiatric Association Publishing Textbook of Psychopharmacology,* 6th ed. Arlington, VA (in press).

Table 26–18 Number Needed to Treat to Harm of Common Side Effects from Antipsychotics Relative to Placebo or Active Control in Bipolar Depression

Medications	Dosage	Patients	Duration (week)	Mean NNH (Number Needed to Treat to Harm)				
				Discontinuation DAEs	Somnolence	≥ 7% WG	Akathisia	Overall EPS
Aripiprazole	5–30 mg/day	Bipolar I	8	14	ns	ns	5	19
Cariprazine	0.75 mg/day	Bipolar I	6	ns	ns	ns	ns	ns
Cariprazine	1.5 mg/day	Bipolar I		ns	30	53	30	21
Cariprazine	3 mg/day	Bipolar I		ns	ns	ns	13	17
Lumateperone	42 mg/day	Bipolar I or II	6	ns	13	ns	n/a	ns
MS + lumateperone	28 mg/day	Bipolar I or II	6	ns	25	ns	ns	ns
MS + lumateperone	42 mg/day	Bipolar I or II		18	20	ns	ns	ns
Lurasidone	20–60 mg/day	Bipolar I	6	ns	ns	27	18	ns
Lurasidone	80–120 mg/day	Bipolar I		ns	ns	ns	12	15
MS + lurasidone	20–120 mg/day	Bipolar I	6	ns	ns	ns	ns	ns
Olanzapine	5–20 mg/day	Bipolar I	8	24	6	5	n/a	ns
Olanzapine–fluoxetine combination	6/25, 6/50, or 12/50 mg/day	Bipolar I		ns	12	5	n/a	ns
Olanzapine	5–20 mg/day	Bipolar I	6-8	32	8	5	n/a	ns
Olanzapine–fluoxetine combination versus Lamotrigine	6/25, 6/50, or 12/50 mg/day 150–200 mg/day	Bipolar I	7	ns	10	4	n/a	n/a
Quetiapine-IR	300 mg/day	Bipolar I or II	8	25	7	29	n/a	29
Quetiapine-IR	600 mg/day	Bipolar I or II	8	12	7	16		22
Quetiapine-XR	300 mg/day	Bipolar I or II	8	9	4	14	n/a	ns
Ziprasidone	40–80 mg/day	Bipolar I	6	ns	10	ns	ns	ns
Ziprasidone	120-160 mg/day	Bipolar I	6	10	7	ns	38	ns

Note: Cariprazine, lumateperone, lurasidone, olanzapine–fluoxetine combination, quetiapine-IR, and quetiapine-XR are approved for bipolar depression. n/a, not available; n/s, not significant different. NNH= 1 ÷ (active response rate–placebo response rate). A positive number of NNH indicates that the response rate in active treatment is higher than that in placebo. A small NNH is indicative of a medication having a larger effect relative to placebo in a side effect compared to a medication for the same side effect with a large NNH relative to placebo.

Abbreviations: DAEs, discontinuation due to adverse events; EPS. Extrapyramidal side effects; IR, immediate release; MS, mood stabilizers (lithium or valproate); WG, weigh gain; XR, extended release.

Gao K, Wu R, Grunze H, et al. Phamarcological treatment of acute bipolar depression. In: Yildiz A, Ruiz P, Nemeroff C, eds. *Bipolar Book: History, Neurobiology, and Treatment.* New York: Oxford University Press; 2015:281–298.

Pinto JV, Saraf G, Vigo D, et al. Cariprazine in the treatment of Bipolar Disorder: a systematic review and meta-analysis. *Bipolar Disord.* 2020;22(4):360–371.

Sanford M, Dhillon S. Lurasidone: a review of its use in adult patients with bipolar I depression. *CNS Drugs.* 2015;29(3): 253–63.

Suppes T, Durgam S, Kozauer SG, et al. Adjunctive lumateperone (ITI-007) in the treatment of bipolar depression: results from a randomized placebo-controlled clinical trial. *Bipolar Disord.* 2023 Feb 13. doi: 10.1111/bdi.13310. Online ahead of print.

iv. Antidepressants

a. Monotherapy—The controversy on the efficacy and safety of antidepressants, especially antidepressant monotherapy, in the acute BPD remains unsettled. Evidence suggests that monotherapy with certain antidepressants for BPD may increase the risk for treatment emergent manic/hypomanic switch (TEM). The possibility of such risk has made regulatory agencies and professional organizations advise clinicians not to use antidepressant monotherapy for BPD. The best data for antidepressant efficacy as monotherapy in BPD are from a RCT of quetiapine-IR and paroxetine in BPI or II depression. In the study, quetiapine-IR 600 and 300 mg/d were significantly more effective than placebo in reducing depressive symptoms, but paroxetine was not (Table 26–17). However, the study has been criticized for the apparent low dosing of paroxetine (20 mg/day) which might have compromised the results.

The finding that paroxetine was not more effective than placebo in reducing depressive symptoms in BPI or II depression confirmed previous speculation that antidepressants at best only have limited efficacy in BPD. Some small RTCs and randomized open-label studies suggest that antidepressant monotherapy including fluoxetine, sertraline, and venlafaxine are effective and safe as lithium, olanzapine monotherapy, or OFC in BPII depression. However, antidepressants are a diverse group. The efficacy of other antidepressant monotherapy in BPD needs to be studied separately. A similar risk for TEM of paroxetine as placebo should not be considered as the evidence of the safety for using antidepressant monotherapy in BPD. Again, the relative low dose of paroxetine might explain the apparent low switch risk. In addition, patients with more frequent cycling courses and recent SUD were excluded from the study. These groups of patients are more likely to have TEM.

b. Adjunctive to or combination with a mood stabilizer—Antidepressant adjunctive therapy to a MS has been recommended as an option for the acute treatment of BPD, but good data supporting this practice are lacking. With the exception of OFC, there is no large RCT demonstrating that an antidepressant is effective in acute BPD. A meta-analysis of 15 RCTs with 2373 patients of antidepressant adjunctive to a MS found that antidepressants were not superior to placebo or other active treatments for BPD (Table 26–17), although an earlier meta-analysis of antidepressants for acute BPD showed that antidepressants were superior to placebo in short-term treatment of BPD. There was no increased risk for TEM or any individual adverse event with antidepressant relative to placebo, but different risk for TEM from different antidepressants was reported. TCAs had higher TEM than other antidepressants combined (10% vs. 3.2%). Venlafaxine adjunctive to a MS also had a higher risk for TEM than sertraline or bupropion adjunctive to a MS in BPD.

c. Monotherapy or adjunctive therapy from non-randomized and/or non-double-blind studies—An early study from the Stanley Foundation Bipolar Network (SFBN) showed that about 15% of patients (84 of 549) who received at least one antidepressant treatment with a MS might benefit from antidepressant treatment. However, among those who completed at least 60-day antidepressant treatment, the remission rate was 44% (84 of 189). High response rates (> 60%) were also reported in open-label studies and other naturalistic studies of antidepressants in BPD. Results from some studies even suggested that patients with BPD, especially with BPII depression, had higher response rates than those with MDD.

One of the main reasons for the discontinuation of antidepressants after acute treatments is fear of manic switching. The majority of studies has shown that antidepressant adjunctive therapy to a MS does not have an increased risk for TEM. However, the data from the SFBN showed that acute or continuation treatment with venlafaxine plus a MS had higher risk for TEM compared to sertraline or bupropion plus a MS. In addition, there are also inconsistent data on the benefit from continuation of antidepressant treatments. The SFBN studies showed that the continuation of antidepressants is beneficial in those who responded initially. A study of the STEP-BD (Systematic Treatment Enhancement Program for Bipolar Disorder) found that antidepressant continuation trended toward less severe depressive symptoms, but there were no benefits in prevalence or severity of new depressive or manic episodes, or overall time in remission. Bipolar II disorder did not predict enhanced antidepressant response, but rapid-cycling course predicted three times more depressive episodes with antidepressant continuation.

d. Guideline recommendation—The International Society for Bipolar Disorder (ISBD) Task Force on Antidepressant in BPD, which consisted of 65 international experts in BDs, found that there was striking disparity between the wide use and the weak evidence base for efficacy and safety of antidepressants in BDs. The Canadian Network for Mood and Anxiety Treatments (CANMAT) and ISBD 2018 guidelines for the management of patients with BD recommend SSRIs/bupropion for BPD as a second-line options after DIV. The first-line medications includes quetiapine monotherapy, lithium monotherapy, lurasidone monotherapy or adjunctive to lithium or VPA, LTG monotherapy or adjunctive to lithium or VPA. OFC was the last option in the second-line medications due its metabolic side effects. Cariprazine and lumateperone in BPD were not available at that time. They should be first-line medications based on their efficacy and safety data.

Altshuler LL, Sugar CA, McElroy SL, et al. Switch rates during acute treatment for bipolar II depression with lithium, sertraline, or the two combined: a randomized double-blind comparison. *Am J Psychiatry*. 2017;174(3):266–276.

Gao K, Wu R, Grunze H, et al. Phamarcological treatment of acute bipolar depression. In: Yildiz A, Ruiz P, Nemeroff C, eds. *Bipolar Book: History, Neurobiology, and Treatment*. New York: Oxford University Press; 2015:281–298.

Tondo L, Baldessarini RJ, Vázquez G, et al. Clinical responses to antidepressants among 1036 acutely depressed patients with bipolar or unipolar major affective disorders.. 2013; 127(5):355–364.

Pacchiarotti I, Bond DJ, Baldessarini RJ, et al. The International Society for Bipolar Disorders (ISBD) task force report on antidepressant use in bipolar disorders. *Am J Psychiatry*. 2013;170(11):1249–1262.

Yatham LN, Kennedy SH, Parikh SV, et al. Canadian Network for Mood and Anxiety Treatments (CANMAT) and International Society for Bipolar Disorders (ISBD) 2018 guidelines for the management of patients with bipolar disorder. *Bipolar Disord*. 2018;20(2):97–170.

Wu R, Gao K, Calabrese JR, et al. Treatment induced mood instability: treatment – emergent affective switches and cycle acceleration. In: Yildiz A, Ruiz P, Nemeroff C, eds. *Bipolar Book: History, Neurobiology, and Treatment*. New York: Oxford University Press;; 2015:417–434.

v. Dopaminergic agents

a. Wakefulness-promoting agent—Modafinil and armodafinil are wakefulness-promoting agents that have been approved by the FDA for improving wakefulness in patients with excessive sleepiness associated with narcolepsy, obstructive sleep apnea, and shift-work sleep disorder. Their antidepressant efficacy in BPD was assessed with RCTs in patients with bipolar I or II depression and inadequately responsive to a MS with or without concomitant antidepressant therapy. One medium size study of modafinil showed superiority over placebo in reducing depressive symptoms. The results of armodafinil on the primary outcome have been inconsistent, although some secondary outcomes demonstrated significant benefit from armodafinil over placebo (Table 26–17). One study found that armodafinil 150 mg/d was superior to placebo in reducing depressive and panic/phobic symptoms and improving increased appetite, concentration/decision-making, and energy level. The most common adverse events were headache, insomnia, and diarrhea. There were no significant differences in the discontinuation DAEs, TEM, electrocardiogram, or metabolic parameters.

b. Dopamine 2/3 receptor agonist—Pramipexole is a dopamine 2/3 receptor agonist that is approved for the treatment of Parkinson disease. A systematic review including five RCTs, three open-label trials, and five observational studies of pramipexole in UPD and BPD found that an overall short-term response rate of 52.2% and remission rate of 36.1%, and an overall long-term response rate of 62.1% and remission rate of 39.6%. In RCTs, pramipexole was superior to placebo in reducing depressive symptoms.

c. Stimulants—A systematic review and meta-analysis of the effects of dopaminergic agents (modafinil, armodafinil, pramipexole, methylphenidate, and amphetamines) on BPD of nine studies (1716 patients) found that treatment with dopaminergic agents for BPD was associated with an increase in both response and remission rates. There was no evidence of an increased risk of mood switch associated with these mediations. A cumulative incidence of mood switch was of 3% during a mean follow-up period of 7.5 months.

Gao K, Wu R, Grunze H, et al. Phamarcological treatment of acute bipolar depression. In: Yildiz A, Ruiz P, Nemeroff C, eds. *Bipolar Book: History, Neurobiology, and Treatment.* New York: Oxford University Press; 2015:281–298.

Tundo A, de Filippis R, De Crescenzo F. Pramipexole in the treatment of unipolar and bipolar depression. A systematic review and meta-analysis. *Acta Psychiatr Scand.* 2019;140(2):116–125.

Szmulewicz AG, Angriman F, Samamé C, et al. Dopaminergic agents in the treatment of bipolar depression: a systematic review and meta-analysis. *Acta Psychiatr Scand.* 2017;135(6):527–538.

vii. Polyunsaturated fatty

—An early meta-analysis of six RCTs of Omega-3 for BD with a total of 291 patients in 2012 revealed a significant effect on reducing depressive symptoms favoring Omega-3 over placebo with a small effect size of 0.34, but the effect on manic symptoms was not significantly different between Omega-3 and placebo. A most recent systematic review of 33 observational trials including 15 on fatty acids, 9 on micronutrients, 5 on specific foods, and 4 on macro- and micronutrients found that dietary intake or supplementation of unsaturated fatty acids, mainly Omega-3 along with seafood, folic acid, and zinc seems to be associated with improved BD symptoms. However, good quality data in this area are still lacking.

Gabriel FC, Oliveira M, Martella BM, et al. Nutrition and bipolar disorder: a systematic review. *Nutr Neurosci.* 2023;26(7):637–651.

McPhilemy G, Byrne F, Waldron M, et al. A 52-week prophylactic randomised control trial of omega-3 polyunsaturated fatty acids in bipolar disorder. *Bipolar Disord.* 2021;23(7):697–706.

viii. Thyroid hormones

—Augmentation with triiodothyronine (T_3) (13–188 mcg/d) was effective in reducing depressive symptoms in patients with BD. Early studies suggested that supraphysiological doses (250–500 mcg/d) of thyroxine (T_4) were effective in the acute and maintenance treatment of bipolar or unipolar patients with TRD. However, a recent large multicenter, 6-week RCT of fixed-dose levothyroxine 300 μg/d versus placebo adjunctive to ongoing treatment in patients with BPI or II depression found a numerically, but not significantly, better in improving depression with levothyroxine compared to with placebo. A subgroup analysis of women ($n = 32$) revealed a significant difference between groups in mean change in depressive symptoms, and a high baseline THS level was a significant predictor for levothyroxine antidepressant effect in women.

Stamm TJ, Lewitzka U, Sauer C, et al. Supraphysiologic doses of levothyroxine as adjunctive therapy in bipolar depression: a randomized, double-blind, placebo-controlled study. *J Clin Psychiatry.* 2014;75(2):162–168.

ix. Glutamatergic modulating agents

—In a small RCT ($n = 19$) of riluzole monotherapy versus placebo in BPD for 8 week, riluzole (50–200 mg/d) was not significantly superior to placebo in reducing depressive symptoms. In contrast, ketamine has shown efficacy in reducing depressive symptoms in BPD. In a recent systematic review of six studies with 135 patients confirmed the previous results that ketamine infusion at 0.5 mg/kg adding to ongoing mood-stabilizing agent(s) was significantly superior to placebo in reducing depressive symptoms in patients with BPD. The overall response rate was 61% for those receiving ketamine and 5% for those receiving a placebo. Ketamine infusion was well tolerated.

Bahji A, Zarate CA, Vazquez GH. Ketamine for bipolar depression: a systematic review. *Int J Neuropsychopharmacol.* 2021;24(7):535–541.

3. Maintenance treatment of bipolar disorder—

Although mania/hypomania is the hall marker of BD, patients with bipolar I or II disorder experience depressive symptoms much more commonly than manic/hypomanic symptoms when they are symptomatic. Studies have shown that moderate to extreme impairment in work, social, and family life occurs more often from depressive than manic symptoms in patients with BD. In addition, significant psychosocial impairment during illness-free periods has been more strongly associated with the number of past depressive episodes than past manias. Importantly, suicide in BD often occurs during depressive episodes, and euthymic bipolar patients have similar quality of life as the general population, suggesting that the prevention of acute MDEs and maintaining a stable mood state is critical to reduce the morbidity and mortality and improve the quality of life associated with BD. However, as the acute treatment of BPD, the prevention of depressive relapse during maintenance treatment is still an urgent unmet need.

As medications for the maintenance treatment of MDD, most FDA-approved medications for bipolar maintenance were studied with relapse-prevention design. A detailed description of pros and cons from a relapse-prevention design is out of the scope of this chapter. However, the clinicians need to understand the basics of study design that can affect the interpretation of the results. There is still little consensus on "standard" methodology for bipolar maintenance studies, but over the years, the methods that have evolved the most include: (1) study enrollment (inclusion and exclusion criteria), (2) study design (crossover vs. parallel), (3) outcome measures (diagnostic instruments vs. rating scales), (4) index episode (mania, hypomania, depression, and/or euthymia), (5) study duration (more than 6 months or less), and (6) statistical analysis (time-to-event analysis with hazard ratio vs. event count analysis with rate).

Lithium is the first medication approved for the maintenance treatment of BD and its efficacy supported by first-generation maintenance studies conducted and published during the 1960s and 1970s. The need for alternatives to lithium for maintenance treatment of BD has led to the development of anticonvulsants and atypical antipsychotics for maintenance treatment of BD. The first relapses-prevention study after a MDE in patients with BD was conducted to assess the efficacy and safety of LTG versus placebo in early 2000s, which led the approval of LTG in 2003 for preferential prevention of depressive episode relapses. However, what should be used for the maintenance treatment after a manic episode remains debatable. The most common practice in the Unites States is the continuation of the medication(s) that resolve an acute manic episode. Similarly, the medication(s) that resolve a depressive episode should continue. However, most currently available medications for maintenance treatment of BD have used mania as an index episode. Currently, lithium, LTG, olanzapine, aripiprazole, quetiapine, ziprasidone, and olanzapine/samidorphan have been approved for the maintenance treatment of BD, but their efficacies in preventing different bipolarities are different (Table 26–19).

i. Lithium—Lithium's approval for bipolar maintenance treatment was based on early maintenance studies that had a number of methodological issues. However, its efficacy as monotherapy or adjunctive therapy in preventing any mood relapse was replicated by most studies using modern study designs and the DSM nomenclature during the development of DIV, LTG, olanzapine, and quetiapine in maintenance treatment of BD. The overall impression was that lithium was as effective as other newer FDA-approved agents in preventing any mood relapse, and more effective preventing manic than preventing depressive relapse (Table 26–18). Standard dosing to achieve blood levels of lithium between 0.8 and 1.0 mEq/L or higher is generally recommended over "low" dosing to levels between 0.4 and 0.6 mEq/L for BPI, especially for preventing manic/hypomanic relapse. Maintenance at "low" lithium levels has been associated with a greater risk of relapse compared to standard dosing into the higher range. However, lithium side effects are more frequent when standard higher dosing is used.

ii. Anticonvulsants

a. Lamotrigine—Two 18-month large RCTs led to the approval of LTG as a maintenance therapy in bipolar I disorder. One used an index episode of a manic, hypomanic, or mixed state, and another used an index episode of depression. In both studies, 50% of patients achieved stabilization criteria allowing for progression into double-blinded maintenance therapy with LTG (50–400 mg/day), lithium (0.8–1.1 mEq/L), or placebo. Both LTG and lithium were superior to placebo in the time to intervention for any mood episode in both studies. LTG, but not lithium, was superior to placebo in the time to a depressive episode in both studies. Lithium, but not LTG, was superior to placebo in the time to a manic, hypomanic, or mixed episode.

b. Divalproex/valproate—VPA is commonly used as both antimanic and maintenance therapy for BD, although it does not carry a labeled indication for maintenance. Early studies suggested that the VPA had comparable efficacy as lithium for maintenance with better tolerability. However, the first maintenance RCT of DIV in bipolar I patients who were after a manic episode did not find significant differences between lithium, DIV, and placebo during 52-week study period. In an olanzapine versus DIV study in patients with acute mania, the reduction in manic symptoms was significantly greater with olanzapine over a 47-week period. However, the rates of symptomatic remission or subsequent relapse were not significantly different between the two groups.

c. Carbamazepine—A 1999 meta-analysis that included 10 RCTs comparing carbamazepine to lithium found no significant difference in relapse rates over a 1–3 year maintenance period (55 vs. 60%, respectively). However, the maintenance

Table 26–19 Relative Efficacy of Medication to Placebo in Preventing Relapse of Different Bipolarities in Maintenance Treatment of Bipolar Disorder as Monotherapy or Combination Therapy

Medication	Index Episode	Bipolar Types	Delay Relapse/Recurrence		
			Any Mood	Manic/Mixed	Depressive
Monotherapy					
Aripiprazole	Manic or mixed	Bipolar I	+++	++++	–
Lithium	Manic or depressive	Bipolar I	++++	++++	+
Lamotrigine	Manic or depressive	Bipolar I	++++	++	+++
Olanzapine	Manic or mixed	Bipolar I	+++	++++	++
Paliperidone	Manic or mixed	Bipolar I	++++	++++	–
Quetiapine	Manic, mixed, or depressive	Bipolar I or II	++++	++++	++++
Quetiapine	Depressive	Bipolar I or II	+++	–	++++
Risperidone LAI	Manic or mixed	Bipolar I	++++	++++	–
Valproate	Manic, partially recovered from mania, or euthymia	Bipolar I	–	–	–
Combination therapy					
Aripiprazole + lamotrigine	Manic or mixed	Bipolar I	++	++	–
Aripiprazole + Val	Manic or mixed	Bipolar I	+	–	+
Aripiprazole + Li or Val	Manic or mixed	Bipolar I	+++	++++	–
Oxcarbazepine+ Li	Euthymia or mild symptoms	Bipolar I or II	_	n/a	n/a
Olanzapine + Li or Val	Manic or mixed	Bipolar I	+++	–	+
Quetiapine + Li or Val	Manic, mixed, or depressive	Bipolar I or II	++++	++++	++++
Risperidone LAI + treatment as usual	Manic, hypomanic, depressed, mixed, or euthymic	Bipolar I	+++	n/a	n/a
Ziprasidone + Li or Val	Manic or mixed	Bipolar I	+++	++++	–

Note: –, not significantly different between active treatment and placebo; + $P > .05$, but $< .1$ or $\geq 25\%$ risk reduction; ++, $P \leq .05$ or $\geq 35\%$ risk reduction; +++, $P \leq .01$ or $\geq 45\%$; ++++, $P \leq .001$ or $\geq 60\%$ reduction. The risk reduction is based on the hazard ratio. If both P value and hazard ratio are available, hazard ratio is used from at least one trial to determine the treatment efficacy.

Abbreviations: LAI, long-acting injection; Li, lithium; n/a, not available; Val, valproate.

Adapted from Gao K, Wu R, Calabrese JR. Pharmacological treatment of the maintenance phase of bipolar depression: efficacy and side effects. In: Parnham M, Bruinvels J, series eds. Milestones in Drug Therapy series; (Zarate Jr CA, Manji HK, eds. Bipolar Depression: Molecular Neurobiology, Clinical Diagnosis and Pharmacotherapy, 2nd ed. Springer International Publishing Switzerland (outside the USA); 2016:213–242.

with carbamazepine monotherapy has produced inconsistent results and consensus based on available data and expert opinion is that carbamazepine monotherapy is inferior to lithium in the maintenance treatment of BD. Its use in combination with other MS for maintenance, especially with lithium, has stronger evidence.

d. Combination of lithium and valproate—In the BALANCE study, lithium was superior to VPA in delaying any mood relapse with a 29% risk reduction. The combination of lithium and VPA was superior to VPA alone in delaying any mood relapse with a 41% risk reduction. There is no significant difference between the combination and lithium alone on any mood relapse. For preventing depression relapse, the combination was significant superior to VPA alone with a 49% of risk reduction, and lithium was superior to VPA with 37% risk reduction. For preventing manic relapse, the combination was superior to VPA with 50% risk reduction, and lithium and VPA did not significantly differ in this measure.

iii. Atypical antipsychotics for maintenance therapy—Olanzapine, aripiprazole, quetiapine, and risperidone/

paliperidone monotherapy have been studied with RCTs and approved in the maintenance treatment of BD. Both quetiapine and ziprasidone adjunctive therapy (lithium or VPA) also received FDA approval for maintenance treatment of BD. Only quetiapine had enrolled patients presenting recently depressed. The olanzapine, aripiprazole, ziprasidone, and risperidone maintenance trials used manic or mixed as an index episode for an initial stabilization phase. Using only manic/mixed as an index episode has important implications to investigate full mood-stabilizing efficacies of these and other medications since it has been demonstrated that the polarity of the index episode tends to predict the same polarity of relapse into a subsequent episode in a ratio of about 2:1 to 3:1.

Olanzapine prevents bipolar I relapse into any mood state for significantly longer periods of time than placebo but prevented patients from relapse into mania more than into depression. Aripiprazole was superior to placebo in delaying the time to any mood relapse that was mainly due to preventing manic relapse, but not depressive relapse. Similarly, ziprasidone was superior to placebo in preventing manic relapse, but not in depressive relapse. Risperidone long-acting therapy also showed differential efficacy in preventing manic/hypo-manic versus depressive relapse with significant difference in preventing manic/hypomanic relapses only compared to placebo. In contrast, quetiapine monotherapy or combination with lithium or VPA was equally and significantly effective in preventing manic/hypomanic and depressive relapses compared to placebo. The results of combination therapies suggest that medications with differential bipolarity efficacies may not be complementary to each other (Table 26–19).

Gao K, Bai Y, Calabrese JR. Lithium and mood stabilizers. In: Nemeroff CB, Rasgon N, Schatzberg AF, Strakowski SM, eds. *The American Psychiatric Association Publishing Textbook of Mood Disorders*, 2nd ed, Washington DC; 2022:271–284.

Gao K, Kemp D E, Wu R, et al. Mood stabilizers. In: Tasman A, Kay J, Lieberman, JA, First MB, Riba MB, eds. *Psychiatry*, 4th ed. Chichester, UK: John Wiley & Sons, Ltd; 2015:2129–2153.

Gao K, Kemp DE, Calabrese JR. Pharmacological treatment of the maintenance phase of bipolar depression: focus on relapse prevention studies and the impact of design on generalizability. In: Parnham M, Bruinvels J, series eds. *Milestones in Drug Therapy Series*; Zarate Jr CA, Manji HK, eds, *Bipolar Depression: Molecular Neurobiology, Clinical Diagnosis, and Pharmacotherapy*. Switzerland: Birkhauser Verlag AG, Springer Science + Business Media; 2009:159–179.

Gao K, Wu R, Calabrese JR. Pharmacological treatment of the maintenance phase of bipolar depression: efficacy and side effects. In: Parnham M, Bruinvels J, series eds. *Milestones in Drug Therapy series*; Zarate Jr CA, Manji HK, eds. *Bipolar Depression: Molecular Neurobiology, Clinical Diagnosis, and Pharmacotherapy*, 2nd ed. Springer International Publishing Switzerland (outside the USA); 2016:213–242.

B. Psychotherapeutic Interventions

1. Acute mania—Patients with acute mania/hypomania, depression or mixed symptoms, or euthymia were enrolled in studies of psychotherapeutic interventions. A systematic review and component network meta-analysis of adjunctive psychotherapy for BD found that CBT, psychoeducation, and family/conjoint therapy were significantly associated with improved manic symptoms in 12 months compared to TAU. Therapies with cognitive restructuring components and regulating daily rhythms were associated with greater stabilization of manic symptoms. In contrast, behavioral activation was associated with lesser mood stabilization. Family/conjoint focused therapy (FFT) and brief psychoeducation were associated significant higher rates of retention than standard length of ≥ 6 sessions. Moreover, the family format appeared to be the only component associated with a higher retention rate.

2. Acute bipolar depression

i. Cognitive behavior therapy—In the same systematic review mentioned above, CBT, FFT, and interpersonal psychosocial rhythmic therapy (IPSRT) were associated with significantly improved depressive symptoms in 12 months compared to TAU. Therapies with cognitive restructuring components, regulating daily rhythms, and communication training were the most potent components for reducing depressive symptoms. The combination of these three components was more effective than TAU. The least potent components for reducing depressive symptoms were behavior activation and individual format. A study of STEP-BD, pharmacotherapy + psychotherapy (CBT, IPSRT, or FFT weekly and biweekly for up to 30 sessions) versus pharmacotherapy + 3 sessions of psychosocial strategy education (collaborative care) included patients with acute BPI or II depression. It found that patients received three intensive therapies (CBT, IPSRT, or FFT) recovered faster than those received the collaborative care. There were no significant differences among CBT, IPSRT, or FFT in recovery rate and the time to recovery. Further analyses found that patients with an AD, especially GAD, benefit more from intensive therapies compared to from collaborative care. The number of lifetime comorbid ADs also moderated the effect of psychotherapy on the recovery for BPD. Specifically, only patients with one lifetime number AD significantly benefited from the intensive psychotherapy compared to from collaborative care.

ii. Interpersonal and social rhythm therapy—IPSRT is an individual psychotherapy designed specifically for the treatment for BD. The IPSRT grew from a chronobiological model of BD that life events (both negative and positive) might cause disruptions in patients' social rhythms that, in turn, perturb circadian rhythms and sleep–wake cycles and lead to the development of bipolar symptoms. Along with medications, IPSRT helps patients regularize their daily routines, diminishes interpersonal problems, and adheres to medication regimens. Early studies showed that participants assigned to IPSRT in the acute treatment phase stayed stable significantly longer without a new affective episode, irrespective of maintenance treatment assignment. The ability to increase regularity of social rhythms during acute treatment was associated with reduced likelihood of recurrence during the maintenance phase. In a real-world study of BD patients who received the IPSRT or TAU, patients from the IPSRT reported a significant improvement in depressive, anxiety and manic symptomatology, global functioning, and response to MS at the assessment of 3 and 6 months. However, a meta-analysis of five independent RCTs with 631 patients found that IPSRT significantly improved overall functioning but did not significantly improve the symptoms.

iii. Family-focused therapy—FFT is a psychoeducational treatment for patients with BD focused on alleviation of mood symptoms, relapse prevention and enhanced psychosocial functioning and usually given in conjunction with pharmacotherapy after a mood episode. The treatment includes conjoint educational sessions regarding bipolar illness, communication enhancement training, and problem-solving skills training. Eight randomized controlled trials with adults and adolescents with BD found that FFT and mood-stabilizing medications hasten recovery from mood episodes, reduce recurrences, and reduce levels of symptom severity compared to briefer forms of psychoeducation and medications over 1–2 years. Several studies indicate that the effects of FFT on symptom improvement are greater among patients with high-expressed emotion relatives. A more recent study of 127 high-risk youths for BD and a median of 98 follow-up weeks (range, 0–255 weeks) did not find significant differences between FFT and enhanced care in time to recovery from pretreatment symptoms but had longer intervals from recovery to the emergence of the next mood episode, especially to next depressive episode relapse.

Deckersbach T, Peters AT, Sylvia L, et al. Do comorbid anxiety disorders moderate the effects of psychotherapy for bipolar disorder? Results from STEP-BD. *Am J Psychiatry*. 2014; 171(2):178–86.

Lam C, Min-Huey Chung MH. A meta-analysis of the effect of interpersonal and social rhythm therapy on symptom and functioning improvement in patients with bipolar disorders: applied research in quality of life, International Society for Quality-of-Life Studies Springer 2021;16(1):153–165.

Miklowitz DJ, Efthimiou O, Furukawa TA, et al. Adjunctive Psychotherapy for bipolar disorder: a systematic review and component network meta-analysis. *JAMA Psychiatry*. 2021;78(2): 141–150.

Miklowitz DJ, Schneck CD, Walshaw PD, et al. Effects of family-focused therapy vs enhanced usual care for symptomatic youths at high risk for bipolar disorder: a randomized clinical trial. *JAMA Psychiatry*. 2020;77(5):455–463.

C. Other Interventions

1. Acute treatment of mania

i. **Electroconvulsive therapy**—Early studies found that ECT monotherapy was as effective as lithium monotherapy for acute mania. However, unlike ECT in BPD, there is no large study to assess the efficacy and safety of ECT monotherapy or adjunctive therapy to MS in acute mania. A recent meta-analysis of 12 randomized controlled trials, mainly from China, found that ECT combination with a MS was significantly more effective than the MS alone in reducing manic symptoms. The significant difference occurred after 3–5 treatments or after a 1-week treatment.

ii. **rTMS**—The efficacy and safety of TMS in mania have less been studied. Current available treatments including MSs and ECT are effective for mania. Considering the less side effects and less logistic requirement from rTMS compared to ECT, there may be a room for TMS in the treatment of acute mania in the future. A meta-analysis of small studies of rTMS in acute mania suggested that rTMS is effective and safe in acute mania.

iii. **Blocking blue lights**—Small studies have shown that dark room therapy is effective in patients with mania less than 2 weeks. Virtual darkness therapy with blocking blue light

(a wave length of 450–470 nm) by wearing glasses found that manic inpatients who received pharmacological treatment and blue-light blocking glasses (BBG) had a higher sleep efficiency and a faster decline in manic symptoms than those received placebo. Large RCTs are needed for BBG being used in routine clinical practice.

Crowe M, Porter R. Inpatient treatment for mania: a review and rationale for adjunctive interventions. *Austr N Z J Psychiatry*. 2014;48(8):716–721.

Hett D, Marwaha S. Repetitive transcranial magnetic stimulation in the treatment of bipolar disorder. *Ther Adv Psychopharmacol*. 2020;10:2045125320973790.

Mylona I, Floros GD. Blue light blocking treatment for the treatment of bipolar disorder: directions for research and practice. *J Clin Med*. 2022;11(5):1380.

Zhang J, Wang G, Yang X, et al. Efficacy and safety of electroconvulsive therapy plus medication versus medication alone in acute mania: a meta-analysis of randomized controlled trials. *Psychiatry Res*. 2021;302:114019.

2. Acute treatment of bipolar depression

i. **ECT**—A few ECT studies solely targeted patients with BPD. Most results of ECT in BPD are from previous studies that included patients with UPD or BPD. An earlier systematic review in 2012 found a similar remission rate with ECT in UPD and BPD, 51% for UPD and 53% for BPD. In a study of right unilateral ECT versus algorithm-based pharmacological therapy in treatment-resistant BPD, the response rates were significantly higher in the ECT group than in the medication group, 74 versus 35%, but the remission rates not significantly different, 35 versus 30%. A systematic review and network meta-analysis of 113 non-surgical brain stimulation trials that randomized 6750 patients with MDD or BPD found that BL ECT and high dose RUL ECT are the two most effective treatments among the 10 strategies with significant efficacy relative to sham therapy.

ii. **TMS**—The safety and efficacy of rTMS in the acute treatment of BPD are ongoing with large RCTs. The results from a meta-analysis of small controlled studies including different coils placement and stimuli frequency found that overall, rTMS is effective in reducing depressive symptoms, but the bilateral is least effective. A more recent systematic review including RCTs, open-label studies, and case series of rTMS in BD concluded that the results, even in BPD, had been inconsistent, and the most effective rTMS protocol for BPD had yet to reach a consensus.

iii. **Light therapy**—The efficacy and safety of light therapy in treatment of BPD are less well studied. A recent systematic review and meta-analysis including seven RCTs with 259 patients found that light therapy was significantly effective in reducing depression symptoms than control. The response rate was also significantly higher with light therapy than with control, 64.3 versus 42.9%, but the remission rate was not significantly different, 40.7 versus 16.9% (*P*=.09). However, light therapy parameters varied widely with intensity ranging from 400 lux to 10,000 lux, duration from 15 to 360 minutes per day, and the time of treatment from the morning, mid-day, to both morning and evening. Another recent meta-analysis of RCTs (*n* = 5) and cohort studies (*n* = 7) of light therapy in BPD with 847 patients also found that significant reduction in depression with light therapy, and a total of less than 10 hours treatment had a large effect than those with more than 10 hours. Morning plus night/evening therapy also yielded a large effect size compared to that of morning only therapy. White light therapy was associated with a larger effect size than the green light therapy. Sleep deprivation, lithium treatment, and light intensity ≥ 5000 lux are also associated with a large effect.

iv. Transcranial current stimulation—The evidence of transcranial current stimulation including transcranial tDCS in BPD is limited. In a randomized, sham-control study of direct current stimulation in patients with bipolar I or II depression who failed at least one pharmacological treatments for the current episode, patients in the active tDCS condition showed significantly superior improvement compared to those receiving sham, with significantly higher response rates 67.6 versus 30.4%. A systematic review including 5 RCTs, 7 open trials with a total of 207 BPD patients found that active tDCS is superior over sham in reducing depression, with changes from baseline ranging from 18 to 92%.

v. Deep brain stimulation—The studies of DBS in treatment-resistant BPD are even sparser. Most bipolar patients in DBS studies are with bipolar II depression and a part of study of MDD. Overall, patients with bipolar II depression have similar benefit as patients with MDD. However, the current evidence of DBS as an add-on or alternative to pharmacological and psychological treatments in patients with BDs is very limited, although DBS may provide opportunity to treat patients who fail medication and less invasive nonpharmacological interventions.

Dierckx B, Heijnen WT, van den Broek WW, et al. Efficacy of electroconvulsive therapy in bipolar versus unipolar major depression: a meta-analysis. *Bipolar Disord*. 2012;14(2):146–150.

D'Urso G, Toscano E, Barone A, et al. Transcranial direct current stimulation for bipolar depression: systematic reviews of clinical evidence and biological underpinnings. *Prog Neuropsychopharmacol Biol Psychiatry*. 2023;121:110672.

Gippert SM, Switala C, Bewernick BH, et al. Deep brain stimulation for bipolar disorder-review and outlook. *CNS Spectr*. 2017;22(3):254–257.

Konstantinou G, Hui J, Ortiz A, et al. Repetitive transcranial magnetic stimulation (rTMS) in bipolar disorder: a systematic review. *Bipolar Disord*. 2022;24(1):10–26.

Lam RW, Teng MY, Jung YE, et al. Light therapy for patients with bipolar depression: systematic review and meta-analysis of randomized controlled trials. *Can J Psychiatry*. 2020;65(5):290–300.

Mutz J. Brain stimulation treatment for bipolar disorder. *Bipolar Disord*. 2023;25(1):9–24.

Nguyen TD, Hieronymus F, Lorentzen R, et al. The efficacy of repetitive transcranial magnetic stimulation (rTMS) for bipolar depression: a systematic review and meta-analysis. *J Affect Disord*. 2021;279:250–255.

Sampaio-Junior B, Tortella G, Borrione L, et al. Efficacy and safety of transcranial direct current stimulation as an add-on treatment for bipolar depression: a randomized clinical trial. *JAMA Psychiatry*. 2018;75(2):158–166.

Schoeyen HK, Kessler U, Andreassen OA, et al. Treatment-resistant bipolar depression: a randomized controlled trial of electroconvulsive therapy versus algorithm-based pharmacological treatment. *Am J Psychiatry*. 2015;172(1):41–51.

Wang S, Zhang Z, Yao L, et al. Bright light therapy in the treatment of patients with bipolar disorder: a systematic review and meta-analysis. *PLoS One*. 2020;15(5):e0232798.

3. Maintenance treatment of bipolar disorder—Non-pharmacological maintenance treatments for BD are scarce. For patients achieving response and/or remission with an acute ECT series, continuation/maintenance ECT is a common practice, although there is no good evidence support this practice. Most psychosocial intervention studies are initiated during an acute depressive episode or shortly after a mood episode and continued for from 6 months to 24 months. As mentioned previously, CBT, FFT, and IPSRT were associated with significantly improved depressive symptoms compared to TAU. In addition, manualized treatments were associated with lower recurrence rates than control treatments, and psychoeducation with guided practice of illness management skills in a family/group format was associated with lower recurrences compared to an individual format. A personalized approach based on the phase of illness, personality traits, comorbidities, and psychosocial factors may be necessary to use different therapeutic methodologies to address acute and long-term mood stability for each individual patient.

Miklowitz DJ, Efthimiou O, Furukawa TA, et al. Adjunctive psychotherapy for bipolar disorder: a systematic review and component network meta-analysis. *JAMA Psychiatry*. 2021;78(2):141–150.

D. Treatment of Psychiatric Comorbidities

1. Anxiety disorders—Anxiety disorders are the most common comorbid conditions in BD, but the evidence for treating anxiety comorbidities in BD is very limited. Unlike patients with MDD, patients with BD are likely to have higher rates of lifetime and current SUD and ADHD, and both can complicate the treatment of comorbid ADs. A history of comorbid SUD increases the risk for abuse/dependence of benzodiazepines and other controlled substances including stimulants. Benzodiazepines are very effective for reducing anxiety symptoms and do not destabilize mood. Antidepressants in comorbid AD in BD have never been systematically studied. The risk of potential switching to mania/hypomania with antidepressants and their limited efficacy in BPD, even with a MS, have make experts and guidelines not recommend antidepressants for BPD and comorbid ADs.

A "step-wise" approach was recommended in the ISBD 2018 guidelines. Mood stabilization is the priority before specific anxiety treatments are considered. CBT is a first-line treatment for comorbid anxiety. Antidepressants, particularly serotoninergic agents, should be employed with caution due to their potential to provoke mood destabilization. Benzodiazepines are an important clinical tool because they can rapidly alleviate anxiety, but clinicians should prescribe them at the lowest possible dose for the shortest period possible, given the concerns about suicide risk, abuse and dependence.

For patients who are euthymic and treated with lithium, adding VPA, LTG, or some atypical antipsychotics with anxiolytic effects may be considered. However, not all antipsychotics have anxiolytic effect. Quetiapine showed some benefit in reducing anxiety symptoms in bipolar patients with comorbid GAD and/or panic disorder, but risperidone, ziprasidone, and DIV did not have significant benefit for reducing anxiety symptoms compared to placebo. A recent systematic review and meta-analysis of 2175 participants with anxiety symptom measures found that compared with placebo, the overall effect size of medications (primarily atypical antipsychotics) on anxiety symptoms was small. For patients taking an antipsychotic, LTG, or VPA/DIV, lithium should be added before considering other medications. Gabapentin reduced anxiety symptoms in patients with BD as an adjunctive therapy in open-label studies. Pregabalin is approved by the European Union for GAD and approved by the FDA for seizure disorder and neuropathic pain. It is a category IV controlled medications but may have less addiction and abuse potential compared to benzodiazepines. As in MDD, antihistamines and a β-blocker can also be considered.

2. Posttraumatic stress disorder—The evidence for pharmacological treatment of patients with BD and PTSD is very limited. A recent systematic review of the impact of PSTD on BD treatment suggested that comorbid PTSD affects treatment response to lithium or quetiapine in patients with BD. Although SSRIs/SNRIs are the first-line medication for PTSD, patients with bipolar and PTSD should follow a "step-wise" approach as recommended for ADs by in the CANMAT and ISBD to minimize the risk of manic/hypomanic switching from SSRIs/SNRIs. Other antidepressants including mirtazapine and amitriptyline may also improve symptoms of PTSD. Prazosin can be added as an adjunctive medication when nightmares are present. There is no convincing evidence on the usefulness of the antipsychotic group compared to placebo as a group in PTSD, but atypical antipsychotics (aripiprazole and quetiapine) have been used in PTSD.

The most compelling evidence for treatment of PTSD is the use of trauma-focused therapies such as cognitive processing therapy, prolonged exposure therapy, EMDR, and others with trauma-focus therapies (Chapter 28). These approaches should be considered in patients with bipolar and PTSD. Additional medication use may be of assistance in treatment of symptomology, but benzodiazepines or other sedative hypnotic medications should be avoided because those medications may increase intrusive thoughts and dissociative symptoms over time. MDMA-assisted therapy may also be useful in BP and PTSD.

3. Obsessive-compulsive disorder—Similar to the treatment of PTSD in BD, patients with bipolar and OCD should follow a "step-wise" approach. SSRIs as the first-line medication for "pure" OCD should be used with caution after mood is stabilized. Adjunctive some second-generation antipsychotics may be beneficial in comorbid OCD. Clomipramine is still a gold standard treatment for non-comorbid OCD and should be considered if SSRIs are ineffective. Previous studies found that 42.1% of comorbid patients required a combination of multiple MS. Adding antidepressants to MS might lead clinical remission of both conditions. Some BD-OCD patients on MS therapy may benefit from adjunctive psychotherapy such as CBT and the ERP (Chapter 30).

4. Attention-deficit-hyperactivity disorder—According to the CANMAT Task Force in 2012, individuals with BD+ADHD, particularly those with BPI disorder, should be prescribed mood-stabilizing medications before initiating ADHD therapies. Bupropion is a reasonable first-line treatment for BD with ADHD, while mixed amphetamine salts and methylphenidate may be considered in patients determined to be at low risk for manic switch. Modafinil and CBT are second-line choices. However, behavioral therapy, cognitive training, neurofeedback, working memory training used in children and adolescents ADHD may also be beneficial to adult patients. For patients with comorbid ADHD and an AD, the ADHD should be treated after the depression and anxiety symptoms are under control although this is no evidence supporting this approach. For patients with ADHD and SUD, non-stimulant ADHD medication such as atomoxetine, guanfacine, and clonidine should be considered first. Literature from children and adolescents suggests that using a stimulant for comorbid ADHD with BD after mood stabilization did not increase the risk for manic or hypomanic switching.

5. Substance use disorder—The efficacy of MS monotherapy (lithium, VPA, LTG, quetiapine, risperidone, and aripiprazole), lithium plus VPA plus LTG, topiramate, naltrexone, acamprosate, and disulfiram was assessed in bipolar patients with comorbid AUD, cocaine use disorder, and/or cannabis use disorder. VPA showed efficacy in reducing alcohol use in euthymic bipolar I patients. Naltrexone may reduce craving for alcohol. Treatment with lithium plus VPA reduced substance use including alcohol, cannabis, and/or cocaine. Quetiapine monotherapy also reduce alcohol and alcohol use in patients with BD comorbid GAD and other psychiatric comorbidities including SUD. A systematic review of 16 studies including 3 with psychotherapy and 13 with pharmacotherapy (lithium, VPA, LTG, topiramate, naltrexone, acamprosate, disulfiram, quetiapine, and citicoline) found that VPA and naltrexone may decrease alcohol use and citicoline may decrease cocaine use and enhance cognition. Integrated psychosocial interventions are helpful in decreasing substance abuse (Chapters 16–23).

Bond DJ, Hadjipavlou G, Lam RW, et al. The Canadian Network for Mood and Anxiety Treatments (CANMAT) task force recommendations for the management of patients with mood disorders and comorbid attention-deficit/hyperactivity disorder. *Ann Clin Psychiatry*. 2012;24(1):23–37.

Catalá-López F, Hutton B, Núñez-Beltrán A, et al. The pharmacological and non-pharmacological treatment of attention deficit hyperactivity disorder in children and adolescents: a systematic review with network meta-analyses of randomised trials. *PLoS One*. 2017;12(7):e0180355.

Cullen C, Kappelmann N, Umer M, et al. Efficacy and acceptability of pharmacotherapy for comorbid anxiety symptoms in bipolar disorder: a systematic review and meta-analysis. *Bipolar Disord*. 2021;23(8):754–766.

Del Casale A, Sorice S, Padovano A, et al. Psychopharmacological treatment of obsessive-compulsive disorder (OCD). *Curr Neuropharmacol*. 2019;17(8):710–736.

Gao K, Wu R, Kemp DE, et al. Efficacy and safety of quetiapine-XR as monotherapy or adjunctive therapy to a mood stabilizer in acute bipolar depression with generalized anxiety disorder and other comorbidities: a randomized, placebo-controlled trial. *J Clin Psychiatry*. 2014;75(10):1062–1068.

Gao K, Arnold JG, Prihoda TJ, et al. Sequential Multiple Assignment Randomized Treatment (SMART) for bipolar disorder at any phase of illness and at least mild symptom severity. *Psychopharmacol Bull*. 202019;50(2):8–25.

Gao K, Ganocy SJ, Conroy C, et al. A placebo controlled study of quetiapine-XR in bipolar depression accompanied by generalized anxiety with and without a recent history of alcohol and cannabis use. *Psychopharmacology (Berl)*. 2017;234(15):2233–2244.

Kemp DE, Gao K, Ganocy SJ, et al. A 6-month, double-blind, maintenance trial of lithium monotherapy versus the combination of lithium and divalproex for rapid-cycling bipolar disorder and co-occurring substance abuse or dependence. *J Clin Psychiatry*. 2009;70(1):113–121.

Russell SE, Wrobel AL, Skvarc D, et al. The impact of posttraumatic stress disorder on pharmacologic intervention outcomes for adults with bipolar disorder: a systematic review. *Int J Neuropsychopharmacol*. 2023;26(1):61–69.

Salloum IM, Brown ES. Management of comorbid bipolar disorder and substance use disorders. *Am J Drug Alcohol Abuse*. 2017;43(4):366–376.

Schrader C, Ross A. A review of PTSD and current treatment strategies. *Mo Med*. 2021;118(6):546–551.

Yatham LN, Kennedy SH, Parikh SV, et al. Canadian Network for Mood and Anxiety Treatments (CANMAT) and International Society for Bipolar Disorders (ISBD) 2018 guidelines for the management of patients with bipolar disorder. *Bipolar Disord*. 2018;20(2):97–170.

B. Treatment of suicidality

As in MDD, suicidality in BD commonly occurs in the depressive phase of the illness and the severity of suicidality is commonly associated with depression severity and psychiatric comorbidities. In addition, the majority of completed suicide in patients with BD occurred when they are depressed. BD has the highest rate of suicide of all psychiatric conditions and is approximately 20–30 times that of the general population. Risk factors for suicide in bipolar patients include severe depression, male gender, living alone, divorced, no children, Caucasian, younger age (< 35 years), elderly age (> 75 years), unemployment, a personal history of suicide attempt, a family history of suicide attempt or suicide completion, a history of rapid-cycling BD, comorbid SUD, and comorbid ADs. Although ketamine treatment may reduce acute suicidality in BPD as in MDD, lithium remains the only medication associated with lowered suicide rates in BD. However, the effect of lithium in reducing suicide risk is a long-term effect. It is not very useful for patients with acute suicidality, and even contraindicated to patients with serious suicide intent. Early intervention and treatment with anti-suicidal medications, such as lithium, along with close observation and follow-up is the best way to mitigate suicidality in patients with BD. Studies have demonstrated that long-term treatment with lithium reduces suicide attempts by about 10% and deaths by suicide by about 20%. It appears crucial for lithium efficacy in suicide prevention to maintain the lithium blood concentrations in the efficient therapeutic zone. In addition, an anti-suicidal effect independent from mood change from lithium was also reported.

Benard V, Vaiva G, Masson M, et al. Lithium and suicide prevention in bipolar disorder. *Encephale*. 2016;42(3):234–241.

Gao K, Bai Y, Calabrese JR. Lithium and mood stabilizers. In: Nemeroff CB, Rasgon N, Schatzberg AF, Strakowski SM, eds. *The American Psychiatric Association Publishing Textbook of Mood Disorders*, 2nd ed. Washington DC; 2022:271–284.

Miller JN, Black DW. Bipolar disorder and suicide: a review. *Curr Psychiatry Rep*. 2020;22(2):6.

▶ Complications/Adverse Outcomes of Treatment

Compared to antidepressants, MSs have much more short- and long-term side effects. Acute sides effects from lithium such as gastrointestinal disturbances and tremor can be mitigated by slower dosing strategies. Worsening psoriasis, acne, and other skin/hair reactions may occur with lithium therapy. The severe adverse outcomes from lithium include polydipsia, polyuria, and toxicity. Acute adverse effects with DIV/VPA are usually mild, transient, and easily managed, but potential serious adverse effects such as irreversible hepatic failure, hemorrhagic pancreatitis, or hyperammonemic encephalopathy may occur. Patients may experience severe abdominal distress, confusion, or delirium. During the treatment with carbamazepine, liver transaminase elevations, rash, hyponatremia, and blood dyscrasias may complicate acute treatment. For LTG, rare cases of Stevens–Johnson syndrome, aseptic meningitis and hemophagocytic lymphohistiocytosis may have severe consequences.

For antipsychotics in acute use, somnolence and sedation are common side effects for most atypical antipsychotics, but akathisia from aripiprazole is the highest among atypicals. Weight gain and metabolic side effects, especially from olanzapine, risperidone, and quetiapine, are a major concern for long-term use. Compared to patients with MDD, patients with BD have a high risk of metabolic syndrome and cardiovascular related death. Tardive dyskinesia is also problematic for a small number of patients. For antidepressants and stimulants, TEM is a concern during the treatment of BPD and comorbidities.

▶ Prognosis

The prognosis of patients with BD based on DSM-5 criteria is not yet available. A study as a part of the NIMH Collaborative Depression Study through measuring the weekly affective symptom severity and polarity in BPI and BPII patients based on Research Diagnostic Criteria for up to 13 years found that both disorders were surprisingly chronic even with ongoing pharmacological and non-pharmacological treatments. About a half of the time were symptomatic with moderate severity (minor depression or hypomania) or subsyndromal affective symptoms. The subsyndromal symptoms were three times more common than symptoms at the syndromal level of MDE or manic/hypomanic episode. The availability of treatments appears to change the length of each episode. With the emergence of early intervention and successful treatment of the illness, the effects of kindling on outcome may have been interrupted, resulting in fewer episodes over time and reduced cycle length. However, longitudinal studies also observed that the availability of antidepressants, especially SSRIs and SNRIs, might significantly affect the length of between episodes, especially in the United States. The shortened intervals between episodes are speculated to be associated with the increased use of antidepressant monotherapy (kindling effect) in the United States as compared to European countries where lithium is still commonly used as the first-line medication for BD.

Early disease onset suggests poor prognosis. Patients who experience their initial episode in their late teens are likely to have a less favorable outcome than patients who experience their initial episode in their early 30s. Patients with early-onset BD should be quickly identified and aggressively treated. Comorbidity with SUD, ADHD, antisocial behavior, and personality disorders often complicates the clinical treatment and outcome. Substantial psychosocial morbidity can affect marriage, children, occupation, and other aspects of the patient's life. Divorce rates are two to three times higher in bipolar patients than in the general population, and occupational status is twice as likely to deteriorate. The suicide risk in BD is the highest among all psychiatric disorders. About 34% of patients attempted suicide and 15–20% completed suicide in their lifetime. On the other hand, patients in euthymia have a similar level of quality of life, enjoyment, and satisfaction as the general population.

Judd LL, Schettler PJ, Akiskal HS, et al. Long-term symptomatic status of bipolar I vs. bipolar II disorders. *Int J Neuropsychopharmacol.* 2003;6(2):127–137.

Anxiety Disorders

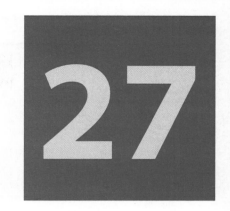

Richard C. Shelton, MD
Akhil Anand, MD

General Considerations

A. Epidemiology

Anxiety disorders are among the most common of psychiatric disorders, affecting up to 15% of the general population at any time (Table 27–1). Individual anxiety disorders occur frequently. Social anxiety disorder has a 13% lifetime prevalence, generalized anxiety disorder (GAD) about 6%, panic disorder about 5%, and agoraphobia about 3%. The comorbidity of anxiety disorders with one another is high. For example, 48–68% of adults with one anxiety disorder have another concurrent anxiety disorder (Lamers et al, 2011). The comorbidity of anxiety disorders with other psychiatric disorders is also high, as about 40% of individuals with primary anxiety disorders will have a lifetime history of major depressive disorder. Clinicians must be familiar with anxiety disorders because clinically significant anxiety is common in clinical practice.

B. Etiology

1. Psychodynamic theory—Traditional psychoanalytic theory describes anxiety disorders as being rooted in unconscious conflict. Freud originally used the term "Angst" (literally, "fear") to describe the simple intrapsychic response to either internal or external threat. He later derived the concept of the pleasure principle, which describes the tendency of the psychic apparatus to seek immediate discharge of impulses. In his earliest organized theory of anxiety, Freud postulated that conflicts or inhibitions result in the failure to dissipate libidinal (i.e., sexual) drives. These restrictions on sexual expression could occur because of external threat and would subsequently result in a fear of the loss of control of the drive. The damming up of the impulses, along with the fear of loss of control, would result in anxiety.

Freud soon began to see the limitations of this theory and later proposed that anxiety was central to the concept of neurosis. He acknowledged that anxiety was a natural, biologically derived response mechanism required for survival. He abandoned the concept of the transformation of sexual drive (energy) into anxiety and accepted the prevailing notion of the time: anxiety was a result of threat. He recognized two sources of such threat. The first, termed **traumatic situations**, involved stimuli that were too severe for the person to manage effectively and could be considered the common or natural fear response. The second, called **danger situations**, resulted from the recognition or anticipation of upcoming trauma, whether internal (by loss of control of drives) or external. The response to these threats resulted in what was called **signal anxiety**, which was an attenuated and therefore more manageable anxiety response not directly related to trauma. Signal anxiety could be seen as anxiety that resulted from the avoidance of threat.

The structural hypothesis of mental function—which includes the id as the seat of drives, the superego as the location of inhibitions, and the ego as the apparatus for managing drives and inhibitions—evolved during this time period. Central to this hypothesis is the concept of **defense mechanisms**. Psychological defenses are thought to be primarily a function of the ego, which uses these defenses to manage id impulses and superego demands. **Repression** is formulated as the primary defense mechanism, in which unacceptable drive states are maintained largely outside of awareness. Failure of repression could result in anxiety and the use of secondary mechanisms to maintain intrapsychic stability.

The concept of the primacy of the defense mechanism to both generate and manage the anxiety has remained central to psychoanalysis for much of its history. Further, psychoanalytic treatment has focused on the need to uncover childhood trauma, releasing unnecessary defensive inhibitions and developing psychological competence. A number of schools of thought have been elaborated from classical Freudian psychoanalysis, including ego psychology, object relations theory, and self-psychology (see Chapter 7).

Table 27–1 Anxiety Disorders

Separation anxiety disorder
Selective mutism
Specific phobia
Social anxiety disorder
Panic disorder
Panic attack (specifier)
Agoraphobia
Generalized anxiety disorder
Substance/medication-induced anxiety disorder
Anxiety disorder due to medical condition
Other specified anxiety disorder
Unspecified anxiety disorder

2. Learning theory—The basic principles of learning theory as they relate to human development are rooted in the work of developmental psychologists, especially Jean Piaget (see Chapter 8). Piaget's observations of children led to an understanding of the progress of development through a series of predictable stages, referred to as epigenesis. Developmental milestones represent an interaction between the maturing brain substrate and environmental influences. Hence, children learn according to both the capacity of the brain to manage incoming stimuli and the nature of the stimuli themselves. Appropriate environmental responses facilitate a normal learning process, and aberrant reactions produce problems in development.

As stimuli are assimilated and processed, learning takes place. Learning theory proposes two forms of learning: classical conditioning and operant conditioning (see Chapter 9). The classical conditioning model depends on the pairing of a stimulus that evokes a response (the unconditioned stimulus) with a neutral environmental object or event (the conditioned stimulus). The repeated pairing of the two stimuli would lead to the ability of the conditioned stimulus to elicit the same response as the unconditioned stimulus (the conditioned response).

Whereas classical conditioning views the organism as a relatively passive participant in the learning process, operant conditioning views stimuli as a series of either positive or negative events that influence subsequent behavior. Positive reinforcement occurs when a particular behavior results in a reward. Alternatively, negative reinforcement results when a specific behavior leads to the successful avoidance of an aversive event (i.e., punishment). Positive or negative reinforcements would then enhance the likelihood that the behavior would be repeated. Reinforcements of behaviors, whether they are achievements of rewards or avoidance of pain, underlie learning.

According to learning theory, an anxiety disorder develops when environmental cues become associated with anxiety-producing events during development. Within the construct

of GAD, for example, worry and fear become conditioned and are repeated in order to avoid intermittent negative reinforcement. Hence, the periodic successful avoidance of a negative outcome reinforces the behavior. For example, an individual's fear (and subsequent avoidance) of air travel would be enhanced by reading about occasional air disasters.

Traditional behavioral therapy of anxiety involves the uncoupling of the unconditioned response from the associated stimulus. Wolpe postulated that actions that inhibited anxiety (i.e., relaxation) in the face of the conditioned stimulus would reduce symptoms. Behavioral treatment of anxiety uses **systematic desensitization** (progressive exposure to an anxiety-evoking stimulus). This type of treatment has been used successfully to treat anxiety disorders such as phobias and obsessive-compulsive disorder (OCD), but it has had limited systematic study in other anxiety disorders.

3. Cognitive theory—In a subsequent elaboration of learning theory, a cognitive theory of the etiology of depressive and anxiety disorders has evolved (see Chapters 4, 9). Although several theories have been advanced, Beck's concept of the cognitive triad has gained the broadest acceptance and application. In this view, abnormal emotional states, such as anxiety and depression, are a result of distorted beliefs about the self, the world, and the future. Anxiety disorders, therefore, involve incorrect beliefs that interpret events in an exaggeratedly dangerous or threatening manner. These fundamental belief systems, or schemata, result in automatic thought responses to external or internal cues that trigger anxiety. As such, anxiety disorders consistently involve abnormalities of information processing that result in symptom formation.

Cognitive–behavioral therapy (CBT) involves elements of classical behavioral approaches such as systematic desensitization; however, treatment is extended to the discovery and correction of distorted cognitive schemata. The absence of exaggerated misinterpretations of cues leads to a reduction in symptom formation. Cognitive–behavioral psychotherapy has been used successfully to treat a variety of anxiety disorders, including panic disorder, phobias, and OCD.

4. Biological theories—From a biological standpoint, anxiety and fear have high adaptive value in all animals because they increase the animal's capacity for survival. The emotion of anxiety drives a number of highly adaptive behaviors, including escape from threat. The normal brain functions that underlie the anxiety response have been elucidated gradually over the past 50 years. The current understanding of the biological nature of anxiety has been prompted in part by an elucidation of the actions of drugs that reduce the symptoms of anxiety disorders. These observations can be divided into three broad areas: the gamma-aminobutyric acid (GABA) receptor/benzodiazepine receptor/chloride channel complex; the noradrenergic nucleus locus coeruleus and related brainstem nuclei; and the serotonin system, especially the raphe nuclei and their projections. Abnormalities in the functioning of these areas have been associated with various anxiety disorders.

Gray and colleagues have developed a general theory of a **neural behavioral-inhibition system** that mediates anxiety. The purpose of this system is to evaluate stimuli—consistent with punishment, non-reward, novelty, or fear—that simultaneously produce behavioral inhibition and increase arousal and attention. Antianxiety drugs inhibit responses in these areas. Using pharmacologic and lesioning studies, researchers have related anxiety to several interconnected anatomical areas. Sensory stimuli activate the hippocampus, especially the entorhinal cortex, which secondarily produces habituation by actions on the lateral and medial septal areas. Behavioral inhibition is achieved by projections to the cingulate gyrus. These areas are then influenced by noradrenergic activity of the locus coeruleus and are modulated both by serotonergic innervations from the raphe and by $GABA_A$-receptor activity. Antianxiety drugs work via mechanisms that influence these areas and receptors. These mechanisms include noradrenergic activation (e.g., tricyclic antidepressants), serotonergic activity (e.g., selective serotonin reuptake inhibitors [SSRIs] or buspirone), or benzodiazepine interactions with GABA receptors.

Acute threat results in fear, activating the "fight or flight" response. This, in turn, is mediated by brain regions such as the locus coeruleus and the amygdala. The amygdalae participate in the encoding of fearful memory and aversive conditioning; they are therefore involved in both acute fear and negative anticipatory expectation (i.e., anxiety).

Acute fear activates the sympathetic nervous system via the locus coeruleus, resulting in physical symptoms such as tachycardia, tremor, and diaphoresis. Awareness of fear occurs in the cortex, especially the frontal cortex that registers fear and responds with adaptive survival behaviors. The cingulate gyrus is also involved in the mediation of information between cortical and subcortical structures.

C. Genetics

Controlled family studies of the major subtypes of anxiety disorders, including panic disorder, phobic disorders, and GAD, reveal that all of these anxiety subtypes are familial, and twin studies suggest that the familial aggregation is attributable in part to genetic factors. Panic disorder and its spectrum show the strongest genetic determinants; half or more of persons with panic disorder have a family history of the disorder. Although there has been a plethora of studies designed to identify genes underlying these conditions, to date no specific genetic loci have been identified and replicated in independent samples. Due to genetic pleiotropy, the comorbidity of anxiety disorders with depressive disorders is high.

▶ Clinical Findings

A. Signs & Symptoms

Anxiety is a normal emotion, a common reaction to the stresses of everyday life. At what point does anxiety become pathologic? In order to make this distinction, one must define the key characteristics of the disorders and recognize that in pathologic anxiety, normal psychological adaptive processes have been overwhelmed to the point that daily functioning has been impaired. Anxiety disorders begin at the point of impairment. For example, everyone worries occasionally. When this worry begins to preoccupy a person's thoughts to the point that psychosocial functioning is impeded, an anxiety disorder may be diagnosed.

Anxiety is commonly associated with other medical or psychiatric conditions. Other conditions that give rise to anxiety have their own diagnostic categories: anxiety disorder due to medical condition and substance-induced anxiety disorder.

B. Psychological Testing

Psychological testing has not been shown to be useful in aiding the diagnosis of anxiety disorders.

C. Laboratory Findings

There are no laboratory findings suggesting or supporting the diagnosis of anxiety disorders, though there is evidence that a family or personal history of panic disorder may convey a liability to experience anxiety with carbon dioxide (CO_2) exposure.

D. Neuroimaging

Structural imaging is not helpful in studying anxiety disorders. However, functional neuroimaging studies in individuals with anxiety disorders have shown neurophysiological abnormalities during symptom provocation tests, implicating limbic, paralimbic, and sensory association regions.

▶ Course of Illness

Anxiety disorders often have a chronic course. They are frequently accompanied with other anxiety disorders and other psychiatric comorbidities; this is discussed in more detail in the paragraphs that follow.

▶ Differential Diagnosis (Including Comorbid Conditions)

These differential diagnoses, along with other psychiatric disorders that can manifest significant anxiety, are listed in Table 27–2.

Table 27–2 Differential Diagnosis of Anxiety Disorders

Medical Illnesses
Cardiac
Angina
Arrhythmias
Congestive failure
Infarction
Mitral valve prolapse
Supraventricular tachycardia
Endocrinologic
Hyperthyroidism
Cushing disease
Hyperparathyroidism
Hypoglycemia
Premenstrual dysphoric disorder
Neoplastic
Carcinoid
Insulinoma
Pheochromocytoma
Neurologic
Huntington disease
Meniere disease
Migraine
Multiple sclerosis
Seizure disorder
Transient ischemic attack
Vertigo
Wilson disease
Pulmonary
Asthma
Embolism
Obstruction
Obstructive pulmonary disease
Other
Porphyria
Psychiatric Disorders
Major depression
Developmental disorders (e.g., autism, Williams syndrome)
Dissociative disorders
Personality disorders
Somatoform disorders
Schizophrenia (and other psychotic disorders)
Substance Use/Misuse
Alcohol/sedative withdrawal
Antidepressants
Caffeine
Hallucinogen
Psychostimulants (e.g., methylphenidate, amphetamine)
Steroids (corticosteroids, anabolic steroids)
Stimulant abuse (e.g., cocaine)
Sympathomimetics (e.g., pseudoephedrine)

PANIC DISORDER AND PANIC ATTACKS

 General Considerations

A. Epidemiology

Panic disorder occurs in 5% of the population and is twice as common in women. Panic attacks are not specific to panic disorder and can occur in other psychiatric and physical conditions. Panic disorder has a bimodal distribution, with a peak onset in late adolescence and then again in the mid-30s. It is rare for panic disorder to start late for the first time in late life; if this is the case, a medical evaluation is warranted. Panic disorder in childhood may be underrecognized or misdiagnosed as conduct disorder or school avoidance. Children with panic disorder often exhibit considerable avoidance behavior with associated educational disability. Panic disorder may flare up in childhood, then become quiescent in the teenage years and early adult life, only to reemerge later.

B. Etiology

Although there have been many theories about the genesis of panic, two dominant (and not mutually exclusive) frameworks have been proposed. There is strong evidence to support a biological foundation. For example, some antidepressant and antianxiety drugs can block the attacks. Further, specific substances known as "panicogens" (e.g., intravenous sodium lactate or inhalation of 5–35% CO_2) can induce panic attacks in persons with panic disorder while sparing those without such a history. These agents collectively activate brainstem nuclei such as the locus coeruleus. Klein and colleagues have postulated that panic attacks are a result of a misperception of suffocation, referred to as a false suffocation response.

There also is support for a cognitive theory of the disorder. Persons with panic disorder often exhibit common cognitive characteristics, with a strong sensitivity to, and misinterpretation of, physical sensations. Cognitive theory suggests that mild physical symptoms are misinterpreted as dangerous. Cognitive–behavioral psychotherapy, with its emphasis on recognizing and correcting catastrophic thoughts, reduces both agoraphobic avoidance and the panic attacks themselves.

C. Genetics

Of all the major subtypes of anxiety disorders, panic disorder and its spectrum have the strongest familial clustering and genetic underpinnings; half or more of persons with panic disorder have a family history of the disorder. First-degree relatives of persons with panic disorder have a three- to fivefold elevation of risk of developing panic disorder, compared to the general population (Ströhle et al, 2018).

Clinical Findings

A. Signs & Symptoms

Although the symptoms of panic disorder have been described for over a century, and effective treatment has been available for more than 35 years, the disorder has been recognized widely for only about the past 30 years. Panic disorder is characterized by recurring, spontaneous, unexpected anxiety attacks with rapid onset and short duration. Because of the physical symptoms of the attacks, individuals are likely to fear that they are experiencing a heart attack, stroke, or the like. Occasionally they will think that they are going "crazy" or are "out of control." Individuals with panic disorder typically fear further attacks, worry about the implications of the attacks (e.g., that the attacks indicate a serious undiagnosed physical illness), and change their behavior as a result.

Panic attacks involve severe anxiety symptoms of rapid onset. These symptoms climb to maximum severity within 10 minutes but can peak within a few seconds. Typical symptoms include shortness of breath, tachypnea, tachycardia, tremor, dizziness, hot or cold sensations, chest discomfort, and feelings of depersonalization or derealization. A minimum of four symptoms is required to meet the diagnosis of panic attack. The symptoms usually last for less than 1 hour and most commonly diminish within 30 minutes. Majority of panic attacks occur during the daytime but nocturnal panic attacks do occur and are related to greater distress and functional impairment (Nakamura et al, 2013).

People who experience a panic attack will usually seek help, often at a hospital emergency room. Although this condition is readily diagnosable by clinical signs and symptoms, most cases are not diagnosed initially. This is unfortunate because early detection and treatment can usually prevent disability. Left untreated, the panic attacks will likely continue.

B. Laboratory Findings

A number of studies have shown that individuals with panic disorder have greater anxiety responses to the inhalation of enhanced CO_2 mixtures than do controls or those with other psychiatric illnesses. There is also evidence that well subjects at high risk for panic disorder (i.e., subjects with a family but no personal history of panic disorder) experience more anxiety following CO_2 exposure than do subjects without such history.

C. Neuroimaging

There is emerging evidence that 5-HT_{1A}-receptor binding is reduced in some patients with panic disorder.

Course of Illness

The course of panic disorder is usually chronic and fluctuating. The long-term prognosis is okay with high rates of symptom improvement at 75% over 3 years. However, over the same period, complete functional recovery is only 12% (Nay et al, 2013). It is important that panic disorder be treated as early as possible and that close attention be given to comorbid disorders, especially depression, as they are known to negatively affect outcome.

Differential Diagnosis (Including Comorbid Conditions)

Panic disorder shares features with other mental disorders. Persons with OCD, specific and social phobias, posttraumatic stress disorder, major depression, psychotic disorders, and some personality disorders (e.g., avoidant, paranoid, dependent, schizoid) exhibit social avoidance. These disorders, however, do not share the features of spontaneous panic attacks. The absence of spontaneous panic attacks also distinguishes other disorders with somatic fears including obsessive–compulsive spectrum disorders (e.g., somatic obsessions and body dysmorphic disorder), GAD, and somatization disorders. Although persons with specific and social phobias may have situationally bound panic attacks, recurring unexpected panic attacks do not occur.

Although the diagnosis is usually straightforward, many patients with panic disorder undergo extensive, unnecessary medical evaluation. Some differential diagnostic possibilities for panic attacks include paroxysmal atrial tachycardia, pulmonary embolus, seizure disorder, Meniere disease, transient ischemic attack, carcinoid syndrome, Cushing disease, hyperthyroidism, true hypoglycemia, and pheochromocytoma. Extensive medical evaluation for these disorders is indicated in older-onset (Giacobbe and Flint, 2018) and only when other features suggest physical disease (see Table 27–2).

Treatment

A. Psychopharmacologic Interventions

Panic in mildly ill patients often requires no medication and can be managed with psychotherapy alone. Behavioral or CBT is the treatment of choice (see also Chapter 10). Medications in combination with psychotherapy should be reserved for more severely ill individuals.

Medication should be considered if the panic disorder impairs functioning, for example, (1) if agoraphobia is present or developing, (2) if major depression (currently or by history) or a personality disorder is present, (3) if the patient reports significant suicidal ideation, or (4) if the patient voices a strong preference for medication management. The last option is intended to strengthen therapeutic alliance and to encourage the patient's involvement in therapy. Many patients with panic disorder fear behavioral therapy because of the need for exposure to the phobic stimuli.

Tricyclic antidepressants are effective for panic. However, the side effect profile is such that they are rarely used.

Table 27–3 Drugs Used for the Treatment of Panic Disorder

Drug	Starting Dosage	Dosing Range	Common Side Effects
Imipramine (or other tricyclic antidepressants)	25 mg at bedtime	50–200 mg	Dry mouth, blurred vision, constipation, urinary hesitancy, orthostasis, somnolence, anxiety, sexual dysfunction
Phenelzine	15 mg twice daily	30–90 mg	Dry mouth, drowsiness, nausea, anxiety/nervousness, orthostatic hypotension, myoclonus, hypertensive reactions
Paroxetine	20 mg	20–60 mg	Nausea, diarrhea, anxiety/nervousness, sexual dysfunction, somnolence
Sertraline	50 mg	50–200 mg	Nausea, diarrhea, anxiety/nervousness, sexual dysfunction
Alprazolam	0.25–0.5 mg	0.25–1.5 mg three times daily	Somnolence, ataxia, memory problems, physical dependence, withdrawal reactions
Clonazepam	0.25–0.5 mg	0.25–2.0 mg twice daily	Somnolence, ataxia, memory problems, physical dependence, withdrawal reactions
Venlafaxine	37.5 mg	37.5–225 mg	Diarrhea, anxiety/nervousness, sexual dysfunction, withdrawal reactions

The physician must warn patients about the potential for the development of transient anxiety, along with other side effects (Table 27–3). The dosage should start low and be titrated upward slowly. High plasma levels appear to worsen outcome.

Imipramine, amitriptyline, and clomipramine have reasonable empirical support for their effectiveness. Other drugs such as nortriptyline or doxepin have limited support. There is some evidence that other antidepressants, such as desipramine, maprotiline, and bupropion, are less effective than imipramine.

The monoamine oxidase inhibitors, especially phenelzine, have relatively strong empirical support. Like tricyclics, phenelzine reduces the frequency and intensity of panic attacks. It also appears to have a substantial antianxiety and antiphobic effect. Unfortunately, the effectiveness of phenelzine is limited by its side effects and safety problems. Besides the side effects listed in Table 27–3, hypertensive reactions can occur when the patient's diet has a high tyramine content. Further, toxicity can be produced when this drug is taken with other agents, such as meperidine or sympathomimetic amines. Although such toxic effects can generally be avoided, those with panic disorder are especially fearful of them.

Research data support the effectiveness of SSRIs antidepressants, including paroxetine, sertraline, and the selective norepinephrine reuptake inhibitor venlafaxine extended release, in the treatment of panic disorder. These drugs have become the standard for pharmacological management and have supplanted other antidepressants and benzodiazepines in the treatment of panic disorder; however, in standard antidepressant dosages, these drugs may not be tolerated because of increased anxiety. Dosages should be started low and titrated upward slowly.

Low-dose benzodiazepine management can be used on an as-needed basis to reduce anticipatory anxiety and to facilitate exposure activities. Though virtually any benzodiazepine can be used successfully in this way, the high-potency benzodiazepines alprazolam and clonazepam have specific antipanic effects. Within the usual dosing range, most patients with panic experience a substantial reduction in both panic attacks and in anticipatory anxiety.

Although the likelihood of benzodiazepine abuse is relatively low if the drug is administered acutely in carefully selected patients, benzodiazepines should be avoided in patients with a history of alcohol or drug abuse. However, nearly all patients eventually develop some degree of physical dependency in the case of continuous use. On taper or discontinuation, classical withdrawal effects can occur, such as a rebound return of panic symptoms. Many patients find it very difficult to withdraw completely. As many as 60% will stay on these medications indefinitely. Moderate- to high-dose benzodiazepine therapy should be reserved for patients who require pharmacotherapy and who have failed on antidepressant treatment, for those who are unable to tolerate antidepressants, or for those for whom antidepressant medications are otherwise inappropriate.

The medications discussed in this section generally reduce the intensity and frequency of panic symptoms as long as they are taken. After discontinuation, most patients relapse. Relapse often occurs during dosage tapering, even with benzodiazepines. As a result, behavioral or CBT with exposure should be combined with pharmacotherapy.

B. Psychotherapeutic Interventions

A variety of therapies have been used to treat panic disorder. Only traditional behavioral treatments and cognitive–behavioral psychotherapy have significant empirical evidence to support their effectiveness. Considerable evidence supports the effectiveness of CBT for treatment of panic disorder. This approach helps patients to recognize the relationships between specific thoughts (i.e., cognitions) and the anxiety that they produce. These thoughts represent misinterpretations of external, or more commonly internal, cues as being threatening. For example, feeling mildly short of breath, slightly tremulous, or having a small increase in heart rate can be misinterpreted as an indication that a catastrophic physical event (e.g., heart attack) is occurring. Successful treatment, then, would help the patient to discover the true relationship between specific internal or external cues and their anxiety and to correctly interpret the cues as benign.

C. Other Interventions

An elaboration of CBT includes **interoceptive exposure** as part of the treatment. This method uses experimental manipulations of physical sensations to induce symptoms that are commonly misinterpreted. Exposure techniques may include spinning in place, hyperventilating voluntarily, or ingesting large amounts of caffeine in order to simulate the physical cues that stimulate anxiety. This technique helps the therapist to uncover the catastrophic cognitions and helps the client to interpret them correctly.

The last component of CBT of panic disorder involves more traditional relaxation and exposure activities, in which patients gradually and systematically expose themselves to situations that induce anxiety, thereby desensitizing themselves.

▶ Complications/Adverse Outcomes of Treatment

Complications and adverse outcomes related to the various biological interventions have been detailed in the preceding paragraphs, where emphasis was given to complications specific to various therapeutic intervention strategies.

▶ Prognosis

Overall, the long-term prognosis for panic disorder is good, although a significant proportion of patients are likely to develop disability if the condition is not treated soon after the occurrence of the first attack. Major depression occurs in about 40% of patients. Although both depression and panic symptoms respond to antidepressant drugs, comorbid depression worsens the outcome of panic disorder and increases the rate of suicide. About 7% of patients with panic disorder commit suicide, and more than 20% of patients with panic disorder and comorbid psychiatric disorders will eventually commit suicide. Substance abuse, especially alcoholism, also occurs at an increased frequency in patients with panic disorder relative to the general population.

Bakker A, van Balkom AJ, Stein DJ. Evidence-based pharmacotherapy of panic disorder. *Int J Neuropsychopharmacol.* 2005;8:473.

Coryell W, Pine D, Fyer A, Klein D. Anxiety responses to CO_2 inhalation in subjects at high-risk for panic disorder. *J Affect Disord.* 2006;92:63–70.

Giacobbe P, Flint A. Diagnosis and management of anxiety disorders. *Continuum (Minneap Minn).* 2018 Jun;24(3, BEHAVIORAL NEUROLOGY AND PSYCHIATRY):893–919. doi: 10.1212/CON.0000000000000607. PMID: 29851884.

Hirschfeld RM. Panic disorder: diagnosis, epidemiology, and clinical course. *J Clin Psychiatry.* 1996;57(Suppl 10):3.

Katon W. Panic disorder: relationship to high medical utilization, unexplained physical symptoms, and medical costs. *J Clin Psychiatry.* 1996;57(Suppl 10):11.

Lamers F, van Oppen P, Comijs HC, et al. Comorbidity patterns of anxiety and depressive disorders in a large cohort study: the Netherlands Study of Depression and Anxiety (NESDA). *J Clin Psychiatry.* 2011;72:341–348. [PubMed: 21294994]

Merikangas KR, Low NC. Genetic epidemiology of anxiety disorders. *Handb Exp Pharmacol.* 2005;169:163–179.

Nakamura M, Sugiura T, Nishida S, et al. Is nocturnal panic a distinct disease category? Comparison of clinical characteristics among patients with primary nocturnal panic, daytime panic, and coexistence of nocturnal and daytime panic. *J Clin Sleep Med.* 2013;9(5):461–467. doi:10.5664/jcsm.2666.

Nay W, Brown R, Roberson-Nay R. Longitudinal course of panic disorder with and without agoraphobia using the National Epidemiologic Survey on Alcohol and Related Conditions (NESARC). *Psychiatry Res.* 2013;208(1):54–61. doi:10.1016/j.psychres.2013.03.006.

Pollack MH, Otto MW. Long-term course and outcome of panic disorder. *J Clin Psychiatry.* 1997;58(Suppl 2):57.

Rosenbaum JF, Pollock RA, Otto MW, Pollack MH. Integrated treatment of panic disorder. *Bull Menninger Clin.* 1995;59(2 Suppl A):A54.

Ströhle A, Gensichen J, Domschke K. The diagnosis and treatment of anxiety disorders. *Dtsch Arztebl Int.* 2018 Sep 14;155(37):611–620. doi: 10.3238/arztebl.2018.0611. PMID: 30282583; PMCID: PMC6206399.

Twelve-month and lifetime prevalence and lifetime morbid risk of anxiety and mood disorders in the United States—PubMed (nih.gov)

AGORAPHOBIA

▶ General Considerations

A. Epidemiology

In DSM-V, agoraphobia was made a distinct anxiety disorder; before this, it was considered a subtype classifier for panic disorder; which meant that agoraphobia could be diagnosed only within the context of panic disorder or as the result of panic attacks or panic-like symptoms.

Because of the recent divergence from panic disorder, there is disparity between the prevalence of agoraphobia; prevalence is estimated between 1.3 and 3%. The prevalence is higher in older adults (>65 years) at 10.4%. The annual incidence rate of agoraphobia is 0.9%. Women are twice as likely as men to experience agoraphobia.

B. Etiology

Individuals with agoraphobia have a high rate of comorbidity with panic attacks and panic disorder. But the relationship between agoraphobia and panic disorder changes throughout the lifetime. Young adults with agoraphobia typically present with panic attacks and panic disorder. Whereas older persons with agoraphobia generally do not have a history of panic disorder or panic attacks, they typically develop agoraphobia following the onset of a physical illness (e.g., vertigo, Parkinson disease) or traumatic event (e.g., fall) (Ritchie et al, 2013). Extraversion is considered a protective factor of agoraphobia, whereas neuroticism is a risk factor. Other personality factors including, anxiety sensitivity, and avoidant and dependent personality traits, are associated with agoraphobia. Other etiologic factors associated with agoraphobia include parental overprotectiveness, traumatic childhood experiences, and early bereavement or grief (Tearnan et al, 1984).

C. Genetics

The estimated heritability for agoraphobia is 61%. A family history of anxiety disorders is associated with earlier onset of agoraphobia; a family history of panic disorder particularly increases the risk of agoraphobia.

▶ Clinical Findings

A. Signs & Symptoms

The essential feature of agoraphobia is fear or anxiety that is out of proportion to the actual specific situation. The fear or anxiety must occur in more than one setting. The amount of fear or anxiety is variable but may become a limited- or full-symptom panic attack. The individual will behaviorally and cognitively avoid these situations, impacting their functioning. The symptoms are persistent and must last for at least 6 months. In severe cases of agoraphobia, the individual may be completely homebound.

▶ Neuroimaging

Functional neuroimaging studies in these individuals reveal hyperactivation of the ventral striatum and insula when they are anticipating agoraphobia specific situations (Wittmann et al, 2014).

▶ Course of Illness

The course of agoraphobia is usually chronic and persisting. Without treatment, remission is rare.

▶ Differential Diagnosis (Including Comorbid Conditions)

Agoraphobia is most associated with specific phobias. The difference is that a specific phobia is fear or anxiety related to one situation. Separation anxiety disorder, social anxiety, panic disorder, acute stress disorder or posttraumatic stress disorder, and major depressive disorder are also in the differential.

▶ Treatment

Making a diagnosis between panic disorder with comorbid agoraphobia and agoraphobia alone is important for clinical management because, unlike panic disorder, there is no effective pharmacotherapy for agoraphobia; the treatment of choice is in vivo exposure and CBT.

▶ Complications/Adverse Outcomes of Treatment

Individuals with agoraphobia are likely to self-medicate to address their symptoms; these individuals are particularly susceptible to misusing sedating agents like alcohol and other anxiolytics and hypnotics. Agoraphobia is also associated with an increased risk of developing comorbid major depression, panic, and other anxiety disorders.

▶ Prognosis

As mentioned earlier, agoraphobia is a persistent and chronic condition. Without treatment, complete remission is rare; the remission rate is 10%. The prognosis is worse if the individual has a more severe form, an earlier onset, another anxiety disorder, a co-occurring mood disorder, and co-occurring substance use disorder.

PHOBIC DISORDERS: SPECIFIC PHOBIA & SOCIAL PHOBIA (SOCIAL ANXIETY DISORDER)

▶ General Considerations

A. Epidemiology

Phobic disorders are among the most common of all psychiatric disorders. Specific phobia affects 5–10% of the general population, and social phobia (also referred to as social anxiety disorder) affects about 3%. The onset is typically in childhood or early adulthood, and the condition is usually chronic. Many people with specific phobias learn to "live around" the feared stimulus. Social phobia is often more disabling.

B. Etiology

Phobic disorders may develop because of a pairing of anxiety with specific environmental events or experiences. For example, emotional trauma accompanying experiences such as riding in a car or speaking in public may produce a phobia. However, most individuals with these problems do not report that particular events have led to the disorder. Under these circumstances, the etiology is unknown.

Clinical Findings

A. Signs & Symptoms

A specific phobia is an intense, irrational fear or aversion to a particular object or situation, other than a social situation. Typical specific phobias are fears of animals (especially insects or spiders); the natural environment (e.g., storms); blood, injection, or injury; or situations (e.g., heights, closed places, elevators, airplane travel). Most people deal with this problem by avoiding the feared stimulus, although this is not always possible. For example, people who fear of insects or spiders may avoid basements, attics, or closets; however, the emotional reactions or avoidance behavior may cause more serious problems. People who fear flying may be unable to perform certain kinds of work. People with blood–injection–injury phobia may experience vasodilation, bradycardia, orthostatic hypotension, or fainting on exposure.

Social phobia is characterized by an extreme anxiety response in situations in which the affected person may be observed by others. People with social phobia usually fear that they will act in an embarrassing or humiliating manner. As with a specific phobia, social situations are avoided or endured with severe anxiety. Common phobic situations include speaking in public, eating in public, using public restrooms, writing while others observe, and performing publicly. Rarely do people with this condition suffer from generalized social phobia, in which most or all social situations are avoided.

Neuroimaging

Functional neuroimaging studies have shown that CBT in patients with phobic disorders resulted in decreased activity in limbic and paralimbic areas; it is noteworthy that similar effects were observed after successful intervention with SSRIs.

Course of Illness

Relatively little is known about the long-term course of phobic disorders; however, untreated phobic disorders often are chronic conditions.

Differential Diagnosis (Including Comorbid Conditions)

In phobic disorders, anxiety or fear is restricted to a particular object or situation. Panic disorder, by definition, is characterized by severe, unexpected anxiety attacks during at least some phase of the disorder. This condition is differentiated by anxiety that occurs in situations in which help might not be available in case of a panic attack.

Avoidant personality disorder shares many features—and is often comorbid—with social phobia. The generalized form of social phobia is especially difficult to distinguish from avoidant personality. An avoidant personality disorder is in many ways equivalent to pathologic shyness; like social phobia, an avoidant personality disorder is usually associated with a fear of being shamed or ridiculed; however, in social phobia the fear is often confined to performance situations, with a relative sparing of other social interactions. For example, a person with social phobia may find it quite impossible to speak or write in public, whereas they could conduct a casual conversation without difficulty. This would not be true of someone with avoidant personality disorder.

People with psychotic disorders may experience abnormal fears and avoid others, but delusional beliefs characterize these. Patients with somatoform disorders (e.g., hypochondriasis) may exhibit anxiety and avoidance that can be confused with phobic disorders. However, unlike patients with somatoform disorder, those with specific or social phobias retain insight into the irrationality of their condition. For example, in major depression, social avoidance is common, but not related to performance anxiety. Persons with OCD may also avoid situations to prevent the stimulation of obsessions and compulsions. However, compulsive behaviors typically do not occur in phobic disorders.

Treatment

A. Psychopharmacologic Interventions

Although treatments for phobic disorders typically are psychotherapeutic, some drug treatments have been used (Table 27–4). Benzodiazepines are sometimes used to reduce the anxiety associated with specific and social phobias. β-Blockers such as propranolol have been used with success to reduce the autonomic hyperarousal and tremor associated with performance situations. β-Blockers can also be helpful in blood–injection–injury phobia. These medications all have attendant side effects and are often unnecessary because behavioral treatments are so effective. Controlled clinical trials have shown antidepressants, particularly the SSRIs, to be beneficial in treating social phobia.

B. Psychotherapeutic Interventions

Behavioral or cognitive–behavioral psychotherapies are the treatments of choice. A typical treatment regimen involves relaxation training, usually coupled with visualization of the phobic stimulus, followed by progressive desensitization through repeated controlled exposure to the phobic cue. This regimen is generally followed by the extinction of the anxiety response. A cognitive–behavioral approach adds the dimension of managing the catastrophic thoughts associated with exposure to the situation.

Table 27–4 Pharmacologic Treatment of Social Phobia

Drug	Starting Dosage	Dosing Range	Common Side Effects
Paroxetine	20 mg	20–60 mg	Nausea, diarrhea, anxiety/nervousness, sexual dysfunction, somnolence
Sertraline	50 mg	50–200 mg	Nausea, diarrhea, anxiety/nervousness, sexual dysfunction

▷ Complications/Adverse Outcomes of Treatment

Specific and social phobias are common and relatively benign conditions compared to panic disorder. Many people experience specific fears but learn to live around them. Most people with phobias avoid situations in which they may be exposed to a phobic stimulus. However, phobias occasionally have a disabling effect. For example, a business executive with a fear of public speaking or flying may find that phobia restricts their ability to benefit from career advancement. Although behavioral treatments may be anxiety provoking, they often produce significant results. Some individuals use substances of misuse, especially alcohol, to endure their anxiety; therefore, a careful alcohol and drug history is important in evaluating patients with phobic disorders.

▷ Prognosis

Relatively little is known about the long-term course of phobic disorders; however, untreated, phobias often are chronic conditions.

American Psychiatric Association. *Diagnostic and Statistical Manual of Mental Disorders* (5th ed., text rev.). 2022. https://doi.org/10.1176/appi.books.9780890425787

Blanco C, Raza MS, Schneier FR, Liebowitz MR. The evidence-based pharmacological treatment of social anxiety disorder. *Int J Neuropsychopharmacol.* 2003;6:427.

Curtis GC et al. Specific fears and phobias. Epidemiology and classification. *Br J Psychiatry.* 1998;173:212.

Marks I. Blood-injury phobia: a review. *Am J Psychiatry.* 1988;145:1207.

Rapaport MH, Paniccia G, Judd LL. A review of social phobia. *Psychopharmacol Bull.* 1995;31:125.

Ritchie K, Norton J, Mann A, Carrière I, Ancelin ML. Late-onset agoraphobia: general population incidence and evidence for a clinical subtype. *Am J Psychiatry.* 2013 Jul;170(7):790–798. doi: 10.1176/appi.ajp.2013.12091235. PMID: 23820832.

Tearnan BH, Telch MJ, Keefe P. Etiology and onset of agoraphobia: a critical review. *Compr Psychiatry.* 1984 Jan-Feb;25(1):51–62. doi: 10.1016/0010-440x(84)90022-1. PMID: 6141894

Wittmann A, Schlagenhauf F, Guhn A, et al. Anticipating agoraphobic situations: the neural correlates of panic disorder with agoraphobia. *Psychol Med.* 2014 Aug;44(11):2385–2396. doi: 10.1017/S0033291713003085. Epub 2014 Jan 7. PMID: 24398049.

GENERALIZED ANXIETY DISORDER

▷ General Considerations

A. Epidemiology

GAD typically begins in early adulthood, is slightly more common in women, and is usually chronic. Although GAD is rather common, it is seen more often in general medical practice than in psychiatry practice. Patients with GAD typically experience persistent worry of variable severity over time, often leading them to their primary care clinician. Continuity of care across time is critical to recognizing and treating this disorder. Further, patients with GAD have a high rate of comorbidity with major depression. GAD comes closest to the classic concept of anxiety neurosis. GAD may be associated with an emotionally reactive temperament (traditionally referred to as neuroticism). The emotionally reactive temperament has a significant genetic component and may predispose to various anxiety or depressive disorders.

B. Genetics

There is emerging evidence from family studies that GAD exhibits a mild to moderate familial aggregation; this holds if subjects are self-selected or are recruited from a clinical or community setting. Twin studies also indicate that GAD is moderately heritable.

▷ Clinical Findings

A. Signs & Symptoms

GAD is a syndrome of persistent worry coupled with symptoms of hyperarousal. Often, patients with GAD do not recognize themselves as having a psychiatric disorder, even though the symptoms can be quite disabling. As a result, these patients are much more likely to present in a general medical setting than in a psychiatrist's office. For this reason, primary care clinicians must be particularly sensitive to patients' emotional needs.

B. Neuroimaging

A study using proton magnetic resonance spectroscopy has demonstrated that GAD can be associated with asymmetric increases in the N-acetyl aspartate–creatine ratio, a suggested marker of neuronal viability, in the (right dorsolateral) prefrontal cortex.

Differential Diagnosis (Including Comorbid Conditions)

Persistent hyperarousal coupled with obsessive thoughts are common to other psychiatric disorders (e.g., major depression). In some ways, GAD could be considered to be major depression without persistently depressed mood or anhedonia (see Chapter 17). In fact, GAD often responds well to treatment with tricyclic antidepressants, as discussed later in this chapter. If the patient worries chronically, depression should always be considered in the differential diagnosis. Other psychiatric disorders with obsessive thinking (e.g., OCD; panic disorder; somatoform disorders; psychotic disorders, especially paranoid subtypes; eating disorders, particularly anorexia nervosa; and many personality disorders) are associated with persistent fear, apprehension, or worry that can be confused with GAD. The focus of the worry should not be related primarily to one of these conditions. For example, if a patient fears the occurrence of a panic attack, the obvious cause of the problem is panic disorder, even if other associated worries (e.g., personal health or well-being of a significant other) are present. Similarly, if the central concern is physical health, without panic attacks, then somatoform disorder is likely to be the primary diagnosis.

Treatment

The management of GAD should consider the longstanding nature of the problem. Treatment should deal with the underlying causes of the condition, such as persistently distorted cognitions. Unfortunately, several factors work against treatment. GAD tends to be under-recognized. Even when it is identified, the problem is often not taken as seriously as the degree of disability associated with the condition would suggest. If treatment is provided, it is likely to be brief. Finally, insurance coverage tends to discriminate against the treatment of GAD. Together, these factors conspire to ensure that most patients with GAD do not get appropriate treatment.

A. Psychopharmacologic Interventions

Patients with GAD are likely to receive benzodiazepines, even though psychotherapies and other medications are clearly beneficial. Although benzodiazepines reduce symptoms, GAD is a chronic condition and benzodiazepines are not curative. If benzodiazepines alone are used, long-term management is required to prevent symptoms from returning. Benzodiazepines generally should not be used alone to treat GAD, but they can be helpful adjuncts to treatment, particularly when the symptoms are severe. Short-term, low-to-moderate dosages of benzodiazepines can facilitate psychotherapy. Benzodiazepines can also be used to reduce symptoms and to return the patient to normal functioning. After a few weeks, the benzodiazepine should be reduced and eventually discontinued.

Most clinicians worry about the potential for benzodiazepine abuse. Epidemiologic studies, however, demonstrate that legitimate clinical use far outweighs any abuse. True abuse is relatively uncommon. Benzodiazepine abuse is seen most often when they are used to (1) counteract the adverse effects of psychostimulants such as cocaine; (2) augment the euphoric effects of other sedative drugs such as alcohol; or (3) self-medicate alcohol or other sedative withdrawal.

Benzodiazepines should not be given to patients who have a personal history or strong first-degree family history of drug or alcohol abuse. Even though the primary abuse of benzodiazepines is uncommon, some patients develop psychological and physiologic dependence. Physiologic dependence becomes an increasing problem when benzodiazepines have been given continuously for 3 months or more, although mild withdrawal reactions can occur after shorter treatment periods. Clinicians who are considering treating GAD with benzodiazepines should first weigh the alternatives (described later in this section). In general, brief, interrupted courses of benzodiazepine treatment should be given as psychotherapeutic management is being initiated; prescription refills should be monitored carefully; and the drug should then be tapered if continuous use exceeds 1 month. Problems can generally be avoided under these circumstances.

Benzodiazepines can produce other adverse effects, such as daytime sedation, ataxia (which can cause dangerous falls in older persons), accident proneness (e.g., motor vehicle accidents), headaches, memory problems (ranging from short-term memory problems to brief periods of profound memory loss), and occasionally, paradoxical excitement or anxiety. These problems are especially prominent in older persons, whose reduced metabolism means that drug metabolites can accumulate, resulting in high plasma levels.

The anxiolytic buspirone, a serotonin$_{1A}$ receptor partial agonist, is an alternative to benzodiazepines (Table 27–5). Buspirone has several advantages. It produces no motor, memory, or concentration impairments. It has no abuse potential, and it does not cause dependency or withdrawal, even after long periods of exposure. It does not produce drug interactions. It appears to be an almost ideal anxiolytic; however, it has some disadvantages. In contrast to the benzodiazepines, which are often experienced by patients as having an immediate effect, buspirone requires at least 3 weeks to mitigate anxiety. Patients with severe anxiety, especially those who previously received benzodiazepines, may have a reduced level of response. Further, buspirone stimulates the locus coeruleus, which may be associated with a paradoxical increase in anxiety in some patients. Despite these disadvantages, buspirone should be considered a practical alternative to benzodiazepines.

The tricyclic antidepressant imipramine and the heterocyclic antidepressant venlafaxine have demonstrated significant benefit in the treatment of GAD. Like buspirone, the therapeutic effect is delayed, but severely anxious patients appear

Table 27–5 Pharmacologic Treatment of Generalized Anxiety Disorder

Drug	Starting Dosage	Dosing Range	Common Side Effects
Buspirone	5 mg three times	15–60 mg daily	Anxiety/nervousness, headache, nausea
Imipramine	25 mg at bedtime	25–200 mg	Dry mouth, blurred vision, constipation, urinary hesitancy, orthostasis, somnolence, anxiety
Venlafaxine	37.5 mg daily	37.5–225 mg daily	Anxiety/nervousness, diarrhea, sexual dysfunction, withdrawal reactions
Benzodiazepines	—	—	Somnolence, ataxia, memory (various) problems, nausea, physical dependence, withdrawal reactions

to improve. Other tricyclic antidepressants or SSRIs may be helpful but have not been tested adequately. β-Blockers and clonidine have been reported to be helpful in treating GAD. Although these drugs can reduce anxiety, side effects of hypotension and depression are prominent. Antipsychotic drugs, such as chlorpromazine or haloperidol, reduce anxiety, but the risk of tardive dyskinesia outweighs the potential benefit.

B. Psychotherapeutic Interventions

Two psychotherapeutic approaches are helpful in treating GAD. Behavioral therapy can teach patients progressive deep muscle relaxation while they imagine anxiety-inducing stimuli. If the patient avoids situations that generate significant anxiety, progressive desensitization can be helpful.

An alternative is CBT. This treatment adds a cognitive component to basic behavioral therapy on the assumption that the anxiety associated with GAD is a result of persistent distortions about the self, other people, and the future. Misinterpretations, especially catastrophic misperceptions of threat or danger, contribute significantly to anxiety. CBT helps patients to recognize the relationships between specific situations and pathogenic distortions of thinking. Further, the treatment helps to elucidate the faulty fundamental belief systems that underlie the distorted thinking. Patients learn to recognize and counter the distortions with alternative thoughts that eventually become automatic.

C. Other Interventions

Other interventions may be needed, such as marital, family, or occupational therapy. Other primary therapies (e.g., psychodynamic, client-centered, or interpersonal therapy) have little or no empirical support.

▶ Complications/Adverse Outcomes of Treatment

GAD is a highly comorbid condition. The most common comorbid diagnosis is major depression. As noted earlier in this chapter, diagnostic primacy may shift frequently across the patient's lifetime in a more chronic neurotic pattern

between the more typical depressive and anxious symptoms. GAD may be comorbid with other conditions, including personality disorders (e.g., obsessive–compulsive, schizoid, histrionic, avoidant) or other anxiety disorders (e.g., OCD, panic disorder). The diagnosis of GAD should be given only if the diagnosis is clearly independent of other Axis I or Axis II disorders. For example, the diagnosis would not be given to a patient who has a history of persistent anxiety or worry occurring only in the context of major depression. Similarly, the diagnosis is excluded if the worries or fears are clearly related to the pattern of OCD, social phobia, or panic disorder. However, the diagnosis can be given if the symptoms of GAD predate the onset of these other conditions or are otherwise definitely temporally independent. Because the frequency of comorbidity is high, the existence of comorbid disorders should be examined whenever the diagnosis of GAD is considered.

▶ Prognosis

Untreated, GAD typically follows a chronic pattern, with waxing and waning severity. Comorbid conditions may contribute to chronicity. Pharmacologic treatments will relieve symptoms, but the syndrome usually reemerges after treatment has been discontinued. Psychotherapeutic management (with or without symptomatic treatment with medications) often is helpful in reducing the chronicity associated with GAD.

Barlow DH, Wincze J. DSM-IV and beyond: what is generalized anxiety disorder? *Acta Psychiatr Scand*. 1998;393(Suppl):23.

Chambless DL, Gillis MM. Cognitive therapy of anxiety disorders. *J Consult Clin Psychol*. 1993;61:248.

Charney DS. Neuroanatomical circuits modulating fear and anxiety behaviors. *Acta Psychiatr Scand Suppl*. 2003;417:38–50.

Erickson TM, Newman MG. Cognitive behavioral psychotherapy for generalized anxiety disorder: a primer. *Expert Rev Neurother*. 2005;5:247.

Gelenberg AJ, Lydiard RB, Rudolph RL, et al. Efficacy of venlafaxine extended-release capsules in nondepressed outpatients with generalized anxiety disorder: a 6-month randomized controlled trial. *JAMA*. 2000;283:3082.

Hettema JM, Neale MC, Myers JM, et al. A population-based twin study of the relationship between neuroticism and internalizing disorders. *Am J Psychiatry*. 2006;163:857.

Mackintosh MA, Gatz M, Wetherell JL, Pedersen NL. A twin study of lifetime Generalized Anxiety Disorder (GAD) in older adults: genetic and environmental influences shared by neuroticism and GAD. *Twin Res Hum Genet*. 2006;9:30–37.

Mathew SJ, Mao X, Coplan JD, et al. Dorsolateral prefrontal cortical pathology in generalized anxiety disorder: a proton magnetic resonance spectroscopic imaging study. *Am J Psychiatry*. 2004;161:1118–1121.

Mitte K, Noack P, Steil R, Hautzinger M. A meta-analytic review of the efficacy of drug treatment in generalized anxiety disorder. *J Clin Psychopharmacol*. 2005;25:141.

Newman SC, Bland RC. A population based family study of DSM-III generalized anxiety disorder. *Psychol Med*. 2006;36:1275–1281.

Rickels K, Downing R, Schweizer E, Hassman H, et al. Antidepressants for the treatment of generalized anxiety disorder. *Arch Gen Psychiatry*. 1993;50:884.

Sellers EM et al. Alprazolam and benzodiazepine dependence. *J Clin Psychiatry*. 1993;54(Suppl):64.

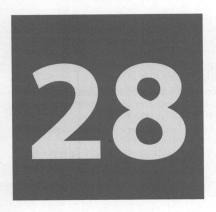

Posttraumatic Stress Disorder and Acute Stress Disorder

Douglas C. Johnson, PhD
John H. Krystal, MD
Steven M. Southwick, MD[†]

POSTTRAUMATIC STRESS DISORDER

General Considerations

It has long been known that traumatic events can have profound effects on memories, cognitions, emotions, and behaviors. However, despite abundant evidence for persisting and sometimes disabling psychological sequelae of exposure to extreme stressors, the evolution of posttraumatic stress disorder (PTSD) as a modern diagnosis is relatively recent. PTSD-like disorders were described in the U.S. Civil War (DaCosta's syndrome, irritable heart of soldiers), following railroad accidents in the late nineteenth century (Railway Spine), and as the tragic consequence of World Wars I and II (shell shock, traumatic neurosis, neurasthenia, and survivor syndrome).

In the 1950s and 1960s, debate revolved around the issue of whether there was anything unique about the psychiatric symptoms that emerged following extreme stress relative to psychiatric symptoms that were expressed in the context of the stresses of everyday life. Thus, the diagnosis of Gross Stress Reaction appeared in the initial *Diagnostic and Statistical Manual of Mental Disorders (DSM)* but was excluded from DSM-II. In 1980, in the wake of clinical research on soldiers of the Vietnam War, studies of victims of physical and sexual assault, and victims of natural disasters, the American Psychiatric Association introduced PTSD diagnostic criteria in a form that is fundamentally similar to current diagnostic schemata. Unlike other disorders, PTSD is predicated on the occurrence of at least one discrete external event, namely a precipitating trauma. DSM-III defined a trauma as "experiencing an event that is outside the range of usual human experience." However, subsequent epidemiologic studies found that traumatic events are common, that greater than half of the population experienced trauma sometime during their life, and that even witnessing trauma could be predictive of PTSD. The DSM-IV-TR stipulated two subcriteria—one objective,

one subjective—to meet formal diagnosis of PTSD: (A1) the person experienced, witnessed, or was confronted with an event or events that involved actual or threatened death or serious injury, or a threat to physical integrity of self or others; *and* (A2) the person's response involved fear, helplessness, or horror. The change in the definition of a traumatic event from DSM-III to DSM-IV resulted in higher rates of PTSD in a number of epidemiologic studies. Critical work on effective therapies, incidence, and cost of PTSD to society are generally based on studies of American military veterans. The fiscal year 2005 report from the Department of Veterans Affairs (VA)n indicated that PTSD was the costliest diagnosis for the VA, and the third most frequently claimed disability, making up 4.2% of all claims. The DSM-5 removed subcriterion A2, rendering individual response to traumatic events irrelevant to diagnosis. Moreover, with DSM-5 and DSM-5-5TR, PTSD is no longer considered an anxiety disorder and is listed under a new category of Stress and Trauma-Related Disorders.

A. Epidemiology

1. Extreme stress exposure—A majority of Americans have been exposure to at least one potentially traumatic (Criterion A) event. The National Comorbidity Study (NCS) surveyed 5877 Americans (2812 men and 3065 women) aged 15–54 years and reported that 60.7% of men and 51.2% of women reported experiencing at least one extremely stressful event in their lifetime (Kessler et al, 1995). Of those who had experienced at least one of these events, 56.3% of men and 48.6% of women reported experiencing multiple extremely stressful events.

The prevalence of exposure to extreme stress has also been examined within specific populations such as women, inner-city residents, and combat veterans. For example, in a sample of 4008 American women, 69% of respondents reported at least one traumatic event in her life (Resnick et al, 1993); in the city of Detroit reported rates of traumatic exposure were 92.2% for men and 87.1% for women (Breslau et al, 1998); and among U.S. Army and Marine Corps personnel serving

[†]Deceased

in Iraq, 70% endorsed "seeing dead or seriously wounded or killed Americans" (Hoge et al, 2004).

2. Prevalence rates of PTSD—In the NCS, 7.8% of Americans met DSM-III criteria for lifetime PTSD despite a 60.6% exposure rate for men and 51.2% for women (Kessler et al, 1995). Similar rates were reported in the National Epidemiologic Survey on Alcohol and Related Conditions, where 6.4% of 34,653 Americans met DSM-IV criteria for lifetime PTSD with an additional 6.6% meeting criteria for lifetime partial PTSD (Pietrzak et al, 2011). As part of the National Comorbidity Survey Replication, lifetime morbid risk for PTSD (i.e., the percentage of Americans who already have a lifetime history of PTSD plus those who do not have a lifetime history of PTSD but who are expected to develop PTSD at some point in their life) has been estimated at 10.1% (Kessler et al, 2012).

Rates of PTSD vary depending on the nature of trauma. For example, rape results in high rates of PTSD in both men (65%) and women (46%), whereas automobile accidents have been associated with lower rates of PTSD (men, 25%; women, 13.8%) (Kessler et al, 1995). Regarding rates of PTSD among veterans of war, the National Vietnam Veterans Readjustment Study (NVVRS) found that 18.7% of Vietnam veterans met lifetime and 9.1% current criteria for PTSD (Dohrenwend et al, 2006). More recently the Institute of Medicine estimated prevalence of PTSD to be between 13% and 20% among U.S. soldiers who served in Iraq and Afghanistan (IOM, 2012).

B. Etiology

Multiple psychological, biological, and environmental factors appear to be involved in the etiology of PTSD. In attempting to understand neural and behavioral mechanisms that contribute to the etiology of PTSD, investigators have highlighted at least four features of PTSD.

1. Fear conditioning and learning—The *Two-Factor* model (Mowrer, 1947) is a combination of classical (Pavlovian) and operant (reinforcement) conditioning. Classical conditioning is the process of pairing together, or associating, two stimuli: the traumatic event (unconditioned stimulus, UCS) and associated sensory stimuli (conditioned stimuli, CS). As a result of this pairing, the formerly neutral CS now elicits the same fear response (conditioned response, CR) and autonomic arousal as the UCS.

In cases of PTSD, there may be modality-specific (i.e., classical conditioning), as well as polymodal (i.e., contextual conditioning), stimuli paired with the CR. Moreover, behavioral neuroscience research has shown that classical and contextual conditioning are partially mediated by different brain regions. Classical conditioning is known to involve thalamo–amygdala pathways, whereas contextual conditioning occurs via input to the hippocampus and amygdala from higher cortical areas. In the case of contextual conditioning, multiple and often complex environmental stimuli that are present during exposure to the feared stimulus (UCS) become associated. For example,

after exposure to a roadside improvised explosive device in Iraq, a veteran while driving in the United States may experience fear and autonomic arousal when exposed to modality-specific (e.g., a loud muffler backfire) or contextual (e.g., hot dirt road, trash in the median, and smell of diesel fuel) stimuli, each of which were previously neutral. Sounds, sights, smells, time of day or year (i.e., anniversary reaction), or other ordinarily neutral stimuli that are present during the frightening event may later trigger fear and physiological arousal.

Typically, fear-conditioned memories extinguish over time if survivors systematically expose themselves to fear-inducing stimuli while in a safe environment. Gradually, the brain learns that these stimuli are no longer dangerous. However, when trauma survivors knowingly or unknowingly avoid traumatic thoughts, triggers, or reminders in order to avoid feeling anxious or afraid, they no longer have the opportunity to extinguish these fear-conditioned memories. Although avoidance generally reduces anxious arousal in the short run, it also creates a powerful reinforcement for continued avoidance with the unintended consequence of perpetuating trauma-related psychopathology.

2. Information processing—Although a stimulus (S) → response (R) model sufficiently explains the acquisition of fear-based conditioning, it is inadequate in that a stimulus does not always produce the same response. Models that involve the processing of information and emotions typically emphasize the role of appraisal or interpretation of trauma-related information/experiences. Individuals are more likely to appraise a situation as threatening or out of their control, and thus are more likely to develop trauma-related psychopathology, when they believe that they do not possess the personal capabilities or external resources to meet the demands of the situation. On the other hand, individuals are more likely to appraise a situation as a challenge when they believe they can successfully deal with it. Whether an individual appraises a stressful situation as a challenge or a threat depends on numerous factors including personality, cognitive, behavioral and emotion regulation skills, prior experiences of success or failure in stressful situations, personal meaning of the event, and quality and degree of social support, among other factors (Southwick & Charney, 2012).

The processing of trauma-related emotions is particularly relevant to avoidance and intrusive memories. According to the Emotion Processing Theory (Foa & Kozack, 1986), memories of traumatic events are stored, along with associated (i.e., conditioned) cues, in information networks called "fear structures." The individual with PTSD avoids encountering or thinking about the trauma, or its cues, in an attempt to avoid activation of the associative network of trauma-related memories. Intrusive memories are believed to occur as a result of implicit exposure to one or more cues that activate the fear structure.

3. Neurobiological systems—A number of neurobiological models have been proposed to explain PTSD or specific aspects of PTSD. Examples include the role of genetic polymorphisms related to stress vulnerability (e.g., polymorphisms of the serotonin transporter gene), sensitization of neurobiological systems (e.g., noradrenergic system) involved in the stress response, exaggerated fear conditioning, overconsolidation of emotional memories, insufficient cortical inhibition of limbic activity, reduced capacity to extinguish fear-conditioned memories, and poor regulation of hypothalamic–pituitary–adrenal (HPA) axis and sympathetic nervous system responses to stress. In one of the most comprehensive causal neurobiological models of PTSD, Admon, Milad, and Hendler (2013) propose that preexisting hyperactivity of the amygdala and dorsal anterior cingulate cortex (dACC) is associated with exaggerated fear responses and with increased likelihood of developing PTSD. They further speculate that traumatic exposure may cause alterations to areas of the medial prefrontal cortex (mPFC) and to structural and functional connections between the mPFC and the hippocampus, resulting in an acquired reduction in capacity to inhibit/regulate the fear response. Currently, it is uncertain to what degree neurobiological alterations are either the cause or consequence of PTSD.

C. Risk

Some people are more likely to develop PTSD than others when exposed to traumatic events. Risk for developing PTSD is likely increased by a variety of genetic, neurobiological, and psychosocial factors. Psychosocial risk factors have typically been classified as pretraumatic, peritraumatic, and posttraumatic (Brewin et al, 2000; Ozer et al, 2003). Common pretraumatic risk factors that have been identified in published research, meta-analyses, and literature reviews include female gender, younger age, lower education, lower intelligence, negative emotionality (i.e., disposition characterized by anxiety, emotional lability, poor interpersonal interactions, and overall negative mood), past history of trauma (e.g., childhood sexual or physical abuse), and past individual or family psychiatric history. Commonly identified peritraumatic factors include high degree of traumatic exposure, pronounced dissociation, and excessive peritraumatic physiological activation (e.g., panic attack). For example, a survey of 1008 adult survivors of the September 11, 2001, World Trade Center attacks found that 7.5% reported symptoms consistent with a diagnosis of PTSD; however, higher rates of PTSD (20%) were found within the larger sample for those living closer to the World Trade Center (Galea et al, 2002). Finally, posttrauma risk factors have included dysfunctional coping strategies (e.g., avoidance), low social support, and subsequent exposure to additional stressors and traumatic events.

D. Resilience

Given that not all individuals exposed to the same traumatic event will develop PTSD, it becomes vital to understand what is different about those individuals who do well under stress and are able to recover from the stress of trauma. In contrast to traditional investigations that seek to determine the causes and catalysts for psychopathology, resilience research, particularly within the field of trauma studies, attempts to explain why some individuals are relatively resistant to the negative impact of trauma, recover rapidly after traumatic exposure, or experience positive growth in response to trauma. Resilience to stress has been investigated from neurobiological (Charney, 2004) and psychosocial perspectives (Southwick et al, 2005; Southwick and Charney, 2012).

1. Neurobiological resilience factors—Numerous genetic factors, developmental influences, brain regions, and endocrine and neurotransmitter systems appear to be associated with resilience to stress. Among the neurobiological factors that recently have received attention are sympathetic nervous system activity that responds robustly to stress but that returns to baseline rapidly, perhaps secondary to regulation by neuropeptide Y (NPY) and galanin; capacity to contain the corticotropin-releasing factor (CRF) response to stress, perhaps in association with DHEA, NPY, and a host of other regulators; a durable dopamine-mediated reward system that might allow traumatized individuals to remain optimistic and hopeful even in the context of extreme or chronic stress; an amygdala that does not overreact to the environment; a hippocampus that provides sufficient inhibition to the HPA axis and that accurately differentiates cues for danger and safety; and ample cortical executive and inhibitory capacity.

Elevated levels of plasma NPY have been found in humans following extreme stressors such as military survival training. Moreover, higher levels of NPY have been correlated with better performance during simulated prisoner of war training with Special Forces soldiers. In contrast, lower baseline and yohimbine-stimulated levels of NPY have been found in combat veterans with a current diagnosis of PTSD, but other studies of combat-related PTSD and female victims of sexual assault (Seedat et al, 2003) have yielded mixed results. Other neurophysiological factors associated with an adaptive response to extreme stress and the ability to physically and mentally recover following trauma are high vagal tone and increased heart rate variability (HRV). HRV is vagally mediated, with efferent projections to heart and lungs, and afferents involved in regulation of blood pressure. Thus, HRV is a measure of the balance between sympathetic and parasympathetic signals and represents overall flexibility to anticipate, respond to, and recover from stress. Higher resting-state HRV is characterized by parasympathetic dominance. A recent meta-analysis of fMRI studies reported a relationship between HRV and activation in prefrontal (mPFC, dACC) and limbic (amygdala) regions (Thayer et al, 2012). In terms of function, higher HRV is associated with increased working memory capacity, greater emotion regulation, and enhanced response inhibition.

2. Psychosocial resilience factors—Resilience to stress has been correlated with *optimism, humor, social support,* and an *active* rather than avoidant *coping style.* Research has also identified *openness to change* and *extroversion* as positive predictors of growth following traumatic experiences. Two closely related constructs associated with resilience are *cognitive flexibility* and *emotion regulation. Cognitive flexibility,* marked by the ability to reframe problems and extract personal meaning from stressful situations, has been associated with reappraisal of events as less threatening and a greater sense of self-efficacy in the face of challenge. Moreover, there is some evidence to suggest that resilience is not a static or stable dimension but is responsive to therapeutic and pharmacological intervention.

Clearly, resilience to stress is associated with a complex set of interactions between neurobiological and psychosocial factors. For example, Kaufman et al (2004) studied the effects of social support networks in children who were at risk genetically (s/s allele of the 5-HTTLPR serotonin transporter gene promoter polymorphism) and environmentally (documented history of maltreatment) and found that strength of social support networks and positive social relationships moderated the risk for depression independent of genetic vulnerabilities and early exposure to overwhelming stress.

E. Genetics

Data from twin studies suggest that risk for PTSD is moderately heritable. A study of 4042 Vietnam-era twin pairs indicates that vulnerability to PTSD has a significant genetic component. After controlling for variability in combat exposure, genetic concordance accounted for 13–30% of the variance in reexperiencing symptoms (Cluster B), 30–34% of the variance in avoidance symptoms (Cluster C), and 28–32% of the variance in the (Cluster D) hyperarousal symptoms (True et al, 1993). Proneness to exposure to traumatic events may also be influenced by familial nongenetic factors.

To date, using a candidate gene approach where genes are selected for analysis based on known underlying molecular pathways, specific genes associated with PTSD have been linked to dopaminergic, serotonergic, noradrenergic, and HPA axis systems. However, in many cases results have been inconsistent or have not been replicated. One of the most promising approaches for studying genetic contributions to risk for PTSD involves genome-wide association studies (GWAS) where the entire genome is analyzed in relation to PTSD. For example, in a series of recent GWAS, Xie and colleagues (2013) reported a significant association between TLL1 rs6812849 and PTSD among European Americans. TLL1rs6812849 is a protein implicated in promoting neurogenesis, which is known to be inhibited by stress.

Recent research in epigenetics has shown that a host of external and internal stimuli, such as social support, fear, and stress, can trigger biochemical reactions that can affect gene expression by either "turning on" or "turning off" genes. This rapidly growing field shows great promise in advancing the understanding of stress vulnerability and stress resilience (Nestler, 2012).

▶ Clinical Findings

A. Signs and Symptoms

PTSD diagnostic criteria were revised in DSM-5 to more closely reflect published clinical evidence. In DSM-5, PTSD was moved from the Anxiety Disorders group into a new category of Trauma and Stressor-Related Disorders that also includes Acute Stress Disorder (ASD) and Adjustment Disorders. Criterion A2 was dropped from DSM-5 because response to trauma (i.e., fear, helplessness, and horror) has been shown to be a poor predictor of subsequent PTSD diagnosis or symptom severity (Pereda & Forero, 2012). In addition, PTSD symptom clusters were revised from three criteria (reexperiencing, avoidance, and hyperarousal) in DSM-IV to four criteria (intrusion, avoidance, negative affect, and hyperarousal) in DSM-5. Most pathognomonic among these four symptom clusters are episodes of reexperiencing (i.e., flashbacks, nightmares, and intrusive memories). Such memories are rarely, if ever, wanted and intrude against the will, sometimes for years or even a lifetime. Individuals with PTSD typically try to avoid these memories, both cognitively and behaviorally, and often rearrange their lives around avoiding potential reminders of the trauma that trigger remembrance. In addition to cognitive and behavioral avoidance, PTSD is marked by significant avoidance of emotional arousal (i.e., emotional numbing); indeed, avoidance and emotional numbing often have debilitating effects on psychosocial function.

Some individuals with PTSD experience amnesia for aspects of the traumatic event. This inability to recall certain trauma-related memories, despite hyperaccessibility of other trauma memories, may be explained in part by selective attention, dissociation, or extreme arousal, which can compromise encoding and consolidation of memory at the time of trauma. Likewise, degree of dissociation has been found to be predictive of PTSD following life-threatening trauma. Emotional numbing can be difficult to identify clinically because it is not necessarily manifest as flat affect, but rather as a restricted range of affect and marked detachment from others. In this regard, collateral reporting sources (e.g., family members, significant others) are often integral to an accurate diagnostic assessment. Moreover, emotional numbing can often appear as indifference toward future plans and general apathy about setting goals such as getting married, owning a home, need for a healthy lifestyle, or career advancement.

Insomnia is a major problem for many trauma survivors with PTSD. They often describe difficulty falling asleep and staying asleep secondary to hypervigilance and/or fear of having nightmares. It is not uncommon for vivid nightmares to violently awaken survivors from their sleep.

B. Specific Behavioral or Physioiogical Findings (Laboratory Findings)

1. Physiological—Exaggerated physiological reactivity has been described among traumatized individuals for centuries. In fact, in the 1940s, PTSD was referred to as "physioneurosis" because unlike other "neuroses," it appeared to have a profound underlying physiological basis. More recently, in a meta-analysis of more than 1000 adults, Pole (2007) found that PTSD was associated with higher resting arousal as well as larger responses to startling sounds, standardized trauma cues, and personal trauma memories compared to individuals without PTSD. One of the most reliable correlates of PTSD was elevated heart rate, which has been shown to prospectively predict PTSD. Such cardiac reactivity may be relatively specific to PTSD, as comparison studies including veterans with anxiety disorders other than PTSD have not shown similar increases in heart rate. Moreover, cardiac reactivity in PTSD does not appear to be a generalized autonomic response to indiscriminate stressors, but rather is associated with trauma-specific cues (Orr et al, 2002).

2. Cognitive—Information-processing biases in PTSD have been studied using various cognitive paradigms. Studies of attentional bias using a dot-probe task and eye tracking indicate that PTSD is associated with increased attention toward trauma-related cues and difficulty disengaging from threat-related words. Emotion regulation and response inhibition have been studied using the emotional Stroop task. The "Stroop effect" is demonstrated by the increased response time needed to inhibit a prepotent (i.e., overlearned) response. The emotional Stroop is a variation of the traditional color-word naming task, but substitutes trauma-related words (e.g., insurgent, amputate) for color words. Relative to age- and education-matched civilian and military controls, veterans of OEF/OIF took longer to respond and were less accurate for combat words (Ashley et al, 2013). Moreover, there were no group differences in response times for noncombat words. Rather than global information processing inefficiencies, these results suggest that individuals with PTSD have a unique processing bias for threat-related information.

There is tentative support for biases in judgment showing that individuals with PTSD interpret ambiguous sentences and words (e.g., homographs) as threatening. Memory biases in PTSD have been less consistently demonstrated. In particular, there is some evidence for a mood-congruent memory effect in PTSD, to wit, individuals with PTSD demonstrate a memory advantage for trauma-related information. However, it remains unclear whether this explicit memory bias is the result of recall advantages inherent in personally salient information, or whether the advantages are due to true mood congruency between internal affective state and emotional valence assigned to the remembered material. Support for implicit memory biases in PTSD, based on implicit priming (i.e., below perceptual awareness threshold) and word stem completion task paradigms, is also limited.

Biases in forgetting, in particular thought suppression and cognitive avoidance, have been explored as an explanation for the inconsistent memory findings in PTSD. It has been hypothesized that individuals with PTSD will attempt to suppress or avoid recall of trauma-related memories. In fact, some studies have indicated a bias away from anxiety-provoking information, suggesting that there is an implicit or strategic effort to avoid aversive thoughts and memories. However, evidence that individuals with PTSD engage in cognitive avoidance strategies or thought suppression during recall of trauma-related information is tentative.

3. Neuropsychological—Individuals with PTSD demonstrate a range of cognitive abnormalities, particularly in the areas of attention (simple, divided, and sustained), concentration, learning, and memory (Vasterling & Brewin, 2005). Combat-related PTSD is also associated with decreased (i.e., quicker) reaction time on stimulus recognition tests. In addition, PTSD is associated with lower full-scale IQ; however, reliance on estimates of premorbid intellectual functioning makes causal inferences difficult. A study of deployed and nondeployed Gulf War–era veterans ($N = 2189$) showed differences in rates of neuropsychological impairment. After adjusting for academic achievement, age, and rank, 3.7% of deployed veterans had definite impairments in sustained attention, and 2.6% had definite impairments in motor speed. In contrast, 1.7% and 1.4% of nondeployed veterans had definite impairments in sustained attention and motor speed, respectively (Toomey et al, 2009).

In a recent comprehensive review of prospective, longitudinal, twin, and cross-sectional studies of executive function, Aupperle and colleagues (2012) report that PTSD is characterized by deficits in executive function, including attention and working memory, sustained attention, and inhibitory functions, as well as flexibility, switching, and planning. Although PTSD has been associated with enhanced attention to threat-relevant stimuli, it has also been associated with dysfunction in ability to subsequently inhibit or disengage from these stimuli. The authors speculate that these deficits might exacerbate reexperiencing and arousal symptoms, which in turn may increase avoidance of arousing stimuli. There is some evidence to suggest that subtle deficits in executive function may predate trauma in some individuals and thus increase the risk of developing PTSD.

Performance of individuals with PTSD on tasks of executive set-switching has been mixed, with some studies showing relative inefficiencies, whereas others show that individuals with PTSD are within normal limits. Of note, cognitive deficits in these domains occur with threat-neutral, nontrauma stimuli. Relative to non-PTSD combat-exposed and nondeployed personnel, individuals with PTSD have been shown to experience increased combat-related thought intrusions during a neutral thought suppression task. Moreover, the neutral thought suppression task was more difficult for individuals with PTSD as measured by physiologic indicators of effort and stress (e.g., galvanic skin conductance; Aikins et al, 2009). Similarly, PTSD research with emotionally neutral list-learning tasks has revealed retrieval deficits for newly learned information. That occurrence of deficits in free recall of recently learned information, but not during recognition trials, suggests that such impairments are not due to encoding impairments but rather indicate a problem with consolidation of new information into long-term storage. Neuropsychological domains that appear to remain intact include visuospatial functioning, language, and psychomotor performance.

4. Psychobiological—Multiple neurobiological alterations or abnormalities have been associated with PTSD. The most extensively studied alterations have involved the HPA axis and the sympathetic nervous system. Alterations in the HPA axis in PTSD include (1) elevated resting cerebrospinal fluid levels of CRF; (2) alterations in 24-hour urine excretion of cortisol, 24-hour plasma cortisol levels, lymphocyte glucocorticoid receptor number, cortisol response to dexamethasone, adrenocorticotropic hormone (ACTH) response to CRF, and β-endorphin and ACTH response to metyrapone; and (3) adrenal androgen abnormalities.

Alterations in sympathetic nervous system reactivity include exaggerated increases in heart rate, blood pressure, and epinephrine in response to traumatic reminders administered in the laboratory; elevated 24-hour plasma norepinephrine; elevated 24-hour urine excretion of norepinephrine and epinephrine; reduced platelet adrenergic receptor number; increased subjective, behavioral, physiological, and biochemical (increased plasma methoxyhydroxyphenylglycol) responses to intravenous yohimbine (an α2-adrenoreceptor antagonist); blunted response to clonidine; and altered yohimbine-induced cerebral blood flow. Alterations in sympathetic nervous system reactivity may contribute to symptoms of reexperiencing and hyperarousal. Neurocognitive and brain imaging studies comparing individuals with PTSD and individuals without psychiatric disorders have reported that subjects with PTSD show biased attention to negative and potentially dangerous information, reductions in hippocampal volume and function, exaggerated amygdala responses to stressful cues, and stress-induced reduction in PFC metabolism.

C. Neuroimaging

PTSD is associated with alterations in both brain structure and function. Consistent with animal research, studies in humans have reported smaller bilateral volume and reduced neuronal density of the hippocampus, smaller volume in prefrontal cortical brain regions including the ventral medial prefrontal cortex (vmPFC) and the anterior cingulate cortex, and alterations in white matter tract integrity in the cingulum bundle among subjects with PTSD compared to controls. In response to trauma-related stimuli, functional neuroimaging studies have found exaggerated activation of the amygdala,

dACC, and insula, as well as decreased activation of areas of the vmPFC among subjects with PTSD compared to controls. Taken together these findings have lead researchers to propose a neurocircuitry model of PTSD that includes overactivation of areas of the brain involved in detection and response to fear and internal body states including arousal (i.e., amygdala, anterior cingulate cortex, insula) in conjunction with decreased activation of brain regions that inhibit negative emotional states and that facilitate extinction of fear (i.e., vmPFC). In addition, evidence suggests that abnormalities reported in hippocampal structure and function may affect memory as well as ability to differentiate safe versus dangerous contextual cues.

Currently there is debate about the temporal relationship between brain structure and function and the development of PTSD. Evidence suggests that structural and functional differences represent both vulnerability factors and maladaptation to trauma. For example, studies of individuals with PTSD and their non–trauma-exposed cotwins suggest that reduced hippocampal volume may be a premorbid risk factor as well as a result of trauma exposure (Kitayama et al, 2005; Gilbertson et al, 2002). Similarly, increased resting-state metabolic activity in the dACC of non–trauma-exposed twins has been associated with symptom severity in combat-exposed cotwins with PTSD (Shin et al, 2009), whereas reduced functional connectivity between hippocampus and vmPFC may be the result of exposure to acute stress (e.g., Admon et al, 2013). Finally, there is emerging evidence that reduction of PTSD symptoms is associated with increased vmPFC activation (Hughes & Shin, 2011).

D. Course of Illness

The course of PTSD is variable. PTSD can occur from very early childhood to late in life. Onset of PTSD symptoms commonly occurs within 3 months following trauma exposure, although symptom manifestation can be delayed for years after the trauma. Common trajectories of PTSD symptoms include chronic elevation, chronic subsyndromal, delayed onset, recovery, and resilience/resistant (Pietrzak et al, 2013). Despite variation in course, epidemiologic studies suggest that the majority of symptoms do attenuate with time. For example, the NCS indicated that PTSD resolves in 6 years in approximately 60% of cases. However, it may be that some symptoms are more likely to decrease than others over time. A study of Israeli military personnel over a 2-year period found that symptoms of reexperiencing and intrusive memories decreased, whereas avoidance and emotional numbing symptoms increased (Solomon & Mikulincer, 1992). Although recovery occurs in most of those diagnosed with PTSD, for those who do not recover PTSD is often markedly detrimental to physical, social, occupational, and interpersonal functioning. Moreover, PTSD can be complicated by recurrent exposure to trauma or trauma-associated cues that trigger reactivation of symptoms.

E. Psychological Testing

A variety of rating scales have been developed for the assessment of PTSD, the nature of certain traumas, and specific responses to stress. Some of these measures have been validated for use in diagnostic and treatment settings; however, some researchers have recommended that reliance solely on self-report checklist should be avoided when possible, especially in cases involving differential diagnosis. For example, in a study of individuals with traumatic brain injury (TBI) ($n = 34$), 44–59% of participants were diagnosed with PTSD based on self-report questionnaires. In contrast, when a structured clinical interview was used, only 3% were determined to meet DSM-IV-TR criteria for PTSD (Sumpter & McMillan, 2005).

1. Self-report measures

i. Combat Experiences Scale (CES)—The CES is an assessment of exposure to stereotypical warfare experiences such as firing a weapon, being fired on (by enemy or friendly fire), witnessing injury and death, and going on special missions and patrols that involve such experiences. The CES, standardized in a Persian Gulf War sample, was developed as a contemporary version of the Vietnam era Combat Exposure Scale.

ii. PTSD Checklist for DSM-5-TR (PCL-5)—The PCL is a 20-item assessment of PTSD symptom severity developed by the National Center for PTSD. Items correspond to 20 PTSD symptom criteria directly adapted from the DSM-5. The PCL-5 can be used for screening, presumptive diagnosis, and monitoring symptom change during and after treatment. The self-report rating scale for each item is 0 (not at all) to 4 (extremely), with total scores ranging from 0 to 80. The increase in number of items and change in rating scale means that scores on the PCL-5 do not correspond to scores on the DSM-IV version of the PCL and should be interpreted separately.

iii. Posttraumatic Diagnostic Scale (PDS)—The PDS is a 49-item measure of PTSD symptom severity and frequency according to the DSM-IV criteria. Symptom severity is anchored to an individual's "most upsetting traumatic event." The PDS is distinct from other PTSD assessments in that it also assesses features Criteria A (trauma) and Criteria F (functioning).

iv. Davidson Trauma Scale (DTS)—The DTS assesses each of 17 PTSD symptoms corresponding to DSM-IV-TR criteria. Symptom frequency and intensity are assessed separately for each symptom on a 5-point Likert scale. Frequency scores range from 0 (not at all) to 4 (every day). Intensity scores range from 0 (not at all) to 4 (extremely distressing).

v. Perceived Stress Scale (PSS)—The PSS is one of the most widely used measures of subjective experiences of stress. The PSS assesses the individual perceptions of stress over the last 30 days across three dimensions: uncontrollability, unpredictability, and overwhelming nature.

vi. Connor-Davidson Resilience Scale (CD-RISC)—The CD-RISC is a 25-item self-report scale assessing stress coping ability. The scale comprises five factors that broadly correspond to tenacity, tolerance of negative affect, acceptance of change, perceived control, and spirituality. The CD-RISC has several potential applications, including identifying individuals at risk for stress-related psychopathology, and as a treatment outcome variable.

vii. Response to Stressful Experiences Scale (RSES)—The RSES is a 22-item measure that assesses how individual typically responds to stressful life events. The scale comprises five protective factors: (1) meaning-making and restoration, (2) active-coping, (3) cognitive flexibility, (4) spirituality, and (5) self-efficacy. The RSES asks respondents, "During and after life's most stressful events, I tend to…. " Responses are measured on a 5-point Likert scale ranging from 0 (not at all like me) to 4 (exactly like me).

viii. Deployment Risk and Resilience Inventory-2 (DRRI-2)—The DRRI-2 is a suite of 17 measures designed to assess psychosocial factors associated with vulnerability to stress before, during, and after military deployment. The DRRI-2 was developed in a national sample of veterans from Operation Enduring Freedom (OEF) and Operation Iraqi Freedom (OIF) (Vogt et al, 2013). Psychosocial factors assessed by the DRRI-2 include unit cohesion, perceived social support, training and readiness, combat exposure, aftermath of battle, and family stressors.

2. Clinician-administered scales

i. Clinician-Administered PTSD Scale for DSM-5-TR (CAPS-5)—The CAPS is a 30-item structured clinical interview measuring the frequency and intensity of the DSM-5 symptoms of PTSD (Weathers et al, 2013). The CAPS-5 comprises standardized questions and probes for each of the 20 DSM-5 symptom criteria. Additional questions assess onset and duration of symptoms, social and occupational functioning, change over time, response validity, and overall symptom severity. There are also specifications for diagnosis of depersonalization and derealization subtypes. The CAPS-5 can be used to make a current (past month) diagnosis of PTSD, make a lifetime diagnosis of PTSD, and assess PTSD symptoms over the last week.

ii. Structured Clinical Interview for DSM Disorders (SCID)—The SCID is a clinician-based structured interview designed to assess the majority of mental health disorders. The PTSD portion of the SCID is found in Module F—Anxiety Disorders. Several versions of the SCID are available for use dependent on the setting (e.g., research, clinical, and nonpatient populations).

TheSCID is also available in several different languages. A new DSM 5 version was scheduled to be released in October 2014. It can reliably be used with DSM-5-TR.

iii. Mississippi Scale for PTSD—The scale consists of 39 self-report items derived from the *Diagnostic and Statistical Manual of Mental Disorders III-R* criteria for PTSD. The first version of the Mississippi Scale contained 35 items, based on the unrevised DSM-III criteria for PTSD. The four added items (items 36–39) assess reexperiencing, psychogenic amnesia, hypervigilance, and increased arousal symptomatology.

iv. Impact of Events Scale (IES)—The IES is a 22-item self-report measure of reaction to stressful events. The IES was created for the study of bereaved individuals and was then adopted for studying the psychological impact of trauma.

v. Trauma Symptom Inventory (TSI)—The TSI is a 100-item evaluation of acute and chronic symptomatology from a wide variety of traumas, including rape, combat experiences, major accidents, and natural disasters, as well as childhood abuse. The various scales of the TSI assess a wide range of psychological impacts. These include not only symptoms typically associated with PTSD or ASD but also those intra- and interpersonal difficulties often associated with more chronic psychological trauma. The TSI does not generate DSM-IV diagnoses; instead, it is intended to evaluate the relative level of various forms of posttraumatic distress.

vi. Morel Emotional Numbing Test (MENT)—The MENT is currently the only clinician-administered tool developed specifically to detect symptom exaggeration in PTSD. The MENT is a 60-item forced choice recognition test and requires the respondent to match various facial expressions with a label that correctly identifies the expressed emotion. Each item comprises one correct response and one foil. Several published studies support the reliability and validity of the MENT in distinguishing individuals with PTSD from individuals feigning PTSD-related cognitive impairment (Messer & Fremouw, 2007; Morel, 1998, 2008).

▶ Differential Diagnosis (Including Comorbid Conditions)

1. Major or mild neurocognitive disorder (NCD) due to traumatic brain injury (TBI)—PTSD and TBI frequently co-occur as a result of trauma, and symptom overlap can make differential diagnosis challenging, particularly in cases of mild TBI. Individuals who have suffered a closed head injury can experience difficulties with attention and concentration, sleep disturbance, posttraumatic amnesia, and negative affect, all of which are also symptoms of PTSD. In cases where head injury was sustained during a life-threatening trauma, formal neuropsychological testing and a structured clinical interview of symptoms can inform differential diagnosis. In cases of potential PTSD and/or NCD due to mild TBI, attention should be given to clinical indicators unique to each condition, such as avoidance and reexperiencing in PTSD, or loss of consciousness, neurological soft signs (i.e., Glasgow Coma Score), and cognitive slowing in mild TBI.

2. Adjustment disorder (AD)—Symptoms that arise from an event that is stressful, but not of the life-threatening nature and intensity of Criterion A events for PTSD, fall under the rubric of AD.

3. Acute stress disorder (ASD)—ASD is differentiated from PTSD on two criteria. The first is that ASD symptoms must occur within 4 weeks of the traumatic event, whereas PTSD may have a delayed onset. The second distinction is that ASD symptoms must remit within 4 weeks of their initial presentation; symptoms that last beyond 4 weeks may indicate PTSD.

4. Obsessive–compulsive disorder (OCD)—OCD and PTSD have overlapping symptoms of intrusive thoughts. However, unwanted thoughts in PTSD are distinct in that they are circumscribed to trauma-related events and memories. Although intrusive thoughts in OCD are often distressing, they are not specific to a traumatic event.

5. Psychotic disorders—Delusions and hallucinations, characteristic of psychotic episodes, are distinct from those that occur during PTSD flashbacks. According to diagnostic criteria, persistent reexperiencing of the trauma may include hallucinations and illusions about specific life-threatening events. Such flashbacks may seem, at the time, real to the individual with PTSD. However, conclusion of the PTSD flashback is frequently followed by an acknowledgment that the event was not really reoccurring, although it felt like it at the time. In contrast, by their nature, delusions and hallucinations are indistinguishable from reality for the person experiencing psychosis.

6. Personality disorders—An emerging literature on the comorbidity of personality disorders with anxiety spectrum disorders requires an understanding of personality disorders that frequently co-occur with PTSD. Retrospective and longitudinal research has identified significant correlations between PTSD and some personality disorders. In particular, there is a close relationship between PTSD and borderline personality disorder (BPD). Longitudinal research documented that a diagnosis of PTSD, rather than a history of mere trauma exposure, was the strongest predictor of features of BPD. Among the personality disorder features most closely associated with PTSD are frantic efforts to avoid abandonment, rejection of help, inappropriate anger, and general impulsiveness.

7. Malingering—PTSD diagnostic evaluations often rely on self-report measures. An accurate diagnosis of PTSD can be complicated by the fact that, by definition, it requires an identifiable (Criterion A) event. As such, issues of secondary gain and remuneration for personal damages make PTSD especially open to legal scrutiny of potential malingering. Thus, ruling out feigned symptoms through collateral reporting sources and psychometrically sound measures is a fundamental component of differential diagnosis for PTSD.

8. Comorbidity—Epidemiological studies indicate that PTSD is rarely a sole diagnosis. In both the NCS and the NVVRS, 50–88% of individuals with a diagnosis of PTSD also had at least one concomitant disorder. In the NVVRS, 99% of those who received a diagnosis of PTSD had at least one other comorbid diagnosis in their lifetime. The most prevalent comorbid diagnoses with PTSD are major depressive disorder (MDD) and alcohol abuse. Although MDD tends to occur equally in males and females as a comorbid diagnosis, alcohol abuse is more frequently found among males with PTSD. Anxiety spectrum disorders such as specific phobias, social phobia, generalized anxiety disorder, and agoraphobia frequently co-occur with PTSD. Results from the NCS also revealed high comorbidity rates for antisocial personality disorder (43% male and 15% female). Other studies of personality disorders and PTSD have been limited by sample size but reveal notable trends. Among these studies, high PTSD comorbidity rates have been found in BPD and paranoid personality disorder.

▶ **Treatment**

A. Psychopharmacologic Interventions

Psychoactive medications play an important role in the treatment of PTSD. A large study of veterans (N = 247,297) diagnosed with PTSD showed that 80% were provided prescriptions for psychotropic medications. Of those prescribed medications for management of PTSD symptoms, 89% were prescribed antidepressants, 61% received anxiolytics, and 34% received antipsychotics (Mohamed & Rosenheck, 2008).

Selective serotonin reuptake inhibitors (SSRIs) are generally considered first-line medications for the treatment of PTSD (VA/DOD Treatment Guidelines, 2010; Watts et al, 2013). Currently, sertraline and paroxetine are the only two medications that have been approved by the U.S. Food and Drug Administration for the treatment of PTSD. Fluoxetine, another SSRI, and venlafaxine, a serotonin–norepinephrine reuptake inhibitor, have also demonstrated efficacy in placebo-controlled trials. SSRIs have been shown to reduce symptoms of all PTSD symptom clusters as well as comorbid mood and anxiety symptoms. There is evidence to suggest that some individuals with PTSD can continue to experience additional symptom reduction when SSRIs are continued beyond 12 weeks.

The investigation and clinical use of monoamine oxidase inhibitors (MAOIs) for the treatment of PTSD has been limited because of potential side effects, particularly in patients with comorbid substance abuse disorders. Although results have been inconsistent in open trials, in a well-designed randomized controlled trial (RCT) involving Vietnam veterans with PTSD, those treated with phenelzine demonstrated significant improvement in reexperiencing and arousal symptoms (Kosten et al, 1991). Tricyclic antidepressants appear to be as effective as MAOIs or SSRIs in treating PTSD. However, like MAOIs, they generally have a more adverse side effect profile than SSRIs. In a recent RCT, desipramine was as effective as sertraline in treating veterans with PTSD and comorbid alcohol dependence (Petrakis et al, 2012).

Prazosin, an adrenergic agent that blocks alpha-1 receptors, has been shown in several RCTs to improve sleep and reduce nightmares in PTSD. In a recent 15-week RTC involving 67 active-duty combat veterans with PTSD, prazosin was found to be effective in reducing traumatic nightmares and other symptoms of arousal as well as improving global functioning (Raskind et al, 2013).

Medications that have not shown consistent positive effects for the treatment of PTSD include atypical antipsychotics (e.g., risperidone), anticonvulsants (e.g., valproate), and benzodiazepines. In fact, there is some evidence to suggest that the prolonged use of benzodiazepines immediately following traumatic exposure may increase the likelihood of developing symptoms of PTSD, perhaps by interfering with extinction and/or the cognitive processing of traumatic memories. In general, RCTs for psychotropic medications have reported small to moderate effect sizes for the treatment of PTSD.

The use of pharmacological agents to prevent the development of PTSD is a topic of great interest (Kearns et al, 2012). Based on preclinical findings, it has been hypothesized that a number of agents might reduce or prevent the likelihood of developing PTSD. Examples include the use of adrenergic agents (e.g., propranolol) and opiates (e.g., morphine) to block encoding/consolidation/reconsolidation of traumatic memories, CRF antagonists to suppress sympathetic and HPA-axis responses to stress, glucocorticoids to downregulate supersensitive glucocorticoid receptors, and antidepressants (e.g., imipramine). Psychotropic medications are often prescribed in combination with cognitive–behavioral psychotherapies, which have been shown to be more effective than medications for the treatment of PTSD.

There is a great need for more effective pharmacologic treatments for PTSD. The medications that are currently approved were not developed to address specific neurobiological alterations seen in PTSD. It is anticipated that pharmacological interventions specifically designed to address underlying pathophysiological alterations in PTSD will enhance treatment efficacy. It is also possible that matching an individual to a specific pharmacologic treatment will enhance efficacy, because biological profiles or subtypes might differ among individuals with PTSD.

B. Psychotherapeutic Interventions

Several psychotherapeutic techniques have been shown to be effective in treating PTSD. A recent meta-analysis of 137 treatment comparisons showed cognitive therapy, exposure therapy, and eye-movement desensitization and reprocessing (EMDR) were among the most effective (Watts et al, 2013). Results also indicate that no single therapy is consistently most effective, and some therapies may not be effective for PTSD.

1. Cognitive–behavioral therapy (CBT)—Although cognitive–behavioral approaches were not developed specifically for PTSD, CBT has become the preferred treatment modality given growing treatment outcome data demonstrating its success with other anxiety disorders. CBT comprises several variations, all of which have a goal of fear extinction and improved coping through conditioning and modifying thoughts.

i. Exposure therapy—Exposure therapy involves reexposing the traumatized individual to sensory stimuli associated with the traumatic event. Exposure can take the form of mental imagery, pictures, role playing, virtual reality, or reinstatement of physiological arousal cues through interoceptive exercises (i.e., sweating, hyperventilation, increased heart and respiratory rates, etc.). The duration of exposure varies and can be as short as a few seconds or as long as 90 minutes (e.g., Prolonged Exposure [PE] therapy). In hierarchical reexposure, trauma cues are introduced systematically, starting with the least threatening stimuli, gradually increasing to exercises of greater intensity as desensitization is achieved. *Systematic desensitization (SD)* occurs over a period of several weeks, though some approaches immediately escalate to the most extreme stressors (e.g., flooding therapy). In either approach, the key to successful exposure therapy is controlling avoidance behaviors and ensuring a positive outcome at the conclusion of each exposure trial. A positive outcome is imperative for each exposure to facilitate extinction of the original feared cue through learning new associations (i.e., cue = positive or tolerable outcome).

ii. Stress inoculation training (SIT)—The principle goal of SIT is to reduce fear reactions that foster operant avoidance and prohibit extinction learning. This goal is accomplished through a three-stage process involving psychoeducation (conditioning theory and psychobiology of fear), cognitive skills training (reframing and relaxation techniques), and application (scenarios, roleplaying, or in vivo exposures).

iii. Cognitive therapy (CT)—CT for PTSD focuses on thoughts and beliefs about the trauma and its associated cues. Targeted thoughts include "the likelihood the trauma will reoccur," "how the individual has responded to trauma," and "what certain reactions to trauma exposure might mean." Individuals are encouraged to identify assumptions and automatic beliefs about the traumatic event (e.g., "I can't handle this," "I'm going crazy," or "PTSD will ruin my life forever"). Individuals then learn to challenge those assumptions through alternative hypothesis generation and reality testing. Other cognitive skills involve learning how to change perspectives (i.e., cognitive reframing or restructuring), decatastrophizing, and relaxation techniques.

iv. Cognitive processing therapy (CPT)—CPT was developed to address the broader range of emotions other than fear that frequently accompany PTSD in victims of rape and crime: anger, guilt, sadness, and shame (Resick & Schnike, 1992). CPT focuses on memories of the traumatic event and exploring associated intense emotions. Trauma memories are explored through the use of diaries and narrative scripts about their trauma, and individuals are encouraged to articulate personal meaning of the traumatic event. Memories of the trauma are reconstructed in narrative format, incorporating as many sensory stimuli into the description as possible. These narratives are then to be read on a daily basis for several weeks. Therapy sessions involve discussion of the trauma narrative and examination of irrational thoughts and unpleasant emotions evoked by remembering. Support for CPT continues to grow, due in part to recent comparison studies that highlight larger treatment effect sizes compared to medication. For example, following a 12-session course of CPT in Vietnam combat veterans, 40% of the intention-to-treat sample no longer met diagnostic criteria for PTSD, a result that was independent of service-connected disability status (Monson et al, 2007).

v. Mindfulness based cognitive therapy (MBCT)—MBCT is a mindfulness-based therapeutic approach that incorporates components of CPT. It is focused on promoting an individual to attain a "decentered" perspective (i.e., thoughts are not facts) (Boyd et al, 2017). This enables individuals with PTSD to better distinguish fear from their current reality.

2. Eye-movement desensitization and reprocessing (EMDR)—EMDR is a controversial technique, not regarding its efficacy, but rather its theoretical underpinnings. EMDR was unintentionally discovered when its originator (Shapiro, 1996) noticed that focusing visual attention on wave movements of tree leaves in the wind provided relief from unpleasant rumination. From this observation, EMDR has evolved as a repetitive lateral eye-movement exercise that facilitates cognitive processing of trauma-related thoughts. EMDR is conducted by the therapist waving the tip of the index finger rapidly back and forth in front of the patient's eyes. The finger tip is held 30–35 cm from the patient's face at a rate of 2 waves per second, for a total of 24 waves. Following each eye-movement trial, the patient is instructed first to attempt to block out the memory, take a relaxing breath, and then return to the memory. Each sequence of EMDR is followed by subjective appraisals of distress precipitated by the memory; the sequence is repeated until subject distress decreases to zero.

3. Mindfulness-based treatments—Since its introduction into Western psychology in the 1980s and 1990s, mindfulness has grown exponentially in its use within the field. Mindfulness-based stress reduction is a commonly used treatment approach. One model of treatment may consist of 8 weeks of 2- to 2.5-hour group sessions. The approach may use mindfulness meditation and yoga. The program encourages nonjudgmental and acceptance of thoughts as they occur in the present (Boyd et Al, 2017).

Several theoretical models have been proposed as to how mindfulness affects brain function and reduces the symptomatology of PTSD. Although mindfulness-based approaches have utility in treating PTSD, more work is needed for them to become first-line approaches. (Boyd et.al 2017)

▶ Complications/Adverse Outcomes of Treatment

The primary complication to psychotherapy for PTSD, especially for cognitive–behavioral-based approaches, is avoidance. Behavioral avoidance can take the form of missed therapy appointments, incomplete treatment homework, or failure to engage trauma cues during in vivo exposures. Cognitive avoidance can also complicate treatment if it is persistent. Sometimes individuals who appear to engage exposure exercises behaviorally may be covertly dissociating from the experience in an effort to attenuate arousal and full exposure to the trauma cue. Avoidance may also take the form of self-medication through the use of alcohol and substance abuse. A complication that has received limited attention is the potential impediment that benzodiazepines present to exposure therapies. The short half-life (i.e., fast action) of some benzodiazepines is a powerful reinforcement to individuals with PTSD who are averse to autonomic arousal. A heavy reliance on benzodiazepines or alcohol interferes with new learning (i.e., extinction conditioning) that is pivotal for extinguishing maladaptive associations with trauma cues. Additional impediments to treatment include sleep irregularities that make new learning more difficult, as well as psychosocial dysfunction that often accompanies chronic, untreated PTSD.

▶ Prognosis

The fact that most individuals with PTSD get better over time does not lessen its psychosocial and functional impact, as subclinical symptom levels can have profound negative consequences. However, the evolution of several promising therapies for PTSD (see section Treatment) suggests that even the most difficult cases are treatable. As is the treatability for those who have strong support networks, fewer comorbid diagnoses, and fully engage in empirically validated treatments. In contrast, individuals with complex PTSD resulting from multiple childhood traumas, poor interpersonal support networks, personality disorders, comorbid substance abuse, and diminished cognitive resources are less likely to recover.

Admon R, Leykin D, Lubin G, et al. Stress-induced reduction in hippocampal volume and connectivity with the ventromedial prefrontal cortex are related to maladaptive response to stressful military service. *Hum Brain Mapp.* 2013;34(11):2808–2816.

Admon R, Milad MR, Hendler T. A causal model of post-traumatic stress disorder: disentangling predisposed from acquired neural abnormalities. *Trends Cogn Sci.* 2013;17(7):337–347.

Aikins DE, Johnson DC, Borelli JL, et al. Thought suppression failures in combat PTSD: a cognitive load hypothesis. *Behav Res Ther.* 2009;47(9):744–751.

American Psychiatric Association: *Diagnostic and Statistical Manual of Mental Disorders*, 4th ed. Washington, DC: American Psychiatric Association; 1994.

American Psychiatric Association. *Diagnostic and Statistical Manual of Mental Disorders*, 4th ed, text revision. Washington, DC: American Psychiatric Association; 2000.

American Psychiatric Association: *Diagnostic and Statistical Manual of Mental Disorders*, 5th ed. Washington, DC: American Psychiatric Association; 2013.

Ashley V, Honzel N, Larsen J, et al. Attentional bias for trauma-related words: exaggerated emotional Stroop effect in Afghanistan and Iraq war veterans with PTSD. *BMC Psychiatry.* 2013;13:86.

Aupperle RL, Melrose AL, Stein MB, et al. Executive function and PTSD: disengaging from trauma. *Neuropharmacology.* 2012; 62(2):686–694.

Baker DG, Ekhator NN, Kasckow JW, et al. Higher levels of basal serial CSF cortisol in combat veterans with posttraumatic stress disorder. *Am J Psychiatry.* 2005;162:992–994.

Boyd J, Lanius R, McKinnon C. Mindfulnes-based treatments for posttraumatic stress disorder: a review of the treatment literature and neurobiological evidence. *J Psychiat Neurosci.* 2018;43(1):7–25.

Breslau N, Kessler RC, Chilcoat HD, et al. Trauma and posttraumatic stress disorder in the community: the 1996 Detroit Area Survey of Trauma. *Arch Gen Psychiatry.* 1998;55(7):626–632.

Brewin CR, Andrews B, Valentine JD. Meta-analysis of risk factors for posttraumatic stress disorder in trauma exposed adults. *J Consult Clin Psychol.* 2000;68:748–766.

Brewin CR, Andrews B, Hejdenberg J, Stewart L. Objective predictors of delayed-onset post-traumatic stress disorder occurring after military discharge. *Psychol Med.* 2012;42(10):2119–2126.

Bryant RA. Post-traumatic stress disorder. In: Stein D, Friedman M, Blanco C, eds. *Psychological Interventions for Trauma Exposure and PTSD.* Chichester, UK: Wiley; 2011:170–202.

Bryant RA, Creamer M, O'Donnell M, et al. A study of the protective function of acute morphine administration on subsequent posttraumatic stress disorder. *Biol Psychiatry.* 2009;65:438–440.

Charney DS. Psychobiological mechanisms of resilience and vulnerability: implications for successful adaptation to extreme stress. *Am J Psychiatry.* 2004;161:195–216.

Dohrenwend BP, Turner JB, Turse NA, et al. The psychological risks of Vietnam for US veterans: a revisit with new data and methods. *Science.* 2006;313:979–982.

Eysenck HJ. *The Biological Basis of Personality.* Springfield, IL: Thomas; 1967.

Foa EB, Kozack MJ. Emotional processing of fear: exposure to corrective information. *Psychol Bull.* 1986;99:20–35.

Friedman MJ. Future pharmacotherapy for post-traumatic stress disorder: prevention and treatment. *Psychiatr Clin North Am.* 2002;25:427–441.

Galea S, Ahern J, Resnick H, et al. Psychological sequelae of the September 11 terrorist attacks in New York City. *N Engl J Med.* 2002;346:982–987.

Galea S, Vlahov D, Resnick H, et al. Trends of probably post-traumatic stress disorder in New York City after the September 11 terrorist attacks. *Am J Epidemiol.* 2003;158:514–524.

Gilbertson MW, Shenton ME, Ciszewski A, et al. Smaller hippocampal volume predicts pathologic vulnerability to psychological trauma. *Nat Neurosci.* 2002;5(11):1242–1247.

Gurvits TV, Metzger LJ, Lasko NB, et al. Subtle neurologic compromise as a vulnerability factor for combat-related posttraumatic stress disorder: results of a twin study. *Arch Gen Psychiatry.* 2006;63:571–576.

Hoge CW, Castro CA, Messer SC, et al. Combat duty in Iraq and Afghanistan, mental health problems, and barriers to care. *N Engl J Med.* 2004;351:13–22.

Holbrook LH, Galarneau MS, Dye JL, et al. Morphine use after combat injury in Iraq and post-traumatic stress disorder. *N Engl J Med.* 2010;362:110–117.

Hidalgo RB, Davidson JRT. Posttraumatic stress disorder: epidemiology and health-related considerations. *J Clin Psychiatry.* 2000;61(suppl 7):5–13.

Hughes KC, Shin LM. Functional neuroimaging studies of posttraumatic stress disorder. *Expert Rev Neurother.* 2011;11:275–285.

Institute of Medicine (U.S.), & National Academies Press (U.S.). Treatment for posttraumatic stress disorder in military and veteran populations: initial assessment. Washington, DC: National Academies Press; 2012.

Jeffreys M, Capehart B, Friedman M. Pharmacotherapy for posttraumatic stress disorder: review with clinical applications. *J Rehabil Res Dev.* 2012;49:703–716.

Kaufman J, Yang BZ, Douglas-Palumberi H, et al. Social supports and serotonin transporter gene moderate depression in mal-treated children. *Proc Natl Acad Sci USA.* 2004;101(49):17316–17321.

Kearns MC, Ressler KJ, Zatzick D, et al. Early intervention for PTSD: a review. *Depress Anxiety.* 2012;29(10):833–842.

Kessler RC, Sonnega A, Bromet E, et al. Posttraumatic stress disorder in the National Comorbidity Survey. *Arch Gen Psychiatry.* 1995;52(12):1048–1060.

Kessler RC, Petukhova M, Sampson NA, et al. Twelve-month and lifetime prevalence and lifetime morbid risk of anxiety and mood disorders in the United States. *Int J Methods Psychiatr Res.* 2012;21(3):169–184.

Kim JJ, Fanselow MS. Modality specific retrograde amnesia of fear. *Science.* 1992;256:675–677.

Kitayama N, Vaccarino V, Kutner M, et al. Magnetic resonance imaging (MRI) measurement of hippocampal volume in posttraumatic stress disorder: a meta-analysis. *J Affect Disord.* 2005;88:79–86.

Kosten TR, Frank JB, Dan E, et al. Pharmacotherapy for posttraumatic stress disorder using phenelzine or imipramine. *J Nerv Ment Dis.* 1991;179:366–370.

Kulka RA, Schlenger WE, Fairbank JA, et al. *Trauma and the Vietnam War Generation: Report of Findings from the National Vietnam Veterans Readjustment Study.* New York: Brunner/Mazel; 1990.

Larson GE, Konoske, P, Hammer, PS, et al. Predeployment and in-theater diagnoses of American military personnel serving in Iraq. *Psychiatr Serv.* 2011;62(1):15–21.

Messer JM, Fremouw WJ. Detecting malingered posttraumatic stress disorder using the Morel Emotional Numbing Test-Revised (MENT-R) and the Miller Forensic Assessment of Symptoms Test (M-FAST). *J Forens Psychol Pract.* 2007;7:33–57.

Mohamed S, Rosenheck R. Pharmacotherapy of PTSD in the U.S. Department of Veterans Affairs: Diagnostic- and symptom-guided drug selection. *J Clin Psychiatry.* 2008;69(6):959–965.

Morel KR. Development and preliminary validation of a forced-choice test of response bias for posttraumatic stress disorder. *J Pers Assess.* 1998;70:299–314.

Morel KR. Comparison of the Morel Emotional Numbing Test for Posttraumatic Stress Disorder to the Word Memory Test in neuropsychological evaluations. *Clin Neuropsychol.* 2008;22(2):350–362.

Monson CM, Schnurr PP, Resick PA, et al. Cognitive processing therapy for veterans with military-related posttraumatic stress disorder. *J Consult Clin Psychol.* 2007;74(5):898–907.

Mowrer OH. On the dual nature of learning: a re-interpretation of "conditioning" and "problem-solving." *Harv Educ Rev.* 1947;17:102–148.

Nestler EJ. Epigenetics: stress makes its molecular mark. *Nature.* 2012;490:171–172.

North CE, Pfefferbaum B, Tivis L, et al. The course of posttraumatic stress disorder in a follow-up study of survivors of the Oklahoma City bombing. *Ann Clin Psychiatry.* 2004;16:209–215.

Orr SP, Metzger LJ, Pitman RK. Psychophysiology of post-traumatic stress disorder. *Psychiatr Clin North Am.* 2002;25:271–293.

Ozer EJ, Best SR, Lipsey TL, Weiss DS. Predictors of posttraumatic stress disorder and symptoms in adults: a meta-analysis. *Psychol Bull.* 2003;129(1):52–73.

Pereda N, Forero CG. Contribution of Criterion A2 to PTSD screening in the presence of traumatic events. *J Trauma Stress.* 2012;25:1–5.

Petrakis IL, Ralevski E, Desai N, et al. Noradrenergic vs serotonergic antidepressant with or without naltrexone for veterans with PTSD and comorbid alcohol dependence. *Neuropsychopharmacology.* 2012;37(4):996–1004.

Phillips RG, LeDoux JE. Differential contribution of amygdala and hippocampus cued to contextual fear conditioning. *Behav Neurosci.* 1992;106:274–285.

Pietrzak RH, Goldstein RB, Southwick SM, Grant BF. Prevalence and Axis I comorbidity of full and partial posttraumatic stress disorder in the United States: results from Wave 2 of the National Epidemiologic Survey on Alcohol and related Conditions. *J Anxiety Disord.* 2011;25:456–465.

Pietrzak RH, Feder A, Singh R, et al. Trajectories of PTSD risk and resilience in World Trade Center responders: an 8 year prospective cohort study. *Psychol Med.* 2013;3:1–15.

Pole N. The psychophysiology of posttraumatic stress disorder: a meta-analysis. *Psychol Bull.* 2007;133:725–746.

Raskind MA, Peterson K, Williams T, et al. A trial of prazosin for combat trauma PTSD with nightmares in active-duty soldiers returned from Iraq and Afghanistan. *Am J Psychiatry.* 2013;170:1003–1010.

Resick PA, Schnicke MK. Cognitive processing therapy for sexual assault victims. *J Consullt Clin Psychol.* 1992;60(5):748–756.

Resnick HS, Kilpatrick DF, Peterson EL, et al. Prevalence of civilian trauma and posttraumatic stress disorder in a representational national sample of women. *J Consult Clin Psychol.* 1993;61:984–991.

Ressler KJ, Mercer KB, Bradley B, et al. Post-traumatic stress disorder is associated with PACAP and the PAC1 receptor. *Nature.* 2011;470:493–497.

Roy-Byrne P, Arguelles L, Vitek ME, et al. Persistence and change of PTSD symptomatology—a longitudinal co-twin analysis of the Vietnam Era Twin Registry. *Soc Psychiatry Psychiatr Epidemiol.* 2004;39:681–685.

Santiago PN, Ursano RJ, Gray CL, et al. A systematic review of PTSD prevalence and trajectories in DSM-5 defined trauma exposed populations: intentional and non-intentional traumatic events. *PLoS One.* 2013;8:e59236.

Seedat S, Stein MB, Kennedy CM, Hauger RL: Plasma cortisol and neuropeptide Y in female victims of intimate partner violence. *Psychoneuroendocrinology.* 2003:28;796–808.

Shalev AY, Gilboa A, Rasmusson AM. Post-traumatic stress disorder. In: Stein D, Friedman M, Blanco C, eds. *Neurobiology of PTSD.* Chichester, UK: Wiley; 2011:89–148.

Shapiro F. Eye movement desensitization and reprocessing (EMDR): evaluation of controlled PTSD research. *J Behav Ther Exp Psychiatry.* 1996;27(3):209–218.

Shin LM, Lasko NB, Macklin ML, et al. Resting metabolic activity in the cingulate cortex and vulnerability to posttraumatic stress disorder. *Arch Gen Psychiatry.* 2009;66(10):1099–1107.

Sofuoglu M, Rosenheck R, Petrakis I. Pharmacological treatment of comorbid PTSD and substance use disorder: recent progress. *Addict Behav.* 2014:39:428–433.

Solomon Z, Mikulincer M. Aftermaths of combat stress reactions: a three-year study. *Br J Clin Psychol.* 1992;31(1):21–32.

Southwick SM, Vythilingam M, Charney DS. The psychobiology of depression and resilience to stress: implications for prevention and treatment. *Annu Rev Clin Psychol.* 2005;1:255–291.

Stein DJ, Isper JC. Post-traumatic stress disorder. In: Stein D, Friedman M, Blanco C, eds. *Neurobiology of PTSD.* Chichester, UK: Wiley; 2011:149–170.

Sumpter RE, McMillan TM. Misdiagnosis of post-traumatic stress disorder following severe traumatic brain injury. *Br J Psychiatry.* 2005;186:423–426.

Thayer JF, Ahs F, Fredickson M, et al. A meta-analysis of heart-rate variability and neuroimaging studies: implications for heart rate variability as a marker of stress and health. *Neurosci Biobehav Rev.* 2012;36:747–756.

Toomey R, Alpern R, Vasterling JJ, et al. Neuropsychological functioning of U.S. Gulf War veterans 10 years after the war. *J Int Neuropsychol Soc.* 2009;15:717–729.

True WR, Rice J, Eisen SA, et al. A twin study of genetic and environmental contributions to liability for posttraumatic stress symptoms. *Arch Gen Psychiatry.* 1993;50(4):257–265.

VA/DoD Clinical Practice Guideline. (n.d.) Retrieved from VA Healthcare System website, http://www.healthquality.va.gov

Vasterling JJ, Brewin CR. *Neuropsychology of PTSD: Biological, Cognitive, and Clinical Perspectives.* New York: Guilford; 2005.

Vogt D, Smith BN, King LA, et al. Deployment Risk and Resilience Inventory-2 (DRRI-2): an updated tool for assessing psychosocial risk and resilience factors among service members and veterans. *J Trauma Stress.* 2013;26:710–717.

Watts BV, Schnurr PP, Mayo L, et al. Meta-analysis of the efficacy of treatments for posttraumatic stress disorder. *J Clin Psychiatry.* 2013;74(6):e541–550.

Weathers FW, Blake DD, Schnurr PP, et al. The Clinician-Administered PTSD Scale for DSM-5 (CAPS-5). 2013. Interview available from the National Center for PTSD at www.ptsd.va.gov.

Xie P, Kranzler H, Yang C, et al. Genome-wide association study identifies new susceptibility loci for posttraumatic stress disorder. *Biol Psychiatry.* 2013:1–8.

ACUTE STRESS DISORDER

▶ General Considerations

ASD was first introduced in DSM-IV. The validity of ASD as a disorder distinct from PTSD has been questioned from its inception and has generated much debate. ASD evolved from an effort to account for symptoms exhibited in the early period following trauma exposure. As such, the primary distinction between ASD and PTSD is the duration of symptoms, with ASD being limited to between 2 days and 4 weeks. In addition, because ASD is circumscribed to 4 weeks following the traumatic event, diagnostic criteria emphasize dissociative symptoms during, or shortly after, exposure. In addition to at least one symptom from each of the three (reexperiencing, avoidance, and arousal) symptom categories required for a diagnosis of PTSD, ASD requires at least three distinct dissociative symptoms: subjective sense of numbing, detachment, or absence of emotional responsiveness; a reduction in awareness of surroundings; derealization; depersonalization; and dissociative amnesia. The presence of dissociative symptoms during or shortly after trauma (i.e., peritraumatic dissociation) has also been a source of contention regarding the validity of ASD, namely the assertion that ASD may pathologize adaptive responses to trauma. Whereas the majority of individuals who meet criteria for ASD do go on to develop PTSD, some individuals with PTSD do not initially meet criteria for ASD (i.e., delayed-onset PTSD).

▶ Clinical Findings

In contrast to the vast literature on PTSD, empirical studies of ASD are few. The dearth of research on ASD may be due to its relatively recent introduction into the DSM-IV, and its inclusion was primarily based on theoretical rather than empirical considerations. Additionally, the majority of data on PTSD come from Veterans Affairs Administration studies. Veterans treated in VA Hospitals traumatic experience occurred long before becoming veterans. This leaves no acute group to study. To date, there are three psychometrically valid metrics for assessing ASD: (1) the Stanford Acute Stress Reaction Questionnaire; (2) the Acute Stress Disorder Interview; and (3) the Acute Stress Disorder Scale.

ASD is a strong predictor of PTSD. Prospective studies have found that between 72 and 83% of individuals with ASD have gone on to develop PTSD at 6 months post trauma and that between 63 and 80% of those with ASD meet criteria for PTSD 2 years following trauma.

Differential Diagnosis

Differential diagnosis can be complicated, as a number of seemingly comorbid disorders are mutually exclusive to a diagnosis of ASD. Further complicating the diagnosis of ASD is our increased understanding of the normal range of reactions to human trauma, many of which are also symptoms of ASD and PTSD. Therefore, as with many other disorders, diagnosis is often predicated on duration of the symptoms and functional impairment. In the case of ASD, symptoms must be present for at least 2 days following trauma exposure and produce significant occupational, social, or functional impairment. If symptoms persist for longer than 30 days, then a diagnosis of PTSD is given.

ASD is also differentiated from disorders that are associated with exposure to trauma, namely substance induced disorder and disorder due to a general medical condition such as TBI suffered from motor vehicle accidents or combat trauma. Individuals who do not meet full criteria for ASD but have impairment of functioning following a trauma or stressor should be given a diagnosis of adjustment disorder instead.

Treatment and Complications/Adverse Outcomes of Treatment

See section in PTSD.

Prognosis

Extant research shows that the vast majority of individuals who meet criteria for ASD following trauma go on to develop PTSD. Of note, however, is that the majority of PTSD cases resolve over time. In this respect, the prognosis for individuals with ASD is parallel to that of PTSD.

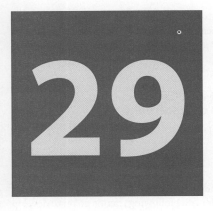

Prolonged Grief Disorder

Sidney H. Weissman, MD

ESSENTIALS ELEMENTS OF DIAGNOSIS

The DSM-5-TR definition of Prolonged Grief Disorder addresses disruptive behavior that interferes on a daily basis with an individual's functioning after the loss of a significant individual in their life at least 12 months after their death. It does not address mourning behaviors. For children and adolescents, the period is 6 months.

Further for an individual's behavior to be labeled prolonged grief, they must experience near-constant psychic pain of enough intensity to be disabling. The experience needs to have been present nearly daily for the month prior to a psychiatric evaluation. The patient must additionally experience either intense yearning or longing for the deceased individual and/or intrusive thoughts or memories of the deceased.

The descriptions of the pathological behaviors or symptoms required for the diagnosis include at least three of the following:

a. Feeling that an element of oneself may have died or is changed since the death
b. Not fully believing the person has died
c. Avoiding artifacts that might remind one of the deceased
d. Intense pain related to the loss
e. Difficulty resuming one's life after the death
f. Difficulty feeling
g. Questioning the meaning of life
h. Feeling alone without the presence of the deceased

▶ Special Considerations

When a new psychiatric disorder is added or deleted from our diagnostic system for Mental Disorders, it is essential to ask why. What have we newly learned to justify adding this new disorder? Is it a new understanding of behavior or new knowledge of brain functioning? When we delete a diagnosis is that because we previously wrongly confused "atypical" behavior as a mental disorder? In the case of prolonged grief disorder (PGD), it may be neither of these. All of us have experienced the loss of a loved one. We have all dealt with that loss in our own unique fashion, which has been shaped by our unique life experiences. Our private experiences of our grief were impacted by our relationship with the deceased. The death of a parent, a spouse, or one's child is particularly painful as experienced uniquely by each of us. Our own learned religious practices contribute to how we respond to a loss. Additionally, the deceased loved one's position in and outside of the family also may have had an impact. Societal behavioral norms also affect us. Mourning is the process of dealing with the grief triggered by the loss. It allows us psychologically to deal with the loss that enables us to resume our unique life activities. Mourning does not remove the experience and sustained memory of a significant loss.

When we have dealt with the losses of differing individuals in our life, we experienced a sense of pain for varied lengths of time for each loss. Initially, we struggled to respond to the world and could not focus on our usual work activities. As time passed, we returned to our previous level of functioning. For some losses, we may have initially blocked out a response and acted as if nothing happened. We observed similar behavior among the members of our family and friends. Observation of the bereaved does not tell us the intensity of their grief and feeling state.

We respond to bereaved individuals by acknowledging their distress with culturally determined responses. Sometimes we offer a silent hug. We may bring them meals or care for family members and initially call them every day. Each of us has unique personal factors that determine our responses.

Losing a loved one, experiencing grief, and mourning the loss are basic human experiences. Today, the American Psychiatric Association and the World Health Organization, in its International Classification of Disease (ICD-11), have concluded that unrelenting grief is not a normal response to loss. Grief while initially disrupting our functioning is a normal response. When it continues to do so in such a manner that it prevents an individual from returning to their normal state is pathological.

However, neither the DSM nor ICD diagnoses prolonged grief on the basis of an individual's behavior alone. The behaviors described in Prolonged Grief Disorder may occur in normal mourning. For the diagnosis of Prolonged Grief Disorder as a mental disorder, these behaviors must occur nearly every day for 6 months after the loss of a loved one according to ICD-11, and 12 months according to DSM-5-TR, significantly interfering with the individual's functioning. After 1 year, these once normal processes are not representative of mourning but of altered thought and feeling processes.

The DSM-5-TR and ICD-11 writers do not designate mourning, which is a complex and at times painful human experience, as a disorder. We have all seen individuals who suffer from what appears as unending, overwhelming pain as they mourn a loss, which interferes with their rerun to their normal functioning. Then at a later date, they resume their prior life, while others, apparently experiencing less severe suffering, do not. The writers of Prolonged Grief Disorder in the DSM and ICD struggled to understand the complex forces that shape how each of us mourns a given loss, how long this process will take, and when mourning becomes a pathological process. This difficulty is underlined by the fact that the DSM suggests it can take twice as long for the mourning process to become pathological and ineffective compared to the ICD. Whether in 6 or 12 months, when sustained grief occurs, it prevents an individual from resuming their normal level of functioning.

EPIDEMIOLOGY

The exact numbers of individuals who have suffered from Prolonged Grief Disorder are difficult to determine. The percentages of sufferers in a population differ when using the criteria from ICD-11 and the DSM-5-TR. Which one gives a better assessment of the frequency of the disorder and the pain it manifests will be determined in the future. Some data suggest that women suffer from the disorder at a higher frequency than men.

ETIOLOGY

The stimulus that leads to an individual developing PGD is the loss of a loved one. The factors that prevent an individual within 6 (ICD-11) or 12 (DSM-5-TR) months after the loss from effectively mourning the loss and resuming their prior level of functioning are unique for each individual. Mourning is a complex human experience in dealing with losses.

Recalling the lost individual wishing they were with you is not a sign of ineffective mourning or any psychiatric morbidity. At times, the bereaved, even years later, will at some moment "experience" the deceased as being with them or experience an intense pain as they think or associate some action or event to the lost person. However, when the pain of the loss and a focus on the lost loved one is experienced daily and prevents a return to previous levels of functioning after 12 months (DSM), we do not consider these responses as an element of mourning. This is now a pathological process, not mourning. We do not know for a given individual what interferes with the mourning process such that the individual experiences sustained grief and cannot return to their previous level of functioning.

While DSM requires the persistence of behaviors focused on the deceased, which exist for a month and interfere with functioning after 12 months after the loss, to be called prolonged grief, individuals may suffer from disabling grief prior to 12 months. Indeed, as previously noted, it is the disabling grief that interferes with mourning, which prevents one from resuming their life. The difficulty in assessing when the persistence of grief is interfering with essential life processes is seen in the differing time frames of ICD-11 and the DSM-5-TR to make the diagnosis.

GENETICS

There are no genetic involvements.

CLINICAL FINDINGS

▶ Signs and Symptoms

The critical factor in making a diagnosis of Prolonged Grief Disorder is that an individual cannot function effectively at their normal level on a daily basis, is preoccupied with the loss of a loved one, and is in near constant psychic pain. They may or not be tearful, but their thoughts and feelings are dominated by preoccupations with the deceased and a connection to them. These personal experiences must occur on a near daily basis for 12 months after the loss and prevent a return to the individual's normal level of functioning. It is assumed in this diagnosis that the pain of a loss should have been effectively dealt with within 1 year. Grieving the loss of a pet or a possession does not allow one to call it Prolonged Grief, even though the responses may be the same.

PSYCHOLOGICAL TESTING

Psychological testing may be helpful in identifying some impaired cognitive functioning or a subtle personality disorder, which may interfere with mourning.

Laboratory Findings

None.

Neuroimaging

No specific diagnostic imaging studies have revealed specific lesions for Prolonged Grief Disorder.

Differential Diagnosis

In assessing individuals with grief responses and pain, it is important not to just consider patients potentially suffering from PGD. An immediate complication of a loss with overwhelming grief complicating an individual's response to the loss is whether it was the result of a suicide or that the survivor was a caretaker. In these situations, some will feel guilt that they should have prevented the death. These life experiences may both create pathological grief but may also precipitate suicidal ideation in the bereaved manifested by a desire to be re-united with the lost loved one. The psychiatrist must be alert to their suicidal risk.

Concurrent with PGD, an individual may also suffer from or develop a number of other mental disorders. Most significant is a major depression. If the death was a violent event in which the individual was a survivor, they may also suffer from PTSD.

The death of a child triggers unique responses some of which are PGD and others are not. Parents for years may keep in their minds the deceased child and frequently speak to others of their thoughts of what the deceased child would be doing if alive. This is not an example of Prolonged Grief Disorder.

The confluence of psychological responses that creates prolonged grief may also precipitate suicidal ideation in the bereaved manifested by a desire to be reunited with the lost loved one. The psychiatrist must be alert to these individuals' suicidal risk.

For some individuals, the behavioral responses observed in PGD will appear similar to those suffering from separation anxiety disorder except that for PGD the separation is for a deceased individual. Strikingly, the time requirement in the DSM for separation anxiety disorder for destructive behaviors is 6 months. However, the DSM gives flexibility to clinicians in making this diagnosis.

The observed and reported symptoms of PGD cannot be explained by any other medical or psychiatric disorder. Further, the length and intensity of the bereavement must exceed the societal, religious, or cultural norms for the bereaved. However, it is important to use the 12-month requirement to make the diagnosis as only a guideline.

TREATMENT

Treatment for a specific behavior, which is determined to meet the criteria of a mental health disorder, is based on the determination that the patient's symptoms and behaviors are at a significant variance from the societal, religious, or cultural norms that are expected for the age of the individual. Treatments are predicated on an understanding of the both the cause of the disorder and the symptomatic behavior that cause pain. The intent of treatment is to reduce a patient's experience of suffering. In the case of PGD, this is complicated by the symptoms and behavior being potentially manifestations of normal mourning when observed within a year of a loss.

Psychotherapy

Before instituting any treatment of PGD, it is essential that the clinician engage in an in-depth psychological assessment of the patient. This must include a close examination of their relationship to the deceased. For example, how frequently did they interact. Did the bereaved look to the deceased for guidance in various aspects of their life and feel they could not function without them? Further, it is also critical to learn how they have dealt with losses in the past, which may have interfered for some time with their functioning. Learning of their culture and religious beliefs and how they impacted on bereavement and their daily life is essential. If available, interviewing family members may be helpful.

In assessing a parent who has lost a child, it is also critical to learn if parenting was shared with a co-parent or another family member. Parents who have lost children frequently continue to maintain a psychological connection to them. For years, they will "in their minds" age them and wonder what they would be like or doing. This need not interfere with another aspect of their lives.

The selection of a therapy where the disorder is similar in many cases to "normal" mourning where many individuals retain powerful memories and pain from a loss throughout their lives is difficult. What in these varied circumstances should be the focus of therapy? With these questions in mind after a careful assessment using a biopsychosocial and societal framework, the clinician must select treatment. Some success is reported with versions of cognitive behavioral therapy. Dynamic psychotherapy would be indicated if it is possible to identify with the patient issues they have not resolved with the deceased. In psychotherapeutic exploration, other characterological issues that impair dealing with the loss may be discovered and addressed.

A number of special considerations confront psychiatrists when addressing patients suffering from pain while mourning. First, the intense pain may not be from the loss of a loved one but from the loss of a pet, an idea, a political cause, or their house or effects. DSM-5-TR PGD only addresses the loss of a person. However, that does not mean that the same experience cannot occur for other losses. Further, DSM-5-TR addresses a condition after 1 year from the loss. Individuals may seek help for intense pain while mourning well before a year. The clinician uses their skills to assess these individuals. If they do not meet the criteria for Prolonged Grief Disorder but still exhibit signs of distress, the clinician develops a treatment plan. In these circumstances, the treatment plans will be difficult and may be developed along the lines of treatment plans for PGD.

In developing treatment plans for these patients, it is necessary to assess for other mental disorders. They may also suffer from PTSD, various forms of depression, as well as from a personality disorder, schizophrenia, and bipolar disorder. Again, the clinician must then be prepared to treat all disorders and how they impact on each other.

Determining treatment for anyone suffering from pain while mourning at any time during the grieving process after a loss requires the clinician to use all of their empathic clinical skills.

▶ **Psychopharmacologic Interventions**

Symptomatic use of benzodiazepines may be useful for the reduction of intense anxiety. Medications may also be required for other psychiatric disorders present.

▶ **Prognosis**

An unweathering experience of disabling grief for an individual would appear to signal a poor outcome of resuming normal functioning. However, we do not know the factors for each individual that triggered the disorder, so it is not possible without working with them to assess a long-term prognosis.

Dietl, Wagner B, Fydrich T. User acceptability of the diagnosis of prolonged grief disorder: how do professionals think about inclusions in ICD11. *J Affect Disord.* 2018;229:306–313.

Eisma N, Janshen A, Lonneke J, Lenferink M. Content overlap analyses of ICD-11 and DSM-5 prolonged grief disorder and prior criteria-sets. *Eur J Psychopharmacol.* 2022;13:2011691.

Freud S. *Mourning and Melancholia.* Standard Edition, Volume X1V. London: Hogarth Press; 1957:1915–1917.

Harrison O, Windmann S, Rosner R, Steil R. Inclusion of the other in the self as a potential risk factor for prolonged grief disorder: a comparison of patients with matched bereaved healthy controls. *Clin Psychol Psychother.* 2022;29(3):1101–1112.

Middleton W, Raphael B, Martinek N, Misso V. Pathological grief reactions. In: *Handbook of Bereavement.* Cambridge, UK: Cambridge University Press; 1993:44–61.

Levy Y. Prolonged grief disorder a new diagnostic entity in DSM-5-TR. *Vertex.* 2022;33(156):51–55.

Stroebe S, Strobe W, Hansson R. *Handbook of Bereavement: Theory, Research, and Intervention.* Cambridge, UK: Cambridge University Press; 1993.

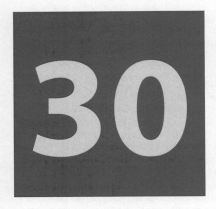

Obsessive–Compulsive Disorder

Sarah B. Abdallah, MD
Thomas V. Fernandez, MD

ESSENTIALS OF DIAGNOSIS

Obsessive–compulsive disorder (OCD) is a psychiatric disorder characterized by disabling obsessions and compulsions that are difficult to control. Obsessions are unwanted, aversive cognitive experiences (thoughts, sensations, or urges) usually associated with feelings of dread, loathing, or a disturbing sense that something is not right. The individual usually recognizes that these concerns are inappropriate in relation to reality and will generally attempt to ignore or suppress them. Compulsions are overt behaviors or covert mental acts performed to reduce the intensity of the aversive obsessions, relieve anxiety associated with the obsession, or achieve a sense of completion. They may occur as behaviors governed by rigid, but often irrelevant, internal specifications. They are inappropriate in nature or intensity in relation to the external circumstances that provoked them.

OCD is diagnosed by clinical evaluation based on the criteria outlined in the *Diagnostic and Statistical Manual of Mental Disorders,* Fifth Edition, Text Revision (DSM-V-TR), listed in Table 30-1. To qualify for the diagnosis, an individual must have time-consuming obsessions or compulsions that cause distress and impairment. Rating scales can be used to assess symptom severity and monitor response to treatment. The most widely applied OCD symptom scales are the Yale–Brown Obsessive Compulsive Scale (Y-BOCS) for adults and the Children's Y-BOCS (CY-BOCS) for children.

▶ General Considerations

A. Epidemiology

1. Population frequencies—Worldwide lifetime prevalence rates of OCD range from 1–3%; they are similar (approximately 2%) in Europe, Africa, Canada, and the Middle East but appear to be lower (0.5–0.9%) in certain Asian countries (i.e., India and Taiwan). Lower prevalence rates in selected U.S. and other national populations could be related to cultural factors resulting in differential reporting of symptoms or biological factors resulting in differential susceptibility. Although OCD is considered a lifetime illness, lifetime prevalence rates in young adults are more than twice than those in older adults. It is unclear whether this observation represents a reporting bias, waning of symptoms with advancing age, shorter life expectancy in individuals with OCD, or changing environmental factors relating to the etiology of the illness.

OCD is usually first seen in childhood or early adulthood: 65% of individuals have their onset before the age of 25 years, 15% after the age of 35 years, and 30% in childhood or early adolescence. In this latter group, there is a 2:1 preponderance of males; in contrast, OCD in the adult population is slightly more predominant in females.

The frequency of specific obsessions and compulsions is consistent across populations. Contamination fears are present in approximately 50% of individuals with OCD, unwarranted fears that something is wrong (called pathologic doubt) in 40%, and other obsessions, including the need for symmetry, fear of harm to self or others, and unwanted sexual concerns, in 25–30%. Checking and decontamination rituals are the predominant compulsions in OCD (50–60%). Other rituals, such as arranging, counting, repeating, and repetitive superstitious acts, occur less frequently (30–35%). Most individuals with OCD (60%) have multiple obsessions or compulsions, and symptom clusters can change over time (e.g., a compulsive hand-washer will lose the fear of contamination and develop fears of harming others).

2. Population subtypes—The DSM-V-TR indicates insight and tic-related specifiers as subtypes of OCD and related disorders. Insight categories include good or fair insight, poor insight, or absent insight (complete conviction in OCD-related thoughts). Tic-related OCD may include compulsions such as touching, tapping, rubbing, blinking, and repetitive behaviors. These compulsions may resemble complex tics but

Table 30–1 Diagnostic Criteria

Presence of obsessions, compulsions, or both:

Obsessions are defined by (1) and (2):

1. Recurrent and persistent thoughts, urges or images that are experienced, at some time during the disturbance, as intrusive, unwanted, and that in most individuals cause marked anxiety or distress.
2. The individual attempts to ignore or suppress such thoughts, urges, or images or to neutralize them with some thought or action (i.e., by performing a compulsion).

Compulsions are defined by (1) and (2):

1. Repetitive behaviors (e.g., hand washing and ordering checking) or mental acts (e.g., praying, counting, and repeating words silently) that the person feels driven to perform in response to an obsession, or according to the rules that must be applied rigidly.
2. The behaviors or mental acts are aimed at preventing or reducing distress or preventing some dreaded event or situation. However, they are either not connected in a realistic way with what they are designed to neutralize or prevent, or they are clearly excessive.

The obsessions or compulsions are time-consuming (e.g., take more than 1 hour per day) or cause clinically significant distress or impairment in social, occupational, or other important areas of functioning.

The disturbance is not better explained by the symptoms of another mental disorder.

The disturbance is not due to the direct physiological effects of a substance (e.g., drug of abuse and a medication) or a general medical condition.

Specify if:

With good or fair insight: the individual recognizes that obsessive–compulsive beliefs are definitely or probably not true or that they may or may not be true.

With poor insight: the individual thinks that obsessive–compulsive disorder beliefs are probably true.

With absent insight/delusional beliefs: the individual is completely convinced that obsessive–compulsive disorder beliefs are true.

Specify if:

Tic related: the individual has a current or past history of a tic disorder.

---

are performed to relieve the distress from an obsession rather than to fulfill a sensory or premonitory urge.

Individuals can also be subtyped into two groups based on experiences of (1) pathologic doubt (e.g., dread and uncertainty) or (2) incompletion or "not-just-right" perceptions. Individuals within these two subgroups appear to share common symptom clusters, coexisting conditions, and treatment prognoses. Finally, a subset of individuals with OCD and schizotypal personality disorder has been characterized. These individuals are more likely to have poor insight and poor social functioning, may require a different treatment regimen, and are often refractory to treatment.

B. Etiology

The etiology of OCD is understood to involve a combination of genetic and environmental factors. As is the case for many psychiatric disorders, the genetics of OCD are complex and not yet well understood. Environmental influences are thought to be multifactorial and may include birth complications, reproductive cycle events, and stressful or traumatic life experiences.

OCD can result from pathologic processes affecting cerebral functioning. For example, severe head trauma and epilepsy have been associated with obsessive–compulsive symptoms. Disorders affecting the functioning of the basal ganglia have also been associated with OCD, and a postinfectious autoimmune-related form of OCD has been described in children. OCD symptoms in children have been observed

after infection with type A β-hemolytic *Streptococcus* bacteria, such that the syndrome has been called Pediatric Autoimmune Neuropsychiatric Disorder Associated with Streptococcal infection (PANDAS). Still, the role of autoimmune illness in the development of OCD remains contested and poorly understood.

C. Genetics

OCD occurs more frequently in family members of individuals with OCD, with an estimated rate in first-degree relatives that is 5- to 10-fold greater than the general population. When combined with subclinical obsessions and compulsions, symptom prevalence rates approach 20% in first-degree relatives. Notably, familial rates of OCD are significantly higher with childhood-onset than adult-onset OCD. This may be related to a heritable tic-related form of OCD with onset in childhood. Twin studies demonstrate the heritability of OCD, with estimates ranging from 27 to 47% for adult-onset and 45 to 65% for childhood-onset cases.

Progress has been made in recent years toward identifying genes and genetic variants associated with OCD. The disorder is understood to be highly polygenic, meaning many genes contribute to the condition, and different individuals with OCD have different combinations of genetic factors contributing to the etiology. Current understanding posits that a combination of small-effect common variants and large-effect rare variants in hundreds of genes and other genomic regions contribute to developing OCD.

Several genome-wide association studies (GWAS) have been conducted to understand the role of common genetic variation (defined as having a frequency in the general population of greater than 5%) in OCD. The largest OCD GWAS to date found genome-wide significant associations at approximately 30 independent genetic loci, including one previously identified locus. Studies examining rare genetic variants have seen a significant association with de novo variants, which arise spontaneously in individuals rather than being inherited from their parents. Studies of whole-exome DNA sequencing in individuals with OCD and their parents have found an increased rate of rare gene-damaging de novo variants in OCD versus control subjects. Examining these variants has implicated two likely OCD risk genes, *CHD8* and *SCUBE1*. Finally, rare copy number variants (deletions or duplications of DNA segments over one kilobase in length) have been implicated in OCD. However, these have not yet identified OCD risk genes or loci.

▶ **Clinical Findings**

A. Signs & Symptoms

The clinical hallmarks of obsessions are aversive experiences of dread and uncertainty or the disturbing sense that something is not right or is incomplete. Obsessive thoughts are the ideas associated with obsessive experiences. They are often bizarre or inadequate explanations for these experiences. Obsessions can take the form of aversive mental images, dread, and disgust related to perceived defilement, feelings that something terrible has happened or is about to happen, or an urgent sense that something that must be done has not yet been completed. A sense of immediacy and urgency is almost always associated with the aversive experiences. Obsessions can be present without compulsions, most frequently when the individual recognizes that no action can alleviate the aversive experience. Under such circumstances, individuals may only seek reassurance that their fears are unfounded or unrealistic.

Compulsions are willed responses to reduce the aversive circumstances associated with obsessive thoughts. They are generally carried out in concordance with the ideation surrounding the obsessions. They can be overt behaviors or silent mental acts such as checking, praying, counting, or other mental rituals. Mental compulsions differ from obsessive experiences in that they are willed mental acts performed for a purpose rather than sensory or ideational experiences. Compulsions are usually carried out in a repetitive or stereotyped fashion, although they can be situation specific, dependent on the content of the obsessive thought. Compulsions can also be carried out in the absence of specific obsessive thoughts. In such cases, they are usually responses to an urgent sense that something is not right or is incomplete.

Most adults with OCD recognize their fears and behaviors as unrealistic or excessive. Insight in OCD can vary from states of total awareness that the symptoms are irrational, with a few lingering doubts, through equivocal acknowledgment, to a delusional state in which the individual is convinced of the validity of their fear and the necessity of the consequent behavior. Some adults lose insight only during exacerbations of their illness. Others, often with schizotypal personalities, may have true insight only early in the illness or transiently when their condition is quiescent.

Avoidance may be a prominent secondary symptom of OCD. Individuals with OCD avoid circumstances that trigger aversive obsessions or lead to time-consuming compulsions. Avoidance, itself, is not a compulsion, but when the illness is severe, it can be a prominent clinical feature. During treatment, as avoidance is reduced, a temporary, paradoxical increase in compulsions can occur because of increased exposure to circumstances that trigger them.

B. Associated Experiences

OCD stands out among psychiatric disorders in the degree to which the individual's thoughts and concerns diverge from their awareness of reality. Most individuals with OCD recognize the irrational nature of their behavior. They are acutely aware of demeaning perceptions that others might have if they knew the degree to which they were affected by their illness. Ashamed and embarrassed, they are often reluctant to disclose their symptoms to anyone who might not understand their condition. As a result, individuals with OCD may be highly secretive about their symptoms.

Early in the illness, individuals with OCD will try to hide their symptoms and may delay seeking treatment until those around them notice their symptoms. Many will not reveal their condition to their primary physicians. Therapists sometimes will care for a patient for several years before discovering that they have OCD. This is particularly true for individuals who experience horrific sexual, blasphemous, or violent thoughts and images. These individuals may fear that their therapist will believe that they want these scenarios to occur and that they might act inappropriately in concordance with their obsessive thoughts. In short, they fear the therapist will confirm their fears and self-condemnation. They may leave a therapeutic relationship if they sense that the therapist does not understand the illness.

The combination of secrecy, avoidance of contact with others, and the time-consuming nature of compulsions may lead to social isolation and secondary depression. Most individuals with OCD also experience heightened internal tension and distress. When their OCD is worse, they will describe feelings of desperation and despair as they cannot relieve their feelings of dread and uncertainty. It is these feelings that may lead the individual to seek initial treatment. Individuals with OCD may also have an unreasonable fear of losing control. These feelings can be exacerbated by a perceived inability to control their compulsive behavior. The individual with OCD may fear that they will lose control of natural inhibitions and act socially or personally maladaptively.

C. Psychological Testing & Instruments for Diagnosis & Measurement

The most commonly used diagnostic measure for OCD is the Y-BOCS. This semi-structured interview includes a symptom checklist, a symptom hierarchy list, and the Y-BOCS. The rating scale evaluates the severity of obsessions and compulsions on an ordinal scale from 0 to 4 (based on time spent, interference, distress, resistance, and degree of control). The maximum score for this scale is 40. Individuals with scores above 31 are considered to have extreme symptoms. Scores of 24–31 indicate severe symptoms, and 16–23 indicate moderate symptoms. Scores below 16 are considered mild to subclinical symptoms that often do not require treatment. Y-BOCS scores for individuals with untreated OCD who enter an OCD clinic are typically 23–25. The Y-BOCS also rates certain ancillary symptoms for informational purposes and provides for global assessments of severity and improvement.

Similarly, the CY-BOCS is a semi-structured interview to assess the severity of symptoms in children and adolescents between the ages of 6 and 17 years, with a similar scoring system. Importantly, while the Y-BOCS and CY-BOCS are often used to assess symptom severity and impact of OCD, these scales are not intended to be independent diagnostic tools on their own. Instead, clinicians diagnose OCD using combined information gathered via structured clinical interviews, clinician-administered inventories, self-report, and parent-report measures. Self-report rating scales used for assessing OCD symptom severity and for tracking changes over time include the Florida Obsessive-Compulsive Inventory, the Obsessive-Compulsive and Related Disorders-Dimensional Scales, and the Brief Obsessive-Compulsive Scale.

D. Laboratory Findings & Imaging

Currently, no clinical laboratory or imaging tests are used to diagnose, monitor, or otherwise inform the treatment of OCD. However, some neuroimaging research studies have shown structural and functional differences in the brain of individuals with OCD compared to unaffected control subjects. One of the most consistent findings across neuroimaging studies in OCD points to dysregulated activity and connectivity in cortico–striatal–thalamocortical (CSTC) circuits. These circuits connect neural pathways between the cerebral cortex and thalamus via the basal ganglia.

Structural imaging studies using magnetic resonance imaging (MRI) or computed tomography (CT) have reported decreased frontal gray and white matter volume bilaterally in OCD. Functional imaging studies, including positron emission tomography (PET) and single photon emission computed tomography (SPECT), have found increased resting metabolic activity in the orbitofrontal cortex. Increased metabolic activity has also been found in the basal ganglia, particularly the caudate nucleus. Hyperactivity in CSTC circuits correlates with OCD symptomatology, and effective treatment of OCD by either pharmacologic or behavioral means has been associated with regionally specific decreases in resting metabolic activity. Currently, imaging procedures are primarily of research interest and have little diagnostic or therapeutic value.

Other studies have found biochemical, neuroendocrine, and physiologic alterations associated with the neurotransmitter serotonin. Again, clinically useful tests have yet to result from this work. Finally, neurologic soft signs, eye-tracking results, and electroencephalogram measurements have sometimes been found to be abnormal in individuals with OCD, and the severity of soft signs may correlate with the severity of OCD.

▶ Differential Diagnoses and Co-Existing Conditions

A. Differential Diagnoses

When considering a diagnosis of OCD, it is important to consider several other conditions that may present with similar symptoms. Differential psychiatric diagnoses for OCD are summarized in Table 30–2.

1. Major depressive disorder—Major depressive disorder (MDD) and related mood disorders can present with features resembling obsessions of OCD. Depressive ruminations involve the persistent cognitive reprocessing of memories and experiences associated with sadness, a sense of loss, or regret. Unlike obsessions, there is no dread, uncertainty, or sense of urgency that the situation must be remedied. Individuals with MDD also can experience pathologic guilt, a heightened experience of responsibility for misfortune or harm. The perceived responsibility is usually excessive for the circumstance and can even be delusional in nature. It is almost always associated with depressed mood. It differs from an obsession in that the individual truly believes they bear responsibility for an adverse circumstance and experiences excessive remorse. Individuals with OCD may fear being responsible for horrific events but usually recognize their fears are unrealistic. Notably, many individuals with

Table 30–2 Differential Psychiatric Diagnosis for Obsessive–Compulsive Disorder

Anorexia nervosa
Body dysmorphic disorder
Excoriation disorder
Generalized anxiety disorder
Illness anxiety disorder
Major depressive disorder
Obsessive–compulsive personality disorder
Specific phobias
Trichotillomania

OCD become depressed, and MDD is the most common co-occurring diagnosis with OCD.

2. Generalized anxiety disorder—Anxious ruminations and excessive worries are common features of generalized anxiety disorder. These persistent, intrusive concerns about adverse circumstances in the future can be confused with obsessions. However, they differ from obsessions in that they are realistic, although they may be excessive. Worries can be fleeting or semiconscious mental experiences associated with feelings of anxiety, whereas anxious ruminations are drawn out in time as the mind reviews potential adverse scenarios. They are not associated with rituals. In contrast to anxious ruminations, obsessions are immediate, aversive sensory experiences; they are often accompanied by incongruous dreadful mental images and specific, unrealistic fears that those circumstances might occur or might have already occurred. Although an individual may take preparatory actions associated with anxious ruminations, the experience lacks the dreadful immediacy of obsessive fears and the sense of urgency that drives the compulsive behaviors.

3. Obsessive–compulsive personality disorder—Obsessive-compulsive personality disorder (OCPD) is a personality disorder with a name that sounds similar to OCD but is associated with meticulousness, persistence, rigidity, and personal isolation. Only a small minority of individuals with OCD have concurrent OCPD. The key difference between the elements of OCPD and OCD is the ego-syntonic nature of the experiences and behavior in OCPD. There is no dread but rather a desire that others conform to the individual's standards.

4. Specific phobias—Specific phobias involve excessive fears of particular situations or circumstances. They often include fears of situations that others might experience as mildly aversive or anxiety provoking (e.g., contact with snakes or spiders), but the phobic individual has an excessive reaction to those circumstances. Avoidance is prominent and effective in allaying anxiety. In OCD, fears can be situation specific; however, there is usually a sense of doubt or uncertainty associated with the dread (e.g., uncertainty about whether germs are present), as the individual cannot be sure they have successfully avoided the aversive circumstance. No rituals are involved in simple phobias.

5. Illness anxiety disorder—Illness anxiety disorder (IAD) is an unreasonable, excessive worry that one has a severe illness. It can lead to repeated requests for medical care or reassurance. It can mimic the obsessions of OCD; however, concerns are limited to the body, and there are no other obsessions and compulsions. The individual is usually not delusional and may recognize that the behavior is excessive. Individuals with IAD usually lack the sense of immediacy that exists in OCD. The individual experiences worry about long-term health rather than short-term immediate dread.

IAD can be associated with abnormal somatic perceptions, which are unusual in OCD.

6. Body dysmorphic disorder—Body dysmorphic disorder (BDD) involves the unreasonable sense that something about the body is malformed, inadequate, or offensive to others. The individual may spend excessive time looking at or seeking medical or surgical treatment for the affected area. BDD differs from OCD in the degree of insight, as the individual with BDD truly believes that the body area is abnormal. There is no sense of incompletion or dread that something terrible will happen. The driven behaviors associated with BDD involve corrective measures to hide or alter an imagined defect and are not carried out because something has not been completed. The distinction between BDD and OCD can be difficult when the individual experiences "just-right" perceptions related to the body or when the individual has a fear of having an offensive body odor. In such cases, the diagnosis of OCD may be warranted.

7. Trichotillomania—Trichotillomania is characterized by urges to pull hairs from the body. The hair is most frequently pulled out singly, and pulling is associated with an experience of pleasure or a release of tension. Binges of hair pulling result in large bald patches. Trichotillomania differs from OCD in that the former involves no obsessions, and the behavior is rewarding.

8. Excoriation disorder—Excoriation disorder or skin-picking disorder can occur as an unconscious habit or response to an exaggerated concern about the skin's texture. The individual may be drawn to the behavior by an attractive process that is hard to overcome. Individuals are typically aware that their actions are destructive; however, they cannot overcome the desire to carry out the behavior. Such picking is similar to trichotillomania in this regard. It differs from OCD in that in pathologic skin-picking, there is no sense of dread, uncertainty, or incompletion, and the behavior is not carried out to prevent something bad from happening. It also differs from OCD in that pathologic skin-picking has a self-destructive or mutilative component rarely seen in uncomplicated OCD.

9. Anorexia nervosa—Anorexia nervosa involves an excessive concern with body image, accompanied by a refusal to eat, with purposeful behavior directed at maintaining a low body weight. In anorexia nervosa, there is a delusional perception that the body is overweight. Unlike in OCD, the individual with anorexia has no insight regarding this concern. Feelings of dread, uncertainty, or incompletion are absent or are not prominent. Driven behaviors are performed to maintain or exacerbate a desired condition. Although hoarding may be observed, no true compulsions are associated with the primary illness. Individuals with OCD can experience significant weight loss in conjunction with fears related to food contamination. These individuals, however, do not typically have concerns about their body image and often acknowledge the absurdity of their condition.

B. Co-Existing Conditions

OCD can co-occur with several other psychiatric disorders, including many described above. These can arise as independent conditions or secondary complications of OCD, as described later in this chapter. Other notable psychiatric diagnoses that are commonly observed alongside OCD are listed below.

1. Attention-deficit/hyperactivity disorder—Attention-deficit/hyperactivity disorder (ADHD) is a neurodevelopmental disorder characterized by inattention and/or hyperactivity-impulsivity, usually arising in childhood, that impairs functioning. Among children and adolescents with OCD, up to 30% also meet the diagnostic criteria for ADHD. Further, studies suggest that children with ADHD are at increased risk of developing OCD.

2. Tic disorders—There is a high prevalence of vocal and motor tics in OCD (20%) and in the families of individuals with OCD (20%). Tourette syndrome (TS) is present in only 5–7% of adult individuals with OCD. More than 60% of children with OCD will experience at least transient tics, and as many as 15% will develop TS. For children with an early onset of symptoms, OCD may be the first manifestation of TS. OCD symptoms occur in 40–70% of individuals with TS and in 12% of family members of TS patients who do not themselves have TS. Complex tics may occur in the setting of a tic disorder and are usually motivated by unwanted urges without rational motivation. Although some complex tics are confined to localized muscle groups, others can mimic the compulsions of OCD. These latter tics often involve "just-right" perceptions, accompanied by urges to order, align, or arrange. Because treatment decisions can be affected by tics, the clinician should always observe the patient for such processes and ask about distinctive habits or mannerisms they might have or might have had previously, particularly in childhood.

3. Stereotypic movement disorder—Stereotypic movement disorder is characterized by perseverative motor behavior that is rhythmic in nature. It may be associated with primary reward or a reduction of anxiety awareness, or another aversive experience. Stereotypic movements may be associated with autism spectrum disorder or other psychiatric disorders, but they also are observed in otherwise typically developing children.

▶ Treatment

Treatment options for individuals with OCD range from behavioral interventions to neurosurgery. Mild forms of OCD (i.e., with Y-BOCS scores of less than 16) that occur with temporary stress may respond to stress reduction and supportive measures. Most patients with OCD seen by psychiatrists, however, require more definitive treatment.

A. Psychotherapeutic Interventions

Behavioral therapy for OCD involves exposure and response prevention. According to learning theorists, individuals with OCD have learned an inappropriate active avoidance response to anxiety associated with circumstances that trigger their OCD symptoms. The clinician must encourage the patient to experience the aversive condition (exposure) without performing the compulsion (response prevention). Chronic exposure alone will reduce the anxiety associated with the exposure, but the compulsions will remain if not specifically restricted. Response prevention is critical. Typically, the individual is asked to order their fears hierarchically. A decision is then made regarding which obsessive–compulsive dyad will be addressed. The patient is exposed by increasing degrees to the feared stimulus and is prohibited from carrying out the compulsive behavior. Anxiety with initial exposure is usually intense and enduring; however, the intensity and duration decrease with repeated exposure. When it is not possible to practice exposures in the office setting, the therapist may accompany the patient to a location, such as the home or the street, where the feared stimuli are more prevalent. In an outpatient session, the patient is typically instructed to repeatedly expose themselves to a specified set of circumstances on a proscribed number of occasions as "homework" between sessions. The patient should be encouraged to assess or question the validity of their obsessive thoughts as an adjunct to treatment. Such a cognitive approach may increase compliance, and when no compulsions are present or exposure is impractical, it may be the primary adjunct to therapy. In other cases, exposure to the actual fear may not be practicable, and the patient must engage in imaginal exposure. Typically, the therapist and patient will work on one symptom complex until the symptom has been reduced to an agreeable level or until a joint decision is made to address another symptom.

Many clinicians have neither the time nor the experience to carry out behavioral therapy and should refer the patient to a specialist in this area. Symptoms most amenable to behavior therapy involve contamination concerns and fears evoking behavior that can be elicited in the office. Behavioral therapy is most challenging for individuals with only obsessions or compulsions involving only mental activities such as counting or mental checking. Individuals with poor insight, and those who cannot tolerate exposure, tend to have more difficulty with this treatment method.

Behavioral therapy is effective in roughly 70% of individuals who agree to undergo the process. However, approximately 30% of individuals with OCD will decline this form of treatment. Behavioral therapy may be better tolerated if the patient has appropriate pharmacologic treatment. In some circumstances, symptoms can disappear completely; however, they often return over six months, and an additional short course of behavioral therapy may be needed to treat the symptoms effectively.

B. Family Therapy

Individuals with OCD frequently have partners or family members involved in the illness who may unwittingly interfere with the success of traditional treatments. Families can facilitate OCD symptoms through a process termed accommodation. The facilitator may perform rituals for the individual or permit them to control the environment, allowing the illness to flourish without constraints. Alternatively, family members who do not understand the disorder may antagonize the individual with OCD by reacting to symptoms with hostility, which further exacerbates the symptoms.

In such cases, family therapy can be helpful. At the very least, education regarding the individual's condition and appropriate responses should be attempted. In general, family members should not assist the individual with OCD rituals, nor should they significantly alter or compromise the quality of their lives to accommodate the symptoms of the illness. The family should be supportive of reductions in symptoms but not critical of exacerbations. Family members should avoid disparaging remarks related to the disorder. More extensive family therapy involves mutually acceptable contracts between the individual and family members regarding behaviors targeted for suppression. OCD behaviors outside the contract that do not compromise the lives of family members should be dealt with only in a positive and constructive manner. Family members should be aware that behavior therapy is a stepwise process and that behavior currently not a part of the contract can be addressed in the future. In addition to interventions targeting OCD, internal family conflicts may need to be addressed in therapy because they can exacerbate OCD symptoms and impair the quality of life of all concerned.

C. Psychopharmacologic Interventions

1. Serotonergic reuptake inhibitors—Selective serotonin reuptake inhibitors (SSRIs), the first-line treatment for OCD, inhibit serotonin uptake into neurons. These medications include fluoxetine, sertraline, paroxetine, citalopram, escitalopram, and fluvoxamine. Another serotonin reuptake inhibitor (SRI), clomipramine, is a tricyclic antidepressant with significant anticholinergic, antihistaminic, and anti-α-adrenergic side effects. Clomipramine is metabolized to desmethyl clomipramine, a metabolite that inhibits noradrenaline uptake. Meta-analyses of efficacy do not demonstrate apparent differences between clomipramine and SSRIs in treating OCD. Further, there is no clear evidence that any SSRI is more effective. Except in the case of fluvoxamine, each multicenter trial for SSRIs showed nonsignificant trends for higher doses being more effective for treating OCD, suggesting that the optimal doses for these medications may be at the higher end of the typical prescription range.

Although SRIs exert their primary effects on depression after 3–6 weeks of treatment, in OCD, they must be administered for up to 12 weeks to determine their full range of benefits. Withdrawal from medication is frequently associated with relapse within 2–3 weeks; therefore, patients should be advised to continue taking their medication regularly to prevent relapse.

Medications used to treat OCD are unlikely to eliminate the OCD syndrome completely; symptoms typically are reduced by 35% in aggregate and 50–70% in most responders. Clinical practice suggests that these figures underestimate patients' full benefits from medications. Although symptom levels may fall by less than half of their baseline levels, such individuals often experience a significant improvement in the quality of their lives, allowing them to function more effectively. Approximately 50–60% of those initiating a trial of an SSRI will achieve a clinically significant response. These medications increase their ability to tolerate obsessions and their urges to carry out compulsions without acting on them. Combining behavioral therapy with medication is often the ideal choice, as up to 25% of patients who fail one modality will respond to combined treatment.

If a patient has no response to medication after 8 weeks or has an inadequate response after 12 weeks, the clinician should consider trying a different SRI. Approximately 20% of patients who do not respond to one SRI will respond to another. If the patient has not responded to a second SSRI, a third SRI trial should be attempted. One of the three SRI trials should involve clomipramine.

2. Adjunctive medications—If a patient does not respond adequately with proper trials of SRI monotherapy, a second medication may be added. Some of the most common and well-studied augmentation options include low doses of antipsychotic medications, including risperidone, haloperidol, aripiprazole, quetiapine, and olanzapine. Such augmentation may be beneficial if the patient has coexisting tics, a family history of tics, or features of a schizotypal personality disorder. The use of antipsychotics should be carefully considered, weighing the risks versus benefits due to the potential for side effects. Another augmentation strategy is the combination of an SSRI and clomipramine; this combination may significantly augment serotonin uptake inhibition because fluvoxamine can inhibit the conversion of clomipramine to its noradrenergic desmethyl metabolite. For patients whose OCD has a significant anxiety component and for patients with a history of seizures, the addition of clonazepam may be considered.

Other medications used as adjunctive treatments and showing promise for SRI-refractory OCD symptom reduction via network meta-analysis include memantine, lamotrigine, ondansetron, and granisetron.

D. Neuromodulation and neurosurgery

Transcranial magnetic stimulation (TMS) and electroconvulsive therapy (ECT) have been studied as noninvasive neuromodulatory approaches to treating OCD. TMS uses a magnetic coil to deliver brief magnetic pulses through the scalp to modulate cortical activity in a targeted brain region. Recently, deep TMS (dTMS) with the H7-coil device received the FDA clearance for the treatment of OCD after multicenter sham-controlled trials demonstrated its safety and efficacy. Real-world dTMS data show an initial treatment response from the first session and a sustained response with additional sessions. ECT is a treatment performed under anesthesia in which an electrical current is passed through the brain to induce a brief seizure. While ECT is an established treatment for other psychiatric disorders, current literature does not demonstrate adequate evidence for the efficacy of ECT in OCD. Still, OCD patients have been shown to respond positively to ECT, and further investigation of this treatment modality may be warranted.

Neurosurgery is the treatment of last resort. Neurosurgical procedures include bilateral cingulotomy, limbic leukotomy, anterior capsulotomy, and subcaudate tractotomy. Estimates of clinically significant improvement range from 25 to 90%. There is some disagreement regarding the optimal site of the lesion. In intractable cases, however, neurosurgery is a treatment that may offer relief from disabling symptoms and extreme psychic pain. Improvement after surgery is not immediate but may occur over a period of up to 1 year. Adverse effects include seizures, disinhibition syndromes, and the attendant risks of general anesthesia.

Individuals should not be referred for surgery unless they have had full trials of at least three SRIs at appropriate dosages, including one trial of clomipramine and trials of neuroleptic and clonazepam as adjunctive medications. A trial of a monoamine oxidase inhibitor should have been attempted. The patient should have had a course of behavioral therapy with a qualified therapist, preferably while receiving optimal pharmacologic treatment. In addition, OCD or its complications should have life-threatening consequences for the patient or cause extreme dysfunction or severe psychic pain. Patients should be referred to centers with stringent presurgical entrance criteria and extensive experience with this treatment modality.

E. Experimental Treatments

Several additional medications and treatments have been tried for OCD with some success, although the evidence base for these options is mixed or developing. As such, they are not to be considered as first-line therapies for OCD but as potential new mechanistic approaches to future treatments. A few are mentioned below.

1. Anti-glutamatergic medications—Riluzole is an anti-glutamatergic agent trialed in smaller studies of treatment-refractory OCD with mixed results. It is currently FDA-approved for neuroprotection in treating amyotrophic lateral sclerosis, but further study is warranted in treating OCD. Similarly, N-acetylcysteine, which reduces synaptic glutamate release, has mixed evidence in its efficacy for OCD. Topiramate is an FDA-approved anticonvulsant that acts as an antagonist at glutamate receptors and activates $GABA_A$ receptors. While there is some evidence of its efficacy in placebo-controlled trials of OCD, it has been found to have poor tolerability.

2. NMDA antagonists—Ketamine is a potent N-methyl-D-aspartate (NMDA) receptor antagonist that has recently been FDA-approved in an intranasal form for treatment-resistant depression and its use as an anesthetic agent at higher doses. Trials of intravenous ketamine in adults with OCD have shown short-term benefits, though further research is needed on its potential sustained efficacy. Memantine is a noncompetitive NMDA receptor antagonist that is FDA-approved for Alzheimer disease. One placebo-controlled trial has shown efficacy in OCD when added to the SSRI fluvoxamine.

3. Immunosuppressant & antistreptococcal treatments—These treatments have been used to treat recurrent, episodic, and postinfectious OCD in children. Immunosuppressant therapies include steroids, plasmapheresis, and immunoglobulin treatment. However, specific clinical recommendations regarding these treatments are not available. These treatments have not demonstrated efficacy in treating OCD in adults.

▶ Complications/Adverse Outcomes of Treatment

A. Psychiatric Complications

Individuals with OCD often have co-occurring psychiatric disorders, with depression being the most common secondary diagnosis. Approximately 50% of individuals with OCD will develop a major depressive episode in their lifetime. Depressive episodes may be triggered when OCD symptoms prevent the individual from engaging in activities important for self-esteem, when attempts to resist the symptoms or adequately meet the demands of the illness inevitably fail, or when symptoms lead to continual conflict with significant others and social isolation. Effective treatment of OCD in these cases often leads to resolution of the depressive episode.

Individuals with OCD also have a high prevalence of panic disorder, secondary agoraphobia, social phobia, and alcohol and other substance misuse. Agoraphobia can result from an individual's attempts to avoid circumstances that may trigger obsessions. There is also a high prevalence of personality disorders with OCD (50–70%). Interestingly, although personality disorder symptoms are thought to be lifelong fixed traits, effective treatment of OCD will eliminate personality disorder symptoms in most individuals with OCD, suggesting that the personality symptoms may, in part, be secondary to stress and tension associated with OCD.

Anxiety can complicate OCD, as the individual worries about both the consequences of having OCD and the consequences of being unable to complete compulsions. Individuals with OCD may describe panic-like attacks that are not true panic attacks. Instead, they are attacks of severe anxiety related to violating an obsessive concern. For example, when an individual with contamination fears discovers that they have been contaminated, they may experience an overwhelming sense of dread, anxiety, and despair related to the impossible task of decontaminating everything they have defiled. This individual might mislabel these experiences as panic attacks. The clinician must be aware of this process to avoid unnecessarily complicating the patient's diagnostic picture.

B. Adverse Effects of Treatment

The treatments used in OCD have known side effects that require monitoring for tolerability and safety. Common side effects of serotonergic agents include sexual dysfunction, drowsiness, weight gain, dry mouth, insomnia, fatigue, and nausea. Rare side effects of SSRIs include increased bleeding risk, akathisia, and suicidal thinking among children and adolescents. Prescribers should avoid prescribing multiple serotonergic agents when possible, and patients should be monitored for serotonin syndrome. Still, these medications are among the best tolerated, and side effects generally improve over time.

Antipsychotics generally have a less favorable side-effect profile than SRIs, and for this reason, are considered second-line in the management of OCD. Typical antipsychotics act predominantly as dopamine-blocking agents. They most commonly produce side effects of sedation and extrapyramidal symptoms, including acute dystonia, parkinsonism akathisia. Long-term use can result in tardive dyskinesia. Through nonspecific action on dopamine circuits, these medications can also induce hyperprolactinemia. Atypical antipsychotics act by blocking both dopamine and serotonin. While they are associated with fewer extrapyramidal side effects, they tend to carry a greater risk of metabolic side effects such as weight gain, hyperlipidemia, and diabetes. Patients requiring antipsychotic treatment should be monitored for extrapyramidal, metabolic, and hormonal side effects. In the case of antipsychotics with a greater risk of cardiac effects, electrocardiogram monitoring should be used with dose titration.

▶ Prognosis

Although OCD tends to persist and become chronic, individuals can experience significant alleviation of symptoms with behavioral therapy and pharmacologic treatment. Serotonergic medications have been shown to reduce symptoms by 30–50% in 60–80% of individuals. Even such partial remission is a welcome relief for individuals plagued by this illness and often allows them to function at full capacity with some effort. 75–85% of individuals seeking treatment will achieve a significant clinical response with optimal combination treatments. Individuals with schizotypal features or neurologic soft signs have a poorer response prognosis, and the former group may not respond to either pharmacotherapy or behavioral interventions. Likewise, individuals who will not or cannot tolerate medications and behavioral measures have a less favorable prognosis. With the recent approval of TMS for OCD, there is a new, noninvasive neuromodulatory approach to treating the disorder. Research on the underlying biology of the disorder and potential novel treatments continues to progress. The clinician should be optimistic that, although at present, there is no outright cure, the future may provide far more effective treatments.

American Psychiatric Association. *Diagnostic and Statistical Manual of Mental Disorders.* 5th ed. *Text Revision (DSM-5-TR).* American Psychiatric Publishing; 2022.

Jenike MA, Baer L, Minichiello WE. *Obsessive-Compulsive Disorders: Practical Management.* 3rd ed. Mosby; 1998:xxii, 885 p.

Scahill L, Riddle MA, McSwiggin-Hardin M, et al. Children's Yale-Brown Obsessive Compulsive Scale: reliability and validity. *J Am Acad Child Adolesc Psychiatry.* Jun 1997;36(6):844–852. doi:10.1097/00004583-199706000-00023

Goodman WK, Price LH, Rasmussen SA, et al. The Yale-Brown Obsessive Compulsive Scale. I. Development, use, and reliability. *Arch Gen Psychiatry.* Nov 1989;46(11):1006–1011. doi:10.1001/archpsyc.1989.01810110048007

Goodman WK, Price LH, Rasmussen SA, et al. The Yale-Brown Obsessive Compulsive Scale. II. Validity. *Arch Gen Psychiatry.* Nov 1989;46(11):1012–1016. doi:10.1001/archpsyc.1989.01810110054008

Karno M, Golding JM, Sorenson SB, Burnam MA. The epidemiology of obsessive-compulsive disorder in five US communities. *Arch Gen Psychiatry.* Dec 1988;45(12):1094–1099. doi:10.1001/archpsyc.1988.01800360042006

Rasmussen SA, Eisen JL. The epidemiology and differential diagnosis of obsessive compulsive disorder. *J Clin Psychiatry.* Oct 1994;55(Suppl):5–10; discussion 11-4.

Geller DA, Biederman J, Jones J, et al. Obsessive-compulsive disorder in children and adolescents: a review. *Harv Rev Psychiatry.* Jan-Feb 1998;5(5):260–273. doi:10.3109/10673229809000309

Bloch MH, Landeros-Weisenberger A, Rosario MC, et al. Meta-analysis of the symptom structure of obsessive-compulsive disorder. *Am J Psychiatry.* Dec 2008;165(12):1532–1542. doi:10.1176/appi.ajp.2008.08020320

Brander G, Pérez-Vigil A, Larsson H, Mataix-Cols D. Systematic review of environmental risk factors for obsessive-compulsive disorder: a proposed roadmap from association to causation. *Neurosci Biobehav Rev.* Jun 2016;65:36–62. doi:10.1016/j.neubiorev.2016.03.011

Pauls DL. The genetics of obsessive-compulsive disorder: a review. *Dialogues Clin Neurosci.* 2010;12(2):149–163. doi:10.31887/DCNS.2010.12.2/dpauls

Endres D, Pollak TA, Bechter K, et al. Immunological causes of obsessive-compulsive disorder: is it time for the concept of an "autoimmune OCD" subtype? *Transl Psychiatry.* Jan 10 2022;12(1):5. doi:10.1038/s41398-021-01700-4

Orlovska S, Vestergaard CH, Bech BH, et al. Association of streptococcal throat infection with mental disorders: testing key aspects of the PANDAS hypothesis in a nationwide study. *JAMA Psychiatry*. Jul 1 2017;74(7):740–746. doi:10.1001/jamapsychiatry.2017.0995

Nestadt G, Samuels J, Riddle M, et al. A family study of obsessive-compulsive disorder. *Arch Gen Psychiatry*. Apr 2000; 57(4):358–363. doi:10.1001/archpsyc.57.4.358

van Grootheest DS, Cath DC, Beekman AT, Boomsma DI. Twin studies on obsessive-compulsive disorder: a review. *Twin Res Hum Genet*. Oct 2005;8(5):450–458. doi:10.1375/183242705774310060

Strom NI, Yu D, Gerring ZF, et al. Genome-wide association study identifies new locus associated with OCD. *medRxiv*. 2021:2021.10.13.21261078. doi:10.1101/2021.10.13.21261078

Mattheisen M. 13.2 Identification and characterization of genome-wide associated loci in OCD. *J Am Acad Child Adolesc Psychiatry*. 2022;61(10):S296.

Cappi C, Oliphant ME, Péter Z, et al. De novo damaging DNA coding mutations are associated with obsessive-compulsive disorder and overlap with Tourette's disorder and autism. *Biol Psychiatry*. 2020;87(12):1035–1044.

Halvorsen M, Samuels J, Wang Y, et al. Exome sequencing in obsessive-compulsive disorder reveals a burden of rare damaging coding variants. *Nat Neurosci*. Aug 2021;24(8): 1071–1076. doi:10.1038/s41593-021-00876-8

Grunblatt E, Oneda B, Ekici AB, et al. High resolution chromosomal microarray analysis in paediatric obsessive-compulsive disorder. *BMC Med Genomics*. Nov 28, 2017; 10(1):68. doi:10.1186/s12920-017-0299-5

McGrath LM, Yu D, Marshall C, et al. Copy number variation in obsessive-compulsive disorder and tourette syndrome: a cross-disorder study. *J Am Acad Child Adolesc Psychiatry*. Aug 2014;53(8):910–919. doi:10.1016/j.jaac.2014.04.022

Gazzellone MJ, Zarrei M, Burton CL, et al. Uncovering obsessive-compulsive disorder risk genes in a pediatric cohort by high-resolution analysis of copy number variation. *J Neurodev Disord*. 2016;8:36. doi:10.1186/s11689-016-9170-9

Hollander E. *Current insights in obsessive compulsive disorder*. J. Wiley; 1994:xiii, 297 p., 1 p. of plates.

Pigott TA, L'Heureux F, Dubbert B, et al. Obsessive compulsive disorder: comorbid conditions. *J Clin Psychiatry*. Oct 1994; 55(Suppl):15–27; discussion 28–32.

Pittenger C, Pittenger C. *Obsessive-Compulsive Disorder: Phenomenology, Pathophysiology, and Treatment*. Oxford University Press; 2017.

de Wit SJ, Alonso P, Schweren L, et al. Multicenter voxel-based morphometry mega-analysis of structural brain scans in obsessive-compulsive disorder. *Am J Psychiatry*. Mar 2014; 171(3):340–349. doi:10.1176/appi.ajp.2013.13040574

Saxena S, Rauch SL. Functional neuroimaging and the neuroanatomy of obsessive-compulsive disorder. *Psychiatr Clin North Am*. 2000;23(3):563–586. doi:10.1016/s0193-953x(05)70181-7

Hollander E, Stein DJ. *Obsessive-Compulsive Disorders: Diagnosis, Etiology, Treatment*. Medical Psychiatry. Dekker; 1997:xiii, 393 p.

Mersin Kilic S, Dondu A, Memis CO, Ozdemiroglu F, Sevincok L. The clinical characteristics of ADHD and obsessive-compulsive disorder comorbidity. *J Atten Disord*. Oct 2020;24(12):1757–1763. doi:10.1177/1087054716669226

Miguel EC, do Rosário-Campos MC, Shavitt RG, et al. The tic-related obsessive-compulsive disorder phenotype and treatment implications. *Adv Neurol*. 2001;85:43–55.

Leckman JF, Grice DE, Barr LC, et al. Tic-related vs. non-tic-related obsessive compulsive disorder. *Anxiety*. 1994;1(5):208–215.

Baer L, Rapoport Judith L. *Getting Control: Overcoming Your Obsessions and Compulsions*. 3rd ed. Plume; 2012:xvi, 268 pages.

Foa EB, Wilson RR. *Stop Obsessing!: How to Overcome Your Obsessions and Compulsions*. Rev. ed. Bantam Books; 2001:xvii, 247 p.

Decloedt EH, Stein DJ. Current trends in drug treatment of obsessive-compulsive disorder. *Neuropsychiatr Dis Treat*. 2010;doi:10.2147/ndt.s3149

Bloch MH, McGuire JF, Landeros-Weisenberger A, et al. Meta-analysis of the dose-response relationship of SSRI in obsessive-compulsive disorder. *Mol Psychiatry*. 2009;doi:10.1038/mp.2009.50

Maiti R, Mishra A, Srinivasan A, Mishra BR. Pharmacological augmentation of serotonin reuptake inhibitors in patients with obsessive–compulsive disorder: a network meta-analysis. *Acta Psychiatr Scand*. 2023;doi:10.1111/acps.13568

Carmi L, Tendler A, Bystritsky A, et al. Efficacy and safety of deep transcranial magnetic stimulation for obsessive-compulsive disorder: a prospective multicenter randomized double-blind placebo-controlled trial. *Am J Psychiatry*. Nov 1, 2019;176(11):931–938. doi:10.1176/appi.ajp.2019.18101180

Roth Y, Tendler A, Arikan MK, et al. Real-world efficacy of deep TMS for obsessive-compulsive disorder: post-marketing data collected from twenty-two clinical sites. *J Psychiatr Res*. May 2021;137:667–672. doi:10.1016/j.jpsychires.2020.11.009

Luyten L, Hendrickx S, Raymaekers S, et al. Electrical stimulation in the bed nucleus of the stria terminalis alleviates severe obsessive-compulsive disorder. *Mol Psychiatry*. Sep 2016; 21(9):1272–1280. doi:10.1038/mp.2015.124

Mindus P, Rasmussen SA, Lindquist C. Neurosurgical treatment for refractory obsessive-compulsive disorder: implications for understanding frontal lobe function. *J Neuropsychiatry Clin Neurosci*. Fall 1994;6(4):467–477. doi:10.1176/jnp.6.4.467

Coric V, Taskiran S, Pittenger C, et al. Riluzole augmentation in treatment-resistant obsessive-compulsive disorder: an open-label trial. *Biol Psychiatry*. Sep 1, 2005;58(5):424–428. doi:10.1016/j.biopsych.2005.04.043

Pittenger C, Bloch MH, Wasylink S, et al. Riluzole augmentation in treatment-refractory obsessive-compulsive disorder: a pilot randomized placebo-controlled trial. *J Clin Psychiatry*. Aug 2015;76(8):1075–1084. doi:10.4088/JCP.14m09123

Paydary K, Akamaloo A, Ahmadipour A, et al. N-acetylcysteine augmentation therapy for moderate-to-severe obsessive-compulsive disorder: randomized, double-blind, placebo-controlled trial. *J Clin Pharm Ther*. Apr 2016;41(2):214–219. doi:10.1111/jcpt.12370

Costa DLC, Diniz JB, Requena G, et al. Randomized, double-blind, placebo-controlled trial of N-acetylcysteine augmentation for treatment-resistant obsessive-compulsive disorder. *J Clin Psychiatry*. Jul 2017;78(7):e766–e773. doi:10.4088/JCP.16m11101

Sarris J, Oliver G, Camfield DA, et al. N-acetyl cysteine (NAC) in the treatment of obsessive-compulsive disorder: a 16-week, double-blind, randomised, placebo-controlled study. *CNS Drugs*. Sep 2015;29(9):801–819. doi:10.1007/s40263-015-0272-9

Mowla A, Khajeian AM, Sahraian A, et al. Topiramate augmentation in resistant OCD: a double-blind placebo-controlled clinical trial. *CNS Spectr*. Nov 2010;15(11):613–617. doi:10.1017/s1092852912000065

Berlin HA, Koran LM, Jenike MA, et al. Double-blind, placebo-controlled trial of topiramate augmentation in treatment-resistant obsessive-compulsive disorder. *J Clin Psychiatry*. May 2011;72(5):716–721. doi:10.4088/JCP.09m05266gre

Bloch MH, Wasylink S, Landeros-Weisenberger A, et al. Effects of ketamine in treatment-refractory obsessive-compulsive disorder. *Biol Psychiatry*. Dec 1 2012;72(11):964–970. doi:10.1016/j.biopsych.2012.05.028

Rodriguez CI, Kegeles LS, Levinson A, et al. Randomized controlled crossover trial of ketamine in obsessive-compulsive disorder: proof-of-concept. *Neuropsychopharmacology*. Nov 2013; 38(12):2475–2483. doi:10.1038/npp.2013.150

Ghaleiha A, Entezari N, Modabbernia A, et al. Memantine add-on in moderate to severe obsessive-compulsive disorder: randomized double-blind placebo-controlled study. *J Psychiatr Res*. Feb 2013; 47(2):175–180. doi:10.1016/j.jpsychires.2012.09.015

Cascade E, Kalali AH, Kennedy SH. Real-world data on SSRI antidepressant side effects. *Psychiatry (Edgmont)*. Feb 2009; 6(2):16–18.

Arana GW. An overview of side effects caused by typical antipsychotics. *J Clin Psychiatry*. 2000;61(Suppl 8):5–11; discussion 12-3.

Ananth J, Parameswaran S, Gunatilake S. Side effects of atypical antipsychotic drugs. *Curr Pharm Des*. 2004;10(18):2219–2229. doi:10.2174/1381612043384088

Somatic Symptom and Related Disorders

Charles V. Ford, MD
Louis Trevisan, MD

Diagnostic criteria for somatic symptom disorder include one or more symptoms that are distressing or result in significant disruption of daily life, such as excessive thoughts, feelings, behaviors related to the somatic symptoms or associated health concerns as manifested by at least one of the following: (1) disproportionate and persistent thoughts about the seriousness of one's symptoms; (2) persistently high level of anxiety about health or symptoms; and (3) excessive time and energy devoted to these symptoms or health concerns. Although any one somatic symptom may not be continuously present, the state of being symptomatic is persistent (typically more than 6 months). Specifiers include the following: *with predominant pain* (previously pain disorder); this specifier is for individuals whose somatic symptoms predominantly involve pain. *Persistent*: a persistent course is characterized by severe symptoms, marked impairment, and long duration (more than 6 months). *Current severity* is also a specifier: *mild*—only one of the symptoms specified in criterion B is fulfilled. *Moderate*—two or more of the symptoms specified in Criterion B are fulfilled. *Severe*—two or more of the symptoms in Criterion B are fulfilled, plus there are multiple somatic complaints (or one very severe somatic symptom) (DSM-5-TR).

Patients who somatize psychosocial distress commonly present in medical clinical settings. Approximately 25% of patients in primary care demonstrate some degree of somatization, and at least 10% of medical or surgical patients have no evidence of a disease process. Somatizing patients use a disproportionately large amount of medical services and frustrate their physicians, who often do not recognize the true nature of these patients' underlying problems. Somatizing patients rarely seek help from psychiatrists at their own initiative, and they may resent any implication that their physical distress is related to psychological problems. Despite the psychogenic etiology of their illnesses, these patients continue to seek medical care in nonpsychiatric settings where their somatization is often unrecognized.

Somatization is not an either–or proposition. Rather, many patients have some evidence of biological disease but overrespond to their symptoms or believe themselves to be more disabled than objective evidence would indicate. Medical or surgical patients who have concurrent anxiety or depressive disorders use medical services at a rate two to three times greater than that of persons with the same diseases who do not have a comorbid psychiatric disorder.

Despite the illusion that somatic symptom and related disorders are specific entities, as is implied by the use of specific diagnostic criteria from the *Diagnostic and Statistical Manual of Mental Disorders*, 5th Edition (DSM-5-TR), the symptoms most of these patients experience fail to meet the diagnostic criteria of the formal somatic symptom disorder. Further, over time, patients' symptoms tend to be fluid, and patients may be best described as having one disorder at one time and another disorder at some other time. Somatization is caused or facilitated by numerous interrelated factors, and for an individual patient a particular symptom may have multiple etiologies. In other words, these disorders are heterogeneous both in clinical presentation and in etiology.

Somatic symptom and related disorders are generally multidetermined, and because they represent final common symptomatic pathways of many etiologic factors, each patient must be evaluated carefully so that an individualized treatment plan can be developed (see Table 31–1).

Ford C. Somatization and fashionable diagnoses: illness as a way of life. *Scand J Work Environ Health*. 1997;3(23 suppl):7–16.

Lowe B, Levenson J, Depping M, et al. Somatic symptom disorder: a scoping review of the empirical evidence of a new diagnosis. *Pschol Med*. 2022;52:632–648

FUNCTIONAL NEUROLOGICAL SYMPTOM DISORDER

The diagnostic criteria for conversion disorder (functional neurological symptom disorder) include one or more symptoms of altered voluntary motor or sensory function. Clinical findings provide evidence of incompatibility between the

Table 31–1 Causes of Somatization

Illness allows a socially isolated person access to an auxiliary social support system.

The sick role can be used as a rationalization of failures in occupation, social, or sexual roles.

Illness can be a means of obtaining nurturance.

Illness can be used as a source of power to manipulate other people or social situations.

Somatic symptoms may be used as a communication or as a cry for help.

The somatic symptoms of certain psychological disorders (e.g., major depression and panic disorder) may be incorrectly attributed to physical disease.

Because physical illness is less stigmatizing than psychiatric illness, many patients prefer to attribute psychological symptoms to physical causes.

Some individuals may be hypersensitive to somatic symptoms and amplify them. Such hypersensitivity is often related to concurrent emotions such as depression and anxiety.

Somatic symptoms can represent behavior learned in childhood, in that some parenting styles may emphasize attention to illness.

The sick role can provide incentives such as disability payments, the avoidance of social responsibilities, and solutions to intrapsychic conflicts.

Trauma, particularly childhood physical or sexual abuse, appears to predispose individuals to the use of somatic symptoms as a communication of psychosocial distress.

Physicians can inadvertently reinforce the concept of physical disease by symptomatic treatment or through so-called fashionable diagnoses, such as multiple chemical sensitivities or reactive hypoglycemia.

symptom and recognized neurological or medical conditions. The symptom or deficit is not better explained by another medical or mental disorder. The symptom or deficit causes clinically significant distress or impairment in social, occupational, or other important areas of functioning or warrants medical evaluation. Specify symptom type: with weakness or paralysis, with abnormal movement, with swallowing symptoms, with speech symptoms, with attacks or seizures, with anesthesia or sensory symptoms. One also needs to specify: acute episode or persistent, with psychological stressor or without psychological stressor (DSM-5-TR).

▶ General Considerations

Functional neurological symptom disorder, previously known as conversion disorder and prior to that known as hysteria or hysterical conversion reaction, is an ancient medical diagnosis, described in both the Egyptian and Greek medical literature. Although often thought to have disappeared with the Victorian age, these disorders continue to the present, but often with more subtlety and sophisticated mimicry than characterized by the dramatic symptoms of the past.

A. Epidemiology

The reported incidence of conversion symptoms varies widely depending on the populations studied. The lifetime incidence of conversion disorder in women is approximately 33%; however, most of these symptoms remit spontaneously, and the incidence in tertiary-care settings is considerably lower. The incidence in men is unknown. Patients with conversion symptoms comprise 1–3% of patients seen by neurologists. Functional neurologic symptom disorder is diagnosed in 5–10% of hospitalized medical or surgical patients who are referred for psychiatric consultation. Functional neurologic symptom disorder symptoms occur in all age ranges from early childhood to advanced age. The disorder occurs with an approximately equal frequency in prepubertal boys and girls, but it is diagnosed much more frequently in adult women than in men.

Functional neurologic symptom disorder symptoms appear to occur more frequently in people of lower intelligence, in those with less education or less social sophistication, and in those with any condition or situation in which verbal communication may be impeded.

B. Etiology

Some authors have viewed conversion as more of a symptom than a diagnosis, with the implication that another underlying psychiatric disorder is usually present. It is likely that conversion is heterogeneous and that for some patients there is more than one cause. Among proposed etiologies are suggestions that the symptoms resolve an intrapsychic conflict expressed symbolically through a somatic symptom. For example, a person with a conflict over anger may experience paralysis of the right arm. Interpersonal issues have also been implicated. That is, the symptom may manipulate the behavior of other persons and elicit attention, sympathy, and nurturance.

Functional neurologic symptom disorder often follows a traumatic event and may be a psychological mechanism evoked to cope with acute stress. Conversion or functional neurologic symptom disorder symptoms are frequently found in patients receiving treatment on neurologic services and in patients with cerebral dysfunction. It seems likely that underlying neurologic dysfunction facilitates the emergence of conversion symptoms, perhaps as a result of impairment in these patients' ability to articulate their distress. Functional neurologic symptom disorder may also be viewed as a learned behavior. For example, a person who has genuine epileptic convulsions may learn that seizures have a profound effect on others and may develop pseudoseizures. In this case, the individual may have both genuine epileptic seizures and pseudoseizures, and distinguishing between the two may be difficult.

Current theories about the etiology of conversion emphasize the role of communication. People who have difficulty in verbally articulating psychosocial distress, for any reason, may use conversion symptoms as a way of communicating their distress.

C. Genetics

According to one nonreplicated Scandinavian study, relatives of patients with conversion disorder were at much higher risk for conversion symptoms. Polygenic transmission was proposed.

▶ Clinical Findings

A. Signs & Symptoms

A functional neurologic symptom disorder symptom, by definition, mimics dysfunction in the voluntary motor or sensory system. Common symptoms include pseudoseizures, vocal cord dysfunction (e.g., aphonia), blindness, tunnel vision, deafness, and a variety of anesthesias and paralyses. On careful clinical examination and with the aid of laboratory investigations, these symptoms prove to be nonphysiologic. A clinical example is the presence of normal deep tendon reflexes in a person with a "paralyzed" arm.

Contrary to popular belief, patients with functional neurologic symptom disorder may be depressed or anxious about the symptom. Some phenomena that have traditionally been associated with conversion, such as symbolism, *la belle indifference* (an inappropriate lack of concern for the disability), and histrionic personality, do not reliably differentiate conversion from physical disease.

B. Psychological Testing

Psychological tests often demonstrate comorbid psychiatric illness associated with tendencies to deny or repress psychological distress. A characteristic finding on the Minnesota Multiphasic Personality Inventory-2 (MMPI-2) is the presence of the "conversion V," in which the hypochondriasis and hysteria scales are elevated above the depression scale, forming a "V" in the profile. However, such a finding is not pathognomonic for conversion.

C. Laboratory Findings

Most functional neurologic symptom disorder symptoms are, by definition, pseudoneurologic. Laboratory examinations, such as nerve conduction speed, electromyograms, and visual and auditory evoked potentials, demonstrate that the sensory and nervous system is intact despite the clinical symptoms. Simultaneous electromyographic and video recording of a patient with pseudoseizures can be diagnostic when the patient has epileptic-like movements, while the simultaneous electroencephalogram tracing demonstrates normal electrical activity in the brain.

D. Neuroimaging

Consistent with observations that conversion symptoms are more likely to involve the nondominant side of the body is the finding that the majority of functional neurologic symptom disorder patients have unilateral right hemisphere structural or physiological abnormalities demonstrated by neuroimaging. Functional neuroimaging has demonstrated decreased activity in cortex and subcortical circuits, reflecting cerebral representation of peripheral symptoms (e.g., decreased activation of visual cortex during "hysterical" blindness). These decreases have been frequently shown to be associated with concurrent activation in limbic regions such as the cingulate or orbitofrontal cortex. In general, there appears to be similarity of functional neuroimaging findings of conversion disorder and hypnosis.

E. Course of Illness

Most functional neurologic symptom disorder symptoms remit quickly, often spontaneously. They are frequently transient reactions to acute psychosocial stressors. Prolonged symptoms are generally associated with environmental reinforcers (e.g., the symptom provides a solution to a chronic family conflict and/or disability payments). Conversion symptoms, either similar to the original symptoms or a new symptom, may occur with recurrence of stressors. This is particularly true with pseudoseizures.

▶ Differential Diagnosis (Including Comorbidity)

The differential diagnosis of conversion disorder always involves the possibility of physical disease. Even when conversion is obvious, the patient may have underlying neurologic or other disease that he or she has unconsciously amplified or elaborated.

Malingering must also be considered. The primary difference between malingering and conversion is that the degree of conscious motivation is higher in malingering. Systematic studies of conversion disorder suggest that it is often accompanied by other psychiatric disorders. Depression is common; and schizophrenia has also been reported, though rarely. Patients with functional neurologic symptom disorder may be responding to overwhelming environmental stressors that they cannot articulate, such as concurrent sexual or physical abuse or the feeling of being overwhelmed with responsibilities. Dissociative syndromes are also often associated with conversion, particularly pseudoseizures (which are regarded by some clinicians as dissociative episodes). Some clinicians have proposed that dissociative disorders and conversion disorders involve the same mechanisms: dissociation reflects mental symptoms and conversion represents somatic symptoms. Functional neurologic symptom disorder is grouped with the dissociative disorders in *International Classification of Disease*, 10th edition (ICD-10).

▶ Treatment

The treatment of functional neurologic symptom disorder is often multimodal and varies according to the acuteness of the symptom. If the symptom is acute, symptom relief often occurs spontaneously or with suggestive techniques. If the symptom is chronic, it is often being reinforced by factors in the patient's environment; therefore, behavioral modification techniques are necessary.

A. Psychopharmacologic Interventions

There are no specific psychopharmacologic interventions for functional neurologic symptom disorder. However, when comorbid conditions are identified (e.g., depression), these conditions must be treated with the appropriate medications.

B. Psychotherapeutic Interventions

Acute conversion symptoms may, on occasion, respond to insight-oriented psychotherapy techniques. On the whole, insight-oriented therapies have not been effective for chronic conversion symptoms, which generally require behavioral modification for symptom relief. Behavioral therapy can be offered in the context of physical or speech therapy, and this offers the patient a face-saving mechanism by which he or she can gradually discard the symptoms. Patients also receive positive reinforcement for symptomatic improvement and are ignored, to avoid reinforcement, at times of symptom expression.

C. Other Interventions

An acute conversion symptom may remit with suggestions through hypnosis or by the use of an Amytal (or lorazepam) interview that creates an altered state of consciousness. Such techniques may be useful in determining underlying psychological stressors, but caution must be exercised so that patients do not incorporate the interviewer's suggestions as a part of their own history.

D. Environmental Manipulation

When the conversion symptom represents "a cry for help" because of environmental pressures, it may be necessary to manipulate these stressors in order to produce symptomatic relief. For example, the pseudoseizures of a teenage girl might be a cry for help because she is involved in an incestuous relationship with her stepfather. Obviously, symptom relief will require attention to the sexual abuse.

E. Treatment of Comorbid Disorders

When identified, comorbid disorders must be treated concurrently. Conversion symptoms may respond, for example, to treatment for an underlying depression.

▶ Complications/Adverse Outcomes of Treatment

Remission, with treatment of a conversion symptom, does not rule out the possibility that the patient has an underlying physical disease to which he or she was reacting with exaggeration or elaboration. Thus, each patient must receive a careful medical evaluation. Conversely, a failure to consider conversion disorder and to continue to provide treatment as though the patient has a physical disease reinforces the symptom and can lead to permanent invalidism.

▶ Prognosis

Most conversion symptoms remit quickly; those that persist are often associated with environmental reinforcers and are more resistant to treatment. Factors associated with a good prognosis are symptoms precipitated by stressful events, good premorbid psychological health, and the absence of comorbid neurologic or psychiatric disorders.

In the past, an underlying neurologic disease would later emerge in about 25% of patients. However, at the present, with more sophisticated neurologic diagnostic tests, the subsequent emergence of previously undetected neurologic disease is uncommon.

Epssy AJ, Aybeck S, Carson A, et al. Current concepts in diagnosis and treatment of functional neurological disorders. *JAMA Neurol.* 2018;75:1132–1141.

O'Neal MA, Baslet G. Treatment for patients with a functional neurological disorder (conversion disorder). *Amer J Psychiatry.* 2018;175:307–317.

SOMATIC SYMPTOM DISORDER

The DSM-5-12 diagnostic criteria for somatic symptom disorder are listed at the beginning of this chapter. The majority (about 75%) of patients previously diagnosed with hypochondriasis as well as somatization disorder would now be diagnosed under this grouping.

▶ General Considerations

The syndrome of multiple unexplained physical symptoms was traditionally known as "hysteria" or "grand hysteria." It also received the eponym "Briquet's syndrome" for a brief time before being defined and renamed Somatization Disorder by the *Diagnostic and Statistical Manual of Mental Disorders*, 3rd Edition (DSM-III) in 1980. There have been repeated efforts to refine diagnostic criteria, but recent phenomenological studies indicate that there is considerable overlap with hypochondriasis.

A. Epidemiology

Reports of the incidence of somatic symptom disorder in the general population vary widely, depending on the populations studied and the techniques used. According to the Epidemiologic Catchment Area studies, the incidence of somatization disorder is 0.1–0.4%. However, in one investigation of an academic family practice, 5% of patients met criteria for somatization disorder. A similarly high incidence has been demonstrated for hospitalized medical or surgical patients. Of note, most patients with somatization disorder are not diagnosed as such, and because of their "doctor-shopping" behavior they see multiple physicians, often simultaneously. The prevalence of undifferentiated somatoform disorder (the subsyndromal form of the disorder) is much higher than that of somatization disorder and may affect as much as 4–11% of the general population. Individuals who meet the full criteria for somatization disorder tend to be female, unmarried, poorly educated, and from rural areas.

B. Etiology

There are no well-accepted theories as to the etiology of somatization disorder. Patients with this disorder often come from chaotic, unstable, and dysfunctional families in which alcohol was abused. These patients often use physical symptoms as a coping mechanism. The high rate of psychiatric comorbidity associated with somatization disorder suggests that the disorder may represent a common final symptomatic pathway for different psychiatric problems, particularly major depression and personality disorder.

C. Genetics

The evidence for a genetic influence in the development of somatization disorder is limited but suggestive of a common genetic tendency associated with criminality. Women are more likely to express this genetic tendency as somatization disorder, and men more likely to express it as antisocial personality disorder. It is difficult to delineate precise genetic mechanisms in the face of massive environmental influences.

▶ Clinical Findings

A. Signs & Symptoms

Patients with somatic symptom disorder, by definition, present to physicians with multiple unexplained physical symptoms. These presentations are often accompanied by a sense of urgency. Thus, these patients are subjected to numerous invasive diagnostic or treatment procedures. Symptoms are multisystemic in nature and frequently involve chronic pelvic pain, atypical facial pain, and nonspecific subjective complaints such as dizziness. Medical care costs for these patients may run as high as two to eight times that of age-matched control subjects. Patients with somatization disorder also have a number of psychological symptoms, including depression, anxiety, suicidal gestures, and substance abuse. They may be addicted to prescribed medications, and at times they may exhibit drug-seeking behaviors.

B. Psychological Testing

There are no specific psychological tests for somatization disorder, but patients with this disorder usually score high on MMPI-2 scales 1 (hypochondriasis) and 3 (hysteria) and on the somatization scale of the Symptom Check List-90, revised version. Because of high comorbidity (see later discussion), psychological testing is not consistent for the group as a whole.

C. Laboratory Findings

There are no specific laboratory findings for somatization disorder. The diagnosis is based on a lack of objective evidence to substantiate physical disease.

D. Neuroimaging

Studies reporting neuroimaging results in patients with somatic symptom disorder have been inconsistent, suggesting that somatic symptom disorder is a poorly defined disorder that may be the final common symptomatic pathway of several different underlying psychiatric disorders.

E. Course of Illness

These patients, by definition, develop multiple unexplained physical symptoms beginning in adolescence or early adulthood. Symptomatic presentation, which can be quite dramatic, is frequently associated with concurrent psychosocial stressors. The number and intensity of symptoms may wax and wane over time, but rarely does a year or two pass without some symptomatic complaints. These patients characteristically undergo numerous invasive diagnostic and therapeutic procedures that, in retrospect, had vague indications. Somatization disorder frequently persists into late life.

▶ Differential Diagnosis (Including Comorbidity)

Organic physical disease is always part of the differential diagnosis for these multisymptomatic patients who often carry poorly documented diagnoses of systemic diseases (e.g., systemic lupus erythematosus). Many of these patients have received one or more "fashionable diagnoses" such as fibromyalgia, dysautonomia, chronic fatigue syndrome, or total allergy syndrome. Few physicians have the means or the energy to make complete reviews of these patients' medical records, but such reviews generally fail to demonstrate objective evidence for any of these diagnoses.

Patients with somatic symptom disorder frequently present with a significant psychiatric diagnosis and almost always meet criteria for at least one personality disorder. Despite the multiplicity of psychiatric signs and symptoms, and a medical history of multiple unexplained physical complaints, patients with somatic symptom disorder are often unrecognized.

▶ Treatment

Patients with somatic symptom disorder perceive themselves as being medically ill and are unlikely to seek psychiatric care for their distress. They may resent any implication that their problems are psychogenic and may reject referrals for psychiatric treatment. Thus, the primary management of these patients falls on the primary care physician and his or her capability to coordinate care with multiple medical specialists.

A. Psychopharmacologic Interventions

There is no specific psychopharmacologic treatment for somatic symptom disorder. These patients do, however, frequently suffer from comorbid psychiatric disorders such as mood or anxiety disorders which should be appropriately treated (see Chapters 26 and 27).

B. Psychotherapeutic Interventions

The provision of group experiences, particularly those that are supportive rather than insight-oriented, may significantly reduce medical care utilization. Group support allows these patients to feel socially connected and reduces their need to reach out to the medical system for assistance.

C. Management Principles

Primary care physicians can use several simple management techniques to significantly lower medical care utilization by patients with somatization disorder. These principles include the following: (1) schedule frequent appointments without requiring development of a new symptom, (2) avoid statements that the symptoms are "all in your head," (3) undertake invasive diagnostic or therapeutic procedures only if objective signs or symptoms are present, and (4) prescribe all medications and coordinate medical care.

▶ Complications/Adverse Outcomes of Treatment

Patients with somatic symptom disorder are at risk for iatrogenic complications of invasive or therapeutic procedures (e.g., peritoneal adhesions resulting from multiple abdominal operations). Habituation to prescribed analgesics or anxiolytics also occurs frequently. Clinicians must exercise caution when prescribing any potentially lethal medication for these patients because they are prone to impulsive acting-out behaviors including suicide attempts. Conversely, an approach that is too confrontational about the basic psychological issues underlying the medical care–seeking behaviors may motivate these patients to find a physician who is less psychologically minded and more accommodating to requests for medications and operations.

▶ Prognosis

Somatic symptom disorder is a chronic problem that continues throughout the patient's life. Management principles are aimed at reducing symptoms and containing medical care costs, not at cure. These patients frequently experience iatrogenic complications from medications and surgical procedures. However, one long-term study found no evidence of reduced longevity, which suggests that these patients do not have any underlying biological disease.

Henningsen P. Management of somatic symptom disorder. *Dialogues Clin.* 2018;20:23–31.

ILLNESS ANXIETY DISORDER

The diagnostic criteria for illness anxiety disorder (as a minority of hypochondriasis cases are now classified) include a preoccupation with having or acquiring a serious illness. The somatic symptoms are not present or, if present, are only mild in intensity. If another medical condition is present or if there is a high risk for developing a medical condition (e.g., if a strong family history is present), the preoccupation is clearly excessive or disproportionate. There is a high level of anxiety about health, and the individual is easily alarmed about personal health status. The individual performs excessive health-related behaviors (e.g., repeatedly checks self for signs of illness) or exhibits maladaptive avoidance (e.g., avoids doctor's appointments and hospitals). Illness-related preoccupation has been present for at least 6 months, but the specific illness that is feared may change over that period of time. The illness-related preoccupation is not better explained by another mental disorder, such as somatic symptom disorder, panic disorder, generalized anxiety disorder, body dysmorphic disorder (BDD), obsessive–compulsive disorder (OCD), or delusional disorder, somatic type. Specifiers include care-seeking type and care-avoidant type.

▶ General Considerations

Hypochondriasis, which literally means "below the cartilage," reflects the abdominal symptoms and concerns of these patients. Hypochondriasis was once considered to be the male equivalent of "hysteria," but it is now recognized as having equal gender distribution. Recent phenomenological research suggests that there is considerable overlap between somatic symptom disorder and illness anxiety disorder.

A. Epidemiology

The incidence of illness anxiety disorder in the general population is not known. The typical age at onset is young adulthood, and the disorder occurs with an approximately equal frequency in men and women. Contrary to popular belief, it is not more prevalent among the elderly. Transient hypochondriasis frequently follows acute illness or injury and may be viewed as a normal hypervigilant scanning of bodily functions for detection of further injury.

B. Etiology

Illness anxiety disorder has been interpreted from a psychodynamic perspective as the turning inward of unacceptable feelings of anger. An alternative explanation is that hypochondriasis is learned behavior resulting from a childhood in which family members were excessively preoccupied with illness and bodily functions. Other proposed etiologies include the view that hypochondriasis is a form of depression or OCD, with a symptomatic focus on bodily function. Illness anxiety disorder is likely a multidetermined disorder.

C. Genetics

Illness anxiety disorder is a familial disorder, but there is no direct evidence of genetic input. The increased incidence in family members can be explained on the basis of learned behavior or the indirect influence of psychiatric disorders that do have genetic input (e.g., major depression) and that occur in both the patient and family members.

▶ Clinical Findings

A. Signs & Symptoms

The illness anxiety disordered patient typically presents with fear and concern about disease rather than with dramatic symptoms. The fears may emanate from the misinterpretation of normal bodily sensations. Sensations regarded as normal aches and pains by most people are interpreted by the hypochondriacal patient as evidence of serious disease. The Illness anxiety disordered patient characteristically relates his or her history in an obsessively detailed manner, often with relatively little affect. These patients tend to be emotionally constricted and are limited in their social, occupational, and sexual functions. Many hypochondriacal patients keep their own personal medical records. They often own the *Physicians' Desk Reference* or the *Merck Manual* and use the internet to obtain medical knowledge or advice. They feel transient relief when reassured that they do not have serious disease but, within hours or days, begin to obsessively doubt that assurance and may return for another visit.

B. Psychological Testing

Psychological testing (e.g., the MMPI-2) generally demonstrates a preoccupation with somatic symptoms in association with underlying depression and anxiety.

C. Laboratory Findings

No laboratory findings are diagnostic of illness anxiety disorder. The diagnosis is often made by exclusion when all tests for physical diseases are normal.

D. Neuroimaging

There are no reported studies of neuroimaging of patients with illness anxiety disorder.

E. Course of Illness

Illness anxiety disorder is a condition that characteristically begins in early adulthood and continues to late life. Symptoms wax and wane and symptomatic exacerbation may occur at times of occupational or interpersonal stress, with learning about an acquaintance's illness, or reading about a disease in a magazine. Worry or concern about relatively minor symptoms such as those associated with irritable bowel syndrome may escalate into an obsessional conviction of having a malignancy. At times, the patient may become so preoccupied with disease fears/conviction that interpersonal relationships are adversely effected. Interestingly, these patients often handle genuine physical disease in an appropriate and realistic manner.

▶ Differential Diagnosis (Including Comorbidity)

The hypochondriacal patient must be reevaluated continually for the possibility that physical disease may underlie each new symptomatic complaint. Hypochondriacal patients may have concurrent relatively benign polysymptomatic illnesses that they interpret as evidence of more severe disease. They also have a higher prevalence of major depression, panic disorder, and OCD than is expected for the general population. These patients may interpret the physiologic symptoms of major depression or panic disorder as evidence of disease.

▶ Treatment

Treatment of illness anxiety disorder falls predominantly to the primary care physician to whom these patients repeatedly return; hypochondriacal patients see their problems as medical, not psychiatric. Although some patients ultimately accept referral to a psychiatrist, premature referral may destroy rapport and make management more difficult.

A. Psychopharmacologic Interventions

Symptomatic improvements of hypochondriacal symptoms have been demonstrated after administration of selective serotonin reuptake inhibitors (SSRIs). This is independent of the effects of treating comorbid psychiatric illness and suggests the possibility that, at least for some patients, hypochondriasis may be a subtype of OCD.

B. Psychotherapeutic Interventions

Illness anxiety disorder patients are usually not good candidates for traditional insight-oriented psychotherapy because they tend to be alexithymic (unable to express feelings in words). However, a recently developed psychotherapeutic intervention based on the principles of cognitive–behavioral therapy (CBT) appears to hold promise. The approach is based on the provision of new information, discussion, and exercises intended to modulate the sensations of benign bodily discomfort that are due to normal physiology and to help patients reattribute these sensations to their appropriate cause rather than to fears of serious illness. This combined behavioral intervention can be used by the primary care physician or by staff working within the medical setting.

Group therapy techniques can also meet these patients' needs for relationships and can be a vehicle by which cognitive–behavioral approaches are used to modify these patients' illness behavior.

C. Treatment of Comorbid Disorders

Illness anxiety disorder is often accompanied by depression, anxiety, or OCD. When one or more of these disorders are present, appropriate treatment should be initiated. Hypochondriacal patients tend to be inordinately sensitive to medication side effects. They continually scan their bodies in a hypervigilant fashion for bodily sensations. It is often necessary to initiate pharmacologic treatment with very low dosages—while encouraging the patient to tolerate side effects—and then to gradually increase the dosage into the therapeutic range as tolerated.

D. Management Principles

Within the primary care setting, patients should be seen at regularly scheduled intervals. Each new complaint or worry should be accompanied by a limited evaluation to ensure that it does not represent the development of organic disease. Invasive procedures should not be undertaken without clear indication. The doctor–patient relationship should be warm, trusting, and empathetic and should gradually enable these patients to express their emotional feelings more openly.

▶ Complications/Adverse Outcomes of Treatment

Failure to recognize illness anxiety disorder may result in needless expense due to exhaustive medical evaluation. Purely medical management may reinforce the symptoms, and iatrogenic complications may result from unneeded invasive procedures.

▶ Prognosis

Illness anxiety disorder is characterized by a chronic fluctuating course. With few exceptions, cure is not to be anticipated for these long-term patients. Patients whose illness anxiety disorder is related to a defined depressive episode or to panic disorder often experience a significant relief of hypochondriacal symptoms when the comorbid condition is treated effectively. A few patients with more severe chronic comorbid depression or OCD will deteriorate; some become invalids for life. Patients with good premorbid psychological health who demonstrate transient hypochondriasis in response to acute illness or life stress have a good prognosis and may show complete remission of symptoms.

Creed F, Barsky F. A systematic review of the epidemiology of somatization disorder and hypochondriasis. *J Psychosom Res.* 2004;56:391–408.

Starcevic V. Hypochondriasis: treatment options for a diagnostic quagmire. *Australas Psychiatry.* 2015;23:369–373

BODY DYSMORPHIC DISORDER

BDD is now listed in DSM-5-TR under Obsessive–Compulsive and Related Disorders. The diagnostic criteria include the following: preoccupation with one or more perceived defects or flaws in physical appearance that are not observable or appear slight to others. At some point during the course of the disorder, the individual has performed repetitive behaviors (e.g., mirror checking, excessive grooming, skin picking, reassurance seeking) or mental acts (e.g., comparing his or her appearance with that or others) in response to the appearance concerns. The preoccupation causes clinically significant distress or impairment in social, occupational, or other important areas of functioning. The appearance preoccupation is not better explained by concerns with body fat or weight in an individual whose symptoms meet diagnostic criteria for an eating disorder. Specifiers include the following: *with muscle dysmorphia*, where the individual is preoccupied with the idea that his or her body build is too small or insufficiently muscular. This specifier is used even if the individual is preoccupied with other body areas, which is often the case. Also specify: *with good insight or fair insight, with poor insight,* or *with absent insight/delusional beliefs.*

▶ General Considerations

Dysmorphophobia was originally described in the nineteenth century and has been regarded as closely related to other monosymptomatic hypochondriacal disorders (e.g., delusions of bromosis). It was first included in the *Diagnostic and Statistical Manual of Mental Disorders*, 3rd Edition, revised (DSM-III-R) in 1987. Patients with BDDs are characterized by their preoccupations with perceived defects in appearance—"imagined ugliness" (a term coined by K. A. Phillips in 1991).

A. Epidemiology

Studies in the general population have found an incidence of BDD in the range of 1–5%. However, there are higher rates among dermatology and cosmetic surgery patients. There is probably a dimensional rather than a categorical quality to BDD that ranges from relatively normal concern with one's body (in a society preoccupied with appearance) to a delusional intensity to the preoccupation that becomes totally incapacitating.

Of those individuals who present for clinical attention, there is a roughly equal distribution between men and women. Most patients are 20–40 years old. A high percentage of these patients have never married or are unemployed.

B. Etiology

Theories of the etiology of body BDD are closely tied to issues of comorbidity (see later section). Many clinicians believe that BDD is a part of obsessive–compulsive spectrum of disorders but it is also closely related to social anxiety disorder and major depression. Cultural values that emphasize personal appearance may also contribute to the development of BDD.

C. Genetics

No studies have reported evidence for a genetic influence in the development of BDD.

▶ Clinical Findings

A. Signs & Symptoms

Patients with BDD are most commonly preoccupied with hair or facial features such as the shape of the nose. Other parts of the body such as breasts or genitalia can also be the source of preoccupation. For example, a man may become preoccupied with the size of his penis. Patients may spend hours each day gazing in a mirror or other reflective surfaces. Fears of humiliation, because of the imagined defect, may cause these patients to become housebound, unable to use public transportation or attend social functions or work. These patients may visit physicians multiple times seeking treatment, particularly surgical intervention to correct defects that are imperceptible to the normal observer. Most patients with BDD spend considerable time, hours per day, in repetitive behaviors attempting to improve or hide the perceived defect. These behaviors may include attempts to camouflage the defect such as engaging in excessive grooming or behaviors such as picking at the skin. Patients with BDD, on the whole, have little insight into their condition, and a considerable proportion can be described as delusional.

B. Psychological Testing

One simple screening question, "Are you concerned about your appearance?" may lead to other questions that confirm the diagnosis. Psychological testing such as the MMPI-2 or projective testing can help determine the presence of comorbid disorders. Tests may indicate depression, OCD, social phobia, or an underlying psychotic process.

C. Laboratory Findings

No specific laboratory findings establish a diagnosis of BDD.

D. Neuroimaging

One study using single-photon emission computed tomography demonstrated a broad range of findings that did not support the view of BDD as being in either the OCD or major depressive disorder (MDD) spectrum of disorders. It did, however, suggest some involvement of parietal regions, consistent with cerebral areas involved in facial recognition.

E. Course of Illness

Patients generally have the onset of BDD in adolescence. In the more extreme forms it is associated with complete social withdrawal and a high incidence of suicide. Because of the pain from their imagined ugliness, persons with BDD are highly impaired in interpersonal relationships and their occupations; often unable to work because they are housebound. They frequently seek multiple consultations from dermatologists or plastic surgeons. The course of BDD is chronic with low rates of remission even with treatment.

▶ Differential Diagnosis (Including Comorbidity)

The differential diagnosis of BDD includes delusional disorder, somatic type, in which the patient has a clear-cut noninsightful distortion of reality; anorexia nervosa, in which the patient has a distorted body image and refuses to maintain body weight at or above a minimally normal weight for age and height; and gender identity disorder, in the which the patient is preoccupied with his or her body, thinking that it reflects the wrong gender (i.e., transsexualism).

The large majority of patients with BDD have a comorbid psychiatric disorder, most commonly MDD, social phobia, psychotic disorders, OCD, substance use disorders, and personality disorders (most commonly cluster C). Persons with BDD have high rates of suicidal ideation and attempts.

▶ Treatment

BDD can best be conceptualized as a syndrome of heterogeneous etiology rather than as a specific entity. As such, one must keep in mind the high incidence of psychiatric comorbidity and the various underlying psychiatric disorders that are manifested as a preoccupation with appearance. Many of these patients seek surgery, and the psychiatrist may be asked to render an opinion as to whether surgery is contraindicated (see later discussion). Physicians must remain alert to the increased risk of suicide in patients with BDD.

A. Psychopharmacologic Interventions

A serotonin reuptake inhibitor (SRI) should be the first choice as an antidepressant medication. The SRIs are of proven efficacy in treating BDD but are, as yet, an "off-label" prescription; there are no FDA-approved medications for BDD. Positive responses to SSRIs have been reported in patients, whose symptoms have a delusional intensity, lending further credence to the opinion that BDD is in the OCD spectrum of disorders. Similar to the treatment of OCD patients being treated with SRIs, treatment response for BDD may require 10–12 weeks, at relatively high dosages.

B. Psychotherapeutic Interventions

CBT provided in either individual or group format has been demonstrated to be an effective treatment for BDD. Techniques emphasize cognitive restructuring, exposure with response prevention (e.g., exposing the perceived defect in social situations and preventing avoidance behaviors), and behavioral experiments such as empirically testing hypotheses involving dysfunctional thoughts and beliefs.

There are no reports concerning psychodynamic psychotherapy, but it is unlikely that this modality would be helpful in patients with so little insight about their disorder.

C. Nonpsychiatric Medical Interventions

Although the majority of BDD patients seek nonpsychiatric treatment from dermatologists and cosmetic surgeons, these treatments are rarely effective and at times may worsen the disorder.

D. Treatment of Comorbid Conditions

Comorbid psychiatric conditions such as major depression and social phobia should be treated.

▶ Complications/Adverse Outcomes of Treatment

It is important to recognize the intensity of the BDD patient's distress. These patients are at risk for suicide or the development of psychosis. Patients who receive surgical interventions are frequently displeased with the result and continue to seek further operations.

▶ Prognosis

The long-term outcome of BDD is unknown. Diagnostic criteria for the disorder have been formulated relatively recently, and data are preliminary. Earlier reports on dysmorphophobia (an earlier described syndrome similar to BDD) suggest that a significant proportion of these patients develop psychotic processes and that most are severely disabled from their disorder. Suicide rates are markedly elevated. Recent reports of success in treating BDD with SSRIs may portend a more favorable long-term prognosis.

Hong K, Nezgovorova G, Schlussel D, et al. Pharmacological treatment of body dysmorphic disorder. *Curr Neurophamacol.* 2019;17:697–707.

Jassi A, Kreb G. Body dysmorphic disorder. *Psychiatr Clin North Am.* 2023;46:197–209.

Phillips KA, Pagano ME, Menaid W, Stout RL. A 12-month follow-up study on the course of body dysmorphic disorder. *Am J Psychiatry.* 2006;163:907–912.

SOMATIC SYMPTOM DISORDER: WITH PREDOMINANT PAIN

Pain disorder is no longer a separate diagnostic heading in DSM-5-TR. It is now located under Somatic Symptom Disorder with the specifier of with predominant pain.

▶ General Considerations

Somatic symptom disorder with predominant pain syndromes are categorized based on whether they are associated primarily with (1) psychological factors, (2) a general medical condition, or (3) psychological factors and a general medical condition. The second categorization is not considered to be a mental disorder but is related to the differential diagnosis. This classification of pain appears to be superior to previous systems because it takes into account underlying physical disease to which the patient may be reacting in an exaggerated form. Thus the clinician can avoid the either–or dualism that prevailed earlier. Most patients probably have some degree of physical disease that initiates painful sensations, and it is the response to these sensations that constitutes abnormal illness behavior.

A. Epidemiology

Pain is the most common complaint with which patients present to physicians. It is estimated that the cost to the U.S. economy (direct and indirect costs) for pain-related disability is in the range of $100 billion. A well-constructed European epidemiologic study found that pain disorder is the most common of the somatoform disorders; the incidence over 1 year was 8.1%, and lifetime incidence was 12.7%. According to one U.S. study, 14% of internal medicine private patients had chronic pain. Those who seek medical care for chronic pain may be a subgroup of those who experience it.

B. Etiology

Pain is a heterogeneous disorder. No single etiologic factor is likely to apply to all patients. Among the proposed etiologies are psychodynamic formulations that pain represents an unconsciously determined punishment to expiate guilt or for aggressive feelings or an effort to maintain a relationship with a lost object. Consistent with psychodynamic theories, some patients with pain syndromes demonstrate masochistic, self-defeating personality characteristics.

Another etiologic theory proposes that pain represents learned behavior. It is hypothesized that the patient's previous experiences of personal pain have led to changes in other persons' behavior, thereby reinforcing the experience of pain and pain behaviors. Consistent with this theory are observations that some pain patients have experienced medical illnesses or injuries associated with pain or lived in childhood homes where disease, illness, and pain were present. It has also been proposed that pain represents a somatic expression of depression. There is a high incidence of depression in pain patients and among their family members, and depression often precedes pain symptoms. Another important dysphoric affect is anger, which often precedes the onset of chronic pain symptoms and/or is an important factor in maintaining the pain complaints.

Because pain is a subjective symptom, it is easy to simulate. A substantial percentage of litigants who claim pain have been shown to exaggerate or outright feign the symptom.

C. Genetics

No studies have related genetic factors to pain disorder.

► Clinical Findings

A. Signs & Symptoms

Patients who repetitively seek treatment for pain may represent a subset of individuals with pain who have certain patterns of illness behavior, rather than reflecting psychological characteristics of all persons who have pain per se. Pain syndromes include fibromyalgia, atypical facial pain, chronic pelvic pain, chronic low back pain, recurrent or persistent headaches, and so on. These patients' descriptions of pain are often dramatic and include vivid descriptions such as "stabbing back pain" or "a fire in my belly."

B. Psychological Testing

Psychological tests such as the MMPI are often used to evaluate pain patients. Common findings include somatic preoccupation, underlying depression or anxiety, and a tendency to deny psychological symptoms. The McGill Pain Questionnaire, a patient self-report test, frequently discloses that the patient uses idiosyncratic and colorful words to describe his or her pain experience.

C. Laboratory Findings

In experimental settings, pain disorder patients often have a lower threshold for pain than do normal subjects. It is difficult to determine if this greater sensitivity is the result of physiologic or psychological differences.

D. Neuroimaging

Elucidation of brain mechanisms involved in pain is evolving rapidly through techniques of functional neuroimaging. Interpretations of findings remain at the investigational stage, but there is promise for future clinical applications. Available information, to date, implies that the anterior cingulate cortex plays a critical role in the emotional component of pain. Chronic pain syndromes have been associated with increased activity in the somatosensory cortices, anterior cingulate cortex, and prefrontal cortex and decreased activity in the thalamus.

E. Course of Illness

No common symptoms or psychological features describe all pain patients. Despite this heterogeneity, pain patients share some features. Pain patients tend to focus on their pain as an explanation for all their problems; they deny psychological problems and interpersonal problems, except as they relate to pain. These patients frequently describe themselves as independent, yet observations of them suggest that they are dependent on others. They frequently demand that the doctor remove the pain, and they are willing to accept surgical procedures in their search for pain relief. "Doctor shopping" is common. Family dynamics are altered in a manner that makes the pain patient the focus of the family's life.

Pain patients often see themselves as disabled and unable to work or perform usual self-care activities. They demand, and often receive, a large number of medications, particularly habituating sedatives and analgesics. The pain persists despite chronic and often excessive use of these medications, on which these patients may become both psychologically and physiologically dependent.

► Differential Diagnosis (Including Comorbidity)

The differential diagnosis of pain disorder inevitably involves underlying disease processes that may cause the pain. The coexistence, however, of such disease does not rule out the diagnosis of pain disorder if psychological factors are believed to exacerbate or intensify the pain experience. Patients with chronic pain have a high frequency of comorbid psychiatric disorders, including depressive spectrum disorders, anxiety disorders, conversion disorder, and substance use disorders. Many of these patients meet diagnostic criteria for a personality disorder, most commonly dependent, passive-aggressive, or histrionic personality disorders.

► Treatment

The treatment of acute pain disorder is generally aimed at reducing the patient's underlying anxiety and the acute environmental stressors that exacerbate the patient's personal distress. Psychiatrists are much more likely to be involved in the evaluation than in the treatment of chronic pain syndromes. Psychiatrists may see patients with these syndromes on referral or as a part of a multidisciplinary pain treatment team. Because patients with chronic pain often resent implications that their pain has psychological causes, psychiatrists are usually most effective when serving as consultants to other health care providers. Chronic pain characteristically leads to changes in behavior that are reinforced by environmental factors. These patients have often assumed an identity as a chronically disabled person and have taken a passive stance toward life. The major objectives for treatment must be to make the patient an active participant in the rehabilitation process, to reduce the patient's doctor shopping, and to identify and reduce reinforcers of the patient's pain behaviors.

A. Psychopharmacologic Interventions

Patients with chronic pain have generally received prescriptions for multiple analgesics, often including opiate medications. These patients may demand increasing dosages of medication if they have become dependent, and they may exhibit considerable resistance to discontinuing or decreasing medications. Clinicians must explain to these patients that medications have not been successful in relieving pain and that other techniques are indicated. Medications may play a limited role as part of the overall treatment. As a general rule, nonsteroidal anti-inflammatory agents rather than opiates should be the first choice in medication. When more potent analgesics are indicated, they should be prescribed on a fixed-dosage schedule rather than on a variable-dosage schedule. Patients who are prescribed medication on an as-needed basis are much more likely to engage in pain behaviors to indicate the need for medication. The use of a fixed-dosage schedule enables the extinction of pain behaviors as a means of communicating the need for more medication. Patients who have been prescribed opiates either over a long period of time or in high dosages may require a detoxification program rather than abrupt discontinuation.

Antidepressant medications are often helpful to pain patients, particularly when symptoms of major depression are present. Clinical experience suggests that dual-reuptake inhibitors (serotonin and norepinephrine) such as duloxetine or venlafaxine are more effective than the serotonin reuptake inhibitors. Tricyclic antidepressants such as nortriptyline continue to have a role in the treatment of chronic pain patients, and patients may have a beneficial response to dosages lower than those used to treat depression. Caution must be used in prescribing potentially habituating medications (e.g., benzodiazepines) for sleep or anxiety because these patients are at high risk for prescription drug abuse/dependency. Anecdotal reports suggest that "off-label" use of the atypical antipsychotic medications (e.g., olanzapine) or antiepileptic medications (e.g., gabapentin) may be useful in some patients.

B. Psychotherapeutic Interventions

Insight-oriented psychotherapy may be helpful for the few patients who have identified unconscious conflictual issues. However, the vast majority of patients with chronic pain are not psychologically oriented, and insight psychotherapy is not efficacious. Supportive psychotherapy may be helpful in reassuring and encouraging these patients and in improving their compliance with other aspects of the treatment program. As a general rule, behavioral therapy is the most effective type of psychotherapy in the treatment of pain disorders. Both operant conditioning and CBT are widely used (see Chapter 10).

Operant conditioning is based on the concept that certain learned behaviors develop in response to environmental cues. Thus the patient has learned a variety of pain behaviors that are elicited in certain situations. Patients often communicate their pain to others (e.g., by grimacing) to elicit responses. Behavioral analysis identifies both the stimuli and the response-altering reinforcements to these behaviors. The behavioral therapist works to substitute new behaviors for previously learned pain behaviors. Patients are praised for increasing their activity and are not rewarded for pain. Behavioral techniques are most useful when the patient's family is included in the overall treatment program, so that pain behavior is not reinforced when the patient returns home.

CBT techniques focus on identifying and correcting the patient's distorted attitudes, beliefs, and expectations. One variety of this treatment involves teaching the patient how to relax or refocus thinking and behavior away from the preoccupation of pain.

C. Pain Clinics & Centers

Chronic pain patients are often disabled and receive fragmented medical care from multiple specialists. A pain clinic provides comprehensive integrated medical care. These clinics seem to work best when a strong behavioral therapy component is associated with a comprehensive evaluation and when treatment interventions include the patient's spouse, family, and, when applicable, employer. The therapeutic focus of pain clinics is to transfer the patient's sense of responsibility for treatment from physicians and medications to the patient himself or herself and to work actively within a rehabilitation program to restore self-care and social and occupational functioning. The focus is on rehabilitation more than it is on pain relief. The message provided is that the patient must learn how to "play hurt." These techniques are often useful for short-term improvement in function. Limited data are available regarding long-term outcome.

D. Treatment of Comorbid Disorders

Treatment of the symptom of pain often involves attention to coexisting or secondary psychiatric disorders. Major depression should be treated pharmacologically, and anxiety disorders should be treated as indicated with relaxation techniques, behavioral therapy, or pharmacotherapy. Substance abuse problems frequently require detoxification and appropriate rehabilitation techniques to maintain abstinence. Patients whose pain appears to be related to symptoms of posttraumatic stress disorder may require treatment for that disorder; specialized treatment programs for the survivors of violent crimes or sexual abuse may be indicated.

▶ Complications/Adverse Outcomes of Treatment

Pain disorder patients are at risk for iatrogenic addiction to opiate compounds or benzodiazepines. These patients often sabotage their treatment programs, proclaim that psychiatric treatment was not successful, and then use this as proof that their pain has a physical cause.

Prognosis

Surprisingly, little information is available concerning prognosis for chronic pain patients. Clinicians may see patients who have complained of chronic pain for many years, even decades, and who, in the interim, have been subjected to multiple surgical procedures and have experienced iatrogenic complications. Factors known to be of poor prognostic significance include ongoing litigation related to the pain (e.g., when the illness or accident that caused the pain was associated with a potentially compensable injury), unemployment, loss of sexual interest, or a history of somatization prior to the onset of chronic pain.

Cohen SP, Vase L, Hooten WM. Chronic pain; an update on burden, best practices and new advances. *Lancet.* 2021;397:2082–2097.

Edwards RR, Dworkin RH, Sullivan MD, et al. The role of psychological processes in the development and maintenance of chronic pain. *J Pain.* 17 (9 suppl):T70–92.

Seminowicz DA, Moayed M. The dorsolateral prefrontal cortex in acute and chronic pain. *J Pain.* 2017;18:1027–1035.

OTHER SPECIFIED SOMATIC SYMPTOM AND RELATED DISORDER

This category applies to patients whose somatic symptom causes significant distress or impairment in social, occupational, or other important areas of function, and they predominate but do not meet the full criteria for any of the disorders in the somatic symptom and related disorders diagnostic class. Some examples of presentations that can be specified using "other specified" include the following: (1) brief somatic symptom disorder: duration less than 6 months, (2) brief illness anxiety disorder, and (3) illness anxiety disorder without excessive health-related behaviors: criterion D for illness anxiety disorder is not met. (4) Pseudocyesis: A false belief of being pregnant that is associated with objective signs and reported symptoms of pregnancy.

UNSPECIFIED SOMATIC SYMPTOM AND RELATED DISORDER

This diagnostic category applies to presentations in which symptoms characteristic of a somatic symptom and related disorder cause clinically significant distress or impairment in societal, occupational, or other important areas of functioning but do not meet the full criteria for any of the disorders in

the somatic symptom and related disorders diagnostic class. This category of disorder should not be used unless there are decidedly unusual situations where there is insufficient information to make a more specific diagnosis.

General Principles for the Treatment of Somatizing Patients

As noted earlier in this chapter, the somatizing disorders display considerable phenomenological overlap and fluidity of symptomatic expression over time. Relatively few somatizing patients fit clearly into one of the somatoform disorder categories described in this chapter. Table 31–2 provides general guidelines for the management of somatizing disorders.

Table 31–2 General Guidelines for the Treatment of Somatizing Disorders

1. The clinician must remain vigilant to the possibility that the patient has covert physical disease and may develop physical disease during the course of treatment for his or her somatization.
2. A patient with somatization should not be conceptualized from an either–or perspective. Most somatizing patients have some degree of concurrent physical disease.
3. To the greatest extent possible, medical or surgical care should be coordinated by one primary care physician. Psychiatric consultation, however, is often valuable in helping the primary care physician formulate a treatment plan for the patient.
4. The somatizing patient frequently has a comorbid psychiatric disorder. When identified, such disorders should be treated because the somatization may represent the symptomatic expression of one of these disorders.
5. The somatizing patient should not be told that his or her symptoms are psychogenic or "all in your head." Such comments are almost inevitably rejected and destroy therapeutic rapport, and they may be inaccurate.
6. Invasive diagnostic or therapeutic procedures for the somatizing patient should be initiated only for objective signs and symptoms, not for subjective complaints.
7. The acute onset of a somatoform disorder may be associated with an acute stressor in the patient's life (e.g., physical or sexual abuse).
8. Chronic somatization is rarely responsive to traditional insight-oriented psychotherapy, but behavioral modification techniques are often useful in modifying the patients' illness behavior.
9. The treatment of somatization disorders generally requires multiple treatment techniques provided by a multidisciplinary treatment team.
10. Somatization is often a chronic condition (i.e., "illness as a way of life"), and cure is improbable. Somatizing patients require ongoing management using techniques that reduce the risk of iatrogenic complications.

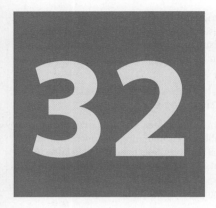

Factitious Disorders and Malingering

Charles V. Ford, MD
Louis Trevisan, MD

The diagnostic criteria for Factitious Disorders now appear and are classified under Somatic Symptom and other Related Disorders in DSM-5-TR.

Factitious Disorder Imposed on Self: falsification of physical or psychological signs or symptoms, or induction of injury or disease, associated with identified deception. The individual presents himself or herself to others as ill, impaired, or injured. The deceptive behavior is evident even in the absence of obvious external rewards. The behavior is not better explained by another mental disorder, such as delusional disorder or another psychotic disorder. Specifiers include single episode and recurrent episodes (DSM-5-TR).

FACTITIOUS DISORDERS

Factitious disorders are consciously determined surreptitious simulations or productions of diseases. Factitious disorder imposed on self is relatively uncommon, but when present it consumes large amounts of professional time and medical costs. The factitious disorder imposed on another is a particularly malignant form of child abuse that physicians must identify and manage in order to save the health or lives of children.

1. Some patients with factitious disorder present with predominantly psychological signs & symptoms— Patients with factitious disorders may simulate psychological conditions and psychiatric disorders. For example, a patient may feign bereavement by reporting that someone to whom he or she was close has died or been killed in an accident. Patients may simulate symptoms of posttraumatic stress disorder or provide false reports of previous trauma (e.g., a civilian accident or combat experience). Closely related to factitious posttraumatic stress disorder is the false victimization syndrome, in which the patient falsely claims some type of abuse. For example, a woman may falsely report that she had been raped. Other simulated

psychological disorders include various forms of dementia, amnesia, or fugue; multiple personality disorder; and, more rarely, schizophrenia.

2. Patients sometime present with predominantly physical signs & symptoms—The production of physical symptoms or disease is probably the most common form of factitious disorder. Essentially, all medical diseases and symptoms have been either simulated or artificially produced at one time or another. Among the most common of these disorders are factitious hypoglycemia, factitious anemia, factitious gastrointestinal bleeding, pseudoseizures, simulation of brain tumors, simulation of renal colic, and more recently, simulation of acquired immunodeficiency syndrome (AIDS). There are a group of patients with factitious disorder who present with Combined Psychological & Physical Signs & Symptoms.

A patient may be admitted to the hospital with factitious physical symptoms and, in the course of hospitalization, perhaps in an attempt to obtain more sympathy or interest, may report or simulate a variety of psychological symptoms such as having experienced the recent loss of a close relative or friend or having been raped in the past.

3. A person may also perpetrate symptoms as another person—This was formerly known as Munchausen by proxy syndrome.

▶ General Considerations

Factitious illnesses have been known since the Roman era and were described in Galen's textbook of medicine. Modern interest in this surreptitious production of symptoms presented to physicians was spurred by Asher's 1951 description and naming of "the Munchausen syndrome"; subsequently more than 2000 articles in professional journals have described, and tried to explain, this perverse form of illness behavior.

A. Epidemiology

The true incidence of factitious illness behavior is unknown, but it is probably more common than is recognized. One Canadian study estimated that approximately 1 in 1000 hospital admissions is for factitious disease. However, another investigation of an entirely different type determined that approximately 3.5% of renal stones submitted for chemical analysis were bogus and represented apparent attempts to deceive the physician. A study of patients referred with fever of unknown origin to the National Institutes of Health found that almost 10% had a factitious fever. One can conclude that the incidence of factitious disorder, except in certain specialized clinical settings, is relatively uncommon but may be more frequent than is recognized.

Age and gender distribution varies according to the clinical syndromes described in the next section. Patients with the full-blown factitious disorder imposed on self syndrome are most frequently unmarried middle-aged men who are estranged from their families. Patients with common factitious disorder are most likely to be unmarried women in their 20s or 30s who work in health service jobs such as nursing. Perpetrators of the factitious disorder imposed on another are most often mothers of small children who themselves may have previously engaged in factitious disease behavior or meet the criteria for somatic symptom disorder.

B. Etiology

Explanations for the apparently nonsensical and bizarre behavior of factitious disorder are largely speculative. Underlying motivations for this behavior are probably heterogeneous and multidetermined. The following explanations have been suggested:

1. The search for nurturance—Individuals in the sick role are characteristically excused from societal obligations and cared for by others. When alternative sources of care, support, and nurturance are lacking, a person may deliberately induce illness as a way of seeking such support. Many patients with factitious disorder are themselves caretakers. Factitious illness behavior allows for a reversal of roles: instead of caring for others, the patient assumes the dependent cared-for role.

2. Secondary gains—Patients with factitious disorders sometimes use illness to obtain disability benefits or release from usual obligations such as working. Their illnesses may elicit from family members attention that might not otherwise be forthcoming. When litigation is involved, the boundary between factitious disorder and malingering becomes blurred or disappears.

3. The need for power & superiority—A person who successfully perpetuates a ruse may have a feeling of superiority in his or her capacity to fool others. This has been described as "putting one over" or "duping delight." Thus, the individual can experience a transformation from feeling weak and impotent to feeling clever and powerful over others. Simultaneously, the individual may devalue others whom he or she regards as stupid or foolish because they have been deceived.

4. To obtain drugs—Some patients have used factitious illness to obtain drugs. Even those patients who have sought controlled substances appear to have done so more for the thrill of fooling the physician than because of addiction.

5. To create a sense of identity—A patient with severe characterological defects may have a poor sense of self. The creation of the sick role and the associated pseudologia fantastica (pathologic lying) may provide the patient with a role by which his or her personal identity is established. Such a person is no longer faceless but rather the star player in high drama.

6. To defend against severe anxiety or psychosis—A patient with overwhelming anxiety due to fears of abandonment or powerlessness may use a factitious illness to defend against psychological decompensation. Through the perpetuation of a successful fraud and the simultaneous gratification of dependency needs, the patient feels powerful, in control, and cared for.

C. Genetics

No information is available regarding a relationship between factitious disorders and heredity.

▶ Clinical Findings

A. Signs & Symptoms

DSM-5-TR diagnostic criteria do not adequately describe the different clinical syndromes of persons who present with factitious disorder. Three major syndromes have been identified, although some overlap may exist.

1. Factitious disorder imposed on self (peregrinating factitious disorder)—The original Munchausen syndrome, as first described by Asher in 1951, consists of the simulation of disease, pseudologia fantastica, and peregrination (wandering). Some patients with this disorder have achieved great notoriety. These patients typically present to emergency rooms at night or on the weekends when they are more likely to encounter inexperienced clinicians and when insurance offices are more likely to be closed. Their symptoms are often dramatic and indicate the need for immediate hospitalization. Once hospitalized, they become "star patients" because of their dramatic symptoms, because of the rarity of their apparent diagnosis (e.g., intermittent Mediterranean fever), or because of the stories that they tell about themselves (e.g., tales of being a foreign university president or a former major league baseball player). These patients confuse physicians because of inconsistencies in their physical and laboratory findings and because of their failure to respond to standard therapeutic measures. They rarely receive visitors, and it is difficult to obtain information concerning prior hospitalizations; their frequent use of aliases makes it difficult to track them. When confronted with their factitious illness behavior, they often become angry, threaten to sue, and sign out of the hospital against medical advice. They then travel to another hospital, where they once again perpetuate their ruses.

Personal historical information about factitious disorder imposed on self-syndrome patients is limited because they are unreliable historians and are reluctant to divulge accurate personal information. What is known may be somewhat selective in that it is derived from a subgroup of patients who have allowed themselves to be studied. These individuals often come from chaotic, stressful childhood homes. They sometimes report that they were institutionalized or hospitalized during childhood, experiences that were not regarded as frightening but rather were considered a reprieve from stress at home. Childhood neuropathic traits (e.g., lying or fire setting) are often reported. Many of these patients have worked in health-related fields (e.g., as a hospital corpsman in the military). Many have a history of psychiatric hospitalization and legal difficulties.

2. Common factitious disorder (nonperegrinating)—
The most common form of factitious disorder is common factitious disorder. Disease presentations may involve dermatologic conditions from self-inflicted injuries or infections, blood dyscrasia from the surreptitious use of dicumarol or self-phlebotomy, hypoglycemia from the surreptitious use of insulin, and other diseases. The patient generally has one primary symptom or finding (e.g., anemia) and is characteristically hospitalized on multiple occasions, but the physician or hospital staff never learns the true nature of the underlying "disease." In the process of their hospitalizations, these patients become the object of considerable concern from physicians, colleagues, and family members, with whom they typically have conflicted relationships.

Patients with common factitious disorder often lie, exaggerate, and distort the truth, but not to the same extent, or with the same degree of fantasy, as those with the factitious disorder imposed on self. Patients with common factitious disorder may perpetuate the ruse for years before being discovered. Unmasked, these patients typically react with hostility, eliciting angry disbelief from treating physicians, nurses, and other staff. Even in the face of incontrovertible evidence, these patients often continue to deny the true nature of their problems.

Patients with common factitious disorder typically come from dysfunctional families and exhibit histrionic or borderline personality characteristics.

3. Factitious disorder imposed on another (previously factitious disorder by proxy)—Falsification of physical or psychological signs or symptoms, or induction of injury or disease, in another, associated with identified deception. The individual presents another individual (victim) to others as ill, impaired, or injured. The deceptive behavior is evident even in the absence of obvious external rewards. The behavior is not better explained by another mental disorder, such as delusional disorder or another psychotic disorder. Note: the perpetrator, not the victim, receives the diagnosis. Specifiers include single and recurrent episodes (DSM-5).

This invidious disorder, in which a mother produces disease in her child, was first described in 1978. Subsequently, hundreds of case reports from all over the world have confirmed this form of child abuse. Every major children's hospital will see several cases per year.

In factitious disorder imposed on another historically referred to as Munchausen syndrome by proxy, the perpetrator (usually the mother) presents a child (usually an infant) for medical treatment of either simulated or factitiously produced disease. For example, the child may have collapsed after the mother surreptitiously administered laxatives or other medications, or the child may have experienced repeated attacks of apnea secondary to suffocation (e.g., by pinching the nostrils). After the child has been hospitalized, the mother is intensely involved in her child's care and with the ward staff. Interestingly, the mother is surprisingly willing to sign consent forms for invasive diagnostic procedures or treatment. The child may inexplicably improve when the mother is out of the hospital for a period of time. The child's father is usually uninvolved or absent.

When the mother is confronted with suspicions (or proof) that she has caused the child's illness, she often reacts with angry denial, and hospital staff may also express disbelief. Reasonable suspicion of factitious disorder imposed on another mandates reporting, as a form of child abuse, to the appropriate child protective services. Children who have been victims of factitious disorder imposed on another have a high mortality rate (almost 10% die before reaching adulthood). Studies of their siblings show a similarly high mortality rate because this disease-producing behavior may be perpetrated on subsequent children. These children may need to be placed outside the home (e.g., with other relatives or in a foster-care setting).

B. Psychological Testing

Approximately 30% of factitious disorder imposed on self-patients have some form of cerebral dysfunction. This dysfunction is most commonly demonstrated by the patient's verbal IQ score being significantly greater than his or her performance IQ score, a finding possibly related to pseudologia fantastica.

Test results of patients with common factitious disorder are consistent with histrionic or borderline personality traits, somatic preoccupation, and conflicts about sexuality.

Test results of the perpetrators of factitious disorder imposed on another may reflect personality disorders (e.g., narcissistic) and concurrent disorders (e.g., major depression). Frequently they demonstrate no clear-cut abnormality.

C. Laboratory Findings

Laboratory testing may disclose inconsistent findings, not typical of known physical diseases (e.g., the pattern of hypokalemia that occurs with surreptitious ingestion of diuretics). The presence of toxins or medications, the use of which the patient denies, may establish the diagnosis of factitious disease behavior. For example, phenolphthalein may be present in the stool of a baby who is experiencing diarrhea as a result of Munchausen syndrome by proxy.

D. Neuroimaging

No neuroimaging studies have been reported specifically for factitious disorder. However, in view of the extensive lying in which these persons engage and some similarities to malingering, it would be reasonable to expect similarities to findings with lying/malingering (see later discussion).

E. Course of Illness

The deceptive nature of persons with factitious illness behavior precludes good data concerning either the course of the disease or the prognosis. We do know that some patients with common factitious disorder imposed on self may persist in their symptom production for years. They may give it up spontaneously or perhaps after being "caught" and confronted. Persons with Munchausen syndrome may perpetrate their simulation of disease for decades, often traveling widely and using aliases to make tracking more difficult. Some patients die as a result of miscalculations in their illness productions. Other patients trade the drama of the hospital for the drama of the courtroom and sue physicians for causing the very disease that the patient him/herself created (e.g., suing a surgeon for postoperative infections that were self-induced).

Differential Diagnosis (Including Comorbidity)

As with all somatic symptom disorders, the diagnosis of factitious disorders involves ruling out the presence of a genuine disease process. Patients with factitious disorder often have physical disease, but the disease is the result of deliberate and surreptitious behavior such as self-phlebotomy. Occasionally, a patient with a genuine physical disease (e.g., diabetes mellitus) will learn how to manipulate symptoms and findings in such a way as to create a combination of physical disease and factitious disorder. In such cases, both the disease process and the behavior will require therapeutic attention.

Factitious disorders must also be distinguished from malingering; the difference here is one of motivation. The person with malingering has a definable external goal that motivates the behavior, such as disability payments from an insurance company, whereas with factitious disorders, the patient's goal is to seek the sick role for the psychological needs it fulfills. Malingering and factitious disorders often overlap.

Patients with factitious disorders may also meet the criteria for other somatic symptom and related disorders, particularly somatic symptom disorder or other disorders such as major depression or, more rarely, schizophrenia. Most patients with factitious disorders are comorbid for one of the cluster B personality disorders (i.e., antisocial, borderline, histrionic, narcissistic).

Treatment

Therapeutic approaches to factitious disorder must be different from those used to treat specific disease states. A factitious disorder represents disordered behavior that is determined by widely varied and often multiple motivations. The clinician must evaluate and develop a separate treatment plan for each patient. Further, because factitious behavior is often associated with severe personality disorders, the clinician must avoid splitting and other manipulative behaviors by the patient. Thus, a multidisciplinary management strategy involving attorneys, nurses, social workers, and other professionals is essential. Unfortunately, for many patients with factitious disorder, the goal must be to contain symptoms and avoid unnecessary and expensive medical care rather than to effect a cure.

A. Psychopharmacologic Interventions

There are no pharmacologic treatments that are specific for factitious diseases.

B. Psychotherapeutic Interventions

The overwhelming majority of patients with factitious illness have severe underlying personality disorders. Despite their superficial confidence and, at times, braggadocio, these patients are fragile. They are not candidates for confrontative insight-oriented psychotherapy and may decompensate in such treatment. The techniques described in this section are suggested for use by either psychiatrists or other members of the medical treatment team as indicated. Many patients completely reject any psychiatric treatment, and therapeutic efforts must be made by nonpsychiatric personnel.

1. Individual psychotherapy—Psychotherapy needs to be supportive, empathic, and nonconfrontative. At times just "being there" and allowing the patient to talk, even if much of the talk consists of pseudologia fantastica, provides sufficient support for the patient to no longer have the immediate need to engage in factitious illness behavior. Such treatment is not curative but helps prevent further iatrogenic complications and high medical utilization.

2. Face-saving opportunities—At times the patient will discard the symptom if he or she does not need to admit the behavior. For example, the patient may be told that the problem will resolve with physical therapy, medications, or other treatment techniques. The patient may use such an opportunity to discard symptoms in a face-saving manner and behavior without ever overtly acknowledging culpability for factitious illness behavior.

3. Inexact interpretations—Insight-oriented psychotherapy is almost always contraindicated. However, it may be useful to make interpretations without direct confrontation. For example, a patient whose factitious illness behavior is tied to losses or separation might be told in a very general way that it seems that he or she has difficulty in dealing with disappointments in life.

4. Therapeutic double-binds—The patient who is suspected of factitious illness behavior might be told that such suspicions exist—and that if symptoms fail to respond to a proposed treatment, then such a failure would be confirmation of factitious illness. Although this technique may be symptomatically effective, there are obvious questions as to its ethical appropriateness. For example, is it ethical to lie to a lying patient in order to effect change?

5. Family therapy—Patients with simple factitious disorder often come from dysfunctional families and are experiencing current conflicted interpersonal relationships. The patient's factitious illness behavior may be a way of controlling or manipulating the family in order to obtain a sense of power or gratification of dependency needs. Family therapy may be one way to address distorted communications in the family and provide for the more appropriate expression of needs.

C. Other Interventions

1. Staff meetings—When factitious disorder is suspected, the treating physician must recruit a multidisciplinary task force to assist with ethics and management. Such a task force, and associated staff meetings, educates all health care personnel as to the nature of the disorder, facilitates communication in such a manner as to defuse attempts by the patient to split staff, and ensures a united front for treatment. The multidisciplinary task force might include hospital administrators, the hospital attorney, a chaplain or ethicist, the patient's primary physician, a psychiatrist, and representatives from the nursing staff. Although this degree of involvement may seem like overkill, it is necessary in order to anticipate medicolegal complications.

2. Confrontation—When factitious disorder is suspected or has been confirmed, the medical staff must confront the patient. Such confrontation is generally best accomplished with several of the multidisciplinary staff members present. The staff should communicate to the patient that they know he or she has been surreptitiously producing or simulating

the disease and that such behavior is indicative of internal distress. The staff should suggest to the patient that it is time to reformulate the illness from a physical disease to a psychological disorder. The patient should be told that the treatment team is concerned and that appropriate help and treatment can be made available. Despite such a supportive approach, many patients will continue to deny that they have contributed to their illness and will angrily reject any referral for psychological help.

3. Treatment of comorbid disorders—Patients must be evaluated carefully for comorbid psychiatric disorders such as major depression or schizophrenia. The presence of another disorder is relatively uncommon, but, when present, it must be treated before proceeding with psychotherapy and other management.

D. Treatment Issues in Factitious Disorder Imposed on Another

When the victim of factitious disorder imposed on another is a child, it may be necessary to place the child in foster care in order to protect his or her health and life. The child will require supportive psychological assistance to deal with separation from the parent and changes in his or her environment.

Perpetrators of factitious disorder imposed on another, usually mothers, generally have severe personality disorders, which are very difficult to treat. This is especially true when the perpetrator continues to deny her behavior. Many psychiatrists believe that return of the child to the mother must depend on the mother's acknowledgment of her behavior, the requirement that she stop it, and her recognition of the needs and rights of the child. These mothers may have severe narcissistic personality disorder. They may view others merely as objects to be manipulated rather than as separate persons with feelings, needs, and rights. When there is a history of an unexplained death of a sibling, extra care must be taken to ensure the safety of the child.

E. Ethical & Medicolegal Issues

Many ethical and medicolegal issues are raised in treating factitious disorders. Some physicians may believe that because patients with these disorders are liars, they can treat them in a cavalier manner. The following discussion demonstrates that this is not the case.

1. Confidentiality—Because a patient with factitious disorder has presented himself or herself to the physician fraudulently, violating the traditional doctor–patient relationship, a legitimate question can be raised as to whether this invalidates the physician's obligation of confidentiality. To what extent should such an individual be allowed to perpetuate fraud, as it may affect family members, friends, and other physicians? This question is not easily answered, but from a medicolegal standpoint any violation of confidentiality must be in the interest of protecting the patient's health or significantly reducing the damage to others. Such violations should not occur capriciously but only after careful consideration and consultation with the multidisciplinary task force.

2. Surreptitious room searches—The medical literature on factitious disorders contains multiple descriptions of searches of patients' rooms after they have been sent off for testing or for other reasons. Syringes and other paraphernalia may have been found, thereby confirming the diagnosis. Such searches, however, violate patients' civil rights and should be undertaken only after careful consideration and consultation with the multidisciplinary task force.

3. Withdrawal of medical care—The physician who finds that he or she has been the object of the fraudulent seeking of medical care is likely to react with anger and possibly rejection. The expenditure of professional time and the use of scarce medical supplies for patients with factitious disorders may be questioned. However, an analogy can be drawn to the question of whether medical care should be withdrawn from a patient with liver cirrhosis who continues to drink alcohol or from a patient with emphysema who continues to smoke cigarettes. The point at which one starts to enter the "slippery slope" is always an issue for debate. Medical care should be withdrawn only after careful consideration of the medicolegal ramifications.

4. Involuntary psychiatric treatment—Many patients with factitious disorder engage in self-injurious behavior that could permanently affect body function or cause death. Involuntary psychiatric treatment has been suggested but is generally rejected by the courts. In one case, a judge provided an "outpatient commitment" for a patient and ordered that all of her (publicly funded) medical care be coordinated by a guardian. Such an approach seems eminently reasonable, but it may be difficult to effect in many states, especially if the patient is covered by private insurance.

5. Malpractice lawsuits—On the surface, one might ask how or why a patient might ever initiate a malpractice lawsuit against a physician when the patient is responsible for the medical illness. Such lawsuits, however, have occurred and can emerge in one of two different forms. One form of lawsuit can occur because many of these patients have severe borderline personality disorder. Such individuals are likely to idealize a physician initially and then later devalue him or her. With such devaluation comes rage and a resort to malpractice suits as a way of inflicting injury. The lay people who comprise juries are not knowledgeable about factitious disorders and may side with the patient.

Another form of lawsuit can occur when the patient admits factitious disorder and sues the physician for failure to recognize it. In other words, "I was lying to you, but this is a recognized medical illness, and you were incompetent not to have recognized my fraudulent behavior." One such lawsuit was settled out of court with a payment to the patient.

6. Reporting requirements—If the health of another individual is involved (particularly that of a child), the clinician is legally required to report his or her suspicions to the appropriate authorities. In the case of children, this is a legal requirement equivalent to that of reporting any suspected child abuse. Insofar as the report is made in good faith, the physician is exempt from prosecution for the violation of confidentiality.

▶ Complications/Adverse Outcomes of Treatment

Patients with factitious disorder have a remarkable ability to obtain hospitalization and to be treated with invasive procedures. As a result, these patients often experience unnecessary operations such as nephrectomies and even pancreatectomies. They are at risk for a number of iatrogenic complications, and physicians may contribute to drug dependence. Hundreds of thousands of dollars, millions in some cases, may be spent in the diagnosis and treatment of surreptitious and self-induced illness. The physician is also at risk. When angered, patients with these disorders may initiate lawsuits and, at the very least, will generally create disarray and dissension among their medical caretakers.

For the victim of the factitious disorder imposed on another, the clinician's failure to recognize the disorder or to take decisive action may result in continued medical treatment, medical complications, or even death.

▶ Prognosis

Relatively little is known about the long-term outcome of factitious disorder. Some patients die as a result of their factitious illness behavior, and others experience severe medical complications including the loss of organs (e.g., pancreas or kidney) or limbs. If the factitious disorder is the outgrowth of, for example, a psychotic depression, the prognosis is better than if the factitious illness results from severe personality disorder, as is usually the case. Although there are reports of successful psychotherapeutic intervention with some patients, there is no evidence of continued remission on follow-up. Factitious disorder imposed on another appears to be relatively refractory to treatment, although the ultimate outcome for most of these patients is unknown. When confronted, some patients with common factitious disorder enter psychotherapy and appear to improve and demonstrate fewer symptoms. Some patients deny their illness and merely change physicians, continuing their factitious illness behavior elsewhere; other patients deny their illness but apparently cease their behavior after being confronted with it.

The long-term prognosis of factitious disorder imposed on another is not encouraging. Victims have a high mortality rate during childhood, and those who survive childhood may develop somatoform disorders or factitious disorders upon reaching adulthood. Because this is a recently recognized disorder, long-term follow-up information is not yet available.

Asher R. Munchausen syndrome. *Lancet.* 1951;1:339–341.

Eisendrath SJ, McNeil DE. Factitious physical disorders, litigation and mortality. *Psychosomatics.* 2004;45:350–352.

Ford CV, Sonnier L, McCollumsmith C. Deception syndromes: factitious disorders and malingering. In: Levenson JL ed. *Textbook of Psychosomatic Medicine and Consultation-Liason Psychiatry*; 3rd ed. American Psychiatric Association Publishing; 2019:323–340.

MALINGERING

Malingering is listed in DSM-5-TR as a Z code (76.5). The essential feature of malingering is the intentional production of false or grossly exaggerated physical or psychological symptoms, motivated by external incentives such as avoiding military duty, avoiding work, obtaining financial compensation, evading criminal prosecution, or obtaining drugs (DSM-5-TR).

General Considerations

Malingering differs from factitious disorder in that it is a deliberate disease simulation with a specific goal (e.g., to obtain opiates). Malingering is underdiagnosed, often because of the physician's fear of making false accusations. However, covert surveillance has indicated that as many as 20% of pain clinic patients misrepresent the extent of their disability.

Malingering may include the deliberate production of disease or the exaggeration, elaboration, or false report of symptoms. The essential diagnostic issue for malingering is the determination that the person is willfully simulating disease for a defined purpose. But no physician is a mind reader. Thus, conscious intent must be inferred from other behaviors and psychological testing.

Malingering is not a medical/psychiatric diagnosis but rather a situation in which someone is deliberately using a bogus illness to obtain a recognizable goal. The goal may be deferment from military service, escape from incarceration (e.g., not guilty by reason of insanity), procurement of controlled substances, or monetary compensation in a personal injury lawsuit.

The judgment of the morality of malingering is largely a matter of the observer and circumstances. Most people would regard the defraudment of an insurance company, through a false injury, as an antisocial act. In contrast, the malingering of a prisoner of war, who is attempting to manipulate his or her captors, would be seen by most compatriots as a skillful coping mechanism.

A. Epidemiology

Malingering is most frequently seen in settings in which there may be an advantage to being sick (e.g., in the military or in front of worker's compensation review boards).

The prevalence of malingering is not known, but it is most likely underdiagnosed.

B. Etiology

Malingering, by definition, is determined by a person's willful behavior to use illness for an external goal. It has been proposed, however, that malingering is one extreme of a continuum of conscious–unconscious motivation that is anchored at the other extreme by conversion symptoms. Many simulated symptoms lie somewhere between these extremes and have both conscious and unconscious components.

Patients with antisocial personality disorder are believed to be more inclined to malinger, using physical symptoms as one of their means to manipulate or defraud others. All personality types, however, have been described in association with malingering, and it can be viewed as a coping mechanism when other coping strategies are ineffective. For example, a malingered symptom may be one mechanism for an exploited laborer to get out of an intolerable work situation.

C. Genetics

There are no reported studies that have linked malingering with heredity.

Clinical Findings

A. Signs & Symptoms

Malingering may involve either exaggeration or elaboration of genuine illness for secondary gain (e.g., continued disability after a mild industrial injury) or the simulation of disease (e.g., faked injuries after a contrived automobile accident). Malingering may be inferred in persons who behave differently and demonstrate different function when they think they are not being observed. For example, insurance companies may make covert video recordings of "disabled workers" who waterski on weekends. Psychiatric disorders may also be malingered. Perhaps the most common of these are posttraumatic stress disorder and postconcussive syndrome. These disorders are characterized by subjective, often difficult to quantify, symptoms and a higher probability of being associated with potential compensable injuries.

B. Psychological Testing

Malingered psychological symptoms can often be detected from psychological testing. The validity scales of the Minnesota Multiphasic Personality Inventory-2 (MMPI-2) may demonstrate changes indicative of false reporting. Mental status examinations and psychological testing may reveal findings that are inconsistent with, or clearly not typical of, the simulated disorder. Forced choice tests may indicate that the suspected malingerer has in a statistically significant manner answered questions in an incorrect way, thereby demonstrating he/she actually knew the correct answer.

C. Laboratory Findings

There are no specific laboratory tests for malingering. Some diagnostic tests may be abnormal if the person is deliberately exacerbating an existing disease or creating a new disease (e.g., surreptitious use of a diuretic).

D. Neuroimaging

Although no specific test utilizing neuroimaging to detect malingering has yet been standardized, there is considerable evidence that deception does induce brain activation. In one recently reported study of feigned memory impairment, findings included bilateral activation of prefrontal cerebral regions with both genders and different mother tongues, suggesting the importance of these regions during malingering and deception in general. This finding is consistent with a number of other studies that suggest attempted deception is associated with greater activation of executive brain functions (anterior cingulate and prefrontal cortices) as compared to truthfulness.

E. Course of Illness

A malingering symptom is generally discarded when the desired goal (e.g., financial compensation) is achieved or if the malingerer suspects that the deception has been detected. On occasion, with longstanding simulated symptoms, the symptom may persist, perhaps to save face or because it has been incorporated into the person's identity.

▶ Differential Diagnosis

The differential diagnosis of malingering includes physical disease; factitious disorder (i.e., with no discernible motive); somatoform disorders, particularly conversion disorder (in which the motive is unconscious); and pseudo-malingering. In the last situation, the patient believes that he or she is in conscious control of a symptom but actually has a disease (e.g., a person who is psychotic pretends to be psychotic in order to hide from himself the fact that he is not in control of his mental processes).

▶ Treatment

"Treatment" of malingering is, in a sense, a contradiction in terms because the "patient" does not want to be well until the desired goal (e.g., financial compensation) is achieved. The physician must be alert in order to avoid becoming an accomplice in the malingerer's manipulations.

A. Psychopharmacologic Interventions

There are no known psychopharmacologic interventions for malingering.

B. Psychotherapeutic Interventions

There are no known psychotherapeutic interventions for malingering.

C. Subtle Confrontation

At times, subtle hints to the malingerer that the ruse has been detected will motivate the malingerer to drop the malingered symptom in a face-saving manner.

▶ Complications/Adverse Outcomes of Treatment

It is commonly believed that malingered symptoms disappear when the malingering has achieved the patient's goal. In the process of the illness, the malingerer may experience iatrogenic complications of diagnostic or therapeutic procedures. A psychological complication occurs when, after years of litigation, the malingerer has come to believe in the illness (i.e., through learned behavior) and does not relinquish the symptom after successful resolution of the lawsuit.

▶ Prognosis

Little is known about the prognosis of malingering. Persons who are successful at perpetuating disease simulations do not come to medical attention.

Bass C, Halligan P. Factitious disorders and malingering in relationship to functional neurological disorders. *HandbClin Neurol.* 2016;139:509–520.

Lee TMC, Liu HL, Chan CCH, et al. Neural correlates of feigned memory impairment. *Neuroimage.* 2005;28:305–313.

McCollumsmith CB, Ford CV. Simulated illness; the factitious disorders and malingering. *Psychiatr Clin N Am.* 2011;34: 621–641.

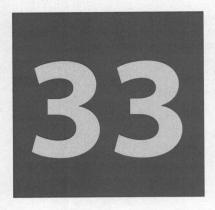

33 Dissociative Disorders

Muhammet Celik, MD
Brian Fuehrlein, MD, PhD

General Considerations

The *Diagnostic and Statistical Manual of Mental Disorders*, 5th Edition, Text Revision (DSM-5-TR) defines dissociation as a disruption, interruption, and/or discontinuity of the normal, subjective integration of potentially any aspect of experience and cognition, including behavior, memory, identity, consciousness, emotion, perception, body representation, and motor control. The cardinal feature of the dissociative disorders is an acute or gradual, transient or persistent, disruption of consciousness, perception, memory or awareness, not associated with physical disease or organic brain dysfunction, and severe enough to cause distress or impairment. The DSM-5 dissociative disorders are dissociative identity disorder (DID), dissociative amnesia, depersonalization/derealization disorder (DDD), other specified dissociative disorders, and unspecified dissociative disorder. The distinction between these types may be blurred, particularly when patients exhibit symptoms from more than one type.

A. Epidemiology

Dissociative amnesia—The lifetime prevalence of dissociative amnesia ranges from 1.8 to 7.3% in various research studies, with an equal likelihood of manifestation in both men and women. According to the ACE study, one of the most comprehensive population studies examining the link between childhood adversities and medical, psychiatric, and behavioral issues later in life, individuals who experienced sexual and physical abuse during childhood were more likely to have deficits in their autobiographical memory.

Dissociative identity disorder—DID has been found to have a lifetime prevalence range of 1.1–1.3% in various community-based epidemiological studies. In North American studies, the ratio of female to male DID cases is estimated to be as high as 8 to 1. The reason behind this gender discrepancy could be attributed to variations in the types, age of onset, and duration of maltreatment encountered by men and women. It may also be due to differences in clinical manifestations, with male cases having a higher probability of remaining undiagnosed. Additionally, it is possible that more male cases of DID may be referred to criminal justice or substance abuse treatment systems instead of mental health services.

Depersonalization/derealization disorder—The lifetime prevalence of DDD in the general population varies between 0.8 and 2.8% in different studies, with no significant differences observed based on age or gender. However, the prevalence of transient depersonalization/derealization is considerably higher. It has been reported that up to 74% of the general population may experience transient depersonalization/derealization at some point in their lifetime, which commonly occurs after experiencing depression, substance abuse, or life-threatening situations.

B. Etiology

Normal dissociation is an adaptive defense used to cope with overwhelming psychic trauma. It is commonly encountered during and after civilian disasters, criminal assault, sudden loss, and war. In normal dissociation, the individual's perception of the traumatic experience is temporarily dulled or dispelled from consciousness. Normal dissociation prevents other vital psychological functions from being overwhelmed by the traumatic experience. The capacity to dissociate, as evidenced by susceptibility to hypnosis, is widely distributed among normal people. However, it is unclear whether pathologic dissociation is an extreme or more enduring form of normal dissociation (i.e., whether there is a continuum of dissociation between normal and abnormal) or whether the pathologic form is distinctive. Recent studies of trauma subjects have found only a low correlation between hypnotizability and measures of dissociation.

Theories concerning the basis of pathologic dissociation can be classified as psychological, neurocognitive, traumagenic, psychosocial, and genetic.

1. Psychological theories—Janet postulated that some people have a constitutional "psychological insufficiency" that renders them prone to dissociate in the face of frightening experiences. At that time, memories associated with "vehement emotions" become separated or dissociated from awareness in the form of subconscious fixed ideas, which are not integrated into memory. Rather, they remain latent and are prone to return to consciousness as **psychological automatisms** such as hysterical paralyses, anesthesias, and somnambulisms (trance states).

Breuer and Freud suggested that hysterical patients harbor inadmissible ideational "complexes" resulting in a splitting of the mind and the emergence of abnormal (hypnoid) states of consciousness. Pathologic associations formed during hypnoid states fail to decay like ordinary memories but reemerge to disrupt somatic processes in the form of hysterical sensorimotor symptoms or disturbances of consciousness. Breuer and Freud disputed Janet's concept that dissociation is a passive process reflecting a hereditary degeneracy. They introduced the concept of an active defensive process that energetically deflects the conscious mind from disruptive ideas. Out of this theory emerged the later psychoanalytic concepts of repression and ego defense.

Dissociative amnesia with and without dissociative fugue characteristically arises in a setting of overwhelming stress, particularly in time of war or civilian catastrophe. Murderers, for example, often claim amnesia for the crime long after it would be legally advantageous to do so. Money problems, the impending disclosure of a sexual misdemeanor, marital conflict, or the death of a loved one are the usual precipitants of amnesia and fugue. Sometimes, the dissociative state is precipitated by an intolerable mood, such as severe depression with intense guilt. Dissociation blots out the unendurable memory; and a fugue represents an attempt to get away and start a new life.

It is unclear whether depersonalization represents a minor variant of global dissociation or a different process. In depersonalization, affect and the sense of being connected is split off from the individual's sense of self and perception of the outside world, giving rise to the feeling of being detached, like a robot or in a dream. Depersonalization may be the subjective component of a biological mechanism that allows an animal to function in a terrifying situation, whereas dissociation is represented by the freezing behavior that enables hunted animals to escape detection. These extreme survival maneuvers are subject to overload. Learned helplessness in animals, for example, may represent a breakdown of those neural circuits that modulate the sensitivity of the brain to incoming stimuli.

2. Neurocognitive theories—**Episodic memory** is a form of explicit memory involving the storage of events, which then have access to conscious awareness. Episodic memory is usually recounted in words, as a narrative. If significant enough, episodic memories become part of **autobiographical memory**, the history of the self. The medial temporal lobe, particularly the hippocampus, is essential to the encoding, storage, and retrieval of episodic memory. Dissociation may represent an interference with the encoding, storage, or retrieval in narrative form of traumatic episodic memories.

The locus coeruleus is an important source of noradrenergic fibers that project to the cerebral cortex, hypothalamus, hippocampus, and amygdala. The amygdala and orbitofrontal cortex select out those stimuli that have been primary reinforcers in the past. The amygdala projects to the hippocampus (via the entorhinal cortex), to the sensory association cortex, and to the hypothalamus and brain stem, coordinating a central alarm apparatus that scans sensory input for stimuli the animal has learned to fear, and sounds an alert when such stimuli are encountered. Evidence indicates that serotonin acts postsynaptically in the amygdala to provoke the synthesis of enkephalins, which modulate or dampen the affect associated with fearful experience and may interfere with the consolidation of traumatic memories. If the amygdaloid alarm system becomes overloaded and breaks down, the animal will be at the mercy of raw fear. Thus, whenever reminders of trauma are perceived in the environment, or whenever fragments of traumatic episodic memory threaten to emerge into awareness, an alarm is sounded and the failsafe, last-resort defense of dissociation must be invoked.

Traumatic memories are stored in two systems: (1) the hippocampal explicit episodic memory system and (2) the amygdaloid implicit alarm system. The amygdaloid system can disrupt storage and retrieval via the hippocampal system. Research suggests that immature animals exposed to early inescapable stress or gross deprivation of cospecies contact are particularly vulnerable to subsequent trauma. In primates, morphine decreases (and naloxone increases) the amount of affiliative calling of an animal separated from its mother, whereas diazepam reduces freezing and hostile gestures in reaction to direct threat, probably through the prefrontal cortex. Animal research has suggested that high circulating corticosteroid levels in stressed juveniles are associated with a reduction in the population of glucocorticoid receptors in the hippocampus. Furthermore, neuroimaging studies of veterans with chronic posttraumatic stress disorder have demonstrated an apparent shrinkage in hippocampal volume.

3. Traumagenic theories—Clinical evidence for the linkage between emotional trauma and dissociation is derived from the following observations: (1) the high prevalence of histories of childhood trauma reported by patients with dissociative disorder; (2) elevated levels of dissociation in people who report child abuse; (3) elevated levels of dissociation in combat veterans with posttraumatic stress disorder; (4) the prevalence of acute dissociative reactions in war or disaster; and (5) the observation that marked dissociation during a traumatic experience predicts subsequent posttraumatic stress disorder. Almost all adults with DID report significant trauma in childhood, particularly incest, physical abuse, and emotional abuse. These patients commonly report repeated abuse, sometimes of an extremely sadistic, bizarre nature.

4. Psychosocial theories—The difficulty of corroborating retrospective accounts of abuse has provoked much controversy. Are these reports false, unwittingly created by clinical interest and the recent explosion of coverage in the media? The possibility of iatrogenic facilitation cannot be excluded. The more dramatic forms of dissociative disorder—particularly fugue and multiple identity—may represent, at least in part, forms of abnormal illness behavior, distorted attempts by emotionally needy patients to elicit care and protection from therapist–parent surrogates, or bids to retain the interest of therapists in the context of an intense transference relationship. Traumagenic and psychosocial theories are not necessarily mutually exclusive.

5. Genetic theories—The relationship between genetics and dissociation symptoms is not yet fully understood. However, there is evidence to suggest that genetic factors may play a role in the development of dissociative disorders. According to twin studies, approximately 50% of the variability in the occurrence of dissociative symptoms can be attributed to genetic factors. Several studies have found a connection between single nucleotide polymorphisms (SNPs) in certain genes and the occurrence of dissociative disorders. In a study investigating the role of the serotonin transporter gene promoter polymorphism (5-HTTLPR) in the development of dissociation, participants with the SS genotype of 5-HTTLPR reported experiencing more dissociative symptoms compared to those with other genotypes. Another study demonstrated that physical neglect experienced during childhood, in conjunction with the SS genotype of the 5-HTT gene, was a significant predictor of dissociation in patients with obsessive–compulsive disorder (OCD). A genome-wide association study conducted to investigate genetic polymorphisms associated with the symptoms that characterize the dissociative subtype of post-traumatic stress disorder (PTSD) identified 10 SNPs that might be linked to depersonalization and derealization symptoms. The most prominent SNP among them was rs263232 located in the adenylyl cyclase 8 (ADCY8) gene which is known to play a role in long-term potentiation and synaptic plasticity. Regarding hypnosis, which can be utilized for the treatment of dissociative disorders, the Val[158]Met polymorphism of the catechol-O-methyltransferase gene has been found to be significantly associated with hypnotizability.

DISSOCIATIVE IDENTITY DISORDER

▶ Clinical Findings

A. Signs & Symptoms

DID is a disruption of identity characterized by two or more distinct personality states, which may be described in some cultures as an experience of possession. The disruption in identity involves marked discontinuity in sense of self and sense of agency, accompanied by related alterations in affect, behavior, consciousness, memory, perception, cognition and/or sensory–motor functioning. These signs and symptoms may be observed by others or reported by the individual. In addition, the person will experience recurrent gaps in the recall of everyday events, important personal information and/or traumatic events that are inconsistent with ordinary forgetting. This disturbance should not be a normal part of a broadly accepted cultural or religious practice.

(DID) is usually not diagnosed until patients are in their late 20s, but retrospective evidence indicates that it begins much earlier, usually in childhood. Some patients with DID have had years of treatment before the correct diagnosis is made. These patients commonly exhibit transient depression, mood swings, sleep disturbance, nightmares, and suicidal behavior. They are often self-injurious and exhibit a host of dissociative symptoms including amnesia, episodes of "lost time" (i.e., amnesia varying from several minutes to several days), depersonalization, fugue, and hallucinations. Anxiety and its somatic concomitants (e.g., dyspnea, palpitations, chest pain, choking sensations, faintness, tremors) commonly herald a switch of alter personalities. Quasineurologic symptoms such as headache, syncope, pseudoseizures, numbness, paresthesia, diplopia, tunnel vision, and motor weakness are sometimes encountered. Symptoms referable to the cardiorespiratory, gastrointestinal, or reproductive systems may dominate the clinical presentation.

Questioning will reveal that most patients have audiovisual hallucinations and quasidelusions. The auditory hallucinations may be fragments of conversations heard during traumatic experiences or metaphoric expressions of self-disgust in the form of hostile voices that revile and derogate the patient or command her to harm herself, commit suicide, or attack others. Other voices may be conversations between people about the patient, people offering solace, and the weeping and crying of distressed children. Some patients report a sense of being controlled, alterations in their body image, or the conviction that they are being followed or that their lives are threatened by shadowy enemies (e.g., the former perpetrators of alleged "ritual abuse"). Occasional discontinuities of thought and thought "slippages" may be the result of alter switching or the intrusion of traumatic themes into the stream of consciousness, causing microdissociations.

As mentioned earlier in this chapter, these patients may have had many medical and neurologic investigations. Many have been treated for mood disorder, anxiety disorder, or schizophrenia. Some wander from job to job, place to place, and doctor to doctor. Many are prone to repeated victimization by virtue of their poor choice of occupation or consorts.

The cardinal feature of DID is multiple personalities, two or more entities, each of which has a characteristic and separate personality, age, gender, sexual orientation, history, affect, values, and function. However, the original personality state is often the dominant presence. The number of alters is usually about 10, though it may be many more. Typically, the alters are somewhat two-dimensional in quality and include such entities as the host personality; a variety of child personalities (e.g., innocent child, traumatized child, "Pollyanna"); a persecutor; a cross-sex alter; an internal helper; a brazen, promiscuous "hussy"; a variety of demons; and "no one." The entities usually first emerge during childhood, in the form of imaginary protectors or companions that help the child cope with recurrent experiences of abuse and fear. The alter personalities often switch abruptly, producing a bewildering change in demeanor, sometimes with anxiety and apparent disorganization of thought. Sometimes one alter or several alters will be unaware of the other alters. Often alters will communicate with each other. The complete dramatis personae usually emerge only after therapy.

It can be difficult to elicit alter personalities. The clinician must have a reasonable suspicion that DID is present (e.g., in a patient who exhibits abrupt changes in demeanor, "lost time," total amnesia for childhood, and many physical symptoms). The exploration of puzzling events or lost time will often elicit an alter. Sometimes the clinician must ask directly to speak to "that part of you" that did something or experienced something.

B. Psychological Testing

See discussion of dissociative amnesia.

▶ Differential Diagnosis (Including Comorbid Conditions)

DID is most likely to be confused with the following conditions: partial complex seizures, schizophrenia, PTSD, bipolar disorder, major depression with psychotic features, Munchausen syndrome, Munchausen syndrome by proxy, and malingering. Partial complex seizures, which usually last no more than a few seconds, may be confused with alter switching; however, other cardinal signs of DID are not seen in epilepsy. Occasionally, telemetry is required.

Patients with DID frequently report the following phenomena: quasidelusions, ideas of being externally controlled, auditory hallucinations involving conversations, comments about the patient cast in the third person, commands, and ideas of thought loss. When these phenomena are associated with the disruption of thinking coincident with alter switching or microdissociation, it is not surprising that patients with DID have often been mistakenly diagnosed as having schizophrenia. DID should be differentiated from schizophrenia by the lack of emotional incongruity; the dramatic, care-eliciting presentation; the history of severe trauma; the alter personalities; and high scores on dissociation scales. Additionally, hallucinations in DID usually start in childhood and follow a fluctuating pattern. However, in schizophrenia variety of psychotic symptoms occur concurrently

and usually patient's functionality deteriorates severely in a later age. Hypnosis is sometimes helpful in distinguishing DID from schizophrenia.

DID and PTSD usually co-occur. These two conditions can be distinguished by lack of hallmark symptoms of PTSD including re-experiencing traumatic events, avoidance of stimuli associated with traumatic events, and hyperarousal. However, PTSD has a dissociative subtype with prominent dissociative symptoms. Therefore, a careful examination is required.

Rapid-cycling bipolar disorder is sometimes confused with the apparent mood swings caused by alter switching in DID. However, in DID mood states switch in response to environment and usually last only from a few seconds to a few hours.

Major depression with psychotic features can be confused with DID if only a superficial diagnostic evaluation has been completed, particularly because many patients with DID have an associated depressive mood. In major depression with psychotic features, the auditory hallucinations and delusions are consistent with the prevailing depressive mood. For example, the patient hears voices derogating him or her for being a bad person and is convinced that he or she has committed an unpardonable sin, is impoverished, is being hounded by tax officials, or is rotting inside. In DID, the hallucinations are often derogatory, but they convey the theme of helpless victimization and command patients to hurt others or themselves.

In some cases of Munchausen syndrome, the pseudopatient has presented himself or herself for medical attention with the symptoms of DID. In some cases of Munchausen syndrome by proxy, a mother presents her child with the symptoms of DID. The imposture is deliberate, but the gain obscure. Satisfaction is apparently obtained from being the center of medical investigations and therapeutic attention, or from being the brave parent of a child with dramatic psychopathology. In malingering, the gain is less enigmatic. The pseudopatient is usually a criminal defendant seeking exculpation on the grounds of insanity.

▶ Treatment

The treatment of DID is the subject of much controversy. Integrative psychotherapy, phasic trauma treatment, and supportive psychotherapy are main psychotherapeutic approaches. While integrative psychotherapy may also involve a phased approach to trauma treatment, it is not the primary focus of the approach. Rather, the therapist may use various therapeutic techniques and modalities throughout the treatment process, depending on the patient's needs and goals. Integrative psychotherapy is a broader approach that seeks to integrate various theoretical and therapeutic modalities into a holistic treatment plan, while phasic trauma treatment is a specific approach that involves dividing the treatment process into distinct phases.

Phasic trauma treatment focuses on trauma recovery, which is also commonly employed in the treatment of complex posttraumatic disorders, and is considered the standard of care. Patients with DID require a significant amount of psychotherapy, which is why care must be carefully designed to reduce the burden on the health care system. Phasic trauma treatment involves a three-staged approach; Stage 1: stabilization and safety, Stage 2: focus on traumatic memories, Stage3: identity integration and rehabilitation.

Individuals with DID often live in a world of ongoing trauma and are at a heightened risk for various co-morbid conditions and self-destructive behaviors. Prioritizing safety is crucial. Safety agreements, hospitalization, and educating patients about the nature of the disease and treatment plan can be effective in achieving this goal.

The second stage involves an intense focus on traumatic experiences and the recall of life history. This stage requires the achievement of goals from previous stages, a strong therapeutic alliance, control of PTSD symptoms, and a good understanding of the risks and benefits of the treatment by the patient. However, it is important to note that there are potential risks associated with this stage, such as the worsening of symptoms and self-destructive behavior. Therefore, ongoing safety measures and stabilization efforts must be maintained throughout this stage of treatment.

The third stage is re-integration into life. This stage is characterized by the achievement of a more unified sense of self, and the dissociative divisions are resolved. While some individuals achieve a complete fusion of identities, others may only attain a therapeutic resolution that enables them to function adequately.

A powerful body of opinion questions the validity of this diagnosis and questions therapeutic approaches that seek to integrate alters. Kluft describes four approaches to treatment: (1) integrate the alters; (2) seek harmony between the alters; (3) leave the alters alone and focus on improving adaptation to the here-and-now; and (4) regard the alters as artifacts, ignoring them and treating other symptoms (e.g., depression). The last of these approaches is adopted by those who believe that DID is a fictive condition generated or reinforced by the clinicians who treat it. The first three approaches are not mutually exclusive and are adopted in accordance with the patient's capacity to tolerate the stress of integrating the alter personalities.

Excessively rapid movement in the assessment or treatment of DID will generate resistance. Once DID is identified and the diagnosis communicated, the patient will experience anxiety. Patients with DID tend to be profoundly distrustful of others and may themselves be deceptive. Patients are likely to be hypersensitive to deceit, impatience, or authoritarianism. Clinicians must be able to tolerate uncertainty, normalize any anomalous experiences that patients divulge, and eschew premature reassurance. Many patients report complete amnesia for early and middle childhood. Most are also confused about current experience and are able to

report the past in only a piecemeal fashion. Clinicians should inquire about instances of lost time, depersonalization, out-of-body experiences, flashbacks, and hallucinations. Most patients with DID are able to suppress alter switching during brief contact, but they are likely to manifest the phenomenon if the interview session extends over an hour.

It can be useful to draw maps, diagrams, or family trees of the internal system of alters, identifying the components by name, age, and sex. These maps must be revised regularly throughout treatment. When a particular alter acknowledges lost time, another alter may have been internally active during that period. The internal helper alter may be the most reliable informant in the clinician's attempt to conceptualize the structure of personality fragments. A number of issues should be considered before embarking on integrative therapy. Table 33–1 lists situations in which integrative therapy is contraindicated.

If supportive therapy is pursued because the patient has a limited potential for integration, the clinician attempts to rehabilitate the patient by strengthening the ego of the host personality and by helping the patient to cope with reality. The emphasis is on stabilization, control of affect and impulse, increased responsibility in everyday behavior, and palliation of distress. Whether the treatment is supportive or integrative, attention must be given to the shame and low self-esteem associated with sexual victimization.

Alters should be directed toward verbal and creative affective expression instead of impulsive, destructive, self-defeating acting out. Each alter represents the expression of a fixed idea: images, thoughts, or associations related to a particular traumatic experience that retains a pristine emotional charge because it has been sequestered from the normal processes of memory decay. The therapist must relate effectively to each of these internal fragments, seeking to improve the contribution

Table 33–1 Contraindications for Integrative Therapy

Severe ego defect related to early neglect and trauma, and a lifelong reliance on dissociative defenses.

Severe, pervasive comorbid pathology, particularly borderline personality disorder, histrionic personality disorder, depression, substance abuse, and eating disorder.

Poor environmental support. If the patient is involved in dysfunctional and nonsupportive relationships, retraumatization is likely to occur. There must be at least a moderate level of environmental stability and support.

The incapacity of the clinician to tolerate devaluation, acting-out behavior, suicidality, self-injury, and deceptiveness.

The inability of patient and clinician to establish and maintain a therapeutic alliance. The therapist must provide a flexible balance between support and interpretation and maintain stable boundaries in interaction with the patient. The patient is likely to test the limits by acting out, seduction, failing to appear for appointments, or devaluing the clinician.

of each fragment to overall functioning. The superordinate aim of integrative therapy is to promote the confluence of the entire system, not to strengthen dissociation between alters. The amount of time devoted to the development of greater general ego strength should exceed the amount of time spent in strengthening separate alters.

Persecutory and malevolent alters are best dealt with by patient rechanneling of hostile impulses in more appropriate directions, particularly by expressing rage in words or artistic productions rather than in deeds. Malevolent alters should be confronted gently with the identity confusion that leads them to consider themselves as part of the abuser rather than as part of the patient.

The internal helper alter is a useful ally in treatment and can serve as a consultant to the therapist, providing information about the total system. The ultimate aim of integrative therapy is to reverse the pervasive attachment disruption and splitting that have accompanied abuse. As the patient improves, he or she may begin to grieve for a lost childhood and for normal attachment experiences that were lost or never provided.

The therapist should help the patient develop effective coping skills, using a gentle, educative approach, modeling accurate perception, management of affect, containment of impulse, and the consideration of alternative responses to stress. Inhibited, withdrawn alters will benefit from the encouragement of self-expression and self-assertion. Shame-based alters require the supportive resolution of shame. As the patient becomes more aware of different traumata, a dialogue may occur between the different alters. The therapist should emphasize the need for cooperation. The aim is toward increased dialogue and mutual cooperation.

The **abreaction of emotion** is an essential component of therapy and is aimed at resolving dissociation and restoring integration. The therapeutic component of abreaction may not be catharsis of feeling but rather the consequent reformulation of traumatic memories. Some patients revert to dissociative trances when they are about to remember and disclose particular traumatic experiences, and spontaneous abreaction may be triggered by reminders of trauma such as anniversaries. However, abreaction without reformulation is unproductive. During abreaction, the therapist's task is to keep the patient safe, nudge him or her toward reality, and keep him or her in the abreaction until it is concluded. Abreaction is followed by debriefing and exploration of the meaning of the experience. Successful abreaction requires full experience of the affect associated with the event, not just a disembodied memory. Premature initiation of abreaction, or the induction of abreaction in patients who cannot tolerate it, is counterproductive. Table 33–2 summarizes the sequential stages in psychotherapy with these patients.

Late in the therapy, the spontaneous fusing of alters signals readiness for personality unification. Usually this proceeds as

Table 33–2 Stages in the Integrative Psychotherapy of Dissociative Identity Disorder

1. Establish a working alliance.
2. Make the diagnosis, inform the patient, and maintain the therapeutic alliance.
3. Make contact with the different alters.
4. Explore the structure of the system of alters.
5. Understand the particular "fixed idea" behind each alter.
6. Work with the problems of particular alter states.
7. Help the patient develop increasing cooperation between alter states.
8. Help the patient develop nondissociative coping skills.
9. Confront dissociation and support the patient's integration of memory, affect, and identity via the abreaction of traumatic experience.
10. Help the patient develop and consolidate a new identity.

two or more alters combine at a time. The therapist must be patient and not press for premature fusion. Full integration involves (1) reduced reliance on the dissociative segregation of experience, (2) the blending of alters into a single nondissociative personality, and (3) the harmonious coexistence of different aspects of the patient's personality. Integration is relative. Some patients are able to tolerate complete fusion and unification. Others are not capable of full unification but benefit from improved functional integration.

Several other types of psychotherapy may be helpful. In group therapy, groups specifically designed for individuals with DID can be helpful in stabilizing these patients. In contrast, groups consisting of general psychiatric patients have been found to be less successful due to potential disruptions caused by the emergence of alters and the traumatic nature of DID patients.

Family and couples therapy are important parts of the treatment process for individuals with DID. Educating family members about the condition and addressing their concerns can promote the development of healthy coping mechanisms and create a supportive environment for the patient. It is important to emphasize that family members should not interact directly with different alters.

Eye-Movement Desensitization and Reprocessing Therapy (EMDR) is a type of therapy that was originally developed for PTSD treatment. While there is no consensus on its effectiveness for DID patients, some believe that if performed by a well-trained clinician, EMDR can be helpful in well-stabilized DID patients with adult trauma.

Hypnotherapeutic interventions can be useful when rapid diagnosis is required, although it may be preferable to allow the alters to emerge spontaneously. The clinician should explore each alter with regard to the following information: name, age, and sex; developmental origin; dominant affect and perceptual style; survival functions; and unique symptoms and dysfunctions. The clinician should ask to speak to

Table 33–3 Medications Used in Dissociative Identity Disorder Treatment

Alpha-Adrenergic Blocking Agents
   PTSD nightmares and daytime symptoms
Selective serotonin reuptake inhibitors
   Affective disorders (no agent preference) and obsessive–
      compulsive disorder (fluvoxamine)
Tricyclic antidepressants
   obsessive–compulsive disorder
Mood stabilizers
   PTSD and anxiety
Atypical neuroleptics
   Thought disorder
Serotonin antagonist and reuptake inhibitors
   Sleep problems (Trazodone)
Opioid antagonists
   Self-injurious behavior and addictions (Naltrexone)

a particular alter identified by name or behavior and should ask for a signal (e.g., a lifted finger) as a signal of the alter's willingness to appear. Rapport must be developed with each alter. After conducting the appropriate interview, the clinician should ask the alter to resubmerge. Although initially the clinician must treat each alter as if he or she is a separate person, it is important to convey the understanding that each alter is but a dissociated element of the client as a whole.

The medications for treating DID are similar to those used for treating PTSD, with the goal of addressing the symptoms of DID. Table 33–3 lists medications used for DID.

Prognosis

The symptoms of DID typically manifest during childhood. In cases where childhood trauma leads to DID, a positive prognosis can be expected with early intervention and treatment. However, some patients develop histrionic or borderline personalities, with a stormy adulthood. Others are introverted, depressed, and socially avoidant. Males are more likely than females to have a history of episodic violence in the correctional system. Many patients with DID manage to conceal their symptoms for years.

DISSOCIATIVE AMNESIA

Clinical Findings

A. Signs & Symptoms

Dissociative amnesia is an inability to recall important autobiographical information, usually of a traumatic or stressful nature, that is inconsistent with ordinary forgetting. It most often consists of localized or selective amnesia for a specific event or events; or generalized amnesia for identity and life history.

The DSM-5-TR considers dissociative fugue as a subtype of dissociative amnesia, while in the ICD-10 classification, dissociative fugue is classified as a separate diagnosis. Dissociative fugue may occur with dissociative amnesia and DID. Dissociative fugue is apparently purposeful travel or bewildered wandering that is associated with amnesia for identity or for other important autobiographical information. Dissociative fugue can last from minutes to months.

The amnesia for distressing events can be localized (i.e., complete amnesia for events during a circumscribed period of time), selective (i.e., failure to remember some but not all events during a circumscribed period of time), generalized (i.e., affecting an entire period of life), or continuous (i.e., failure to remember anything after a particular date). Patchy amnesia is prevalent among people exposed to military or civilian trauma. A common sequence is for the patient to progress from a first stage, characterized by an acute altered state of consciousness (mental confusion, headache, and preoccupation with a single idea or emotion), to a second stage in which he or she loses the sense of personal identity. At this point, the patient may be found wandering in a fugue state, unable to give an account of himself or herself. Rarely, the patient enters a third stage in which he or she assumes a new identity, usually one more gregarious and uninhibited than previously. During the first stage of confusion and altered consciousness, some patients report audiovisual hallucinations and a preoccupation with quasidelusional ideas. This condition, originally known as hysterical twilight state, lacks the disorganization of thought processes and affective incongruity found in schizophrenia. The patient operates at a higher level of consciousness than is associated with epilepsy or other organic brain dysfunctions.

B. Psychological Testing

Table 33–4 lists tests that are useful screens in the diagnosis of dissociative disorders.

Differential Diagnosis (Including Comorbid Conditions)

Differential diagnosis is based on a full history, a detailed mental status examination, physical and neurologic examination, and when appropriate, special investigations such as a toxicology screen, laboratory testing, electroencephalography, brain imaging, and neuropsychological testing.

Nonpathologic amnesia: the typical presentation of dissociative amnesia, which has a well-defined boundary, onset, and offset, is distinct from the recall gradient observed in normal memory. For example, it can be demonstrated by an inability to remember a specific age, a difficulty in recalling a particular person, activity, or time of year. Memory lapses that are considered harmless and do not stem from stressful events are a regular occurrence in human memory function.

Table 33–4 Screening Tests for Dissociative Disorders

Test	Description
Dissociative Disorders Interview Schedule (DDIS) has been updated for DSM-5	A 132-item yes–no format structured interview that examines for dissociative disorder, somatoform disorder, depression, borderline personality disorder, substance abuse, and physical and sexual abuse
Revised Structured Clinical Interview for the DSM Dissociative Disorders (SCID-D-R) being updated for DSM-5	A semi-structured clinician administered interview derived from the SCID. Assesses the symptom severity and considered gold standard for research purposes
Dissociative Experiences Scale (DES)	A 28-item self-report questionnaire that screens for dissociative symptoms in adults (age ≥18 years)
Adolescent Dissociative Experiences Scale (A-DES)	A 30-item self-report screening questionnaire for adolescents (age 12–20 years)
Child Dissociative Checklist (CDC)	A 20-item screening checklist to be completed on children (age 5–12 years) by a parent or adult observer
Structured Interview for Reported Symptoms (SIRS)	A structured interview designed to detect the malingering of psychosis
Cambridge Depersonalization Scale (CDS)	A 29-item test characterizes the quality, frequency, and duration of dissociative symptoms over the last 6 months

Table 33–5 Mental Status Examination Questions for Dissociative Amnesia

Do you ever have blackouts? Blank spells? Memory lapses?
Do you have gaps in your experience of time?
Do you have any knowledge of what happened during these periods?
Are there behaviors that you cannot recall but you may have done?
Do you find objects in you possession?
Do you find that your relationships change in a way that you cannot explain?
Do you find that sometime your hand skills fluctuate?
Do you have gaps in your memory of your life?
Do you sometimes see yourself from a distance as if you watching a movie of yourself?
Do you feel like your body does not belong to you?

Modified from Loewenstein RJ. An office mental status examination for chronic complex dissociative symptoms and multiple personality disorder. *Psychiatry Clin North Am.* 1991;14(3):567–604.

impairment is generally more specific than in dissociative amnesia and is often limited to certain aspects of the traumatic event.

Substance use-related amnesia: amnesia can be caused by various substances. To differentiate between substance-induced amnesia and dissociative amnesia, a comprehensive timeline of memory impairment and instances of substance intoxication can be useful in many cases.

Feigned or malingered amnesia: there are currently no tests available to differentiate between malingering and dissociative amnesia. Malingering can occur when an individual attempts to avoid a situation that involves legal, financial, or personal difficulties. In some cases of dissociative amnesia, both genuine memory loss and feigning can be present at the same time.

Treatment

Patience and the expectation that memory loss will soon clear are usually enough to help the amnestic patient recover. Most cases resolve spontaneously following the removal of stressful situation. The key to treatment is a safe environment (e. g., hospitalization) removed from the source of stress and a trusting therapeutic relationship.

The psychotherapeutic approach for dissociative amnesia usually involves the three-staged phasic trauma psychotherapy that is also utilized in treating DID. The primary objectives are to achieve stability, ensure patient safety, and reduce symptoms.

Hypnotherapy or narcoanalysis (e.g., using amobarbital, benzodiazepines, or methylamphetamine) is sometimes required to facilitate recall. There are no medications that are specifically indicated for treating dissociative amnesia. Antidepressants can be used to address the co-occurring depression.

Delirium and dementia: typically, dementia causes notable cognitive decline in various domains. As a result, it is uncommon to observe loss of personal identity memory in the absence of significant cognitive impairment. Dissociative amnesia typically does not impact a person's capacity to learn new cognitive information or carry out tasks. When it comes to elderly patients, physicians may tend to primarily associate memory impairments with neurological conditions or commonly occurring psychiatric disorders. Therefore, a thorough evaluation and careful examination are necessary for an accurate diagnosis (Table 33–5).

Transient epileptic amnesia: the defining features of epileptic amnesia include recurring, temporary episodes of isolated memory loss that generally lasts less than an hour. This condition typically affects middle-aged and elderly populations. The diagnosis of epileptic amnesia can be established through various methods, including administering neuropsychological tests, EEG scans, and evaluating the patient's response to anticonvulsant medication.

Post traumatic amnesia: amnesia is commonly associated with trauma disorders. In cases of PTSD, memory

Prognosis

Dissociative amnesia and dissociative fugue are usually short lived. However, several case series on chronic disease course with generalized, continuous, or severe localized amnesia exist. Short symptom duration and comorbid depression have been proposed as favorable prognostic indicators for dissociative amnesia. After the restoration of memory and identity, the patient must deal with the source of the problem.

DEPERSONALIZATION/DEREALIZATION DISORDER

Clinical Findings

A. Signs & Symptoms

DDD is defined as the presence of persistent or recurrent experiences of depersonalization, derealization or both in the presence of intact reality testing. Depersonalization is defined as experiences of unreality, detachment or being an outside observer with respect to one's thoughts, feelings, sensations, body or actions (e.g., perceptual alterations, distorted sense of time, unreal or absent self, emotional and/or physical numbing). Derealization is defined as experiences of unreality or detachment with respect to surroundings (e.g., individuals or objects are experienced as unreal, dreamlike, foggy, lifeless, or visually distorted).

The onset is usually sudden and typically occurs in a setting of anxiety. Patients feel numb and out of touch with their feelings, bodies, and surroundings. Sometimes they feel as if they are observing themselves or as though they are automatons in a dream. Depersonalization is difficult to describe, and patients may express concern about "going crazy," particularly if the condition is accompanied by déjà vu experiences and distortions in the sense of time and in patients who were raised in homes with a mentally ill family member. Depression and anxiety are commonly associated with depersonalization.

B. Psychological Testing

See discussion of dissociative amnesia.

Differential Diagnosis (Including Comorbid Conditions)

Dissociative disorders in which depersonalization or derealization is the cardinal symptom probably merge imperceptibly with other disorders in which depersonalization is a subsidiary symptom. For example, depersonalization is likely to be elicited from patients with anxiety disorders (particularly panic disorder), other dissociative disorders, depressive disorder, and borderline personality disorder.

DDD can be distinguished from depressive disorders by the absence of major symptoms of MDD. Individuals with personality disorders may experience depersonalization or derealization symptoms, but their behaviors are typically inflexible and pervasive, and consistent across various personal and social situations.

Depersonalization has been reported in 11–42% of patients with schizophrenia. Depersonalization in schizophrenia often becomes incorporated into the individual's delusions, contributing to their distorted perception of reality. Conversely, DDD patients typically have intact reality testing.

Depersonalization may also be encountered in substance use, particularly with alcohol, marijuana, hallucinogens, cocaine, phencyclidine, methylamphetamine, narcotics, and sedatives. Depersonalization has also been reported after medication with indomethacin, fenfluramine, and haloperidol. In the majority of cases, depersonalization resulting from drug use is temporary.

In epilepsy, particularly temporal lobe epilepsy, depersonalization may be encountered as an aura, as part of the seizure itself, or between seizures. Depersonalization in epilepsy is more likely to be associated with stereotypic movements (e.g., lip smacking), senseless words or phrases, and loss of consciousness than in dissociative disorders, in which it is likely to be more highly elaborated. Depersonalization may also be evident in postconcussive disorder, Meniere disease, cerebral atherosclerosis, and Korsakoff syndrome.

To differentiate DDD from other dissociative disorders like DID and dissociative amnesia, certain factors need to be considered. DDD does not involve distinct personality states like DID does. Furthermore, DDD patients usually do not suffer from extensive gaps in their autobiographical memory, which distinguishes it from dissociative amnesia.

Due to a variety of conditions associated with depersonalization, it is essential to conduct a thorough medical and neurological evaluation that encompasses standard laboratory studies, EEG, and, if appropriate, drug screen.

Treatment

Early diagnosis of DDD is the key for successful treatment of this disorder. Helping patients achieve a state of comfort and stability by removing them from any traumatic situations or interactions is the most appropriate approach for treating this disorder. Due to significant delays in diagnosis, interventions for the disease often take place years after its onset. When there is uncertainty in diagnosis or patients have atypical symptoms, brain imaging can be useful in facilitating diagnosis.

Various types of psychotherapy, including psychodynamic, cognitive, behavioral, hypnotherapeutic, and supportive therapies, can be utilized in the treatment of DDD. However, there is currently no research that directly compares the effectiveness of these therapies. The relative effectiveness of supportive psychotherapy, hypnosis, exploratory psychotherapy, family therapy, and cognitive–behavioral therapy (CBT) is not known. Psychotherapy focuses on the recovery of the traumatic experience from which the pathologic dissociation is thought to have arisen. Hypnosis may help in this regard. Cognitive–behavioral desensitization, flooding, and exposure have also been used.

CBT for DDD focuses on altering the cognitive perception of symptoms to make them seem less threatening, reducing avoidance behaviors, creating safety behaviors, and decreasing symptom monitoring. Some experts believe that CBT should be the first line psychotherapy for DDD patients. However, based on limited number of trials testing CBT in this patient population, efficacy of CBT seems limited by itself. Hence, it is crucial to consider using different treatment modalities together.

The primary focus of psychodynamic psychotherapy is to identify the root causes of threats to self-constancy that result in emotionally intolerable feelings and to integrate these emotions with the core sense of self to facilitate the transition from an "unreal" self to a more "real" owned self. Currently, there are no clinical trials available in the literature that examine the effectiveness of psychodynamic psychotherapy in treating DDD. Nevertheless, several case reports have demonstrated successful implementation of this treatment approach.

In terms of pharmacologic treatment of DDD, there are currently no known psychiatric medications that have been proven to be effective. However, there is some limited evidence supporting the use of clomipramine for addressing co-occurring depression and anxiety in DDD. Additionally, naltrexone has been demonstrated to be partially effective in treating depersonalization that is resistant to other forms of treatment. Transcranial Magnetic Stimulation targeting the temporal–parietal junction has shown promising results in reducing DDD symptoms in these patients

▶ Prognosis

DDD commonly follows a chronic course. It commonly occurs in late adolescence and early adulthood, and it rarely develops as late as 50s. Depersonalization that is associated with intoxication, trauma, or other psychiatric conditions often resolves after the removal of the underlying cause and appropriate treatment. Patients with chronic depersonalization may experience significant and prolonged functional impairment.

OTHER SPECIFIED DISSOCIATIVE DISORDER

▶ Clinical Findings

A. Signs & Symptoms

This category applies to presentations in which symptoms characteristic of a dissociative disorder that cause clinically significant distress or impairment predominate but do not meet the full criteria for any of the disorders. The other specified dissociative disorder category is used in situations in which the clinician chooses to communicate the specific reason that the presentation does not meet the criteria for any specific dissociative disorder. The specific reason is provided. Examples include:

Chronic and recurrent syndromes of mixed dissociative symptoms include identity disturbance associated with less-than-marked discontinuities in sense of self and agency, or alterations of identity or episodes of possession in an individual who report no dissociative amnesia.

Identity disturbance due to prolonged and intense coercive persuasion affects individuals who have been subjected to intense coercive persuasion (e.g., brainwashing, thought reform, indoctrination while captive, torture, long-term political imprisonment, recruitment by sects/cults or by terror organizations) and presents with prolonged changes in, or conscious questioning of, their identity. The risk of persistent depersonalization and substantial shifts in identity in addition to various dissociative symptoms including amnesias, trance-like behaviors, diminished environmental responsiveness, and emotional numbing is very high in these patients.

Acute dissociative reactions to stressful events refer to acute, transient conditions that typically last less than 1 month, and sometimes only a few hours or days. These conditions are characterized by constriction of consciousness, depersonalization, derealization, perceptual disturbances (e.g., time slowing, macropsia), micro-amnesias, transient stupor, and/or alterations in sensory–motor functioning (e.g., analgesia, paralysis). Although this condition usually is precipitated by traumatic or nontraumatic stressors, unlike acute stress disorder, a specific stressor is not necessary to diagnose this condition. Some cultural syndromes like ataques de nervios (attacks of nerves) might meet the diagnosis criteria of this condition. However, cultural syndromes are extremely complicated and need to be assessed in an individual basis.

Dissociative trance disorder is a temporary, marked alteration in the state of consciousness or loss of the customary sense of personal identity without alteration or change of identity. There is an acute narrowing or complete loss of awareness of immediate surroundings that manifests as profound unresponsiveness or insensitivity to environmental stimuli. The unresponsiveness may be accompanied by minor stereotyped behaviors (e.g., finger movements) of which the individual in unaware and/or that he/she cannot control, as well as transient paralysis or loss of consciousness. The dissociative trance is not a normal part of a broadly accepted collective cultural or religious practice.

Ganser syndrome, although was considered a "dissociative disorder not otherwise specified" in the DSM-IV, is not listed in DSM-5-TR. Cardinal symptoms of this syndrome include approximate answers, clouding of consciousness, somatic conversion symptoms, and hallucinations. Ganser syndrome is a poorly understood condition with a very low prevalence, and its underlying etiology is unknown.

B. Psychological Testing

See discussion of dissociative amnesia.

▶ Differential Diagnosis (Including Comorbid Conditions)

These syndromes must be differentiated from schizophrenia, substance-induced psychosis, major depression with psychotic features, and epilepsy.

▶ Treatment

Identity disturbance due to prolonged and intense coercive persuasion: no specific treatment has been developed for this condition. The primary approach to managing patients with this disorder is to employ the phasic trauma treatment model.

Acute dissociative reactions to stressful events: there is no established treatment specifically targeting this disorder. The treatment plan should prioritize pharmacological interventions for managing symptoms, alongside psychotherapy.

Dissociative trance disorder: treatment is focused on patient education about the condition and symptoms. In appropriate cases, hypnosis and supportive expressive psychotherapy may be utilized.

Ganser syndrome: due to clouding of consciences and dissociation, psychiatric hospitalization may be needed in acutely presenting patients. The exploration of potential stressors may be beneficial, but confrontation of the patient's approximate responses is not productive. Supportive psychotherapy and low dose antipsychotics can be used. Usually, patients return to normal function within days.

▶ Prognosis

The prognosis is generally good but varies. However, the long-term outlook depends on the quality of family support and the patient's personality.

UNSPECIFIED DISSOCIATIVE DISORDER

This category applies to presentations in which symptoms characteristic of a dissociative disorder that cause clinically significant distress or impairment predominate but do not meet the full criteria for any of the disorders in the dissociative disorders diagnostic class. The unspecified classification is used in situations in which the clinician chooses not to specify the reason that the criteria are not met for a specific dissociative disorder and includes presentations for which there is insufficient information to make a more specific diagnosis.

American Psychiatric Association. *Diagnostic and Statistical Manual of Mental Disorders*, 5th ed., text rev.; 2022.

Briere J. Dissociative symptoms and trauma exposure: specificity, affect dysregulation, and posttraumatic stress. *J Nerv Ment Dis.* 2006;194:78–82.

Enoch MD, Trethowan WH. The Ganser syndrome. *Uncommon Psychiatr Syndr.* 1979:50–62.

Gabbard GO, ed. *Gabbard's Treatment of Psychiatric Disorders*. 5th ed. Washington, DC: American Psychiatric Publishing; 2014:471–478.

Guralnik O, Simeon D. Depersonalization: standing in the spaces between recognition and interpellation. *Psychoanal Dial.* 2010; 20(4):400–416.

Hornstein NL, Putnam FW. Clinical phenomenology of child and adolescent dissociative disorders. *J Am Acad Child Adolesc Psychiatry.* 1992;31:1077.

Hunter EC, Baker D, Phillips ML, Sierra M, David AS. Cognitive-behaviour therapy for depersonalisation disorder: an open study. *Behav Res Ther.* 2005;43(9):1121–1130.

International Society for the Study of Trauma and Dissociation. Guidelines for treating dissociative identity disorder in adults, third revision. *J Trauma Dissoc.* 2011;12(2):115–187.

Isaac M, Chand PK. Dissociative and conversion disorders: defining boundaries. *Curr Opin Psychiatry.* 2006;19:61–66.

Jang KL, Paris J, Zweig-Frank H, Livesley WJ. Twin study of dissociative experience. *J Nerv Ment Dis.* 1998;186(6): 345–351.

Lochner C, Seedat S, Hemmings SM, Moolman-Smook JC, Kidd M, Stein DJ. Investigating the possible effects of trauma experiences and 5-HTT on the dissociative experiences of patients with OCD using path analysis and multiple regression. *Neuropsychobiology.* 2007;56(1):6–13.

Loewenstein RJ. An office mental status examination for complex chronic dissociative symptoms and multiple personality disorder. *Psychiatr Clin North Am.* 1991;14(3):567–604.

Lowenstein RJ, Putnam FW. Dissociative disorders. In: Sadock BJ, Sadock VA, eds. *Comprehensive Textbook of Psychiatry*, 8th ed. Philadelphia: Lippincott, Williams & Wilkins; 2005:1844–1901.

Mantovani A, Simeon D, Urban N, Bulow P, Allart A, Lisanby S. Temporo-parietal junction stimulation in the treatment of depersonalization disorder. *Psychiatry Res.* 2011;186(1):138–140.

McHugh PR, Putnam FW. Resolved: multiple personality is an individually and socially created artifact. *J Am Acad Child Adolesc Psychiatry.* 1995;34:957.

McKay Gavin, Michael D Kopelman. Psychogenic amnesia: when memory complaints are medically unexplained. *Adv Psychiatr Treat.* 2009;15:152–158.

Michelson LK, Ray WJ. *Handbook of Dissociation: Theoretical, Empirical and Clinical Perspectives.* New York: Plenum Publishing Corp; 1996.

Nurcombe B. Dissociative hallucinosis and allied conditions. In: Volkmar F, ed. *Psychoses of Childhood and Adolescence.* Washington DC: American Psychiatric Press; 1996:107–128.

Orrù G, Bertelloni D, Cesari V, Conversano C, Gemignani A. Targeting temporal parietal junction for assessing and treating disembodiment phenomena: a systematic review of TMS effect on depersonalization and derealization disorders (DPD) and body illusions. *AIMS Neurosci.* 2021;8(2):181–194.

Pieper S, Out D, Bakermans-Kranenburg MJ, van Ijzendoorn MH. Behavioral and molecular genetics of dissociation: the role of the serotonin transporter gene promoter polymorphism (5-HTTLPR). *J Trauma Stress.* 2011;24(4):373–380.

Putnam FW. *Dissociation in Children and Adolescents.* New York: Guilford Press; 1997.

Sadock, Benjamin J, et al. *Kaplan and Sadock's Comprehensive Textbook of Psychiatry.* 10th ed., Wolters Kluwer; 2017.

Simeon D, Abugel J. *Feeling Unreal: Depersonalization Disorder and the Loss of the Self,* 2nd ed. Oxford University Press.

Simeon D, Knutelska M, Nelson D, Guralnik O. Feeling unreal: a depersonalization disorder update of 117 cases. *J Clin Psychiatry.* 2003;64(9:90–997.

Simeon D, Knutelska M. An open trial of naltrexone in the treatment of depersonalization disorder. *J Clin Psychopharmacol.* 2005;25(3):267–270.

Smith CN, Frascino JC, Kripke DL, McHugh PR, Treisman GJ, Squire LR. Losing memories overnight: a unique form of human amnesia. *Neuropsychologia.* 2010;48(10):2833–2840. doi: 10.1016/j.neuropsychologia.2010.05.025.

Szekely A, Kovacs-Nagy R, Banyai EI, et al. Association between hypnotizability and the catechol-O- methyltransferase (COMT) polymorphism. *Int J Clin Exp Hypn.* 2010;58(3):301–315.

Wolf EJ, Rasmusson AM, Mitchell KS, Logue MW, Baldwin CT, Miller MW. A genome-wide association study of clinical symptoms of dissociation in a trauma-exposed sample. *Depress Anxiety.* 2014;31(4):352–360. doi: 10.1002/da.22260.

34 Sexual Dysfunctions and Paraphilic Disorders

Richard Balon, MD
R. Taylor Segraves, MD, PhD

INTRODUCTION

Sexual dysfunctions and paraphilic disorders are disorders of either disturbance of processes in sexual functioning (sexual dysfunctions) or sexual behavior(s) (paraphilic disorders). Human sexuality presents a very complex interaction of biology and psychology, which is reflected in complex physiological responses. A seemingly very simple event, such as erection, is regulated on the central nervous system and peripheral nervous system level, modified by various hormones, affected by vascular changes, and influenced by various expectations, interpersonal issues, and intrapsychic processes, not to mention the influences of medications and substances of abuse, the aging processes, diseases, and personal habits. Although there is a substantial body of literature on human sexuality in general and sexual dysfunctions and paraphilias in particular, good evidence-based literature on most aspects of these disorders is mostly lacking. The focus has definitely moved from psychology to biology and medicalization of human sexuality. The biological sciences, such as pharmacology, have contributed enormously to developments in this area. However, an exclusive focus on biology and medical aspects of human sexuality is unwarranted and may trivialize a very complex area of human behavior. Even the clearly "biological" treatment approaches to sexual dysfunction may fail in certain situations due to various psychological factors. Thus, we caution the reader to always consider all factors, biological and psychological, in making the diagnosis and in planning treatment. In most cases, the judicious combination of biological and psychological treatment approaches will yield the most satisfactory results.

The diagnoses of sexual dysfunctions and paraphilic disorders are mostly descriptive; no diagnosis-specific tests or examinations are usually available. The classification of sexual dysfunctions was historically based on the notion of connected yet separate and clearly defined phases of the sexual response cycle—desire, arousal/excitement, orgasm, and resolution. However, this model of sexual response is not considered as truly reflecting the intricacies of female sexual response and thus has been replaced by a different, more complicated circular model. As the linearity of sexual response in women was abandoned, the entire classification/listing of sexual dysfunctions in DSM-5 was changed, and the dysfunctions are listed alphabetically. Sexual dysfunctions in males are still diagnosed according to impairments of one of the first three "phases" (no impairment of the resolution phase has been identified). In females (in a simplistic way of explanation), the former female desire and arousal are combined into the diagnosis of female sexual interest/arousal disorder (FSIAD), and the diagnosis of female orgasm disorder is kept. However, clinically these disturbances are not so clearly separated and frequently overlap or coexist (e.g., lack of libido with impaired erection or orgasm). In addition, the previous diagnoses of painful sexual dysfunctions of dyspareunia and vaginismus are replaced with a single diagnosis of genito-pelvic/penetration disorder; and sexual aversion has been removed as a full-fledged diagnosis (could be diagnosed as other specified sexual dysfunction). Interestingly, the present classification defines and uses only one end of the sexual functioning spectrum, the "lack" of functioning (e.g., lack of libido), though imprecisely and vaguely. Hypersexuality is not well defined and not conceptualized as a dysfunction, but rather at times (if at all) as related to addiction, compulsivity, or impulsivity. Another important point in classifying and diagnosing sexual dysfunctions and paraphilic disorders is the use of clinically significant distress or impairment as one of the defining criteria of some these disorders (sexual masochism disorder, fetishistic disorder, transvestic disorder). Thus, if the lack of sexual desire does not cause any distress or impairment, one should not qualify it as a dysfunction. Similarly, if a paraphilic behavior does not cause any distress or impairment in cases of sexual masochism, fetishism and transvestism, it should not be classified as paraphilic disorder, but as paraphilia. In the remaining five major paraphilic disorders (voyeuristic disorder, exhibitionistic disorder, frotteuristic disorder, sexual sadism disorder, and pedophilic disorder), either the person must act on these urges with a nonconsenting person (in case of pedophilic disorder, no matter whether consenting or nonconsenting) or the urges or fantasies must cause clinically significant distress or impairment. There seem to be some individuals who have no interest in sex and are not distressed by it; thus, they do not suffer from any sexual disorder according to the currently used diagnostic systems (they may present just one end of the spectrum of certain behavior, similar to premature/rapid versus absent ejaculation, discussed later). The diagnoses of sexual dysfunction also include two newly introduced criteria—defined frequency of symptomatology (on almost all or all occasions, usually defined as 75–100% of the time) and defined duration of symptomatology (~6 months). Both these changes intent to increase the "homogeneity" of the diagnosis, and the duration criterion makes diagnoses of sexual dysfunctions consistent with the rest of the DSM-5-TR. It is also known from previous studies that many patients who meet the diagnostic criteria of sexual dysfunction initially do not meet these criteria at 6 months or a later time point.

The DSM-5-TR diagnostic system employs same subtypes and specifiers for sexual dysfunctions—lifelong, acquired, generalized, and situational—and thus sexual dysfunctions may be further subclassified, for instance, to lifelong generalized or acquired generalized and other subtypes. The use of specifiers may be relevant to prognosis, course, or treatment selection. One exception is specifiers of substance/medication-induced sexual dysfunction—with onset during intoxication; during withdrawal; and after medication use. Paraphilic disorder specifiers are usually based on the type of attraction and behavior (e.g., age or gender of the person the behavior is connected to) and whether the behavior occurs in a controlled environment or is in remission. The subtypes and specifiers may be useful to consider in formulating the diagnosis and especially the treatment plan.

The DSM-5-TR also provides severity specifiers for each sexual dysfunction—mild, moderate, or severe (as to the intensity of distress; or time to occurrence in case of premature ejaculation (PE); or frequency in case of substance/medication-induced sexual dysfunction).

American Psychiatric Association. *Diagnostic and Statistical Manual of Mental Disorders.* 5th ed. Text Revision. Washington, DC: American Psychiatric Association; 2022.

▼ SEXUAL DYSFUNCTIONS

DELAYED EJACULATION (DE) (FORMERLY MALE ORGASMIC DISORDER)

▶ General Considerations

DE refers both to marked delay in ejaculation and absence of ejaculation/orgasm. The symptoms must be experienced on almost all or all occasions (approximately 75–100%) of partnered sexual activity, must be distressing, and should persist for a minimum duration of approximately 6 months. A variety of terms have been used in the literature to refer to this disorder. They include retarded ejaculation, inhibited ejaculation, *ejaculatio retarda, impotencia ejaculandi*, anejaculation, among others. A time-based definition of an intravaginal latency time of 25 minutes has been proposed for this diagnosis as it corresponds to two standard deviations above the man ejaculatory latency time found in population-based studies.

A. Epidemiology

The exact prevalence is unknown. Only 75% of men report always ejaculating during sexual activity. In a national epidemiological study, approximately 8% of U.S. males aged 18–59 years complained of an inability to reach orgasm. However, less than 1% of men complain of problems reaching ejaculation lasting more than 6 months.

B. Etiology

The etiology of DE may be due to psychological factors, drug-induced, or due to a general medical condition (e.g., hypothyroidism). Substance-induced DE may be caused by tricyclic antidepressants (TCAs), monoamine oxidase inhibitors (MAOIs), selective serotonin reuptake inhibitors (SSRIs), drugs causing alpha-adrenergic blockade, dopamine D-2 blockers, and benzodiazepines. Diseases, accidents, or surgical procedures that interrupt the nerve supply of the ejaculatory apparatus can interfere with the ability to reach orgasm. Spinal cord lesions and pelvic surgery as well as peripheral neuropathies can cause anorgasmia. Difficulty reaching orgasm can be part of the presentation of severe depression. Anger at women in general or to the sexual partner in specific has been hypothesized to be responsible for male anorgasmia due to psychological factors. This hypothesis is unproven. Some have suggested association with orthodoxy of religious belief. There is minimal evidence concerning the etiology and treatment of this disorder when it is due to psychological factors. It has also been proposed that ejaculatory latency may be a neurobiological variant and not necessarily indicative of a pathologic process.

C. Genetics

A population-based study of Finnish twins found no evidence of a genetic contribution to delayed ejaculation in young men.

▶ Clinical Findings

A. Signs & Symptoms

The typical patient reports that either he is unable to ejaculate or it takes an inordinately long period of sexual stimulation in order to ejaculate. Some men may struggle so hard to ejaculate that they deny sexual pleasure to both themselves and their partners.

B. Psychological Testing

Psychological testing is not available for this disorder.

C. Laboratory Testing

If a neurological etiology is suspected, pudendal nerve conduction studies and evoked potential studies can be ordered.

D. Neuroimaging

One MRI study with a small sample size found increased activation in the right fusiform gyros of the occipital lobe and right hippocampus in 3 men with lifelong delayed ejaculation as compared to 6 normal controls.

▶ Course of Illness

DE due to psychological factors is rarely encountered in clinical practice, and there is minimal evidence regarding its clinical course. Most clinicians regard this as a chronic condition.

▶ Differential Diagnosis

A careful medical history is taken to rule out DE due to a general medical condition such as multiple sclerosis, diabetes mellitus, or surgical lesion affecting the nerve supply to the genitalia. A careful pharmacological history should focus on the use of opioid drugs, benzodiazepines, serotonergic drugs, or drugs with significant alpha or dopamine D-2 blockade.

A thorough review of the presenting symptoms may indicate probable etiologies. For example, if the difficulty is situational (i.e., partner or sex specific), one should suspect psychological factors. If the problem is acquired and global, one should carefully rule out DE due to a general medical condition and substance-induced DE.

▶ Treatment

Treatment of DE should be tailored and etiology specific and may include patient/couple psychoeducation and/or psychosexual therapy, pharmacotherapy, or integrated treatment.

A. Psychopharmacological Treatment

There is no pharmacological treatment for DE due to a general medical condition. Substance-induced DE can be reversed depending on the offending agent. Serotonergic antidepressants can be replaced with antidepressants with a decreased likelihood of causing orgasm delay. Buspirone at a dose of 60 mg/d can be used as an antidote. Other possible antidotes include cyproheptadine (2–16 mg) and amantadine. If DE is due to antipsychotic agents, one can substitute aripiprazole, quetiapine, or olanzapine.

B. Psychotherapeutic Treatment

There is no evidence-based therapy for DE due to psychological factors. Most clinicians would attempt behavioral therapy using a vibrator for intense stimulation. Once ejaculation can be reliably achieved in solitary masturbation homework assignments, the clinician might try to gradually phase this new skill into partner-related activities. Different approaches may be selected based on subtyping (lifelong vs. acquired, situational vs. generalized).

C. Other Treatment

If infertility is a primary concern in DE due to a general medical condition, sperm can be obtained by the stimulation of the internal ejaculatory organs by a transrectal electrical probe.

▶ Complications/Adverse Outcomes of Treatment

In cases of substance-induced DE, drug substitution carries the risk of recurrence of the psychiatric disorder being treated.

▶ Prognosis

The prognosis in substance-induced DE is good. The prognosis of DE due to psychological or medical conditions is poor.

Althof S. Psychological interventions for delayed ejaculation/orgasm. *Int J Impot Res.* 2012;24:131–136.

American Psychiatric Association. *Diagnostic and Statistical Manual of Mental Disorders.* 5th ed. Text Revision. Washington, DC: American Psychiatric Association; 2022.

Flannigan R, Heier L, Voss H, et al. Functional magnetic resonance imaging detects between-group differences in neural activation among men with delayed orgasm compared with normal controls: preliminary report. *J Sex Med.* 2019;16:1246–1254.

Holstege G, Georgiadis J, Paans A, et al. Brain activation during human male ejaculation. *J Neurosci.* 2003;23:9185.

Jenkins C, Mulhall J. Delayed orgasm and anorgasmia. *Fertil Steril.* 2015;104:1082–1088.

Jern P, Santtila P, Witting K, et al. Premature and delayed ejaculation: genetic and environmental effects in a population-based sample of Finnish twins. *J Sex Med.* 2007;4:1739–1749.

Laumann EO, Paik A, Rosen RC. Sexual dysfunction in the United States: prevalence and predictors. *JAMA.* 1999;281:537–544.

McMahon C, Abdo C, Incrocci L, et al. Disorders of orgasm and ejaculation in men. In: Lue T, Basson R, Rosen R, et al., eds. *Sexual Medicine. Sexual Dysfunctions in Men and Women.* Plymouth, UK: Health Publications; 2004:409.

McMahon CG, Jannini E, Waldinger M, Rowland D. Standard operating procedures in disorders of orgasm and ejaculation. *J Sex Med.* 2013;10:204–229.

Martin-Tuite P, Shnidel A. Management options for premature and delayed ejaculation in men. *Sex Med Rev.* 2020;8:473–485.

Shindel A, Althof S, Carrier S, et al. Disorders of ejaculation: an AUA/SMSNA Guideline. *J Urol.* 2022;207:504–512.

Waldinger M. Male ejaculation and orgasmic disorders. In: Balon R, Segraves RT, eds. *Handbook of Sexual Dysfunction.* New York: Taylor & Francis; 2005:215.

Waldinger MD. Delayed and premature ejaculation. In: Balon R, Segraves RT, eds. *Clinical Manual of Sexual Dysfunction.* Arlington, VA: American Psychiatric Publishing; 2009:273–304.

ERECTILE DISORDER (ED)

General Considerations

A. Epidemiology

The prevalence of problems with erections is 1–9% below the age of 40 years, increasing to as high as 20–40% after the age of 60 years. Major correlates of erectile problems include age, depression, smoking, diabetes, cardiovascular disease, and lower urinary tract disease.

B. Etiology

Major depressive disorder, social anxiety, and posttraumatic stress disorder (PTSD) may be associated with ED. Embarrassment and apprehension about possible erectile failure in the future after an initial episode of erectile failure are felt to be involved in the genesis of psychogenic erectile disorder. After an episode of failure, a negative cognitive set and unwitting self-distraction from erotic cues may perpetuate the problem. Neurotic personality traits and alexithymia have also been described as associated with erectile problems.

A variety of diseases including diabetes mellitus, multiple sclerosis, vascular disease, and hypogonadism may be associated with organic erectile problems. Endothelial dysfunction is assumed to be involved in most cases or organic erectile dysfunction. Various medications (namely, antihypertensives, and psychiatric) may be associated with erectile problems.

Multiple studies found that anxiety and depression were common in men with erectile dysfunction. Most cases of ED are assumed to be multifactorial with contributions from both psychological and biological factors.

One study reported an association between recreational use of erection-enhancing medications in young men and the development of insecurity regarding erectile function.

C. Genetics

Twin registry studies indicate that heredity accounts for approximately 30% of ED. Genome-wide studies have found possible loci near SIM1 suggesting involvement of the melanocortin signaling system.

Clinical Findings

A. Signs & Symptoms

The major symptom of ED is the failure to obtain erections in a situation in which they were anticipated. This is usually accompanied by embarrassment, self-doubt, and loss of self-confidence. The DSM-5 specifies that at least one of the following must be experienced on almost all or all (75–100%) occasions for sexual activity for minimum duration of 6 months: (1) marked difficulty in obtaining erection during sexual activity; (2) marked difficulty in maintaining an erection until the completion of sexual activity; and (3) marked decrease in erectile rigidity.

B. Psychological Testing

The most commonly employed questionnaire used to measure improvement over time is the International Inventory of Erectile Function. Other questionnaires commonly used are the International Inventory of Erectile Function-5, the Male Sexual Health Questionnaire, and the Brief Male Sexual Inventory.

C. Laboratory Testing

Standard laboratory testing includes serum free testosterone and serum prolactin, especially if complaints of libido are also present. Other commonly ordered screening laboratory examinations include fasting glucose, lipids, and thyroid function tests. Nocturnal penile tumescence (NPT) testing is sometimes used to differentiate psychogenic from organic impotence. Some clinicians have employed waking erections to erotic audiovisual material to try to distinguish between ED due to psychological factors and ED due to a general medical disorder. However, both of these procedures are used infrequently because of the lack of specificity. Evaluation of erection after intracavernosal injection of erectogenic drugs is sometimes used as a general screening procedure. However, the specificity of this procedure is also unclear. Specialized assessment of vascular function involves dynamic infusion cavernosography, duplex Doppler penile ultrasound, and arteriography. Specialized neurological testing might include dorsal nerve conduction latency and bulbocavernosus reflex latency testing.

D. Neuroimaging

Neuroimaging studies are not useful in diagnosis at this time. Several studies of brain processing during penile erections in response to visual sexual stimuli have found that the claustrum had one of the highest activations. Other activations occurred in the paralimbic areas, striatum, and hypothalamus. Studies using direct stimulation of the penis found that activation of the insula is prominent. A complex neural circuit associated with sexual arousal involving the anterior cingulate, insula, amygdala, hypothalamus, and secondary somatosensory cortices has been proposed. Based on some imaging studies, it has been suggested that atrophy of the nucleus accumbens may play an important role in psychogenic erectile dysfunction. A recent neuroimaging study found that men with psychogenic ED could be discriminated from normal men by abnormal representations at different levels in the right anterior cingulate gyrus and left precuneus. Abnormalities at other brain levels as well suggest that psychogenic ED involves multilevel aberrant brain representations.

Course of Illness

The natural history of lifelong ED is unknown.

Brief episodes of erectile failure in sexually inexperienced males frequently remit without intervention. A small number of cases of chronic psychogenic erectile dysfunction will remit without intervention.

In a study of a stratified population sample of British individuals ages 18–44, approximately 6% complained of erectile problems lasting 1 month or less, whereas less than 1% complained of problems lasting 6 months or more. Prospective studies have also found evidence that some cases of erectile dysfunction remit without medical intervention.

Differential Diagnosis

The major issue in differential diagnosis is to establish whether the disorder is due to another mental disorder or whether it is exclusively substance-induced or exclusively due to a general medical condition. Although a variety of laboratory assessments are available, the most important element in the differential diagnosis is a careful psychiatric evaluation, including a sexual history. If the erectile problem is part of the symptomatic presentation of a major depressive disorder, one would diagnose it as a separate disorder. The next major element in the differential diagnosis is to rule out a substance-induced disorder. Many drugs such as antidepressants and antipsychotics have been reported to be associated with erectile dysfunction. If the history establishes that the disorder began after a drug was administered or after a dose adjustment, a trial off the suspected drug is in order. Erectile dysfunction may be associated with hyperprolactinemia or hypogonadism, both of which can be detected by laboratory assays. In general, these causes of erectile dysfunction are also associated with a complaint of decreased libido. By history, one would establish the presence or absence of diseases likely to cause erectile problems. For example, erectile dysfunction is common in diabetes mellitus and multiple sclerosis. It also can be a result of pelvic surgery or radiation therapy.

Cases with a situational or lifelong pattern are suggestive of a psychogenic etiology. Most organic etiologies are global and acquired. The presence of erections under any circumstances, especially erections upon awakening, is suggestive of a psychogenic etiology. Since the advent of safe oral therapies, extensive laboratory examinations to determine the etiology of erectile complaints are uncommon.

Treatment

Modification of risk factors/lifestyle may be useful as the first step (or in combination with any treatment) in management and even prevention of ED. This could include increased physical activity, weight loss, cessation of smoking, diet (Mediterranean), diabetes control, treatment of hypertension (though some antihypertensives may be associated with ED), and treatment of depression (though some antidepressants may be associated with ED).

A. Psychopharmacological Treatment

First line pharmacological interventions include avanafil, sildenafil, tadalafil, and vardenafil, all phosphodiesterase type 5 (PDE-5) inhibitors. These agents have been used with success in both psychogenic and organic impotence. In psychogenic impotence, indications for the use of oral vasoactive drugs include (1) failure of psychotherapy, (2) low self-confidence, (3) chronicity, (4) alexithymia, and (5) a coexisting contributing biological factor. Oral yohimbine, L-arginine, apomorphine, and bremelanotide may also be effective.

B. Psychotherapeutic Treatment

Psychological treatment is usually behavioral and involves graduated sexual homework assignments, a temporary cessation of attempts at coitus, modification of unrealistic expectations and cognitions, and supportive psychotherapy. The preferred technique is conjoint couple behavioral psychotherapy.

C. Other Treatment

Vacuum erection devices and intracavernosal and intraurethral prostaglandins E1 have been used in men with both psychogenic and organic impotence. As a last resort, vascular surgery or microsurgery, or penile prosthesis implantation can be employed.

Treatment modalities could and should be tailored and combined (e.g., PDE-5 inhibitors with various therapies). Low intensity shock wave therapy, platelet-rich plasma, and stem cell therapy are all considered experimental.

Complications/Adverse Outcomes of Treatment

PDE-5 inhibitors may have the following side effects: priapism, facial flushing, nasal stuffiness, visual disturbances, dyspepsia, and syncope. These drugs are contraindicated with the use of nitrates and should be used in caution in individuals with unstable angina or who are on multiple antihypertensive drugs.

Both intraurethral and intracavernosal prostaglandins E1 can be associated with pain at the site of injection as well as the risk of priapism. There are operative risks with penile prosthesis implantation, including hemorrhage and infection.

Prognosis

The prognosis in acquired psychogenic erectile dysfunction is excellent. The prognosis in lifelong global erectile dysfunction is poor. In organic problems of mild to moderate severity, the prognosis is good with the use of oral agents. In ED with combined psychological and organic features, the prognosis for return of sexual activity is less promising unless psychotherapy is combined with pharmacotherapy.

Althof S. Erectile dysfunction: psychotherapy in men and couples. In: Leiblum SR, Rosen R, eds. *Principles and Practice of Sex Therapy.* New York: Guilford; 2000:133.

Althof S. Therapeutic weaving: the integration of treatment techniques. In: Levine S, Risen C, Althof S, eds. *Handbook of Clinical Sexuality for Mental Health Professionals.* New York: Brunner-Mazel; 2003:359.

American Psychiatric Association. *Diagnostic and Statistical Manual of Mental Disorders.* 5th ed. Arlington, VA: American Psychiatric Association; 2013.

Burnett A, Nehra A, Breau R, et al. Erectile dysfunction: AUA Guideline. *J Urol.* 2018;200;633–641.

Fagan P. Psychogenic impotence in relatively young men. In: Levine S, Risen C, Althof S, eds. *Handbook of Clinical Sexuality for Mental Health Professionals.* New York: Brunner-Routledge; 2003:217.

Ferretti A, Caulo M, DelGratta C, et al. Dynamics of male sexual arousal: distinct components of brain activation revealed by fMRI. *Neuroimage.* 2005;26:1086.

Georgiadis J, Holstege G. Human brain activation during stimulation of the penis. *J Comp Neurol.* 2005;493:33.

Glina S, Sharlip ID, Hellstrom WJG. Modifying risk factors to prevent and treat erectile dysfunction. *J Sex Med.* 2013; 10:115–119.

Jern P, Gunst A, Sandnabba K, Santtila P. Are early and current erectile problems associated with anxiety and depression in young men? A retrospective self-report study. *J Sex Marit Ther.* 2012;38;349–364.

Lewis R, Fugl-Meyer K, Bosch R, et al. Epidemiology of sexual dysfunction. In: Lue T, Basson R, Rosen R, et al., eds. *Sexual Medicine. Sexual Dysfunctions in Men and Women.* Plymouth, UK: Health Publications; 2004:37.

Mercer C, Fenton K, Johnson A, et al. Sexual function problems and help seeking behavior in Britain: national probability sample survey. *Br Med J.* 2003;327:426.

NikAhd F, Shindel A, Pharmacotherapy for erectile dysfunction in 2021 and beyond. *Urol Clin North Am.* 2022;49:209–217

Patel D, Pastuszak A, Hotaling J. Genetics and erectile dysfunction: leveraging early foundations for new discoveries. *Int J Impot Res.* 2022;34;252–259.

Porst H, Burnett A, Brock G, et al. SOP conservative (medical and mechanical) treatment of erectile dysfunction. *J Sex Med.* 2013;10:130–171.

Redoute J, Stoleru S, Greguire M, et al. Brain processing of visual sexual stimuli in human males. *Hum Brain Mapp.* 2000; 11:162.

Rosen R, Cappelleri J, Gendrano N. Erectile function (IIEF): a state of the science review. *Int J Imp Res.* 2002;14:226.

Rosen R, Hatzichristou D, Broderick G, et al. Clinical evaluation and symptom scales: sexual dysfunction assessment in men. In: Lue T, Basson R, Rosen R, et al., eds. *Sexual Medicine. Sexual Dysfunctions in Men and Women.* Plymouth, UK: Health Publications; 2004:173.

Santtila P, Sandnabba K, Jern P, et al. Recreational use of erectile dysfunction medications may decrease confidence in the ability to gain and hold erections in young men. *Int J Impot Res.* 2007;19:591–596.

Segraves RT. Recognizing and reversing sexual side effects of medication. In: Levine S, Risen C, Althof S, eds. *Handbook of Clinical Sexuality for Mental Health Professionals.* New York: Brunner-Routledge; 2003:377.

Segraves R. Considerations for diagnostic criteria for erectile dysfunction in DSM. *J Sex Med.* 2010;7:654–671.

Stoleru S, Gregoire MC, Gerard D, et al. Neuroanatomical correlates of visually evoked sexual arousal in human males. *Arch Sex Behav.* 1999;28:1–21.

Towe M, Peta A, Saltzman R, et al. The use of combination regenerative therapies for erectile dysfunction: rationale and current status. *Int J Impot Res.* 2022;34:735–738.

Wylie K, MacInnes I. Erectile dysfunction. In: Balon R, Segraves RT, eds. *Handbook of Sexual Dysfunction.* New York: Taylor & Francis; 2005:155–191.

Yafi A, Huynh L, Ahlering T. What is a validated questionnaire? A critical review of erectile function assessment. *J Sex Med.* 2020;17:849–860

Zhang X, Guan M, Chen X, et al. Identifying neuroimaging biomarkers for psychogenic erectile dysfunction by fusing multi-level brain information: a resting-state functional magnetic resonance imaging study. *Andrology.* 2022;10:1398–1410.

FEMALE ORGASMIC DISORDER

General Considerations

In the past, female orgasmic disorder (FOD) has been referred to as inhibited sexual orgasm or anorgasmia.

A. Epidemiology

In a national epidemiology study of U.S. females aged 18–59 years, approximately 24% of U.S. females complained of difficulty reaching orgasm. In a study of a stratified probability sample of British individuals aged 18–44 years old, 14.4% of women complained of anorgasmia lasting 1 month or less, whereas only 3.7% complained of this problem lasting 6 months or more. The rates of prevalence vary widely (10–42%), depending on multiple factors such as age and culture. One study found that approximately 49% of newly wed women report consistently experiencing orgasm.

B. Etiology

The etiology may be psychogenic, drug-induced (e.g., antidepressants), or due to a general medical condition. Orgasmic capacity appears to be a learned response, with a lower rate in younger women. Lack of an advanced degree and report of religious affiliation is related to a lower frequency of orgasm attainment during masturbation. There is some evidence that early separation from the father may be related to problems achieving orgasm in heterosexual activities. Substance-induced orgasmic disorder may be caused by TCAs, SSRIs, alpha-blockers, D-2 blockers, and benzodiazepines. Diseases, accidents, or surgical events that affect the nervous innervation of the genitalia, such as spinal cord lesions, multiple sclerosis, diabetes mellitus, surgical lesions, and alcoholic peripheral neuropathies, may cause FOD. Anorgasmia may be part of the symptomatic presentation of severe depression or social anxiety.

C. Genetics

Twin studies indicate that genetics probably account for 31% of the variance in the frequency of orgasm during coitus and 51% of the variance in the frequency of orgasm during masturbation. The higher percentage of the variance in the frequency of orgasm explained by genetic factors during masturbation than coitus may be due to the absence of relationship variables during masturbation.

▶ Clinical Findings

A. Signs & Symptoms

The typical patient will complain of normal libido and sexual excitement without the capacity to reach orgasm. The DSM-5 specifies presence of either of the following symptoms experienced on all on almost all (75–100%) of sexual activity for approximately 6 months: (1) marked delay in, marked infrequency of, or absence or orgasm; (2) marked reduced intensity of orgasmic sensations.

B. Psychological Testing

Psychological testing is rarely required to make this diagnosis. Psychometric instruments that can be used to measure progress in treatment include the Changes in Sexual Functioning Questionnaire, the Female Sexual Function Index, the Orgasm Rating Scale and the Bodily Sensations of Orgasm Questionnaire.

C. Laboratory Testing

Laboratory testing is rarely indicated in the investigation of FOD. Nerve conduction studies can be obtained if one has reason to suspect neurogenic anorgasmia. Several studies have found that women who have difficulty achieving orgasm may have higher sensory thresholds for perceiving sensory stimuli.

D. Neuroimaging

One study in women with spinal cord injury found that orgasm elicited by self-stimulation of the vaginal-cervical region included the hypothalamic paraventricular nucleus, medial amygdala, anterior cingulate, frontal, parietal, and insula cortices as well as the cerebellum. Female orgasm differed from male ejaculation in that the amygdala was not deactivated and the periaqueductal gray area was activated. Other studies suggested the association of deep cerebellar nuclei with orgasm-specific muscle contractions, while other dopamine-containing brain structures were also involved. The neuroimaging findings during orgasm are so far nonspecific and not clinically or otherwise useful.

▶ Course of Illness

Most women who have difficulty reaching orgasm in early sexual experiences gain better orgasmic capacity after sexual experience in a long-term committed relationship.

▶ Differential Diagnosis

A careful sexual history will usually establish the presence or absence of disease capable of causing FOD—for example, another mental disorder (e.g., major depressive disorder), or medical condition (e.g., multiple sclerosis). A careful pharmacological history may reveal a probable substance-induced FOD. Serotonergic antidepressants such as paroxetine, sertraline, fluoxetine, citalopram, and escitalopram may be associated with FOD. It is less common with bupropion, nefazodone, and duloxetine. Both traditional and atypical antipsychotics may be associated with anorgasmia because of either alpha-adrenergic blockade or dopamine D-2 blockade. Benzodiazepines may also cause orgasmic delay. FOD may also be associated with relationship discord.

If FOD is global and lifelong, a psychological etiology is probable. If the problem is acquired and situational, relationship discord is a probable etiology. If the problem is acquired and global, one should carefully rule out FOD due to a general medical condition and substance-induced FOD.

▶ Treatment

A. Psychopharmacological Treatment

There are no known therapies for FOD due to a general medical condition. In substance-induced FOD, change of medication or the use of antidotes may reverse the disorder. If the patient is on an SSRI, one can substitute bupropion, nefazodone, or duloxetine or use high-dose buspirone (60 mg/d) as an antidote. It is unclear whether sildenafil can reverse SSRI-induced orgasmic delay (it has in small studies). If the patient is on a typical antipsychotic or risperidone, one can try substituting aripiprazole, quetiapine, or olanzapine. One unreplicated, controlled study found that sildenafil had a significant positive effect in orgasm attainment in young women with high libido who were in committed long-term relationships. Another unreplicated, controlled study found that bupropion improved orgasmic capacity in women with hypoactive sexual desire disorder (HSDD). It is unclear whether bupropion is effective in women with a primary diagnosis of FOD. Hormone treatment may help in postmenopausal women with low testosterone and low estrogen levels. Melanocortin receptor agonists may also facilitate achieving orgasm.

B. Psychotherapeutic Treatment

Cognitive–behavioral therapy (CBT) appears to be effective in the treatment of lifelong FOD due to psychological factors, but not in acquired FOD. CBT involves changing of negative sexual thoughts and attitudes. Directed masturbation homework assignments are commonly employed. Most women can learn to achieve orgasm by self-stimulation. A smaller number learn to transfer this to partner-related activities. Mindfulness, yoga, sensate focus therapy, and coital alignment may be considered as possible adjunct management modalities.

C. Other Treatment

There is some anecdotal evidence that the use of mechanical clitoral vacuum device (EROS Clitoral-Therapy Device, basically a small battery-operated vacuum pump over the clitoris) may augment orgasmic capacity in women with FOD.

▶ Complications/Adverse Outcomes of Treatment

The use of buspirone with serotonergic antidepressants may increase the risk of a serotonin syndrome. Bupropion lowers the seizure threshold. Drug substitution always carries the risk of relapse or emergence of comorbid psychiatric illness.

▶ Prognosis

The prognosis for FOD due to psychological factors is good. CBT combined with masturbation homework assignments is usually successful in teaching women how to achieve orgasm through masturbation. A smaller number of women are able to transfer this skill to partner-related activities.

American Psychiatric Association. *Diagnostic and Statistical Manual of Mental Disorders*. 5th ed. Text Revision. Washington, DC: American Psychiatric Association; 2022.

Caruso S, Intelsano G, Lupo L, et al. Premenopausal women affected by sexual arousal disorder treated with sildenafil: a double-blind, cross-over, placebo-controlled study. *BJOG*. 2001;108:623.

Cervilla O, Vallejo-Medina C, Gomez-Berrocal C, et al. Validation of the Orgasm Rating Scale in the context of masturbation. *Psicothema*. 2022;34:151–159.

Dawood K, Kirk KM, Bailey JM, et al. Genetic and environmental influences on the frequency of orgasm in women. *Twin Res Hum Genet*. 2005;8:27–33.

Ellison C. Facilitating orgasmic responsiveness. In: Levine S, Risen C, Althof S, eds. *Handbook of Clinical Sexuality for Mental Health Clinicians*. New York: Brunner-Routledge; 2003:167.

Graham C. The DSM criteria for female orgasmic disorder. *Arch Sex Behav*. 2010;39:256–270.

Gruenwald I, Lauterbach R, Gartman I, et al. Female orgasm dysfunction and genital sensation deficiency. *J Sex Med*. 2020;17:273–278.

Keller A, McGarvey E, Clayton A. Reliability and construct validity of the changes in sexual functioning questionnaire short form (CSFQ-14). *J Sex Marital Ther*. 2006;32:43–52.

Komisaruk BR, Whipple B, Crawford A, et al. Brain activation during vaginocervical self-stimulation and orgasm in women with complete spinal cord injury: fMRI evidence of mediation by the vagus nerves. *Brain Res*. 2004;1024:77–88.

Laan E, Rellini AH, Barnes T. Standard operating procedures for female orgasmic disorder; consensus of the International Society for Sexual medicine. *J Sex Med*. 2013;10:74–82.

Leonhardt N, Willoughby B, Busby D, et al. The significance of the female orgasm: a nationally representative, dyadic study of newlyweds' orgasm experience. *J Sex Med*. 2018;15:1140–1148.

Laumann E, Gagnon J, Michael R, et al. *The Social Organization of Sexuality*. Chicago: University of Chicago Press; 1994.

Marchard E. Psychological and behavioral treatment of female orgasmic disorder. *Sex Med Rev*. 2021;9:194–211.

Mercer C, Fenton K, Johnson A, et al. Sexual function problems and help seeking behavior in Britain: national probability sample survey. *Br Med J*. 2003;327:426–427.

Meston CN, Levine R. Female orgasm dysfunction. In: Balon R, Segraves RT, eds. *Handbook of Sexual Dysfunction*. New York: Taylor & Francis; 2005:193.

Rellini AH, Clifton J. Female orgasmic disorder. *Adv Psychosom Med*. 2011;31:35–56.

Salonia A, Briganti A, Rigatti P, et al. Medical conditions associated with female sexual dysfunction. In: Goldstein I, Meston C, Davis S, et al., eds. *Women's Sexual Function and Dysfunction*. New York: Taylor & Francis; 2006:263.

Segraves R. Role of the psychiatrist. In: Goldstein I, Meston C, Davis S, eds. *Women's Sexual Function and Dysfunction*. New York: Taylor & Francis; 2006:696.

Webb A, Reissing E, Huta H. Orgasm Rating Scale and Bodily Sensations of Orgasm Scale: validation for use with pre, peri and post -menopausal women, *J Sex Med*. 2022:19:1156–1172.

Wise N, Frangos E, Komisaruk B, et al. Brain activity unique to women in orgasm: an fMRI study. *J Sex Med*. 2017;14:1380–1391.

FEMALE SEXUAL INTEREST/AROUSAL DISORDER

▶ General Considerations

Sexual desire and sexual arousal frequently coexist and are elicited in response to adequate sexual cues or stimulation. The relationship between desire and arousal in women is fairly complex, and at times, some women may become aroused without preceding sexual desire and the sexual desire may develop during the response to partner (responsive desire).

FSIAD is diagnosed when the lack of or significantly reduced sexual interest/arousal is manifested by at least three of the following six symptoms: absent/reduced interest in sexual activity; absent/reduced sexual/erotic thoughts or fantasies; no/reduced initiation of sexual activity, and typically unreceptive to a partner's attempt to initiate sex; absent/reduced sexual excitement/pleasure during sexual activity in almost all or all (approximately 75–10%) sexual encounters; absent/reduced sexual interest/arousal in response to any internal or external sexual/erotic cues (written, verbal, visual); and absent/reduced genital or nongenital sensations during sexual activity in almost all or all (approximately 75–100%) sexual encounters. The symptoms must be distressing and last at least 6 months.

It is important to note that the interpersonal context must be taken into account in evaluating FSIAD—the fact that a woman has a lower sexual desire for sexual activity than her partner is not sufficient for making the diagnosis of FSIAD. The patient may agree to sexual activity in the absence of desire in order to stabilize a relationship.

A. Epidemiology

The prevalence of FSIAD as defined by the DSM-5 is unknown. Seventy-five per cent of women diagnosed with HSDD meet criteria for FSIAD. Thus, prevalence data for HSDD can be used to approximate the prevalence of FSIAD. Epidemiological studies from different countries around the world found that the prevalence of low sexual desire in females is approximately 25–30%, although these estimates did not use the 6-month duration criterion. The 1-year prevalence of problems with lubrication in U.S. females aged 18–59 years is approximately 20%. Epidemiological studies in European populations have reported a 10–15% prevalence increasing to 25–35% after age 50 years, suggesting a positive relationship between problems of lubrication and aging. Problems with arousal lasting 1 month or less are much more common than problems lasting 6 months or more.

B. Etiology

The etiology of FSIAD is unknown and is probably complex. Low sexual desire may be due to general medical conditions such as hypothyroidism, hyperprolactinemia, or post oophorectomy. Low sexual desire may be also associated with substance use or medications, or due to other psychiatric disorders such as depressive disorders, anxiety disorders, or schizophrenia. Oral contraceptives have been reported to be associated with low sexual desire, although evidence from controlled studies is inconclusive. Other etiological factors in low sexual desire could be social anxiety, interpersonal conflict, partner factors (partner's sexual and general health), individual vulnerability (poor body image, history of sexual abuse), stressors (job loss), cultural/religious issues, negative attitudes toward sexuality, and problems with sexual intimacy. Various psychological factors also interfere with

sexual arousal. Problems with lubrication in perimenopause and menopause are due to a hypoestrogenized vaginal vault. Radiation therapy and cancer chemotherapy often result in diminished lubrication. Any lesion to the nervous innervation of the genitalia (e.g., spinal cord lesion, multiple sclerosis, alcoholic neuropathy) may result in decreased vaginal lubrication. Pelvic vascular disease can also result in diminished vaginal lubrication. Isolated complaints of difficulties with arousal in premenopausal women who have normal libido are rare.

C. Genetics

There is no information concerning the genetics of this disorder. Interestingly, a recently published twin study suggested that female sexual dysfunction is not etiologically homogenous. Sexual desire shared the least amount of genetic association with lubrication and orgasm, and environmental factors contributed more to desire.

▶ Clinical Findings

A. Signs & Symptoms

The symptomatology of FSIAD includes symptoms of female sexual desire and female arousal as described in previous editions of the DSM. Female sexual desire, erotic/sexual thoughts, fantasies and sexual excitement, pleasure feelings, vasocongestion in the genital area, and lubrication frequently overlap. FSIAD is also frequently associated with difficulties in achieving orgasm, pain during sexual activity, and lower frequency of sexual activity. It is important to differentiate among lifelong, acquired, generalized, and situational subtypes of FSIAD. If a lifelong lack of sexual desire is better explained by one's self-identification as "asexual," then, according to the DSM-5, a diagnosis of FSIAD should not be made.

B. Psychological Testing

No specific psychological testing is required for establishing the diagnosis of FSIAD. The Female Sexual Function Index was specifically developed to assess female arousal impairment. A validated instrument used in the study of treatment outcomes in this disorder is the Sexual Event Diary. The Sexual Interest and Desire inventory, although validated in a HSDD population, contains items reflecting both interest and arousal.

C. Laboratory Findings

No useful, reliable laboratory tests are available for this disorder. Endocrinological tests (e.g., thyroid-stimulating hormone, prolactin levels) may help if endocrinopathy is suspected.

D. Neuroimaging

Neuroimaging does not contribute to the diagnosis of this disorder.

Course of Illness

Normative changes in sexual interest and arousal across the life span are not known. Vaginal dryness developing in some older females may contribute to the worsening of symptomatology of FSIAD. The course of the lifelong subtype of FSIAD is, per its definition, chronic. However, most sexual problems present in women who are relatively inexperienced sexually will improve over time in a stable, committed relationship.

Differential Diagnosis

Differential diagnosis of FSIAD includes nonsexual mental disorders (e.g., major depression, PTSD), substance use disorders, treatment with various medications (e.g., SSRIs), various medical conditions (diabetes mellitus, thyroid dysfunction, endothelial disease, multiple sclerosis, arthritis, irritable bowel syndrome, vaginitis), other sexual dysfunctions (e.g., genito-pelvic pain penetration disorder [GPPPD]), interpersonal difficulties, and inadequate or absent sexual stimuli.

FSIA could be comorbid with other sexual dysfunctions, various mental disorders (including those just mentioned and urinary incontinence), sexual and physical abuse, alcohol use, and other complex problems.

In postmenopausal women not on estrogen replacement, one needs to consider FSIAD due to hypogonadism as the primary diagnosis.

Treatment

A. Psychopharmacological Interventions

Dopamine receptor agonists (e.g., apomorphine) have been minimally studied in women with arousal problems to date. Topical lubricants and moisturizers may also facilitate coital activities. Various pharmacological treatments could also be implemented based on prevailing symptomatology or underlying cause. These may include testosterone patches (especially in women with bilateral oophorectomy), other hormones (local and systemic estrogens), L-arginine, and PDE-5 inhibitors. None of these preparations have been approved by the FDA for this indication (understandably). Nasal testosterone is currently being investigated.

Estrogen treatment can reverse sexual symptoms related to menopause. Estrogen can be applied locally in the form of vaginal creams or by the use of vaginal rings containing estrogen. Estrogen can also be administered systemically either orally or by transdermal patches. Testosterone patches, as mentioned, could be useful in women after oophorectomy. Subcutaneous testosterone with either sildenafil or buspirone have been shown to be effective in the treatment of FSIAD. Flibanserin and bremelotide may also be effective.

B. Psychotherapeutic Treatment

Both group mindfulness-based cognitive therapy and group supportive sex education and therapy appear to be effective interventions, An online version of mindfulness therapy also appears to be effective.

C. Other Treatment

There is some evidence that a small battery-operated device that is applied to the clitoris causing increased blood flow into the clitoris and labia is effective in the treatment of female arousal difficulties. One double-blind, controlled study found that a botanical massage oil applied to the genitals improved sexual arousal.

D. Complications/Adverse Outcomes of Treatment

Systemic estrogen therapy is associated with an increased risk of breast cancer and cardiovascular disease. Local irritation can be produced by the use of the mechanical vacuum device or botanical oils. Pharmacological interventions have potential side effects.

Prognosis

Psychiatric comorbidity and marital conflict could probably predict a poor outcome.

Altman C, Deldon-Saltin D. Available therapies and outcome results in transition and postmenopausal women. In: Goldstein I, Meston C, Davis S, et al., eds. *Women's Sexual Function and Dysfunction.* New York: Taylor & Francis; 2006:539.

American Psychiatric Association. *Diagnostic and Statistical Manual of Mental Disorders.* 5th ed. Arlington, VA: American Psychiatric Association; 2013.

Basson R. Female hypoactive sexual desire disorder. In: Balon R, Segraves RT, eds. *Handbook of Sexual Dysfunction.* Boca Raton, FL: Taylor & Francis; 2005:43.

Billups KL, Berman L, Berman J, et al. The role of mechanical devices in treating female sexual dysfunction and enhancing the female sexual response. *World J Urol.* 2002;20:137–141.

Both S. Recent developments in psychopharmacological approaches to treating female sexual interest and arousal disorder. *Curr Sex Health Rep.* 2017;9:192–199.

Brotto L, Stephenson K, Zippan N. Feasibility of an online mindfulness-based intervention for women with sexual interest/arousal disorder. *Mindfulness.* 2022;13:647–659.

Brotto L, Zdaniuk B, Chivers M, et al. A randomized trial comparing group mindfulness-based cognitive therapy with group supportive sex education and therapy for the treatment of female sexual interest/arousal disorder. *J Consult Clin Psychol.* 2021;84:626–639.

Burri A, Greven C, Leupin, M, et al. A multivariate twin study of female sexual dysfunction. *J Sex Med.* 2012;9:2671–2681.

Davis A, Castano P. Oral contraceptives and sexuality. In: Goldstein I, Meston C, Davis S, et al, eds. *Women's Sexual Function and Dysfunction.* New York: Taylor & Francis; 2006:290.

Davis A, Guay A, Shifren J, et al. Endocrine aspects of female sexual dysfunction. *J Sex Med.* 2004;1:82–86.

Dennerstein L. The sexual impact of menopause. In: Levine S, Risen C, Althof S, eds. *Handbook of Clinical Sexuality for Mental Health Professionals.* New York: Brunner-Routledge; 2003:187.

Ferguson D, Steidle C, Singh C, et al. Randomized, placebo-controlled, double-blind, crossover design trial of the efficacy and safety of Zestra for women in women with and without female sexual arousal disorder. *J Sex Marital Ther.* 2003;29(suppl 1):33–44.

Fourcroy J. Female sexual dysfunction: potential for pharmacotherapy. *Drugs.* 2003;63:1445–1457.

Fugl-Meyer A, Fugl-Meyer K. Prevalence data in Europe. In: Goldstein I, Meston C, Davis S, et al, eds. *Women's Sexual Function and Dysfunction.* New York: Taylor & Francis; 2006:34.

Kang J, Laumann E, Glasser D, et al. Worldwide prevalence and correlates. In: Goldstein I, Meston C, Davis S, et al., eds. *Women's Sexual Function and Dysfunction.* New York: Taylor & Francis; 2006:42.

Laan E, Both S. Sexual desire and arousal in women. *Adv Psychosom Med.* 2011;31:16–34.

Laan E, Everaerd W, Both S. Female sexual arousal disorder. In: Balon R, Segraves RT, eds. *Handbook of Sexual Dysfunction.* New York: Taylor & Francis; 2005:123.

Laumann EO, Nicolosi A, Glasser D, et al. Sexual problems among women and men aged 40–80 years: prevalence and correlates identified in the global study of sexual attitudes and behaviors. *Int J Impot Res.* 2005;17:39–57.

Laumann EO, Paik A, Rosen RC. Sexual dysfunction in the United States: prevalence and predictors. *JAMA.* 1999;281:537–544.

Maravilla K. Blood flow magnetic resonance imaging and brain imaging for evaluating sexual arousal in women. In: Goldstein I, Meston C, Davis S, et al., eds. *Women's Sexual Function and Dysfunction.* New York: Taylor & Francis; 2006:368.

Mercer C, Fenton K, Johnson A, et al. Sexual function problems and help seeking behavior in Britain: national probability sample survey. *BMJ.* 2003;327:426–427.

O'Loughlin J, Basson R, Brotto L. Women with hypoactive sexual desire disorder versus sexual interest desire disorder. An empirical test of raising the bar. *J Sex Res.* 2018;55:734–746.

Paik A, Laumann E. Prevalence of women's sexual problems in the USA. In: Goldstein I, Meston C, Davis S et al., eds. *Women's Sexual Function and Dysfunction.* New York: Taylor & Francis; 2006:23.

Parish S, Simons J, Davis S, et al. International Society for the Study of Women's Sexual Health clinical practice guidelines. *J Sex Med.* 2021;18:840–847.

Rosen R, Brown C, Heiman J, et al. The Female Sexual Function Index (FSFI): a multidimensional self-report instrument for the assessment of female sexual function. *J Sex Marital Ther.* 2000;26:191–208.

Rossouw J, Anderson G, Prentice R, et al. Risks and benefits of estrogen plus progestin in healthy postmenopausal women: principal results from the Woman's Health Initiative randomized controlled trial. *JAMA.* 2002;288:321–333.

Sills T, Wunderlich G, Pyke R, et al. The Sexual Interest Desire Inventory-Female (SIDI-F). *J Sex Med.* 2005;2:801–818.

Utian W, MacLean D, Symonds T, et al. A methodological study to validate a structured diagnostic method used to diagnose female sexual dysfunction and its subtypes in postmenopausal women. *J Sex Marital Ther.* 2003;31:271–283.

Van Nes Y, Bloemers J, Kessels R, et al. Psychometric properties of the Sexual Event Diary in a sample of Dutch women with female sexual interest/arousal disorder. *J Sex Med.* 2018;15:722–731.

GENITO-PELVIC PAIN/PENETRATION DISORDER

▶ General Considerations

Previously, two diagnostic categories were used to describe various pain and difficulties during intercourse—dyspareunia and vaginismus. In addition, a number of other terms have been used to describe dyspareunia in females, including chronic pelvic pain, vulvodynia, vulvovestibulitis, vestibulodynia, and provoked vestibulodynia. These terms do not have precise definitions. Vulvar vestibulitis refers to pain experienced in the vulvar vestibule upon contact, whereas vulvodynia usually refers to chronic vulvar pain that may occur with or without sexual contact. However, many patients cannot describe the location of their pain with precision. The diagnoses of dyspareunia and vaginismus lack solid reliability, overlap, and are difficult to differentiate. These concerns led to a creation of a new diagnosis that in a way combines these two entities into a simpler diagnostic entity of GPPPD. This diagnosis is descriptive and is intended to provide a framework for clinical assessment and diagnosis of women suffering from pain and penetration difficulties. The diagnosis of GPPPD is, per definition, given only to women. According to the DSM-5, this diagnosis requires one of four commonly comorbid symptom dimensions: (1) difficulty having intercourse; (2) genito-pelvic pain; (3) fear of pain or vaginal penetration; and (4) tension of the pelvic floor muscles. GPPPD may be lifelong or acquired after a period of normal sexual functioning.

A. Epidemiology

This relatively new diagnostic entity has broad coverage and we have minimal evidence regarding its prevalence. Studies of vulvodynia have reported a lifetime prevalence of 9.9% and 16% in the United States. In an Australian representative population study, 17% complained of pain during coitus. One population study of GPPD reported a prevalence of 10% in Iranian women. Eleven percent of women in Spanish primary care settings were diagnosed with this disorder.

B. Etiology

Risk factors for vestibulodynia (acquired GPPPD) include recurrent yeast infections, endometriosis, and post-menopausal vaginal atrophy. Risk factors for vaginismus (lifelong GPPPD) include low education, conservative religious views, relationship factors, and a history of sexual assault. Sexual guilt has bene found to be an associated factor in college aged women.

One study found a much higher incidence of GPPPD in African American females than in white or Hispanic females.

C. Genetics

One study found an increased incidence of vestibulectomy in first, second, and third degree relatives of women who had been treated by vesiculectomy.

Clinical Findings

A. Signs & Symptoms

The symptomatology of GPPPD includes persistent or recurrent difficulties with at least one of the following: (1) vaginal penetration during intercourse; (2) marked vulvovaginal or pelvic pain during vaginal intercourse or penetration attempts; (3) marked fear or anxiety about vulvovaginal or pelvic pain in anticipation of, during, or as a result of vaginal penetration; (4) marked tensing or tightening of the pelvic floor muscles during attempted vaginal penetration. These symptoms must cause distress and must persist for at least 6 months. Pain could be characterized as superficial (vulvovaginal) or deep (occurring during deep penetration). The intensity of the pain may be related to distress. Pain may persist after intercourse and may occur during urination.

B. Psychological Testing

Psychological testing is not helpful in establishing this diagnosis.

C. Laboratory Findings

Yeast cultures, testing for venereal disease, and evaluation for endometriosis may be performed by gynecologists prior to referral to the mental health professional. Hormonal assays and cytological examination may also be performed. Most gynecologists will use a cotton swab during the pelvic examination to locate areas where touch elicits pain. Many but not all women with this disorder may have spasm of the vaginal musculature during a gynecological examination. Some women may actually try to avoid gynecological examination and/or use of tampons.

D. Neuroimaging

One study found similar patterns of neural activation in women with provoked vestibulodynia as controls. However, the patient group had greater activation than controls to the same stimulus intensity.

Course of Illness

The course of GPPPD has not been appropriately studied and is unknown. Prognosis may be better in lifelong GPPPD (ex vaginismus) than in acquired GPPD (dyspareunia).

Differential Diagnosis

Differential diagnosis of GPPPD includes various medical conditions (endometriosis, infections—e.g., candidiasis, lichen sclerosus, pelvic inflammatory disease, vaginal dryness, vulvovaginal atrophy), other sexual dysfunctions, and somatic symptom disorder. Inadequate sexual stimulation may play some role in the development of GPPPD—inadequate arousal or foreplay may lead to difficulties in penetration accompanied by pain and/or avoidance.

Treatment

Treatment of genito-pelvic pain is usually difficult, requires a multidisciplinary approach, and should be handled by a specialist to whom patients should be referred. The discussion of the GPPPD treatment is a bit theoretical, because no treatments for this new diagnosis have been established and tested. A combination of treatment approaches used for dyspareunia and vaginismus seems to be the most appropriate approach. The cornerstone of each treatment is an adequate and appropriate assessment that should also be multidisciplinary (including psychiatric, gynecological, and urological examinations). Treatment should be individualized.

A. Psychopharmacological Interventions

There are no specific pharmacotherapies for this disorder. Antidepressants (e.g., duloxetine) may hypothetically help if depression accompanies GPPD. Individual case reports suggest that benzodiazepine-assisted systematic desensitization may be successful in reversing vaginal spasms. Hormone replacement therapy may alleviate dyspareunia secondary to postmenopausal vaginal atrophy.

B. Psychotherapeutic Treatment

Both CBT and mindfulness-based CBT have proven efficacy. Pelvic floor physical therapy is often utilized. Anxiety-reduction techniques involving graduated vaginal penetration exercises are frequently employed when fear of vaginal penetration in the predominant symptom. Internet-based therapies are also available.

C. Other Treatment

GPPPD associated with atrophic vaginitis can be alleviated by vaginal creams, and nonhormonal vaginal lubricants may be helpful. Treatment of yeast infections may be necessary. Acupuncture and hypnotherapy have been advocated for dyspareunia. For idiopathic dyspareunia, gynecologists may suggest sitz baths, topical lidocaine, corticosteroid creams, or physical therapy. Vestibulectomy may be performed in cases of severe pain.

D. Complications

The risks and complications are not known and are probably related to the treatment modality used. There are no known risks of psychotherapeutic modalities suggested for the management of GPPPD.

Prognosis

Prognosis of GPPD is unknown. Sexual and/or physical abuse have been cited as poor prognostic factors of sexual pain, but the literature is not clear in regard to this issue. Interpersonal problems, partner factors, stress, individual vulnerability, and untreated medical conditions (e.g., vaginal infections) could play a significant role in the prognosis of this disorder.

Alizadeh A, Farnam F, Raisi F, et al. Prevalence of and risk factors for genito-pelvic pain/penetration disorder: a population-based study of Iranian women. *J Sex Med.* 2019;16:1068–1077.

American Psychiatric Association. *Diagnostic and Statistical Manual of Mental Disorders.* 5th ed. Arlington, VA: American Psychiatric Association; 2013.

Azim K, Happel-Parkins A, Moses A, et al. Racialized differences across experiences of pain in genitopelvic pain/penetration disorder. *J Sex Med.* 2022;20:224–228.

Basson R, Schultz W, Binik Y, et al. Women's sexual desire and arousal disorders and sexual pain. In: Lue T, Meston C, Davis S, et al., eds. *Sexual Medicine. Sexual Dysfunction in Men and Women.* Plymouth, UK: Health Publications; 2005:851.

Berenguer-Soler M, Navarro-Sanchez A, Compan_Rosique A, et al. Genito-pelvic/pain penetration disorder (GPPPD) in Spanish women-clinical approach in primary health care: review and metanalysis. *J Clin Med.* 2022;11(9):2340. doi:10.3390/jcm11o92340

Bergeron S, Meana M, Binik Y, et al. Painful genital sexual activity. In: Levine S, Risen C, Althof S, eds. *Handbook of Clinical Sexuality for Mental Health Professional.* New York: Brunner-Routledge; 2003:131.

Binik Y. The DSM diagnostic criteria for vaginismus. *Arch Sex Behav.* 2010;39:278–291.

Binik Y. The DSM diagnostic criteria for dyspareunia. *Arch Sex Behav.* 2010;39:292–303.

Boyer SC, Goldfinger C, Thibault-Gagnon S, et al. Management of female sexual pain disorders. *Adv Psychosom Med.* 2011;31:83–104.

Brotto L, Zdanivk B, Rietchel L, et al, Moderators of improvement from mindfulness-based versus traditional cognitive behavioral therapy for provoked vestibulodynia. *J Sex Med.* 2020;17:2247–2259.

Fugl-Meyer KS, Bohm-Starke N, Damsted Petersen C, et al. Standard operating procedures for female genital sexual pain. *J Sex Med.* 2013;10:83–93.

Goldstein I. Medical management: perspective of the sexual medicine physician. In: Goldstein I, Meston C, Davis S, et al., eds. *Women's Sexual Function and Dysfunction.* New York: Taylor & Francis; 2006:508.

Herman H. Physical therapy for female sexual dysfunction. In: Goldstein I, Meston C, Davis S, et al., eds. *Women's Sexual Function and Dysfunction.* New York: Taylor & Francis; 2006:496.

Liu M, Juravic M, Mazza G, et al. Vaginal dilators: issues and answers. *Sex Med Rev.* 2021;9:212–220.

Meana M, Binik, Y. The biopsychosocial puzzle of painful sex. *Annu Rev Clin Psychol.* 2022;18:471–495.

Morgan J, Allen-Brady K, Monson M, et al. Familiarity analysis of provoked vestibulodynia supports genetic predisposition. *Am J Obstet Gynec.* 2018;214:609.e1–7. doi10/1016/j.ajog.2015.11.019

Payne K, Bergeron S, Khalife J, et al. Assessment, treatment strategies and outcome results: perspective of pain specialists. In: Goldstein I, Meston C, Davis S, et al., eds. *Women's Sexual Function and Dysfunction.* New York: Taylor & Francis; 2006:471.

Pukall C, Payne K, Kao A, et al. Dyspareunia. In: Balon R, Segraves RT, eds. *Handbook of Sexual Dysfunction.* New York: Taylor & Francis; 2005:249.

Richter J, Yeung A, Rissel C, et al. Sexual difficulties, problems, and help-seeking in a national representative sample: the second Australian study of health and relationships. *Arch Sex Behav.* 2022;51:1435–1446.

Schultz WCM, Van de Wiel HBM. Vaginismus. In: Balon R, Segraves RT, eds. *Handbook of Sexual Dysfunction.* New York: Taylor & Francis; 2005:273.

Stewart E. Physical examination in female sexual dysfunction. In: Goldstein I, Meston C, Davis S, et al., eds. *Women's Sexual Function and Dysfunction.* New York: Taylor & Francis, 2006:347.

Sutton K, Yessic L, Wild C, et al. Exploring the neural correlates of touch and pain in women with provoked vestibulodynia. *Pain.* 2020;161:926–937.

Weinberger B, Houman J, Caron A, et al. Female sexual dysfunction. A systematic review of outcomes across various treatment modalities. *Sex Med Rev.* 2019;7:223–250.

Zarski A, Berking M, Ebert D. Efficacy of internet-based treatment for genito-pelvic/penetration disorder results of a randomized clinical trial. *J Consult Clin Psychol.* 2021;89:909–924.

MALE HYPOACTIVE SEXUAL DESIRE DISORDER

▶ General Considerations

Generally, the lack of sexual desire and absence of erotic thoughts must be persistent or recurrent and must occur for at least 6 months. Interpersonal context and factors must be taken into account. The clinician should take into consideration such factors as the patient's age and life circumstance and use clinical judgment whether a problem should be diagnosed as a psychiatric disorder. If the individual is not stressed by the absence of libido and it does not cause interpersonal distress, a disorder cannot be diagnosed. The report of a high frequency of coital activity does not rule out the presence of low sexual desire in one member of a couple. The patient may agree to sexual activity in the absence of desire in order to stabilize a relationship. In the past, male hypoactive sexual desire disorder (MHSDD) has been labeled inhibited sexual desire, generalized sexual dysfunction, and frigidity. The etiology of lifelong MHSDD is usually unknown. Situational MHSDD is suggestive of interpersonal discord.

A. Epidemiology

Epidemiological studies in Europe, the United States, South America, and Asia have found the prevalence of complaints of low sexual desire in males to be approximately 12–25%; the prevalence was highest in Southeast Asia. The number meeting the diagnostic criteria of this causing marked distress is probably less. Transient problems with low sexual desire are far more common than those lasting 6 months or more—about 6% of younger males (ages 18–24 years) and 41% of older males (ages 66–74 years) have some problems with sexual desire, but persistent lack of sexual desire lasting 6 months or more occurs in only about 1.8% of men between ages 16 and 44 years.

A Danish population-based study found that 23% of sexually experienced males reported absence of sexual activity with a partner in the preceding year. A prevalence of MHSDD of 4.7% in German males and 3.4% in Danish males has been reported.

B. Etiology

MHSDD may due to a general medical condition such as hypothyroidism, hyperprolactinemia, or hypogonadism. Substance-induced MHSDD may be related to the use of SSRIs and antipsychotic drugs. MHSDD may be due to other psychiatric disorders such as depressive and anxiety disorders as well as schizophrenia and PTSD. Psychological factors such as social anxiety, depression, self-directed homophobia, interpersonal conflict, negative attitudes toward sexuality, and problems with sexual intimacy may be etiological factors. Alcohol and other substance use may negatively affect sexual desire.

Lifelong MHSDD may represent a normal variation and thus may not be indicative of pathology.

C. Genetics

There is no information concerning the genetics of this disorder.

▶ Clinical Findings

A. Signs & Symptoms

The major symptom is the absence of desire for sexual activity. The DSM-5 specifies the persistently or recurrently deficient (or absent) sexual/erotic thoughts or fantasies and desire for sexual activity of a minimum duration of 6 months. The judgment of deficiency is made by the clinician, who should take into account factors affecting sexual desire such as age and cultural context.

B. Psychological Testing

Psychological testing is not required to make this diagnosis. A structured diagnostic method has been shown to have good reliability between expert diagnosticians in sexual medicine and novices in this area, and well-validated psychometric instruments may help to validate the diagnosis and monitor progress in treatment.

C. Laboratory Findings

In hypogonadism, serum free testosterone will be low. MHSDD may be a sign of hypothyroidism or hyperprolactinemia.

D. Neuroimaging

Neuroimaging does not contribute to the diagnosis of this disorder.

▶ Course of Illness

Lack of desire related to environmental factors such as transient stress or transient interpersonal conflict may resolve as the conflict resolves. Lack of desire, which is lifelong or chronic, has a poor prognosis for recovery. There is a normative age-related decline in sexual desire.

▶ Differential Diagnosis

In general, if the disorder is situational as opposed to global, MHSDD due to psychological factors is suspected.

Low sexual desire may be part of the symptomatic presentation of mood disorder, various anxiety disorders, and schizophrenia. Substance-induced sexual disorder should be ruled out. Many pharmacological agents such as anticonvulsants, narcotics, antipsychotics, TCAs, MAOIs, and SSRIs may be associated with low sexual desire. Bupropion, duloxetine, and nefazodone have lower incidence of sexual dysfunction than the SSRIs. Among antipsychotics, olanzapine and aripiprazole appear to have lower rates of sexual dysfunction. Low desire for sexual activity with the designated partner may also reflect the presence of a paraphilia. In such cases, a careful history would reveal normal libido for paraphilic behavior but decreased desire for nonparaphilic behavior. In such cases, the specific paraphilia would be the diagnosis. If an organic etiology is found, the diagnosis would be HSDD due to a specified medical condition (e.g., hypogonadism). There is some evidence that thyroid disorders and temporal lobe lesions may be associated with disorders of desire. A chronic debilitating or painful medical condition may be associated with low sexual desire. Desire discrepancies, in which both members of a relationship have normal libido but one member wishes that the other had higher libido, obviously would not meet diagnostic criteria. Relationship discord must always be considered in the differential diagnosis.

▶ Treatment

A. Psychopharmacological Interventions

Bupropion has been reported to increase various indices of sexual responsiveness in women with low sexual desire. There have been no controlled trials of bupropion in males with this disorder and thus its role in MHSDD is unknown. It is unclear whether flibanserin is effective in this condition. Nutraceuticals are ineffective. One study suggests that kisspeptin, a key endogenous hypothalamic activator, may increase sexual desire in men,

B. Hormonal Interventions

If hypogonadism is detected in male patients, hormone replacement therapy is indicated (the goal is a physiological level of testosterone). Testosterone could be administered using various formulations. The easiest administration is transdermally, using testosterone in gel, cream, or patches. Testosterone may be also administered via bioadhesive buccal testosterone, or in intramuscular injection of testosterone cypionate (weekly, or up to every 2–3 weeks) or testosterone undecanoate every 10–14 weeks. There is no evidence supporting the efficacy of dehydroepiandrosterone in this disorder. Testosterone supplementation in eugonadal men has minimal effect on libido.

C. Psychotherapeutic Interventions

Psychological treatment usually involves CBT combined with behavioral sex therapy. Negative cognitions are challenged. The patient may be taught how to not distract himself from erotic stimuli. The patient may be taught how to develop sexual fantasies. A major goal will be to educate the patient how to communicate his sexual preferences to the partner. Sensate focus is usually employed to decrease sexual anxiety. Psychodynamic psychotherapy, group therapy, psychodrama, and sex therapy have also been used for MHSDD.

▶ Complications

Bupropion lowers the seizure threshold. Rarely, changing libido in one member of a relationship may destabilize the relationship. The risks of androgen therapy include polycythemia, exacerbation of sleep apnea, and altered serum lipids. The presence of breast or prostate carcinoma is a contraindication to androgen therapy. Thus, treatment with testosterone requires routine follow-up of prostate-specific antigen, hematocrit, testosterone levels, and lipids.

Methylated testosterone may cause liver toxicity. This is rarely an issue with transdermal testosterone preparations.

▶ Prognosis

The prognosis for idiopathic MHSDD is poor. Prognosis of MHSDD due to hypogonadism is usually good.

American Psychiatric Association. *Diagnostic and Statistical Manual of Mental Disorders*. 5th ed. Text Revision. Washington, DC: American Psychiatric Association; 2022.

Brotto L. The DSM diagnostic criteria for hypoactive sexual desire disorder in men. *J Sex Med*. 2010;7:2015–2030.

Castillo O Jr, Chen I, Amini E, et al. Male sexual health related complications among combat veterans. *Sex Med Rev*. 2022;10:591–597.

Laumann EO, Nicolosi A, Glasser D, et al. Sexual problems among women and men aged 40–80 years: prevalence and correlates identified in the global study of sexual attitudes and behaviors. *Int J Impot Res*. 2005;17:39–57.

Levine SB, Hasan S, Boraz M. Male hypoactive sexual desire disorder. In: Balon R. Segraves RT, eds. *Clinical Manual of Sexual Disorders*. Arlington, VA: American Psychiatric Publishing; 2009:161–184.

McCabe MP. Evaluation of a cognitive behaviour therapy program for people with sexual difficulties. *J Sex Marital Ther*. 2001;27:259–271.

Meissner V, Schroeter L, Kohn F, et al. Factors associated with low sexual desire in 45 year old men: findings from the German Male Sex Study. *J Sex Med*. 2019;16:981–991.

Mercer C, Fenton K, Johnson A, et al. Sexual function problems and help seeking behavior in Britain: national probability sample survey. *BMJ*. 2003;327:426–427.

Mills E, Ertl N, Wall M, et al. Effects of kisspeptin on sexual brain processing and penile tumescence in men with hypoactive sexual desire disorder. A randomized clinical trial. JAMA Netw Open. 2023;6(2):2254313. doi:10.1001/jamanetworkopen.2022.54313.

Morales A, Buvat J, Gooren I, et al. Endocrine aspects of sexual dysfunction in men. *J Sex Med*. 2004;1:69–81.

Nimbi F, Tripodi F, Rossi R, et al. Expanding the analysis of psychosocial factors of sexual desire in men. *J Sex Med*. 2018; 15:230–244.

Rubio-Aurioles E, Bivalacqua TJ. Standard operational procedures for low sexual desire in men. *J Sex Med*. 2013;10:94–107.

Segraves RT, Clayton A, Croft H, et al. Bupropion sustained release for the treatment of hypoactive sexual desire disorder in premenopausal women. *J Clin Psychopharmacol*. 2004;24:339–342.

PREMATURE (EARLY) EJACULATION

▶ General Considerations

In general terms, PE is ejaculation that occurs prior to or shortly after vaginal penetration. The DSM-5 diagnostic criteria specify "A persistent or recurrent pattern of ejaculation occurring during partnered sexual activity within approximately 1 minute following vaginal penetration and before the individual wishes it." This symptom must be present for at least 6 months, must be experienced on almost all or all (approximately 75–100%) occasions of sexual activity, must be distressing, and must not be explainable by another mental (nonsexual!) disorder or attributed to the effect of a substance/medication or medical condition. The diagnosis of premature or early ejaculation may apply to individuals involved in nonvaginal sexual activities, but the duration for these activities has not been established.

A. Epidemiology

Approximately 28% of U.S. males aged 18–59 years complained of problems with rapid ejaculation in the preceding year. In epidemiological studies, significant correlations have been found between measures of anxiety and PE. In one Scandinavian study, only 2–3% of men reported that they had a problem with rapid ejaculation. In contrast, 18–22% of the women reported that their male partners had problems with rapid ejaculation. Interestingly, two thirds of the men surveyed stated that their partners took too long to reach orgasm. Later cohorts of women reported rapid ejaculation in their partners more often that earlier cohorts, suggesting that changing societal expectations may play a role in defining when rapid ejaculation is considered to be a problem.

However, with the new definition requiring the ejaculation to occur within approximately 1 minute, only about 1–3% of men would probably meet the diagnostic criteria for PE.

B. Etiology

There are several major hypotheses concerning the etiology and patterns of lifelong PE. Psychoanalytically oriented clinicians hypothesized that unconscious anger toward women was an etiological factor. Cognitive–behavioral clinicians posited that rapid ejaculation is a pattern learned in adolescence and then maintained by performance anxiety. In spite of the wide acceptance of the cognitive–behavioral hypothesis, there is minimal evidence to support it. Other clinicians have hypothesized that PE is the result of abnormalities in either spinal or central nervous system mechanisms controlling ejaculatory threshold. Waldinger postulated that ejaculatory speed is hereditarily determined, is normally distributed in the general population, and represents a normal variation and thus is not a psychiatric disorder. He further hypothesized that the set point of the ejaculatory threshold is related to hyposensitivity of the serotonin 5HT2^C receptor and hypersensitivity of the 5HT1^A receptor. This hypothesis is consistent with the effect of various pharmacological influences on ejaculatory latency. There is some evidence that premature (early) ejaculation is more common in men with panic disorder and social anxiety.

There is minimal evidence concerning the etiology of acquired PE. There appears to be a higher incidence of acquired PE in men with chronic prostatitis and after certain brain and spinal cord injuries. PE is also associated with hyperthyroidism, and its prevalence decreases with normalization of thyroid-stimulating hormone. PE has been report to occur on heroin and methadone withdrawal.

C. Genetics

Population-based twin studies have found evidence for a moderate (28%) genetic influence on PE. Studies have found that both serotonin and dopamine transporter gene polymorphism may be associated with PE. Other genetic polymorphisms have been reported.

▶ Clinical Findings

A. Signs & Symptoms

Men with lifelong PE will report ejaculating rapidly since their first experience with a sexual partner. They may be able to delay ejaculation during masturbation but not with a sexual partner. Often, they seek treatment at the insistence of their sexual partner.

B. Psychological Testing

Psychological testing is not required to establish this diagnosis.

C. Laboratory Testing

The most frequent diagnostic procedure used in clinical trials is intravaginal ejaculatory latency, measured by stopwatch during sexual activities at home. The partner is the one who uses the stopwatch. How much this procedure influences ejaculatory latency is unknown.

If a neurological lesion is suspected, specialized procedures are possible, such as measurement of pudendal nerve latency and the characteristics of cortical evoked potentials from pudendal nerve stimulation or urethral stimulation. These procedures are rarely used in the evaluation of men with complaints of rapid ejaculation.

D. Neuroimaging

Neuroimaging is not useful in diagnosis of PE.

▶ Course of Illness

The pattern of PE in the absence of treatment is considered to be lifelong. There is no evidence of improvement with aging. Not much is known about the course of acquired PE.

▶ Differential Diagnosis

Cases of lifelong generalized PE are predominantly devoid of organic pathology. One should establish if the problem is secondary to a panic disorder or social anxiety disorder. If the man reports rapid ejaculation with one partner and not another, one obviously would investigate the differences in sexual patterns with the two partners.

If the problem is acquired, the possibility of a relationship issue or an organic pathology should be considered.

▶ Treatment

A. Psychopharmacological Treatment

Many clinicians employ serotonergic drugs in the treatment of rapid ejaculation. The two agents used most frequently are paroxetine (strongest ejaculation delay) and clomipramine. Paroxetine usually requires regular, daily dosing at 20 mg. An occasional patient will respond to as-needed dosing after 2 weeks of daily dosing. Clomipramine can be used on an as-needed basis, ingesting the drug 4–6 hours prior to sexual activity. Other serotonergic drugs such as fluoxetine and sertraline are used less frequently. Based on data from studies by Waldinger and colleagues, citalopram and fluvoxamine are considered less useful in this indication. Dapoxetine (structurally similar to fluoxetine), a compound specifically developed for the treatment of PE, has been used in some countries. Dapoxetine is not approved for use in the United States. Some investigators have reported success with benzodiazepines or tramadol. Topical anesthetics such as lidocaine and or prilocaine (cream, gel, or spray) have also been used to delay ejaculation. A dose-metered lidocaine–prilocaine topical spray has been approved in Europe. PDE-5 inhibitors have minimal efficacy in this disorder.

B. Psychotherapeutic Treatment

Behavioral approaches are usually employed. These include the "start–stop" and squeeze technique. Both techniques involve repeated episodes of manual penile stimulation stopped prior to ejaculatory inevitability. The "squeeze technique" involves a firm squeeze of the frenulum before the next episode of stimulation. Clinical experience suggests that the technique requires the participation of the sexual partner to be successful. The mechanism by which these techniques work is unclear. It is assumed that in the absence of performance pressure, the man learns to monitor his level of sexual stimulation and thus modulate his level of excitement. Behavioral treatment of PE has been shown to be more effective than a waiting-list control and equally as effective as sertraline therapy.

C. Other Treatment

Psychodynamic psychotherapy is rarely utilized in the treatment of this condition. The role of PDE-5 inhibitor as a possible treatment modality of PE is not clear. Patient and couple counseling, guidance, and/or relationship therapy could also be used in the management of PE.

▶ Complications/Adverse Outcomes of Treatment

Use of serotonergic drugs with short half-life can result in a withdrawal syndrome. This has been most often reported with the immediate-release form of paroxetine. The incidence of side effects of SSRIs is usually low in patients with PE. Topical anesthetics can result in penile anesthesia, and there is a risk of vaginal absorption.

▶ Prognosis

The short-term prognosis with behavioral therapy and pharmacotherapy is excellent. However, the problem recurs if the drug is stopped, and there is a high relapse rate after successful behavioral therapy.

Abdel-Hamid IA, El Naggar E, Gilani A. Assessment of an as needed use of pharmacotherapy and the pause-squeeze technique in premature ejaculation. *Int J Impot Res.* 2001;13:41.

American Psychiatric Association. *Diagnostic and Statistical Manual of Mental Disorders.* 5th ed. Arlington, VA: American Psychiatric Association; 2013.

Atikeler M, Gecit I, Senol F. Optimum use of prilocaine-lidocaine cream in premature ejaculation. *Andrologia.* 2002;34:356–359.

Butcher M, Zubert T, Christianson K. Topical agents for premature ejaculation. *Sex Med Rev.* 2020;8:92–99.

Chen T, Mulloy E, Eisenberg M. Medical treatments of disorders of ejaculation. *Urol Clin N Am.* 2022;49:219–230.

Dunn KM, Croft P, Hacket G. Association of sexual problems with social, psychological and physical problems in men and women in a cross sectional population survey. *J Epidemiol Commun Health.* 1999;53:144–148.

Figeira I, Possidente E, Arques C, et al. Sexual dysfunction: a neglected complication of panic disorder and social phobia. *Arch Sex Behav.* 2001;30:369–377.

Gao M, Geng B, Jannini T et al. Thalamocortical dysconnectivity in lifelong premature ejaculation: a functional MRI study. *Urology.* 2022;159:133–138.

Haaviola-Mannila E, Kontula O. *Sexual Trends in the Baltic Sea Area.* Helsinki: Family Federation of Finland; 2003.

Jannini E, Burri A, Jern P, et al. Genetics of human sexual behavior: where we are, where we are going. *Sex Med Rev.* 2015;3:65–77.

Janssen P, Bakker S, Rethelyi J, et al. Serotonin transporter promoter region (5-HTTLPR) polymorphism is associated with the intravaginal ejaculation latency time in Dutch men with lifelong premature ejaculation. *J Sex Med.* 2008;6:276–284.

Jern P, Santtila P, Witting K, et al. Premature and delayed ejaculation: genetic and environmental effects in a population-based sample of Finnish twins. *J Sex Med.* 2007;4:1739–1749.

McCabe M, Sharlip I, Lewis R, et al. Incidence and prevalence of sexual dysfunction in women and men: a consensus statement from the Fourth International Consultation on Sexual Medicine 2015. *J Sex Med.* 2016;13:144–152.

McMahon CG, Jannini E, Waldinger M, Rowland D. Standard operating procedures in disorders of orgasm and ejaculation. *J Sex Med.* 2013;10:204–229.

Nkangineme I, Segraves RT. Neuropsychiatric aspects of sexual dysfunction. In: Schiffer R, Rao S, Fogel B, eds. *Neuropsychiatry,* 2nd ed. Philadelphia: Lippincott Williams & Wilkins; 2003: 338.

Patrick D, Althof S, Pryor J, et al. Premature ejaculation: an observational study of men and their partners. *J Sex Med.* 2005;2:358.

Porst H, Burri A. Novel treatments for premature ejaculation in the light of currently used therapies: a review. *Sex Med Rev.* 2019;7:129–140.

Santtila P, Jern P, Westberg L, et al. The dopamine transporter gene (DAT1) polymorphism is associated with premature ejaculation. *J Sex Med.* 2010;7:1538–1546.

Screponi E, Carosa E, Di Stasi M, et al. Prevalence of chronic prostatitis in men with premature ejaculation. *Urology.* 2001; 58:198–202.

Segraves R. Considerations for an evidence based definition of premature ejaculation in the DSM. *J Sex Med.* 2010;7(2 pt 1): 672–679.

Simpson G, McCann B, Lowy M. Treatment of premature ejaculation after traumatic brain injury. *Brain Inj.* 2003;17:723–729.

Tannenbaum J, Youssef M, Attia A. Hyperthyroidism as an underlying cause of premature ejaculation. *Sex Med Rev.* 2922;10:108–112.

Waldinger M. Rapid ejaculation. In: Levine S, Risen C, Althof S, eds. *Handbook of Clinical Sexuality for Mental Health Professionals.* New York: Brunner-Routledge, 2003:257.

SUBSTANCE/MEDICATION-INDUCED SEXUAL DYSFUNCTION

Substance/medication-induced sexual dysfunction is a condition in which a significant disturbance in sexual function is in the clinical picture and there is evidence (from the history, physical examination, or laboratory findings) that (1) the symptoms developed during or soon after substance intoxication or withdrawal or after exposure to a medication and (2) the involved substance/medication is capable of producing these symptoms. The symptoms have to be distressing and not explained by sexual dysfunction that is not substance/medication-induced. This dysfunction should not occur during the course of delirium. The clinician should specify whether the dysfunction is "With onset during intoxication," "With onset during withdrawal," or "With onset after medication use." Prevalence varies based on implicated substance (numerous medications, namely SSRIs, TCAs, MAOIs, antipsychotics, but also antihypertensives, hormones and others; and substances of abuse such as alcohol, heroin, methadone and others).

Management of this dysfunction may be a complex matter, unless a simple removal of the offending substance is possible. There are numerous strategies for antidepressant–associated and other medication-associated sexual dysfunctions, such as waiting for a spontaneous remission, starting with or switching to an antidepressant with a lower incidence of associated sexual dysfunction, reduction to a minimal effective dose, or use of numerous "antidotes." Substance-induced sexual dysfunction in cases of using substances of abuse may need to be treated as one would treat specific sexual dysfunction not induced by this substance, if the removal of the substance is not possible (e.g., in case of opioid-induced sexual dysfunction when the patient is on methadone maintenance and continues to have firmly established opioid-induced sexual dysfunction).

American Psychiatric Association. *Diagnostic and Statistical Manual of Mental Disorders.* 5th ed. Text Revision. Washington, DC: American Psychiatric Association; 2022.

Segraves RT, Balon R. *Sexual pharmacology. Fast facts.* New York: WW Norton; 2003.

OTHER SPECIFIED SEXUAL DYSFUNCTION

This category includes symptom presentation of a sexual dysfunction that causes clinically significant distress but does not meet full criteria of any of the disorders in this class.

Specific reasons may be present—for example, sexual aversion could be classified as "other specified sexual dysfunction, sexual aversion."

American Psychiatric Association. *Diagnostic and Statistical Manual of Mental Disorders.* 5th ed. Text Revision. Washington, DC: American Psychiatric Association; 2022.

▼ PARAPHILIC DISORDERS

A paraphilic disorder according to the DSM-5 is a paraphilia that is currently causing distress or impairment in various areas of person's functioning or a paraphilia that entails harm or risk of harm to oneself or others. The DSM-5_TR specifies that the term *paraphilia* denotes any intense and persistent sexual interest other than sexual interest in genital stimulation or preparatory fondling with phenotypically normal, physically mature, consenting human partners. The term paraphilia literally means love (philia) beyond the usual (para). The essential features of paraphilias are recurrent, intense, sexually arousing fantasies, sexual urges, or behaviors involving non-human objects; or the suffering or humiliation of oneself or one's partner; or children or other nonconsenting persons; or also any combination of urges or behaviors over a period of at least 6 months and causing significant distress or impairment in social and other functioning. A paraphilia is necessary but not sufficient condition for having a paraphilic disorder, and a paraphilia by itself does not necessarily justify or require clinical intervention (DSM-5-TR, p 780).

The wide category of paraphilias not otherwise specified includes, among others, rare entities such as telephone scatophilia (obscene phone calls), necrophilia (sexual acts with corpses), partialism (exclusive focus on one body part), zoophilia (sexual activity involving animals), coprophilia (including feces), urophilia (urine, urination), klismaphilia (enemas), and others.

Studies of paraphilias/paraphilic disorders, especially treatment studies, are difficult to conduct, as (1) paraphilias/paraphilic disorders are rare and are not socially acceptable (and thus, treatment is usually not sought by individuals with paraphilias), (2) comorbidity with other disorders is high, and (3) ethical considerations frequently do not allow for rigorous studies. There is no FDA-approved treatment for paraphilic disorders.

Men with paraphilias/paraphilic disorders seem, in general, to have difficulties with attachment and intimacy; they tend to be self-centered and antagonistic and have higher levels of neuroticism, lower agreeableness, and lower conscientiousness.

Treatment of paraphilic disorders is challenging, as no good data exist and patients usually avoid treatment unless forced by law. Treatment should always include both pharmacotherapy (when evidence is available) and psychotherapy. There is no evidence that either of these two modalities is better than the other. Treatment should progress from modalities associated with fewer side effects and complications, such as CBT and relapse prevention and later antidepressants, to treatments with a higher risk of severe complications, such as antiandrogens and other hormones.

This chapter presents paraphilic disorder following the DSM-5-TR classification and listing of these disorders, starting with disorders based on *anomalous activity preference*. These disorders are divided into two subgroups: (1) *courtship disorders*, resembling distorted components of human courtship behavior (voyeuristic disorders, exhibitionistic disorder, and frotteuristic disorder), and (2) *algolagnic disorders*, which involve pain and suffering (sexual masochism disorder and sexual sadism disorder). The second group of paraphilic disorders includes disorders with *anomalous target preference*, one directed at other humans (pedophilic disorder) and two directed elsewhere (fetishistic disorder and transvestic disorder).

American Psychiatric Association. *Diagnostic and Statistical Manual of Mental Disorders*. 5th ed. Text Revision. Washington, DC: American Psychiatric Association; 2022.

VOYEURISTIC DISORDER

▶ General Considerations

The diagnosis of voyeuristic disorder requires recurrent and intense sexual arousal from observing an *unsuspecting* person who is naked, disrobing, or involved in sexual activity. Over the period of 6 months, the person must act on these urges/fantasies with a nonconsenting person, or these must cause significant distress or impairment. The act of looking is for the purpose of achieving sexual excitement, and sexual activity with the observed person is usually not sought. Sexual satisfaction is achieved via masturbation, either during looking or later in response to the memory of whatever was witnessed.

A. Epidemiology

There are no solid data on the epidemiology of voyeuristic disorder. The highest cited estimate of lifetime prevalence is 12% in men. It is the most common of potentially law-breaking behaviors. It is also very rare among females.

B. Etiology

The etiology of voyeurism/voyeuristic disorder is unknown. As noted, some experts view voyeurism as a disorder of courtship (finding a partner phase).

C. Genetics

There is no evidence regarding heritability of this condition.

▶ Clinical Findings

A. Signs & Symptoms

Sexual satisfaction is achieved via masturbation either during observation of the unsuspecting individual, or later in response to the memory of the observation. The victim's lack of suspicion and the risk of being caught are central to the person's arousal.

B. Psychological Testing

There is no psychological testing available for diagnosing voyeuristic disorder.

C. Laboratory Findings

There are no voyeuristic disorder-specific laboratory findings.

D. Neuroimaging

There are not known neuroimaging studies of voyeuristic disorder.

▶ Course of Illness

The onset of voyeuristic disorder is usually before age 15, though it should be diagnosed only in persons 18 years old or older to differentiate it from the age-appropriate adolescent sexual curiosity and activity. The course tends to be chronic.

▶ Differential Diagnosis (Including Comorbid Conditions)

The differential diagnosis of voyeuristic disorder includes other paraphilic disorders, voyeurism (no significant distress, not acting on the urges), personality disorders (namely antisocial one), psychosis, schizophrenia, manic episode, major neurocognitive disorder, intellectual developmental disorder, personality change due to another medical condition, conduct disorder, and substance use disorders. Voyeuristic disorder may be comorbid with other paraphilic disorders, bipolar disorder, depressive and anxiety disorders, attention deficit/-hyperactivity disorder, and personality disorders.

▶ Treatment

A. Psychopharmacological Interventions

Successful treatment of voyeuristic disorder with antidepressants such as paroxetine and fluoxetine has been reported. Hormonal therapy should be reserved for cases resistant to other pharmacotherapy and psychotherapy.

B. Psychotherapeutic Interventions

CBT, individual psychotherapy, relapse prevention, and behavioral modification may be useful in the treatment of voyeuristic disorder. No solid data are available on their usefulness in this condition.

C. Other Interventions

No other interventions have been reported for this condition.

▶ **Complications/Adverse Outcomes of Treatment**

Antidepressant side effects such as diarrhea, headaches, or prolonged ejaculation may occur when these medications are used in voyeurism.

▶ **Prognosis**

Prognosis of untreated voyeurism is probably poor.

Balon R. Voyeuristic disorder. In: Balon R, ed. *Practical Guide to Paraphilia and Paraphilic Disorders*. Springer; 2016:63–75.

EXHIBITIONISTIC DISORDER

▶ **General Considerations**

The arousal is derived from the exposure of one's genitals to an unsuspecting person and is manifested by fantasies, urges, or behaviors. Over the period of 6 months, the person must act on these urges/fantasies with a nonconsenting person, or these must cause significant distress or impairment. The onset is usually before the age of 18 years, but it can begin at an older age. Most persons suffering from exhibitionism are heterosexual. The DSM-5-TR requires that it be specified whether the person becomes sexually aroused by exposing the genitals to prepubertal children, or physically mature individuals, or to prepubertal children and to physically mature individuals.

A. Epidemiology

The incidence and prevalence of exhibitionistic disorder is unknown (highest estimates are 2–4%). Exhibitionistic disorder, like most paraphilic disorders, is more frequent among males.

B. Etiology

The etiology of this disorder is unknown. Some have speculated that males suffering from exhibitionism/exhibitionistic disorder are shy and unable to establish a normal sexual relationship. In the psychoanalytical view, male exhibitionism is associated with a dominant, seductive mother and a distant father. The assault on masculinity and adequacy is resolved in feelings of power and gratification when a female reacts to his genital displays. Deviant arousal may also play a role in the etiology of exhibitionism. According to the courtship theory, exhibitionism is an impairment of the pretactile interaction of courtship.

C. Genetics

There is no information about the genetics of exhibitionistic disorder.

▶ **Clinical Findings**

A. Signs & Symptoms

Persons suffering from exhibitionistic disorder usually display their genitals hoping to shock or excite the victim. They are usually unable to control the urge to expose themselves. They expose themselves in various places, for example, while driving, or in parks and parking lots, and contrary to the popular beliefs, could occur in crowded areas, too. The exposure is usually accompanied or followed by masturbation. Various triggers (stress, interpersonal conflict, boredom) may elicit the urge to expose oneself. The exposure may make the subjects feel excited, turned on, wanted, desired, and calm.

B. Psychological Testing

Psychological testing is not helpful in establishing the diagnosis of exhibitionistic disorder.

C. Laboratory Findings

There are no specific laboratory tests for exhibitionistic disorder.

D. Neuroimaging

Neuroimaging is not useful in the diagnosis of exhibitionistic disorder.

▶ **Course of Illness**

The duration of exhibitionistic disorder is long, usually with no asymptomatic periods, and the course is chronic if untreated. The disorder possibly becomes less severe after the age of 40, though not much is known about its persistence over time.

▶ **Differential Diagnosis (Including Comorbid Conditions)**

The differential diagnosis includes other paraphilias, manic episode, major neurocognitive disorder, intellectual developmental disorder, personality change due to another medical condition, substance intoxication, schizophrenia, conduct disorder, antisocial personality disorder, and exhibitionism (no significant distress, not acting on urges). Exhibitionism should be distinguished from nudism—persons with exhibitionism do not usually have interest in exposure at nudist places.

Comorbidity of exhibitionism with other disorders is high (up to 92%), especially with current and lifetime sexual disorders, other paraphilias, impulse-control disorders, conduct disorder, and substance use disorders. Major depression and substance use appear largely secondary to exhibitionism.

Treatment

A. Psychopharmacological Interventions

Serotonergic antidepressants (e.g., fluvoxamine, paroxetine, clomipramine) have been found helpful in some cases. More severe cases (e.g., repeat offenders, failure with other treatments) may be helped with hormonal preparations, such as long-acting agonists of luteinizing hormone-releasing hormone (LHRH) and antiandrogens in special settings. Treatment with LHRH agonists and other antiandrogens requires appropriate initial and follow-up laboratory testing, as serious side effects are not uncommon (discussed later). Buspirone hydrochloride has also been successfully used in a case of exhibitionism.

B. Psychotherapeutic Interventions

Psychotherapy is important in fostering compliance and ameliorating attitudinal problems. CBT, group therapy, relapse prevention, private exposure and covert sensitization, and even aversion approaches have been recommended as useful in this condition.

Complications/Adverse Outcomes of Treatment

Side effects of treatment using antidepressants include headaches, gastrointestinal disturbances, and prolonged ejaculation. Antiandrogens can produce more serious side effects, including feminization, fatigue, liver damage, and decreased bone density, among others. Comorbid or secondary depression and substance abuse need to be treated vigorously.

Prognosis

Prognosis of treated exhibitionism is probably fair to good. Untreated exhibitionism is usually chronic.

Balon R. Exhibitionistic disorder. In: Balon R, ed. *Practical Guide to Paraphilia and Paraphilic Disorders.* Springer; 2016:77–91.

Grant JE. Clinical characteristics and psychiatric comorbidity in males with exhibitionism. *J Clin Psychiatry.* 2005;66:1367–1371.

Lamontagne Y, Lesage A. Private exposure and covert sensitization in the treatment of exhibitionism. *J Behav Ther Exp Psychiatry.* 1986;17:197–201.

Osborne CS, Wise TN. Paraphilias. In: Balon R, Segraves RT, eds. *Handbook of Sexual Dysfunction.* New York: Taylor & Francis; 2005:293.

Segraves RT, Balon R. Sexual Pharmacology. Fast Facts. New York: WW Norton; 2003.

FROTTEURISTIC DISORDER

General Considerations

The behavior usually occurs in crowded places (e.g., public transportation), which are conducive to this behavior and from which escape of arrest is easier. The hallmark of this disorder is the recurrent, intense sexual arousal from touching or rubbing against a nonconsenting person, as manifested by fantasies, urges, or behaviors. Again, over the period of 6 months, the person must act on these urges/fantasies with a nonconsenting person, or these must cause significant distress or impairment. Frotteuristic disorder tends to be a crime of opportunity or an example of social incompetency and is rarely preferred over other sexual activities. It occurs frequently in crowded public places (public transportation, concerts). In some countries there are "women only" spaces in public transportation vehicles.

A. Epidemiology

There are no data on the epidemiology of frotteuristic disorder and the estimates vary significantly, depending on the setting. Frotteuristic acts may occur in up to 30% of adult males in the United States and Canadian general population. Again, frotteuristic disorder occurs more frequently in males.

B. Etiology

The etiology of frotteuristic disorder is unknown. Frotteurism is viewed by some as a disturbance of the tactile interaction phase of courtship.

C. Genetics

There are no data available on genetics of frotteuristic disorder.

Clinical Findings

A. Signs & Symptoms

The person suffering from frotteurism/frotteuristic disorder usually rubs his or her genitalia against the victim's thighs or buttocks or fondles the victim's genitalia or breasts with hands ("toucherism"). The person usually fantasizes about an exclusive relationship with the victim.

B. Psychological Testing

Psychological testing is not useful in diagnosing frotteuristic disorder.

C. Laboratory Findings

No specific laboratory findings have been reported in frotteuristic disorder.

D. Neuroimaging

There are no reports of neuroimaging in individuals with frotteuristic disorder.

Course of Illness

Frotteuristic disorder peaks between 15 and 25 years of age and then gradually declines in frequency.

Differential Diagnosis (Including Comorbid Conditions)

Differential diagnosis includes other paraphilic disorders, social phobia, manic episode, major neurocognitive disorder, intellectual developmental disorder, personality change due to another medical condition, substance abuse, conduct disorder, conduct disorder, antisocial personality disorder, schizophrenia, and frotteurism (no distress, not acting on urges).

Frotteuristic disorder is frequently associated with autistic spectrum disorder behavior.

Treatment

A. Psychopharmacological Interventions

Little is known about the pharmacological treatment of frotteuristic disorder. SSRIs (fluoxetine) may be helpful in frotteuristic disorder. One study of a case refractory to other treatments used leuprolide acetate, a gonadotropin-releasing hormone agonist.

B. Psychotherapeutic Interventions

No good data on the use of psychotherapeutic interventions exist. CBT may be useful, as persons with frotteuristic disorder frequently use cognitive distortions in justification of their behavior. Supportive therapy and self-help texts may also be useful.

Complications/Adverse Outcomes of Treatment

If hormones are used, their side effects (in case of leuprolide acetate erectile dysfunction, decreased bone mineral density) may occur.

Prognosis

The prognosis, especially in cases of comorbidity with conditions such as autistic spectrum disorder, is poor.

Balon R Frotteuristic disorder. In: Balon R, Ed. Practical Guide to Paraphilia and Paraphilic Disorders. Springer; 2016:93–106.

SEXUAL MASOCHISM DISORDER

General Considerations

The sexual arousal in this disorder is derived from the act of being humiliated, beaten, bound, and made to suffer. It must be accompanied by distress and/or impairment and last for at least 6 months. Sexual masochism is frequently linked to sexual sadism. Sigmund Freud was the first one to combine these two terms into sadomasochism, though the term masochism was invented by Richard von Krafft-Ebing, derived from the name of Leopold von Sacher-Masoch. Individuals with masochism frequently do not seek help, unless they have marital problems or concerns about being harmed.

A. Epidemiology

The prevalence of sexual masochism disorder in the general population is unknown, though masochistic fantasies are not uncommon. Some suggest that sexual masochism occurs more often among middle and upper socioeconomic class individuals. Earlier studies suggested that sexual masochism could be more common among women.

B. Etiology

The etiology of sexual masochism disorder is unknown. Various psychoanalytical explanations exist, entertaining childhood trauma and abuse; nevertheless, none provides a satisfactory explanation.

C. Genetics

There are no data regarding the genetics of sexual masochism disorder.

Clinical Findings

A. Signs & Symptoms

The behavior of sexual masochists may range from mild forms (such as being spanked) to more severe ones (such as being bound and beaten, whipped, receiving electrical shocks, being cut, and having objects inserted in the orifices). Other forms of humiliation, such as being urinated or defecated on or being forced to crawl and bark like a dog, may also be involved. Some individuals may just invoke masochistic fantasies during masturbation or intercourse. Hypoxyphilia or asphyxiophilia (sexual arousal by oxygen deprivation by strangling, mask, etc.; a DSM-5-TR sexual masochism disorder specifier) is considered the most extreme and the most dangerous variation of masochism.

B. Psychological Testing

Psychological testing is not helpful in establishing the diagnosis of sexual masochism disorder.

C. Laboratory Findings

There are no laboratory findings specific to sexual masochism disorder.

D. Neuroimaging

There are no specific neuroimaging studies of sexual masochism disorder.

Course of Illness

Masochistic fantasies are likely present during childhood. Sexual masochism behavior usually starts during early adulthood. The course is usually chronic, with repetition of the same sexual behaviors. Yet, these behaviors may diminish with advancing age.

Differential Diagnosis (Including Comorbid Conditions)

The differential diagnosis of sexual masochism disorder includes other paraphilic disorders and sexual masochism (no distress). Sexual masochism frequently coexists with sexual sadism, fetishism, hypersexuality, transvestic fetishism, and substance use disorders.

Treatment

A. Psychopharmacological Interventions

Not much information on psychopharmacology of sexual masochism is available. There have been cases of sexual masochism treated with lithium and with leuprolide acetate, and serotonergic antidepressants may be helpful.

B. Psychotherapeutic Interventions

Individual psychotherapy and CBT could be used in treatment of sexual masochism disorder, but no specific data are available.

C. Other Interventions

No other treatments are available.

Complications of Treatment

Hormonal treatment of paraphilic disorders could be associated with side effects specific to a selected hormone mentioned before (see "Pedophilic Disorder" section).

Prognosis

Prognosis is unknown and is probably poor.

Wylie RA, Wylie KR. Sexual masochism disorder. In: Balon R, ed. *Practical Guide to Paraphilia and Paraphilic Disorders*. Springer; 2016:107–122.

SEXUAL SADISM DISORDER

General Considerations

The central feature of sexual sadism/sexual sadism disorder is sexual arousal due to physical or psychological suffering of the victim. Over the period of 6 months, the person must act on these urges/fantasies with a nonconsenting person, or these must cause significant distress or impairment, to meet the criteria for a *disorder*. Some individuals may fantasize sadistic acts during sexual activity and do not act on them. Sexual sadism may occur with a consenting partner (e.g., in sadomasochism) (not necessarily a disorder) or with a nonconsenting partner (disorder). Sexual sadism may vary from mild forms, such as spanking, to much more severe acts, such as beating and humiliation of the victim, and may involve rape or killing of the victim.

A. Epidemiology

No reliable data on the prevalence of sexual sadism disorder are available. The estimates vary, are close to 2%. It is especially difficult to estimate the prevalence of sadism because of the legal consequences of this disorder. Serious forms of sexual sadism disorder attract a lot of media and general public attention but are relatively rare.

B. Etiology

As with other paraphilic disorders, the etiology of sexual sadisms is unknown. There are various psychoanalytic theories of sadism. Sexual sadists frequently meet the criteria for personality disorder(s). None of the theories or associations explains the etiology of sexual sadism disorder.

C. Genetics

There are no genetic studies of sexual sadism disorder.

Clinical Findings

A. Signs & Symptoms

Sexual sadists' behavior, parallel to sexual masochism, may vary from mild forms, such as spanking the partner, to more severe, such as tying and beating, whipping, cutting, stabbing the partner, sensory deprivation (e.g., using blindfolds), dominance-submission role-play, and inserting objects into partner's orifices. Other forms of humiliation, such as forcing the victim to crawl and bark like a dog or keeping the victim in a cage, may also be involved. Some individuals may only invoke sadistic fantasies during masturbation or intercourse.

B. Psychological Testing

Psychological testing is not helpful in diagnosing sexual sadism disorder. Homicidal sexual offenders scored higher on Psychopathy Checklist—Revised and portrayed themselves better in the areas of sexual functioning (Derogatis Sexual Functioning Inventory) and aggression/hostility (Buss–Durkee Hostility Inventory).

C. Laboratory Findings

No specific laboratory tests for sexual sadism disorder are available. It is unclear whether phallometric testing can help in diagnosing sexual sadism/sexual sadism disorder. However, one phallometric study demonstrated that sadists responded more to cues of violence/injury in the laboratory.

D. Neuroimaging

There are no neuroimaging findings specific to sexual sadism disorder and no known neuroimaging studies of sexual sadism disorder.

▶ Course of Illness

The age of onset of sexual sadism disorder varies, but it usually starts during early adulthood. Sadistic fantasies are likely to occur in childhood. The course of sexual sadism, especially untreated, is usually chronic. The advancing age may be associated with decreasing sadistic preferences and behavior.

▶ Differential Diagnosis (Including Comorbid Conditions)

The differential diagnosis of sexual sadism includes other paraphilic disorders, hypersexuality, personality disorders (especially antisocial personality disorder), psychosis, substance use disorders, intellectual developmental disorder, organic brain syndrome, and infliction of physical or psychological suffering during the commission of sex crime (e.g., rape) unless there is evidence that the perpetrator derives pleasure from inflicting the pain and from the suffering of the victim. Sexual sadism (urges to make another person to suffer are not acted on and there is no distress or impairment) should also be ruled out.

▶ Treatment

A. Psychopharmacological Interventions

Treatment of sexual sadism disorder should be carried out in specialized settings involving a team of specialists familiar with the treatment of this paraphilic disorder (especially in cases involving legal issues). Serotonergic antidepressants (e.g., fluoxetine) have been occasionally used in the treatment of sexual sadism. Hormonal preparations such as cyproterone acetate (not available in the United States), leuprolide acetate, triptorelin, and medroxyprogesterone acetate have been used in the treatment of sexual offenders. These hormones are useful in reducing sexual drive, erotic fantasies,

sexual activity, possibly aggressiveness, and NPT. In the past, some antipsychotics were also used in the treatment of sexual sadism disorder.

B. Psychotherapeutic Interventions

Individual psychotherapy has been used in many cases of sexual sadism disorder. A cognitive–behavioral approach with a focus on control and management of problematic thoughts, urges, and behaviors, modification of paraphilic arousal, amelioration or management of comorbid conditions, resolution of other life issues, and relapse prevention may also be useful. Various techniques described for the treatment of pedophilia (discussed later) could also be useful. Evidence for psychotherapy of this condition in an organized fashion is lacking.

C. Other Interventions

Surgical castrations of sexual sadists have been performed in other countries but are not condoned in the United States.

▶ Complications/Adverse Outcomes of Treatment

Hormonal treatment of paraphilias could be associated with side effects specific to the selected hormone (see section on "Pedophilic Disorder").

▶ Prognosis

The prognosis of sexual sadism disorder is unknown, but is probably poor, especially in untreated cases.

Briken P, Bourget D, Dufour M. Sexual sadism in sexual offenders and sexually motivated homicide. *Psychiatr Clin North Am.* 2014;37:215–230.

Firestone O, Bradford JM, Greenberg DM, Larose MR. Homicidal sex offenders: psychological, phallometric and diagnostic features. *J Am Acad Psychiatry Law.* 1998;26:537–552.

Liu A, Zhang E, Leroux EJ, Benassi P. Sexual sadism disorder and coercive paraphilic disorder: a scoping review. *J Sex Med.* 2022;19:496–506.

Seto MC, Lalumiere ML, Harris GT, Chivers ML. The sexual response of sexual sadists. *J Abnormal Psychol.* 2010;12:739–753.

Thibaut F. Pharmacological treatment of paraphilias. *Isr J Psychiatry Relat Sci.* 2012;49:297–305.

PEDOPHILIC DISORDER

▶ General Considerations

The central features of this disorder are recurrent, intense, sexually arousing fantasies, sexual urges, or behaviors that include sexual activity with a prepubescent child or children generally involve children 13 years or younger. Over the period of 6 months, the person must act on these urges/fantasies, or these must cause significant distress or impairment. The diagnosis of pedophilic disorder should specify whether the patient is attracted to males, female, or both, and whether it is limited to incest. Other subtyping includes exclusive type (attracted only to children) and nonexclusive type. Pedophilic disorder usually develops during adolescence/puberty, though it could start at any age. The frequency of pedophilic behavior fluctuates and worsens with stress. It is important to note that the diagnosis of pedophilic disorder cannot be assigned to a child. Also, the perpetrating person should be at least 16 years old and at least 5 years older than the child or children he/she is sexually involved with. Not all child sexual offenses are necessarily pedophilic; some of them could be indiscriminate in partner choice due to excessive drive, poor impulse control, intoxication, dementia, intellectual developmental disorder, and other causes.

A. Epidemiology

The prevalence of pedophilic disorder in the general population is unknown but is likely less than 3%. Pedophilic disorder has also been reported in women but is a small fraction of the prevalence in men.

B. Etiology

The etiology of pedophilia/pedophilic disorder is unknown. Numerous factors such as brain abnormalities (e.g., attention-deficit/hyperactivity disorder, dementia, intellectual disability disorder, seizure disorder), biological abnormalities (hormonal levels, or neurotransmitter changes), comorbidity and clinical similarities (e.g., with obsessive–compulsive disorder), developmental (sexual abuse during childhood, etc.), environmental, psychological (psychodynamic theories), and other factors have been considered in the etiology of pedophilia/pedophilic disorder. However, none of these factors can fully explain pedophilia/pedophilic disorder or any other paraphilic disorder, and neither can the response to treatment modality (e.g., SSRIs, hormones).

C. Genetics

Though the possibility of familial transmission of pedophilic disorder has been suggested, there are no solid data on the genetics of pedophilia/pedophilic disorder available. There are reports of association between pedophilic disorder and Klinefelter syndrome.

▶ Clinical Findings

A. Signs & Symptoms

Sexual arousal by children—whether in sexual fantasies, by watching child pornography, by contacting children via the Internet, or by sexually abusing children—is the central behavioral manifestation of pedophilic disorder.

B. Psychological Testing

Differences between pedophiles and other subjects on various psychological tests (e.g., Millon, neuropsychological batteries, Rorschach) have been reported. However, no psychological test is useful in diagnosing pedophilic disorder.

C. Laboratory Findings

Phalloplethysmography has been used in diagnosing pedophilia/pedophilic disorder. It is a psychophysiological technique in which the person's penile blood volume is monitored during exposure to a standardized set of sexual stimuli involving, among others, male and female children and adolescents. The sensitivity of this test in detecting pedophilia (studies done prior to the DSM-5 diagnostic criteria of disorders established) in nonadmitters is ≥55%, and the specificity is around 95%. Nevertheless, its usefulness is still considered questionable and is limited to research or comprehensive assessment of pedophiles, which includes other testing. It is probably more reliable and useful than psychological testing.

Viewing time (using photographs of nude or minimally clothed persons as visual stimuli and measuring the differences in time persons spends watching the individual pictures) could be used to diagnose pedophilic disorder, especially in combination with self-report measures. The problem in using this test is (and phalloplethysmography) that possession of certain pictures used here (children) may violate American law regarding possession of child pornography, even when this is used solely for diagnostic purposes!

Other laboratory testing (though occasional abnormalities may occur) has not been found useful in diagnosing pedophilic disorder.

D. Neuroimaging

There are no solid neuroimaging data of pedophilic disorder, though altered brain activity was detected in the frontal area in some studies.

▶ Course of Illness

The course of pedophilic disorder is usually chronic, especially in those attracted to males. The course of this disorder may fluctuate. Pedophilic disorder appears to be a lifelong condition, whether remission occurs is not clear. Advanced age is likely to diminish frequency of this behavior.

▶ Differential Diagnosis (Including Comorbid Conditions)

Other paraphilic disorders, personality disorders, obsessive–compulsive disorder, psychosis, substance use disorders, dementia, intellectual developmental disorder, brain injury, and seizure disorder should be considered in the differential diagnosis of pedophilic disorder. Pedophiles frequently meet the criteria for personality disorder(s), namely, antisocial personality disorder. Nevertheless, the diagnosis of personality disorder does not explain or supplant the diagnosis of pedophilic disorder. Pedophilia (sexual urges not acted on, no marked distress or interpersonal difficulty) should also be ruled out.

Treatment

Treatment of pedophilic disorder is usually done in a specialized setting. It is recommended that the treatment be comprehensive and designed to

1. reduce pedophilic interests,
2. establish adult sexual interests, and
3. decrease attitudes and beliefs supportive of pedophilic behaviors.

These goals could be achieved by psychopharmacological, psychological, or, in extreme cases, partially by surgical approaches.

A. Psychopharmacological Interventions

Various serotonergic antidepressants (e.g., fluoxetine, sertraline), antipsychotics (e.g., chlorpromazine, risperidone), and mood stabilizers (e.g., carbamazepine, lithium) have been reported as useful in the treatment of pedophilia/pedophilic disorder, mostly in case reports or small series of patients. Serotonergic antidepressants are especially useful in reducing compulsive urges.

Interestingly, naltrexone, a competitive antagonist of opioid receptor, was reportedly useful in the treatment of adolescent pedophiles and other sexual offenders.

Hormones such as cyproterone acetate (CPA, not available in the United States), methylprogesterone acetate (MPA), and leuprolide acetate (LPA) have been successfully used in the treatment of pedophilic disorder. CPA and MPA are available in IM and oral forms, LPA only in an IM form. These hormones are useful in reducing sexual drive, erotic fantasies, sexual activity, possibly aggressiveness, and NPT.

B. Psychotherapeutic Interventions

Numerous psychological interventions have been used in pedophilia/pedophilic disorder with more or less success. Covert sensitization, olfactory aversion, satiation strategies (e.g., masturbation till orgasm to nondeviant fantasies with continuing masturbation focusing on pedophilic fantasies), and imaginal desensitization have been used to reduce pedophilic interests. Fading (gradual replacement of pedophilic visual stimulus with adult sexual stimulus), exposure, and masturbatory conditioning have been used to establish adult sexual interests. Finally, cognitive restructuring, externalization of cognitive distortions, victim empathy training, and developing a prosocial behavior have been used to decrease attitudes and beliefs supportive of pedophilic behavior.

Individual psychodynamic psychotherapy was used in pedophilia/pedophilic disorder in the past. CBT may be useful in cognitive restructuring, but also in ameliorating or management of comorbid conditions, resolution of other life issues, and relapse prevention.

C. Other Interventions

Surgical castration and/or stereotactic neurosurgery have been successfully used in the treatment of pedophilic disorder, with recidivism rates below 5%. However, these interventions are not usually used in the United States for ethical reasons.

Complications/Adverse Outcomes of Treatment

Antidepressant treatment could be complicated by the usual side effects of antidepressants (nausea, headaches, and others), including prolonged ejaculation or anorgasmia. Hormonal treatment could be complicated by numerous side effects such as weight gain, thrombophlebitis, pulmonary embolism, changes in sperm count and motility, hypertension, nausea, liver damage, erectile failure, elevated risk for depression, diabetes, insomnia, and others. Thus, various tests (blood pressure, blood glucose, weight, complete blood count, liver function tests, hormonal levels, bone density) should be done before treatment and monitored through the treatment.

Prognosis

The prognosis of untreated pedophilic disorder is poor.

Abel GG, Osborn C, Phipps AM. Pedophilia. In: Gabbard GO, ed. *Treatment of Psychiatric Disorders*. 3rd ed. Washington, DC: American Psychiatric Press; 2001:1981.

American Psychiatric Association. *Diagnostic and Statistical Manual of Mental Disorders*. 5th ed. Text Revision, Washington, DC: American Psychiatric Association; 2022

Bebbington PE. Treatment of male sexual deviation by use of vibrator: case report. *Arch Sex Behav*. 1977;6:21–24.

Bradford JM. Organic treatment for the male sexual offender. *Ann N Y Acad Sci*. 1988;528:193–202.

Freund K, Blanchard R. Phallometric diagnosis of pedophilia. *J Consult Clin Psychol*. 1989;57:100–105.

Gaffney GR, Lurie SF, Berlin FS. Is there familial transmission of pedophilia? *J Nerv Ment Dis*. 1984;172:546–548.

Perilstein RD, Lipper S, Friedman LJ. Three cases of paraphilia responsive to fluoxetine treatment. *J Clin Psychiatry*. 1991;52:169–170.

Ryback RS. Naltrexone in the treatment of adolescent sexual offenders. *J Clin Psychiatry*. 2004;65:982–986.

Schober JM, Kuhn PJ, Kovacs PG, et al. Leuprolide acetate suppresses pedophilic urges and arousability. *Arch Sex Behav*. 2005;34:691–705.

Wiebking C, Northoff G. Neuroimaging in pedophilia. *Curr Psychiatry Rep*. 2013;15:351.

FETISHISTIC DISORDER

General Considerations

Fetishistic disorder is usually considered relatively harmless. It frequently occurs in the frame of other paraphilic disorders (e.g., sadomasochism). The diagnosis requires recurrent, intense sexual arousal from either the use on nonliving objects or from a highly specific focus on non-genital body part(s) (partialism) manifested by fantasies, urges, or behavior. Again, it must be accompanied by distress and/or impairment and last at least 6 months.

A. Epidemiology

The incidence and prevalence of fetishistic disorder are unknown, partially because a large number of fetishism/fetishistic disorders do not reach *clinical* significance. Fetishistic disorder is more common among males, and in clinical samples it is nearly exclusively reported in men.

B. Etiology

The etiology of fetishistic disorder is unknown. According to psychoanalytical theories, a male child experiences anxiety about his mother's missing penis, for which he finds a symbolic object, and thus resolves this fear. The fetish may be linked to someone else whom the person was close to during childhood.

C. Genetics

No genetic findings regarding fetishistic disorder are available.

Clinical Findings

A. Signs & Symptoms

Fetishistic disorder is frequently ego-syntonic. There are numerous objects that could serve as a fetish. Frequent fetishes include women's underpants, bras, shoes, and other apparel. Highly eroticized body parts associated with fetishism include feet, toes, and hair. The person usually either masturbates while holding, rubbing, or smelling the fetish, or asks the sexual partner to wear it.

B. Psychological Testing

Psychological testing is not helpful in establishing the diagnosis of fetishistic disorder.

C. Laboratory Findings

There are no laboratory findings specific to fetishistic disorder.

D. Neuroimaging

There are no known imaging studies of fetishistic disorder.

Course of Illness

The course of fetishistic disorder tends to be fluctuating and chronic.

Differential Diagnosis (Including Comorbid Conditions)

Differential diagnosis includes transvestic disorder, sexual masochism disorder and other paraphilic disorders. Fetishism, that is, the use of fetish without any associated distress or impairment should also be ruled out. Fetishistic disorder is frequently comorbid with other paraphilic disorders (e.g., sexual masochism disorder) and hypersexuality.

Treatment

A. Psychopharmacological Interventions

Very little is known about psychopharmacological treatment of fetishism, as many people with fetishism live healthy, happy lives and consider their sexual interest or preoccupation to be a "gift." Several case reports describe treatment of fetishism with either antidepressants (fluoxetine, clomipramine) or antiandrogens and anxiolytics. Interestingly, one case report described treatment of fetishism with naltrexone.

B. Psychotherapeutic Interventions

Again, very little is known about psychotherapy of fetishism. Possibly useful modalities include psychoeducation, CBT, and individual psychodynamic psychotherapy, if distress is present.

C. Other Interventions

A classical conditioning paradigm with erections elicited by vibrator was used in one case.

Complications/Adverse Outcomes of Treatment

If antidepressants or antiandrogens are used, their various side effects mentioned previously may occur.

Prognosis

Prognosis is unknown, as most patients do not seek treatment and there are no outcome studies.

Bebbington PE. Treatment of male sexual deviation by use of a vibrator: a case report. *Arch Sex Behav.* 1977;6:21–24.

Fedoroff JP. The paraphilic world. In: Levine S, Risen C, Althof S, eds. *Handbook of Clinical Sexuality for Mental Health Professionals.* New York: Brunner-Routledge; 2003:333.

Firoz K, Sankar VN, Rajmohan V, et al. Treatment of fetishism with naltrexone: a case report. *Asian J Psychiatry.* 2014;8:67–68.

TRANSVESTIC DISORDER (FORMERLY TRANSVESTIC FETISHISM)

▶ General Considerations

The diagnostic consideration should be focused on whether transvestic disorder is associated with gender dysphoria, that is, discomfort with one's gender role or identity. Transvestic disorder is not necessarily heterosexual. The majority of transvestites who have been treated or volunteered for research are white, well-educated, currently or previously married, in their 40s, and began cross-dressing before the age of 12. The major feature of this disorder is recurrent and intense sexual arousal from cross-dressing that is clinically distressing (or causing impairment) and lasts at least 6 months. It should be specified whether it is transvestic disorder with fetishism (sexually aroused by fabrics, materials, garments, etc.) or with autogynephilia (sexually aroused by thoughts or images of self as female).

A. Epidemiology

The prevalence of transvestic disorder is unknown. In a random sample general population study from Sweden, 2.8% of males and 0.4% of females reported at least one episode of transvestic fetishism. No similar data from the United States are available. Transvestic disorder is more common among males.

B. Etiology

The etiology of transvestic disorder is unknown. The psychoanalytic explanation of this paraphilia frequently entertains the idea of unconscious fantasy of merging or identification with the mother.

C. Genetics

No genetic studies of transvestic disorder are available. There is some evidence for familial occurrence of transvestic disorder.

▶ Clinical Findings

A. Signs & Symptoms

Cross-dressing not only leads to sexual arousal but also decreases anxiety and elevates the mood of the person with transvestic fetishism. Transvestites may pass as a woman for a short period of time. Cross-dressing is a complex psychosexual phenomenon, and orgasm does not necessarily occur during all cross-dressing activities. The initial cross-dressing may be total or partial, with partial cross-dressing later progressing into full cross-dressing.

B. Psychological Testing

Psychological testing does not contribute to the diagnosis of thisdisorder.

C. Laboratory Findings

There are no laboratory tests useful for the diagnosis of transvestic disorder.

D. Neuroimaging

No neuroimaging findings specific to transvestic disorder are available.

▶ Course of Illness

Transvestic disorder usually begins during the first decade of life. The course is fluctuating and chronic. Some cases of transvestic disorder may progress into gender dysphoria.

▶ Differential Diagnosis (Including Comorbid Conditions)

The differential diagnosis includes other paraphilic disorders, namely fetishistic disorder, gender dysphoria, and personality disorders. Transvestic disorder frequently occurs together with fetishistic disorder and sexual masochism disorder. Other comorbid conditions include erectile disorder, alcohol use disorder, marital discord, persistent depressive disorder (dysthymia), major depression, and, infrequently, psychosis. It is important to note that unless the fantasies, urges, or behaviors involving cross-dressing are accompanied by distress or impairment, the diagnosis of fetishistic should not be made and this condition should be diagnosed as transvestism.

▶ Treatment

A. Psychopharmacological Interventions

Various psychotropic medications (e.g., buspirone; serotonergic antidepressants such as fluoxetine and sertraline; lithium) have been successfully used in cases of transvestic disorder. Hormones such as estrogens and antiandrogens (diethylstilbestrol, medroxyprogesterone acetate) have also been successfully used in some cases of this paraphilia. However, no studies of any treatment modality are available.

B. Psychotherapeutic Interventions

Psychodynamic psychotherapy has been the treatment of choice for transvestic disorder for a long time. It still remains an important part of a comprehensive treatment plan. CBT could probably be useful in transvestic disorder, too, but reports on its usefulness in this paraphilic disorder are not available. Marital therapy may be useful in cases of marital discord. Attendance at self-help groups and treatment of the spouse should also be included in the treatment of transvestic disorder.

C. Other Interventions

Electrical aversion techniques to apply operant conditioning were used in the past but are no longer considered ethical. Posthypnotic suggestion has also been used in transvestic disorder.

▶ Complications/Adverse Outcomes of Treatment

Complications of treatment include the various side effects of antidepressants and hormones (see "Pedophilic Disorders" section).

▶ Prognosis

The prognosis of transvestic disorder, especially untreated, is rather poor.

American Psychiatric Association. *Diagnostic and Statistical Manual of Mental Disorders.* 5th ed. Text Revision, Washington, DC: American Psychiatric Association; 2022.

Brown GR. Transvestism and gender identity disorder in adults. In: Gabbard GO, ed. *Treatment of Psychiatric Disorders.* 3rd ed. Washington, DC: American Psychiatric Press; 2001:2007.

Fedoroff JP. Buspirone hydrochloride in the treatment of transvestic fetishism. *J Clin Psychiatry.* 1988;49:408–409.

Langstrom N, Zucker KJ. Transvestic fetishism in the general population: prevalence and correlates. *J Sex Marital Ther.* 2005;31:87–95.

OTHER SPECIFIED PARAPHILIC DISORDER

This category, as noted in DSM-5-TR, applies to presentations in which symptoms are characteristic of a paraphilic disorder that cause distress and/or impairment in various areas of functioning, but do not meet full diagnostic criteria for any of the paraphilic disorders discussed in the group of paraphilic disorders. Some examples include telephone scatophilia (obscene phone calls), necrophilia (corpses), zoophilia (animals), olfactophilia (odors), coprophilia (feces), urophilia (urine), klismaphilia (enema), somnophilia (sleeping partner), abasiophilia (lame or crippled partner), apotemnophilia (own amputation), troilism (observing partner having sex with another person), and others.

American Psychiatric Association. *Diagnostic and Statistical Manual of Mental Disorders.* 5th ed. Text Revision. Washington, DC: American Psychiatric Association; 2022.

Eating Disorders

Griffin A. Stout, MD
Michael H. Ebert, MD

INTRODUCTION

Eating disorders are a complex, common, and multifactorial set of illnesses that have high mortality, morbidity, and poor quality of life. Nearly 30 million Americans will suffer from an eating disorder in their lifetime (Deloitte, 2020). Eating disorders affect at least 9% of the worldwide population (Arcelus et al, 2011). Those who suffer with eating disorders are at higher risk for death, suicide, and poor quality of life. Someone dies every 52 minutes from an eating disorder. Anorexia nervosa (AN) has the second highest mortality of all psychiatric illnesses, second only to opioid overdose. Approximately, one-quarter of patients with eating disorders attempt suicide (Arcelus et al, 2011). Since the COVID-19 pandemic, there has been an increase in disordered eating struggles and an increase in patients requiring both inpatient and outpatient care (Hartman et al, 2022).

Changes in the DSM-5 (American Psychiatric Association, 2013) with eating disorders include increasing inclusive language across the lifespan, sexes, and accounting for developmental changes in childhood and adolescents. Specific changes include the addition of binge eating disorder (BED), Avoidant Restrictive Food Intake Disorder, eliminating Eating Disorder Not Otherwise Specified in place of Otherwise Specified Feeding and Eating Disorder. These changes helped to diagnose patients of all genders, sexes, ages, and body sizes more accurately with the correct eating disorder. Accurate diagnosing helps patients receive the best possible treatment. Less than 6% of patients diagnosed with an eating disorder are also diagnosed as being "underweight" (Flament et al, 2015). Black, Indigenous and People of Color with eating disorders are half as likely to be diagnosed or to receive treatment (Deloitte 2020). Black teenagers are 50% more likely than white teenagers to struggle with binging and purging behaviors (Becker et al, 2015). Nearly 9 of 10 LGTBQ youth report being dissatisfied with their bodies (Trevor Project, 2023). Therefore, these changes to the DSM-5 are helpful in appropriately diagnosing and treating clients with disordered eating patterns.

One common potential precipitating factor of eating disorders is dieting behavior. Unfortunately, body dissatisfaction and dieting is common in society and youth. Forty-two percent of 1st and 3rd graders reported wanting to be thinner (Collins, 1999). Eighty-one percent of 10-year-old children are afraid of being fat (McNutt et al, 1997). Nearly half of 9–11-year-olds are "sometimes" or "very often" on diets (Gustafson-Larson et al, 1992). Around half of adolescent girls report crash dieting, fasting, self-induced vomiting, diet pills, or laxative use to control their body size (Boutelle et al, 2020). There are links to dieting behavior and eating disorder behaviors. By the time a youth is 15 years old, if they have engaged in dieting behaviors, they are 8 times more likely to develop an eating disorder (Patton et al, 2019).

Early detection is important to decrease the duration of illness. Eating disorders often start in childhood and adolescents; therefore, pediatricians and primary care providers should be aware and screen for these illnesses often and consistently, regardless of a patient's gender, sexuality, race, or ethnicity. The SCOFF or Eating Disorder Screen for Primary Care (ESP) can evaluate for the need for a further eating disorder assessment.

ESP

1. Are you satisfied with your eating patterns?*

2. Do you ever eat in secret?

3. Does your weight affect the way you feel about yourself?

4. Have any members of your family suffered with an eating disorder?

5. Do you currently suffer with or have you ever suffered in the past with an eating disorder?

---

*An answer of no on question 1 is abnormal, yes for questions 2–5 is abnormal. Two or more abnormal responses shows a sensitivity of 100% and a specificity of 71% (Cotton et al, 2003).

SCOFF

1. Do you make yourself **S**ick because you feel uncomfortably full?
2. Do you worry you have lost **C**ontrol over how much you eat?
3. Have you recently lost more than **O**ne stone (6.35 kg or 14 lbs) in a 3-month period?
4. Do you belief yourself to be **F**at when others say you are too thin?
5. Would you say **F**ood dominates your life?

Score of two or more "yes" indicates the need for further screening, sensitivity of 84.6% and specificity of 89.6% (Hill et al, 2010)

If screening positively, linking with treatment is important. Given the nutritional and medical concerns associated with these illnesses, multidisciplinary assessment and treatment is recommended per NICE guidelines. A treatment team should include a team that is trained in eating disorders, including a therapist, registered dietitian, medical provider, and psychiatrist. Together, the team can address all aspects and challenges associated with those who struggle with disordered eating. We will discuss these assessments and treatments in this chapter.

American Psychiatric Association. *Diagnostic and Statistical Manual of Mental Disorders.* 5th ed. Arlington, VA: American Psychiatric Association; 2013.

Arcelus J, Mitchell AJ, Wales J, Nielsen S. Mortality rates in patients with anorexia nervosa and other eating disorders: a meta-analysis of 36 studies. *Arch Gen Psychiatry.* 2011;68(7):724–731. doi:10.1001/archgenpsychiatry.2011.74

Becker AE, Franko DL, Speck A, Herzog DB. Ethnicity and differential access to care for eating disorder symptoms. *Int J Eating Disorders.* 2003;33(2):205–212. doi:10.1002/eat.10129

Boutelle K, Neumark-Sztainer D, Story M, Resnick M. Weight control behaviors among obese, overweight, and nonoverweight adolescents. *J Pediatr Psychol.* 2002;27(6):531–540. https://doi.org/10.1093/jpepsy/27.6.531

Collins ME. Body figure perceptions and preferences among preadolescent children. *Int J Eat Disord.* 1991;10:199–208. https://doi.org/10.1002/1098-108X(199103)10:2<199::AID-EAT2260100209>3.0.CO;2-D

Cotton MA, Ball C, Robinson P. Four simple questions can help screen for eating disorders. *J Gen Internal Med.* 2003;18(1):53–56.

Deloitte Access Economics. *The Social and Economic Cost of Eating Disorders in the United States of America: A Report for the Strategic Training Initiative for the Prevention of Eating Disorders and the Academy for Eating Disorders;* 2020. Available at: https://www.hsph.harvard.edu/striped/report-economic-costs-of-eating-disorders/.

Flament MF, Henderson K, Buchholz A, Obeid N, Nguyen HNT, Birmingham M, Goldfield G. Weight status and DSM-5 diagnoses of eating disorders in adolescents from the community. *J Am Acad Child Adolesc Psychiatry.* 2015;54(5):403–411.e2, ISSN 0890-8567, https://doi.org/10.1016/j.jaac.2015.01.020.

Gustafson-Larson AM, Terry RD. Weight-related behaviors and concerns of fourth-gradechildren. *J Am Dietetic Assoc.* 1992;92(7):818–822. https://pubmed.ncbi.nlm.nih.gov/1624650/

Hartmann-Munick SM, Lin JA, Milliren CE, Braverman PK, Brigham KS, Fisher MM, Golden NH, Jary JM, Lemly DC, Matthews A, Ornstein RM. Association of the COVID-19 pandemic with adolescent and young adult eating disorder care volume. *JAMA Pediatrics.* 2022;176(12):1225–1232.

Hill LS, Reid F, Morgan JF, Lacey JH. SCOFF, the development of an eating disorder screening questionnaire. *Int J Eat Disord.* 2010;43:344–351. https://doi.org/10.1002/eat.20679

LGBTQ Youth and Body Dissatisfaction; 2023. Retrieved February 6, 2023 from https://www.thetrevorproject.org/research-briefs/lgbtq-youth-and-body-dissatisfaction-jan-2023/

McNutt SW, Hu Y, Schreiber GB, Crawford PB, Obarzanek E, Mellin L. A longitudinal study of the dietary practices of black and white girls 9 and 10 years old at enrollment: the NHLBI Growth and Health Study. *J Adolesc Health.* 1997;20(1):27–37. https://doi.org/10.1016/S1054-139X(96)00176-0

Patton GC, Selzer R, Coffey CCJB, Carlin JB, Wolfe R. Onset of adolescent eating disorders: population-based cohort study over 3 years. *Bmj.* 1999;318(7186):765–768.

ANOREXIA NERVOSA

General Considerations

AN is a serious medical and psychological illness that involves a strong drive for thinness, intentional restriction of food intake, significant fear of gaining weight, and behaviors that interfere with weight restoration (F50.02). Malnutrition or a body weight that is below what is expected based on previous growth trajectories is a crucial piece of the diagnosis. This malnutrition can cause serious medical harm, and medical evaluations are important in the assessment and appropriate treatment of AN. AN has the second highest mortality rate (second to opioid use disorder) with a mortality rate of 5.6% per decade of illness (Moore and Boker, 2022). Mortality in AN is related to both medical malnutrition and increased risk of suicide. One out of five patients who die, die by suicide. The rate of death for 15–24-year-olds is 5 times higher than same age peers.

Etiology/Epidemiology

Lifetime prevalence of AN is 0.9% in females and 0.3% in males. Most cases of AN occur prior to the age of 25 (Hoek and Hoeken, 2003). The median age of onset is 12.3 years old (Swanson et al, 2011). There have been studies to show high heritability with AN, ranging from 16 to 74%, depending on if strict DSM or subthreshold criteria are used (Watson et al, 2019). Twin studies estimate heritability between 50 and 60% (Yilmaz et al, 2015).

Clinical Findings

Patients with AN typically present in teenage years to young adulthood. Often there is a presentation of an anxious, people-pleasing child who is introduced to the idea of weight loss or being "healthier" by an adult. Patients with AN may also have experienced bullying for their body size or shape or potentially even a traumatic event. Typically, a patient starts to make small "healthy" changes to their intake, for instance decreasing "junk food," eating less fast food, and increasing intake of fruit and vegetables. Unfortunately, this can turn into more severe dietary restriction, rigidity with how and what they eat and around whom they eat. They may restrict previously enjoyed foods or entire food groups related to "health" concerns. Patients may become preoccupied with discussing, preparing, and consuming food. Often patients may become more isolated or not join in social eating opportunities. Patient may attempt to hide their weight loss from others, at times wearing big, bulky clothes. If a physician or parent notes significant weight loss, often the patient is resistant to increasing intake, which can cause significant conflict and stress in the family system.

Potential signs and symptoms associated with AN may include weight loss, hypothermia, amenorrhea, lanugo, hypotension, bradycardia, hair loss, presyncope/syncope, cyanosis in extremities and cold intolerance/hypothermia. As mentioned above, given the potentially severe malnutrition that can occur, a medical evaluation is important through the assessment and treatment of AN. Medical complications of malnutrition can affect every body system. Most acutely is the cardiovascular system. Bradycardia is a common precipitator to the patient requiring inpatient medical stabilization and renourishment. Patient may also present with orthostatic hypotension, which should be monitored, and patient may require medical attention. Patients with AN often struggle with significant gastrointestinal concerns, including but not limited to decreased motility, constipation, increased abdominal pain, and bloating. In severe cases of malnutrition, a patient may experience superior mesenteric artery syndrome, which requires urgent medical attention and renourishment is the treatment. Please see Table 35–1 for laboratory abnormalities common in AN.

In patients who are severely malnourished, when renourishment occurs, it is important to monitor for the potentially deadly condition of refeeding syndrome. Refeeding syndrome occurs related to the shift of electrolytes related to insulin/glucose release after the body has experienced significant starvation. Refeeding syndrome can occur in patients of any age and weight. Factors that elevate a patient's risk of refeeding include chronic malnutrition, little to no energy intake for more than 10 days, severe malnutrition of less than 75% median BMI, rapid weight loss of greater than 10–15% of weight loss within 3–6 months, and significant alcohol intake. Prevention of refeeding includes medical hospitalization to monitor patient closely, baseline and daily evaluation of electrolytes with replacement, as necessary. Monitoring blood glucose and replacing as

Table 35–1 Laboratory Abnormalities in Anorexia Nervosa

Category	Common	Uncommon/Rare
Hematology	Leukopenia	Thrombocytopenia
Chemistry	Abnormal luteinizing hormone (LH) release	Hyperamylasemia
	Elevated cortisol	Hypomagnesemia
	Elevated liver functions	Hypophosphatemia
	Elevated serum bicarbonate	Metabolic acidosis
	Hypercarotenemia	
	Hypercholesterolemia	
	Hypochloremia	
	Hypokalemia	
	Hypozincemia	
	Low estrogen (females)	
	Low normal thyroxine (T^4)	
	Low triiodothyronine (T^3)	
Miscellaneous	Positive stool for occult blood	
Electrocardiogram	Sinus bradycardia	Arrhythmias
Electroencephalogram	Diffuse abnormalities	
Resting energy expenditure	Significantly reduced	
Brain imaging	Increased ventricular/brain ratio Widened cortical sulci	

necessary, daily multivitamin, potentially with thiamine in those at risk of Wernicke encephalopathy. With nutritional rehabilitation it is important to be thoughtful and not too aggressive. It is recommended to start at 1600–2400 kcal per day with increases of 200–500 kcal per day every 1–3 days. Caloric goal may be 3500–4000 kcal/day given their state of malnutrition, so a low and slow increase will be important (AED Report, 2021).

Neurologic changes are common for those with AN. Walter Kaye has theorized that there are traits that may affect serotonin modulation, which affects the dysregulation of reward pathways, so those with AN do not experience the pleasurable aspects of eating and misinterpret dietary restraint as either harm avoidant (avoiding the more dysphoric mood) or pleasurable. Patients with AN while acutely underweight have shown reduced gray matter volume and cortical thinning, which improves after treatment (King et al, 2018). Malnourished individuals with AN have shown to have altered concentrations of CRH, NPY, beta-endorphin, and leptin, which normalizes after recovery.

Differential Diagnosis/Comorbidities

Important medical causes to malnutrition and weight loss are important to rule out, as they have an organic etiology and should be treated medically. In a patient who presents with decrease appetite and weight loss, it is important to rule out diabetes mellitus, inflammatory bowel disease, celiac disease, thyroid disease, Addison disease, pregnancy, and malignancies (Campbell and Peebles, 2014). Those with AN often present with other psychiatric illnesses. Major depressive disorder in up to half of the patients. Half to three-quarters of patients with AN may struggle with major depressive disorder, and 30–65% may have anxiety as a comorbidity (Table 35–2). For those with AN, one-quarter may have obsessive–compulsive disorder. Substance abuse is less likely in those with AN compared to bulimia nervosa (BN), those with AN, specifically the binge eating/purging type 12–18% may struggle with substance abuse as well (Swanson et al, 2011).

Treatment

Early identification and intervention improve the overall prognosis and treatment for AN. Treatment for AN should include medical assessments, nutritional restoration, psychoeducation, and involve the patient's supports when appropriate (NICE guidelines). There are various levels of care in which a client with AN may be treated. The most restrictive, highest level of care is inpatient medical or psychiatric treatment. If a client is medically or psychiatrically unstable, they may require this close 24×7 monitoring. Next is residential level of care, which is also 24 hours a day; however, it does not incorporate the intensity of daily medical assessments and treatment. Partial Hospitalization Programs are often 5–7 days per week, allowing patient to be outside of programming in the evening hours. Intensive outpatient programs are often 3–5 hours per day, several days per week to continue to allow clients more freedom outside of treatment. Least restrictively is outpatient treatment where a client meets with multiple providers 1–2 times per week.

Nutritional restoration is critical. Without consistent and appropriate nutrition, the patient will not recover medically or psychologically. Weight restoration of 0.5–1 kg per week is important as many physical and psychological symptoms improve once malnutrition resolves.

For psychological treatment, in adolescents with AN, family-based therapy (FBT) is the recommended treatment. This treatment relies on the caregivers to assume all food-related decisions for the patient. This places nutritional restoration appropriately as the main initial goal of treatment. There are three phases with FBT. Phase 1 is focused on weight restoration, phase 2 slowly transitions control of eating back to the adolescent while maintaining weight/consistent nutrition, and phase 3 resolves any other comorbid psychological concerns, relapse prevention, and termination (Lock and LeGrange, 2013).

For adults and adolescents who are not able to participate in FBT, enhanced cognitive behavioral therapy (CBT-E) is an appropriate treatment. This treatment focuses on self-monitoring, psychoeducation on the harms of disordered eating patterns that helps the patient work on increasing nutrition and challenging negative cognitive distortions and misperceptions of their dietary intake and body (Linardon et al, 2017).

Psychopharmacologic treatments for AN are extremely limited. There is no evidence for the use of any psychotropic medication for weight recovery, anxiety, or depression in acute phase AN (Cassioli et al, 2020). As discussed above, psychiatric symptoms associated with AN, including but not limited to the obsessive nature and perseveration around eating, anxiety, depression, and suicidal thoughts, often resolve with weight restoration. Medications have potential side effects, especially in those who are malnourished. In these patients, it is important to keep in mind cardiac effects of psychotropics, including but not limited to delayed repolarization of ventricle, measured by the QT interval, orthostatic hypotension, and the potential decrease of the seizure threshold in malnourished clients. The World Federation of Societies of Biological Psychiatry (WFSBP) found olanzapine to be grade B (limited positive evidence) to help with symptoms associated with AN including weight restoration, improved depression anxiety, and obsessions. Other antipsychotics received a grade C (evidence from uncontrolled studies or case reports/expert opinion) (Aigner et al, 2011).

Complications/Adverse Outcomes of Treatment

It is important to remember that AN has the second highest mortality rate of any psychiatric illness (second only to opioid use disorder), and AN has a 5% mortality rate per decade from either medical complications or suicide (Moore and

Table 35–2 Comorbidity of Anorexia Nervosa

Disorder	Percentage
Anxiety disorders	60–65
Phobia	40–61
Obsessive–compulsive disorder	26–48
Mood disorders	36–68
Substance abuse	23–35
Personality disorders	23–35
Cluster A	<5
Cluster B	15–55
Cluster C	15–60

Bokor, 2021). Other potential long-term concerns of clients with AN are low bone mineral density, especially in clients with amenorrhea; however, it can occur in males and females who suffer from severe malnutrition.

Prognosis

Overall prognosis improves when effective, multidisciplinary treatment occurs as quickly as possible. Recovery from AN can be difficult to measure and quantify as the symptoms affect not only the nutritional state but also the mental state. Emotional recovery includes improved self-esteem, less obsession/worry about eating and body size/shape, and eating with significantly more freedom. Physical recovery includes weight restoration, return of typical pubertal progression. While many may achieve weight restoration, some individuals continue to struggle with pervasive disordered eating behaviors or beliefs. However, research shows that approximately 47% can recover with the return of menses and improved weight gain at 4–10 year follow-up and potentially as many as three-quarters can reach recovery beyond 10 year follow-up. Approximately 21% may struggle with chronic disordered eating (Steinhausen, 2002).

Academy for Eating Disorders. *Eating Disorders: A Guide to Medical Care Report*. 4th ed; 2021. 2120_AED_Medical_Care_4th_Ed_FINAL.pdf (higherlogicdownload.s3.amazonaws.com)

Aigner M, Treasure J, Kaye W, Kasper S, Disorders WTFOE. World Federation of Societies of Biological Psychiatry (WFSBP) guidelines for the pharmacological treatment of eating disorders. *World J Biol Psychiatry*. 2011;12(6):400–443. doi:10.3109/15622975.2011.602720

Campbell K, Peebles R. Eating disorders in children and adolescents: state of the art review. *Pediatrics*. 2014;134(3):582–592. 10.1542/peds.2014-0194

Cassioli E, Sensi C, Mannucci E, Ricca V, Rotella F. Pharmacological treatment of acute-phase anorexia nervosa: evidence from randomized controlled trials. *J Psychopharmacol*. 2020;34(8):864–873. doi:10.1177/0269881120920453

Hoek HW, van Hoeken D. Review of the prevalence and incidence of eating disorders. *Int J Eat Disord*. 2003;34(4):383–396. doi:10.1002/eat.10222. PMID: 14566926.

King JA, Frank GK, Thompson PM, Ehrlich S. Structural neuroimaging of anorexia nervosa: future directions in the quest for mechanisms underlying dynamic alterations. *Biol Psychiatry*. 2018;83(3):224–234.

Linardon J, Wade TD, de la Piedad Garcia X, Brennan L. The efficacy of cognitive-behavioral therapy for eating disorders: a systematic review and meta-analysis. *J Consult Clin Psychol*. 2017;85(11):1080–1094. https://doi.org/10.1037/ccp0000245

Lock J, LeGrange D. *Treatment Manual for Anorexia Nervosa: A Family Based Approach*., 2nd ed. New York: The Guilford Press; 2013.

Moore CA, Bokor BR. Anorexia nervosa. In: StatPearls [Internet]. Treasure Island (FL): Stat Pearls Publishing; 2022.

Steinhausen HC. The outcome of anorexia nervosa in the 20th century. *Am J Psychiatry*. 2002;159(8):1284–1293. doi: 10.1176/appi.ajp.159.8.1284. PMID: 12153817.

Swanson SA, Crow SJ, Le Grange D, Swendsen J, Merikangas KR. Prevalence and correlates of eating disorders in adolescents: results from the National Comorbidity Survey Replication Adolescent Supplement. *Arch Gen Psychiatry*. 2011;68(7):714–723. doi:10.1001/archgenpsychiatry.2011.22

Watson HJ, Yilmaz Z, Thornton LM, et al. Genome-wide association study identifies eight risk loci and implicates metabo-psychiatric origins for anorexia nervosa. *Nat Genet*. 2019;51(8):1207–1214.

Yilmaz Z, Hardaway JA, Bulik CM. Genetics and epigenetics of eating disorders. *Adv Genomics Genet*. 2015;5:131–150.

BULIMIA NERVOSA

General Considerations

Patients who suffer with BN share similarities with those with AN in that they have a strong drive for thinness, significantly negative body image and value the "thin ideal" and notice significant psychic distress if perceived to have gained weight or eaten inappropriately. Those with BN suffer with a cycle of restriction, binge, and purge episodes that lead to significant guilt and shame. One clinical difference is that those with BN have not suffered from significant weight loss and growth trajectories either indicate maintenance of body weight or potentially weight gain over time (insert DSMV criteria).

Etiology/Epidemiology

Lifetime prevalence of BN is 1.5% in females and 0.5% in males. Adolescent prevalence of BN is 0.9%. Similar to AN, the median age of onset for BN is 12.4 years old (Swanson et al, 2011). Genetic factors predispose approximately 28–83% for those with BN (Munn-Chernoff et al, 2021) (Table 35–3).

Clinical Findings

There are many similarities in patients who struggle with BN compared with AN. Those with BN are similarly driven to

Table 35–3 Prevalence Rate Estimates for Bulimia Nervosa

	Mean	Range
Binge eating	36%	7–75%
Weekly binge eating	16%	5–39%
DSM-III bulimia	9%	3–19%
DSM-III-R bulimia nervosa	2%	1–3%

Data from Devlin MJ et al. Is there another binge eating disorder? A review of the literature on overeating in the absence of bulimia nervosa. *Int J Eating Dis*. 1992;11:333; Fairburn CG, Beglin SJ. Studies of the epidemiology of bulimia nervosa. *Am J Psychiatry*. 1990;147:401; and Mitchell JE. *Bulimia Nervosa*. Minneapolis: University of Minnesota Press; 1990.

restrict and attempt to lose weight. However, for many reasons, the ability to consistently restrict throughout the day is not possible for patients with BN. They will suffer with binges, likely worsened by the fact they restrict throughout the day. These binges can cause such severe distress and shame, leading to the use of compensatory behaviors in an attempt to repair and avoid weight gain. Compensatory behaviors can include self-induced vomiting, compensatory and obsessive exercise, or inappropriate medication use (including but not limited to laxatives, diuretics, insulin, and stimulants).

Patients may present to providers with the desire to lose weight. A thorough and sensitive clinical examination and screening should occur as patients are not likely to self-disclose these behaviors due to the guilt and shame associated with them. Pertinent clinical signs that may raise suspicion for purging behaviors can include frequent weight fluctuations, increased time in bathroom after meals, salivary gland hypertrophy, erosion of dental enamel, calluses on knuckles of dominant hand (Russell's sign), petechiae, or hematemesis.

In fMRI studies of patients with BN, insular functioning and interoceptive networking are abnormal (Klabunde et al, 2017). Those with BN have higher measures of impulsivity, sensation seeking, novelty seeking, extremes of intense affect, impulse dysregulation, and lower distress tolerance (Frank, 2007).

Laboratory examination is important in the assessment of clients with BN due to the electrolyte shifts that can occur with self-induced vomiting. Comprehensive metabolic panel with calcium, magnesium, and phosphorus will evaluate for any electrolyte shifts that may indicate self-induced vomiting as well as requiring medical treatment. Sodium may be depleted in patients who abuse laxatives or are water loading to falsely elevate their weight. Potassium may be depleted with purging. Chloride may be decreased with vomiting or elevated due to laxative use. Blood urea nitrogen may be increased in dehydrated state, as well as creatinine may be elevated in patients with dehydration or potentially with renal failure. A low phosphate may be present in those with poor nutrition state or potentially in refeeding syndrome. Magnesium may be depleted in those abusing laxatives, or in refeeding syndrome. Patients may have low glucose or potentially elevated glucose depending on binge frequency. Amylase can be elevated in patients with self-induced vomiting and may be an indicator of a behavior if patient denies such behavior. A complete blood count with differential can evaluate for any anemia or potential blood loss. It is important to evaluate electrocardiogram (EKG) as well for those who are purging to evaluate for cardiac arrhythmias, bradycardia, or prolonged QTC interval (Gaudiani et al, 2014). It is important to recall that patients who are purging frequently may also be at risk for refeeding so nutritional rehabilitation should start low and go slow as described above. Monitoring lab work regularly is important (Table 35–4).

Table 35–4 Medical Complications of Bulimia Nervosa

Cardiovascular
Cardiomyopathy (with ipecac abuse)
Electrocardiogram changes and arrhythmias
Orthostatic hypotension

Dehydration and electrolyte abnormalities
Hypokalemia
Metabolic acidosis
Metabolic alkalosis

Dental
Increased caries
Upper incisor erosions

Dermatologic
Hand abrasions (Russell sign)
Petechial hemorrhages

Endocrine
Irregular menses and amenorrhea

Gastrointestinal
Cathartic colon (with laxative abuse)
Constipation
Esophageal/gastric perforations
Esophagitis/gastritis
Gastrointestinal bleeding
Salivary gland hypertrophy

Neurologic
Increased seizure frequency

▶ Differential Diagnosis/Comorbidities

Medical illnesses causing repetitive vomiting or overeating need to be considered when evaluating a patient suspected to have BN. Potentially these clients may have gastric outlet obstruction, rumination, hyperemesis gravidarum, cyclic vomiting, or inflammatory bowel disease. Clinical history, examination, and blood work can help differentiate BN from other illnesses.

Psychiatric comorbidities are common in patients with BN; 88% of youth and 94.5% of adults have at least one psychiatric comorbidity. Among adolescents with BN, 27% had three or more classes of comorbid disorders. Mood disorders were highly comorbid, including 18.5% reporting bipolar disorder type I or II, 26% reporting PTSD, and 22.1% reporting substance abuse disorder; a higher rate in those reporting any substance abuse or dependence (66.2%) (Swanson et al, 2011) (Table 35–5).

▶ Treatment

Treatment for BN requires multidisciplinary care as the symptomatology affects patient's physical and mental state. The disordered eating patterns in those with BN are often

Table 35–5 Comorbidity of Bulimia Nervosa

Disorder	Percentage
Mood disorders	24–88
Anxiety	2–3
Obsessive–compulsive disorder	3–80
Substance abuse	9–55
Personality disorders	
Cluster A	<10
Cluster B	2–75
Cluster C	16–80

amenable to cognitive behavioral therapy, which utilizes support, psychoeducation, and close monitoring to help decrease and eventually arrest the restrict, binge, and purge cycle. In younger children who have a supportive and available support system, family behavioral therapy has a treatment module for those with BN. This again places the caregiver in the decision-making role of dietary intake as well as closer supervision to decrease any purging behaviors that may occur. In patients who do not respond to these methods, interpersonal therapy, dialectical behavior therapy, and integrative cognitive-affective therapy may also be considered.

While medication should not be the sole treatment for BN, fluoxetine 60mg/day is FDA-approved in adults to help decrease urge to purge (Hagan and Walsh, 2021). Fluoxetine has been shown to be helpful for the symptoms of BN even in the absence of comorbid depression. Fluoxetine has a grade A from the WFSBP with good risk–benefit ratio in adults. However, current clinical guidelines continue to not recommend psychiatric medication for BN due to the lack of positive published studies (Gorrell and LeGrange, 2019). There has been one open-label trial of fluoxetine 60mg in 10 adolescents over 8 weeks (Kotler et al, 2003); however, more studies will help determine the safety and efficacy of this medication in the youth population.

Tricyclic antidepressants and topiramate have been studied in clients with BN and while it has shown a decrease in binge and purging behaviors, there are concerns related to the potential side effects including cardiac arrhythmias, toxicity in overdose, the risk of cognitive slowing, and kidney stones, so these medications are typically not recommended.

Complications/Adverse Outcomes of Treatment

Similar to patients with AN, medical complications can occur in all the organ systems. In clients who struggle with self-induced vomiting, laxative or diuretic use, monitoring electrolytes is important as hypokalemia and hypophosphatemia can occur. Cardiac arrhythmias may occur as well as orthostatic hypotension. The gastrointestinal system can be significantly affected with the persistent purging behaviors including esophagitis, Mallory–Weiss tears, constipation, cathartic colon, and rarely esophageal rupture. Patients with chronic self-induced vomiting are at risk for cardiomyopathy. Potentially ipecac abuse can lead to irreversible cardiomyopathy (Brotman et al, 1986).

Prognosis

There can be varied recovery for clients with BN. Often it can be nonlinear, affected by life events, stressors, trauma, and comorbidity. The highest recovery rates occur between years 4 and 9 of the disease. Around half can achieve full recovery, one-quarter have improved considerably, whereas another quarter have a chronic and protracted course of illness. There is a mortality rate of 0.32% per year (Steinhausen, 2009)

Frank GK, Bailer UF, Meltzer CC, et al. Regional cerebral blood flow after recovery from anorexia or bulimia nervosa. *Int J Eat Disord*. 2007;40(6):488–492.

Gaudiani JL, Sabel AL, Mehler PS. Low prealbumin is a significant predictor of medical complications in severe anorexia nervosa. *Int J Eat Disord*. 2014;47(2):148–156.

Gorrell S, Le Grange D. Update on treatments for adolescent bulimia nervosa. *Child Adolesc Psychiatr Clin N Am*. 2019;28(4): 537–547. doi:10.1016/j.chc.2019.05.002

Hagan KD, Walsh BT. State of the art: the therapeutic approaches to bulimia nervosa. *Clin Ther*. 2021;43(1):40–49. ISSN 0149-2918, https://doi.org/10.1016/j.clinthera.2020.10.012.

Isner JM. Effects of ipecac on the heart. *N Engl J Med*. 1986; 314(19):1253–1253.

Klabunde M, Collado D, Bohon C. An interoceptive model of bulimia nervosa: a neurobiologicalsystematic review. *J Psychiatr Res*. 2017;94:36–46. ISSN 0022-3956. https://doi.org/10.1016/j.jpsychires.2017.06.009.

Kotler LA, Devlin MJ, Davies M, Walsh BT. An open trial of fluoxetine for adolescents with bulimia nervosa. *J Child Adolesc Psychopharmacol*. 2003;13(3):329–335. doi:10.1089/104454603322572660

Munn-Chernoff MA, Johnson EC, Chou YL, et al. Shared genetic risk between eating disorder-and substance-use-related phenotypes: evidence from genome-wide association studies. *Addict Biol*. 2021;26(1):e12880.

Steinhausen HC. The outcome of anorexia nervosa in the 20th century. *Am J Psychiatry*. 2002;159(8):1284–1293. doi: 10.1176/appi.ajp.159.8.1284. PMID: 12153817.

Swanson SA, Crow SJ, Le Grange D, Swendsen J, Merikangas KR. Prevalence and Correlates of eating disorders in adolescents: results from the national comorbidity survey replication adolescent supplement. *Arch Gen Psychiatry*. 2011;68(7): 714–723. doi:10.1001/archgenpsychiatry.2011.22

BINGE EATING DISORDER

BED is a serious medical illness, the most common eating disorder that can affect individuals of all genders, body sizes, and socioeconomic status. As it was a new diagnosis in the DSM-V, long-term data are lacking. Clients can present similar to those with BN, as they can tend to struggle with a similar restrict and binge cycle; however, they do not participate in purging. Part of the clinical criteria includes guilt, shame, and embarrassment around these eating patterns. Therefore, self-disclosure or seeking care primarily for the binge behavior is rare. Patients often seek care to assist with weight reduction. In these clients, it is important to screen for binge eating behaviors. It is critical to recall that there is not a criteria of weight or BMI in BED. While some larger patients may struggle with binge eating, patients of any size may struggle with binge behaviors. A confounder in research on BED is often the frequent focus on weight loss as a studied outcome and if weight loss does not occur, the intervention is not effective; however, decreasing binge episodes is of utmost importance. Another diagnostic consideration is the difficulty in making this diagnosis in growing youth. There can be many factors that affect their dietary intake, pubertal development, activity, social norms and may make it difficult to obtain a clear history of "eating more than most would eat" or the feeling of loss of control.

Etiology/Epidemiology

BED is the most prevalent eating disorder with lifetime prevalence of 2.6% (Kessler et al, 2013). The male-to-female ratio is higher than with other eating disorders, with male-to-female ratio of 4 to 6 (Bohon, 2019). Median age of onset is higher than in other eating disorders, late teens to early 20s (Kessler et al, 2013). BED has shown to be highly heritable with studies suggesting 41–57% heritability, independent of obesity (Yilmaz et al, 2015). Prevalence of BED in youth is estimated to be 1–3% (Smink et al, 2014).

Clinical Findings

Often a patient with BED may present in a larger body, approximately two-thirds have a BMI greater than 30. However, it is critical to remember that not every obese individual suffers from BED and not every person who suffers from BED is obese. Again, weight is not a criterion for BED; the symptoms are related to eating behaviors and the emotional and physical feelings associated with eating larger portions of food than intended. Clients with BED compared to those in larger bodies without BED had more chaotic eating habits, higher levels of eating disinhibition, and higher levels of eating disorder psychopathy (Wilfley et al, 2000). Clients with BED suffer as greatly with body image disturbances as those with AN and BN. Often patients are in a cycle of restricting throughout the day in order to control their body size; however, they lose control towards the end of the day or when they can eat in secret. At times, a binge can be used to cope with or numb psychic distress. At times patient can describe a near dissociation and lose control of what they are eating. The foods chosen tend to be "high value" foods that a patient attempts to restrict typically to attempt to lose weight.

Potential risk factors for developing BED include adverse childhood experiences, negative comments about shape/weight and eating, experiencing weight stigma or weight-based bullying, parental depression (Fairburn et al, 1998).

Given potential weight fluctuations, patients may be at higher risk for metabolic syndrome, abnormalities in blood glucose, elevated lipids, and higher blood pressure. It is important to know that weight cycling itself (gaining weight, losing weight, gaining weight) is an independent risk factor for cardiovascular disease, inflammation, high blood pressure, and insulin resistance. So patients can decrease risk by consistently fueling their body rather than utilizing extreme diets that are not feasible for the patient long term.

Differential Diagnosis/Comorbidities

In terms of differential diagnosis, it is important to rule out other medical causes for excessive eating including Klein–Levin syndrome, Prader Willi. The highest comorbidity with BED is major depressive disorder reported in 50–60%. Patients with BED also report elevated rates of alcohol use disorder and anxiety disorders. It is noted that males with BED have higher rate of substance use disorders (57%) than females (28%) (Grilo, 2002). Neurobiological findings show impairments in reward processing, inhibitory control, and emotion regulation (Giel et al, 2022).

Treatment

As with all eating disorders, a multidisciplinary team is necessary. Nutritional adequacy and consistency is important with all clients, especially those with BED who, if in a larger body, may have been told to restrict throughout the day, which can increase the risk for binges later in the day, especially in secret related to shame. Patients with BED often are amenable to treatment, primarily with self-help programs as well as CBT-E (Hilbert, 2020). If CBT-E is not possible, patients may respond to IPT (Hilbert, 2012).

There are very limited studies on treating BED in youth; however, there is one FDA-approved medication for adults, lisdexamfetamine dimesylate (LDX) for moderate to severe BED. LDX is most effective at dose of 50–70 mg/day and is effective for decreasing binge episodes, symptoms, and obsessive–compulsive features of BED (Citrome et al, 2015; McElroy et al, 2015). LDX is a controlled substance; therefore, it is important to monitor its use carefully not only as it is a stimulant, but one that can be used inappropriately to decrease appetite as a potential compensatory purging behavior. Topirimate has also been studied and Claudino et al (2007) determined that there was benefit in using this medication to augment CBT treatment. It is important to keep in mind topiramate's side effect profile, and the studies with this medication had higher dropout rates.

Complications

If untreated, patients with BED may continue to struggle with uncontrolled eating, attempts at weight loss, weight cycling, and increased stress. If a patient struggling with BED is in a larger body, it is also possible they may have experienced weight stigma. Weight stigma is prevalent, especially during medical appointments. It has been theorized that a client who experiences weight stigma, notes increased stress, cortisol production, perpetuated restrict/binge cycle, and therefore increased weight gain (Tomiyama, 2014). There is also a well-established association of patient's experiencing weight stigma and increasing disordered eating patterns (Vartanian and Porter, 2016).

Prognosis

Following patients over 5 years, one study showed that the disease remits over time. In this study, only 18% of patients received eating disorder treatment (Fairburn, 2000). However, a more stringent 4-year study that did not include subthreshold cases showed that 38% continued to struggle with full criteria at 1 year follow-up and 55% met criteria for eating disorder not otherwise specified (Crow, 2002). Therefore, prognosis improves if clients are linked with treatment. Clinicians should consistently and nonjudgmentally assess for disordered eating patterns in individuals of all shapes/sizes so as to not undertreat those with disordered eating patterns.

Bohon C. Binge eating disorder in children and adolescents. *Child Adolesc Psychiatr Clin N Am.* 2019;28(4):549–555. doi:10.1016/j.chc.2019.05.003

Citrome L. Lisdexamfetamine for binge eating disorder in adults: a systematic review of the efficacy and safety profile for this newly approved indication—what is the number needed to treat, number needed to harm and likelihood to be helped or harmed? *Int J Clin Pract.* 2015;69(4):410–421. doi:10.1111/ijcp.12639

Claudino AM, de Oliveira IR, Appolinario JC, et al. Double-blind, randomized, placebo-controlled trial of topiramate plus cognitive-behavior therapy in binge-eating disorder. *J Clin Psychiatry.* 2007;68(9):1324–1332. doi:10.4088/jcp.v68n0901

Crow SJ, Agras WS, Halmi K, Mitchel, JE, Kraemer HC. Full syndromal versus subthreshold anorexia nervosa, bulimia nervosa, and binge eating disorder: a multicenter study. *Int J Eat Disord.* 2002;32:309–318.

Fairburn CG, Doll HA, Welch SL, Hay PJ, Davies BA, O'Connor ME. Risk factors for binge eating disorder: a community-based, case-control study. *Arch Gen Psychiatry.* 1998;55(5):425–432.

Fairburn CG, Cooper Z, Doll HA, Normal P, O'Connor M. The natural course of bulimia nervosa and binge eating disorder in young women. *Arch Gen Psychiatry.* 2000;57:659–665.

Giel KE, Bulik CM, Fernandez-Aranda F, et al. Binge eating disorder. *Nat Rev Dis Primers.* 2022;8:16. https://doi.org/10.1038/s41572-022-00344-y

Hilbert A, Bishop ME, Stein RI, et al. Long-term efficacy of psychological treatments for binge eating disorder. *Br J Psychiatry.* 2012;200(3):232–237. doi:10.1192/bjp.bp.110.089664

Hilbert A, Petroff D, Herpertz S, et al. Meta-analysis on the long-term effectiveness of psychological and medical treatments for binge-eating disorder. *Int J Eat Disord.* 2020;53(9):1353–1376. doi:10.1002/eat.23297

Kessler RC, Berglund PA, Chiu WT, et al. The prevalence and correlates of binge eating disorder in the World Health Organization World Mental Health Surveys. *Biol Psychiatry.* 2013;73(9):904–914. doi:10.1016/j.biopsych.2012.11.020

McElroy SL, Hudson JI, Mitchell JE, et al. Efficacy and safety of lisdexamfetamine for treatment of adults with moderate to severe binge-eating disorder: a randomized clinical trial. *JAMA Psychiatry.* 2015;72(3):235–246. doi:10.1001/jamapsychiatry.2014.2162

Smink FR, van Hoeken D, Oldehinkel AJ, Hoek HW. Prevalence and severity of DSM-5 eating disorders in a community cohort of adolescents. *Int J Eat Disord.* 2014;47(6):610–619. doi:10.1002/eat.22316

Tomiyama AJ. Weight stigma is stressful. A review of evidence for the Cyclic Obesity/Weight-Based Stigma model. *Appetite.* 2014;82:8–15. ISSN 0195-6663, https://doi.org/10.1016/j.appet.2014.06.108.

Vartanian LR, Porter AM. Weight stigma and eating behavior: a review of the literature. *Appetite.* 2016;102:3–14. ISSN 0195-6663, https://doi.org/10.1016/j.appet.2016.01.034.

Wilfley DE, Friedman MA, Dounchis JZ, Stein RI, Welch RR, Ball SA. Comorbid psychopathology in binge eating disorder: relation to eating disorder severity at baseline and following treatment. *J Consult Clin Psychol.* 2000;68(4):641.

Yilmaz Z, Hardaway JA, Bulik CM. Genetics and epigenetics of eating disorders. *Adv Genomics Genet.* 2015;5:131–150. doi:10.2147/AGG.S55776

AVOIDANT RESTRICTIVE FOOD INTAKE DISORDER

Essentials of Diagnosis

Avoidant Restrictive Food Intake disorder (ARFID) is a reconceptualization from DSM-IV Feeding Disorder of Infancy and Early Childhood, which was a diagnosis for children 6 years old and younger. This new diagnosis incorporates multiple potential drivers for restriction, including low drive for food, picky eating, sensory struggles with eating, or negative consequences from eating. Patients who struggle with ARFID do not struggle with body image issues or a drive for thinness. They often express wanting to gain weight and restore to their previous body size or shape. (F50.82).

General Considerations

Patients with ARFID tend to present at younger ages, often presenting at 11–14 years old. Overall prevalence is unclear and varies from less than 1–15% depending on the studies (Bourne et al, 2020). Similar to BED, males have a higher prevalence of this disorder compared with AN and BN; however, females more commonly present with this disorder.

Etiology is multifactorial and can be affected by medical and psychiatric comorbidities. For example, one retrospective case-controlled study looked at 712 individuals aged 8–18 with ARFID, 28.7% had selective eating from early childhood, 21.4% had generalized anxiety, 19.4% presented with gastrointestinal symptoms that negatively impacting eating, 4.1% had food allergies, and 13.2% had other reasons for their restrictions (Fisher et al, 2014).

▶ Clinical Findings

Often younger children present with significant weight loss, restricted appetite, and food choices. Patients often tend to prefer higher calorie/higher value foods such as pasta, chicken nuggets, pizza. Patients often can be significantly particular about the type or brand of food they prefer. Often patients may refuse or restrict fruits or vegetables, especially as their taste and texture can vary. For instance, two grapes from the same bunch may taste very different; however, one brand of chicken nuggets may stay consistent.

It is important to evaluate for any aversive experiences with food, including but not limited to stressful eating environments, choking or near choking experiences, fear of vomiting, pain, or negative physical experiences with food.

▶ Differential Diagnosis

When diagnosing ARFID, it is important to rule out other illnesses including organic gastrointestinal diseases such as GERD, IBD, iron deficiency, food insecurity, or culturally sanctioned processes such as religious fasting.

Psychiatric comorbidities are higher in this population including higher rates of OCD, GAD, autism, learning disorders, and cognitive impairment.

▶ Treatment

There are limited studies on treatment for ARFID. A multidisciplinary treatment approach is recommended as well as parental psychoeducation on the illness and support to help with nutritional restoration. It appears patients with ARFID are amenable to CBT. There are two case studies on utilization of Risperidone. (Pennell et al 2020) (Naguy et al, 2022). As the rate of comorbidities is common, treating any psychiatric comorbidities can be helpful for treating the ARFID as well, especially anxiety illnesses.

▶ Complications

Complications are primarily related to the malnutrition that can be present. Prognosis of this illness is unknown; however, the longer a patient struggles with this pattern of eating, the more difficult it tends to be to see significant improvement.

Bourne L, Bryant-Waugh R, Cook J, Mandy W. Avoidant/restrictive food intake disorder: a systematic scoping review of the current literature. *Psychiatry Res.* 2020;288:112961. doi:10.1016/j.psychres.2020.112961

Fisher MM, Rosen DS, Ornstein RM, et al. Characteristics of avoidant/restrictive food intake disorder in children and adolescents: a "new disorder" in DSM-5. *J Adolesc Health.* 2014;55(1):49–52.

Naguy A, Al-Humoud AM, Pridmore S, Abuzeid MY, Singh A, Elsori D. Low-dose risperidone for an autistic child with comorbid ARFID and misophonia. *Psychopharmacol Bull.* 2022;52(1):91–94.

Pennell A, Couturier J, Grant C, Johnson N. Severe avoidant/restrictive food intake disorder and coexisting stimulant treated attention deficit hyperactivity disorder. *Int J Eat Disord.* 2016;49(11):1036–1039.

Sleep Disorders

Camellia P. Clark, MD
Polly J. Moore, PhD
J. Christian Gillin, MD[†]

This chapter primarily focuses on sleep and sleep disorders in adults. Although many basic and clinical aspects are similar in children, developmental issues and some disorders not present in adults, such as sudden infant death syndrome, are beyond the scope of this chapter. For further information, the reader is referred to *Principles and Practice of Pediatric Sleep Medicine*. 2nd Ed. (Sheldon, Kryger, Gozal & Ferber 2014).

GENERAL APPROACH TO THE PATIENT

▷ Office Evaluation

Clinicians should ask routinely about sleep and wakefulness. A thorough sleep history lays the foundation for accurate diagnosis and effective treatment of sleep disorders (Table 36–1). Patients' sleep complaints will usually fall into four general categories: complaints of difficulty initiating sleep or staying asleep (insomnia); difficulty staying awake during the day (hypersomnia); abnormal movements or behavior during sleep (parasomnia); timing of the sleep–wake cycle at undesired or inappropriate times over a 24-hour day (circadian rhythm disorder); or a combination of the above.

During the evaluation, the patient's bed partner or other informants should be included whenever possible. Because the patient may be unaware of sleep and wakefulness difficulties, bed partners often initiate the sleep evaluation for sleep apnea, periodic limb movements (PLMs) during sleep, or excessive daytime sleepiness (EDS). Sleep disorders can be disruptive to a household, not just the patient (e.g., sleepwalking, loud snoring).

The clinician should take a thorough history of all pertinent medical and psychiatric problems and family history; review medications, personal relationships, and environmental stressors; conduct a review of systems; and complete a physical examination including a thorough neurologic examination.

[†]Deceased

▷ Sleep Laboratory Evaluation

Most sleep complaints can be managed by the nonspecialist, with the motivation and cooperation of the patient, through behavioral modification, treatment of underlying and comorbid diagnoses, and appropriate use of medication for symptomatic relief of sleep-related symptoms. For sleep apnea, PLMs during sleep, narcolepsy, parasomnias with potential for serious injury, or intractable insomnia, referral to a sleep disorder center should be considered.

Nocturnal polysomnography (PSG) records the patient's sleep overnight in a sleep laboratory. Polygraphic sleep recordings are obtained in a quiet, dark, comfortable laboratory environment. Surface electrodes are affixed to the skin to monitor the electroencephalogram (EEG), bilateral eye movement activity or electrooculogram (EOG), and chin muscle tonus or electromyogram (EMG). Sleep staging is determined by a scanning of these tracings visually. The anterior tibial EMG reflects PLMs when present. Additional physiologic monitoring includes respiratory effort monitoring of the chest and abdomen, airflow such as end tidal CO_2 or nasal–oral thermistor, blood O_2 saturation, and electrocardiogram.

Changes in EEG frequencies discriminate waking and non–rapid eye movement (non-REM) sleep stages; the concurrent presence of eye movements in the EOG. A dramatic decrease in muscle tone in the EMG and a desynchronized EEG distinguish rapid eye movement (REM) sleep. Table 36–2 defines terms commonly used in sleep studies.

OVERVIEW OF SLEEP

▷ Sleep Stages & Architecture

Normal sleep involves two states: REM sleep and non-REM sleep. REM sleep is often associated with dreaming.

Table 36–1 Office Evaluation of Chronic Sleep Complaints

1. Detailed history and review of the sleep complaint, as well as predisposing, precipitating, and perpetuating factors
2. Review of the difficulties falling asleep, maintaining sleep, and awakening early
3. Timing of sleep and wakefulness over the 24-h day
4. Evidence of excessive daytime sleepiness and fatigue
5. Bedtime routines, sleep setting, preoccupations, anxiety, beliefs about sleep and sleep loss, fears about consequences of sleep loss, nightmares, enuresis, and sleepwalking
6. Medical and neurologic history and examination and routine laboratory examinations
7. Review of use of prescription and nonprescription medications, hypnotics, alcohol, and stimulants
8. Evidence of sleep-related breathing disorders: snoring; orthopnea, dyspnea; headaches; falling out of bed; nocturia; obesity; short, fat neck; enlarged tonsils; narrow upper oral airway; and foreshortened jaw (retrognathia)
9. Abnormal movements during sleep; "jerky legs," leg movements, myoclonus, "restless legs," leg cramps, and cold feet
10. Psychiatric history and examination
11. Social and occupational history, marital status, living conditions, financial and security concerns, and physical activity
12. Sleep environment—ambient noise, light, and temperature
13. Sleep–wake diary for 2 weeks
14. Typical exposure to light (sunlight and artificial) and darkness across a 24-h day
15. Interview with bed partners or persons who observe the patient during sleep
16. Recording of respiratory sounds during sleep to screen for sleep apnea

Adapted from Gillin JC, Ancoli-Israel S. The impact of age on sleep and sleep disorders. In: Salzman C, ed. *Clinical Geriatric Psychopharmacology.* 4th ed. Baltimore: Lippincott Williams & Wilkins; 2005:492.

Non-REM sleep is a period of decreased physiologic and psychological activity and is further divided into stages 1, 2, 3, and 4 on the basis of visually scored EEG patterns.

Sleep normally begins with non-REM stage 1, before progressing successively into non-REM stages 2 through 4, during which the EEG generally declines in frequency and increases in amplitude. Stages 3 and 4 of sleep, also called slow-wave sleep (SWS), are typically most intense early in the sleep period. The amount of SWS declines across the night. REM sleep is characterized by high-frequency, low-amplitude EEG; loss of muscle tone in the major antigravity muscles; and REMs (Figure 36–1).

The Neurobiology of Sleep

The neurophysiologic underpinnings of sleep and wakefulness are incompletely understood. Aspects of REM sleep such as periodic REMs and atonia are generated within the

brainstem. Non-REM sleep is partially controlled by rostral brain regions such as the hypothalamus, basal forebrain, and thalamus.

A variety of neurotransmitter systems and brain regions appear to regulate sleep and wakefulness. The arousal network involves the activity of neurons containing acetylcholine, norepinephrine, serotonin, orexin (hypocretin), and dopamine (DA), whereas gamma-aminobutyric acid (GABA)-ergic mechanisms figure prominently in initiating non-REM sleep.

Sleep & Circadian Rhythms

The rhythm of sleep and wakefulness is governed by one or more internal biological "clocks," by environmental stimuli, and by a host of processes that promote or inhibit arousal (Table 36–3). In the absence of *zeitgebers* (time cues such as social activities, meals, and bright lights), humans tend to self-select a sleep–wake cycle of about 25 hours from wake time to wake time. In other words, if a person lives in an experimental environment free of time cues and is allowed to go to bed and arise at will, that person will tend to go to sleep about an hour later each "night" and wake up about an hour later each "morning." For this reason, shifts in the sleep–wake cycle activity are usually easier when the cycle is lengthened rather than shortened—in traveling west rather than east, for example—or when rotating from an afternoon to an evening work shift, rather than from an afternoon to a morning work shift.

Normally, the circadian oscillator is entrained to the 24-hour environment by zeitgebers such as social activities and meals, and especially by environmental light. Information about light reaching the retina is conveyed to the suprachiasmatic nuclei (SCN) in the anterior hypothalamus. The SCN are important oscillators that maintain the circadian rhythm of sleep–wakefulness.

In addition to synchronizing the circadian oscillator with the environment, the timing of light exposure can also shift the phase position of the oscillator (i.e., the temporal relationship between rhythms or between one rhythm and the environment). Bright light (1500 lux) in the evening hours (6–9 PM) coupled with darkness from 9 PM to 9 AM tends to cause a phase delay in sleep–wake and other biological oscillators (i.e., one would go to bed later and wake up later). In contrast, exposure to bright light in the early morning hours (5–7 AM) coupled with darkness in the evening tends to advance the phase position of the oscillator (i.e., one would go to bed earlier and wake up earlier). Furthermore, bright light during daylight hours can enhance the amplitude of the circadian rhythm, thereby demarcating the periods of both nocturnal sleep and daytime wakefulness. Bright light has been reported to have antidepressant effects in seasonal depressions occurring in the winter and in some patients with major depressive disorder or premenstrual depression.

Table 36–2 Glossary of Terms Used in Sleep Studies

Term	Definition
Polysomnography (PSG)	Multichannel physiologic recording of sleep
REM sleep	Rapid eye movement sleep, characterized by bursts of rapid eye movements, low-voltage fast EEG, and atonia; associated with dreaming
Non-REM (or NREM) sleep	Non–rapid eye movement sleep; consists of four stages
Stage 1	A transitional state of lighter sleep between wakefulness and full sleep; characterized by low voltage, mixed frequency EEG and slow rolling eye movements
Stage 2	Sleep characterized by EEG waveforms called K-complexes and spindles, usually around 50–75% of TST
Stage 3	Sleep characterized by 20–50% high-amplitude slow EEG waves
Stage 4	Sleep characterized by >50% high-amplitude slow EEG waves
Total sleep time (TST)	Total minutes of non-REM sleep + total minutes REM sleep
Sleep latency	Elapsed time from "lights out" to onset of sleep
REM latency	Elapsed time from sleep onset to REM onset; normally varies from 70–100 min (in young adults) to 55–70 minutes (in elderly); may be abnormally short in narcolepsy, depression, and other conditions
Sleep efficiency (SE)	Time asleep divided by total time in bed; usually expressed as a percentage, normally ≥90% in young adults; decreases somewhat with age
Wakefulness after sleep onset (WASO)	Time spent awake after sleep onset
Respiratory disturbance index (RDI)	Respiratory events (apneas + hypopneas) per hour of sleep; sometimes referred to as apnea-hypopnea index (AHI)
Apnea	A cessation of airflow of 10 seconds or longer
Hypopnea	A reduction by 50% in airflow of 10 seconds or longer
Multiple Sleep Latency Test (MSLT)	An objective measure of EDS in which sleep latency and REM latency are measured during four to five 20-minute nap opportunities spaced 2 hours apart across the day
Periodic limb movements (PLMs)	Intermittent (every 20–40 seconds) leg jerks or leg kicks during sleep

Adapted from Salzman C. *Clinical Geriatric Psychopharmacology*, 4th ed. Baltimore: Lippincott Williams & Wilkins; 2005.

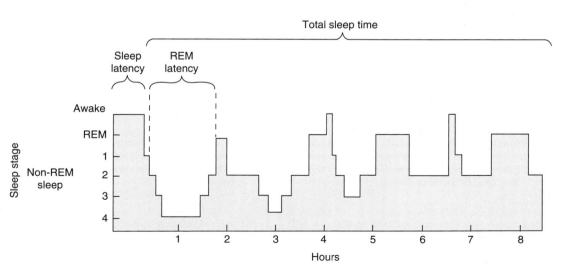

▲ **Figure 36–1** Hypnogram of sleep stages in young versus old. (Adapted with permission from Ancoli-Israel S. *All I Want Is a Good Night's Sleep*. Philadelphia: Mosby Books; 1999.)

Table 36–3 Glossary: Terms Commonly Used in the Study of Circadian Rhythms

Term	Definition
Chronobiology	The study of circadian rhythms
Circadian rhythms	Refers to biological rhythms having a cycle length of about 24 hour. Derived from Latin: *circa dies*, "about 1 day." Examples include the sleep–wake cycle in humans and temperature, cortisol, and psychological variation over the 24-hour day. Characterized by exact cycle length, amplitude, and phase position.
Phase position	Temporal relationship between rhythms or between one rhythm and the environment. For example, the maximum daily temperature peak usually occurs in the late afternoon.
Phase-advanced rhythm	Patient retires and arises early.
Phase-delayed rhythm	Patient retires and arises late.
Zeitgebers	Time cues such as social activities, meals, and bright lights.

Adapted with permission from Salzman C. *Clinical Geriatric Psychopharmacology*, 4th ed. Baltimore: Lippincott Williams & Wilkins; 2005.

Sleep Changes with Development & Aging

Sleep–wake states change dramatically across the life span, not only with regard to the amount of sleep but also to circadian timing. With advancing age, REM latency tends to decrease and the length of the first REM period tends to increase.

The amount of time spent each night in SWS is high in childhood, peaks in early adolescence, and gradually declines with age until it nearly disappears around the sixth decade of life. Young adults typically spend about 15–20% of total sleep time (TST) in SWS. Sleep tends to be shallower, more fragmented, and shorter in duration in middle-aged and elderly adults compared to young adults. In addition, daytime sleepiness increases. The relative amount of "shallower" stages 1 and 2 sleep tends to increase as the "deeper" stages 3 and 4``````` sleep tend to decrease. Men tend to lose SWS at an earlier age than women do.

After the age of 65, about one in three women and one in five men report that they take over 30 minutes to fall asleep. Wakefulness after sleep onset (WASO) and number of arousals increase with age, an increase that may be due at least in part to the greater incidence of sleep-related breathing disorders, PLMs, and other physical conditions in these age groups. WASO may also increase with age because older people are more easily roused by internal and external stimuli.

Changes in the circadian rhythm may lead to daytime fatigue, napping, and poor nocturnal sleep. Related to a phase-advanced temperature rhythm, elders tend to retire and arise earlier than younger adults. Psychosocial alterations can disrupt zeitgebers and light exposure. Napping also increases with age, but the TST per 24 hours does not change with age.

▼ CLINICAL SYNDROMES

This section follows the system in the *International Classification of Sleep Disorders*, Revised (ICSD-2), which groups sleep complaints by primary symptomatology: insomnia, or disorders of initiating and maintaining sleep; hypersomnia, or disorders of EDS (Excessive Daytime Sleep); parasomnias; and circadian rhythm disorders. The section also comprises a brief discussion of sleep alterations associated with psychiatric disorders, substance use, medical conditions, and the reproductive cycle.

INSOMNIA

▶ General Considerations

Insomnia is the complaint of difficulty initiating or maintaining sleep or of nonrestorative sleep (not feeling well rested after sleep that is adequate in amount). Insomnia is more common in women than in men; more common with age; and often associated with medical and psychiatric disorders or use of alcohol, drugs, and medication.

▶ Clinical Findings

Transient insomnia is much more common than chronic (>1 month) insomnia. It generally results from acute stress. Many such cases resolve without intervention. PSG abnormalities have been documented in acute bereavement. However, persistent insomnia should raise the consideration of depression, adjustment disorder, or other psychiatric disorders. Psychophysiologic insomnia is a "disorder of somatized tension and learned sleep-preventing associations that result in a complaint of insomnia" (ICSD-2 1997). All patients with chronic insomnia probably develop learned sleep-preventing associations, such as marked overconcern with the inability to sleep. The frustration, anger, and anxiety associated with trying to sleep or maintain sleep serve only to arouse them further as they struggle to sleep. These patients can acquire aversive associations with their bedrooms, often sleeping better in other places such as in front of the television set, in a hotel, or in the sleep laboratory. Psychophysiologic insomnia can become chronic.

Table 36–4 Stimulus-Control Treatment

Keep bedtimes and awakening constant, even on the weekends.
Do not use the bed for watching television, reading a book, or working. If sleep does not begin within a period of time, say, 30 minutes, leave the bed and do not return until drowsy.
Avoid napping.
Exercise regularly (3–4 times per week) but try to avoid exercising in the early evening if this tends to interfere with sleep.
Discontinue or reduce alcohol, caffeine, cigarettes, and other substances that may interfere with sleep.
"Wind down" before bed with quiet or relaxing activities.
Maintain a cool, comfortable, and quiet sleeping environment.

Differential Diagnosis

Because chronic insomnia is so commonly caused by medical, psychiatric, or substance use comorbidity or in association with medication, the clinician should always look carefully for other conditions and treat the primary disorder. Although 780.59 Breathing-Related Sleep Disorder is classified as a hypersomnia, apneic episodes can cause insomnia. Insomnia can also be associated with sleep-related movement disorders, for example, restless legs syndrome (RLS) and PLMs (discussed separately).

Treatment

Nonpharmacologic treatment includes education about sleep hygiene (Table 36–4, Stimulus-Control Treatment) as well as identifying and correcting faulty beliefs—for example, the fear of not being able to function at all without 8 hours of uninterrupted sleep.

Sleep restriction therapy involves gradually improving sleep consolidation (minimizing interruptions of the nocturnal sleep period) by limiting the time patients spend in bed. Many insomniac patients underestimate actual sleep time ("sleep state misperception") and have poor sleep efficiency (SE). If the patient reports sleeping 6 hours per night, he or she is required to limit time in bed to 6 hours or slightly

more. This simple maneuver usually produces mild sleep deprivation, shortens sleep latency, and increases SE. As sleep becomes more consolidated, the patient is allowed gradually to increase time in bed. It may be helpful to counsel for acute stressors and break the "vicious cycle" of psychophysiological insomnia.

Weighted blankets are popular, but safety concerns have been raised about small children and the elderly.

Meditation is good for sleep problems. The author (C.P. Clark) does not endorse a particular cell phone "app" but has many patients who like Calm. The author encourages looking at the meditation videos on YouTube in the Generation Calm series on anxiety, sleep, physical symptoms (intended for those produced by anxiety but useful for other problems such as side effects, and chronic pain) and recommends the wholesome newsletter as well. (Clare Roberts, PhD, ongoing)

Psychopharmacologic Interventions

Benzodiazepines (BZDs) have been for many years the most widely prescribed true sedative–hypnotics, being safer than barbiturates. They generally reduce sleep latency, minutes awake after sleep onset, SWS, and REM while increasing stage 2. The choice of BZD depends on onset and duration of action (in relation to the timing of sleep complaints) and anxiolytic properties if needed. In the absence of substance abuse history or concomitant abuse of other substances, short-term use of BZDs to treat insomnia is usually safe and effective. The long-term efficacy is not clear; physiologic tolerance can occur.

Non-BZD hypnotics include zolpidem, zaleplon, eszopiclone (the *S*-isomer of zopiclone), ramelteon, and suvorexant (Table 36–5). Compared to BZDs, these drugs tend to have less risk of misuse, rebound insomnia, and withdrawal symptoms and can generally be given to recovering addicts. Zolpidem can be taken in doses larger than described. Aside from ramelteon, these are $GABA_A$ receptor agonists, which probably explains their less marked motor and cognitive side effects. Onset and duration of action should be considered. Some non-BZDs can cause

Table 36–5 Non-benzodiazepine Hypnotics

Generic	Trade	Half-life (h)	Onset	Dose, Adult (mg)	Mechanism
Zolpidem	Ambien	1.5–2.4	Fast	5–10	$GABA_A$ agonist
Zaleplon	Sonata	1	Fast	5–10	$GABA_A$ agonist
Eszopiclone	Lunesta	5–7	Medium	2–3	$GABA_A$ agonist
Ramelteon	Rozerem	1–2.6	Fast	8	Melatonin agonist
Suvorexant	Belsomra	8	Medium	5,10,15,20	Inhibitor of Orexin A and B

morning "hangovers" if taken too late in the night. Controlled-release zolpidem has been approved by the U.S. Food and Drug Administration (FDA) and has shown efficacy in long-term use as well.

Ramelteon, a selective melatonin (MEL) agonist (active at MT1 and MT2 sites), does not bind to GABA receptors, nor does it possess activity within the brain reward system. It is being marketed as "addiction proof"; if this claim stands the test of time, it will provide an important option for many patients in recovery. Its rapid onset of action and melatonergic mechanisms appear promising for initial insomnia, especially in the context of a delayed circadian phase.

Suvorexant is an inhibitor of orexin A and orexin B. Orexin, aka hypocretin, is a hormone that promotes wakefulness. There is concern that suvorexant may be habit forming.

Other medications prescribed for insomnia in the absence of psychiatric comorbidity include trazodone, other sedating antidepressants, and the more sedating atypical antipsychotics.

Over-the-counter (OTC) sleeping pills usually consist of or contain histamine 1 antagonists (e.g., diphenhydramine). Their efficacy is dubious. "Natural" remedies include valerian and MEL; the latter has been used for many years and probably does have some efficacy.

More recently, particularly in some jurisdictions, some cannabis products (cannabidiol [CBD], cannabinol [CBN], and cannabigerol [CBG]) have sedative, anxiolytic, and analgesic properties, although one internet site describes CBN as "mildly intoxicating." Contamination of cannabis products, especially with tetrahydrocannabinol (THC, which produces the "high") is a big problem, and labels must be read cautiously. CBD is FDA-approved as Epidiolex, which is used in two types of epilepsy in small children.

The author wishes to thank Amrit Ahluwalia, MD for his recommendation of www.lazarusnaturals.com, a highly pure source of cannabidoids. The author (C.P. Clark) does not recommend THC or CBN because of the risks of severe psychiatric problems. Caution: any cannabinoid will potentially show as positive on a tox screen. While laws and interpretation of the law are changing throughout the nation, there is no protection for workers taking medicinal cannabinoids of any type under national law. This may affect VA workers, federal contractors, etc. The author thanks Marian Birge, Esq, of Garcia and Birge for her scholarly review of the current legal situation.

Complications/Adverse Outcomes of Treatment

The liability for tolerance, withdrawal, and abuse must be considered in regard to all the BZDs, although many patients with anxiety disorder and insomnia take them long-term without misuse, particularly after proper patient education and supervision. However, withdrawal from prolonged high-dose BZDs can cause seizures, psychosis, delirium, or even death. Rebound insomnia can also occur even with well-planned tapering.

The "war on drugs" increasingly leads many clinicians to prescribe medication with less favorable safety profiles than BZDs (e.g., risk of priapism with trazodone and metabolic complications with atypical antipsychotics). Elderly patients are particularly vulnerable to the anticholinergic side effects of antihistamines.

Many people think "natural" products are safer, not knowing that the FDA classifies them as dietary supplements and does not regulate them as closely as "manufactured" pharmaceuticals. Serious problems have resulted from unsafe processing (e.g., L-tryptophan byproducts causing an eosinophilia-myalgia syndrome). Recently, an analysis of MEL tablets bought at "reputable" pharmacies, supermarkets, and health food stores found widely varying actual doses of MEL as well as adulterants such as CBD. Potential drug interactions are less well known for complementary medicine products, particularly in regard to botanicals, which contain multiple chemical compounds. Recent evidence suggests that MEL can harm the balance of the "gut microbiome" and potentially cause or at least worsen inflammation. The authors recommend avoiding MEL in patients with inflammatory bowel disease; prudence might suggest caution in patients with gastrointestinal symptoms (Luiz da Silva et al, 2023).

▶ Prognosis

Prognosis depends on the underlying cause of insomnia as well as the prevention of secondary complications such as substance misuse in the context of self-medication.

RESTLESS LEGS SYNDROME/PLMS IN SLEEP

▶ General Considerations/Clinical Findings

Restless leg syndrome (RLS) and PLMs are often discussed together because they overlap in presentation and symptoms. RLS is an uncomfortable "creeping, crawling" sensation or "pins and needles feeling" (described as similar to akathisia by patients who have had both) in the limbs, especially in the legs. RLS tends to occur during waking and at sleep onset, whereas PLMs occur during sleep. Patients with RLS sometimes also have PLMs, but patients with PLMs often do not have RLS. For most patients with RLS, being recumbent increases leg discomfort and leads to difficulty sleeping. Further sleep disruption may occur if movement of the affected limb becomes the only way to relieve the dysesthesia.

PLMs are involuntary, rhythmic (roughly every 20–40 seconds over periods up to hours) twitches, typically ankle dorsiflexion. Each movement may lead to a brief arousal; PLMs can provoke tremendous sleep fragmentation, yet patients commonly are not consciously aware of the movements and may present with hypersomnia alone. They may present after accidentally kicking their bedmates or drastically disarranging the bed linens. PLMs increase with age, the prevalence being about 30% over 50 years and 50% over 65.

Differential Diagnosis

The differential diagnosis of RLS and PLMs includes akathisia, neurologic diseases (e.g., neuropathies, myelopathies, spinal cord problems) as well as systemic illness (e.g., anemia, nutritional/metabolic disturbances, cancer, and particularly chronic renal disease with dialysis). Similar symptoms can result from the discontinuation of illicit substances or medications, particularly antidepressants.

Treatment

Treatment should include correcting underlying disorders (e.g., iron deficiency anemia) and (if possible) discontinuing the medications that cause RLS and PLMs. Most treatments reduce either the muscle activity or the sleep disruption. Treatment generally involves one of three drug categories: dopaminergic agents (e.g., ropinirole, pramipexole), GABAergic agents (e.g., baclofen, gabapentin and other anticonvulsants); while BZDs and opiates are effective, they are simply not prudent given the current war on drugs situation. It is not uncommon to have to switch from one drug class to another after a previously effective medication loses efficacy; conversely, it can be helpful to switch to a previously effective medication in a different drug class.

Some sleep experts consider dopaminergic agents the treatment of choice for RLS, although their long-term effects have not been well studied, even in nonpsychiatric populations. Ropinirole (the only FDA-approved RLS treatment) and pramipexole (previously used in Parkinson disease [PD]) have more benign side effects than older agents (e.g., levodopa/carbidopa) and fewer peripheral side effects. Anticonvulsants may be an option, particularly if psychiatric comorbidity (e.g., psychosis) is a relative contraindication to dopaminergic agents.

Prognosis

Prognosis depends on the underlying cause, the degree of sleep disruption, and the extent to which treatment complications can be prevented.

HYPERSOMNIAS

General Considerations/Clinical Findings

The term hypersomnia encompasses pathologically increased sleep duration (e.g., the patient with atypical depression who sleeps 14 hours a day), "sleep attacks" (abrupt involuntary

onset of sleep), EDS, or a combination of these. It is important to note that hypersomnia or EDS can also be associated with poor nocturnal sleep (such as sleep disrupted by PLMs in sleep or other parasomnias) and with circadian rhythm disorders. The most common cause of EDS in the general population is chronic lack of sleep. It is important to differentiate between fatigue and EDS.

Treatment

The treatment of hypersomnia depends on diagnosis. When possible, treatment should attempt to correct an aspect of the pathophysiology itself. Supportive therapy may help patients adjust to the illness and its social sequelae (e.g., being fired for falling asleep on the job).

Prognosis

Prognosis depends on the nature of the underlying disorder, neurological causes of hypersomnia other than narcolepsy being generally more difficult to treat. Early diagnosis and treatment is vital for all hypersomnias to minimize psychosocial sequelae and potentially fatal results (e.g., falling asleep at the wheel of a vehicle).

BREATHING-RELATED SLEEP DISORDER

General Considerations

This disorder is defined as sleep disruption due to abnormal ventilation during sleep, usually presenting as EDS but sometimes as insomnia. This category includes sleep apnea and central alveolar hypoventilation. Obstructive sleep apnea, the most common pathological cause of EDS, is present in 1–2% of the general population.

Because snoring is a common symptom and can cause significant sleep disturbance (with arousals on PSG) even if criteria for sleep apnea are not met, it is described in this section.

Clinical Findings

Sleep apnea is manifested as abnormal breathing during sleep, commonly associated with snoring (often loud enough to disturb bed partners or people in other rooms) and gasping or other evidence of increased respiratory effort. PSG involves apneas (actual cessations of breathing) and hypopneas (shallow, ineffective breaths). The apnea–hypopnea or respiratory disturbance index consists of the total of these events per hour: 10 is abnormal, and 15 almost invariably requires treatment. Based on thoracic and abdominal strain gauges, each period of apnea or hypopnea can be classified as central, obstructive, or mixed, sleep apnea being diagnosed according to the preponderance and pattern of events. PSG often also reveals dysrhythmia and decreased oxygen saturation. Untreated patients are at increased risk of pulmonary hypertension, right-sided heart failure, stroke, myocardial infarction, sudden death, impotence, cognitive problems, and a depressive syndrome that generally remits with treatment. .

In central sleep apnea, respiratory drive governed by the brainstem "shuts off" during sleep. This condition may occur in a variety of neurologic and cardiovascular disorders.

Central alveolar hypoventilation, which occurs with "mechanically normal" lungs, produces hypoxia and often hypercarbia even if apneas or hypopneas are not present. It is often encountered in the morbidly obese.

Snoring may be associated with conditions causing airway turbulence (e.g., deviated septum). The upper airway resistance syndrome entails nonocclusive airway collapse associated with negative intrathoracic pressure; PSG confirmation requires the use of an esophageal pressure transducer. Sleep apnea should be ruled out.

▶ Differential Diagnosis (Including Comorbid Conditions)

The differential diagnosis includes other respiratory disorders that can worsen with the physiologic changes of sleep (e.g., asthma), comorbid neurological disorders, and some anxiety disorders. Comorbid PLMs are also common and require disorder-specific treatment if they do not resolve with treatment of apnea.

▶ Treatment

Treatment focuses on achieving and maintaining airway patency. The treatment of choice for obstructive sleep apnea (OSA) is continuous positive airway pressure (CPAP) delivered through a mask. This treatment "props" open the airway with room air delivered at low pressures (typically 5–15 cm H_2O). Numerous variations help make this as comfortable as possible for the patient, including a variety of nasal and oral masks, humidifiers, variations on pressure control and timing (e.g., bilevel positive airway pressure [BiPAP]), which provides different pressures for inhalation and exhalation).

A number of dental devices have been developed to hold the tongue forward and the airway open. Surgical procedures have been developed, including the uvulopalatopharyngoplasty, which enlarges the upper airway by removing soft tissue. Bony dysmorphology can be corrected surgically. Obese patients should be encouraged to lose weight; weight loss, even if much less than that required to reach ideal weight, can be very helpful.

If snoring is positional, devices such as pillows to discourage the patient from sleeping in a supine position may be helpful. Laser-assisted uvulopalatoplasty (LAUP), which can be performed under local anesthesia as an outpatient and can be repeated as necessary, may control snoring.

Theophylline, medroxyprogesterone, and some antidepressants have been recommended as respiratory stimulants for central apnea with mixed results.

▶ Complications/Adverse Outcomes of Treatment

The risks of cardiovascular and respiratory sequelae (as well as EDS-related accidents) are obvious. Although CPAP is very effective, noncompliance is common. Many patients, especially those with concomitant anxiety, feel "claustrophobic." They may benefit from a supportive, behavioral desensitization as well as the correction of faulty beliefs.

When a LAUP is performed without prior PSG, OSA may go undiagnosed when snoring resolves. However, unresolved silent apnea will continue to disrupt sleep and lead to persistent EDS as well as cardiovascular comorbidity.

▶ Prognosis

Early treatment can prevent cardiovascular comorbidity.

NARCOLEPSY

▶ Clinical Findings

Narcolepsy is associated with uncontrollable sleep attacks in inappropriate, embarrassing, and even dangerous situations (e.g., while driving). Although sleep attacks have been described as brief (e.g., lasting 15–20 minutes) and refreshing, this is not always true. Most narcoleptics experience related symptoms, particularly *cataplexy* (a sudden loss of muscle tone), *hypnagogic hallucinations* (dreamlike experiences while falling asleep), and sleep paralysis (brief paralysis associated with the onset of sleep or wakefulness). However, only 10–15% of narcoleptic patients have all four major symptoms. Many narcoleptic patients report having performed complex behavior (such as walking from one place to another or writing) without recalling it.

Even in the absence of serious consequences, these symptoms can be frightening and frustrating for patients and vexing for family members, coworkers, and others. Cataplexy (which can involve the whole body but at times is confined to one area, such as the hand) is often associated with emotions such as surprise or anger. The symptoms can be misinterpreted or misidentified by lay people and unwary clinicians. For example, mild episodes of cataplexy (dropping a cup upon hearing a joke) may be attributed to carelessness or clumsiness. A patient may be misdiagnosed as psychotic if the doctor mistakenly assumes the hypnagogic hallucinations have occurred during full wakefulness or have the same significance as waking hallucinations.

Narcolepsy is associated with defective REM sleep regulation. Cataplexy and sleep paralysis can be thought of as atonia without REM, whereas hypnagogic hallucinations and sleep attacks have been likened to REM intrusion. Though the absolute risk of developing narcolepsy is only 1–2% in first-degree relatives of accurately diagnosed probands, an increased prevalence of certain histocompatibility locus antigen subtypes has been reported. Recently, animal models of narcolepsy have shown hypocretin neuron deficiencies. Decreased cerebrospinal fluid hypocretin levels have been reported in human narcolepsy.

The diagnosis of narcolepsy is confirmed by a positive Multiple Sleep Latency Test (MSLT) (with the finding of REM onset during two daytime nap opportunities) following a night of PSG ruling out other causes for abnormal MSLT. Sleep-onset REM periods are often present on nocturnal PSG.

▶ Differential Diagnosis (Including Comorbid Conditions)

Sleep attacks and cataplexy-like episodes have been reported in neurological disorders such as traumatic brain injury (e.g., Harriet Tubman). Experts believe that narcolepsy-like syndromes without cataplexy are almost always produced by comorbid neurologic disorder. When no such neurologic disorder is found, such a syndrome would be referred to as Primary Hypersomnia.

Narcolepsy patients are not exempt from other causes of hypersomnia. If narcolepsy worsens in a patient with previously well-controlled symptoms, careful questioning should be conducted about other possible causes of hypersomnia (medications, sleep apnea, and PLMs). Some patients fabricate a history of narcolepsy to obtain stimulants. Obtaining PSG confirmation or previous medical records will protect against this.

▶ Treatment

Although some patients with narcolepsy achieve reasonable control of sleep attacks with scheduled naps, many require medication. Modafinil is the treatment of choice for EDS and may be helpful for EDS related to neurologic comorbidity, medications (e.g., sedating antipsychotics such as clozapine), and OSA in which EDS persists despite optimization of all disorder-specific treatments. Armodafinil is also used. The exact mechanisms by which modafinil is effective are unknown. It is not related to the amphetamines and appears to have less risk of side effects (e.g., insomnia, psychosis) and misuse than "scheduled" stimulants, (e.g., methylphenidate, amphetamines), which are still used. Sodium oxybate (gamma-hydroxybutyrate [GHB]), an endogenous GABA metabolite, is the only medication for cataplexy approved by the FDA. Its exact anticataplectic mechanisms are unknown, although other anticataplectic medications (tricyclic antidepressants [TCAs], monoamine oxidase inhibitors [MAOIs], selective serotonin reuptake inhibitors [SSRIs]) may act via serotonergic mechanisms or by increasing norepinephrine through decreased reuptake or increased release. GHB also alleviates sleep attacks somewhat, perhaps indirectly by alleviating disturbed nocturnal sleep by inducing SWS and consolidating sleep. Because of frequent use as a "club drug" with catastrophic consequences (neurological sequelae and death from intoxication and life-threatening withdrawal not treatable with BZDs), GHB is scheduled and available only through a tightly regulated distribution program. A longer acting version was in trials at the time of the latest revision.

Pitolisant is a histamine 3 inverse agonist effective against EDS in narcolepsy and idiopathic and symptomatic hypersomnia. Solriamfetol, a DA and norepinephrine reuptake inhibitor, is used for EDS in narcolepsy and OSA, although the underlying cause of the OSA should definitely be treated as well as possible.

The treatment of cataplexy and the other cardinal symptoms of narcolepsy was previously based on REM sleep inhibition, which is still useful.

▶ Complications/Adverse Outcomes of Treatment

Although the misuse of stimulants is rare in the absence of a comorbid substance abuse history, withdrawal symptoms, physiological tolerance, and, occasionally, psychosis can develop, particularly with amphetamines and sometimes with methylphenidate. Dramatic cataplexy rebound is to be expected if any anticataplectic agent is stopped, with TCAs being generally more dangerous than SSRIs in this regard.

PARASOMNIAS

See Table 36–6.

▶ General Considerations/Clinical Findings

Parasomnias are sleep-related disorders characterized by unusual events or behavior occurring either during sleep or during sleep–wake transitions. Parasomnias occurring during non-REM sleep are more often associated with being difficult to arouse, confusion upon awakening, and a lack of memory for the event. REM parasomnias generally involve waking clearly and rapidly, with recall for the event. These features are important in obtaining a proper diagnosis.

▶ Differential Diagnosis (Including Comorbid Conditions)

Frequent nightmares should always raise the possibility of psychiatric comorbidity (particularly mood or anxiety

Table 36–6 A Comparison of Parasomnias by Symptoms and Findings

Characteristic	Nightmare Disorder	Sleep Terror Disorder	REM Behavior Disorder	Sleepwalking Disorder
Sleep stage	REM	NREM	REM	NREM
Dream recall	Yes	No	Yes	No
Motor activity	No	Screaming, motoric agitation	Yes	Yes
On awakening	Alert	Confused, disoriented	Alert	Confused, disoriented
Time of night	Last third	First third	Second half	First half
Prevalence	Children 20%, adults 5–10%	Children 5%, adults <1%	Unknown	Children 1–20%, adults <1%
Autonomic activation	Slight, secondary to fear	Extreme, with sweating and vocalizations	Associated with REM and motor activity	Not present
Danger to self	No	No	Patient acts out dream, may accidentally injure bed partner	Patient walks anywhere
Treatment	Monitor; symptoms usually decrease with age; if severe consider psychotherapy and/or suppress REM (MAOIs or other antidepressants)	Monitor; symptoms usually decrease with age; if severe consider low dose tricyclic or BZD	Safe environment for all; clonazepam; consider if triggered by antidepressants; treat neurological comorbidity (common) or watch for future development; not uncommon in narcolepsy	Maintain a safe environment and monitor symptoms; if severe consider suppression of SWS (BZDs, TCAs)

Data from Salzman C. *Clinical Geriatric Psychopharmacology*, 2nd ed. Baltimore: Williams & Wilkins; 1992.

disorder). REM sleep behavior disorder can present as a reversible complication of several antidepressants; otherwise, it is generally associated with current or future neurologic comorbidity, such as narcolepsy and PD. Criminal defendants may allege REM behavior disorder as a defense, particularly for violent or egregious actions; however, it is believed that REM behavior disorder cannot be simulated on PSG.

► Treatment

Treatment depends on the particular disorder. The reassurance that children do not suffer during sleep terrors or recall them afterward can be very helpful for families. It is especially important in sleepwalking and REM behavior disorder to maintain a safe environment for the patient and others. Lock balcony doors. Use special precautions when sleeping in unfamiliar surroundings such as hotels. Move the bedmate into a separate room if needed. Careful instruction in sleep hygiene is important in all parasomnias. Bruxism (tooth grinding) can be treated with dental devices.

Some authorities believe that sudden infant death syndrome is a parasomnia. Parents should be aware that the risks of sudden infant deaths are reduced when infants are put to bed supine (e.g., the "Back to Sleep" campaign).

► Complications/Adverse Outcomes of Treatment

These are often the result of inadequate treatment but may result from medication side effects.

► Prognosis

Prognosis depends on the underlying disorder and the prevention of accidents.

CIRCADIAN RHYTHM DISORDERS

See Table 36–3.

► General Considerations/Clinical Findings

In disturbances of circadian rhythm, there is a misalignment between the timing of sleep–wake patterns and the desired or normal pattern. These patients may complain of either insomnia or hypersomnia (or both at different times of the 24-hour day). Two processes appear to mediate the propensity to sleep: a homeostatic process by which the propensity to sleep is related directly to the duration of prior wakefulness, and a circadian process that regulates the propensity across a 24-hour day. In persons living on a normal sleep schedule, the circadian sleep propensity is greatest at night and mid-afternoon.

DELAYED SLEEP PHASE TYPE

The major symptoms are prolonged sleep latency and difficulty waking up at the desired time. Most common in adolescence, it can also be encountered with "jet lag" and shift work.

THE JET LAG TYPE

This type is characterized by sleepiness and alertness out of synchrony with the "new" time zone. It may be encountered with delayed or advanced sleep phase. Eastward travel (entailing a phase advance of the biological clock) usually takes longer to adjust to than does westward travel (which entails a phase delay).

THE SHIFT WORK TYPE

This type involves insomnia, hypersomnia, or both, at inappropriate times, in relationship to work schedules (e.g., rotating or permanent shift work, or irregular work hours). Complications include gastrointestinal or cardiovascular symptoms, increased use of alcohol, disruption of family and social life, low morale and productivity, and high absenteeism. Many individuals never adjust completely to the work schedule because they try to revert back to a normal sleep–wake schedule on weekends and holidays in order to participate in family and social activities.

UNSPECIFIED TYPE

Unspecified type includes *advanced sleep phase syndrome* and *non-24-hour sleep–wake syndrome*. Common in older persons, advanced sleep phase syndrome is characterized by early evening sleepiness, early sleep onset, and early morning awakening. In non-24-hour sleep–wake syndrome, patients live on a free-running rest–activity cycle continuously shifting in and out of phase with real-world time. This disorder can complicate chronic poor sleep–wake hygiene. It is usually found in the blind, probably because light does not properly synchronize the SCN with the environment.

Differential Diagnosis

Includes other disorders involving circadian disruption (e.g., depression) but is usually not difficult given the history.

Treatment

Involves patient education, the promotion of sleep hygiene, and an attempt to synchronize sleep and wakefulness with

the underlying phase position of the circadian clock. Because the natural cycle length of the circadian clock is longer than 24 hours, it is usually easier to phase-delay the clock than to phase-advance it. Shift workers, for example, tend to do better when shifting in a "clockwise direction" (i.e., from day to evening to night work schedules) than when shifting in a counterclockwise direction. This kind of schedule shift should be implemented in personnel planning for shift workers as much as possible. Many schools are starting later in the morning to minimize tardiness, accidents driving to school, and suboptimal performance related to the near-ubiquitous delayed sleep phase in teenagers.

Appropriate time cues (zeitgebers and timed exposure to bright light) can be very helpful in readjusting and synchronizing the sleep–wake rhythm and the internal clock.

Bright light in the evening produces a phase delay (e.g., retiring later and arising later) and can be very helpful for advanced sleep phase syndrome. In contrast, early-morning bright light phase advances the sleep–wake cycle and is helpful in delayed sleep phase syndrome. It is important to maintain darkness during the desired sleep period: blackout curtains and sunglasses may be helpful. Light administration using sunlight and additional indoor lighting is very useful even if a proper light box is not available. In addition, it is important to maintain the desired sleep–wake schedule and prevent a rapid "relapse" to the previous pattern.

MEL is more effective as a "resynchronizing" agent than as a soporific per se. It can be administered in carefully timed doses to ameliorate jet lag, but unforeseen changes in travel plans can bring severe discomfort. Treatment with both bright light and MEL must be carefully timed, because the sensitivity of the biological clock undergoes a circadian variation.

Treatment of Shift Work Sleep Disorder depends on the individual's symptoms and timing. It may involve judicious use of bright light, MEL, hypnotics, caffeine, and modafinil in any combination. In general, bright light promotes alertness and should be utilized in shift work environments where possible.

Complications/Adverse Outcomes of Treatment

Include the potential "overcorrection" of the circadian phase, "overtreatment" of a given symptom (e.g., if the patient drinks coffee at the end of the shift in order to stay awake long enough to drive home, sleep latency is prolonged), and maladaptive behaviors (e.g., using alcohol as a hypnotic) arising from attempts to self-treat. Excessive doses of MEL have been reported to trigger free running, which is very difficult to treat.

Prognosis

Depends on the underlying disorder and the minimization of safety risks (e.g., preventing drowsy driving during jet lag).

SLEEP & PSYCHIATRIC DISORDERS (SLEEP DISORDERS RELATED TO ANOTHER MENTAL DISORDER)

MOOD DISORDERS

▶ General Considerations

It is important to note that sleep disturbances (particularly insomnia) are often the earliest symptoms of depressive, hypomanic, or manic episodes and are also common in cyclothymia, dysthymia, and episodes of minor depression. Approximately 70% of depressed patients complain of insomnia, which involves initial, middle, or terminal insomnia and subjectively nonrestorative sleep in any combination. Mania can be precipitated by seemingly minor amounts of sleep deprivation or by jet lag. Thus, insomnia and jet lag must be treated aggressively or avoided in bipolar patients.

In unipolar patients, sleep disturbance is often the earliest sign of an impending recurrence or relapse as well as one of the most persistent and distressing residual symptoms during periods of remission. There is evidence that insomnia may be a risk factor for subsequent depressive episodes even in those with no previous history of depression.

▶ Clinical Findings

Most patients are able to report symptoms of sleep disturbance. One possible exception is subjective hypersomnia, common in atypical and bipolar depression. The few polysomnographic studies of depression with hypersomnia have not shown decreased sleep latency on the MSLT or a longer TST, although time in bed is increased.

Mania is characterized by diminished TST and other abnormalities on PSG. In major depression, PSG abnormalities reported include shortened REM latency and increased amounts of REM as well as prolonged sleep latency, reduced TST and SE, and decreased SWS.

▶ Differential Diagnosis

Comorbid anxiety and substance use are common in unipolar and especially bipolar patients; together with medication side effects, these are the most common other causes of insomnia and hypersomnia.

▶ Treatment

A. Psychopharmacologic Interventions

Antidepressants are the pharmacological mainstay of treatment for unipolar depression. They are used in bipolar depression together with mood stabilizers or atypical antipsychotics.

Most antidepressants suppress REM sleep; many affect SWS and sleep continuity measures. Virtually all antidepressants have been reported to exacerbate RLS and PLMs.

Sedating antidepressants can be helpful in treating depression associated with severe insomnia. "Activating" antidepressants are used for hypersomnic or anergic depressions. "Activating" antidepressants can exacerbate insomnia and are generally given early in the day; they include bupropion, most SSRIs, MAOIs, and venlafaxine. Sedating antidepressants are taken at bedtime and include trazodone, mirtazapine, maprotiline, and TCAs, particularly the tertiary amines.

All mood stabilizers except lithium are anticonvulsants and can cause EDS, especially in combination with other medication; however, they generally have few effects on PSG. Lithium, like many antidepressants, may increase REM latency and decrease REM; it also may increase SWS in mania. Atypical antipsychotics (see later discussion) are increasingly used as mood stabilizers to augment antidepressants.

B. Psychotherapeutic Interventions

Careful attention to regular scheduling and optimization of zeitgebers (social rhythm therapy) is very helpful, especially in bipolar disorders.

▶ Complications/Adverse Outcomes of Treatment

It is important to remember that any psychotropic agent can cause unwanted sedation in a given patient. Many effective antidepressants worsen insomnia and are frequently given in conjunction with anti-insomnia drugs, sedating antidepressants (particularly trazodone), and the more sedating atypical antipsychotics. Given the risks of priapism and other cardiovascular complications with trazodone, and the risks of diabetes and weight gain with atypical antipsychotics, these decisions must be made carefully.

▶ Prognosis

It is well known that manic episodes are best treated early with aggressive prescription of sedating medications, especially atypical antipsychotics and BZDs. For mood disorders in general, prognosis is a function of treatment compliance, the presence or absence of comorbidities, and the aggressive treatment of prodromal or residual symptoms (e.g., insomnia).

ANXIETY DISORDERS

▶ General Considerations

Patients with anxiety disorders commonly complain of insomnia. Nightmares are common in posttraumatic stress disorder (PTSD) (civilian or military); some PTSD patients develop a phobic avoidance of sleeping that further aggravates the disorder. In panic disorder, panic attacks are not uncommon during SWS. If sleep panic attacks are mistaken for dangerous cardiac events, the patient may become very afraid of sleep.

Clinical Findings

Most patients with anxiety disorder report symptoms of insomnia and panic attacks directly. However, many patients have faulty beliefs that may be elicited only by direct questioning or after psychoeducation. They may fear that they will die or "go crazy" if they do not get enough sleep. Polysomnographic abnormalities have been found in generalized anxiety disorder (GAD), panic disorder, PTSD, and obsessive–compulsive disorder (OCD).

Differential Diagnosis

Mood disorders and substance use disorders are commonly comorbid. PLMs and sleep-disordered breathing are common in PTSD. Obstructive sleep apnea and other respiratory disorders should be considered in cases involving sleep panic attacks.

Treatment

Appropriately tailored psychotherapy can be extremely helpful and may be absolutely necessary in anxiety disorders. Patient education and brief cognitive–behavioral interventions around sleep are used.

Among the most common medications prescribed for anxiety disorders are the SSRIs and venlafaxine. BZDs are also helpful in many cases, although the best choice for anxiety symptoms may not resolve insomnia. Buspirone is a nonsedating anxiolytic that is not associated with dependence. Atypical antipsychotics are increasingly used in treatment-resistant anxiety disorders.

Complications/Adverse Outcomes of Treatment

Liability for tolerance, withdrawal, and abuse must be considered for all the BZDs, although many anxiety disorder patients take them long term without misuse, particularly with proper education and supervision. Unfortunately, the "war on drugs" has led to a reluctance to prescribe and take BZDs. Many patients, particularly those with anxiety disorders, are terrified of "getting hooked"; the author of this chapter (C.P. Clark) has seen severe consequences of anxiety disorder patients taking less than the prescribed dose, stopping "cold turkey," etc.

Prognosis

As with most psychiatric disorders, prognosis is best with early diagnosis and treatment. Disorders such as OCD, PTSD, and panic disorder (especially with agoraphobia) can cause major suffering and disability. Untreated anxiety (whether as part of an anxiety disorder or not) is increasingly recognized as a risk factor for suicide.

PSYCHOTIC DISORDERS

General Considerations

Sleep disturbance is common in schizophrenia and schizoaffective disorder, often becoming increasingly severe as an acute episode develops. The effective treatment of insomnia can help agitation and positive symptoms to some extent.

Clinical Findings

Disorganized patients may have difficulty reporting their symptoms; in this case information from caregivers can be helpful. The most common PSG findings in schizophrenia are decreased SWS measures and evidence of sleep disruption.

Differential Diagnosis (Including Comorbid Conditions)

Comorbid substance misuse is common and can frequently exacerbate or mimic psychotic disorders. The author (C.P. Clark) has seen one patient on depot medications who remained abstinent from illegal drugs but repeatedly induced psychotic mania with very large amounts of caffeine and "energy drinks" (e.g., 7–8 cans of Red Bull per day).

Comorbid anxiety disorders are common in psychotic patients. Anxiety symptoms in this population are often underdiagnosed and improperly treated; many clinicians assume that anxiety reflects paranoia or worsening psychotic symptoms. Increasing the dose of antipsychotic medication is not particularly helpful for panic attacks. In fact, severe anxiety can be related to akathisia, which can be worsened by increasing the dose of an antipsychotic drug. Careful questioning is required to determine the exact nature of symptoms; patients may not recognize akathisia as a side effect or realize that its characteristic "physical restlessness" is different from "pure" anxiety or agitation. Patients may complain of "paranoia" when they have fear or pathological worry like that in GAD (e.g., that their car will break down and require expensive repairs) rather than believing that someone is persecuting them.

Finally, bizarre complaints of "dying several times every night" may reflect apneic episodes. OSA is common in psychotic patients, who may have special difficulties tolerating and complying with CPAP.

Treatment

Antipsychotic medications are the cornerstone of treatment, although psychotherapy and psychosocial rehabilitation are often necessary as well. Other classes of medication are utilized for augmentation or treatment of specific symptoms (e.g., lithium for chronic suicidality).

Complications/Adverse Outcomes of Treatment

The risks of extrapyramidal side effects (EPSE) and tardive dyskinesia (TD) with conventional antipsychotics has led to more frequent use of atypical antipsychotics that are associated with weight gain, onset or worsening of diabetes mellitus, and other metabolic sequelae. Patients have suffered severe exacerbations after unilaterally discontinuing medication such as olanzapine based on TV ads for malpractice suits.

For conventional antipsychotics, sedation generally increases with decreasing potency. Atypical antipsychotics, particularly olanzapine, quetiapine, and clozapine, can be sedating; clozapine is also associated with enuresis and drooling during sleep.

Prognosis

Prognosis is generally guarded but can be improved by treatment compliance, sobriety, quality of treatment, and the availability of social supports and services.

DEMENTIA

General Considerations

Dementia is one of the most common health problems in older people, and Alzheimer disease (AD) is the most common type of dementia. Given the neural pathophysiology of dementing disorders (e.g., cholinergic degeneration and dysfunction in AD), it is not surprising that sleep disturbance is a common feature. Related problems such as disruptive nocturnal behavior are a common precipitant of institutionalization.

Clinical Findings

Recognizing the presence of dementia is generally not difficult; however, all demented patients should be regularly screened for sleep–wake symptoms. Profound sleep fragmentation and disruption of the sleep–wake cycle have been documented by activity. PSG may show prolonged sleep latency; lowered SE; and decreased TST, SWS, and non-REM sleep. In severe dementia (e.g., AD), the EEG may be so abnormal (e.g., slow waves during waking) that it is difficult to score PSG.

Differential Diagnosis (Including Comorbid Conditions)

Efforts should be made to rule out treatable causes of dementia (e.g., some cases of normal pressure hydrocephalus) and to look for related neurological disorders (e.g., PD). Many demented patients will have comorbid symptoms of anxiety, depression, and/or psychosis. Sudden onset of symptoms and a fluctuating sensorium are cues to rule out delirium.

Sleep-disordered breathing and PLMs are common in dementia. Untreated sleep apnea can worsen symptoms and accelerate neuronal degeneration; CPAP can improve functioning, particularly if applied with special measures to improve tolerability by patients who have early AD.

Treatment

A. Psychopharmacologic Interventions

Cholinesterase inhibitors mitigate deficient cholinergic activity in AD; they are being used increasingly in other dementias as well. Other agents are used to target specific symptoms (e.g., antipsychotics for hallucinations, SSRIs for comorbid depression or anxiety, sedative medications for insomnia).

B. Psychotherapeutic Interventions

It is crucial to intervene to preserve remaining cognition and help maintain socialization and independence (e.g., with adult day programs). Behavioral measures can be very helpful even in advanced disease and decrease the risks of "overmedication." Support and counseling are crucial for caregivers, who are at increased risk for medical and psychiatric disorders.

C. Chronotherapeutic Interventions

Regular routines and schedules are important, with the provision of a sleep-conducive environment at night and appropriate activities and stimulation to enhance daytime wakefulness. Evening bright light and MEL can partially restore a normal circadian rhythm and improve sleep consolidation and behavior.

Complications/Adverse Outcomes of Treatment

Medication side effects are of particular concern. In some studies, BZDs and other sedating medications have been associated with increased falling. On the other hand, such agents may help keep the patient sleeping through the night, indirectly decreasing the risk of falling by preventing night wandering. Cholinergic agents commonly carry sleep–wake and other side effects. Donepezil can worsen insomnia; rivastigmine can produce somnolence.

Demented patients are especially prone to EPSE and TD, yet atypical antipsychotics have been linked to cardiovascular sequelae. The latter risk is especially difficult to determine given the high prevalence of cardiovascular disease in dementia, especially mixed and vascular types. No medication is FDA-approved for treatment of psychosis or agitation in dementia.

▶ Prognosis

The overall poor prognosis may improve gradually with improved treatment.

Terminal dementia patients need to be palliated no less than patients dying from cancer, heart failure, or other "medical" disorders.

SOMATOFORM & RELATED DISORDERS

Chronic fatigue syndrome (CFS) and fibromyalgia involve disturbed or nonrestorative sleep, loss of energy, severe fatigue, tiredness, and easy fatigability. In PFS, pain may be the predominant symptom; in CFS, fatigue and cognitive impairment are predominant. Both disorders have a high comorbidity with depression, yet these PSG patterns are distinct from those observed in major depression.

SLEEP & SUBSTANCE USE

Because of their common features, substance-induced sleep disorders are discussed in general, with further information pertinent to specific substances described below.

▶ General Considerations

Any psychoactive compound will generally affect sleep, particularly in pathologic use, abuse, or dependence. The effects of a drug on sleep are multifaceted and determined by drug type, frequency, dosage and duration of (chronic or acute) use, degree of intoxication, and comorbidity with medical or psychiatric disorders, as well as by possible gradual changes in the brain in response to the drug(s). A systematic description of sleep disturbances associated with substance abuse is complicated because polysubstance abuse is common and can involve drugs with different or opposite effects on sleep. An example is acute intoxication with alcohol while withdrawing from cocaine. In general, the effects of withdrawal are roughly opposite those for intoxication or current use (e.g., hypersomnia in caffeine withdrawal). Within a particular class of drugs, substances with a faster onset of action generally convey greater risk of misuse and withdrawal symptoms than those with a slower onset.

Many people without a substance use disorder use substances (particularly alcohol, nicotine, and caffeine) in ways that affect the sleep–wake cycle. They are often unaware of the effects these substances can have. For example, many people may use alcohol as a hypnotic without realizing it can disrupt sleep later in the night. Sleep disturbances can also occur following appropriately prescribed medication taken as directed.

In general, the sleep–wake effects of withdrawal are roughly opposite those for intoxication or current use of the particular substance (e.g., hypersomnia in caffeine discontinuation).

▶ Clinical Findings

Clinical findings depend on the substance(s) used and its amount, timing, and chronicity.

▶ Differential Diagnosis (Including Comorbid Conditions)

The drinking of alcohol with recreational (or misused/diverted prescription) drugs or the simultaneous use of multiple illicit drugs is very common. Even during prolonged abstinence, many patients with substance abuse or dependence have psychiatric comorbidity such as mood, anxiety, or psychotic disorder. Caffeine commonly produces or exacerbates anxiety. Nicotine use is more common in mood, anxiety, and psychotic disorders than in the general population and is common in patients who use drugs or alcohol.

▶ Treatment

Continued abstinence is the ultimate goal. A variety of psychotherapeutic interventions are aimed at relapse prevention or preventing a "slip" from developing into prolonged use. Twelve-step groups (e.g., Alcoholics Anonymous [AA], Narcotics Anonymous [NA]) can be extremely helpful. SMART Recovery may be helpful for patients who feel AA and NA are too "churchy" and/or are willing to participate in harm reduction but not total abstinence. The treatment of true comorbid disorders (and in some cases other substance-induced disorders such as psychosis) is important to improve the chances of abstinence.

▶ Complications/Adverse Outcomes of Treatment

Risks of treatment are small compared to the risks of untreated substance use or dependence.

▶ Prognosis

Depending on the type of symptoms and the substance that caused them, substance-induced sleep disorders can persist long into abstinence and be associated with considerable morbidity. For example, chronic insomnia is a risk factor for relapse into alcohol abuse.

ALCOHOL

Alcohol is probably the most frequently used sleeping aid in the general population. In normal controls, alcohol at bedtime shortens sleep latency, increases non-REM sleep, and reduces REM sleep. However, when alcohol is metabolized in the middle of the night, a "mini-withdrawal" ensues, with shallow, disrupted sleep and REM rebound, often with indigestion and nocturia. Nightly alcohol use produces some tolerance to REM suppression and initial sedation. Sleepiness potentiates the sedative effects of alcohol, increasing risks of motor vehicle accidents.

At different stages of the illness, alcoholics may experience insomnia, hypersomnia, parasomnias, and even circadian rhythm disturbances. Sleep-disordered breathing and PLMs are especially common long into abstinence.

BZDs are used to treat withdrawal and patients in detoxification programs, but are rarely used otherwise because of the increased risk of abuse and dependence in patients with a history of substance use disorder. Disulfiram, naltrexone, and acamprosate have been used to treat alcoholism.

AMPHETAMINE, OTHER STIMULANTS, AND COCAINE

Cocaine and stimulants such as the amphetamines activate the dopaminergic arousal system. Withdrawal is usually characterized by hypersomnia and depression. PSG shows increased TST as well as depression-like findings (increased REM and shortened REM latency). Insomnia as a side effect, tolerance, and physiological withdrawal can occur with the appropriate use of amphetamine and methylphenidate (e.g., for narcolepsy and attention-deficit/hyperactivity disorder [ADHD]). Even modified-release amphetamine and methylphenidate can be abused (e.g., by snorting the crushed capsule content). Despite frequent concerns by parents, ample evidence shows that appropriately treating ADHD in children and adolescents, even with amphetamine or methylphenidate, decreases rather than increases the risk of abusing substances (perhaps by enhancing impulse control and reducing the risk of school dropout).

CAFFEINE

There are large interindividual differences regarding the effects of caffeine. The extent of caffeine's effects may last 8–14 hours; thus, afternoon intake can disturb sleep. Many OTC analgesics and cold remedies contain caffeine.

NICOTINE

Chronic nicotine use is associated with increased SL and arousals in smokers. Withdrawal may be associated with initial insomnia or hypersomnia, although these are generally minor compared to other symptoms. An exception is heavy dependence, in which withdrawal symptoms awaken the smoker until more nicotine is smoked. Nicotine patches have been associated with increased dreaming and insomnia. Smoking accelerates the metabolism of many drugs. Evidence suggests that smoking increases the risk of sleep-disordered breathing.

OPIOIDS

Though the acute administration of morphine, heroin, and other opioids to normal subjects or abstinent addicts reduces TST, SE, SWS, and REM sleep, opioids can indirectly improve sleep by their analgesic effect in patients with painful conditions. Methadone can be used in detoxification programs, although chronic use of methadone disrupts sleep and can increase the frequency of central apneas. Methadone, buprenorphine, and naltrexone are also used in the long-term treatment of opioid dependence.

SEDATIVES, HYPNOTICS, & ANXIOLYTICS

BZD abuse and dependence generally occurs with simultaneous misuse of alcohol or other drugs, particularly stimulants. Patients with history of abuse or dependence are at increased risk for addiction to BZDs. Barbiturate misuse and withdrawal are sometimes seen in migraine patients taking combination products; withdrawal is generally more severe than BZDs.

BZDs shorten sleep latency, improve sleep continuity, elevate stage 2 sleep, and decrease SWS and REM sleep. True withdrawal may produce long-lasting effects on anxiety and sleep. Withdrawal must be differentiated from rebound or the reemergence of anxiety or insomnia symptoms. Patients should be cautioned not to stop BZDs abruptly or without medical guidance, although this still occurs iatrogenically in general hospitals with surprising frequency.

For short-term use (e.g., acute treatment of insomnia) and when used for PLM/RLS, patients should avoid taking BZDs for several consecutive nights. Even the tapering of chronic BZDs often produces insomnia and should be undertaken gradually whenever possible, with individualized dose adjustment. Switching to longer acting BZDs may facilitate taper in some settings and is best when it becomes necessary to detoxify a patient from barbiturates and BZDs. Although anticonvulsants generally prevent seizures during BZD withdrawal, they are not helpful for the associated autonomic dysregulation.

Table 36–7 Symptoms and Disorders That May Cause Sleep Disturbance

Seizures
Involuntary movements
Dyspnea/respiratory symptoms
Palpitations
Nocturia
Gastroesophageal reflux
Chronic hemodialysis (severe PLMs in sleep)
Trauma (even concussion) or neurological disorders disrupting circuits regulating sleep and wakefulness

SLEEP & MEDICAL CONDITIONS

General Considerations

Sleep complaints are often encountered in a variety of medical-surgical conditions, especially in the hospital. Virtually any type of pain, anxiety, or discomfort can cause insomnia, as can the restriction of normal movement (e.g., in traction), lack of normal circadian zeitgebers in an intensive care unit, noisy monitors, round-the-clock neurologic checks, and so on (Tables 36–7 and 36–8).

Clinical Findings

These disorders can present with insomnia, hypersomnia, parasomnias, or a mixture of these and are coded accordingly in the DSM-5.

Differential Diagnosis (Including Comorbid Conditions)

Patients with medical disorders may have comorbid depression, anxiety, or substance use disorder. Adjustment disorders can also cause insomnia. Furthermore, almost any class of medication can be associated with insomnia, hypersomnia, or sedation. Medications exert their effects through direct effects on sleep stages (e.g., pindolol-associated nightmares), through effects on sleep disorder (e.g., aggravation of PLMs caused by the DA antagonist metoclopramide), and through seemingly unrelated physiologic effects (e.g., diuretic medication leading to nocturia).

Treatment

Behavioral measures for insomnia and in some cases supportive psychotherapy can be helpful. Diagnosing the underlying disorder and optimizing its treatment is crucial. For remaining symptoms, medications otherwise useful for insomnia, hypersomnia, and some parasomnias may be helpful.

Complications/Adverse Outcomes of Treatment

As in patients without comorbid disorders, drugs used to treat insomnia, hypersomnia, and parasomnias can have side effects. Patients with sleep apnea or heavy snoring must not be given drugs that depress respiration.

Prognosis

Prognosis depends primarily on that of the underlying medical disorder.

SLEEP & THE REPRODUCTIVE CYCLE

General Considerations

Physical discomfort disrupts sleep at any stage of pregnancy. The first trimester (with its increased progesterone) is generally associated with daytime sleepiness. The mechanical, physiologic, and hormonal effects of

Table 36–8 Effects of Sleep and Wakefulness on Medical Disorders

Respiratory	Position Decreased respiratory drive Decreased airway tone
Cardiovascular	Position Sleep-related autonomic changes in blood pressure, heart rate Dysrhythmias in susceptible patients Myocardial infarction (MI), sudden death more common in morning (high REM propensity)
Epilepsy	Sleep deprivation may trigger seizures REM may be somewhat protective
Headache	Sleep deprivation may trigger migraines, cluster headaches

pregnancy are also associated with an increased incidence and severity of snoring. Obstructive sleep apnea develops in some cases. Many gravid women develop PLMs or experience an aggravation of it.

Babies disrupt parental sleep. The postpartum period is a time of potential risk for more serious conditions (e.g., affective disorder and psychosis) that can be triggered by sleep loss. Little research has attempted to separate the physical and hormonal effects of lactation on sleep or to examine the implications of sleeping arrangements (e.g., infant cosleeping) on the mother's sleep. Infant cosleeping is discouraged because concerns about possible suffocation of the baby.

During menopause, hot flashes can disrupt sleep. The PSG may show decreased REM and TST and increased sleep latency.

Impulse-Control Disorders

John W. Thompson, Jr., MD
George E. Sayde, MD, MPH

Although impulse-control disorders are often thought to be rare conditions, a recent replication of the National Comorbidity Study demonstrated a 12-month prevalence rate of 8.9%. This percentage, however, also included disorders such as oppositional defiant disorder (1%), conduct disorder (1%), and attention-deficit/hyperactivity disorder (ADHD) (4.1%). Intermittent explosive disorder was reported at 2.6% of the surveyed population. Intermittent explosive disorder and pathological gambling (0.2–3.3% of populations surveyed) are much more common than the other disorders in this group. The impulse-control disorders tend to be more common in males than females, with first onset typically emerging in childhood or adolescence. Comorbid substance use disorders and antisocial personality disorder are common. The characteristic symptoms that comprise impulse-control disorders, namely poor emotional and behavioral modulation, also occur to some degree along the trajectory of healthy character development. Therefore, particular attention should be given to the frequency, persistence, pervasiveness across multiple life contexts, and the degree of psychosocial and functional impairments when considering the presence of a true disorder.

American Psychiatric Association. Disruptive, impulse-control, and conduct disorders. In: *Diagnostic and Statistical Manual of Mental Disorders*. 5th ed. Text Rev.; 2022. https://doi.org/10.1176/appi.books.9780890425787xl5_Disruptive_Impulse Control.

Kessler RC, Chiu WT, Demler O, Walters EE. Prevalence, severity, and comorbidity of 12-month DSM-IV Disorders in the National Comorbidity Survey Replication. *Arch Gen Psychiatry*. 2005;62:617–627.

INTERMITTENT EXPLOSIVE DISORDER

▶ General Considerations

A. Epidemiology

The National Comorbidity Study Replication reported a 12-month prevalence rate of 2.6%. The lifetime prevalence is 4.0%. This is more common than previously realized. Prevalence appears higher in individuals younger than 40 years and in those with a high school education or less.

B. Etiology

The outbursts associated with intermittent explosive disorder (sometimes referred to as episodic dyscontrol) were initially viewed as the result of heightened limbic system discharge, dysfunction, or even as interictal phenomena. The *Diagnostic and Statistical Manual of Mental Disorders*, 5th Edition, Text Revision (DSM-5-TR), excludes those patients in whom an aggressive episode was thought to be related to a general medical condition (e.g., head trauma, temporal lobe seizures, delirium) or to the direct psychological effects of a substance, whether a drug of abuse or a prescribed medication. Serotonergic abnormalities of the limbic system (anterior cingulate) and orbitofrontal cortex are present in individuals with intermittent explosive disorder. Disorders that can be identified as resulting from neurological insult or a seizure disorder are now classified elsewhere. Nevertheless, neurological soft signs, nonspecific electroencephalogram (EEG) anomalies, or mild abnormalities on neuropsychological testing are associated with intermittent explosive disorder.

Psychodynamic explanations have also been proposed. Childhood abuse, including physical and emotional trauma during the first 20 years of life, is thought to be a risk factor for the development of this disorder. Disruptions in attachment to caregivers, such as displacement from home and separation from family members, also appear to potentiate risk. Others postulate narcissistic vulnerability as a possible mechanism that triggers these attacks. Thus, one can conceptualize the "explosive" episodes as resulting from a real or perceived insult to one's self-esteem or as a reaction to a perceived threat of rejection, abandonment, or attack.

C. Genetics

Little is known about the genetics of intermittent explosive disorder. Family studies of individuals with this disorder have shown high rates of mood and substance use disorders in first-degree relatives.

Clinical Findings

A. Signs & Symptoms

Aggressive outbursts are impulsive, occur in discrete episodes, and are grossly out of proportion to any precipitating event or subjectively experienced provocation (e.g., psychosocial stressor). Furthermore, there is often a lack of premeditation, rational motivation, or clear-cut gain to be realized from the aggressive act itself. The patient expresses embarrassment, guilt, and remorse after the act and is often genuinely perplexed as to why they behaved in such a manner. Some patients have described periods of exhaustion and sleepiness immediately after these acts of violence.

B. Psychological Testing

Neuropsychological testing may reveal minor cognitive difficulties such as letter reversals. A careful history may reveal developmental difficulties such as delayed speech or poor coordination.

A history of febrile seizures in childhood, episodes of unconsciousness, or head injury may be reported.

C. Laboratory Findings

Laboratory findings are nonspecific. Nonspecific EEG findings may be noted. Several research projects have found signs of altered serotonin metabolism in cerebrospinal fluid or platelet models.

Differential Diagnosis

If the behavior can be better explained by an underlying neurological insult (e.g., delirium and neurocognitive disorder), then the correct diagnosis should be personality change due to general medical condition, aggressive type. The clinician must also decide whether the aggressive or erratic behavior would be better explained as a result of a personality conduct disorder, oppositional defiant disorder, or ADHD. Disruptive mood dysregulation disorder includes periods of impulsive aggressive outbursts beginning before age 10 years and yet is largely defined by a persistently negative mood state. Purposeful behavior with subsequent attempts to malinger must be distinguished from intermittent explosive disorder, especially in the context of litigation. Recent studies suggest a high rate of combined lifetime mood (depressive and anxiety disorders) and substance use disorders in patients with this disorder.

Treatment

Both psychotherapy and pharmacotherapy have been described as treatments for intermittent explosive disorder; however, no double-blind, randomized, controlled trials have been conducted. There are case reports or open trials of the use of anticonvulsants, antipsychotics, antidepressants, benzodiazepines, β-blockers, lithium carbonate, stimulants, and opioid antagonists. Novel anxiolytics such as buspirone have been efficacious in individual cases. Current scientific data are insufficient and inconclusive regarding treatment of the disorder; therefore, clinicians must proceed with individualized treatment plans based on their best clinical judgment.

Complications/Adverse Outcomes of Treatment

Intermittent explosive disorder can be complicated by legal difficulties, job loss, difficulties with interpersonal relationships, and divorce. Although patients may have been prone to lose their temper repeatedly over a long period of time, they may not seek medical attention until a major life disruption has resulted from one of these outbursts. Intermittent explosive disorder comorbid with posttraumatic stress disorder appears to heighten risk for suicidal thoughts and behaviors.

Adverse outcomes of treatment are related to the side effects of particular medications used to treat this disorder.

Prognosis

Intermittent explosive disorder is thought to have its onset in adolescence or young adulthood and to run its course by the end of the third decade of life. Here again, the data for such conclusions are quite limited.

Coccaro EF, McCloskey MS. Phenomenology of impulsive aggression and intermittent explosive disorder. In: *Intermittent Explosive Disorder: Etiology, Assessment, and Treatment.* London: Academic Press; 2019:37–65.

Fanning JR, Lee R, Coccaro EF. Comorbid intermittent explosive disorder and posttraumatic stress disorder: clinical correlates and relationship to suicidal behavior. *Compr Psychiatry.* 2016; 70:125–133.

Kim SW. Opoid antagonists in the treatment of impulse-control disorders. *J Clin Psychol.* 1998;59:159.

Kessler RC, Üstün TB. *The WHO World Mental Health Surveys: Global Perspectives on the Epidemiology of Mental Disorders.* New York: Cambridge University Press; 2008.

McElroy SL, Soutullo CA, Becman DA, et al. DSM-IV intermittent explosive disorder: a report of 27 cases. *J Clin Psychol.* 1998; 59:203.

New AS, Hazlett EA, Buchsbaum MS, et al. Blunted prefrontal cortical 18fluorodeoxyglucose positron emission tomography response to meta-chlorophenylpiperazine in impulsive aggression. *Arch Gen Psychiatry.* 2002;59(7):621–629.

Siever LJ, Buchsbaum MS, New AS, et al. d,l-Fenfluramine response in impulsive personality disorder assessed with [18F]fluorodeoxyglucose positron emission tomography. *Neuropsychopharmacology.* 1999;20(5):413–423.

Tay AK, Rees S, Chen J, et al. The coherence and correlates of intermittent explosive disorder amongst West Papuan refugees displaced to Papua New Guinea. *J Affect Disord.* 2015;177:86–94.

KLEPTOMANIA

▶ General Considerations

Although kleptomania has been recognized since the early nineteenth century as an ego-dystonic impulse to steal, little systematic study has been undertaken to understand this disorder. The individual with kleptomania often feels guilty and fears apprehension and prosecution. Several psychiatric disorders have been linked to kleptomania; the most recent studies point to eating disorders and compulsive spending.

A. Epidemiology

Because most shoplifters steal for profit, fewer than 5% of shoplifters meet criteria for kleptomania. It appears to be a rare disorder (0.3–0.6% prevalence in the United States) that requires further epidemiological investigation. Kleptomania is reported to be more common in women than in men (at a ratio of 3:1) and typically emerges between ages 16 and 20.

B. Etiology

The etiology of kleptomania is unknown. It may be a symptom rather than a disorder. Neurotransmitter reward pathways associated with serotonin, dopamine, and opioid systems appear to be implicated in kleptomania.

C. Genetics

Little is known about the genetics of kleptomania. Family studies have demonstrated high rates of mood, substance use, and anxiety disorders in first-degree relatives.

▶ Clinical Findings

A. Signs & Symptoms

The hallmark of kleptomania is the repetitive failure to resist the impulse to steal useless objects that have little monetary value. This behavior is not usually purposeful but is performed to relieve a sense of inner tension. There is often a sense of relief upon completion of the theft. The theft usually occurs in retail stores or work locations or from family members. Some patients report feeling high or euphoric while stealing. Most feel guilty after the act, and may donate stolen items to charity, return items to the location from which they were stolen, or pay for the stolen items.

A comprehensive history may reveal other compulsive behavior that does not meet full criteria for obsessive–compulsive disorder (OCD). Symptoms of mood disorders, substance use disorders, anxiety disorders, and eating disorders may also be common in this population.

B. Psychological Testing & Laboratory Findings

Neuropsychological testing and laboratory data are nonspecific.

▶ Differential Diagnosis

The diagnosis of kleptomania should not be given if the patient's behavior is better accounted for by antisocial personality disorder, bipolar disorder, or conduct disorder; or if stealing occurs as a result of anger or vengeance, due to the usefulness or monetary worth of the object, or as a result of a hallucination or delusional belief. Other important diagnoses to consider include major depression, anxiety disorder, and substance use disorders (which are often comorbid).

▶ Treatment

Psychotherapy and pharmacotherapy have been found useful in a small body of evidence. Selective serotonin reuptake inhibitors and lithium are the agents used most frequently to treat kleptomania. One small clinical trial did not show efficacy with use of escitalopram during a 17-week period. Grant et al demonstrated a reduction in stealing behavior with the use of naltrexone compared to placebo. Response rates are confounded by the high rates of comorbid mood and eating disorders.

▶ Complications/Adverse Outcomes of Treatment

The majority of patients with kleptomania have a lifetime diagnosis of a major mood disorder (36–100%). Anxiety disorder (34–80%) is also common as are substance use (22–50%) and eating disorders. Complications include apprehension, arrest, and conviction for stealing with shame and embarrassment to the patient, friends, and family members. Other risks might include self-destructive behavior associated with major mood disorders and substance use. Adverse outcomes of treatment are related to the side effects of medication and failure to recognize comorbid conditions that may be treated easily.

▶ Prognosis

Kleptomania is thought to begin in adolescence and can continue into the third or fourth decades of life. The course is not well studied and includes a spectrum from brief and episodic to chronic.

Black DW. Compulsive buying: a review. *J Clin Psychol.* 1996; 57(Suppl 8):50.

Goldner EM, Geller J, Birmingham CL, Remick RA. Comparison of shoplifting behavior in patients with eating disorders, psychiatric control subjects, and undergraduate controls. *Can J Psychiatry.* 2000;45(5):471–475.

Grant JE, Kim SW, and Odlaug BL. A double-blind, placebo-controlled study of the opiate antagonist, naltrexone, in the treatment of kleptomania. *Biol Psychiatry.* 2009;65:600–606.

Grant JE, Odlaug BL, Kim SW. Kleptomania: clinical characteristics and relationship to substance use disorders. *Am J Drug Alcohol Abuse*. 2010;36(5):291–295.

Koran LM, Aboujaoude E, Solvason B, et al. Escitalopram for compulsive buying disorder: a double-blind discontinuation study. *J Clin Psychopharmacol*. 2007;27:225–227.

McElroy SL, Keck PE Jr, Phillips KA. Kleptomania, compulsive buying, and binge-eating disorder. *J Clin Psychol*. 1995; 56(Suppl 4):14.

Talih FR. Kleptomania and potential exacerbating factors: a review and case report. *Innov Clin Neurosci*. 2011;8(10):35–39.

PYROMANIA

General Considerations

Pyromania strikes fear in the hearts of mental health professionals due to the serious potential for harm to the patient and society. The therapist must balance carefully the issues surrounding confidentiality and the duty to protect third parties from the danger presented by these patients.

A. Epidemiology

The epidemiology of pyromania is unclear. After other causes of fire-setting are ruled out, only a small population of pyromaniac individuals remains. Pyromania is thought to be rare. In clinical populations, however, fire-setters are not uncommon. Between 2 and 15% of psychiatric inpatients are fire-setters. The peak age of fire-setters is 13 years, and 90% of fire-setters are male. Many are from emotionally and economically deprived families.

B. Etiology

The etiology of pyromania is not well understood. There is little research to support any leading set of hypotheses.

C. Genetics

Little is known about the genetics of pyromania.

Clinical Findings

A. Signs & Symptoms

The signs and symptoms of true pyromania may be indistinguishable from other forms of fire-setting. Diagnosis is by exclusion. The motivation for the fire-setting should be elucidated, as an act not otherwise explained by aggression or vengeance, monetary reward, sociopolitical expression, or due to a distortion in perception of reality. Typically, a feeling of relief follows the act, which relieves internal intension (as in kleptomania). Most fire-setting cannot be classified as an impulse-control disorder, but impairment in the ability to control impulses is recognized in most cases of arson. Patients are usually identified after legal charges have been filed.

B. Psychological Testing

Psychological testing of fire-setters reveals a significant amount of psychiatric comorbidity; however, studies on pure populations of pyromaniacs are not available. Among fire-setters, suicidal behavior has been reported. Screening for suicide is warranted for this population.

C. Laboratory Findings

Lower cerebrospinal fluid concentrations of 3-methoxy-4-hydroxyphenylglycol and 5-hydroxyindoleacetic acid have been reported in fire-setters as compared to control subjects.

Differential Diagnosis

The diagnosis of pyromania should not be given if fire-setting can be accounted for more appropriately by motives of profit, crime concealment, or revenge, or as a symptom of another psychiatric disorder. Fire-setting has been found in over half of children with conduct disorder. It may be a harbinger of adult antisocial personality disorder.

Treatment

Early intervention programs with adolescent fire-setters have reported success in deterring fire-setting. Other comorbid psychiatric disorders such as schizophrenia and bipolar disorder should be treated aggressively.

Complications/Adverse Outcomes of Treatment

A significant number of fire-setters will repeat this behavior. While they are working with such patients, therapists must be constantly aware of the potential for harm to third parties. Little is known about the comorbidity of pyromania with other psychiatric disorders. Fire-setting is quite common among psychiatric inpatients: the most common associations are psychotic disorders, mood disorders, substance use disorder, and antisocial personality disorder. Two-thirds of fire-setters are intoxicated at the time of the index offense. Female fire-setters have a high degree of psychiatric comorbidity, as high as 92% in one study.

Prognosis

The prognosis and course of illness are unclear. Early detection and the treatment of comorbid psychiatric disorders are recommended.

Barnett W, Richter P, Sigmund D, et al. Recidivism and concomitant criminality in pathological firesetters. *J Forensic Sci.* 1997;42:879.

Geller JL. Arson in review. From profit to pathology. *Psychiatr Clin North Am.* 1992; 15:623.

Lindberg N, Holi MM, Tanip, Virkkunen M. Looking for pyromania: characteristics of a conservative sample of Finish male criminals with histories of fire-setting between 1973 and 1993. *BMC Psychiatry.* 2005;5:47.

Puri BK, Baxter R, Cordess CC. Characteristics of fire-setters. A study and proposed multiaxial psychiatric classification. *Br J Psychiatry.* 1995;166:393.

TRICHOTILLOMANIA

▶ General Considerations

A. Epidemiology

The incidence of trichotillomania in the general population is unknown, but estimates have placed its prevalence in the United States as high as 8 million people. A survey of 2579 college freshmen indicated that 0.6% would have met criteria for trichotillomania at some point in their lifetimes. Trichotillomania appears to be more prevalent in females (although males may predominate in patients under age 6 years).

B. Etiology

The etiology of trichotillomania is unknown; however, different theories have been proposed about the pathogenesis of this complex disorder. Psychoanalytic theory views pathologic hair pulling as a manifestation of disrupted psychosexual development, often due to pathologic family constellations. In contrast, behavioral theory conceptualizes hair pulling as a learned habit similar to nail biting or thumb sucking. Recently, a biological theory has been postulated as several researchers have proposed a serotonergic abnormality in trichotillomania and have suggested that the disorder may be a pathologic variant of species-typical grooming behaviors. Neuropsychological abnormalities, treatment response to some antidepressants, and frequent comorbidity with OCD have led to speculation regarding a neurobiological etiology, perhaps involving frontal lobe or basal ganglia dysfunction. Of note, trichotillomania is now included in the DSM-5-TR section on Obsessive Compulsive and Related Disorders. Our conceptualization of this disorder is ever-evolving and dynamic; its nosology has expanded to include both elements of impulse-control and OCD.

C. Genetics

Family studies are suggestive of a genetic predisposition for trichotillomania but may reflect environmental learning and are inconclusive. Trichotillomania appears more common in patients with OCD and their first-degree relatives than in the general population.

▶ Clinical Findings

A. Signs & Symptoms

Patients, particularly young ones, frequently deny that they pull their hair intentionally. Others typically describe pulling their hair when alone, but they may pull it openly in front of immediate family members. These episodes tend to occur during sedentary activities such as watching television, reading, studying, lying in bed, or talking on the telephone, and they may be more frequent during periods of stress. Patients may be unaware that they are pulling their hair until they are in the middle of an episode. Some patients report being in a trancelike state when they pull their hair. These episodes may last a few minutes or a few hours. Patients may pull a few hairs or many hairs per episode. Many patients do not feel pain when the hair is pulled; some patients report that it feels good.

Patients frequently engage in oral manipulation of the hair once it is pulled including nibbling on the roots or swallowing the hair. The later behavior can lead to a rare but serious complication, a trichobezoar (hair ball) in the gastrointestinal tract. The consequences of a trichobezoar can be life threatening: obstruction, bleeding, perforation, pancreatitis, and obstructive jaundice.

Patients typically pull hair from their scalp, causing diffuse hair thinning or virtual baldness.

The typical patient demonstrates patchy areas of alopecia without inflammation that spare the periphery. Many patients are adapt at hiding areas of hair loss by judicious hair styling, but may ultimately resort to hairpieces and wigs when the areas become too large or too numerous to hide. Patients may also pull hair from other parts of their body, including eyelashes, eyebrows, pubic region, or from face, trunk, extremities, or underarms.

B. Psychological Testing & Laboratory Findings

Although psychological testing may not be useful in confirming a diagnosis of trichotillomania, a punch biopsy may be of some help in this regard. The biopsy results typically reveal increased catagen hairs along with melanin pigment casts and granules in the upper follicles and infundibulum.

▶ Differential Diagnosis

According to DSM-5-TR diagnostic criteria, a diagnosis of trichotillomania is not warranted if the condition can be better accounted for by another mental disorder or is due to a general medical condition. For example, if a patient has another significant psychiatric disorder (e.g., a condition with delusions or hallucinations) that might account for the hair pulling, then the diagnosis of trichotillomania would not be warranted. When patients deny that they pull their hair intentionally, dermatologic consultation may be required to rule out other causes of hair loss. Most notable among these conditions is alopecia areata, but tinea capitis, traction alopecia, androgenic alopecia, monilethrix, and other dermatologic conditions should also be considered. A punch biopsy may be indicated particularly when one of these disorders is suspected.

Treatment

An initial double-blind crossover trial compared clomipramine to desipramine in 13 patients with trichotillomania screened to rule out neurologic disorder, mental retardation, primary affective disorder, psychosis, and OCD. Clomipramine produced improvement in clinical symptoms (33–53% reduction in severity scores) on each of three rating scales designed to assess trichotillomania symptomatology and clinical improvement; scores on two of the three scales were statistically significant. Two subsequent placebo-controlled, double-blind crossover studies failed to show efficacy for fluoxetine. Small clinical trials show positive preliminary evidence with the use of naltrexone, N-acetyl cysteine, and olanzapine as well.

Little rigorous research has been conducted concerning the differential effectiveness of treatments for trichotillomania. Clomipramine and cognitive behavioral therapy likely constitute the current treatments of choice, but this conclusion is tempered by the paucity of treatment outcome studies. Habit renewal training is the most effective form of behavioral therapy. Trichotillomania occurs with variable levels of severity in terms of hair pulling and comorbid psychopathology. As a result, response to treatment is highly variable and rather unpredictable.

Complications/Adverse Outcomes of Treatment

Although hair loss is self-induced, patients often suffer with low self-esteem and are particularly sensitive to comments about their appearance and go to great lengths to hide their disfigurement. These patients are often fearful that their shameful "secret" will be discovered and that they will be ridiculed in public. If the disorder is protracted, the patient's self-esteem can suffer drastically. Some individuals develop avoidant behavior and become socially withdrawn in order to avoid exposure. Trichobezoar is a rare complication. Little is known about the comorbidity of trichotillomania; however, major depressive disorder and excoriation (skin-picking) disorder commonly accompany this condition. Aside from the possibility that the disorder may be related to anxiety or mood disorder, there has been much speculation that it is a variant of OCD. Some research lends support to this hypothesis; however, the studies that failed to show efficacy for fluoxetine may argue against such a relationship.

Trichotillomania in preadolescents (particularly in those younger than 6 years of age) is thought to be associated with little psychopathology. In adolescent and adult patients, however, an association with other mental disorders has been demonstrated. In a study of 60 adult chronic hair-pullers (50 of whom met strict criteria for trichotillomania), only 18% did not demonstrate a current or past diagnosis of a psychiatric disorder other than trichotillomania. The lifetime prevalence of mood disorders was 65%, and 23% met criteria for current major depressive episode. Lifetime prevalence of anxiety disorders was 57%, and 10% demonstrated a current diagnosis of OCD and 5% a history of OCD. Another 18% endorsed present or past obsessions and compulsions not meeting the full criteria for OCD. Lifetime prevalence of panic disorder with or without agoraphobia was 18%, generalized anxiety disorder 27%, simple phobia 32%, eating disorder 20%, and substance abuse disorder 22%.

A smaller study that used standardized assessment techniques found that 45% of the trichotillomania patients studied met criteria for current or past major depression, 45% had generalized anxiety disorder, 10% had panic disorder, and 35% had alcohol or substance abuse. Unfortunately, patients with OCD were excluded from the study.

Adverse outcomes of treatment are limited to the usual side effects experienced with clomipramine or other antidepressants. Although there might be adverse consequences of psychodynamic psychotherapy or a behavioral treatment approach, such adverse outcomes are generally thought to be rare and unpredictable.

Prognosis

The prognosis and course of illness generally can be predicted from the age at onset. Trichotillomania begins most often in childhood or young adolescence. Hair pulling in very young children is frequently mild and remits spontaneously. Patients with a later age at onset tend to have more severe symptoms that run a chronic course. These patients are thought to have a higher incidence of comorbid anxiety and depressive disorders.

Bienvenu OJ, Samuels JF, Wuyek LA, et al. Is obsessive-compulsive disorder an anxiety disorder, and what, if any, are spectrum conditions? A family study perspective. *Psychol Med.* 2012;42(1):1–13.

Keuthen NJ, O'sullivan RL, Goodchild P, et al. Retrospective review of treatment outcome for 63 patients with trichotillomania. *Am J Psychiatry.* 1998;155:560.

Minichiello WE, O'Sullivan RL, Osgood-Hynes D, et al. Trichotillomania: clinical aspects and treatment strategies. *Harv Rev Psychiatry.* 1994;1:336.

Schreiber L, Odlaug BL, Grant JE. Impulse control disorders: updated review of clinical characteristics and pharmacological management. *Front Psychiatry.* 2011;2:1.

IMPULSE-CONTROL DISORDERS NOT OTHERWISE SPECIFIED

This category is for disorders of impulse control (e.g., skin picking) that cause clinically significant distress or impairment in psychosocial functioning but do not meet the full criteria for any specific impulse control disorder or other mental disorder having features involving impulse control described elsewhere in the DSM-5-TR (e.g., substance dependence, a paraphilia).

American Psychiatric Association. Disruptive, impulse-control, and conduct disorders. In: *Diagnostic and Statistical Manual of Mental Disorders*, 5th ed. Text Rev.; 2022. https://doi.Org/10.1176/appi.books.9780890425787.xl5_Disruptive_Impulse_Control.

Grant TE, Levin L, Kim D, Polenta MN. Impulse control disorders in adult psychiatric inpatients. *Am J Psychiatry*. 2000; 162(11):2184–2188.

McElroy SL, Hudson JI, Pope HG Jr, et al. The DSM-III-R impulse control disorders not elsewhere classified: clinical characteristics and relationship to other psychiatric disorders. *Am J Psychiatry*. 1992;149:318.

38 Adjustment Disorders

Ronald M. Salomon, MD
Rebecca E. Salomon, PhD

▶ Essentials of Diagnosis

The diagnosis of adjustment disorders should be relatively straightforward provided the clinician considers a wide range of stressors and other mental health diagnoses. However, challenging diagnostic situations can arise when the stressor is subtle. For example, a change in a previously stable life situation may occur without the patient complaining of an obvious stressor. The clinician should exclude any specified symptom complex that meets diagnostic criteria for another disorder even if it may be related to a specific stressor. In general, other diagnoses should be recorded only if their criteria are met. However, when a discrete recent stressor is identifiable, an adjustment disorder diagnosis may be more appropriate than, for example, anxiety disorder not otherwise specified or depressive disorder not otherwise specified.

The need to establish an adjustment disorder diagnosis is sometimes underestimated because of the disorder's generally mild, transient clinical course, relatively high incidence, and relatively low prevalence in psychiatric settings (see later discussion). Although its symptoms usually come and go without presenting significant treatment challenges, in some individuals the acute consequences may be quite severe. Because adjustment disorders are very common in primary care settings, even the very small percentage showing severe symptoms account for a significant portion of suicides (see later discussion). An absence of major mood disorder or other major disorder does not rule out acute suicide risk. Although such extreme outcomes are extraordinarily rare compared to the frequency of these disorders, they are noted here to emphasize the essential nature of making adjustment disorder diagnoses, educating patients about responses to stress, and justifying recommendations and reimbursements for treatment.

The normal challenges of life and its stages are usually taken in stride with socially and culturally prescribed ranges of expected responses and adjustments. However, even commonly encountered events can disrupt an unusually crucial part of an individual's self-view (Table 38–1) and provoke symptoms outside of expected norms. Stressors leading to adjustment disorders are often termed "problems in coping." Children and adolescents may not clearly connect stressful recent events with their emotional symptoms or behavior, requiring clinical assessment to establish chronologic relationships. Among adolescents, adjustment disorders frequently emerge following disappointment(s) in relationships with family members or friends. Especially complex difficulties may be encountered among homosexual or gender nonconforming teens. In adult crime victims, early detection of adverse responses has been shown to improve outcome, showing the value of diagnosis and intervention.

A psychiatric hospitalization, or a treatment for another, otherwise unrelated, psychiatric disorder may precipitate an adjustment disorder at any age. For example, after being hospitalized for severe obsessive–compulsive disorder (OCD), a patient may express a conduct disturbance that is otherwise atypical for OCD. Retirement and aging can bring feelings of loss, depleted health and vigor, and fear of the future. The elderly commonly express somatic complaints in response to event-related distress. It may then be appropriate to add the diagnosis of adjustment disorder. Exceptionally severe or extreme stressors, while shy of the exceptional stressors in acute traumatic reactions or posttraumatic stress disorder (PTSD), may still precipitate maladaptive responses. If the symptoms and gravity of the stressor are less than those required for acute stress disorder, the diagnosis of adjustment disorder may be appropriate.

▶ Diagnostic Validity

The diagnostic label of adjustment disorder offers a broad set of behavioral and emotional criteria, the validity of which is sometimes questioned. Still, there are compelling reasons for using it when appropriate. Diagnostic recording allows communication with patients, insurers, and other clinicians. It assists in disease control by focusing research and guiding therapeutic selection. Contemporary knowledge of

Table 38–1 Commonly Observed Precipitants for Adjustment Disorders

College or university adjustments
Conscription into military service
Death of parent or companion
Natural disaster
New marriage or cohabitation
Pregnancy
Recent or anticipated combat
Recent or anticipated loss
Retirement
Terminal illness in self, parent, or companion

differential diagnosis, prognosis, course, and future risks may be illuminated by naming a disorder. Helpfully, research attention suggests that the adjustment disorder diagnosis does fulfill these goals and provides the therapist with criteria that are easily met, defensible, and practical.

At the same time, the adjustment disorder diagnosis must not become a conciliatory label aimed to avoid controversies. A diagnostic label cannot reconcile societal and individual standards of response to a stressor. For example, rational requests for death in terminal cancer patients with otherwise normal behavior and appropriate mood may be less likely to attract an adjustment disorder moniker now than for generations past. Similarly, the adjustment disorder diagnosis may now be used less often to differentiate between biological and functional (purely psychological) disorders than in the past, as the biological basis for symptoms is more widely understood. Still, foci of controversy remain challenging. Various societies' views of substance abuse and alcoholism, often comorbid in patients with adjustment disorders, may affect thresholds for the diagnosis of substance abuse. Adjustment disorder diagnoses should not take the place of understanding individual norms in the setting of societal discomfort with delineating underlying psychopathology. When used with poor specificity or to evade controversy, the application of a diagnosis of adjustment disorder effectively undermines psychological and organic pathological correlates and diminishes the credibility of psychiatric nosology.

While clinical use of the diagnosis of adjustment disorder diagnosis may be less prevalent in other countries, true prevalence appears to be similar across study sites (with minor differences attributable to selections of distressed study populations). Historically vague symptom criteria may also contribute to variance in usage. In the latest revision of the *International Classification of Diseases*, 11th edition (ICD-11[1]), adjustment disorder is now described as a maladaptive reaction to one or more identifiable psychosocial stressors. As a stress-response syndrome, it joins PTSD, complex PTSD, and prolonged grief disorder. Symptoms are categorized as an excessive preoccupation with the stressor or its consequences, in association with a failure to adapt to the stressor with consequences impairing personal, family, social, educational, occupational, or other important functions. Exclusions remain in place when symptom specificity or severity justify other mental disorders in general, while listing several specific disorders for careful differentiation: separation anxiety in childhood, depressive disorders, prolonged grief, uncomplicated bereavement, burnout, and acute stress reaction. The criteria retain a large overlap with adjustment disorder in the *Diagnostic and Statistical Manual of Mental Disorders*, 5th Edition, Text Revision (DSM-5-TR). This DSM rendition recognizes external contexts and cultural factors influencing symptoms in response to the stressor(s) and extends the criteria for impairments beyond social or occupational (academic) functioning to include "other important areas" of function. The specifiers (acute, chronic) have been eliminated while the adjustment disorder subtypes are described more clearly. Both diagnostic systems allow up to 3 months between exposure to a stressor and onset of symptoms. ICD-11 still requires a retrospective view in that the symptoms must resolve within 6 months of the stressor and its consequences having resolved, so that the diagnosis is ostensibly provisional; a revised diagnosis may be needed if this criterion is not met; this issue is not present in the DSM. There are other possible reasons for intercultural differences in the use of the diagnosis of adjustment disorder. In some European countries, reimbursement for treatment does not cover extensive care for minor conditions. Culture-specific syndromes, such as the Latino ataque de nervios, apply to a variety of symptom presentations, many of which do not come to psychiatric attention. Note that Appendix I of DSM-IV-TR was devoted to culture-bound syndromes, which was rejected, replaced, or redefined in DSM-5. Terms now include "cultural syndromes," "cultural idioms of distress," and "cultural explanation/perceived causes." These are viewed as "ways cultural groups experience, understand, and communicate suffering, behavioral problems, or troubling thoughts and emotions." An international standardization of the diagnosis may be difficult to achieve.

Fernández A, Mendive JM, Salvador-Carulla L, et al. DASMAP investigators. Adjustment disorders in primary care: prevalence, recognition and use of services. *Br J Psychiatry*. 2012;201: 137–142.

▶ General Considerations

A. Epidemiology

In the United States, adjustment disorder diagnoses are quite common. Among psychiatric admissions, one estimate

[1]https://icd.who.int/browse11/l-m/en#/http://id.who.int/icd/entity/264310751

suggests that 7.1% of adults and 34.4% of adolescents were diagnosed with adjustment disorders. Among adults in France seen in general practice settings, a similar rate of 13.7% of those with psychological problems was observed, which was 1% of all patients consecutively seen with or without psychological problems. Many of these individuals also merit substance abuse or conduct disorder diagnoses. The newly released ICD-11 criteria (see below) were evaluated in life stress-exposed Lithuanian adults, finding a prevalence of 16.8%. Among university students receiving psychiatric assessments, a very high proportion were diagnosed as having adjustment disorders. Population studies using the older Epidemiologic Catchment Area tools did not assess adjustment disorders because of low sensitivity in the diagnostic instrument used (the Diagnostic Interview Schedule). More recent studies show an improved sensitivity and understanding of cultural, reimbursement, and records-confidentiality influences on true population rates and clinician utilization rates for the adjustment disorder diagnosis.

B. Etiology

Adjustment disorders appear to occur more often in individuals who are at risk for other psychiatric disorders, implying that etiologic factors may be shared. As may also be seen in PTSD, neurobiological characteristics (e.g., elevated corticosteroid blood levels in response to stress) have been associated with the development of adjustment disorders.

A commonplace stressor may not be immediately recognized, or the individual may perceive it as paradoxical. Adaptation difficulties in marriage, pregnancy, or childbirth can provoke feelings of guilt because the experience "should" be welcomed, without emotional distress or discomfort. Natural preferences for lifestyle stability may be difficult to reconcile with goals requiring change. For example, a stably married individual unexpectedly confronted by parenthood faces role change, increased responsibility, and loss of freedom. Improved coping may result if the individual develops insight into a longstanding fear of being thrust into the role of single parent, as may have happened in their own family.

C. Genetics and Other Risk Factors

Small twin studies have not revealed a genetic heritability for adjustment disorders. Other than a global suggestion that a family history of psychiatric disorder is a risk factor for adjustment disorder, little is known about genetic inheritance or determinants of this condition. This is not surprising given the potential heterogeneity of a disorder defined more by a multitude of stressors rather than symptoms. Adjustment disorders may be commonly observed in patients enduring the stresses of other genetically determined illnesses (e.g., Huntington disease) but the relationship between those genes and the adjustment pathophysiology is assumed to be entirely secondary.

1. Risk factors for the general population—Major early risk factors include prior stress exposure, stressful early childhood experiences, and a history of mood or eating disorder. Family unity disruptions or frequent family relocations predispose children to adjustment disorders. The incidence of adjustment disorders is greater in children of divorced families following a subsequent, independent stressor. The death of a parent predisposes children to adjustment disorders, with which a high suicide risk has been reported especially after a loss of the father. Adjustments to living with the extended family (e.g., in-laws, stepparents) are additional predisposing factors. The outlet of symptom expression—be it depressed mood, conduct disturbance, or anxiety—may be determined by prior experience or biological constitution. Prior exposure to war, without meeting criteria for PTSD (see Chapter 28), is a risk factor.

Factors that increase susceptibility in one situation can decrease it in another. For example, a high educational level can protect an individual who faces one stressor, but it can pose as a risk factor for adjustment disorders in another context. A study using ICD-11 criteria noted female gender, greater age, and university education as risk factors. Small-town life can predispose individuals by providing too much shelter from stress while also limiting supportive social networks.

2. Risk factors in special populations—Immigrant populations are at risk for adjustment disorder. It is simplistic to regard the entire immigration process as a precipitant; rather, precipitant stressors should be identified separately. For example, among new immigrants to Israel, an individual's stress responses to missile attacks during the Gulf War could be predicted by their cultural adaptation prior to the attacks. Laotian Hmong immigrants in Minnesota were the focus of highly informative investigations that showed the need for preventive intervention during the acculturation period. Acculturation may be like other novel situations in many ways, but it also presents many unique difficulties, all at the same time (Table 38–2). Any or all these factors may require attention in treatment.

Among prison populations, adjustment disorder contributes heavily to suicide, which is frequently preceded by

---

Table 38–2 Stressors Among Immigrant Populations

Isolation from family and ethnic supports

Longing for familiar environments, all the while teaching hosts about the culture

Novel cognitive styles, task expectations

Reordering of developmental sequences, social expectations, and milestone assessments

Social and language challenges

Trauma of the journey for self and immigrant cohort

Unfamiliar time concepts and spatial orientation

Data from Williams CL, Westermeyer J. *Refugee Mental Health in Resettlement Countries*. New York: Routledge; 1986.

inmate-to-inmate conflict, disciplinary action, fear, physical illness, and the receipt of bad news. For a substantial number, the provision of mental health services within 3 days of the event was not sufficient to prevent suicide.

Chronic illness increases the need for medical contact and may constitute a major challenge to usual coping. Illness appears to be a precipitant rather than a predisposing factor. Adjustment disorders are not more prevalent among those with medical illnesses. On the other hand, should an adjustment disorder occur, it will often affect the clinical course of a somatic illness. The detection of adjustment disorder is remarkably poor, even on oncology services. It might improve with universal screening on admission. Early psychiatric consultation is associated with shorter length of stay. The course of asthma, chronic obstructive pulmonary disease, diabetes mellitus, end-stage renal disease, systemic lupus erythematosus, stroke, coronary artery disease, HIV/AIDS, chronic pain or headache, or cancer and even a COVID-19 illness can be affected by the individual's adjustment and illness acceptance. Illness behavior, the give and take between patient and caregiver, and secondary gain all affect assessments of adjustment. The distinction between lifestyle and coping style as well as the setting of expectations for treatment compliance require skilled clinical judgment. For example, the asthmatic adolescent who rebels by skipping a scheduled inhaler dose may not need as rigid a guideline as one with "brittle" diabetes who skips insulin shots.

Finally, as also observed in the medical setting, complaints or lawsuits against physicians frequently result in adjustment disorder.

▶ Clinical Findings

A. Signs & Symptoms

In the primary care setting, distress reported by individuals, friends, or family members must be carefully assessed. Individual distress is variably reported and interpreted. Adjustment disorder diagnoses derive solely from expressed emotional and behavioral symptoms, which may not be expressed clearly or may be minimized, masking distress. The ICD-11 notes a resemblance to PTSD in that symptoms may worsen upon encountering reminders of stressor(s), and avoidance of such stimuli may be seen. Symptoms themselves may contribute further to the individual's loss of confidence and disrupted sense of safety and well-being. Maladaptive behavior, fear, and uncertainty arise from losing control as customary defenses fail. Symptoms of adjustment disorder may include depressive, anxious and impulsive features, or behavioral expressions such as increased use of tobacco, alcohol, or other substances. The gravity of the stressor is interpreted in a context of past encounters with similar events and cannot be evaluated solely by the therapist's or society's standards. Stress must be evaluated in terms of the individual's subjective perception, giving perceptions a degree of validity.

Adjustment will be facilitated when the diagnostic evaluator (and, later, the therapist) shows flexibility and accepts the individual's needs and distress. Careful listening and sensitivity are required because, with its paucity of somatic symptoms, individuals with adjustment disorder can masquerade as stable, hiding high fragility and even suicide risk. Clinicians may not appreciate the importance of a seemingly minor stressor, but they must give utmost respect to the individual, scheduling an interview that is long enough to understand the patient's subjective perceptions.

The distress experienced with adjustment disorder may include dissimilar emotions and behaviors. Such distress is beyond the expected response to the identified stressor(s). Professional psychiatric assessment and treatment are needed when there is suspicion of heightened severity, intensity (e.g., suicide risk), or duration beyond that manageable by the primary care clinician, or when supportive intervention fails. Symptoms can be delayed, especially in women, and may change over time. Chronic stress can elicit chronic adjustment disorders noting that duration criteria apply only after resolution of the stressor(s) and their consequences. Clinical observation of the course of adjustment disorder reveals a strong association with suicidality, personality disorder, and drug use. A lack of suicide attempt in a first episode does not protect from future attempts. Completed suicide appears to be more frequent after an earlier attempt, or in the presence of personality disorder. The severity and lethality of suicide attempts often increase over time. Individuals with adjustment disorder are no less a suicide risk than those with major depressive disorder.

B. Psychological Testing

Psychological testing (e.g., using the Minnesota Multiphasic Personality Inventory) has documented adjustment disorder risk factors (see "General Considerations" section earlier in this chapter) and comorbidity with type A personality style and other personality disorders (especially cluster B). Psychological testing can help the clinician to identify suicidal individuals and the severity of their depression and hopelessness. Testing suggests that adjustment disorders are more likely in individuals with socially obligatory perfectionism—a tendency toward the exaggerated perception that others have inordinately high expectations of them. On neuropsychological testing, no impairment is observed in patients with adjustment disorders, whereas impairments are often found in patients with depression and other disorders.

C. Laboratory Findings

Pathophysiologic studies of adjustment disorders show little evidence of somatic involvement, although different mechanisms may be involved among different symptom groups. Patients with adjustment disorders resemble normal control subjects in most physiologic studies, with the nonspecific exceptions of elevated cortisol response to stress, decreased sensitivity to pain, and a decrease in delta sleep (e.g., following marital separation or soon after divorce). In comparison to patients with adjustment disorder and controls, individuals with major depressive episodes exhibit more physiologic markers of change (e.g., event-related potentials, decreased heart rate variability, and cortisol and adrenocorticotropin suppression following dexamethasone).

D. Neuroimaging

Treatment-refractory adjustment disorder may be an indication for imaging with a goal of differential diagnosis. Life events are common, so that it may be tempting to ascribe symptoms to one or another unfortunate circumstance. One case report, for example, revealed temporal lobe epilepsy after the patient had 2 years of failed psychotherapy for adjustment disorder. In another case, Hallervorden–Spatz disease was revealed by magnetic resonance imaging in a presentation initially presumed to be a severe adjustment disorder.

E. Course of Illness

The symptoms of adjustment disorder usually resolve quickly, with or without resolution of the stressors. Precipitous onsets with shorter symptomatic periods are often seen following acute and intense stressful events, while chronic stressors often witness onset delays with longer symptomatic courses. Generally, inpatient stays are shorter for adjustment disorders than for depression, and improvement takes place during the first few weeks. Long-term outcome surveys suggest cautious optimism in the prognosis for treated children and adults. Adjustment disorders may reoccur in children and adolescents with greater frequency than in adults. Adolescence, especially, is fraught with many somatic changes and social adjustment requirements. For a first-time diagnosis, most adults will fare very well after suicide risks abate. Data suggest that an adjustment disorder in a child or adolescent predicts future episodes of adjustment disorder but does not predict future major affective episodes. Recovery is not greatly affected by comorbidity; the prognosis of an adjustment disorder alone is like an adjustment disorder with a comorbid diagnosis.

▶ Differential Diagnosis (Including Comorbid Conditions)

A. Relationship to Other Entities

When symptoms do not resolve quickly and therapy reveals other psychopathology or personality disorder, the initial diagnosis of adjustment disorder is often revised. When the diagnosis is uncertain, a provisional diagnosis may accommodate individuals who may otherwise resist treatment because of preconceived expectations or fears of psychiatric labeling. Patients may accept more readily a temporary and minimal diagnosis, one that permits further assessment.

Also, it is often appealing to view a new patient as healthy, with a milder diagnosis. Emergency room diagnoses of adjustment disorder are often changed to conduct disorder or substance abuse. This broadly inclusive diagnosis allows symptoms to be addressed while relatively mild, before a major syndrome develops, such as a major depressive episode. Given these properties, some vagueness and ambiguity are unavoidable.

B. Reactions to Stress

Normal grief reactions or bereavement may show cultural variability and be difficult to differentiate from adjustment disorders. Suicide risks may be present following bereavement no matter which diagnosis is ultimately given. If the reaction to the stressor is within expectable and culturally acceptable norms, a nonpathological reaction to stress should be recorded.

The diagnoses of acute stress disorder and PTSD are appropriate only following extremely threatening or horrific stressors, where adjustment disorder can follow stressors of any severity. An adjustment disorder diagnosis remains appropriate following less serious stressors even if the response is extreme. Conversely, the adjustment disorder diagnosis is also appropriate when responses do not reach severity criteria for PTSD, even if the stressor is sufficient to meet the PTSD stressor criterion.[2] Acute stress disorder follows an extreme stressor (more severe than stressors in adjustment disorder) and is associated with severe, specific symptoms (see Chapter 28). Acute stress disorder differs from PTSD in that the former remits within 1 month. The adjustment disorder diagnosis differs from both stress disorder diagnoses in that it is applicable to a wider range of presentations in onset, severity, and duration than these very specific and severe disorders. Furthermore, the emotional and behavioral responses in adjustment disorder are out of proportion to the stressor. In PTSD, the stressor leads to symptoms that are specific, severe, enduring, and handicapping, and more in proportion to the stressor (see Chapter 28).

In the impulse-control disorders, particularly intermittent explosive disorder, the precipitant stressor is minute in significance.

C. In Medical Settings

Adjustment disorder diagnoses may be applicable when the psychological stress of a physical illness causes psychiatric symptoms. For example, implantable cardioverter defibrillators have been associated with considerable psychological stress. In a way, adjustment disorder is the converse of the diagnosis of psychological factors affecting physical illness,

[2]https://icd.who.int/browse11/l-m/en#/http://id.who.int/icd/entity/264310751

in which a defensive coping style (e.g., repression) might worsen a systemic problem (e.g., peptic ulcer). It may be appropriate to give both diagnoses.

General medical conditions can cause psychiatric symptoms physiologically (and not psychologically as in adjustment disorder) and should be reported as such (e.g., mood disorder due to general medical condition). Individuals with chronic medical conditions may merit a second diagnosis of psychological factors affecting physical condition, reflecting both directions of the mind–body interaction.

D. Comorbidity

The symptoms of cluster B personality disorders often overlap with those of adjustment disorder, so that an adjustment disorder diagnosis may be redundant in some cases. Behavioral and emotional disturbances are excessive in personality disorders; these individuals would almost all be diagnosed as having adjustment disorder. However, adjustment disorder may be specified when the observed adjustment disorder is atypical for that personality disorder type.

Other, often comorbid, diagnoses that may need to be assessed include substance or alcohol abuse or dependence, somatoform and factitious disorders, and psychosexual disorder.

▶ Treatment

Individuals who have adjustment disorder will often appear relatively healthy compared to others with psychiatric disorders, sometimes deceptively so. Although successful treatment rates are greater than 70% in adjustment disorders, about one-third of patients do not fare well. Timely intervention can prevent later, more serious problems and point to underlying vulnerabilities that can be a focus of treatment. As with patients with almost any psychiatric diagnosis, and possibly especially so for adjustment disorders, effective referral for follow-up care has a greater impact on frequency of emergency visits than the diagnosis itself.

According to the patient's capacities, different therapeutic techniques can be chosen that may challenge erroneous beliefs and help the patient develop a psychological understanding of the problem. Adjustment difficulties worsen in the face of novel stressors when strong emotions are harbored but are poorly recognized or awkwardly expressed. Early intervention is probably more important than a particular therapeutic approach. As in other disorders, the building of an alliance during diagnostic interviewing is critical to the success of future therapy. The prudent interviewer will patiently avoid judgmental inflection and allow the individual wide latitude for emotional expression. An expeditious identification of the stressor in a permissive environment, allowing open expression of the fears and perceived helplessness, helps build an alliance focused on management of emotions resulting from the stressor. Table 38–3 summarizes

Table 38–3 Treatment of Adjustment Disorders

Treatment Approach	Primary Method	Secondary Methods
Behavioral	Psychodynamic psychotherapy	Cognitive–behavioral, interpersonal, or supportive psychotherapy
Pharmacologic	Antidepressant (e.g., sertraline, 25–75 mg daily)	Caution if patient has history of alcohol abuse: hypnotics (e.g., zolpidem, 5–10 mg at bedtime for 10 days) or anxiolytics (e.g., clonazepam, 0.5 mg at bedtime for 10 days)

psychotherapeutic and pharmacologic approaches to the treatment of adjustment disorders.

The financing of treatment for adjustment disorders will depend increasingly on the recognition that treatment improves outcome and quality of life, prevents more serious reactions from developing, and reduces the risk of recurrences. There is little to be gained by waiting for the advent of disorders that are difficult to treat. Adjustment disorder should be treated actively, ensuring restored premorbid functioning. Even so, brief therapies will need to be used. To justify treatment, third-party payers typically require information about symptoms that indicate risk, treatment goals, therapeutic methods, and outcome monitoring.

A. Psychotherapeutic Interventions

1. Psychoanalytic & psychodynamic approaches— Numerous viewpoints are used to model psychological disturbances in the effort to create treatment approaches. Historically, psychoanalytic and psychodynamic approaches have taken a leading role in the interpretation of behavior and emotion. In this view, individuals with adjustment disorder struggle unsuccessfully with effects of a stressor that most would manage more adaptively. Different forms of stress, difficult as they are to quantify, affect individuals in markedly different ways. Everyone has coping skills and mechanisms, some of which are used out of habit. Patients may adapt more easily to currently unmanageable stress when a history of similar difficulties is brought to light. Such a history can be examined in the transference, where perceptions of the relationship between the patient and the therapist are contaminated by attributes from prior relationships despite therapeutic neutrality. As therapy unfolds, the therapist becomes a target for misdirected anger and resentment, which is pointed out and examined as a means of exploring the problem. The work of therapy is to help the patient recognize and understand the unconscious struggle that arises when the pursuit of pleasure and relief from irritants (the pleasure principle) stands in the way of grasping reality (the reality principle), as pursued within the transference relationship.

Trauma or loss may be perceived as an assault on a strongly developed self-perception, too noxious to be accessible to grief-coping mechanisms. Inflated perceptions of the self and unreasonable expectations of others are usually strongly guarded secrets. In analytic treatment, transference may harbor the perception that the therapist is a steward of these demands. The overburdening superego (internal conscience) can then be revealed as the true aggressor, alleviating the exaggerated sense of the loss. Although the loss remains a reality, its importance then diminishes to a more acceptable level. Being able to project the cause of discomfort away from inappropriate self-blame onto a realistic outside agent will relieve the patient's sense of responsibility for the loss. For example, irrational guilt can arise over having been away on a trivial errand when a parent dies of cancer. The patient, after expressing a feeling that even the therapist blames him or her, can examine the need to accept cancer as the cause of loss.

Other, briefer types of therapies are encouraged in the current managed care environment. Although good comparison studies are lacking, certain individuals will probably do as well with briefer approaches. Psychodynamic, crisis-focused, time-limited psychotherapies require careful patient selection based on strong past interpersonal relationships, good premorbid functioning, and the absence of personality disorder. Some authors limit the use of these more confrontational techniques to situations in which there is a circumscribed focus, high motivation and capacity for insight, and a powerful degree of involvement in the interview. The time structure of this technique is set out clearly at the beginning, with planned termination emphasized and treated as a new stressor to be managed throughout. Goals must be defined clearly. For example, self-deprecating patients may perceive parents as simultaneously irreproachable yet harsh and over-demanding. Such patients may have recurrent, severe (but brief) emotional disturbances after any confrontation with their bosses. They may benefit from a better understanding of emotional similarities to maladaptive but customary rules of relationships from childhood. Such therapy allows recognition of relationship patterns without focusing primarily on the transference. Brief dynamic therapy has been shown to be effective compared to other therapies.

2. Cognitive–behavioral approaches—Cognitive–behavioral therapy provides the patient with tools for the recognition and modification of maladaptive beliefs regarding the stressor and the patient's ability to cope with it. Adjustment disorders can be addressed in this way because the importance of the stressor is often unrealistically overestimated in the patient's perception. In cognitive–behavioral therapy, the patient learns to recognize connections between emotions and maladaptive perceptions or beliefs and then learns to challenge those beliefs. Cognitive–behavioral therapy has demonstrated utility for adjustment disorders in occupational health. It has been successfully used in telepsychiatry for adjustment disorders in patients with cancer.

3. Interpersonal psychotherapy—Some clinicians prefer interpersonal therapy, especially for patients who have chronic medical illness or HIV infection. Many patients with severe medical illness shun intrapsychic introspection and benefit more from a psychoeducational approach. This is true for many adolescents. Discussion remains in a here-and-now about the sick role, which is a complicated balance of needs, independence, and becoming a willing target for the caring of other individuals. Open discussions ensue about who does what for whom in which way, and about how the illness and its consequences will affect the self and others. The modeling of coping mechanisms can be helpful. Humor can be effective, if introduced carefully. Death and dying become more approachable. These individuals often benefit from a reframing of problems from an interpersonal perspective and welcome discussions of ways to change dysfunctional behavior. The therapist may be able to address issues inaccessible to a medical–surgical team. For example, the patient may be reluctant to seem ungrateful to, and fearful of losing a relationship with, the primary care physician. Such a patient may regard the medical caregiver's purpose as one that provides medical treatment alone.

4. Supportive therapy—Supportive therapy is sometimes erroneously written off as hand-holding and comforting, whereas "real therapy" involves confrontation, analysis, and intellectualization. Supportive therapy should involve specific strategies and careful planning. Interventions have the goal of shoring up inadequate defense mechanisms. Problem-solving therapy may shorten time to partial return to work after 1 year. Intervention gently guides the individual to a verbalization of emotions regarding the stress. Communication, relaxation, and anger control (e.g., "counting to 10") are emphasized. In an acute crisis involving loss, or in medical settings where new information brings acute distress, a skilled supportive intervention can be eminently appropriate and effective.

Arends I, Bruinvels DJ, Rebergen DS, et al. Interventions to facilitate return to work in adults with adjustment disorders. *Cochrane Database Syst Rev.* 2012;12:CD006389.

5. Family therapy—Family therapy is often recommended. It can be among the most effective approaches to alleviating adjustment disorder by identifying the role the family plays in promoting a maladaptive coping response. However, some families are ill prepared to participate in treatment for the "identified" patient. In family sessions, lines of support can be examined and reestablished by skillful work to minimize distortions, blame, and isolation.

B. Psychopharmacologic Interventions

Pharmacotherapy is often used to assist in treatment of adjustment disorders. It may be useful when specific symptoms merit a medication trial. Drug selection is based on symptoms; for example, a short course of a benzodiazepine may be considered for adjustment disorder with anxious mood, but supporting data are few and risks of dependency must be monitored. The treatment goal is rapid symptom relief and prevention of a chronic problem, such as generalized anxiety disorder or PTSD. Antidepressants are used even more frequently now, especially in primary care with the advent of direct-to-consumer marketing. Selective serotonin reuptake inhibitors are generally well tolerated and appear to be beneficial for some patients, but double-blind, placebo-controlled studies are lacking. They are probably under prescribed for adolescents, males, those on welfare, and those in rural areas. Short-term trials of benzodiazepines and alprazolam are often prescribed, for example, for adjustment disorder involving anticipatory anxiety prior to chemotherapy. Hypnotics such as zolpidem, and calming preparations such as hydroxyzine should be considered for short-term use. The use of herbal preparations such as St. John's wort may merit further study.

Casey P, Doherty A. Adjustment disorder: implications for ICD-11 and DSM-5. *Br J Psychiatry*. 2012;201:90–92.

C. Nontraditional Approaches

In association with other treatments, nontraditional approaches can provide added benefit. Relaxation techniques, yoga, massage, and progressive muscle relaxation have been reported as helpful. Guided exposure or guided imagery can help with anticipatory stressors. Acupuncture has been used to treat adjustment disorders, but the results are unclear. Sleep deprivation, effective in treating endogenous and reactive depressions, may be useful in treating adjustment disorders.

▶ Complications/Adverse Outcomes of Treatment

Recovery from adjustment disorders can be complicated by a variety of poor outcomes. It is all too easy to overlook risk factors in the clinical setting. For example, persistent denial of the importance of a stressor may result in masked or displaced anger with an elevated risk of suicidality. In the patient's distorted view, denial will sometimes justify deceit to conceal issues such as physical safety and suicidality. Highly ambivalent, mixed emotional struggles (e.g., terminal illness in an unfaithful spouse, relationship problems among adolescents) require the clinician to be extra attentive and cautious. Among adolescents with adjustment disorder, suicidal ideation, threat, or attempt is associated with previous psychiatric treatment, poor psychosocial functioning, suicide

as a stressor, dysphoric mood, and psychomotor restlessness. Notably, the suicidal process—evolution of ideation to completion—is short and rapid in adjustment disorder and often comes with little warning in the form of prior emotional or behavioral problems. Adolescents in urban areas who were diagnosed as having adjustment disorder made more serious suicidal attempts than those with other disorders. Assessing suicide risk in the presence of adjustment disorder is extremely important.

In the presence of a comorbid personality disorder, adjustment disorder episodes frequently recur to the point where diagnosing them separately is not necessary. However, it is still necessary to treat adjustment disorder in this common context. According to one study, 15% of individuals with adjustment disorder also meet criteria for one of the cluster B personality disorders (antisocial, histrionic, borderline, or narcissistic personality disorders). A personality disorder diagnosis predicts poor acute outcome and the likelihood of chronic impairment in social support among individuals with an adjustment disorder.

Comorbid substance abuse is common in individuals with a primary diagnosis of adjustment disorder. Although alcoholism may "protect" people from stress (see discussion on cultural norms, earlier in this chapter), it clearly diminishes coping skills, promotes social isolation, and adds a suicide risk factor often considered "accidental" (e.g., motor vehicle accident or overdose).

Some adverse outcomes are iatrogenic. Although helpful for some patients, the risks of somatic treatment must be explained carefully. Medications carry side effects and other risks (e.g., suicide by overdose of tricyclic antidepressants), and for these disorders the potential for benefit has not been demonstrated against placebo. Hypomanic or manic switches occur occasionally even with modern antidepressants, and individual risk for this response cannot be predicted reliably. Movement disorder has been reported after single doses of neuroleptics. Benzodiazepines may impair judgment and pose risks of abuse and dependence and long-term neurotoxicity.

▶ Prognosis

Although short-term prognosis is quite good in adjustment disorder, an increased frequency of subsequent diagnoses may be of concern in the longer term. Further research is needed to identify individual prognostic factors and appropriate treatments.

Al-Ansari A, Matar AM. Recent stressful life events among Bahraini adolescents with adjustment disorder. *Adolescence*. 1993;28:339.

Chess S, Thomas A. *Origins and Evolution of Behavior Disorders*. New York: Brunner/Mazel; 1984.

Greenberg WM, Rosenfeld DN, Ortega EA. Adjustment disorder as an admission diagnosis. *Am J Psychiatry*. 1995;152:459.

Gur S, Hermesh H, Laufer N, et al. Adjustment disorder: a review of diagnostic pitfalls. *Isr Med Assoc J.* 2005;7(11):726–731.

Kovacs M, Gatsonis C, Pollock M, Parrone PL. A controlled prospective study of DSM-III adjustment disorder in childhood. Short-term prognosis and long-term predictive validity. *Arch Gen Psychiatry.* 1994;51:535.

Leigh H. Physical factors affecting psychiatric condition. *Gen Hosp Psychiatry.* 1993;15:155.

Newcorn JH, Strain J. Adjustment disorder in children and adolescents. *J Am Acad Child Adolesc Psychiatry.* 1992;31:318.

Oquendo MA. Differential diagnosis of ataque de nervios. *Am J Orthopsychiatry.* 1995;65:60.

Rickel AU, Allen L. *Preventing Maladjustment from Infancy Through Adolescence.* Thousand Oaks, CA: Sage; 1987.

Schatzberg AF: Anxiety and adjustment disorder: a treatment approach. *J Clin Psychiatry.* 1990;51(Suppl 11):20.

Semaan W, Hergueta T, Bloch J, et al. Cross-sectional study of the prevalence of adjustment disorder with anxiety in general practice. (French) *Encephale.* 2001;27:238.

Speer DC. Can treatment research inform decision makers? Nonexperimental method issues and examples among older outpatients. *J Consult Clin Psychol.* 1994;62:560.

Strain J, Hammer JS, Huertas D, et al. The problem of coping as a reason for psychiatric consultation. *Gen Hosp Psychiatry.* 1993;15:1.

World Health Organization. *International Statistical Classification of Diseases and Related Health Problems,* 11th rev. World Health Organization; 2020.

Personality Disorders

39

Sidney H. Weissman, MD

PERSONALITY DISORDERS IN GENERAL

General Considerations

Every individual has their own "unique" patterns of thinking, perceiving, feeling, and relating to themselves and to others. These patterns are maintained with limited modifications throughout an individual's life. Their development begins in childhood. These unique patterns are referred to as personality traits. These "traits" may lead to an individual experiencing disruption in their interactions with others with resultant personal pain. They may also adversely affect others and disrupt personal relationships. When either a disruption of self-experience or disruption of relationships with others occurs, individuals manifesting this behavior are described as having a personality disorder.

We develop our own unique traits through our interaction with the world from birth. Observations of infants reveal that at an infant's early age they are unique. These early life responses, shaped partially by our care takers and our unique nervous systems, are with us throughout our lives. Later experiences, some of which we can recall in later childhood and adolescence, also affect these traits.

In assessing an individual for the presence of a personality disorder, it is essential to perform an in-depth assessment utilizing a bio-psycho-social societal framework. The assessing mental health professional must be aware of their own personality traits and culture and be able to distinguish their own expectations of the expressions of traits from acceptable "learned" traits in others. Personality disorders may represent variants of behavioral traits that may merge imperceptibly from normal behavior into personality disorders. Additionally, clinician must note that the existence of traits that are elements of mental disorders does not mean the individual suffers from a personality disorder.

To address these difficulties, the authors of DSM-5 developed an alternative model of personality disorders defined in terms of personality functioning and pathological expression of personality traits. The alternative model addresses a reality that personality disorders are objectively distinct from other mental disorders. This awareness was addressed in earlier versions of the DSM by placing personality disorders in a unique diagnostic axis, Axis 2, separate from other mental disorders.

Although the alternative model addresses these concerns, operationalizing it is difficult to clinically implement. It includes two critical tables. It's table 2 is a table of levels of personality functioning with 60 potential responses. Its third table is "Definitions of DSM-5 personality disorder trait domains and facets." This scale includes 34 items. These scales might be useful in a psychological test but not in an exploratory clinical interview.

A. Epidemiology

The prevalence of diagnosable personality disorders in the general population has been estimated at 10–20%. This rate is much higher in mental health treatment settings, with as many as 50% of psychiatric patients meeting criteria for one or more personality disorders.

Some personality disorders are diagnosed more frequently in men, and some are more prevalent in women. Thus, for example, borderline personality disorder appears to be more common in women. Antisocial personality disorder predominates in men.

B. Etiology

The life experiences that lead to the development of personality disorders are not well understood. As with essentially every other type of psychiatric disorder, they involve various combinations of biologic, temperamental, and social etiologies. Historically, classic psychoanalytic theory suggests that personality disorders may develop from interactions between infants and parents in infancy. Early developmental relationships with family member as a child are also thought to be potential factors.

Related to the foregoing focus, developmental and environmental problems are a major focus of interest to scholars of personality. This is in part because the onset of behavior which become aspects of personality disturbance can be observed early in life. They are frequently associated with real and perceived disruptive childhood experiences. Of particular interest has been the extremely high rate of reported neglect and childhood sexual, physical, or emotional abuse in patients with certain personality disorders, especially borderline personality disorder and histrionic personality disorder.

C. Genetics

Genetic factors are influential in the etiology of some personality disorders. For example, family, twin, and adoption studies suggest that schizotypal personality disorder is linked to a family history of schizophrenia. Similar studies have delineated genetic factors related to antisocial and borderline disorders.

▶ Clinical Findings

A. Signs & Symptoms

Personality diagnoses be may coexist in one individual with other mental disorders. Personality disorders in DSM-5-TR as previously noted are described as "an enduring manifestation of inner experience and behavior that deviates markedly from the expectations of the individual's culture, is pervasive and inflexible becomes clearly evident in early adulthood and are stable over time, and may lead to distress or impairment."

For purposes of DSM-5-TR classification, there are 10 personality disorders, grouped into three major categories referred to as clusters. Cluster A (paranoid, schizoid, and schizotypal) is composed of individuals who are generally odd or eccentric. They may have abnormal cognitions, such as being overly suspicious or exhibiting peculiar expressions or odd speech, and they have difficulty relating to others. Cluster B personality disorders (antisocial, borderline, histrionic, and narcissistic) consist of individuals with dramatic, acting-out behaviors. Cluster C disorders (avoidant, dependent, and obsessive–compulsive) include those personality disorders generally marked by prominent anxiety and avoidance of novelty.

Several personality disorders may occur in a given individual within a given cluster is common or across clusters. Furthermore, a patient meeting criteria for one particular personality disorder may also have features of other disorders within the same cluster, as well as across clusters without meeting all criteria for the additional personality disorder diagnosis.

DSM-5-TR includes criteria for three other personality disorder diagnoses: Personality Change Due to Another Medical Condition, Other Specified Personality Disorder, and Unspecified Personality Disorder.

As a group, personality disorders are one of the most difficult and complicated emotional disorders to diagnose and to treat. Diagnosis is difficult in part because the disorders are often difficult to differentiate from each other, due to overlapping symptoms, and because the boundary between normality and psychopathology for each diagnosis is not distinct. Treatment of personality disorders is also difficult. Almost by definition, they are well-established behaviors and/or ways of thinking that are not perceived by the afflicted individual as abnormal or aberrant.

Manifestations of behavior diagnosed later in life as personality disorders are frequently evident early in life. Some behaviors in children, such as aggressiveness and stealing may predict later personality problems, such as antisocial personality disorder. However, other behaviors, such as childhood social isolation and shyness seem to be of little value in predicting later cluster C disorders.

B. Psychological Testing

A number of psychological tests have been developed to assess personality traits and disorders. Of particular prominence are the Millon Clinical Multiaxial Inventory (MCMI) and the Minnesota Multiphasic Personality Inventory (MMPI).

The MCMI is a self-administered, true–false inventory that provides information on personality style, significant personality patterns, and associated clinical disorders. The inventory includes 344 items, grouped into 22 overlapping scales. These consist of 4 validity scales, 11 clinical scales, 5 treatment issue scales, and 2 interpersonal scales. Unlike the MCMI, the MMPI was developed to aid in the diagnosis of mental disorders. However, it is often used to describe individuals more globally. It consists of more than 500 items and includes nine basic clinical scales (i.e., hypochondriacal depression, hysteria, psychopathic deviance, masculinity/femininity, paranoia, anxiety, schizophrenia, and mania). Validity scales are also included. Other assessment instruments have been developed, as have various semi-structured interview protocols such as the Structured Clinical Interview initially for DSM-IV, which can also be used to diagnose personality disorders.

C. Laboratory Findings

There are no proven biological markers that are highly specific to identify patients with personality disorders. Recent research is focusing on attempting to identify certain genetic profiles as being related to specific personality disorders.

▶ Differential and Coexisting Diagnoses

Personality disorders frequently are associated with mental disorders of nearly all types. Mood, anxiety, and substance use disorders are the most common correlates. Conversely, it has been reported that over 50% of patients hospitalized with major depressive disorder also have a diagnosable personality disorder. In some cases, a personality disorder is thought to predispose the individual to the recurrence and greater intensity of another mental disorder, thus indicating a poorer prognosis. Also, the presence of another diagnosis can complicate the process of establishing a personality disorder diagnosis, because common symptoms of personality disorders (e.g., interpersonal withdrawal or dependency) can be influenced by mood state. Furthermore, personality disorders are not mutually exclusive. The majority of patients meeting criteria for one personality disorder will also meet criteria for other personality disorders.

Treatment

Personality disorders are difficult to treat, in part because they often do not cause personal distress. Because personality traits are experienced as a fundamental part of each of us, an individual manifesting a personality disorder may not experience any distressing symptoms. Consequently, the affected individual often has limited awareness of the nature of his or her problems. Therefore, people with personality disorders are likely to present for treatment only during times of crisis or with the emergence of major psychiatric symptoms such as depression or anxiety, or when others such as family or coworkers are disturbed by their behavior.

Patients with personality disorders tend to be challenging treat for therapists. They are often angry, manipulative, demanding, or defensive. However, improvement in personality disorders often occurs over time.

Specific psychotherapy techniques, either in individual or group settings, including expressive, dynamic, behavioral, cognitive, or interpersonal therapies may be effective. As in all psychotherapies, the alliance and collaboration between therapist and patient or patient and group appear to be a critical component of successful treatment.

Prognosis

Personality disorders in general are highly associated with disability in the general population, and generally, when coexistent, with serious mental disorders worsen their prognosis.

For some individuals, the behavior and symptoms of their personality disorder remain disruptive for extended periods of time. However, for several personality disorders (borderline personality disorder, antisocial personality disorder) behavioral changes can occur with aging such that they no longer meet the diagnostic criteria for the disorder. Impulsivity and anger, observed in borderline and antisocial personality disorders, tend to show some reduction when the individual reaches middle age.

INDIVIDUAL PERSONALITY DISORDERS DEFINED IN DSM-5-TR

CLUSTER A PERSONALITY DISORDERS

PARANOID PERSONALITY DISORDER

General Considerations

A. Epidemiology

The prevalence of paranoid personality disorder has been estimated at 0.5–4.5% of the general population. It is relatively common in clinical settings, particularly among psychiatric inpatients. Individuals with a paranoid personality disorder rarely seek treatment on their own. They are usually referred by family members, coworkers, or employers. The disorder appears to be slightly more common in women than in men.

B. Etiology

Although the etiology of paranoid personality disorder is uncertain, both genetic and environmental aspects are thought to play an etiologic role. For example, the risk of developing the disorder is somewhat enhanced in families with a history of schizophrenia and delusional disorders. Developmentally, the risk for this disorder appears to be increased if the individual's parents exhibited irrational outbursts of anger and pain. It is thought that the anger the individual experienced or perceived as a child is now seen as coming from others later in life.

C. Genetics

Patients diagnosed with paranoid personality disorder may have biological relatives with higher incidence of schizophrenia than do controls. The link between paranoid personality disorder and schizoid personality disorder is observed but while weak is measurable.

Clinical Findings

Signs & Symptoms

The cardinal feature of paranoid personality disorder is the presence of generalized distrust or suspiciousness. Individuals feel that they have been treated unfairly, are resentful of this mistreatment, and bear long-lasting grudges against those who have slighted them or who they feel have slighted them. They place a high premium on autonomy and react in a hostile manner to others who seek, or they feel seek to control them, and they can become violent. These patients are often unsuccessful in intimate relationships because of their suspiciousness and aloofness.

When interviewed, patients with a paranoid personality disorder are formal, businesslike, skeptical, and mistrustful and may exhibit either poor or fixated eye contact. They consistently project blame for their difficulties onto others, externalizing their own emotions while paying keen attention to the emotions and attitudes of others. Underlying their formal and at times moralistic presentation is considerable hostility and resentment.

▶ Differential Diagnosis

There is considerable overlap among patients with paranoid personality disorder, patients with schizoid personality disorder, and those with schizotypal personality disorder. Of those patients with schizoid personality disorder, 47% were also diagnosed as having a paranoid personality disorder. In addition, the disorder often appears in combination with schizotypal personality disorder, although this in part is because of the shared diagnostic feature of paranoid ideation. Other common personality disorder comorbidities include the borderline and narcissistic personality disorders. When paranoid personality disorder is comorbid with narcissistic personality disorder, the paranoid elements serve to enforce the patient's overvalued ideas. Paranoid personality disorder has features similar to several other mental disorders. These include delusional disorder—persecutory type and schizophrenia, particularly when paranoid delusions are present. Paranoid personality disorder is distinguished from delusional disorder and schizophrenia by the absence of delusions, hallucinations, and defective reality testing, although differentiation is not always easy.

▶ Treatment

A. Psychopharmacologic Interventions

There are little available data to suggest that pharmacologic interventions are of significant benefit in paranoid personality afflicted individuals. Although not supported by controlled clinical trials, it is felt that low-dose antipsychotic medications may decrease the patient's paranoia and anxiety. Under some stressful situations, some patients' paranoid ideation may reach delusional proportions. In such cases, antipsychotic medication can be of benefit.

B. Psychotherapeutic Interventions

1. Group and marital interventions—Group therapy can be quite difficult for patients with paranoid personality disorder. Their lack of basic trust caused by their suspiciousness often prevents them from being integrated fully into groups. Their wariness and suspiciousness may make other group members uncomfortable and rejecting. Paranoid personality disorder patients sometimes present for treatment with family members or as marital couples. Working with them in this context is also difficult, because such patients often feel that the therapist and family members are working against them. It is not advisable to see family members of paranoid patients without their written consent.

2. Individual psychotherapies—Patients with paranoid personality disorder represent a unique challenge to the psychotherapist. Because they lack trust, they rarely enter treatment unless there is another coexisting emotional disorder, such as a mood or anxiety disorder, or coercion from a family member or employer. Because of the suspiciousness, they may not tolerate perceived ambiguity associated with imprecise interventions. Among behavioral techniques used, social-skills role-playing, particularly involving appropriate expression of assertiveness, has been employed. Clinical wisdom suggests that cognitive techniques that focus on the patient's overgeneralizations (e.g., "That person didn't talk to me; therefore, he hates me") and their propensity to dichotomize the social world into trustworthy and hostile are useful. With psychodynamic and interpersonal approaches, interpretations are used sparingly and cautiously because they may be experienced as attacks. Treatment focuses on the gradual recognition of the origins and negative consequences of the patient's mistrust.

▶ Prognosis

Little is known about the long-term outcome of paranoid personality disorder. Although the disorder is difficult to treat, patients generally appear to have a greater adaptive capacity than do those who have personality disorders associated with severe social detachment. As previously noted, under stressful situations, patients with paranoid personality disorder usually withdraw and avoid interpersonal attachments. This perpetuates their mistrust, and they may become overtly psychotic.

SCHIZOID PERSONALITY DISORDER

▶ General Considerations

A. Epidemiology

Estimates of the prevalence of schizoid personality disorder in the general population vary with the criteria used, ranging from 0.5 to 7%, and individuals with this disorder are relatively uncommon in clinical settings. The disorder occurs more often in men than in women and may be more severe in men. The general withdrawal of patients with schizoid personality disorder from social situations means that they rarely disturb others, and in part this accounts for their rare appearance in treatment settings.

B. Etiology

The diagnosis of schizoid personality disorder applies to individuals with a profound defect in the ability to establish and develop personal relationships and to respond to others in a meaningful way.

The causes of schizoid personality disorder are not well understood. Genetic factors are suspected, and some reports suggest that patients with this disorder often come from environments that were deficient in emotional nurturing.

C. Genetics

Although symptoms of schizoid personality disorder resemble the negative symptoms of schizophrenia, an increased prevalence of schizoid personality disorder among individuals with a family history of schizophrenia might have been expected.

However, schizoid personality disorder does not appear to have a strong genetic relationship to schizophrenia. However, it does have some of the features of autism spectrum disorder. This creates the possibility of a relationship to autism exists between them.

Clinical Findings

A. Signs & Symptoms

In the case of schizoid personality, the individual is not necessarily distressed or disturbing to others. Thus, the life history of patients with schizoid personality disorder is typically characterized by a preference for solitary pursuits. These individuals may have none or only a few intimate relationships and show little apparent interest in people, outside of internal fantasy. Social detachment and restricted emotional expressivity, that is, affective constriction, make these patients appear aloof, distant, and difficult to engage. Individuals with schizoid personality disorder are more likely to demonstrate interest when describing abstract pursuits that require no emotional expression. Although reality testing is generally intact, schizoid personality disorder patients' lack of social contact may preclude the correction of their somewhat idiosyncratic interpretations of social transactions.

B. Differential Diagnosis

Patients with schizoid personality disorder resemble individuals with avoidant personality disorder (described later). They can be distinguished from those with avoidant personality disorder by their indifference to others. They also may be confused with patients with schizotypal personality disorder. In contrast to schizotypal personality disorder, the schizoid personality disorder patient is affectively flat and unresponsive, rather than behaviorally eccentric, with odd thoughts, behaviors of both disorders may be seen in the same individual. Finally, the schizoid personality disorder patient may share a number of symptoms in common with patients with autism spectrum disorder.

Treatment

A. Psychopharmacologic Interventions

Little is known about the effective pharmacologic treatment of schizoid personality disorder. Thus far, effective pharmacotherapy has not been demonstrated for the disorder as such, although associated anxiety and depression, when it occurs, may be treated with antidepressants and other medications.

B. Psychotherapeutic Interventions

1. Group and family techniques—Often individuals with schizoid personality disorder come to treatment at the request of family members. In some cases, family-based interventions may be helpful in clarifying for the patient the family's expectations, and perhaps in addressing any intolerance and invasiveness on the part of the family that could be worsening the patient's withdrawal.

Group therapy can also be helpful as a source of directed feedback from others that would otherwise be missed or ignored. Such a setting can also allow for the modeling and acquisition of needed social skills. However, the initial participation of the schizoid personality disorder patient will invariably be minimal, and the therapist may sometimes need to act to prevent the patient from being the hostile target of other group members. However, as with so many therapies, these assertions are based on clinical wisdom and have not been proven experimentally.

2. Individual psychotherapies—Psychotherapeutic interventions tend to be difficult to accomplish in the patient with schizoid personality disorder. Such patients typically experience little perceived distress and are often not psychologically minded. The tendency of these patients to intellectualize and distance themselves from emotional experience can also restrict the impact of treatment.

It is difficult to develop a therapeutic relationship because individuals with schizoid personality disorder do not seek affective connections. For this reason, clinical wisdom suggests that more cognitively based treatment approaches may receive greater initial acceptance. This allows distorted expectancies and perceptions about the importance and usefulness of relationships to be explored.

Prognosis

Patients with schizoid personality disorder display problems more frequently in early childhood than those with other personality disorders. Social disinterest tends to self-perpetuate isolation, as does flattened affect. However, relative to patients with other personality disorders, those with schizoid personality disorder are less likely to experience anxiety or depression, particularly if they are not in social, educational, or occupational situations that tax their limited social skills. Also, the number of individuals with schizoid personality disorder who are not in mental health care may be large, and such individuals may be relatively well adjusted to their lives.

SCHIZOTYPAL PERSONALITY DISORDER

General Considerations

A. Epidemiology

The prevalence rate of schizotypal personality disorder has been estimated at approximately 3–5% of the general population. Furthermore, up to 30% of general psychiatric outpatients have one or more traits associated with schizotypal personality disorder. Comorbidity exists with mood, substance use, and anxiety disorders. Men are slightly more likely to have the disorder.

B. Etiology

Schizotypal personality disorder occurs significantly more frequently among the biological relatives of schizophrenic individuals than in the general population. This finding, together with the results of twin studies, supports a genetic relationship to schizophrenia. Of all of the personality disorders, schizotypal personality disorder most strongly demonstrates a potential continuum with schizophrenia. Thus, it is likely that some of the etiologic factors that induce schizophrenia are similar to those that induce schizotypal personality disorder.

C. Genetics

The concept of schizotypal personality disorder was originally developed because the relatives of schizophrenic patients often had symptoms similar to schizophrenia. There is also evidence that biologic and neurocognitive markers of schizophrenia are shared with patients with schizotypal personality disorder. Schizotypal personality disorder includes behaviors manifested in schizophrenia spectrum disorders (which include schizoaffective disorder, schizophreniform disorder, and psychotic mood disorders). Because of its genetic links to schizophrenia, the factors that lead to it are more likely different than for other personality disorders.

▶ Clinical Findings

Signs & Symptoms

Schizotypal personality disorder is characterized by peculiar behavior, odd thoughts, odd speech, unusual perceptive experiences, and peculiar or "magical beliefs."

These patients usually demonstrate negative or poor rapport and additionally show social dysfunction, social anxiety, and a lack of motivation. They are frequently underachievers with regard to cognitive abilities status.

The disorder may be manifested during childhood or adolescence as social isolation and peculiar behavior or language. Although the features of the disorder resemble schizophrenia, rates of depression and anxiety are also quite high among such patients. The latter features often constitute the presenting complaint, rather than the ongoing cognitive anomalies.

▶ Differential Diagnosis

Schizotypal personality disorder is considered by some investigators to be a form of schizophrenia spectrum disorder.

The relatives of patients with schizophrenia who display schizotypal personality disorder frequently tend to exhibit social isolation and poor rapport, rather than psychotic-like symptoms and ideas of reference. Thus, although the schizotypal personality disorder appears with relatively greater than expected frequency in the relatives of schizophrenic patients (i.e., 10%), it is not necessarily merely a milder form of schizophrenia. With respect to other cluster A disorders, 70% of patients with schizotypal personality disorders have been found to have one or more cluster A personality disorders. Furthermore, comorbidity with major mental disorders involving mood, anxiety, and substance use disorders is also common.

▶ Treatment

A. Psychopharmacologic Interventions

Low-dose antipsychotic medications are sometimes prescribed to treat the cognitive peculiarities, depression, odd speech, anxiety, and impulsivity of patients with schizotypal personality disorder. Antipsychotic medications are particularly useful in patients with moderately severe schizotypal symptoms and in mild transient psychotic episodes. It is unknown whether antipsychotic medications have a prophylactic benefit for this disorder. In addition, some anecdotal evidence suggests that lithium and mood stabilizers may be helpful in treating selected schizotypal patients.

B. Psychotherapeutic Interventions

1. Group and marital interventions—Group therapy, especially social skills training, is believed to be helpful to patients with schizotypal personality disorder. This form of therapy addresses the associated social anxiety and awkwardness. However, patients with more severe symptoms may prove disruptive to the cohesiveness of the group, particularly if paranoid ideation is present. Patients with overtly eccentric behavior may inadvertently make other group members uncomfortable.

2. Individual psychotherapies—Patients with schizotypal personality disorder are generally thought to be poorly suited for nondirective psychotherapies. They have a propensity to decompensate and become disorganized in unstructured interspersal situations. Often a supportive approach is recommended with an emphasis on reality testing and attention to interpersonal boundaries; this may be combined with directive approaches focused on problematic behavior. A cognitive focus also appears useful, with attempts made to help the patient recognize cognitive distortions, such as referential, paranoid, or magical thinking. This can be accomplished through educative interventions that teach patients to corroborate their odd ideas and thoughts with environmental evidence rather than with personal impressions.

Prognosis

Estimates of the proportion of patients with schizotypal personality disorder who go on to develop overt schizophrenia are variable. The proportion is generally thought to be relatively low, possibly around 10% or less, although some estimates are as high as 20–25%. Paranoid ideation, social isolation, and magical thinking when associated with cognitive functional decline are most predictive of a patient eventually meeting the criteria for schizophrenia. These symptoms are also most associated with a poor prognosis and a more chronic outcome.

CLUSTER B PERSONALITY DISORDERS

ANTISOCIAL PERSONALITY DISORDER

General Considerations

A. Epidemiology

Antisocial personality disorder appears to be reasonably common in the general population, with its rate estimated at 2–4% of men and 0.5–1.0% of women. However, because individuals manifesting the symptoms and behaviors of antisocial personality disorder rarely seek treatment voluntarily and generally come to treatment only when interventions are mandated, these numbers are approximate. Finally, there is a strong correlation between having conduct disorder as a child and developing antisocial personality disorder as an adult.

B. Etiology

It appears that both biological and environmental factors are involved as causes of antisocial personality disorder. Individuals are at increased risk for this disorder if they had an antisocial or alcoholic father (even if they were not raised by that person). Other associated variables occurring in childhood include living in a nonintact family, low parental education, conduct problems and bullying at home or in school, and adult criminal offenses in the family. The primary environmental deficiency appears to be the lack of a consistent person to give emotional, loving support, and clear direction as a young child. Living in a high-crime area does not in and of itself increase the risk of antisocial personality disorder. The presence of untreated attention-deficit/hyperactivity disorder by interfering with self-regulation when coupled with distressful life experiences may further relate to the development of antisocial disorder.

C. Genetics

Family studies of individuals with antisocial personality disorder reveal an increased incidence of this disorder in family members. This need not be an indication of genetic causality since the family members live in a common environment. However, individuals are at increased risk for this disorder if they had an antisocial or alcoholic father (even if they were not raised by that person). Twin studies also support a genetic component to the etiology of antisocial personality disorder.

Clinical Findings

Signs & Symptoms

As described in the DSM-5-TR, antisocial personality disorder consists of a pattern of recurrent antisocial, delinquent, and criminal behavior that begins in childhood or early adolescence and basically pervades all aspects of an individual's life. Negative job performance and marital instability are also hallmarks of the antisocial personality disorder patient.

A major feature of antisocial personality disorder is a disregard for the rights and feelings of others. This is a characteristic that leads to a variety of unacceptable behaviors, often noted during adolescence or childhood as a conduct disorder. Thus, beginning earlier than 15 years of age, patients have histories of impulsive behavior, aggression toward others, school discipline problems, and breaking the law. Individuals with antisocial personality disorders are deficient in meeting social roles and occupational obligations. Relationships are generally superficial and short-lived. Use of illegal substances is common. These individuals tend to be easily bored and impulsive. They seek novelty in their lives and seem unable to avoid behavior that has a high probability of leading to punishment. They may exploit others for personal benefit or at times for no good reason. They often rationalize their antisocial behavior as necessarily defensive, believing others are trying to exploit them.

Differential Diagnosis

Substance use disorders is comorbid in two-thirds of patients with antisocial personality disorder. Other comorbid conditions include the following: other personality disorders, sexual dysfunction, paraphilias, mood disorders, and anxiety disorders. Patients with antisocial personality disorder have high premature rates of death from natural causes and suicide.

With respect to personality traits and temperament, antisocial personality disorder patients often score low in harm avoidance, low in reward dependence, and high in novelty seeking. These characteristics are associated with risk taking without fear, lack of concern for others, and impulsivity.

Treatment

A. Psychopharmacologic Interventions

Overall, there is little evidence that the pharmacologic treatment of antisocial personality disorder is effective. However, treatment of coexisting symptoms may be useful.

Psychostimulants may be used to treat symptoms of attention-deficit disorder. Although efficacy has not been demonstrated by controlled clinical trials, selective serotonin reuptake inhibitors (SSRIs), bupropion, and antipsychotic agents have been used to reduce impulsive aggression.

B. Psychotherapeutic Interventions

1. Group, marital, and community programs—Because these patients' lack of insight into their behavioral difficulties, placing them into groups with individuals with similar behavioral problems has been tried. Clinical practitioners often consider socially based interventions, particularly with others of similar temperaments and problems, to be the treatment of choice for patients with antisocial personality disorder. It is thought that in group contexts, rationalization and evasion can be confronted by others who recognize these patterns. Group membership and associated caring for and from others presumably allow patients with antisocial personality disorder to experience feelings of belonging that many never previously experienced from their families. Similarly, family therapy may be useful when the family system is contributing to or perpetuating antisocial behavior. Also, it can address destructive attachments with a spouse, parenting issues, and the experience of aggressiveness that can lead to abuse.

Intensive community-based group treatment programs may be helpful. A decrease of 20–40% in criminal behavior and recidivism, a probable marker of antisocial personality disorder, occurs with such treatment. Usually, such treatments focus on improving social skills, treating substance use, managing impulse control, and diminishing antisocial attitudes.

2. Individual psychotherapeutic interventions—The literature generally considers individual psychotherapy to be of limited effectiveness. These patients in individual psychotherapy are frequently manipulative evasive. Dropout rates may be as high as 70%. It is frequently difficult for these patients to develop a treatment relationship with a therapist.

Cognitive–behavioral psychotherapy has been used with some success in treating antisocial personality disorder. The patient's distorted cognitive constructs and attitudes toward social groups and individuals are analyzed. Specifically, cognitive approaches involve addressing distortions that are typically self-serving or that minimize the future consequences of the individual's behavior.

▶ Prognosis

Antisocial personality disorder, as it appears in young adults, is thought to be among the most treatment refractory of the personality disorders. However, the behavioral problems associated with antisocial personality disorder tend to peak in late adolescence and early adulthood, and 30–40% of these individuals show significant improvement in their antisocial behaviors by the time they reach their mid-30s and 40s and may not meet criteria for the diagnosis.

During their later years individuals with antisocial personality disorder are at risk for developing chronic alcoholism and late-onset depression. They often continue to be irresponsible, but without the dramatic aggressiveness of their earlier years. Possibly of significance, the core personality traits of conscientiousness and agreeableness naturally increase with age, and this change has been suggested to be responsible for the "improvement" in individuals with antisocial personality disorder over time.

BORDERLINE PERSONALITY DISORDER

▶ General Considerations

A. Epidemiology

The prevalence of borderline personality disorder in the general population is about 1–2%. However, the disorder is particularly common among psychiatric inpatients, on related medical units, and patients seen in emergency rooms. Borderline personality disorder is identified more commonly in women than in men, although evidence suggests that it may be under identified in men. The features of the disorder are more common among young adults.

B. Etiology

Borderline personality disorder patients are quite common in psychiatric settings, typically accounting for one third or more of clinical personality disorder diagnoses. The causes of the disorder are uncertain. Psychoanalytic thinking commonly focuses on either disturbance in the early relationship between the child and their mother which interferes with autonomous self-development of the child.

Further effecting the child's emotional growth are reported experiences by these patients of reports of childhood sexual, physical, and/or emotional abuse. It is likely that such abuse or their perception has etiologic significance. This purported abuse may have led to the patient to develop strategies to reduce pain. This in turn may lead to a patient developing dissociation, splitting, repression, mood lability, and identity problems. Other forms of parental actions either such as neglect or difficulty in the expression of affection, over criticism, or invalidating communication have been proposed to be of etiologic importance. For a given patient, these actions may be experienced as traumatic.

C. Genetics

The potential genetic influences leading to borderline personality disorder are not well understood. However, some investigators speculate that a genetic factor may lead to the development of emotional lability. This in turn leads to enhanced anxiety, and instability that are characteristic of borderline personality disorder.

Borderline personality disorder occurs relatively more often in the families of patients with the disorder. There is also some evidence from family studies that bipolar disorder and/or major depression occurs more often in families with individuals with borderline personality disorder. This can be understood as either personality traits (i.e., aggression, impulsivity, affective instability) present in the family or genetically determined. Additionally, the potentially altered family dynamics created by individuals with bipolar or depressive disorders may negatively impact on some developing children. It is also possible that the use MRIs of the brains effected individuals will reveal a site that accounts for emotional lability.

Clinical Findings

Signs & Symptoms

Borderline personality disorder as now defined in DSM-5-TR represents a pervasive pattern of mood instability associated with unstable but intense interpersonal relationships. Commonly impulsivity, inappropriate or intense anger, recurrent suicidal threats and gestures, and self-mutilating behavior occur. There is a persistent identity disturbance, chronic feelings of emptiness or boredom, and an exaggerated attempt to avoid real or perceived abandonment. Transient paranoid ideation or dissociative symptoms may also occur. In addition, primitive defense mechanisms such as splitting (exaggerated dichotomies of good and evil, worthy and unworthy, etc.) are often present. A general overall deficit in the ability to test reality in situations of special meaning is also characteristic of patients with borderline personality.

Borderline personality disorder patients are also characterized by a poorly established self-image that is heavily dependent for validation on relationships, but at times these are experienced with an expectation of mistreatment or exploitation. This combination of features makes those with the disorder extremely concerned about close relationships and highly sensitive to changes in these relationships. Reaction to interpersonal conflicts is characterized by dramatic emotional changes, often associated with impulsive self-destructiveness.

The patient with borderline personality disorder mood often switches between rage, despair, and anxiety over the course of a single day or less. Multiple suicidal gestures and self-mutilation and self-injurious behaviors are among the most striking actions of these patients. As described earlier, such behavior is noted primarily after interpersonal turmoil, often the experience of rejection by a close friend or family member. Suicidal gestures such as cutting often tend to increase in lethality as they recur, and completed suicide occurs in up to 10% of borderline personality disorder patients.

Adding to the complexity of understanding borderline personality disorder, self-injurious behavior, often beginning in childhood or adolescence, may not be a sign of suicidal intent as such. Such cutting, burning, and associated attempts to cause pain are often due to attempts to regulate dysphoric affective states including, guilt, tension, and dissociative symptoms, and/or to communicate emotions. These self-injurious behaviors are especially associated with a self-reported history of childhood sexual abuse.

The assessment of borderline personality disorder patients is complicated by the cognitive style that these patients manifest. Although positive comments can be found, patients' evaluations of themselves and their surroundings often are negative in the extreme. Alternatively, their life situation, and relationships can be overidealized. However, the borderline personality patient's tendency to evaluate his or her mental status negatively (i.e., more depressed or anxious) leads to self-reported clinical pictures that are more pathologic than they outwardly appear.

Patients with the borderline personality symptoms may admit to an observer that they exaggerate a wide variety of behavioral syndromes, including severe depression and anxiety, psychotic features, paranoid ideation, and somatic concerns.

Understanding Signs and Symptoms

The characteristics of the borderline personality disorder patient are considered on a spectrum between the normal and severely symptomatic. Borderline personality disorder patients can be classified with respect to either their temperaments or core personality traits. On the five-factor model of personality scale, they often show high neuroticism, low agreeableness, and low conscientiousness, with no special relationship to extraversion reported. Similarly, for the Tridimensional Personality Questionnaire and its derivative, the cluster for borderline personality disorder consists of high novelty seeking (seen primarily in males), fairly high harm avoidance (primarily in females), low reward dependence, and low self-directedness.

The clinician must determine the severity of the borderline personality disorder behavioral symptoms before determining treatment interventions.

Differential Diagnosis

Borderline personality disorder is frequently associated with a variety of personality disorders, especially those in cluster B. Major depression is commonly comorbid with borderline personality disorder. Substance abuse disorder, alcoholism, posttraumatic stress disorder, and anxiety disorders are frequently diagnosed in patients with borderline personality disorder.

Treatment

A. Psychopharmacologic Intervention

A number of psychopharmacologic strategies are useful in treating borderline personality disorder. Controlled clinical trials demonstrate the efficacy of lithium carbonate in diminishing anger, irritability, and self-mutilation in some patients. A more limited body of evidence indicates that carbamazepine increases behavioral control and diminishes anger and impulsivity. Sodium valproate has been used to treat irritability and aggressiveness in borderline patients. In open-label studies olanzapine reduces paranoid and other psychotic ideation, impulsive aggression, and depression. Similarly, chlorpromazine, clozapine, risperidone, aripiprazole and quetiapine have a similar therapeutic profile to olanzapine in open-label studies. Several SSRI antidepressants (fluoxetine and fluvoxamine) have therapeutic efficacy with regard to mood fluctuations, aggression, and overall adaptive behavior.

Finally, any medication administered to a borderline disorder patient should be monitored carefully and prescribed cautiously because of the enhanced risks for noncompliance, development of substance abuse, and use in suicide attempts or gestures.

B. Psychotherapeutic Intervention

1. Group and family approaches—Group therapy has been reported to be a useful format to address the interpersonal problems of borderline personality disorder patients. In such groups patients can form attachments to the group as such or to individual group members, rather than focusing their positive and negative feelings and transferences on a single therapist. Having peers available who can present alternative accounts of the inevitable conflicts that develop with other group members is also helpful. Similarly, family therapy, used especially to untangle dependency issues and issues of dramatic acting out, has been reported to be helpful.

2. Individual psychotherapies—Generally, psychotherapy with borderline patients is made difficult by the severity and nature of the borderline personality disorder patients' behaviors. The therapist must contain their own responses to the borderline patient's actions. However, there are several structured therapies that have proven useful in the treatment of borderline personality disorder patients.

Dialectical behavior therapy (DBT) is a commonly used and effective form of treatment. In the initial stages of treatment, a supportive approach is used to establish a therapeutic alliance. Over time, the therapist focuses on identifying the patient's ineffective behaviors and the patient is aided in developing alternate responses. The emphasis of the therapy is on stress tolerance, coping skills development, emotional regulation and self-management. This aids the patient in the suppression of secondary gain from acting-out behavior.

With treatment, patients come to recognize the pattern of self-destruction, instability, and projection that have characterized their lives and to understand their origins. Patients also explore with their therapist their rigid good-versus-bad view of others. They can then learn to, recognize that others' motivations, like their own, are more complex than they appear. Their sensitivity to others' untrustworthiness is often a distortion arising out of their own experience.

In controlled trials, DBT has been demonstrated to be effective in reducing self-injurious behavior and anger, resulting in fewer days of inpatient hospitalization. Patients treated with effective psychotherapy have less drug and alcohol use, and depressive symptoms were improved.

Mentalization-based psychotherapy is a type of supportive intervention that aids in focusing as how they think and feel. In treating borderline patients, the therapist and patient must reach agreement about the role of the therapist and how they deal with phone calls, cancelations, and how emergencies are addressed. All of these issues are potentially difficult for these patients. In controlled clinical trials, individuals engaged in mentalization-based therapy showed improvement in anxiety, social adjustment, and organizational skills.

▶ Prognosis

Patients with borderline personality disorder repeatedly engage in self-destructive behaviors that can be lethal. Patients sometimes act in a fashion that disrupts treatment even when it appears to be going well. In part, their difficult treatment course relates to the extreme adverse reactions to the actions of their therapists and varied life events. Undoubtedly related, the consistent stable of disruptive behaviors of many borderline patients is their affective instability and anger. Their behavior tends to become more dramatic and dangerous as others, such as family, therapists, and significant others, are experienced as rejecting or dismissing their needs. As a result, the prognosis can be poor. Patients' over-involvement in family relations, antisocial behaviors, chronic anger, and overuse of medical facilities predict a poor outcome. Conversely, impulsive and dangerous behaviors seem to diminish as these patients approach middle age. A better outcome is associated with higher intelligence, superior social support, and increased self-discipline.

HISTRIONIC PERSONALITY DISORDER

▶ General Considerations

A. Epidemiology

The overall prevalence of histrionic personality disorder has been estimated as about 1.0% in the general population. Rates of the disorder are much higher in psychiatric and general medical settings, because these patients often actively pursue treatment.

Histrionic personality disorder tends to be diagnosed more frequently in women; it is however, likely that the disorder may be overlooked in men. For younger adults, men and women have been reported to be equally likely to receive a diagnosis of histrionic personality disorder, whereas in middle age, women appear to predominate. Nevertheless, epidemiologic studies indicate that overall, the gender differences in prevalence may be slight.

B. Etiology

As with most personality disorders, the etiology of histrionic personality disorder is not well understood. Some researchers speculate that problems in early parent–child relationships lead to the development of associated low self-esteem. It is thought that as a child the patient needed to use dramatic behavior and other similar means to engage others. This behavior seems to both mask and compensate for the patient's low self-concept for and obscures their fears in effectively engaging others.

C. Genetics

There is potential evidence for a genetic component to histrionic personality disorder. There appears to be some connection in families with some members having either a histrionic or antisocial personality disorder.

This could be related to a shared neuropsychiatric vulnerability that is genetically transmitted. Alternatively, the association could relate to shared disruptive family dynamics.

▶ Clinical Findings

Signs & Symptoms

The cardinal feature of histrionic personality disorder is the deliberate use of what is perceived by others excessive emotionality and sexuality to draw attention to themselves and to control others. Histrionic personality disorder patients' experience their self-esteem as highest when they are the center of attention. They feel mistreated and may become petulant when not the center of attention. Their emotions are experienced by others as characteristically labile. They may exhibit temper tantrums, tearful outbursts, or behave in a dramatic fashion when not responded to as they feel entitled. These displays are often used to provoke a reaction such as guilt, sympathy, or acquiescence from those around them.

Patients with histrionic personality disorder are often quite concerned with their physical appearance and attractiveness and may dress and carry themselves in a seductive or provocative manner. Interactions may be dominated by flirtatious banter, interspersed with dramatic anecdotes about the patient's life and circumstances.

Unlike some other personality disorder diagnoses, patients with histrionic personality disorder place a premium on interpersonal relationships, and the quality of these relationships. Frequently to the observer, these relationships appear superficial. There is often a pattern of sequential unsuccessful relationships, with a seemingly capricious flight from relationship to relationship. Although descriptions of events may be passionate and colorful, they tend to be imprecise and lack detail, with the information obtained being more impressionistic than specific.

Also prominent in those with histrionic personality disorder is the repression of anger and other disturbing affects. Anger tends to be expressed either fleetingly or indirectly. They are more comfortable with the expression of physical rather than psychological symptoms, these patients may present with somatic entities such as somatization disorder or conversion disorder.

▶ Understanding Signs and Symptoms

Considered from the perspective of character traits and temperaments, histrionic personality disorder patients are found to be characterized by focusing high levels of energy on social relationships which bring them praise. They are also easily disappointed and experience affective shifts and are described as experiencing high levels of neuroticism. Their behavior leads to scoring high on novelty seeking and reward dependence.

▶ Differential Diagnosis

Histrionic personality disorder especially requires differentiation from the cluster B disorders, narcissistic personality disorder, borderline personality disorder, and less so with antisocial personality disorder. Aspects of this diagnosis also resemble and overlap with symptoms of bipolar spectrum disorders, eating disorders, and substance abuse disorders. In ruling in or out these disorders, a careful diagnostic assessment is critical.

▶ Treatment

A. Pharmacologic Interventions

There is little or no evidence that pharmacologic treatment is effective in altering histrionic personality disorder symptoms not associated with another disorder. However, individuals with this disorder may suffer from depressive disorders and/or an anxiety disorder. For these patients, antidepressants and anxiolytics can be quite effective. Because these patients frequently misuse prescription medications, caution is warranted when prescribing such medications in general, and drugs which may be misused or become addictive.

Psychotherapeutic Interventions

1. Group and marital interventions—It has been suggested that patients with histrionic personality disorder may derive particular benefit from group therapy, especially from groups made up of similar patients. Such groups provide a mirror of the histrionic patient's own behavior and can serve to confront emotional displays rather than accepting or ignoring them. Moreover, histrionic personality disorder patients have considerable need for approval from others and thus are more likely to accept confrontations in order to avoid being rejected.

Histrionic personality disorder patients can be challenging to work in couples or marital therapy. Their commitment for potentially altering the basis of their marital relationship is often limited. They may be unwilling or unable to risk relinquishing the degree of control they maintain in the relationship.

2. Individual psychotherapies—There are no controlled clinical trials that identify the best psychotherapeutic strategies for treating histrionic personality disorder. Clinical consensus indicates that the psychotherapy should be empathic and interactive. Limit setting and identifying acting-out behavior are desirable therapeutic topics.

Histrionic personality disorder is most commonly treated with psychodynamic psychotherapy, supportive psychotherapy, and cognitive–behavioral therapy. Operationally, regardless of the therapy, the tumultuous relationship history of the patient with others will likely be repeated within the psychotherapeutic relationship. Identifying and exploring the patient's feelings toward their therapist triggered in the therapeutic relationship may be a critical aspect of therapy. In this context, delineating the self-perpetuating quality of these emotions and their subsequent behaviors is an important part of the therapy. Focusing on the links between thoughts and feelings increases the patient's capacity for reflection, thereby decreasing the likelihood that impulsive destructive behaviors will occur.

▶ Prognosis

The prognosis for histrionic personality disorder patients is relatively good. These patients tend to be reasonably effective in social settings. This allows them to be the beneficiaries of social feedback and support. In the face of abandonment, they are vulnerable to feeling depressed, but as with many of their other complaints, the dysphoria can be short-lived, and it is highly reactive to external circumstances. The prognosis is more pessimistic if the patient meets criteria for other cluster B personality disorders.

Over time, histrionic personality disorder patients tend to improve regardless of treatment. Significantly, decreases in extraversion and neuroticism often occur as one ages, and these changes have been suggested as an explanation for the improvement that tends to occur over time.

NARCISSISTIC PERSONALITY DISORDER

▶ General Considerations

A. Epidemiology

Narcissistic personality disorder occurs in less than 1% of the general population. It is frequently comorbid in populations of psychiatric patients, being estimated at 2–16%. The disorder maybe somewhat more common in men than in women.

B. Etiology

Although the cause of narcissistic personality disorder is unknown, one hypothesis is that during childhood, parents either significantly overreacted or underreacted to the child's behavior or accomplishments. This behavior is thought to lead the child, and later the adult, to continually seek adoration in order to attain and sustain their self-esteem at realistic levels.

▶ Clinical Findings

Signs & Symptoms

The hallmarks of an individual with the narcissistic personality disorder are grandiosity, a notable lack of empathy, a lack of consideration for others, and a hypersensitivity to evaluation by others. Narcissistic individuals exaggerate their accomplishments, act egotistical, and are manipulative of those around them. They have an exaggerated sense of entitlement, being convinced that they deserve special treatment and admiration. Thus, individuals with narcissistic personality disorder are frequently boastful of their accomplishments and often appear haughty and irritating, although they can be experienced as outwardly charming. Usually, they have little insight into their narcissistic behavior. They have an exaggerated sense of uniqueness and show devaluation, disdain, contempt, and deprecation of others when they cannot control a relationship.

Narcissistic personality disorder patients are prone to attribute and externalize the source of any difficulties they have in relationships. Others they believe may not appropriately appreciate, support, or defer to them. Because they are highly vulnerable to criticism, any negative statements about them provoke anger, disdain, counterarguments, and devaluation of the person making the statement. Some narcissistic individuals react to criticism by becoming enraged, sometimes with acute paranoid ideation and marked deterioration in judgment.

Given the narcissistic personality disorder patient's view of life, they may be vulnerable to depressive episodes and social withdrawal following a self-perceived injury to their self-image. Linked to this, envy of others is a major feature characteristic of narcissistic personality disorder patients. Such envy makes it difficult for these patients to appreciate what they actually have acquired or accomplished. Individuals with narcissistic personality disorder are especially vulnerable to loss of any abilities or changes in appearance in aging. They are prone to become more depressed and demanding during the fourth, fifth, and later decades of life.

▶ Dimensional Consideration

With regard to the core personality or temperamental structure of narcissistic personality disorder patients, such individuals score high on engaging others for self needs and low on cooperativeness. They also score high on novelty seeking and low on harm avoidance and reward dependence.

Differential Diagnosis

Patients with narcissistic personality disorder can be easily confused with patients with hypomania because of the grandiosity common to both disorders. Indeed, bipolar manic patients demonstrate most of the identifying criteria of narcissistic personality disorder, but generally only when manic. Although difficult to differentiate, patients with narcissistic personality disorder, rather than being overly involved in a whirl of activities, are usually more selective, participating only in those tasks that they think merit their special talents and unique abilities, and for which they can be recognized and rewarded.

Patients with narcissistic personality disorder share aspects of behavior with individuals with antisocial personality disorder. Some scholars have suggested that the former is merely a less aggressive version of the latter. Both disorders are characterized by interpersonal exploitiveness and a lack of empathy. However, the patient with narcissistic personality disorder is less likely to be thrill seeking and impulsive, and more likely to exaggerate his or her talents and to be grandiose. It is also difficult to distinguish between patients with narcissistic personality disorder and those with borderline personality disorder. However, the obvious independence and the compulsion to exert interpersonal control in narcissistic personality disorder patients contrasts with the neediness and dependency of many patients with borderline personality disorder. Substance use disorders and hypochondriasis are often comorbid with narcissistic personality disorder.

Treatment

A. Psychopharmacologic Interventions

There is little evidence to suggest that psychopharmacotherapy is effective in the treatment of narcissistic personality disorder, except when comorbid conditions occur such as depression, anxiety, and suicidality. Under such conditions, appropriate antidepressant or other symptom-specific therapies are indicated.

B. Psychotherapeutic Interventions

1. Group and marital interventions—Although controlled studies are lacking, there is a large body of clinical experience regarding the psychotherapy of narcissistic personality disorder. With respect to the group therapies, patients with narcissistic personality disorder can be disruptive if criticized by other group members. To prevent this, the therapist must ensure and provide some support for the patient in order to render the inevitable confrontations more palatable. However, treatment in a homogeneous group of narcissistic personality disorder patients is thought to help

these patients to increase their understanding of themselves through the observation in others of their own maladaptive patterns of behavior.

Patients with narcissistic personality disorder choose to participate in couples therapy with some frequency. Even when noting egregious behavior by the narcissistic patient, the therapist must guard against unilaterally blaming the patient for the disruptions in the relationship. The maladaptive behavior patterns noted between the couple are often complementary and self-sustaining. In such cases role-playing and role-reversal techniques have been considered particularly useful.

2. Individual psychotherapeutic interventions—As with group and marital treatments, psychotherapy with patients with narcissistic personality disorder is usually challenging. These patients often develop expectations of the therapist that are grandiose or expansive. They may not be able to build a trusting or working alliance. Furthermore, they usually seek treatment only following pressure from others, and thus, unless they are depressed or otherwise symptomatic, they are poorly motivated to participate in psychotherapy.

There are certain pitfalls in treating narcissistic personality disorder patients in a psychodynamic or behavioral therapy approach. The therapist to avoid the extremes either of joining the patient in his or her self-admiration, or of strongly criticizing the patient must concurrently monitor their feelings toward the patient. Although confronting the patient is often necessary, it needs to be carefully timed and presented with a tone of support and empathic acceptance.

Cognitive interventions can be directed at the cognitive distortions of self and others that are typical in these patients. Such distortions often involve a magnification of the differences between the patient and other people whereby the difference favors the patient, and others are viewed with contempt. Conversely, if the difference favors another, the patient feels worthless and humiliated. This situation can be addressed by helping the patient to modify their standards and goals to an internal frame of reference, rather than a comparison with others.

Prognosis

Little is known about the long-term prognosis of patients with narcissistic personality disorder. In the absence of treatment, and possibly with treatment, the features of the disorder are unlikely to diminish. Indeed, they tend to worsen during middle age and become more strongly associated with depression and despair.

The features of the disorder tend to self-perpetuate, with the patient's devaluation of others eventually driving away those who might have provided the expected admiration. The significant depression resulting from such rejections is typically resolved by an increase in defensive self-aggrandizement that repeats the cycle.

CLUSTER C PERSONALITY DISORDERS

AVOIDANT PERSONALITY DISORDER

▶ General Considerations

A. Epidemiology

The prevalence of avoidant personality disorder has been estimated at 0.5–2.4% in the general population, with larger numbers occurring in women than in men.

B. Etiology

As with all other personality disorders, the etiology of avoidant personality disorder is uncertain. Because shyness, the experience of discomfort and fear of strangers is a normal component of certain developmental stages, some theorists have speculated that patients with this disorder may be stagnated in their emotional growth in this regard, while other young people may "outgrow" their social awkwardness. Shyness is a personality temperament that evolves and diminishes over age and must be distinguished from avoidant personality disorder in diagnosing this disorder in children or adolescents.

▶ Clinical Findings

Signs & Symptoms

Avoidant personality disorder patients possess a persistent behavioral pattern of avoidance, created by anxiety, which leads to a restricted lifestyle and limited social interactions.

Individuals with avoidant personality disorder are described as introverted, inhibited, and anxious. They tend to have low self-esteem and are sensitive to rejection. They tend to be awkward, have social discomfort, and are very afraid of being embarrassed or acting or looking foolish.

Avoidant personality disorder patients show anxiety and discomfort when discussing their problems. Their excessive concern with evaluation by others is particularly apparent during personal questioning, during which they may interpret innocuous questions as criticism. The social anxiety associated with avoidant personality disorder leads to interpersonal withdrawal and avoidance of unfamiliar or novel social situations, primarily because of fears of rejection rather than because of disinterest in others. In those relationships that are maintained, patients tend to adopt a passive, submissive role, as they are particularly uncomfortable in situations in which there is a great deal of public scrutiny and failures are likely to be observed or widely known.

Temperamentally, patients with avoidant personality disorder score extremely high on neuroticism and extremely low on extraversion scales, thereby being highly introverted.

▶ Differential Diagnosis

There has been a debate as to whether avoidant personality disorder is in the spectrum of anxiety disorders or is a separate psychopathological entity. Avoidant personality disorder has been shown in familial studies to be related to chronic anxiety.

Clearly many features of avoidant personality disorder are indistinguishable from those of social anxiety disorder (social phobia). Indeed, the two diagnoses may actually be alternative names for the same condition. If there is a difference, the primary distinction lies in the continuing nature of avoidant personality disorder symptoms, with characteristics such as low self-esteem and an intense desire for acceptance reflecting an enduring part of the personality rather than a transient condition. Similarly, avoidant personality disorder and generalized anxiety disorder have symptoms in common, as do avoidant personality disorder and major depression. Comorbidity therefore exists with major depressive disorder, dysthymia, social phobia, panic disorders, and related anxiety disorders.

▶ Treatment

A. Psychopharmacologic Interventions

There is some support in the literature for the use of β-blocking agents for controlling the symptoms of social phobia. This suggests that these medications may also be helpful in treating avoidant personality disorder, although controlled studies have not been performed. These medications theoretically may facilitate early efforts at increasing social risk taking and thus allow the patient some successful experiences that can be built upon by enhancing their self-esteem. Other forms of anxiolytic medication (i.e., buspirone, benzodiazepines) may also be helpful for this purpose, although the risk of abuse or addiction with benzodiazepines clearly exists.

B. Psychotherapeutic Interventions

1. Group and marital therapies—Group therapy, either supportive or cognitive in focus, may be of particular use in helping patients with avoidant personality disorder to have contact with strangers within a generally accepting and supportive environment. This helps the patient to overcome social anxiety and to develop interpersonal trust. In such group encounters, the apprehensions that invariably emerge can assist avoidant personality disorder patients in understanding the effect that their rejection sensitivity has on others. Family or couples therapy may also be of particular benefit for patients who are involved in an environment that perpetuates avoidant behavior by undermining self-esteem.

2. Individual psychotherapeutic interventions—Patients with avoidant personality disorder often seek psychotherapy for assistance with their symptoms. However, such patients may be initially reluctant to disclose personal information out of fear of being rejected or humiliated by their therapist. Early psychotherapeutic efforts are typically directed at establishing trust through provision of empathic support and reassurance. Subsequent efforts may be directed at encouraging assertive behavior via assertiveness training, social skills training, and cognitive therapy. In dynamic psychotherapy, distorted thoughts, attitudes, and overvalued assumptions that maintain social withdrawal can be explored. Similarly, behavioral desensitization using gradual exposure to social tasks that have increasing potential for provoking anxiety can lead to positive experiences that enable patients to tolerate social risk taking.

Prognosis

Little is known about the natural course and outcome of avoidant personality disorder. The most consistent and continuing symptoms are feelings of inadequacy and social ineptitude. The social anxiety and withdrawal associated with avoidant personality disorder is obviously longstanding and generalized. However, many patients with this disorder manage to adapt to their problems and show little impairment, assuming they exist in a favorable interpersonal and occupational environment. The prognosis tends to be worse if other personality disorders are present, or if the patient is in a fixed, unsupportive environment that maintains avoidance behaviors.

DEPENDENT PERSONALITY DISORDER

General Considerations

A. Epidemiology

The prevalence of dependent personality disorder has been estimated at 0.5–3.0% in the general population. Furthermore, this disorder is heavily represented in mental health treatment settings because of the general propensity that such patients have to demonstrate help-seeking behavior. The disorder appears to be more common in women than in men. Individuals presenting for treatment with dependent personalities tend to be somewhat older than those with other personality disorders.

B. Etiology

Theories about the cause of dependent personality disorder often suggest a childhood environment in which dependent behaviors were directly or indirectly rewarded, and independent activities were discouraged. Increasing evidence from twin studies may suggest possible, but poorly defined, genetic influences.

Clinical Findings

Signs & Symptoms

The hallmark of dependent personality disorder is a lifelong interpersonal submissiveness. This submissiveness can be

within a particular relationship, but more commonly is a generalized style of relating to others. Dependency arises from poor self-esteem and feelings of inadequacy that drive those afflicted to rely heavily on others to get their needs met. Because abandonment is greatly feared, any expression of displeasure or anger is inhibited so as not to endanger the relationship.

Understanding Signs and Symptoms

Not surprisingly, dependent personality disorder patients have been found to combine increased neuroticism with agreeableness.

Differential Diagnosis

Patients with dependent personality disorder often submerge their identity within the context of a dependency relationship, in a way that is similar to borderline personality disorder. However, patients with dependent personality disorder lack the history of turbulent relationships that characterizes the borderline personality disorder patient. The rage and manipulativeness of the patient with borderline personality disorder contrast with the appeasement behavior that is characteristic of patients with dependents personality disorder.

Many individuals, particularly those with mood and anxiety disorders, as well as those with general medical disorders, can appear quite dependent and can present with low self-esteem. For these individuals, the features may be limited to the duration of the primary disorder and do not reflect a longstanding personality pattern. Dependent personality disorder commonly co-occurs with panic disorder and agoraphobia, as well as with other major mental disorders and other personality disorders.

Treatment

A. Psychopharmacological Interventions

Patients who have dependent personality disorder often experience fatigue, malaise, and vague anxiety. For these symptoms, SSRI or tricyclic antidepressant therapy can be useful. Anxiolytic medication may also be useful, especially during crises that emerge after efforts at establishing autonomy, because fears of abandonment and separation may be exacerbated at these times. However, as with many other disorders, use of antianxiety medications should be time limited and focused on specific target symptoms.

B. Psychotherapeutic Interventions

1. Group and marital interventions—Patients with dependent personality disorder have been reported to derive considerable benefit from group therapy, as it offers an opportunity for the development of supportive peer relations with a low risk for abandonment. Group members can reinforce the patient's efforts at establishing autonomy and

provide a protected arena in which to try out new and more constructive interpersonal behaviors.

Family or couples therapy can also be useful. It may, however, present the challenge of working within a family system in which the patient's dependency may play an important functional role in maintaining the family's equilibrium. It is therefore critical to address the family dynamics and attain the support of other family members. Lest the patient's quest for autonomy will be undermined or met with rejection or withdrawal by other family members that will perpetuate the patient's dependency.

2. Individual psychotherapeutic interventions—Patients with dependent personality disorder are generally receptive to psychological treatment as part of a more general pattern of seeking assistance and support from others. The primary goal of such interventions is to make the patient become more autonomous and self-reliant. As with the other personality disorders, a variety of individual treatments of dependent personality disorder are reported useful. Cognitive–behavioral psychotherapy is reported to be very helpful in assisting in developing assertiveness and effective decision making. Negative, cognitive constructs are challenged. Assertiveness training is a typical component of treatment. Role-playing, focusing on communication skills, particularly around negative feelings allow the patient to practice assertive behaviors. In more psychodynamic oriented treatments, exploration of past separations and their impact on current behaviors is critical. Exploration of the current long-term effects of dependent behavior can be useful. They can help the patient arrive at a greater understanding of how their feeling state and behavioral have adversely affect their views of their self and are as steps toward autonomy.

Prognosis

The prognosis of dependent personality disorder, in the absence of comorbid diagnoses, is generally good. Individuals with this disorder are likely to have had at least one supportive relationship in the past and generally have a capacity for empathy and trust exceeding that observed in most of the other personality disorders. The primary obstacles to improvement may involve the exacerbation of anxieties, Efforts toward establishing autonomy may lead to the emergence of severe depression. The patient may desperately cling to behaviors. Their attempts at autonomy may lead to rejection.

OBSESSIVE–COMPULSIVE PERSONALITY DISORDER

General Considerations

A. Epidemiology

The prevalence of obsessive–compulsive personality disorder has been estimated at roughly 1% in the general population.

Although it is more common in clinical settings, it is seen less often there than are many other personality disorders. This maybe because people with this disorder often view the traits in question as desirable, rather than as a problem. The disorder appears to be more common in men than in women.

B. Etiology

Psychoanalytic theories as to the etiology of obsessive–compulsive personality disorder suggest a developmental focus in various phases of childhood where the child feels they need to perform to please their parents to attain acknowledgement and warmth in order to sustain a positive experience of self and be loveable.

C. Genetics

Genetic components underlying this disorder are uncertain and have hardly been explored. However, there is evidence that first-degree relatives of individuals with obsessive–compulsive disorder have relatively higher rates of obsessive–compulsive disorder. This could be due to a shared genetic relationship or shared life experiences.

Clinical Findings

Signs & Symptoms

Obsessive–compulsive personality disorder is characterized by affective constriction, inflexibility, obstinacy, a penchant for orderliness and quest for the "right" answer. Characteristically, there is a strong pattern of perfectionism. The disorder is typically associated with behavior seen as a times over-conscientiousness. Patients with obsessive–compulsive personality disorder tend to have difficulty in personal relationships because they do not like to submit to others' ways of doing things because they are not the best. This can lead to occupational problems, because these individuals often will simply refuse to work with others they see as not as good as they are. In a diagnostic interview, they are frequently not interested in the feeling state quality of the treatment. They will often describe their life in a solemn and intellectualized manner. Their emotional tone is likely to be muted. They often provide unneeded exceptionally detailed responses to questions.

Differential Diagnosis

Obsessive–compulsive personality disorder was once considered a prelude to obsessive–compulsive disorder. Obsessive–compulsive personality disorder differs from obsessive–compulsive disorder in that diagnosis of obsessive–compulsive disorder is typically associated with marked distress concerning interruptions in the ability to carry out obsessions or compulsions. The patient with obsessive–compulsive personality disorder experiences no such distress, aside from a tendency to worry in general. Indeed, the patient with obsessive–compulsive personality disorder typically views his or her preoccupation with order and perfectionism as a positive characteristic, and one that makes him or her superior to others. As a result, the relationship between the obsessive–compulsive disorder and obsessive–compulsive personality disorder is imperfect at best, and the available evidence suggests that fewer than half of patients with obsessive–compulsive disorder also have an obsessive–compulsive personality disorder. Other personality disorders, such as avoidant and dependent personality disorders, are just as common in patients with obsessive–compulsive disorder. Major depressive disorder, dysthymia, and generalized anxiety disorder are often comorbid with obsessive–compulsive personality disorder. Patients with anorexia nervosa and bulimia are sometimes diagnosed with obsessive–compulsive personality disorder.

▶ Treatment

A. Psychopharmacologic Interventions

Pharmacotherapy has not been demonstrated to be effective in the treatment of obsessive–compulsive personality disorder. Serotonergic drugs, such as clomipramine and other SSRIs, have not been shown to have the degree of usefulness seen with the treatment of obsessive–compulsive disorder. However, these drugs are thought by of limited helpfulness in decreasing the perfectionism and the ritualizing that can occur in individuals with obsessive–compulsive personality disorder. These drugs including benzodiazepines, however, may also be useful during crises in which anxiety and depression are prominent.

B. Psychotherapeutic Interventions

1. Group and marital interventions—Group therapy is difficult to conduct in patients with obsessive–compulsive personality disorder. These patients typically attempt to ally themselves with the therapist and to treat the other group members, whom they often perceive as having the "real" problems. One advantage of treatment in using the group format is that the intellectualized explanations offered by the patient are interrupted by the other group members. This increases anxiety, but also leaves the obsessive–compulsive patient more open to new experiences.

In family or couples therapy, a major challenge involves having the patient relinquish control over other family members by accepting they also have ideas. This process can be assisted by prescribing homework tasks in which various roles, including decision making, are reassigned within the family. The patient's desire to conform to demonstrate their superior ability to the authority of the therapist can be used to facilitate the loosening of control over others, as well as over him or herself.

2. Individual psychotherapeutic interventions—Obsessive–compulsive personality disorder patients are often difficult to treat because they rarely come to psychotherapeutic treatment except when urged to do so by others. They have difficulty seeing that their personality features are maladaptive. When they do come to psychotherapy on their own, they usually do so because of their associated depression, anxiety, or somatic complaints.

The individual with obsessive–compulsive personality disorder desires to perform well as a patient, consistent with his or her general pattern of perfectionism in other life areas. However, the general constriction and distrust of affective expression creates a number of resistances for the therapist to overcome. Patients may be highly critical of themselves or of the therapy, demanding justification for every intervention offered. A central part of the treatment will involve exploring the source and the unreasonable nature of the harsh and rigid standards the patient has set for both self and others.

Given the rationalizing and intellectualizing nature of obsessive–compulsive personality disorder patient, cognitive interventions are often relatively well received. Such efforts usually focus on the inaccuracy of key assumptions held by the patient (i.e., that one must be perfectly in control of the environment, or that any failure is intolerable). Consequences of such beliefs can be explored and ways to refute the beliefs discussed. In controlled clinical trials, cognitive-behavioral psychotherapy has the most efficacy in treating obsessive–compulsive symptoms.

▶ Prognosis

Little is known about the prognosis of obsessive–compulsive personality disorder. The most stable characteristics are rigidity and problems in delegating. In the absence of co-occurring disorders, the outlook is probably favorable for such patients. The patient's capacity for self-discipline and order precludes many of the problems typical of other personality disorders. However, not a few of these patients go on to develop anxiety disorders, and their self-criticism and barren emotional life leave them particularly vulnerable to developing depression.

OTHER PERSONALITY DISORDERS

PERSONALITY CHANGE DUE TO ANOTHER MEDICAL CONDITION

▶ Clinical Findings

In order to diagnose a personality disorder due to another medical condition, the personality disturbance is understood to be caused by the direct pathophysiological effects of the medical condition. In children the changes must alter the course of normal development. The diagnosis is not given if the disturbance is better explained by another mental disorder or if the disturbance occurs only during a period of delirium., The disturbance must also cause disruption in social or occupational functioning.

Signs & Symptoms

Personality change due to another medical condition may include affective lability, poor impulse control, inappropriate aggression or apathy, and suspiciousness and paranoid behavior. The diagnosis is not given if the personality change is caused by an essential behavioral or psychological reaction to a specific medical condition such as the development of dependent behaviors in response to a stroke.

► Treatment

Treatment is focused on the underlying medical condition and the use of supportive psychotherapy and behavioral therapy to address the pathological behaviors.

ADDITIONAL PERSONALITY DISORDER DIAGNOSES

DSM-5-TR includes two additional personality disorders. The diagnosis of Other Specified Personality Disorder is used when behavioral or psychological symptoms characteristic of a personality disorder cause significant distress in varied situations but do not meet the full criteria for personality disorders, but where the clinician desires to indicate the reasons that the patient's presentation does not meet full diagnostic criteria for a specific personality disorder.

The diagnosis of Unspecified Personality Disorder is used when the clinician does not elect to indicate the reasons their presentation does not meet full criteria for a specific personality disorder or for patient presentations where there is not enough data to make a more specific diagnosis.

▼ FUTURE DIAGNOSTIC MODELS TO THE DIAGNOSIS OF PERSONALITY DISORDERS

Section III of DSM-5-TR presents an alternative approach to the criteria that are addressed in this chapter, "Alternative DSM-5-TR Model for Personality Disorders" for a clinician to diagnosis a personality disorder. The alternative approach utilizes a complex set of factors and personality performance scales to assess personality functioning. It assesses personality from a dimensional perspective. The alternative model more clearly addresses and describes personality from a developmental framework than the criteria described in DSM-5-TR do. Its potential clinical implementation with its scores of scales, however, does not address how clinicians think in the limited time available to assess their patients.

American Psychiatric Association. *Diagnostic and Statistical Manual of Mental Disorder*. 5th ed. Text Revision DSM-5-TR. Washington DC; 2022.

Benjamin LS. *Interpersonal Diagnosis and Treatment of Personality Disorders*. New York: Guilford Press; 1993.

Black DW Ed. Andreasen NC. *Introductory Textbook of Psychiatry*. 5th ed. Washington DC: American Psychiatric Press; 2011.

Cloninger RC. *Personality and Psychopathology*. Washington, DC: American Psychiatric Press; 1999.

Coccaro EF. Psychopharmacologic studies in patients with personality disorders: review and perspective. *J Personal Disord*. 1993;7(Suppl):181.

Grinker R, Werble B, Drye B. *The Borderline Syndrome: Behavioral Study of Ego Function*. New York: Basic Books; 1968.

Hubbard JR, Saathoff GB, Barnett BL, Jr. Recognizing borderline personality disorder in the family practice setting. *Am Fam Physician*. 1995;52:908.

Livesley WJ. *The DSM-IV Personality Disorders*. New York: Guilford Press; 1995.

Maj M, Akiskal HS, Mezzich JE, Okasha A. *Personality Disorders*. New York: Wiley; 2005.

Millon T. *Disorders of Personality: Introducing a DSM/ICD Spectrum from Normal to Abnormal*. New York: Wiley; 2011.

Morey LC. *An Interpretative Guide to the Personality Assessment Inventory (PAI)*. Psychology Resources; 1996.

Oldham JM, Skodol AK, Bender DS. Textbook of Personality Disorders. Washington, DC: American Psychiatric Publishing; 2005.

Waldinger RJ. *Psychiatry for Medical Students*. 3rd ed. Section IV. Techniques & Settings in Child & Adolescent Psychiatry. Washington, DC: American Psychiatric Press; 1997.

Intellectual Disability (Intellectual Developmental Disorder)

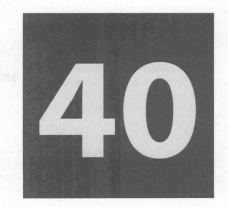

Kerim M. Munir, MD, MPH, DSc, MD
Sandra L. Friedman, MD, MPH
Elizabeth L. Leonard, PhD

INTELLECTUAL DISABILITY (MENTAL RETARDATION*)

ICD-10 Diagnostic Criteria

*Intellectual Disability (ID) has gained universal usage replacing the term Mental Retardation (MR). In this chapter and table we refer to ID as synonymous to MR under the World Health Organization (WHO) International Statistical Classification of Diseases and Related Health Problems 10th Revision (ICD-10). and consistent with the 11th revision (ICD-11), adopted in 2022.

ID represents a group of conditions characterized by impairment of skills manifested during the neurodevelopmental period, skills which contribute to the overall level of intelligence, i.e. cognitive, language, motor, and social abilities. ID can occur with or without any other mental or physical condition.

Intellectual abilities and social adaptation may change over time, and, however poor, may improve as a result of training and rehabilitation. Diagnosis should be based on the current levels of functioning. Degrees of ID are conventionally estimated by standardized intelligence tests. These can be supplemented by scales assessing social adaptation in a given environment. These measures provide an approximate indication of the degree of ID. The diagnosis will also depend on the overall assessment of intellectual functioning by a skilled diagnostician.

If desired, additional codes are used to identify associated conditions such as autism, other developmental disorders, epilepsy, conduct disorders, or severe physical handicap.

A fourth-character subdivision is used to further signify ID categories in order to identify the extent of impairment (or severity):

.0 With the statement of no, or minimal, impairment of behavior

.1 Significant impairment of behavior requiring attention or treatment

.8 Other impairments of behavior

.9 Without mention of impairment of behavior

6A00.1 Mild

Approximate IQ range of 50 to 69 (in adults, mental age from 9 to under 12 years). Likely to result in some learning difficulties in school. As adults individuals will be able to work and maintain good social relationships and contribute to society.

6A00.1 Moderate

Approximate IQ range of 35 to 49 (in adults, mental age from 6 to under 9 years). Likely to result in marked developmental delays in children but most can learn to develop some degree of independence in self-care and acquire adequate communication and academic skills. As adults they will need varying degrees of support to live and work in the community.

6A00.2 Severe

Approximate IQ range of 20 to 34 (in adults, mental age from 3 to under 6 years). Likely to result in continuous need of support.

6A00.3 Profound

IQ under 20 (in adults, mental age below 3 years). Results in severe limitation in self-care, continence, communication and mobility.

6A0Y Other

6A00.Z Unspecified

Individuals who have an age of onset after 18 qualify for the diagnosis qualify for F78 Other, and in those IQ range is not known, it is referred to as F79 Unspecified.

Adapted with permission from International Statistical Classification of Diseases and Related Health Problems, 10th Revision (ICD-10). World Health Organization; 2010.

▶ Essentials of Diagnosis

Intellectual Disability and Intellectual Developmental Disorder (ID/IDD) is the new terminology for **Mental Retardation (MR)** introduced into clinical nosology by the American Psychiatric Association (APA) *Diagnostic and Statistical Manual of Mental Disorders,* Fifth Edition (DSM-5) in May 2013. This definition represents not only a change in terminology but a conceptual shift that characterizes MR as a disability as well as a set of medical disorders as exemplified by their inclusion in a "manual of mental disorders." The content model for this change was originally proposed by the *Working Group on the Classification of Intellectual Disability* reporting to the *World Health Organization (WHO) International Advisory Group for the Revision of ICD-10 Mental and Behavior Disorders* in a landmark meeting in Italy in December 2010. The proposal was followed by an important position article published in *World Psychiatry* in 2011. The preliminary aspects of the proposal had already been presented in publications by keynote members of the World Psychiatric Association Section on Intellectual Disability.

The term MR, adopted by the earlier APA classification in the *Diagnostic and Statistical Manual,* Fourth Edition, Text Revision (DSM-IV-TR), had already been renamed **Intellectual Disability (ID)** by the American Association on Intellectual and Developmental Disabilities (AAIDD) in the intervening period. The new definition of ID/IDD as a group of neurodevelopmental disorders therefore does not necessarily reflect a disavowal of ID, nor does it reflect an alteration in its prevalence, nor a change in the legal status of affected individuals by these neurodevelopmental conditions. The passage of Rosa's Law in October 2010 now requires the federal government in the United States to recognize all instances of ID. The addition of the new IDD terminology as proposed by the WHP Working Group and adopted by the APA brings greater elaboration to these conditions and is already gaining broad acceptance. It provides a framework for early screening, diagnosis, and interventions for these conditions. This framework also combines a public health policy with social and family-oriented interventions and supports.

The overarching terminology **Developmental Disabilities (DD)** is a federal usage in the United States defined by the *Developmental Disabilities Assistance and Bill of Rights Amendments* in 1996 and is commonly referred to in various entitlement statutes. The DD category encompasses broader group of individuals not only with ID/IDD but also those with severe and chronic physical disabilities, manifest before the age of 22. These conditions are all envisioned as lifelong circumstances resulting in substantial functional limitations in three, or more, major life activities in: self-care, receptive and expressive language, learning, mobility, self-direction, capacity of independent living, and economic self-sufficiency. The DD wrap-around category therefore includes ID/IDD. The DD definition is highly useful in that it extends the legislative framework for social inclusion and helps promote funding supports for purposes of early identification, intervention, advocacy, research, and training of the interdisciplinary group of professionals caring for affected individuals and their families. A major federal program in existence since the 1960s includes the Association of University Centers for Excellence in the United States. The psychiatric training of professionals who will take care of individuals with complex ID/IDD needs across the life span ought therefore to be "nested" and nurtured within the DD framework.

A. Evolving Definition

In both the ICD-11 and DSM-5, the ID/IDD is placed under the meta-section **Neurodevelopmental Disorders**, which comprise a group of conditions with their onset in the developmental period. The developmental period no longer construes the period between birth and the 18th birthday. It implies that developmental milestones that characterize an individual's neurodevelopment from conception to young adulthood include a set of cognitive, social, emotional, and physical skills that are both age-specific and influenced by their adaptive circumstances. They have variable etiologies and are characterized by significant impairments in both intellectual and adaptive functioning considered below the levels expected for a person's age, education, and sociocultural context. As in other mental disorders, the ID/IDD conditions can occur in the context of specific medical and genetic/metabolic as well infectious, traumatic, psychosocial, and environmental exposures. This conceptual change identifies ID/IDD as a set of health conditions and reflects an evolution in the definition of MR as a disability over a half-century.

The prior definition of MR in the DSM-IV-TR had three major elements that included:

1. Significant impairments in intellectual functioning, as measured by intellectual quotient (IQ) testing (defined as an IQ score of two standard deviations or more below the mean of an individually administered instrument);

2. Deficits in adaptive behavior and functioning (in conceptual, social, and practical skills);

3. Onset of the disability before age 18, or before the individual became an adult.

For all practical purposes, the role of "IQ testing" had come to underscore a diagnosis of MR in psychiatric practice with MR viewed as a disability and placed on a separate axial classification in prior DSM editions. The impairment in intellectual and adaptive abilities that fell short of the requirement of two standard deviations below the mean was felt insufficient to support a conclusion that an individual had MR. An important contribution of the AAIDD revision of

MR was the emphasis that sub-average intellectual functioning may indeed be necessary but it is also in and of itself an insufficient criterion to establish a diagnosis of ID.

B. DSM-5 Changes

The structure of the ID/IDD in the DSM-5 carries the "tripartite" distinction of the DSM-IV-TR but introduces significant conceptual changes:

- As a **neurodevelopmental disorder**, ID/IDD is now brought onto par with Communication Disorders, Autism Spectrum Disorder (ASD), Specific Learning Disorders (LD), Motor Disorders, and Attention-Deficit Hyperactivity Disorder (ADHD), all with origins in the developmental period as highlighted earlier. The DSM-IV-TR umbrella category of *Disorders Usually First Diagnosed in Infancy, Childhood, or Adolescence* is forfeited.

- ID/IDD is referred to as a mental disorder and no longer envisioned *primarily* as a disability.

- An important distinction from the definition of MR in the DSM-IV-TR, the DSM-5 ID/IDD does not specify an *IQ score of approximately 70 or below on an individually administered IQ test* as a necessary criterion for the diagnosis to be endorsed. Instead it underscores the need for "clinical judgment," although it does not define the requisite training and experience in the field.

- A fundamental consideration for a diagnosis of ID/IDD is now the use of guidelines for established deficits in adaptive functioning across multiple environments.

- The ID/IDD definition suspends any requirement of *age of onset before age 18 years*; instead intellectual and adaptive deficits inherently emerge in the *developmental period*.

- The four severity levels of ID/IDD (*mild, moderate, severe, and profound*) are no longer defined by IQ scores but are considered based on the individual's adaptive skills and behaviors because it is adaptive functioning that determines the supports required by individuals.

- The validity of IQ measures, especially for the lower end of the IQ range, is brought into question.

C. Importance of the Role of Adaptive Functioning

The endorsement of the diagnosis of ID/IDD needs to be accompanied by substantial deficits in adaptive functioning; measurement of IQ is no longer considered sufficient to justify a diagnosis. This approach needs to be explicit in the training of all mental health professionals, as it is intended to ensure that individuals are not misclassified as ID/IDD based on inaccuracies of IQ scores leading to inappropriate labeling, or in an opposite direction, that individuals with ID/IDD are not excluded from services by virtue of "borderline" IQ scores with significant deficits in adaptive functioning. After all, although neurocognitive deficits in ID/IDD

may emerge early, functional impairments in intellectual and adaptive functioning as observed by parents, caregivers, and teachers raise suspicion of ID/IDD before any IQ test can be administered. This is particularly salient in low- and middle-income country (LMIC) settings where standardized IQ measures and/or trained professionals to administer them may not be available. Whatever the sequence in arriving at a diagnosis of ID/IDD in an individual, it is the functional impairment in adaptive functioning that is central to our understanding of ID/IDD, and central to why any such diagnosis matters. As the DSM-5 states, IQ scores do not necessarily translate directly to functioning. Individuals with a certain IQ score may have more difficulty with adaptive and day to day functioning when compared to another individual with the same score. It is important to understand and assess the behavioral, adaptive and social capacity of individuals in addition to IQ.

As the AAIDD definition has long emphasized, although the IQ tests had become more refined and sophisticated, the interpretation of their results required experienced and knowledgeable clinical judgment by psychologists or other clinicians with expertise in assessing them across all domains of functioning. The intent of using approximately two standard deviations below the mean in IQ scores was an implicit need to reflect on the role of such professional judgment and to buffer factors that might contribute to lowering the validity and precision of a diagnostic decision. The framework proposed by the WHO Workgroup on the Revision of ICD-10 and adopted by the APA in the DSM-5 diagnostic framework therefore cannot be fully implemented in the absence of improved clinical judgment and training of professionals in the field. Indeed, this is true not only for ID/IDD but for all neurodevelopmental disorders, in order to accurately interpret test results and assess both adaptive skills and behaviors, and intellectual performance.

It cannot be overstated that the assessment of intellectual functioning through sole reliance on IQ scores is fraught with both the legacy of abuse and the potential for misuse if consideration is not given to measurement errors. A fixed-point cutoff IQ score cannot be psychometrically justifiable. Likewise, adaptive behaviors and skills also need to be assessed clinically and systematically with the use of structured adaptive behavior scales within ranges of measurement error. The AAIDD definition was unique in specifying scores on such scales of two standard deviations or more below an instrument's mean. For example, if a person has an IQ score near the cutoff (within the error range of the instrument, usually ±5 points), the AAIDD specified diagnosis is to be determined by the level of adaptive functioning. In the DSM-5, this rule can no longer solely apply to IQ ranges but needs to consider adaptive functioning as a *sine qua non* that outdoes IQ, irrespective of the measurement range. A person may qualify for the diagnosis of ID/IDD during the school-age years when learning is impaired by poor academic skills, but may lose their diagnosis later, with the acquisition of work and adaptive skills important for an adult.

D. Summary of Key Concepts

- A comprehensive approach to ID/IDD is essential because a single cause is unlikely to explain deficits in intellectual and adaptive functioning.

- The ID/IDD diagnosis represents a group of neurodevelopmental disorders with underlying medical, genetic/metabolic, environmental, and/or psychosocial determinants. Any associated conditions, if known, can now be differentiated as *specifiers*.

- Individuals with ID/IDD present with a cluster of behavioral syndromes and phenotypes, with developmental deficits and impairments in intellectual and adaptive functioning; the deficits in cognitive functioning occur before the acquisition of adaptive skills through learning.

- The various levels of severity of ID/IDD are defined on the basis of adaptive functioning because it is adaptive functioning that determines the level of supports required.

- ID/IDD cannot to be diagnosed by subaverage IQ scores alone.

- Diagnosis of ID/IDD must consider a person's sociocultural and linguistic diversity and associated disabilities.

- ID/IDD may result from an acquired insult during the developmental period during which the associated neurocognitive disorder can also be diagnosed. Maladaptive behaviors should not be automatically seen as part of ID/IDD; such behaviors may be related to life experiences or may reflect psychiatric comorbidity.

- The neurodevelopmental approach to ID/IDD has implications not only for early diagnosis but also in terms of early intervention and prevention.

American Association of Intellectual and Developmental Disabilities. *User's Guide: Intellectual Disability: Definition, Classification and Systems of Supports 9*. Washington, DC: AAIDD; 2012.

American Association on Intellectual and Developmental Disabilities. *Intellectual Disability: Definition, Classification and Systems of Support*. 11th ed. Washington, DC: AAIDD; 2010.

Bertelli MO, Salvador-Carulla L, Scuticchio D, et al. Moving beyond intelligence in the revision of ICD-10: specific cognitive functions in intellectual developmental disorders. *World Psychiatry*. 2014;13(1):93–94.

Bertelli MO, Munir K, Salvador-Carulla L. Fair is foul, and foul is fair: reframing neurodevelopmental disorders in the neurodevelopmental perspective. *Acta Psychiatr Scand*. 2016;134(6): 557–558.

Bertelli MO, Munir K, Harris J, et al. "Intellectual developmental disorders": reflections on the international consensus document for redefining "mental retardation-intellectual disability" in ICD-11. *Adv Ment Health Intellect Disabil*. 2016;10(1):36–58.

Boyle CA, Boulet S, Schieve LA, et al. Trends in the prevalence of developmental disabilities in US children, 1997-2008. *Pediatrics*. 2011;127(6):1034–1042.

Harris, J.C. *Intellectual Disability: Understanding Its Development, Causes, Classification, Evaluation and Treatment*. New York: Oxford University Press; 2006.

Harris JC. New terminology for mental retardation in DSM-5 and ICD-11. *Curr Opin Psychiatry*. 2013;26(3):260–262.

Hassiotis A, Munir K. Developmental psychiatry and intellectual disabilities: an American perspective. *Br J Learn Disabil*. 2004;32:39–42.

Maulik PK, Mascarenhas MN, Mathers CD, et al. Prevalence of intellectual disability: a meta-analysis of population-based studies. *Res Dev Disabil*. 2011;32(2):419–436. Erratum in: *Res Dev Disabil*. 2013;34(2):729.

Munir K, Beardslee WR. Developmental psychiatry: is there any other kind? *Harvard Rev Psychiatry*. 1999;6(5):250–262.

Munir K. Psychiatry of intellectual and developmental disability in the US: time for a new beginning. *Psychiatry (Abingdon)*. 2009;8(11):448–452.

Salvador-Carulla L, Reed GM, Vaez-Azizi LM, et al. Intellectual developmental disorders: towards a new name, definition and framework for "mental retardation/intellectual disability" in ICD-11. *World Psychiatry*. 2011;10(3):175–180.

Sparrow SS, Balla DA, Cicchetti DV. *Vineland Adaptive Behavior Scales*. Circle Pines, MN: American Guidance Series; 1984.

▶ General Considerations

A. Epidemiology

Estimates of the prevalence of ID/IDD have changed over time depending on its definition. With the current definition, it is thought to be about 0.7–1% of the general population in high-income countries and about 2–4% in the LMIC settings. It is estimated that two-thirds of individuals with ID/IDD fall in the mild severity. Individuals with ID/IDD are at increased risk for comorbid mental disorders than expected for the general population; prevalence estimates of comorbidity range between 16 and 71%, with virtually all diagnostic categories represented.

Individuals with ID/IDD represent high economic costs for the health care system in particular and for society in general. There is a need to study the untreated prevalence of ID/IDD beyond the surveillance studies of treated and identified cases in the care system, to examine geographic, gender, and ethnic/racial disparities. Based on the results of the National Health Interview Survey Disability Supplements, the estimated prevalence of ID in the United States is 0.78%. Among school-age children, ID/IDD is more likely to be identified when the child cannot meet the expectation for academic learning. The U.S. Department of Education indicated the prevalence rate of ID/IDD to be 1.14% with variations reported by different states. However, the prevalence based on administrative data, that is, attendance in special education classes, is not necessarily representative and does not also reflect disparities that may exist in the general population in terms of nonidentified cases.

B. Etiology

Etiologic consideration of ID/IDD requires a comprehensive approach that takes into account the timing of insults or risks to developing brains and their impact on developmental and adaptive functioning. There are multiple factors that contribute to the etiology of ID/IDD, with occurrence in the prenatal, perinatal, and postnatal periods. ID/IDD has many different causes, and sometimes biologic, social, behavioral, and educational factors interact to affect how a person functions. There may be similarities in the type of exposures across all three of the developmental time frames, such as infection, toxins, and deprivation of nutritional, environmental, and chemical substances. The timing of these exposures often determines the severity of ID/IDD. In addition, the more significant the etiologic insult, the more likely it is that other types of ID/IDD will result, such as in motor functioning and communication, as well as socialization and development of self-help skills.

1. Perinatal insults—Perinatal insults associated with birth asphyxia have been noted to be the etiology for children with a range of ID/IDD with and without co-occurring cerebral palsy. Events associated with hypoxia and ischemia can be causative also in preterm as well as full-term infants. Other perinatal events, such as infections and their consequences, may also contribute to developmental outcome.

2. Postnatal causes—Postnatal causes are those that are acquired. Mild ID/IDD has been associated with postnatal environmental deprivation, with lack of adequate nutritional and social support. In addition, infections, anoxia, trauma, cerebral vascular events, and malignancy and the effects of its treatment may all influence the level of cognitive function. Risk factors for mild ID/IDD have been associated with multiple births, nutritional and social deprivation, low maternal education, and teen pregnancy. Although male gender has been noted to be a risk factor, this high male-to-female ratio difference is less apparent as the severity of ID/IDD increases. Other risk factors that have been associated with ID include low birth weight and older maternal age (see Table 40–1).

C. Genetics

Most diagnoses of ID/IDD are felt to have prenatal causes. Genetic and metabolic disorders, central nervous system malformations, congenital infections, toxic exposures, deprivation of essential elements in utero, and many idiopathic etiologies are all considered to be potential prenatal etiologic factors. Severe to profound ID/IDD is more likely associated with genetic etiologies, although genetics certainly may play a role in those with moderate and mild ID/IDD. A larger percentage of children with mild ID/IDD are also felt to have idiopathic causes.

Chapman DA, Scott KG, Mason CA. Early risk factors for mental retardation: role of maternal age and maternal education. *Am J Ment Retard*. 2002;107(1):46–59.

Crocker AC, Nelson RP. Mental retardation. In: Levine MD, Carey WB, Crocker AC, eds. *Developmental–Behavioral Pediatrics*. 2nd ed. Philadelphia: WB Saunders; 1992.

Durkin M. The epidemiology of developmental disabilities in low-income countries. *Ment Retard Dev Disabil Res Rev*. 2002;8:206–211.

Lakhan R, Ekúndayò OT, Shahbazi M. An estimation of the prevalence of intellectual disabilities and its association with age in rural and urban populations in India. *J Neurosci Rural Pract*. 2015;6(4):523–528.

Larson SA, Lakin KC, Anderson L, et al. Prevalence of mental retardation and developmental disabilities: estimates from the 1994/1995 National Health Interview Survey Disability Supplements. *Am J Ment Retard*. 2001;106:231–252.

Leonard H, Wen X. The epidemiology of mental retardation: challenges and opportunities in the new millennium. *MRDD Res Rev*. 2002;8:117–134.

Manning M, Hudgins L; Professional Practice and Guidelines Committee. Array-based technology and recommendations for utilization in medical genetics practice for detection of chromosomal abnormalities. *Genet Med*. 2010;12(11):742–745.

Massey PS, McDermott S. State-specific rates of mental retardation—United States, 1993. *MMWR Morbid Mortal Weekly Rep*. 1995:45:61–65.

McLaren J, Bryson SE. Review of recent epidemiological studies of mental retardation: prevalence, associated disorders, and etiology. *Am J Ment Retard*. 1987;92:243–254.

Miller DT, Adam MP, Aradhya S, et al. Consensus statement: chromosomal microarray is a first-tier clinical diagnostic test for individuals with developmental disabilities or congenital anomalies. *Am J Hum Genet*. 2010;86(5):749–764.

Moeschler JB, Shevell M; Committee on Genetics. Comprehensive evaluation of the child with intellectual disability or global developmental delays. *Pediatrics*. 2014;134(3):e903–e918.

Munir KM, Friedman SL, Szymanski LS. Neurodevelopmental disorders: intellectual disability/intellectual developmental disorders. In: Tasman A, Kay J, Lieberman JA, First MB, Riba M, eds. *Psychiatry*. Vol 1. 4th ed. Hoboken, NJ: Wiley-Blackwell; 2015:672–705.

Pescosolido MF, Gamsiz ED, Nagpal S, et al. Distribution of disease-associated copy number variants across distinct disorders of cognitive development. *J Am Acad Child Adolesc Psychiatry*. 2013;52(4):414–430.

Rubin IL. Prematurity and its consequences. In: Rubin IL, Crocker AC, eds. *Medical Care for Children and Adults with Developmental Disabilities*. 2nd ed. Baltimore: Paul H. Brookes; 2006:217–232.

Srour M, Shevell M. Genetics and the investigation of developmental delay/intellectual disability. *Arch Dis Child*. 2014;99(4):386–389.

▶ Clinical Findings

A. Signs & Symptoms

Children with ID/IDD often present with delay in receptive and expressive language skills. Language delays often

Table 40–1 Behavioral Phenotypes

Syndrome	Genetic Findings	Cognitive Features	Behavioral Features	Psychopathology
Fragile X	Full mutation: >200 CGG repeats in FMR1 on Xq27.3	IQ correlated with number of CGG repeats. Males: Mild to severe ID/IDD; females: Borderline IQ to mild ID/IDD	Gaze aversion, perseverations, repetitive speech, social withdrawal	ADHD-like, ASD-like, prone to anxiety
Smith-Magenis	Deletion on 17p11.2	Moderate ID/IDD	SIB, aggression, self-hugging, tantrums	ADHD-like, SMD
Prader–Willi	Either 15q11-q13 deletion on paternal chromosome 15 or maternal uniparental disomy of chromosome 15	Borderline IQ to mild ID/IDD (higher IQ with maternal disomy). Learning disability.	Compulsive hyperphagia, tantrums, aggressive behavior, skin picking	OCD, anxiety, psychotic and affective disorder, ADHD
Angelman	15q11-q13 deletion on maternal chromosome 15, disomy	Severe ID/IDD	Appear happy, sociable, episodic laughter	ASD-like, ADHD-like
Williams	Deletion at 7q11.23	Borderline IQ to moderate ID/IDD	Over-friendly, social disinhibition, excessive empathy	Anxiety, ADHD, sleep disorder
Down syndrome	Trisomy 21(in 92%), translocation	Moderate-severe ID/IDD	Friendly, affectionate, some stubborn, overactive	Depression may occur; early-onset Alzheimer
Rett	X-linked dominant, MECP2 mutation	Severe ID/IDD	Central "hand-wringing," poor social interaction	Early ASD features
Cornelia de Lange	No genetic marker	Severe ID/IDD	Self-injurious, compulsive, overactive aggression	ADHD
CHARGE	Chromosome 8; CHD7 (some patients)	Mild-Moderate ID/IDD to average	Socially withdrawn, need for order	OCD, ADHD
VCFS (DiGeorge)	22q11.2 deletion	Moderate ID/IDD to average	↓ social interaction, blunt affect, poor self-esteem	ADHD, ASD, psychosis (in 25%), bipolar, schizoaffective

CGG: trinucleotides; IQ: intelligence quotient; ADHD: attention-deficit/hyperactivity disorder; ASD: autism spectrum disorder; ID/IDD: intellectual disability (intellectual developmental disorder); SIB: self-injurious behavior; OCD: obsessive–compulsive behavior; FM: fine motor; exec fx: executive function.

become apparent during the second year of life, with motor delay being the more common developmental concern during the first year. Language and cognition are closely associated; children with severe ID/IDD are more apt to have more significant language delays. Children with more significant adaptive and cognitive delays also usually present earlier than those with milder cognitive deficits.

Tests of developmental functioning in the very young child are not felt to be predictive of later cognitive skills, unless there are profound delays. The diagnosis of ID/IDD is generally made after infancy, usually before the child is enrolled in school. Sometimes the diagnosis is made later if an optimal assessment of the child's adaptive and cognitive abilities had not been performed earlier. To make the diagnosis, consideration also needs to be given to the environment in which a child lives, and the manner in which he or she interacts with others on a daily basis.

There are times when the exact level of a child's adaptive and cognitive functioning cannot be determined with certainty. Sometimes a child has not yet received the needed intensive educational support and it is unclear how he or she will respond to these services. Other times, testing cannot be completed or is not felt to reflect a child's potential. In those instances, further testing is required at a future date to more accurately determine the child's level of functioning.

In addition to language delays, children may present with delays in play, social, and adaptive skills. Gross motor skills generally develop well, except in certain disorders associated with significant hypotonia. Fine and oral motor skills may also be affected. Developmental milestone acquisition is generally slow but steady. A child may also display developmental plateaus or regression of developmental skills. In those instances, assessment may be required to rule out the presence of a specific genetic, metabolic, neurodegenerative, or neurophysiologic disorder.

Children with ID/IDD continue to learn, albeit at a rate slower than typically developing peers. It is important to obtain a thorough medical history, which often provides etiologic information. Parental concern has been shown to be an important indicator of the presence of developmental problems. In this respect, the parental level of education is an important driver of early help seeking and ability to deal with social stigma, especially in resource-poor settings and global regions.

The developmental history should include information about pregnancy, delivery, and the perinatal period. Information needs to be obtained regarding past and present medical issues, including any illnesses and injuries. A child's response and recovery from illness also needs to be explored. The history should include milestones in the various developmental domains, as well as the child's overall developmental trajectory. The social environment, with potential stressors, needs to be explored. Family medical history, going back three generations, is needed in the evaluation of potential genetic factors. In addition to psychological and psychiatric assessment, the child requires a physical examination that includes a thorough neurological assessment. This examination should include assessment of growth parameters, including head circumference. Dysmorphology should be identified, as it may point to prenatal contributing factors. Other physical findings are important, such evaluation of integument for neurocutaneous lesions, coarse facies and/or enlarged liver and spleen for certain storage diseases, muscle distribution, bulk, or asymmetries in certain neurological disorders.

B. Psychological Testing

1. Indications for psychological assessment—Psychological assessment measures include both adaptive and cognitive functioning, as well as behavior and academic achievement. It aids in diagnosis, determining disabilities as well as abilities, treatment plan formulation, and eligibility for habilitative services. The selection of specific tests is tailored to the age and ability of each individual. Obtaining collateral information from parents, caregivers, teachers, vocational counselors, and job coaches, as well as employers, is essential for accurate assessment, because nonverbal individuals (irrespective of chronological age) are unable to construct an adequate developmental and behavioral history.

The psychologist must have the requisite developmental training to understand an individual child's ability to sustain attention and comprehend tasks required by a particular test. This is necessary in order to make an informed decision based on interpretation of tests that yield the greatest information about cognition and behavior. Specific instruments have been developed to measure intelligence and associated cognitive abilities, including attention, memory, motor function, receptive and expressive language, and executive functions (planning, sequencing, organization, and task management). Tests administered during childhood may be restricted to a single domain of function. With an individual's evolving maturity, it is possible to measure additional areas of cognition, adaptation, and behavior with a greater degree

of reliability and validity. In a comprehensive assessment, a standardized battery of tests is employed to measure multiple domains of cognition and behavior.

The personality testing is neither useful nor appropriate for individuals with significant ID/IDD, who often lack the language and cognitive skills necessary for exploring intrapersonal dynamics through tests such as the Rorschach, personality inventories (Minnesota Multiphasic Personality Inventory-2), or projective measures like picture Thematic Apperception Test.

2. Measurement of intelligence—The measurement of intelligence on a standardized test, two or more standard deviations below the mean, with an IQ below 70, is necessary but not sufficient in establishing the diagnosis of ID/IDD. To gain an accurate appraisal of the person's function, the individual's adaptive functioning needs also to be appraised. All testing should occur in a quiet and comfortable place free from distraction. Adequate time should be allocated to pace the testing to the comfort level and ability of the individual. It may be necessary to provide for frequent breaks. Testing may often require sessions over different days. The person being tested should not be fatigued. If they become hyperaroused or extremely anxious, test data will not be valid, and testing should be discontinued and administered at a later time. Tests are used for diverse populations stratified by socioeconomic status, culture, language, geographic location, and gender. Individuals of low socioeconomic status may test less well than more affluent and educated persons. The low scores in such situations should not be automatically attributed to mild intellectual impairment. This is one reason why in individuals with suspected ID/IDD, measures of adaptive behavior are critical in order not to confound lack of education, poverty, or inexperience with ID/IDD. If necessary, an interpreter should be used for persons with lack of fluency in English. The validity of test results can be significantly affected by translation and the interpretation of results and ought to be viewed with the caveat that tests have been normed on native English speakers.

Psychological tests of intelligence that are standardized are based on a normal distribution of scores with a mean of 100 and a standard deviation of 15 points. Normal scores range from 85 to 115, representing one standard deviation from the mean. Abnormal scores on standardized tests fall within 1.5–2.0 standard deviations below the mean. Subtests on intelligence tests have scores measured in scaled points ranging from 1 to 18 with a mean of 10 and a standard deviation of 3. Standardized tests are constructed to enable valid comparisons between scores. For example, an IQ of 85 corresponds to a scaled score of 7 on a subtest that might measure a variable such as fund of knowledge (e.g., Information on the Wechsler scales) and a Z score of -1.0 standard deviation. All of these scores are at the 16th percentile and equivalently scaled for comparison.

3. Interpretation of test results—The report prepared by the psychologist on completion of testing ought to list all tests administered, the raw scores as well as the standard scores for test comparisons across time. It is important to stress that the summary scores, such as full scale IQ, do not adequately capture individual differences enumerated by testing. The clinician needs to be aware that summary scores combine data and may lead to a false impression because they represent a mean of all tests administered. The psychologist should look at all scores, and their ranges, to gain an accurate impression of an individual's profile, defining patterns of strengths and weaknesses across all domains evaluated. For IQ tests this means examining index or cluster scores where subtests are divided into similar constructs. Different clusters measure verbal comprehension, perceptual organization, working memory, and processing speed.

Following are other key areas of importance to consider:

- Gross and fine motor skills and coordination.
- Language including vocabulary, syntax, pragmatics, fluency, and articulation.

- Memory including visual and verbal domains for encoding and retrieval.
- Motor strength.
- Visual-motor and perceptual abilities.
- Executive skills involving planning, organization, task management, and cognitive flexibility.
- Achievement testing including reading, arithmetic, and writing.
- Commonly used psychological tests are listed in Tables 40–2 to 40–4.

4. Assessment of adaptive behavior—An understanding of the measurement of adaptive functioning is critical for all psychiatrists and mental health practitioners because of its central role in understanding of ID/IDD. This is critical for enabling appropriate diagnosis of ID/IDD. It is also useful in providing a framework for planning education and habilitative interventions. Adaptive

Table 40–2 Representative Tests Used to Evaluate Different Cognitive Functions at Various Ages

Name of Test	Age		
	Infant/ Preschool	Child	Adult
Ability measured: development/intelligence			
1. Bayley Scales of Infant and Toddler Development—III	•		
2. Miller Assessment of Preschoolers	•		
3. Wechsler Preschool and Primary Scale of Intelligence—III	•		
4. Wechsler Intelligence Scale for Children—IV		•	
5. Stanford-Binet 5		•	•
6. Wechsler Adult Intelligence Scale—III			•
Ability measured: language			
1. Preschool Language Scale—4	•		
2. Peabody Picture Vocabulary Test—4		•	•
3. Expressive One-Word Picture Vocabulary Test		•	•
4. Reynell Developmental Language Scales	•	•	
5. Receptive-Expressive Emergent Language Test—3	•		
6. California Verbal Learning Test		•	•
7. Boston Diagnostic Aphasia Examination—3			•
Ability measured: motor function			
1. Grip Strength		•	•
2. Purdue Pegboard Test		•	•
3. Grooved Pegboard Test		•	•
4. Finger Tapping Test		•	•
Ability measured: adaptive behavior			
1. Vineland Adaptive Behavior Scales-III	•		•
2. AAMR Adaptive Behavior Scales—2		•	•
Ability measured: executive function			
1. NEPSY-II		•	
2. Delis–Kaplan Executive Function System		•	•
Ability measured: achievement			
1. Woodcock–Johnson III NU Tests of Achievement		•	•
2. Wechsler Individual Achievement Test—II			•

Table 40–3 Tests for Special Populations

Nonverbal Tests	Tests for Autism and Related Disorders
Test of Nonverbal Intelligence—3	Autism Diagnostic Interview—Revised
Leiter International Performance Scale—Revised	Autism Diagnostic Observation Scales
Raven's Progressive Matrices	Childhood Autism Rating Scale
Wechsler Nonverbal Scale of Ability	Gilliam Asperger Disorder Scale

behavior ought to be assessed through most recent versions of standardized instruments. These include the Vineland Adaptive Behavior Scales (VABS) or the Adaptive Behavior Assessment Scales (ABAS). Additional adaptive behavior scales are currently in development to address the new ID/IDD diagnostic guidelines. Assessment of adaptive behavior quantifies function in the major domains of development with regard to what an individual can and cannot do in comparison to age-matched peers. The VABS measures the social skills of individuals from birth to 19 years of age. It is administered to parents or primary caregivers familiar with the child. The test contains four sections: communication, daily living skills, socialization, and motor skills. Daily living activities are hierarchically evaluated to include chronological age and maturation that is the hallmark of development. For example, communication skills required for a 3-year-old take into account the complexity of vocabulary development for expression, comprehension, and nonverbal abilities, such as gestural skills, whereas requisite skills for adolescents would include the ability to read, write, and follow written instructions. The ABAS measures three main categories of adaptive behavior skills: conceptual, social, and practical life skills. It is helpful for

Table 40–4 Screening Tests for Office or Bedside Evaluation

Test	Purpose	Age
Denver Developmental Screening Test—II	Overall screen for development for infants and preschool children for language, motor skills, social interaction	Birth to 6 yr
Bayley Infant Neuro-Developmental Screener	Evaluation of infant development including motor, cognitive, social/emotional skills	3–24 months
Folstein Mini-Mental State Examination	Screens various mental functions involved in cognition	Adults

determining the supports needed to maximize independent functioning and quality of life.

C. Laboratory Findings

A number of factors are considered when making the decision to perform laboratory tests. The individual's presentation, medical history, developmental history, family history (family pedigree), physical examination, and the results of psychological testing may all influence which tests are recommended. The workup should be guided by the child's presentation and working hypothesis of etiologic factors and may be done over time as certain medical disorders are ruled out. The lower the level of adaptive and cognitive functioning, the greater the likelihood of finding associated genetic or medical conditions.

1. Genetic testing—The need to provide up-to-date genetic testing in assessment of individuals with ID/IDD (appropriate to the availability of local resources within a given country) is an important priority. Identifying an underlying genetic etiology has implications beyond treatment; it can provide important guidance on life course and prognosis of illness. The American Academy of Pediatrics provides guidelines on genetic testing information on the newest screening modalities. High-resolution karyotyping and fragile-X testing and fluorescence-in-situ-hybridization (FISH) studies are frequently done to confirm or rule out a suspected genetic disorder. Because of the predominance of genetic causes of ID/IDD, the chromosome microarrays, which look at the DNA at the gene level, have become standard testing because they can detect copy-number changes (duplications and deletions) across the genome. There are two types of chromosomal microarrays: the comparative genomic hybridization (CGH), spanning the length of all chromosomes with enrichment in known areas of copy-number variation; and the single-nucleotide polymorphism (SNP) genotyping that examines multiple sites in the genome. The SNP allows for analysis of homozygosity and heterozygosity as well as identification of duplications or deletions. The SNP can also detect consanguinity. It has been estimated that on average the CGH and SNP arrays will yield 10–30% positive findings, whereas the G-banded karyotyping can detect abnormalities in 2–4% of cases, and FISH in 2.4–3.5%. The karyotyping, in addition to or instead of chromosomal array, is useful in aneuploidy syndromes such as trisomy 21 (Down), 18, or 13, or Turner (45,X) or Klinefelter (47,XXY). Whenever parental chromosomal abnormality is suspect, karyotyping of the parents is also recommended for further characterization and for genetic counseling.

2. Metabolic screening tests—These tests are recommended by some practitioners for all children in whom etiology is unclear. Others obtain metabolic testing when the developmental trajectory is characterized by regression, particularly with common illnesses, or there is prolonged recovery from such illnesses. Children with metabolic disorders may also present with a number of signs or symptoms, including but not limited to cyclic vomiting, hearing or visual impairments, enlarged liver or spleen, and coarse facies.

3. Electrophysiological testing—This testing is not a part of a routine workup for children with ID/IDD. However, these children have a higher incidence of seizures disorders compared to the general population and it increases significantly in the presence of severe ID/IDD. An electroencephalogram study should be obtained if there are staring episodes, paroxysmal outbursts with no identifiable precipitants, developmental regression, or behaviors consistent with seizures.

4. Evaluation of hearing acuity—This should be performed on any child with language delay, including those with ID/IDD, even in the context of a normal neonatal hearing test. If routine audiologic assessment using headphones is not feasible, visual reinforcement audiometry, in a sound field without the use of headphones, may be used to make sure that hearing acuity is adequate for language development. If this test is felt to be unreliable or provides insufficient information, neurophysiologic assessment, such as auditory brainstem response or brainstem auditory evoked response, may be performed.

5. Ophthalmologic assessment—This assessment is also important to identify specific medical conditions associated with ID and to rule out reduced visual acuity.***

D. Neuroimaging

Neuroimaging is not indicated for all children with the diagnosis of ID/IDD. It should be considered in the context of an abnormal neurologic examination, such as asymmetry of motor findings or abnormal reflexes. Disproportionate head growth signals a need for neuroimaging. The more severe the ID/IDD, the more likely it is that positive findings will be identified on neuroimaging studies. A magnetic resonance imaging (MRI) study is specifically warranted in the presence of abnormal head size (macrocephaly, microcephaly) or facial abnormalities suggestive of brain malformation. A history of focal or intractable seizures, progressive neurologic deterioration, or movement abnormalities may also suggest that an MRI may be useful. Nevertheless, it ought to be noted that abnormal MRI findings may not always provide clues as to etiology but only help characterize a process.

MRI provides better resolution of brain tissue compared to the computed tomography (CT) scan. CT scan is preferred to identify osseous structures and is a quicker test, but it provides exposure to radiation. Magnetic resonance spectroscopy may also be used in the evaluation of metabolic disorders. Positron emission tomography and single-photon emission computed tomography scans use radioactive tracers, based on glucose metabolism and blood flow, respectively, and may be used in the evaluation of seizure foci.

E. Course of Illness

The life course of ID/IDD depends on its degree, associated disabilities, and etiology, as well as on salient psychological factors (comorbid psychopathology and associated behavioral traits), environmental factors (including the attitudes and stigma experienced from people in the immediate environment and society at large), and the services the person with ID/IDD receives. Across communities and society, however, there are common features in the lives of people who have this diagnosis. To a large extent, they have been shaped by the *normalization principle* and its contemporary prospect involving *social and community inclusion*. These approaches hold that people with ID/IDD should have life opportunities as close as possible to the norms of the society at large and that people with ID/IDD should be included to maximum extent possible in the normative life within society. They should be given the supports necessary for such inclusion to be realized to the optimal extent possible.

The institutionalization of a person with ID/IDD, and children in particular, is no longer an acceptable option, and large state institutions have closed and are in the process of attenuating worldwide. In the United States, by federal law (Individuals with Disabilities Education Act, first enacted in 1975 and amended since), all children with ID/IDD are entitled to special education in their local educational jurisdiction, mostly in regular classrooms, with all necessary ancillary services, through age 21. Adults with ID/IDD usually receive vocational training; many have "regular" or at least sheltered jobs and live in their communities, with their families, in small group homes, or independently.

Allovay TP. Working memory and executive function profiles of individuals with borderline intellectual functioning. *J Intellect Disabil Res.* 2010;54:448–456.

Bayley N. *Bayley Scales of Infant and Toddler Development.* 3rd ed. San Antonio, TX: Psychological Corporation; 2005.

Brown L, Sherbenou R, Johnson S. *Test of Nonverbal Intelligence.* 3rd ed. San Antonio, TX: Psychological Corporation; 1997.

Brownell R, ed. *Expressive One-Word Picture Vocabulary Test.* 2000 ed. Novato, CA: Academic Therapy Publications; 2000.

Bzoch KR, League R, Brown V. *Receptive-Expressive Emergent Language Test.* 3rd ed. Austin, TX: Pro-ed; 2003.

Cohen M. *Children's Memory Scale.* San Antonio, TX: Psychological Corporation; 1997.

Delis D, Kramer J, Kaplan E, Ober B. *California Verbal Learning Test—Children's Version.* San Antonio, TX: Psychological Corporation; 1994.

Delis D, Kramer J, Kaplan E, Ober B. *California Verbal Learning Test.* 2nd ed. San Antonio, TX: Psychological Corporation; 2000.

Delis D, Kaplan E, Kramer J. *Delis-Kaplan Executive Function System.* San Antonio, TX: Psychological Corporation; 2001.

Dunn LM, Dunn LM. *Peabody Picture Vocabulary Test.* 4th ed. Circle Pines, MN: American Guidance Service; 2006.

Dykens E, ed. Special issue on behavioral phenotypes. *Am J Ment Retard.* 2001;106(1):1–107.

Ewing-Cobbs L. Early brain injury in children: development and reorganization of cognitive functions. *Dev Neuropsychol.* 2003;24:669–704.

Folstein M, Folstein S, McHugh P, Fanjiang G. *Mini-Mental State Examination.* Lutz, FL: Psychological Assessment Resources; 2001.

Frankenburg WK, Dodds J, Archer P, et al. *Denver Developmental Screening Test.* 2nd ed. Denver, CO: Denver Developmental Materials; 1990.

Gilliam J. *Gilliam Asperger Disorder Scale.* Austin, TX: Pro-ed; 2001.

Glascoe FP. Parents' concerns about children's development: prescreening technique or screening test? *Pediatrics.* 1997;99(4): 522–528.

Goodglass H, Kaplan E. *Boston Diagnostic Aphasia Examination.* 3rd ed. San Antonio, TX: Psychological Corporation; 2000.

Graham JM Jr, Superneau D, Rogers RC, et al. Clinical and behavioral characteristics in FG syndrome. *Am J Med Genet.* 1999;85(5):470–475.

Graham JM Jr, Rosner B, Dykens E, Visootsak J. Behavioral features of CHARGE syndrome (Hall-Hittner syndrome) comparison with down syndrome, Prader-Willi syndrome, and Williams syndrome. *Am J Med Genet.* 2005;133(3):240–247.

Harrison, PL, Oakland, T. *Adaptive Behavior Assessment System, Manual, and Intervention Planner.* 3rd ed. Torrance, CA: Western Psychological Services; 2015.

Kazuo N, Leland H, Lambert N. *AAMR Adaptive Behavior Scales.* 2nd ed. Lutz, FL: Psychological Assessment Resources; 1992.

Korkman M, Kirk U, Kemp S. *For the NEPSY.* 2nd ed. San Antonio, TX: Psychological Corporation; 2007.

La Malfa G, Lassi S, Bertelli M, et al. Emotional development and adaptive abilities in adults with intellectual disability. A correlation study between the Scheme of Appraisal of Emotional Development (SAED) and Vineland Adaptive Behavior Scales (VABS). *Res Dev Disabil.* 2009;30:1406–1412.

Lord C, Rutter M, DiLovore P, Risi S. *Autism Diagnostic Observation Schedule.* Los Angeles: Western Psychological Services; 1999.

Miller LJ. *Miller Assessment for Preschoolers.* San Antonio, TX: Psychological Corporation; 1982.

Moldavsky M, Lev D, Lerman-Sagie T. Behavioral phenotypes of genetic syndromes: a reference guide for psychiatrists. *J Am Acad Child Adolesc Psychiatry.* 2001;40(7):749–761.

Rauch A, Ruschendorf F, Huang J, et al. Molecular karyotyping using an SNP array for genomewide genotyping. *J Med Genet.* 2004;41:916–922.

Raven JC. *Raven's Progressive Matrices.* San Antonio, TX: Psychological Corporation; 2003.

Reynell JK, Gruber CP. *Reynell Developmental Language Scales.* U.S. ed. Los Angeles: Western Psychological Services; 1990.

Roid GH. *Stanford-Binet Intelligence Scales.* 5th ed. Itasca, IL: Riverside; 2003.

Roid GH, Miller L. *Leiter International Performance Scale—Revised.* Woodale, IL: Stoelting; 1997.

Royal College of Psychiatrists. *DC–LD, Occasional Paper OP 48.* London: Gaskell; 2001.

Rutter M, Le Couteur A, Lord C. *Autism Diagnostic Interview—Revised.* Los Angeles: Western Psychological Services; 1994.

Schopler E, Reichler R, Renner B. *Childhood Autism Rating Scale.* Los Angeles: Western Psychological Services; 1998.

Sparrow S, Cicchetti D, Balla D. *Vineland Adaptive Behavior Scales.* 2nd ed. New York: Pearson Assessments; 2006.

Su CY, Chen CC, Wuang YP, et al. Neuropsychological predictors of everyday functioning in adults with intellectual disabilities. *J Intellect Disabil Res.* 2008;52:18–28.

Tassé MJ1, Schalock RL, Balboni G, et al. The construct of adaptive behavior: its conceptualization, measurement, and use in the field of intellectual disability. *Am J Intellect Dev Disabil.* 2012;117(4):291–303.

Taylor RW, Turnbull DM. Mitochondrial DNA mutations in human disease. *Nat Rev Genet.* 2005;6:389–402.

Velagaleti GVN, Robinson SS, Rouse BM, et al. Subtelomeric rearrangements in idiopathic mental retardation. *Ind J Pediatr.* 2005;72:679–685.

Wechsler D. *Wechsler Intelligence Scale.* 3rd ed. San Antonio, TX: Psychological Corporation; 1997.

Wechsler D. *Wechsler Preschool and Primary Scale of Intelligence.* 3rd ed. San Antonio, TX: Psychological Corporation; 2002.

Wechsler D. *Wechsler Intelligence Scale for Children.* 4th ed. San Antonio, TX: Psychological Corporation; 2003.

Wechsler D, Naglieri J. *Wechsler Nonverbal Scale of Ability.* San Antonio, TX: Psychological Corporation; 2006.

Williams-Costello D, Friedman H, Minich N, et al. Improved survival with increased neurodevelopmental disabilities for extremely low birth weight infants in 1990s. *Pediatrics.* 2005;115:997–1003.

Woodcock RW, McGrew KS, Mather N. *Woodcock-Johnson III,* Normative Update. Itasca, IL: Riverside; 2006.

Zimmerman I, Steiner V, Pond R. *Preschool Language Scale.* 4th ed. San Antonio, TX: Psychological Corporation; 2002.

▶ Differential Diagnosis (Including Comorbid Conditions)

In dementia, including juvenile-onset forms, there is a decline in cognitive functioning from a premorbid level, especially in memory. The onset may be at any age. If the onset is postnatal but premorbid development was normal, both dementia and ID/IDD may theoretically be diagnosed, but because it may be difficult to document that the premorbid development was normal, both the ICD and DSM classification systems do not recommend diagnosing dementia during the early developmental period, or if the neurodevelopmental condition is otherwise sufficiently described by a diagnosis of ID/IDD. The hallmark of ASD is a qualitative impairment in social interaction as well as repetitive behaviors and interests. In contrast, individuals with ID/IDD are able to relate to others in a manner corresponding to their developmental level. With the increasing prevalence of ASD in recent decades, the rate of co-occurrence with ID/IDD has decreased. Now it is estimated that a third of individuals with ASD have co-occurring ID/IDD and about a quarter are nonverbal.

By definition, individuals with LD and Communication Disorders do not present with global intellectual impairment but have deficits in skills in a specific domain that are below level expected for the age, intelligence level, education, and adaptive function. In many other mental disorders, such as in schizophrenia, there may be decline in both intellectual and adaptive functioning. If this occurs during neurodevelopment, a co-occurring diagnosis of ID/IDD ought to be endorsed. If the onset is beyond the early neurodevelopmental period, the history of premorbid normal development sought from informants will be able to rule out the diagnosis of ID/IDD.

Individuals with ID/IDD in the general population are at much higher risk for developing co-occurring mental disorders than those without ID/IDD. The co-occurring disorders include those classified under the neurodevelopmental metacategory (as in autism and attention deficit hyperactivity disorder) as well as in other domains; their manifestations may differ, being modified by the level and nature of the individual's ID/IDD. The standard for classifying a co-occurring disorder should be used and interpreted in the context of a person's communication skills, past experiences, culture, and education, as well as adaptive and cognitive functioning. These will be discussed later in sections on individual disorders. In most situations a clear-cut diagnosis can be established, but often unspecified symptoms or dimensional categories can be endorsed (e.g., in terms of mood regulation, level of agitation), implying a degree of diagnostic atypicality. The higher rate of endorsement of unspecified categories reflects the degree to which the categorical classification systems have not been able to adjust for diagnostic elaboration

in the context of ID/IDD. The Royal College of Psychiatrists in the United Kingdom has published a manual of psychiatric criteria for use with adults with ID/IDD complementary to ICD-10. Clinicians should be aware of phenomenon of "diagnostic overshadowing": if a person has an ID/IDD, clinicians tend to ignore symptoms of a comorbid psychopathology or see it as a manifestation of ID/IDD.

The generic terms "behavior disorder" in the context of ID/IDD are not infrequently encountered, they do not denote a specific diagnostic category. Persons with ID/IDD with such diverse symptomatic behaviors may in fact present with underlying comorbid mental disorders that may go undiagnosed. This sets the stage for significant error rates in treatment of these "challenging behaviors," especially with psychopharmacological agents; for example, aggressive behavior may be exhibited by persons who have diverse comorbid disorders such as mood, psychosis, or posttraumatic stress disorder (PTSD). "Behavior disorder" ought to be used to describe nonspecific behaviors that occur in certain situations only (such as in a classroom), while the diagnosis of an underlying mental disorder is being ruled out in the clinical setting.

A. Comorbid Mental Disorders & Behavioral Problems

Professionals and general public have had many misconceptions about behavior of persons with ID/IDD (Table 40–5). Individuals with ID/IDD often have comorbid neuropsychiatric conditions that may often include atypical problems with affective regulation, anxiety, and attention. They may exhibit disruptive behaviors, impulsivity, overactivity,

Table 40–5 Misconceptions About Psychopathology in People with ID/IDD

Misconception	Reality
Sub-average IQ sufficient for diagnosis	Impairments in both intellectual and adaptive skills and onset in the developmental period all required
ID/IDD is lifelong	Some individuals may lose diagnosis with improvement in adaptive skills
People with ID/IDD sooner or later stop learning	Learning is lifelong (like everyone else) and with appropriate services and supports their lives will improve
People with ID/IDD have unique personalities (e.g., uninhibited, aggressive)	Full range of "personality types" may be seen. Certain traits are more common in certain syndromes but these are characterized as "behavioral phenotypes" (see Table 40–1), but not unique. Low self-image and dependency are common because of societal and environmental factors and experiences
People with ID/IDD are too impaired to have mental disorders	ID/IDD represent a group of neurodevelopmental disorders characterized by impairments in intellectual and adaptive functioning; in turn this group of individuals have an increased morbidity risk for other mental disorders
People with ID/IDD have mental disorders unique to them	Full spectrum of comorbid mental disorders may be experienced and their manifestations may be modified by impairments in communication and cognition skills as well as environmental experiences and available supports
Professionals should focus on person's deficits	Treatment and habilitation should focus on developing person's inherent strengths and abilities (rather than disabilities) with compensatory strategies to overcome impairments and removing barriers if possible

distractibility, mood or anxiety symptoms, and more extreme and aberrant behaviors such as self-injury or stereotypical motor mannerisms.

These behaviors can be evaluated during an informal observation, clinical interview, formal testing, school or work observation, or home visit. There are also instruments that are used to measure behaviors associated with psychiatric and behavioral problems in individuals with ID/IDD. These usually consist of checklists identifying behaviors such as attentional problems. They can be completed by parents, caregivers, or health professionals and are useful in alerting the clinician to more severe problems requiring more comprehensive evaluation.

If available, detailed behavioral data recorded at the individual's school, work or residence should be reviewed. They typically include tabulation of the frequency of behaviors in question in various settings and events that precede and follow the behaviors (antecedents and consequences). For example, temper tantrums that result in being sent out of the classroom may indicate a person's wish to avoid a difficult classroom task. At the end of the assessment the diagnostician should be able to answer the following questions:

a. Does the person have an ID/IDD?
b. Is there a mental disorder warranting a comorbid diagnosis?
c. What is the profile of individual's strengths and impairments?
d. What are the factors causing/maintaining the problem? (These include biomedical, psychological, and environmental considerations)
e. Is intervention necessary?
f. What are the interventions with best benefit/risk ratio?
g. What is the predicted outcome without treatment?

In order to answer these questions, the assessment should be based on a bio-psycho-social and developmental model. Even if he or she may not be responsible for the direct care of a person with ID/IDD, the psychiatrist consulting in the educational and/or vocational habilitation settings needs to conduct the assessment in the context and with understanding of the person's abilities, impairments, and functioning in all domains. An original schema developed by the AAMR in 2002 suggested five dimensions that ought to be considered:

1. Intellectual functioning and adaptive skills.
2. Adaptive behavior skills: conceptual (language, reading and writing, money concepts, self-direction); social (such as interpersonal, responsibility, following rules and laws); practical (daily living, housekeeping, transportation, occupation, safety).
3. Participation, interaction, and social roles.
4. Health (physical and mental, etiology of ID/IDD).
5. Context (environments, culture).

Thus, the first step is to review past medical, psychological, and other assessments. If these are unavailable or unreliable (e.g., only group IQ testing had been done) or outdated (e.g., old genetic testing could not diagnose an underlying ID/IDD), the patient should be referred for psychological, medical, and other appropriate consultations. The psychiatric evaluation follows usual principles, but the techniques have to be modified according to the person's developmental level and communication skills, as described in Tables 40–6 and 40–7.

In the majority of people with ID/IDD who have a mild/moderate cognitive and communication impairment, the usual DSM-5 diagnostic criteria can be used, although they

Table 40–6 Psychiatric Assessment in ID/IDD: History

Informants	Multiple including family, teachers, work counselors ("job coaches"), and therapists
Background history	Critically review and update: past psychological, medical, etiological, environmental assessments, school/work records
Referral history	Overt reasons for referral; why referred now (was it prompted by environmental factors); expectations of various caregivers
Presenting symptoms	Longitudinal history of symptoms, their variability with time, place, caregivers, when/where symptoms do not occur? Concrete description and examples of problem behaviors as well as strengths. Past management of problem behaviors and its effectiveness
Past history, personality	Strengths, adaptive skills, unusual behaviors, communication patterns
Psychiatric history	Evaluations, diagnoses, hospitalizations, treatments, their results and side effects, alternative treatments
Education/work	Settings, programs, supports, results
Health	Health and developmental history, medical problems known to be associated with underlying etiology
Family history (parents, siblings, extended)	Family constellation, medical, psychiatric, and genetic history, understanding of attitudes and feelings about patient's disability, appropriateness of expectations
Environmental	Current and past services and their adequacy (medical, psychiatric, educational, work and other supports, entitlements); family's ability to advocate
Legal and cultural	Guardianship status if over 18; cultural context, disability status, language environment; status of legal affidavit to administer antipsychotic medications if so prescribed

Table 40–7 Psychiatric Assessment in ID/IDD: Patient Interview

Setting	If possible, natural, (home, school, work, unobtrusive observation in waiting room); alone and jointly with caregivers; provide sufficient time
Verbal techniques	Assess patient's skills: observe communication with caregivers; use clear language, avoid leading questions or those requiring yes–no answers, ascertain that questions are understood, encourage spontaneous expression
Nonverbal techniques	Observe general appearance and behavior, activity level, distractibility, eye contact, joint attention, stereotypical and other unusual behaviors, nonverbal social communication, physical clues (e.g., callus from hand-biting)
Content (if verbal)	Strengths, preferences, friendships, functioning in various settings, understanding of the evaluation and of own disability
Mental status	As much as possible avoid standard MS; preferably assess within context of general conversation

may have to be modified to reflect the person's understanding and life context. In those whose communication skills are too low, the diagnosis is made primarily on the basis of history from caregivers and observation of the patient's behavior. Modifications pertaining to more common disorders are discussed next, beginning with disorders emerging in infancy and childhood.

1. ASD—A significant number of individuals with ASD also have ID/IDD. In nonverbal individuals with severe/profound ID/IDD, an ASD diagnosis was more frequently endorsed, especially on the basis of predominance of stereotypical repetitive behaviors and lack of language. However, in more recent years, with greater awareness of ASD, individuals with milder ID/IDD with ASD are also being recognized. A 2014 surveillance report by the Centers for Disease Control and Prevention, on the prevalence of ASD among 8-year-old children in the United States ascertained from professional provider registries and school sources across 11 communities, showed that 31% of children with ASD were also classified as having ID/IDD (based on IQ scores of 70 or below); 23% were in the borderline range (IQ 71–85), and 46% in the average or above average range (IQ >85). The co-occurrence of ID/IDD with ASD was reported for 48% of Black non-Hispanic children, 38% of Hispanic children, and 25% of White non-Hispanic children. The median age of earliest

ASD diagnosis was 53 months and did not differ significantly by sex or race/ethnicity. The increase in ASD prevalence in the United States is disproportionately represented by children with average or above-average IQ scores.

Much of this reported higher prevalence of ASD is among White non-Hispanic children without co-occurring ID/IDD. Co-occurrence of ASD with ID/IDD is disproportionately overrepresented among Black and Hispanic non-White children. Yet, no data are available to support etiologic differences in ASD by race/ethnicity. Likewise, an overrepresentation of nonverbal children with ASD has been reported in referred settings in Africa, suggesting that these children with co-occurring ID/IDD are more likely to be referred to hospitals when their condition is severe and medical attention is not otherwise adequately sought for children with milder forms of ASD without co-occurring ID/IDD, perhaps in view of perceived stigmatization. It is therefore that reported surveillance rates of ASD are significantly biased and underreported among Black non-Hispanic and Hispanic children without ID/IDD compared to White non-Hispanic children without ID/IDD. The data on ASD prevalence with and without ID/IDD therefore point to major disparities in the identification of ASD by racial/ethnic groupings.

2. LD—In the United Kingdom the term "learning disability" was synonymous with ID/IDD, but this term has no scientific validity. Individuals with ID/IDD have significant limitations in learning that mitigate their ability to adjust to their environment. There is sparse literature directly addressing issues of learning in ID/IDD, and most are concerned with cognitive processes. Individuals with ID/IDD learn through repetition and reinforcement and by constant interactions with their external stimulation. Individuals with ID/IDD lack emotional maturity, and this in turn may prevent them from learning adequate social skills. Learning involves a threefold process under the influence of motivation and emotion, cognitive processes, and social adaptation. In the United States, under special circumstances, a co-diagnosis of learning disability can be endorsed in persons with milder forms of ID/IDD or among individuals with borderline intellectual functioning, provided that the impairments in question cannot be adequately explained by the ID/IDD alone and the associated impairments are below the level expected for the person's age, education, and intelligence level.

3. Feeding and eating disorders of infancy or early childhood—Pica (persistent ingestion of nonnutritive substances) is seen sometimes in children and adults with severe/profound ID/IDD and may be life threatening, as is rumination disorder. Medical assessment is essential, including testing for trace metal deficiency (which may be associated with pica), for gastroesophageal reflux disease, and for *Helicobacter pylori* infection.

4. Stereotypic movement disorder (SMD)—Significant ID/IDD is often associated with variety of stereotypic movements, which appear to be self-stimulatory and sometimes lead to self-injury or Self-Injurious Behavior (SIB), in which case a specifier with SIB is added and is an important reason for referral to a psychiatrist. These may also be part of behavioral phenotypes such as Lesch–Nyhan syndrome or may be caused by a painful, undiagnosed medical condition (Table 40–1). The SIB can also be a response to adverse environmental stimuli or related to an activation as a side effect of a medication such as antihistamines or stimulants. It may also be a person's response to pain such as a headache, earache, or dental caries. SIB can lead to severe injury (such as loss of sight) or can even be life threatening. SMD is diagnosed on the basis of observable behaviors, also denoting their frequency, intensity, and location (usually caudal). SIB manifest behaviors often include head banging and hitting, self-biting, and eye poking, as well as aerophagia.

5. ADHD—Hyperactive and impulsive behaviors are a frequent problem in children with ID/IDD in both the home and school settings. The children may fare better in a structured and behaviorally managed classroom setting. The diagnosis of ADHD should not be made readily unless the presentation is persistent and its severity inconsistent with the child's developmental level. Because most of DSM-5 criteria for ADHD are based on observable behaviors, the standard diagnostic approaches are used. Inappropriate classroom placement and other environmental anxiety-producing factors are often the cause of ADHD-like symptoms in individuals with ID/IDD. They may also be a part of a behavioral phenotype, for example, in Fragile-X and in Fetal Alcohol Syndrome.

6. Conduct disorder—One must ascertain that the individual is aware that the inappropriate behaviors are prohibited by societal rules (the same applies to diagnosis of Antisocial Personality Disorder in adults). This may be difficult in persons with low or no language skills. It is difficult to elicit malicious intent among adults with severe/profound ID/IDD. Furthermore, persons discharged from institutions without preparation might not be aware of social rules that are expected of them in the community. Children and adults with ID/IDD are also vulnerable to pressures from others and might be induced by them to break rules and laws. Sometimes they are quite willing to do it, believing that in this way they can make friends. Hence, it is felt that this category is rather difficult to endorse among individuals with ID/IDD with any degree of validity. The same limitations apply also to the category of oppositional defiant disorder.

7. Aggression and other challenging behaviors—The term "challenging behavior" is often applied nonspecifically to any behavior that is inappropriate by a caregiver's standards. Irritability and aggressive behavior are common reasons for referral complaints. There is no single diagnostic category, or treatment, for irritability and aggression. It may be a part of the presentation of virtually any mental disorder in individuals with ID/IDD, including mood disorder, depression, anxiety, PTSD, and psychosis. Comprehensive diagnostic assessment is required, including information about whether aggression is limited to certain persons or situations. Detailed descriptions of the actual behavior are necessary, because some caregivers tend to label any resistance they encounter as aggressive. Nonspontaneous incidents of aggressive behavior may be more characteristically associated with incident seizure disorder, which individuals with ID/IDD may present across the life span. A more complex aggressive behavior, targeted at a specific person(s), is usually not linked to seizures.

In assessing these behaviors, one should differentiate between factors that caused them and factors that maintain them. For example, a painful middle ear infection might lead to intractable head banging and self-injury. The pain may subside after a course of antibiotics, but the SIB may continue if the individual has learned that it provided him with increased attention by the staff.

8. Psychotic disorders—Schizophrenia occurs in people with ID/IDD at least as often as in the general population, and probably more often if one considers individuals with mild ID/IDD and borderline intellectual functioning. In persons with mild ID/IDD and good verbal skills, the manifestations are similar to those in individuals without ID/IDD and the same diagnostic criteria may be used. However, the verbal productions (e.g., description of delusions) may be simpler and more concrete. The diagnosticians must be sure that their questions are understood: for example, when asked about "hearing voices" many patients will assume that they are being asked about their hearing ability. Training of psychiatrists in making such phenomenological distinctions is therefore critical to avoid misclassification of symptoms as psychosis, leading to greater stigmatization and overly zealous use of antipsychotic medications. Careful interviewing and "interpreting" by a caregiver may help in differentiating poor language skills from psychotic verbalizations. In people with severe/profound ID/IDD, often with poor or no language skills, the diagnosis of psychosis or schizophrenia needs to rely on careful observations of behavior and documentation of mood changes, such as behaviors becoming bizarre and moods becoming increasingly paranoid. In many such cases diagnosing a specific category of psychotic illness may not be possible, and the general diagnosis of Psychotic Disorder not otherwise specified might be more appropriate. Solitary, preoccupied, and self-stimulatory bizarre behaviors often observed in individuals with ID/IDD should not be construed as evidence of psychosis. People with velocardiofacial syndrome (often associated with the mild form of ID/IDD) are at increased risk for developing a psychotic disorder as well as a mood disorder. Presentation corresponding to a Brief Psychotic Disorder has been seen in persons with ID/IDD who were subjected to very stressful situations beyond their control and understanding.

9. Mood disorders—People with ID/IDD are at increased risk for depressive disorders. Unfortunately they often remain undiagnosed, because depressed individuals tend to be quiet and not disruptive and may not have language abilities to verbalize depressed mood, anhedonia, or thoughts of death. Manifestation of depression often involves refusal to attend activities they once liked; they may even engage in irritable and oppositional behaviors, or exhibit SMD with SIB. Suicidal behavior has also been described among individuals with ID/IDD. Aggressive behavior is not infrequent, especially if depressed persons with ID/IDD are forced to attend activities required as part of their program. Their complaints may be simpler—for example, that they feel sick—or they may report somatic concerns and/or resistance to doing activities of daily living. The clinician will have to rely on behavioral observations, familiarity of the individual's living situation and routines, looking for presence of vegetative signs, and mood changes as observed by caregivers. An important differential diagnosis is dementia, as in older persons with or without ID/IDD, and especially in adults with Down syndrome. These latter individuals are at high risk for developing Alzheimer dementia. Although neuropathological changes may occur by age 40, clinical dementia is usually not seen before 50, or even later. It is a common mistake for clinicians to begin to diagnose dementia in a younger person with Down syndrome who may be experiencing regressive changes associated with depression or mood disorder. A common rule of thumb is that a person with dementia usually tries to perform a task but fails, whereas one with depression may not even attempt it. Persons with Down syndrome can also have an exaggerated response to losses and complicated grief reactions. Persons with bipolar disorders comorbid with ID/IDD may exhibit irritability, aggression, and hyperactivity; they may masturbate excessively, laugh incongruently, and often appear inappropriately happy or unusually excited. The changes in behavior and mood need to be usually observed and reported by caregivers familiar with the individual.

10. Anxiety disorders—The full spectrum of anxiety disorders has been reported in people with ID/IDD. Once again, poor communication skills may interfere with assessing subjective feelings of anxiety, obsessive thoughts, discomfort, panic, and worry. However, in most anxiety and related disorders, the diagnosis may be made on the basis of behavioral observation. It may be difficult to decide whether perseverative and self-stimulatory behaviors often seen in people with significant ID/IDD are part of an obsessive–compulsive disorder, because in nonverbal persons it is unclear whether they are related to obsessions and whether the person recognizes that they are unreasonable. Anxiety disorders are also part of various behavioral phenotypes (Table 40–1). PTSD is often missed if individuals cannot report a traumatic event (such as an abuse) or are not believed if they report it. On the other hand, persons with ID/IDD are at risk for abuse and victimization, and PTSD should always be considered as a differential diagnosis and if otherwise unexplained behavioral changes occur. An event not considered traumatic by an average person may be traumatic for a person with ID/IDD. The modifications of DSM-5 diagnostic criteria for PTSD that are aimed at children are also relevant for people with significant ID/ID.

Brickell C, Munir K. Grief and its complications in individuals with intellectual disability. *Harv Rev Psychiatry*. 2008;16(1):1–12.

Cooper S-A, Smiley E, Morrison J, et al. Mental ill-health in adults with intellectual disabilities: prevalence and associated factors. *Br J Psychiatry*. 2007;190:27–35.

Cooper S-A, Smiley E, Jackson A, et al. Adults with intellectual disabilities. Prevalence, incidence, and remission of aggressive behavior, and related factors. *J Intellect Disabil Res*. 2009;53: 217–232.

Developmental Disabilities Monitoring Network Surveillance Year 2010 Principal Investigators. Prevalence of autism spectrum disorder among children aged 8 years—Autism and Developmental Disabilities Monitoring Network, 11 sites, United States, 2010. *MMWR Surveill Summ*. 2014;63(Suppl 2):1–21.

Einfeld SL, Ellis LA, Emerson E. Comorbidity of intellectual disability and mental disorder in children and adolescents: a systematic review. *J Intellect Dev Disabil*. 2011;36(2):137–143.

Einfeld SL, Tonge BJ. The Developmental Behavior Checklist: the development and validation of an instrument to assess behavioral and emotional disturbance in children and adolescents with mental retardation. *J Autism Dev Disord*. 1995;25(2):81–104.

Felce D, Kerr M, Hastings RP. A general practice-based study of the relationship between indicators of mental illness and challenging behavior among adults with intellectual disabilities. *J Intellect Disabil Res*. 2009;53:243-254.

Fletcher RJ, Havercamp SM, Ruedrich SL, et al. Clinical usefulness of the diagnostic manual-intellectual disability for mental disorders in persons with intellectual disability: results from a brief field survey. *J Clin Psychiatry*. 2009;70:967–74.

Harris JC. *Intellectual Disability*. New York: Oxford University Press; 2006.

Moldavsky M, Lev D, Lerman-Sagie T. Behavioral phenotype of genetic syndromes: a reference guide for psychiatrists. *J Am Acad Child Adolesc Psychiatry*. 2001;40:749–761.

Munir KM. The co-occurrence of mental disorders in children and adolescents with intellectual disability/ intellectual developmental disorder. *Curr Opin Psychiatry*. 2016;29(2):95–102.

Patja K, Iivanainen M, Raitasuo S, et al. Suicide mortality in mental retardation: a 35-year follow-up study. *Acta Psychiatr Scand*. 2001;103:307–311.

Reid AH. Schizophrenic and paranoid syndromes in persons with mental retardation: Assessment and diagnosis. In: Fletcher RJ, Dosen A, eds. *Mental Health Aspects of Mental Retardation*. New York: Lexington Books; 1993:98–110.

Reiss A, Levitan GW, Szyszko J. Emotional disturbance and mental retardation: diagnostic overshadowing. *Am J Ment Defic*. 1982;86:567–574.

Rojahn J, Matson JL, Naglieri JA, Mayville E. Relationships between psychiatric conditions and behavioral problems among adults with mental retardation. *Am J Ment Retard*. 2004;109:21–33.

Royal College of Psychiatrists. DC-LD: *Diagnostic Criteria for Psychiatric Disorders for Use with Adults with Learning Disabilities/Mental Retardation*. London: Gaskell Press; 2001.

Shattuck PT. The contribution of diagnostic substitution to the growing administrative prevalence of autism in U.S. special education. *Pediatrics*. 2006;117:1028–1037.

Shevell M. Office evaluation of a child with developmental delay. *Semin Pediatr Neurol*. 2006;13:256–261.

Sovner R, Hurley AD. Do the mentally retarded suffer from affective illness? *Arch Gen Psychiatry*. 1983;40:61–67.

Smiley E, Cooper S-A, Finlayson J, Jackson A, et al. The incidence, and predictors of mental ill-health in adults with intellectual disabilities. Prospective study. *Br J Psychiatry*. 2007;191:313–319.

Stein DS, Munir K, Karweck AJ, et al. Developmental depression, regression, and psychosocial stress in an adolescent with Down syndrome. *J Dev Behav Pediatr*. 2013;34(3):216–218.

General Treatment

A. Planning for Treatment & Education

Once the level of the individual's adaptive and cognitive functioning is determined, it is important for the clinician to use this information to develop a plan of intervention that allows persons with ID/IDD to achieve their optimal potential. Therefore, the treatment team will take test information and interpret it to formulate a treatment and education plan to enhance developmental strengths and determine accommodations or remedial methods to strengthen weaker skill areas. Except in individuals with severe/profound ID/IDD where impairment is substantive, individuals are likely to have a profile of developmental strengths and weaknesses for which an individualized treatment plan can be more readily developed. Individuals with severe impairments often require highly specialized programs to alleviate further deterioration. For preschool and latency children, this may include referral for early intervention or special education. For adolescents and young adults, in addition to special education, assessment aids in planning for prevocational and vocational training and preparation for independent or supported employment and living.

B. Pharmacologic Interventions

Medical problems are more common in people with severe ID/IDD. Seizure disorders may present with behavioral problems or developmental regression. Their identification therefore greatly affects the type of treatment that is required. The aim is to treat individuals with the fewest anticonvulsant medications to have the best seizure control without excessive sedation. Adverse reactions to anticonvulsant medications need to be monitored with vigilance. For seizures that are refractory to more conventional treatment, treatments such as the ketogenic diet, vagal nerve stimulator, and even surgery may be considered. The psychopharmacological interventions for comorbid mental disorders are discussed later.

C. Other Interventions

Cerebral palsy is commonly associated with severe ID/IDD. Spasticity has significant impact on the spine, hips, and joints. There needs to be aggressive management to prevent or reduce contractures and to enhance mobility. These individuals generally require physical and occupational therapy. They may also require orthotic and adaptive seating devices. Muscle relaxants may be needed and sometimes orthopedic surgery. Individuals with associated abnormal motor function may have problems with feeding, which may be due to difficulties with swallowing, chewing, gastric motility, and/or gastrointestinal reflux. Determination needs to be made regarding the source of the problem, which will affect recommendations for change in consistency of foods, need for medications, and/or tube feeding to avoid aspiration and promote adequate weight gain.

In terms of educational services and developmental treatments, children less than 3 years of age are eligible for Early Intervention services. With the passage of the Individuals with Disabilities Act (IDEA; PL 101–476) and its subsequent amendments, educational services in the least restrictive environment are now mandated for all children until age 21. In addition to specialized educational curricula, children often require different types of therapy. Occupational therapy addresses fine motor, sensory processing, and adaptive skills. Speech therapy works on receptive and expressive language, articulation, and oromotor problems. Both occupational therapists and speech pathologists may provide feeding therapy. Adaptive physical education may be provided for children with motor difficulties. Resource room assistance may be provided to children who are integrated into a regular classroom but require additional services for certain subjects.

Alvarez N. Neurology. In: Rubin IL, Crocker AC, eds. *Medical Care for Children and Adults with Developmental Disabilities*. 2nd ed. Baltimore: Paul H. Brookes; 2006:249–271.

Friedman S. Nursing homes. In: Rubin IL, Crocker AC, eds. *Medical Care for Children and Adults with Developmental Disabilities*. 2nd ed. Baltimore: Paul H. Brookes, 2006:94–103.

Giangreco MF. Interactions among programs, placement, and services in educational planning for students with disabilities. *Ment Retard*. 2001;39(5):341–350.

Munir KM, Friedman SL, Szymanski LS. Neurodevelopmental disorders: intellectual disability/intellectual developmental disorders. In: Tasman A, Kay J, Lieberman JA, First MB, Riba M, eds. *Psychiatry*. Vol 1. 4th ed. Hoboken, NJ: Wiley-Blackwell; 2015:672–705.

Szymanski LS. Happiness as a treatment goal. *Ment Retard*. 2000;105:352–362.

Szymanski LS. Individual psychotherapy with retarded persons. In: Szymanski LS, Tanguay PE, eds. *Emotional Disorders of Mentally Retarded Persons*. Baltimore: University Park Press; 1980:131–147.

Winter S, Kiely M. Cerebral palsy. In: Rubin IL, Crocker AC, eds. *Medical Care for Children and Adults with Developmental Disabilities*. 2nd ed. Baltimore: Paul H. Brookes; 2006:233–246.

Treatment for Mental Disorders in People with ID/IDD

The common mistake in treatment of mental disorders in this population is to rely only on psychotropic drugs. Yet, principles of treatment are the same as of corresponding disorders in people who do not have ID/IDD. The major modifications are based on the fact that persons with ID/IDD and comorbid mental illness have impairments in multiple domains, have complex needs, and usually depend on others. Therefore, an effective treatment program must be coordinated with treatment approaches in all domains in order to address the person's comprehensive needs.

A. Principles

A comprehensive diagnostic assessment (as delineated earlier) should be made of needs, strengths, and required supports in all areas.

1. Clear goals of treatment, beyond ameliorating inappropriate behaviors that trouble the caregivers, and toward helping the patient to achieve optimal feasible quality of life.

2. Ensuring that the patient receives comprehensive treatment, of which the psychiatric therapies are a part, and which may include medical treatment, education, and habilitation, appropriate school or work, and living arrangements.

3. Collaboration between professionals on treatment team.

4. Full range of psychiatric interventions, including psychotherapies, family therapy, behavior therapy, and psychopharmacology, as needed.

5. Systematic, evidence-based follow-up on patient's progress and adverse effects.

6. Consideration of human rights and legal requirements.

B. Psychotherapeutic Treatment

Persons with ID and comorbid mental disorders can be good candidates for psychotherapy, if they possess sufficient language skills to engage in interactive communication with the therapist, even on a simple level (similar to children) (Table 40–8).

Group psychotherapy follows similar guidelines, but emphasis is given to helping the patients to learn from one another. In multiple-family group therapy, several families, including patients and their siblings, participate and learn from one another's experience.

Standard techniques of behavioral therapy are used. The focus in individuals with ID/IDD should be on rewards for appropriate behaviors and minimizing what they can see as punishment (e.g., "time out"). For some individuals the latter might actually be a reward if it leads to avoiding tasks they dislike. To be effective, a behavioral plan has to be generalized to all situations (such as home and school) and implemented consistently by all caregivers. Baseline behavioral assessment and detailed follow-up are necessary. Aversive techniques are not used, except very rarely by some,

Table 40–8 Guidelines for Psychotherapy with Persons with ID/IDD

Requirements of the therapist	Motivated, experienced with people with ID/IDD, flexible, serving as role model, supportive but not paternalistic, respectful
Requirements of the patient	Willingness, basic communication skills
Verbal techniques	Adapt language level to patient's understanding; avoid too complex or too simple language; ensure that the patient understands (beyond asking "do you understand?"); avoid questions requiring "yes" or "no" answers, encourage spontaneous verbalizations; explain abstract concepts using concrete examples
Verbal content	Focus on patient's strengths first; explore understanding of own behavior and others' feelings about it; if necessary teach through concrete examples; teach understanding of own strengths and disability using examples (e.g., presence and absence of "talent"); if necessary teach concrete scripts of appropriate behavior and communication
Nonverbal techniques	Use games, other activities to create model situations for interpersonal interactions: for example, losing in a game; managing anger. Guide the patient to recognize appropriateness/inappropriateness of own behavior from video or audio recordings of self
Family counseling	Involve family through separate, later joint, sessions; model how to communicate and manage patient's behavior, how to create opportunities to succeed; gradually increase their active participation while decreasing therapist's; teach them to promote patient's self-image and independence; provide them with behavior management plan; help to see patient's strengths and to receive gratification from him/her
School/caregivers collaboration	Obtain ongoing behavioral data on follow-up: collaborate on implementing and generalizing behavioral program; promoting patient's self-image, strengths and independence; providing opportunities to succeed (e.g., meaningful jobs, friendships, and functions at school)

as a last resort, for a brief time, in case of intractable SIB/aggression, in well-controlled situations, and only if markedly effective.

C. Psychopharmacological Treatment

The same principles of rational psychopharmacology as with people without ID/IDD should be followed:

a. Other treatable reasons for inappropriate behaviors should be ruled out (e.g., medical disorder, or painful condition underlying a SIB).

b. If a comorbid mental disorder has been diagnosed, it should be treated appropriately using the same psychopharmacological agents as for typically developing individuals.

c. The least intrusive intervention should be tried first (e.g., behavioral management, environmental changes) and medications added later as needed.

d. Initially, the lowest dose regimen should be used and each dose increase closely monitored.

e. Behavioral data should be collected at baseline and in a regular follow-up.

f. The lowest effective dose should be employed.

g. A drug should be used only if documented effective and with good risk-to-benefit ratio. One should avoid a "Christmas tree" approach of adding new drugs to ineffective ones.

h. Polypharmacy should be avoided unless augmenting the effect of a medication is clearly documented.

i. Adverse effects should be carefully monitored, bearing in mind that a person with limited language skills may not be able to report them. Drug–drug interactions should be considered, as people with ID/IDD often are on multiple medications for medical reasons.

j. An overall goal must be kept in mind: maximizing the person's quality of life, rather than eliminating "challenging" behaviors solely for caregivers' convenience.

k. Legal requirements should be followed, such as obtaining informed consent of the individual or the guardian or court in states that require it (e.g., Massachusetts).

Aman MG, Collier-Crespin A, Lindsay RL. Pharmacotherapy of disorders in mental retardation. *Eur Child Adolesc Psychiatry*. 2000;9(Suppl 1):98–107.

American Academy of Child and Adolescent Psychiatry (AACAP). Practice parameters for the assessment and treatment of children, adolescents, and adults with mental retardation and co-morbid mental disorders. *J Am Acad Child Adolesc Psychiatry*. 1999;38(suppl 12):5S–31S.

Browder DM, Xin YP. A meta-analysis and review of sight word research and its implications for teaching functional reading to individuals with moderate to severe disabilities. *J Spec Educ*. 1998;32(3):130–153.

Deb S, Kwok H, Bertelli M, et al. International guide to prescribing psychotropic medication for the management of problem behaviours in adults with intellectual disabilities. *World Psychiatry*. 2009;8:181–186.

Health Care Financing Administration (HCFA). *General Safety Precautions for Psychopharmacological Medications in ICFs/MR*. Washington, DC: HCFA; 1996:3.

Kwok H, Chui E, Tang A. Prescribing psychotropic medication for problem behaviors in adults with intellectual disabilities in a specialist psychiatric unit in Hong Kong. *Adv Ment Health Intellect Disabil*. 2010;4:27–33.

Meltzer LJ, Zadig JM. Educational assessment. In: Levine MD, Carey WB, Crocker AC, Gross RT, eds. *Developmental-Behavioral Pediatrics*. Philadelphia: WB Saunders; 1983.

Reiss S, Aman MG. *Psychotropic Medications and Developmental Disabilities: The International Consensus Handbook*. Columbus: The Ohio State University; 1998.

Szymanski LS, Kiernan WE. Multiple family group therapy with developmentally disabled adolescents and young adults. *Int J Group Psychother*. 1983;33:521–534.

Yan EG, Munir K. Regulatory and ethical principles in research involving children and individuals with developmental disabilities. *Ethics Behav*. 2004;14:31–49.

▶ Complications & Adverse Outcomes of Treatment

The mortality rate for people with ID/IDD is generally considered to be comparable to the general population under resource-rich care conditions. Persons with severe to profound ID/IDD with medical comorbidity, although now living longer than previously, still have a higher mortality rate than the general population. These individuals may be non-ambulatory and dependent on others for their daily needs, suffer from seizure disorders or other physical impairments, and may require tube feeding. They may have problems handling oral secretions, with increased risk for aspiration, or maintaining a patent airway. Chronic pulmonary problems, such as reactive airway disease or recurrent lower respiratory tract infections, may occur. Other medical problems more commonly seen in severe ID include sleep disorders, vision impairment, and hearing loss.

Botsford A. Status of end of life care in organizations providing services for older people with a developmental disability. *Am J Ment Retard*. 2004;109:421–428.

Chaney RH Eyman RK. Patterns of mortality over 60 years among persons with mental retardation in a residential facility. *Ment Retard*. 2000;38:289–293.

▶ Prognosis

All children with ID/IDD need the love and support of their families and to be included in family life. With ongoing support to meet each individual's needs, the functioning of a person with ID/IDD can be expected to improve over time. Children do best with early identification of their developmental problems, and appropriate services and interventions. The etiology and severity of ID/IDD also influence the level of functioning. Approximately 80–85% of children with ID/IDD fall within the mild range. They generally are able to read, write, and perform math between the third- and sixth-grade levels. Individuals with mild ID/IDD usually live independently within the community as adults, and often the diagnosis is no longer used. Moderate ID/IDD affects about 10% of children with ID/IDD. They may learn some basic reading and writing, as well as a number of functional skills. As adults, they usually require some type of oversight or supervision. Approximately 3–5% of children with ID/IDD are in the severe range. They generally are not able to learn basic academics, although may be able to perform some self-help skills and routines. They will require supervision in their daily activities and living environment. Profound ID/IDD affects about 1–2% of children. Children with profound retardation will need intensive support for the rest of their lives. They may or may not be able to communicate by verbal or other means.

Strauss DJ, Shavelle RM, Anderson TW. Life expectancy of children with cerebral palsy. *Pediatr Neurol.* 1998;18:143–149.

Williams-Costello D, Friedman H, Minich N, et al. Improved survival rates with increased neurodevelopmental disability for extremely low birth weight infants in the 1990s. *Pediatrics.* 2005;115(4):997–1003.

▶ Resources

Organization of families and advocates for children and adults with intellectual and developmental disabilities:

American Association on Intellectual and Developmental Disabilities, at www.aaidd.org

The ARC of the United States, at www.thearc.org

National Association of Individuals with Developmental Disabilities and Mental Health Needs, at www.thenadd.org

National Down Syndrome Society, at www.ndss.org

National Organization for Rare Disorders, at www.rarediseases .org

United Cerebral Palsy, at www.ucp.org

Learning Disorders

41

Michael G. Tramontana, PhD

DEFINITION

Terms such as learning disorder and learning disability often are used interchangeably. The International Statistical Classification of Diseases and Related Health Problems–10th Revision (ICD-10) uses the term *Specific Developmental Disorders of Scholastic Skills* in referring to this category of Disorders of Psychological Development. It is further subdivided into disorders having to do with specific scholastic skills such as reading, spelling, and math. There will be reference to ICD-10 definitions and diagnostic criteria at various points in the discussion of learning disorders in this chapter. However, the coverage of the topic will be broader than that and will incorporate conceptual, empirical, and historical perspectives as well.

A major stride in the definition of learning disabilities came in 1981 from the National Joint Committee on Learning Disabilities (NJCLD). The NJCLD defined learning disability as "a generic term that refers to a heterogeneous group of disorders manifested by significant difficulties in the acquisition and use of listening, speaking, reading, writing, reasoning, or mathematical abilities. These disorders are intrinsic to the individual and presumed to be due to central nervous system dysfunction. Even though a learning disability may occur concomitantly with other handicapping conditions (e.g., sensory impairment, mental retardation, social and emotional disturbance) or environmental influences (e.g., cultural differences, insufficient/inappropriate instruction, psychogenic factors), it is not the direct result of those conditions or influences" (Hammill et al, 1981).

This definition went further than the earlier one contained in the Education for All Handicapped Children Act of 1975 (P.L. 94–142) by stipulating specifically that a learning disability must be *presumed to be due to central nervous system dysfunction*. Although this was implied in previous definitions, never before had it been made explicit. Accordingly, the later definition helped to resolve a good deal of confusion and ambiguity involving identification and differential diagnosis. Deficiencies in academic achievement can arise from a variety of factors, operating alone or in combination. To say that there is a learning disability, however, means that there must be a basis for inferring that some form of brain dysfunction is involved.

ESSENTIALS OF DIAGNOSIS

ICD-10 Diagnostic Criteria for Disorders of Scholastic Skills

The International Statistical Classification of Diseases and Related Health Problems–10th Revision (ICD-10) identifies three types of *Specific Developmental Disorders of Scholastic Skills* including *Specific Reading Disorder* (F81.0), *Specific Spelling Disorder* (F81.1), and *Specific Disorder of Arithmetical Skills* (F81.2). The category is further broken down to include *Mixed Disorder of Scholastic Skills* (F81.3), *Other Developmental Disorders of Scholastic Skills* (F81.8), and *Developmental Disorder of Scholastic Skills, Unspecified* (F81.9).

In each disorder, the diagnosis depends on documentation that:

▶ There is a disturbance in the normal patterns of skill acquisition evident from early stages of development and which are not due to any form of acquired brain trauma or disease

▶ There is significant impairment in the affected skill(s) that is not simply due to low mental age, lack of opportunity, inadequate schooling, or because of specific factors such as problems with visual acuity

The classification further specifies that:

▶ Each disorder can be further described in terms of the particular sub-skills affected (e.g., reading word recognition, reading comprehension, oral reading, and so forth)

- There is continuity in the development of skill deficiencies, as in the case of *Specific Reading Disorder* which is viewed as commonly preceded by a history of disorders of speech or language development
- Spelling problems are frequently associated with a *Specific Reading Disorder* and do not necessarily constitute a separate disorder
- The diagnosis of a *Specific Disorder of Arithmetical Skills* involves deficits in the mastery of basic computational skills rather than more abstract math reasoning skills

Adapted with permission from International Statistical Classification of Diseases and Related Health Problems, 10th Revision (ICD-10). World Health Organization; 2010.

Hammill DD et al. A new definition of learning disabilities. *Learn Disabil Q.* 1981;4:336.

General Considerations

A. Epidemiology

Estimates have varied, but about 2–8% of all school-aged children in the United States are thought to have a learning disability (Goldstein S, Schwebach A. 2009). The estimates are arbitrary to some extent, as they are based on the adoption of an agreed-upon cutoff in a continuous distribution of proficiency levels in learning skills. These estimates are influenced not only by debates over what the objective criteria for identification should be (see later discussion) but also by public policy considerations having to do with the allocation of special services.

B. Etiology

The issue of etiology is addressed, at least in broad terms, by the NJCLD definition of learning disabilities. In one form or another, brain dysfunction is the source of a learning-disabled individual's deficit(s) in reading, spelling, mathematics, or written expression (Hynd GW, Connor RT, Nieves N. 1998). The dysfunction may stem from genetic or congenital factors, arising especially during middle to later stages of fetal brain development. Neuropathologic studies suggest the presence of relatively subtle irregularities (e.g., focal dysplasia, abnormal cortical layering, and polymicrogyria), often clustering in the left perisylvian region, although the precise pattern will vary with the type of learning disability involved. This observation accounts for the specific nature of learning disabilities, in that earlier or more widespread abnormalities in brain development typically would give rise to more generalized disorders such as intellectual disability. Insults occurring after birth may be a factor, provided that they affect the acquisition rather than loss of a particular skill. Although similar deficits may arise, the convention is to regard a learning disability as a neurodevelopmental disorder rather than stemming from an acquired brain injury.

There have been a number of misconceptions regarding the cause of learning disabilities. One misconception has suggested that children with disabilities are not disordered but rather delayed on certain developmental dimensions, their difficulties presumably reflecting a slower rate of maturation of an otherwise normal brain. This would explain why a fairly severe disability can exist in the absence of documented brain impairment, at least when gross indices are used. However, current research does not support such a hypothesis. There is no evidence that the brains of learning-disabled individuals are immature, or unfinished, in some way. Rather, newer and more detailed investigations have documented specific structural abnormalities. Nor is there any indication that the disabled learner's performance resembles that of a normal younger child or that the disability is eventually outgrown. The child with learning disabilities is not merely delayed but rather deviant in the performance of processes necessary for normal reading, spelling, math, or writing. The disability may be "silent" in earlier years, giving the false impression of normal brain development, only to become evident when the child enters school.

Goldstein S, Schwebach A. Neuropsychological basis of learning disabilities. In: Reynolds R, Fletcher-Janzen E, eds. *Handbook of Clinical Child Neuropsychology.* 3rd ed. New York: Springer; 2009:187–202.

Clinical Findings

A. Identification

Clear operational criteria are needed in order to identify learning disabilities. For example, how does one decide whether an individual's academic skills fall below those expected for an individual's chronological age or whether they cannot be better accounted for by other factors such as limited intelligence (diagnostic requirements in ICD-10)? This determination has usually been based on discrepancy criteria that stipulate the minimum difference that must exist between scores obtained on a standardized test of the individual's intelligence quotient (IQ) and scores obtained on one or more areas on an achievement test (Barnes MA, Fletcher J, Fuchs L. 2007).

IQ-achievement comparisons are made using standard scores (which are converted scores based on age norms). Different school systems set their own cutoffs, although the minimum discrepancy is typically one to two standard deviations (SDs) or 15–30 points for standard scores with a mean of 100 and an SD of 15. For example, for an individual with a measured IQ of 105, an achievement test score of 90 or less would be needed to meet discrepancy criteria at 1 SD, 75 or less at 2 SDs, and so forth. The problem with this method is that it does not correct for what is typically the moderate correlation between IQ and achievement test scores. There is also the issue of regression to the mean so that a high score on one test will often be accompanied by a less extreme (lower) score on the other and vice versa. As a result, high-IQ individuals tend to be overidentified, and low-IQ individuals tend to be underidentified, as having a learning disability (Stone LA, Benoit L, Martin A, Hafler J. 2023).

A better approach uses regression-based criteria that adjust the standard test score comparisons for the correlation between IQ and achievement. A regression equation is derived for each achievement measure based on its obtained correlation with IQ (this correlation is usually available in the published test manual). This approach allows for an examination of any discrepancy between actual achievement and expected achievement predicted by the IQ measure. A cutoff between 1 and 2 standard errors of prediction (SE_{pred}) typically would be used in determining whether the discrepancy is significant.

Critics of the discrepancy model argue that there is a lack of evidence that IQ-achievement discrepancies are clear indicators of learning disabilities. Also, it is not necessarily the case that low achievers respond to treatment interventions differently depending on whether or not a significant IQ-achievement discrepancy is present.

A different diagnostic approach in identifying learning disabilities is a model based on response to intervention (RTI). Put simply, a learning disability is implied more strongly the more a learning problem persists despite the provision of appropriate initial interventions. This model goes further than ICD-10 diagnostic criteria, which simply require that Disorders of Scholastic Skills must involve a disturbance in normal skill acquisition not solely because of "a lack of opportunity" or "inadequate schooling." In the RTI approach, nonresponders to initial levels or *tiers* of corrective instruction are identified as having a learning disability and requiring more intensive special education. A potential benefit of this approach is that interventions can be provided early on, without waiting for a child to be far behind. On the other hand, at least early on, the educational interventions are not designed according to particular underlying neuropsychological factors contributing to learning problems in the individual child.

Barnes MA, Fletcher J, Fuchs L. *Learning Disabilities: From Identification to Intervention.* New York: Guilford Press; 2007.

Stone LA, Benoit L, Martin A, Hafler J. Barriers to identifying learning disabilities: a qualitative study of clinicians and educators. *Acad Pediatr.* 2023 Aug;23(6):1166–1174. doi: 10.1016/j.acap.2022.12.008. Epub ahead of print. PMID: 36584937.

B. Subtypes

Learning disabilities occur singly or in combination. Obviously, the underlying pattern of cognitive deficits will vary depending on how many types of learning disability are involved.

Each type of learning disability also can be further differentiated or subtyped based on the pattern of underlying deficits. To date, much of the research has focused mainly on reading and has identified two especially robust patterns of reading disability or dyslexia: an auditory–linguistic subtype and a visual–spatial subtype. For example, the problems with letter reversals and other perceptual distortions that are commonly thought to characterize dyslexia are associated with the visual–spatial subtype of reading disability. However, the auditory–linguistic subtype of reading disability is the more prevalent subtype. A common feature of most poor readers (and spellers) is a weakness in phonologic processing, which makes it difficult for the reader to phonemically segment spoken or printed words. Poor fluency in extracting words from printed material (and vice versa) is the result. Unfortunately, the ICD-10 description of Specific Reading Disorder does not fully incorporate the research on subtyping. It indicates that spelling problems are often associated with it and that it is commonly preceded by a history of disorders in speech or language development (features linked with the auditory–linguistic subtype), but there is no reference to the visual–spatial pattern of disability noted earlier.

Another important category or subtype of learning disorder not included in ICD-10 has to do with the syndrome of nonverbal learning disability (NLD). Rather than referring to a subtype in a particular academic skill area, such as reading, NLD refers to a pattern of cognitive impairment contributing to specific impediments in learning and behavior. This is an empirically derived model involving deficits in various aspects of nonverbal processing (perceptual reasoning, spatial organization, and comprehension of nonverbal visual and auditory cues). These, in turn, can give rise to academic learning deficits (especially in math, in visual–motor skills, and in "getting the picture" in learning new material of any kind). Moreover, it may contribute to social skills deficiencies (missing nonverbal cues in conversation, being overly literal) and to subsequent problems in social–emotional adjustment.

Hynd GW, Connor RT, Nieves N. Learning disabilities subtypes: perspectives and methodological issues in clinical assessment. In: Tramontana MG, Hooper SR, eds. *Assessment Issues in Child Neuropsychology.* New York: Plenum; 1988:281–312.

Lagae L. Learning disabilities: definitions, epidemiology, diagnosis, and intervention strategies. *Pediatr Clin North Am.* 2008 Dec;55(6):1259–1268, vii. doi: 10.1016/j.pcl.2008.08.001. PMID: 19041456.

Rourke BP. *Nonverbal Learning Disabilities: The Syndrome and Model.* New York: Guilford Press; 1989.

C. Assessment Procedures

The most commonly used measure of general intelligence for school-aged children is the Wechsler Intelligence Scale for Children, Fifth Edition (WISC-V). For measuring academic achievement, many individually administered standardized measures are available. Comprehensive or broadband batteries include the Wechsler Individual Achievement Test, Third Edition (Psychological Corporation), and the Woodcock–Johnson Tests of Achievement, Fourth Edition. Both of these tests include specific subtests that assess skills in reading, mathematics, and written expression.

Psychological Corporation. *Wechsler Individual Achievement Test.* 3rd ed. New York: Harcourt Brace Jovanovich; 2010.

Wechsler D. *Wechsler Intelligence Scale for Children.* 5th ed. New York: Psychological Corporation; 2014.

Woodcock RW, Johnson MB. *Woodcock-Johnson Tests of Achievement.* 4th ed. Itasca, IL: Riverside Publishing; 2014.

▶ Differential Diagnosis

A key issue to consider is whether an individual's poor achievement in one or more areas is merely the result of low intelligence. That is, a child's reading skills may be poor not because of a specific processing disorder but because of generally low aptitude or learning ability. Although similar underlying deficits (e.g., poor phonology) may be involved in disabled readers with and without intellectual disability, the requirement for specificity would not be met in the case of the individual with intellectual disability. By definition, discrepancy-based criteria for learning disabilities would help to make this differentiation.

Similarly, other exclusionary criteria pertaining to the diagnosis of learning disabilities (e.g., sensory impairment, cultural differences, and inadequate instruction) must be considered. If such factors are present, it must be assumed that, whether operating alone or in combination, they cannot fully account for deficits exhibited by a particular child.

One of the more common differentiations to be made is between learning disabilities and attention-deficit/hyperactivity disorder (ADHD) (Barkley RA. 2006). In both disorders, poor school achievement is likely, although the underlying mechanisms differ. In ADHD, the problems have to do more with the disruptive effects of inattention and poor task persistence that result in poor learning or skill acquisition. The child's performance is generally more variable in ADHD than in learning disabilities, and close observation often will reveal that the child is capable of processing the material but becomes unfocused or distracted at times. In learning disabilities, the processing deficits persist even when attention is optimal. Of course, some children have both conditions, with estimates of comorbidity being about 25%.

Emotional factors also must be distinguished from learning disabilities. School functioning can become impaired by a significant emotional disturbance, which makes it essential for the clinician to gather a careful history of the onset of academic symptoms. Emotional factors tend to exert a generalized or nonspecific effect, usually by impeding concentration or motivation. Although not the direct cause of specific disabilities, emotional factors may often worsen or compound them. In some cases, phobic reactions may occur to certain types of material, causing significant avoidance and further decreases in achievement. Careful evaluation will often document an underlying pattern of relatively lower aptitude on which specific anxiety reactions may become superimposed.

Barkley RA. *Attention-Deficit Hyperactivity Disorder, Third Edition: Handbook for Diagnosis and Treatment.* New York: Guilford Press; 2006.

Fletcher JM, Grigorenko EL. Neuropsychology of learning disabilities: the past and the future. *J Int Neuropsychol Soc.* 2017 Oct;23(9–10):930–940. doi: 10.1017/S1355617717001084. PMID: 29198282; PMCID: PMC6249682.

▶ Treatment

Generally speaking, there are three types of treatment or intervention for learning disabilities: remedial approaches, compensatory approaches, and interventions for secondary social–emotional problems.

A. Remedial Approaches

Remedial approaches are aimed directly at improving specific skills. For example, a child with poor phonologic processing may receive intensive instruction and practice with phoneme-grapheme correspondence to improve word-attack skills in reading (Al Otaiba S, Rouse AG, Baker K. 2018). Although there is no age cutoff per se, remedial interventions tend to have more of an impact earlier on, usually before the child reaches about 10 years of age. Effectiveness also depends on whether the interventions appropriately target the child's particular pattern of underlying deficits. A child with dyslexia may receive intensive help with visual tracking, even though visual problems may have nothing to do with why he or she is unable to read fluently (as would be true in the vast majority of cases). There has been a proliferation of therapies for learning disabilities, many of which lack empirical validation of their effectiveness.

B. Compensatory Approaches

Compensatory approaches help the individual to compensate, or work around, a particular deficit rather than to change it directly. These approaches are usually deferred until after an adequate course of remediation has been tried but the deficit persists. The individual should be assisted in developing strategies for containing the problem and managing to go on despite it. For example, the person with poor phonology may be taught to rely more on whole word recognition to improve reading fluency. In more severe cases, the individual may have to learn how to adapt without being a proficient reader—concentrating efforts instead on developing minimal "survival skills" (e.g., recognizing common phrases and reading a menu) while emphasizing other areas.

C. Interventions for Secondary Social–Emotional Problems

Children with learning disabilities are at increased risk for problems with frustration, performance anxiety, negative peer interactions, school avoidance, and low self-esteem. Services may include education of parents on how to manage common emotional reactions, school-based interventions that teach positive coping skills, and individual psychotherapy for when more significant emotional problems have emerged. Pharmacotherapy should be considered when more pronounced or persistent anxiety or depressive symptoms are present and when ADHD is also present.

Al Otaiba S, Rouse AG, Baker K. Elementary grade intervention approaches to treat specific learning disabilities, including dyslexia. *Lang Speech Hear Serv Sch*. 2018 Oct 24;49(4):829–842. doi: 10.1044/2018_LSHSS-DYSLC-18-0022. PMID: 30458544.

Newby RF, Recht D, Caldwell J. Empirically tested interventions for subtypes of reading disabilities. In: Tramontana MG, Hooper SR, eds. *Advances in Child Neuropsychology*, Vol 2. New York: Springer; 1994:201–232.

Pratt HD, Patel DR. Learning disorders in children and adolescents. *Prim Care*. 2007 Jun;34(2):361–374; abstract viii. doi: 10.1016/j.pop.2007.04.014. PMID: 17666232.

▶ Prognosis

Children generally do not outgrow learning disabilities. As noted earlier in this chapter, one of the common misconceptions regarding learning disabilities was that they merely reflect a delay—the implication being that the child will catch up eventually and exhibit normal functioning. Children with learning disabilities do improve, but except in the mildest cases, a relative weakness in the affected skill will persist. A child may even improve to roughly average levels, although the achievement would still fall below the expectations for an otherwise bright individual (Spreen O. 1989).

Reviews of research on adult outcomes suggest that, as a group, individuals with learning disabilities attain lower educational and occupational levels. Outcomes are poorer in persons with more severe learning disabilities, lower IQ, frank neurologic impairment, and lower socioeconomic status. Evidence regarding the long-term benefits of early educational intervention is inconclusive.

Spreen O. Learning disability, neurology, and long-term outcome: some implications for the individual and for society. *J Clin Exp Neuropsych*. 1989;11:389–408.

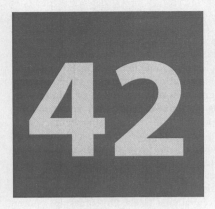

42

Motor Disorders & Communication Disorders

Michael G. Tramontana, PhD

Barry Nurcombe, MD[†]

In this chapter, we focus on two broad categories of developmental disorder—motor disorders and communication disorders. For each, the diagnostic criteria set forth in the International Statistical Classification of Diseases and Related Health Problems—10th Revision (ICD-10) are outlined in the sections below. Our coverage goes beyond that, however, and will incorporate discussion of a broader range of conceptual issues, empirical findings, and diagnostic considerations relevant to each of these categories of disorder.

MOTOR DISORDERS

 ESSENTIALS OF DIAGNOSIS

ICD-10 Diagnostic Criteria for Specific Developmental Disorder of Motor Function

Specific Developmental Disorder of Motor Function (F82) is defined as:

► A disorder in which the main feature is a serious impairment in the development of motor coordination that is not solely explicable in terms of general intellectual disability or of any specific congenital or acquired neurological disorder

► There are neurodevelopmental immaturities such as choreiform movements of unsupported limbs, or mirror movements and other associated motor features, as well as impaired fine and gross motor coordination

The classification includes:

► *Clumsy child syndrome*
► *Developmental coordination disorder*
► *Developmental dyspraxia*

[†]Deceased

Exclusions:

► *Abnormalities of gait and mobility* (R26)
► *Lack of coordination* (R27)

Adapted with permission from International statistical classification of diseases and related health problems-10th revision. 5th ed. Geneva: World Health Organization (WHO); 2016.

The ICD-10 criteria for *Specific Developmental Disorder of Motor Function* include *clumsy child syndrome, developmental coordination disorder,* and *developmental dyspraxia.* Other conditions, such as stereotyped movement disorders, tic disorders, and Tourette disorder, are also touched on briefly later.

► General Considerations

A. Epidemiology

It is estimated that 6% of schoolchildren have developmental coordination disorder. It is about 4 times more common in boys than in girls. General prevalence estimates on stereotyped movement disorder are lacking, but it is more common in boys and among children with intellectual disability.

B. Etiology

Motor development involves the gradual acquisition of central control over reflex movement. There is controversy over whether this acquisition involves the suppression of the reflexes and spontaneous cyclic movements of early infancy or whether infantile movements are incorporated into the elements that become voluntary motor skills.

Skilled movement requires a program of action with a specified objective or set goal. The program is composed of a sequence of hierarchically organized subroutines under executive control. Once acquired, motor skills are flexible.

For example, the child who has learned to walk can do so on smooth, rugged, soft, or hard surfaces. The adaptation to different situations of the programmed subroutines requires accurate perception, central processing, executive control, and progressive feedback. Feedback monitors the approximation of the program to the set goal and allows the modification of timing, speed, force, and direction of movement until the desired endpoint is achieved. Initially, movements are clumsy, as the child struggles to master the skill. Eventually, the skill is regulated centrally and the subroutines automated. A variety of skills can be built up from a limited number of practiced subroutines deployed in accordance with combinatorial rules. The combinatorial rules act as a kind of grammar, organizing the subroutines in hierarchical fashion. Skilled performance can be delayed or disrupted if basic reflexes are not suppressed or incorporated into the program or if the following functions are delayed, defective, or disrupted: perception, central processing and programming, motor function, and feedback.

Developmental coordination disorders involve some form of underlying brain dysfunction arising from various levels (cortical, subcortical, or cerebellar). The cause of stereotyped movement disorder is unclear.

C. Genetics

Like many other neurodevelopmental disorders, it is likely that multiple vulnerability genes are associated with motor disorders. For Tourette disorder, epidemiologic studies suggest that the vast majority of cases are inherited, although the exact mode of transmission is not yet known and no specific gene has been identified (see Chapter 53).

▶ Clinical Findings

A. Signs & Symptoms

Developmental coordination disorders are manifested in clumsiness, slowness, and inaccuracy of performance. The clumsy child is slow, awkward, and inefficient in motor performance. Motor milestones are delayed. The child drops things, tends to lose his or her balance, and has poor eye–hand coordination. The problems may involve gross motor control and/or fine motor control. Associated problems may involve verbal dyspraxia affecting expressive output and motor control of speech. The deficits can interfere with a broad range of activities and affect academic performance and vocational preparation as well as leisure and play. The child's social development is also likely to be affected, particularly if clumsiness is associated with trouble participating in normal physical activities.

Stereotyped movement disorders consist of repetitive and seemingly purposeless motor behavior (e.g., rocking and hand flapping) that interferes with normal activities. They often may reflect motor overflow actions stimulated by excitement. An important distinction has to do with whether self-injurious behavior is involved (e.g., biting, head banging).

Tic disorders involve sudden, rapid, recurrent, non-rhythmic motor movements or vocalizations. For a complete review of *Tourette disorder* and *motor or vocal tic disorders*, see Chapter 53.

B. Assessment Procedures

An essential aspect of assessment entails taking a careful history, which includes questions directed at elucidating the timing and quality of motor skill development. The examination should include direct observation of the child performing age-appropriate motor activities (e.g., walking, hopping, throwing and catching a ball, doing simple drawings) that may reveal problems with motor clumsiness or dyspraxia.

Where indicated, formal test measures can be incorporated in the evaluation of developmental coordination disorders, such as:

- *Movement Assessment Battery for Children—Second Edition*
- *Peabody Developmental Motor Scales—Second Edition*
- *Bruininks-Oseretsky Test of Motor Proficiency—Second Edition*

There currently are no formal testing procedures for assessing stereotyped movement disorder. Assessment of these depends on the careful review of the child's history and presenting symptoms together with direct observation.

Additional psychological testing should be undertaken if there are concerns regarding intellectual capacity, attentional difficulties, or learning disability.

C. Laboratory Findings

Laboratory tests are seldom necessary in the evaluation of clumsiness unless there are abnormal findings on neurologic examination or a history of recent changes in motor skills. However, creatine kinase and lactate dehydrogenase should be measured in children who have reduced muscle mass or limited capacity for physical exertion. There are no definitive laboratory tests for stereotyped movement disorders. However, tests may be ordered to rule out other conditions. For example, a urine drug screen can test for cocaine or stimulants (which can produce or aggravate tics), especially in cases with an abrupt onset of symptoms. An electroencephalogram (EEG) is indicated in some cases to assess whether uncontrolled movements reflect seizures.

D. Neuroimaging

Patients with neurological findings suggestive of a focal brain abnormality should have magnetic resonance imaging or computed tomography as part of their evaluation. Neuroimaging should also be done if there is concern about a degenerative decline. Brain imaging sometimes helps to elucidate underlying impairments with a direct or indirect role in the symptoms for example, a frontal lobe abnormality causing fundamental problems with self-regulatory controls, not just motor execution). However, motor disorders in most cases can be adequately diagnosed without imaging studies.

E. Course of Illness

Typically, mild and moderate degrees of clumsiness in early childhood improve over time. Children with motor deficits that continue into adolescence and adulthood are more likely than their peers to have poor social competence, less academic motivation, lower self-esteem, obesity, and poorer physical fitness due in part to a reluctance to engage in physical activity. The prognosis for children with stereotyped movement disorders depends on the severity of the problems and the presence of comorbid conditions (e.g., intellectual disability). The outcome is probably worse when self-injurious behaviors are involved, especially in the case of repetitive head-banging with traumatic brain injury.

▶ Differential Diagnosis

Clumsiness is observed in chronic intoxication with neuroleptic and anticonvulsant drugs, neuromuscular disorders (e.g., Charcot-Marie-Tooth disease, Duchenne disease), and upper motor neuron disorders (e.g., cerebral palsy, degenerative disorders). Children with Down syndrome, autism spectrum disorder (ASD), specific dyslexia, and attention-deficit/hyperactivity disorder (ADHD) are sometimes more clumsy than is appropriate for their mental age.

As for repetitive behaviors, these can be seen in a variety of conditions besides stereotyped movement disorders, especially ASD. They may also be present in obsessive-compulsive disorder (OCD), although actions in OCD would tend to be part of an organized, ritualistic pattern rather than isolated and nonfunctional as in stereotyped movements. There may be a resemblance to tics, but stereotyped movements are often more intense, less jerky, and more affected by excitement. Sometimes a seizure disorder must be ruled out in accounting for abrupt, purposeless acts, especially if accompanied by blank staring and unresponsiveness. Tourette disorder is often comorbid with OCD. For a complete review of Tourette disorder and OCD, see Chapter 53.

▶ Treatment

Proper intervention for children with developmental coordination disorders is essential. It is important not only to address the primary deficits in motor skills but also to limit their impact on other aspects of the child's functioning (academic, social, recreational) as well as on his or her sense of mastery and self-esteem. Primary interventions directed to the motor skills themselves can be implemented by physical therapists and occupational therapists who offer guidance and graduated exercises aimed at improving coordination and control in a range of age-appropriate motor activities. The interventions

may focus instead on particular areas, such as motor writing skills. There often is a need for school accommodations, with curriculum modifications as well as extra time, support, and assistance to address the motor impediment and limit its effect on other areas of learning and achievement. Psychotherapeutic services may also be indicated to treat any performance anxiety, negative self-esteem, or avoidance that has arisen due to clumsiness and motor incoordination.

Behavior therapy can be used to treat stereotyped movement disorders, especially if self-injurious behavior is involved. Key aspects of this include identifying stimulus antecedents (the behaviors may be seemingly random but, on closer scrutiny, have specific triggers) as well as identifying less disruptive or injurious behavior that can be shaped as a replacement. Medication targeting anxiety or excitability can lessen the frequency or intensity of severe stereotyped movements.

Cools W, Martelaer KD, Samaey C, Andries C. Movement skill assessment of typically developing preschool children: a review of seven movement skill assessment tools. *J Sports Sci Med.* 2009;8;154–168.

Deuel RK. Motor skills disorders. In: Hooper SR, Hynd GW, Mattison RE, eds. *Developmental Disorders: Diagnostic Criteria and Clinical Assessment.* Hillsdale, NJ: Erlbaum; 1992:239–281.

Freeman RD, Soltanifar A, Baer S. Stereotypic movement disorder: Easily missed. *Dev Med Child Neurol.* 2010;8;733–738.

Wilson PH. Practitioner review: approaches to assessment and treatment of children with DCD: An evaluative review. *J Child Psychol Psychiatry.* 2005;46:806–823.

COMMUNICATION DISORDERS

The breakdown of ICD-10 categories pertaining to *Specific Developmental Disorders of Speech and Language* includes *specific speech articulation disorder, expressive language disorder, receptive language disorder, acquired aphasia with epilepsy (Landau-Kleffner), other developmental disorders of speech and language,* and *developmental disorder of speech and language, unspecified.*

 ESSENTIALS OF DIAGNOSIS

ICD-10 Diagnostic Criteria for Specific Developmental Disorders of Speech and Language

Specific Developmental Disorders of Speech and Language (F80) are defined as:

▶ Disorders in which normal patterns of language acquisition are disturbed from the early stages of development. The conditions are not directly attributable to neurological or speech mechanism abnormalities, sensory impairments, intellectual disability, or environmental factors.

▶ These disorders are often followed by associated problems, such as difficulties in reading and spelling, abnormalities in interpersonal relationships, and emotional and behavioral disorders.

This category is subdivided into the following specific disorders:

▶ *Specific speech articulation disorder* (F80.0)
A specific developmental disorder in which the child's use of speech sounds is below the appropriate level for his/her mental age, but in which there is a normal level of language skills.

▶ *Expressive language disorder* (F80.1)
A specific developmental disorder in which the child's ability to use expressive spoken language is markedly below the appropriate level for his/her mental age, but in which language comprehension is within normal limits. There may or may not be abnormalities in articulation.

▶ *Receptive language disorder* (F80.2)
A specific developmental disorder in which the child's understanding of language is below the appropriate level for his/her mental age. In virtually all cases, expressive language will also be markedly affected and abnormalities in word-sound production are common.

Other conditions include:

▶ *Acquired aphasia with epilepsy,* or Landau-Kleffner syndrome (F80.3)
A disorder in which a child with previously normal language development loses both receptive and expressive language skills with the onset of epileptic seizures

▶ *Other developmental disorders of speech and language* (F80.8)

▶ *Developmental disorder of speech and language, unspecified* (F80.9)

Adapted with permission from International statistical classification of diseases and related health problems-10th revision. 5th ed. Geneva: World Health Organization (WHO); 2016.

General Considerations

The ICD-10 breakdown of developmental speech and language disorders does not assign a separate category for speech fluency problems specifically involving stuttering. However, included within *specific speech articulation disorder* is a condition known as *lalling,* a form of stammering in which speech is virtually unintelligible.

Another category of speech/language dysfunction not included in ICD-10 has to do with social (pragmatic) language disorder. The term "pragmatic" refers to the use of language in a social context, with respect to either the understanding or the expression of intended meaning. "Getting the message" entails more than a simple literal decoding of words and their processing according to syntactic rules. It relies on the incorporation of a broader range of features, many of them nonverbal, such as prosodic and gestural cues. The interpretation of indirect meaning, humor, or sarcasm often depends heavily on these features. The same is true with respect to effective expression within a social context. It is an especially important dimension of language functioning from a psychiatric standpoint, as it often relates to problems with interpersonal relationships and social skills development.

Different problems with language use may stem from deficits primarily involving comprehension versus production. Accordingly, ICD-10 incorporates the convention of distinguishing between *receptive language disorder* and *expressive language disorder.* However, in making that distinction, it is recognized that a young child generally does manifest receptive language problems alone. Any disorder affecting receptive language, which would interfere with a child's ability to process and understand spoken input, will also necessarily impede the child's ability to produce spoken language.

The ICD-10 criteria for developmental speech and language disorders stipulate that the conditions are not directly due to impairments in sensory functioning or specific motor mechanisms affecting speech, intellectual disability, or environmental factors. Speech and language impairments due to neurological conditions are also excluded, although that distinction is somewhat arbitrary, given that some form of underlying neurodevelopmental abnormality is presumably involved. The ICD-10 criteria are not clear on this. Speech and language impairment can be due to genetic or congenital factors or due to acquired brain injury or disease. In most cases, the precise causation is unknown. However, for it to be a *developmental* disorder, it must be presumed that any underlying brain dysfunction would have occurred early enough to affect the *acquisition,* and not just the loss, of speech and language ability. Problems of the latter type are classified as acquired aphasias.

A. Epidemiology

Prevalence rates for childhood speech and language deficits vary according to the classification criteria and cutoff points used in defining abnormality. Such deficits can be defined on purely statistical grounds, as when impaired performance is defined as falling below a particular score on a standardized test. For example, if the cutoff is set at two standard deviations (SDs) below the mean, then, by definition, 2% of the reference group fall in the impaired range. This impairment rate rises to roughly 7% if the cutoff is set at 1.5 SDs and so forth. Shrinkage in the estimates results if exclusionary criteria are considered.

There also appears to be an elevated rate of comorbidity with childhood psychopathology. For example, in one study, 60% of children with language disorder met diagnostic criteria for ADHD.

B. Etiology

Speech and language disorders have multiple etiologies, some genetic, some congenital, and some arising from perinatal trauma such as prematurity and anoxia. A form of underlying brain dysfunction is generally assumed, even in disorders of the so-called developmental variety, although evidence for this assumption is often lacking. Many studies of children with language disorders—especially earlier studies—failed to document the presence of any central nervous system abnormality.

New and important insights have unfolded with technological advances in the study of brain function. For example, electrophysiologic features in the newborn—specifically, auditory evoked responses in the left hemisphere—predict language skills at 3 years of age. Further insights have come though advances in functional brain imaging. Such findings support a general presumption of left-hemispheric dysfunction in many speech and language disorders. Pragmatic language functions, and their dependence on various nonverbal abilities, are thought to be influenced strongly by right-hemispheric processes.

C. Genetics

Language disorders occur more frequently in families with a history of language problems or learning disabilities than in the general population. They are about 4 times more likely in boys than girls. As with any genetically complex disorder, it is likely that interactions among multiple genetic loci must be understood in order to predict the degree of affectedness within specific domains of disability. However, an autosomal dominant gene, FOXP2 (Forkhead box protein P2), on chromosome 7q31 has been identified through the study of three generations of one family with a severe communication disorder.

▶ Clinical Findings

A. Signs and Symptoms

Communication disorders is a broad term referring to a variety of developmental disorders in which speech and language skills are affected. Specific disorders must be distinguished because of important differences in prognosis and the approach to treatment.

B. Psychological Testing

Several key issues must be addressed in the diagnosis and evaluation of communication disorders. First, a child's speech or language functioning must be assessed through the use of standardized, individually administered tests. Basing the

Table 42–1 Assessments for Specific Speech and Language Capabilities

Capabilities Measured	Tests
Word comprehension	Peabody Picture Vocabulary Test—Fourth Edition
Expressive vocabulary, or naming abilities	Expressive Vocabulary Test—Third Edition
Listening comprehension for spoken instructions of increasing length and complexity	Token Test for Children—Second Edition
Multifaceted measures of language	Clinical Evaluation of Language Fundamentals—5th Edition
Speech articulation	Goldman-Fristoe Test of Articulation—Third Edition
Pragmatic language functions	Pragmatic Language Skills Inventory

diagnosis on clinical observations alone is generally insufficient, except when the nature or severity of the disorder prevents formal testing. Table 42–1 describes sample measures and instruments.

Second, cutoff points should be set in determining abnormality or impairment on specific measures. In other words, what constitutes a significant deficit? As noted earlier, this is somewhat arbitrary, although the cutoff is typically set at about 2 SDs below the mean on any particular measure. A slightly higher cutoff may be used (e.g., 1–1.5 SDs) if the goal is screening rather than diagnosis. A more liberal cutoff may also be used when it reflects a level of performance that is clearly discrepant with the child's general functioning. Thus, a score of 85 on a standardized language measure—which technically falls in a low average range—could be viewed as reflecting a significant problem in a child with an intelligence quotient of 115 or more.

Finally, it is often important to incorporate an appraisal of nonverbal intellectual capacity in order to obtain an unbiased estimate of a child's global abilities. This is because many intelligence measures depend heavily on verbal abilities, and their results would be unduly lowered when language impairment is involved. That would have the effect of blurring the distinctive nature of the language problems. Measures of nonverbal intelligence include the Test of Nonverbal Intelligence (Brown L, Sherbenou RJ, Dollar SJ. 1982), the Leiter International Performance Scale, and the Perceptual Reasoning section of the Wechsler Intelligence Scales.

C. Laboratory Findings

All children with a communication disorder should have a complete medical evaluation and formal audiologic testing to detect medical conditions or hearing loss that may contribute to their condition.

D. Neuroimaging

Children with abnormal findings on neurological examination suggestive of a focal brain abnormality should have magnetic resonance imaging studies or computed tomography. Functional neuroimaging has also accelerated in recent years. Typically, dyslexic children exhibit altered patterns of brain activation in a variety of brain regions, especially the left parietotemporal cortex and frontal regions. However, the value of these studies for diagnosis has yet to be established.

E. Course of Illness

Communication disorders are usually detectable before 4 years. Severe forms may be apparent by 2 years of age. Children with communication disorders are at high risk of developing learning disabilities and experiencing academic difficulty when they enter school. Parents must advocate for their children in order to ensure that they receive the services they need.

▶ Differential Diagnosis

The valid diagnosis of a communication disorder requires that it be differentiated from other conditions that could interfere with communication. Language acquisition can be impeded by environmental deprivation, although such deprivation would rarely constitute the primary cause of a language disorder. Hearing-impaired children and children with neuromotor dysfunction may exhibit slow oral language growth and control of speech. However, specific language impairment can still be inferred if the degree of impairment exceeds what would be expected due to sensory or sensorimotor deficit alone. The same is true with respect to intellectual disability. Anxiety can aggravate problems with speech fluency or stuttering but is unlikely to result in persistent major disturbance without an underlying vulnerability involving fluency.

It is especially difficult to distinguish communication disorders from ASD. Indeed, the presence of particular communication impairment is one of the defining characteristics of autism. There may be impairment in the various basic language areas noted earlier, although problems in *nonverbal* processing are especially relevant. Social (pragmatic) communication problems are prevalent in ASD. Important differences that distinguish the abnormalities in autism include the idiosyncratic use of words, aprosodic features, deviant eye contact, echolalia, and an apparent disinterest in communication as reflected in the absence of gestural language or other nonverbal means of communication. Also, unlike the poor auditory memory often observed in language-impaired children, children with ASD often have good memory for rote or repetitive material.

It is also sometimes difficult to distinguish language impairment and ADHD. In both disorders, the child may have difficulty following spoken language or expressing ideas in a focused and goal-directed manner. In ADHD, however, problems with efficient focusing are not be limited to verbal areas. The two disorders may coexist (indeed, the comorbidity rate appears fairly high), in which case attention problems may be especially pronounced when verbal processing is involved.

Many forms of learning disabilities can be viewed as the extension of language processing problems into the school-age period, especially when skills such as reading, spelling, and writing are involved. These problems can be considered language-based forms of learning disorder, particularly if accompanied by broader problems with language comprehension or production. The range of learning disabilities is varied, however, if nonverbal learning disability is also present.

▶ Treatment

Therapeutic services for communication disorders are provided by speech and language pathologists. Services may focus on speech impediments, particularly problems with voice quality, oral-motor control, and phonologic and fluency weaknesses. Receptive and expressive language processing problems can also be addressed, with exercises to improve word comprehension, naming ability, syntactic awareness, and higher-order listening comprehension and formulation skills.

Depending on the therapist's qualifications, services can be directed toward facilitating pragmatic language ability such as interpreting indirect meaning, utilizing nonverbal cues, and applying the associated skills necessary for effective social communication (e.g., taking turns, maintaining eye contact). Treating pragmatic deficits is a more specialized aspect of language intervention that is closely related to behaviorally oriented treatment approaches dealing with social skills development. Not all speech and language pathologists have this skill. The same is true with respect to speech and language pathologists who are suited for remedial work in such areas as mnemonics and language-based learning disabilities.

Although not a formal part of speech and language therapy, the management of the emotional and behavioral characteristics of the child is often a key aspect of effective intervention. For example, treatment of problems with speech fluency or stuttering often entails helping the child to cope with anxiety and its effects on the pace or level of pressure accompanying speech. Likewise, helping the child with ADHD to limit distraction or hurried responding is essential in promoting better listening comprehension or more focused expression of thoughts.

Brown L, Sherbenou RJ, Dollar SJ. *Test of Nonverbal Intelligence.* Austin, TX: Pro-Ed; 1982.

Crary MA, Voeller KKS, Haak NJ. Questions of developmental neurolinguistic assessment. In: Tramontana MG, Hooper SR, eds. *Assessment Issues in Child Neuropsychology.* New York: Plenum; 1988:249–279.

Dunn L, Dunn D. *Peabody Picture Vocabulary Test, Fourth Edition (PPVT-4)*. Minneapolis, MN: NCS Pearson PsychCorp, 2007.

Gilliam JE, Miller L. *Pragmatic Language Skills Inventory (PLSI)*. Austin, TX: Pro-Ed; 2006.

Goldman R, Fristoe M. *Goldman-Fristoe Test of Articulation—Third Edition (GFTA-3)*. San Antonio, TX: Pearson Education; 2015.

Hammill DD, Newcomer PL. *Test of Language Development*. Austin, TX: Pro-Ed; 1988.

McGhee R, Ehrler D, DiSomoni F. *Token Test for Children—Second Edition (TTFC-2)*. Austin, TX: Pro-Ed; 2007.

Molfese DL. The use of auditory evoked responses recorded from newborn infants to predict language skills. In: Tramontana MG, Hooper SR, eds. *Advances in Child Neuropsychology*. Vol 1. New York: Springer; 1992:1–23.

Paul R, Cohen DJ, Caparulo BK. A longitudinal study of patients with severe developmental disorders of language learning. *J Am Acad Child Psychiatry*. 1983;22:525.

Phelps-Terasaki D, Phelps-Gunn T. *Test of Pragmatic Language Second Edition (TOPL-2)*. Austin, TX: Pro-Ed; 2007.

Wechsler D; *Wechsler Intelligence Scale for Children*. 4th ed. New York: Psychological Corporation; 2003.

Wiig EH. *Let's Talk: Developing Prosocial Communication Skills*. Columbus, OH: Merrill; 1982.

Wiig EH, Semel E, Secord WA. *Clinical Evaluation of Language Fundamentals, Fifth Edition (CELF-5)*. San Antonio, TX: Pearson Education; 2013.

Williams K. *Expressive Vocabulary Test, Second Edition (EVT-2)*. Minneapolis, MN: NCS Pearson; 2007.

Autism and Autism Spectrum Disorders

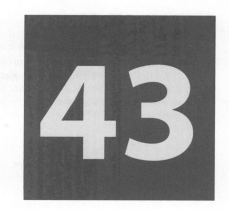

Molly McVoy, MD
Fred R. Volkmar, MD

International Statistical Classification of Diseases and Related Health Problems— 10th Revision (ICD-10) Diagnostic Criteria

Reproduced with permission from Diagnostic Descriptions and Criteria for Autism and Related Pervasive Developmental Disorders from International Classification of Diseases. 10th Ed. Geneva, Switzerland; World Health Organization (WHO); 2003.

Childhood Autism (F84.0)

A. Abnormal or impaired development is evident before the age of 3 years in at least one of the following areas:
   1. receptive or expressive language as used in social communication;
   2. the development of selective social attachments or of reciprocal social interaction;
   3. functional or symbolic play.
B. A total of at least six symptoms from (1), (2), and (3) must be present, with at least two from (1) and at least one from each of (2) and (3).
   1. Qualitative impairments in social interaction are manifest in at least two of the following areas:
      a. failure adequately to use eye-to-eye gaze, facial expression, body postures, and gestures to regulate social interaction;
      b. failure to develop (in a manner appropriate to mental age and despite ample opportunities) peer relationships that involve a mutual sharing of interests, activities, and emotions;
      c. lack of socio-emotional reciprocity as shown by an impaired or deviant response to other people's emotions, or lack of modulation of behavior according to social context, or a weak integration of social, emotional, and communicative behaviors;
      d. lack of spontaneous seeking to share enjoyment, interests, or achievements with other people (e.g., a lack of showing, bringing, or pointing out to other people objects of interest to the individual).
   2. Qualitative abnormalities communication as manifest in at least one of the following areas:
      a. delay in, or total lack of, development of spoken language that is not accompanied by an attempt to compensate through the use of gestures or mime as an alternative mode of communication (often preceded by a lack of communicative babbling);
      b. relative failure to initiate or sustain conversational interchange (at whatever level of language skill is present), in which there is reciprocal responsiveness to the communications of the other person;
      c. stereotyped and repetitive use of language or idiosyncratic use of words or phrases;
      d. lack of varied spontaneous make-believe play or (when young) social imitative play.
   3. Restricted, repetitive, and stereotyped patterns of behavior, interests, and activities are manifested in at least one of the following:
      a. an encompassing preoccupation with one or more stereotyped and restricted patterns of interest that are abnormal in content or focus, or one or more interests that are abnormal in their intensity and circumscribed nature, though not in their content or focus;
      b. apparently compulsive adherence to specific, nonfunctional routines or rituals;
      c. stereotyped and repetitive motor mannerisms that involve either hand or finger flapping or twisting or complex whole-body movements;
      d. preoccupations with part-objects or nonfunctional elements of play materials (such as their odor, the feel of their surface, or the noise or vibration they generate).

C. The clinical picture is not attributable to the other varieties of pervasive developmental disorders; specific development disorder of receptive language (F80.2) with secondary socio-emotional problems, reactive attachment disorder (F94.1), or disinhibited attachment disorder (F94.2); mental retardation (F70–F72) with some associated emotional or behavioral disorders; schizophrenia (F20) of unusually early onset; and Rett syndrome (F84.12).

F84.1 Atypical Autism

A. Abnormal or impaired development is evident at or after the age of 3 years (criteria as for autism except for age of manifestation).
B. There are qualitative abnormalities in reciprocal social interaction or in communication; or restricted, repetitive, and stereotyped patterns of behavior, interests, and activities. (Criteria as for autism except that it is unnecessary to meet the criteria for number of areas of abnormality).
C. The disorder does not meet the diagnostic criteria for autism (F84.0). Autism maybe atypical in either age of onset (F84.10) or symptomatology (F84.11); the two types are differentiated with a fifth character for research purposes. Syndromes that are typical in both respects should be coded F84.12.

F84.10 Atypicality in Age of Onset

A. The disorder does not meet criterion A for autism (F84.0); that is, abnormal or impaired development is evident only at or after age 3 years.
B. The disorder meets criteria B and C for autism (F84.0).

F84.11 Atypicality in Symptomatology

A. The disorder meets criterion A for autism (F84.0); that is, abnormal or impaired development is evident before age 3 years.
B. There are qualitative abnormalities in reciprocal social interactions or in communication, or restricted, repetitive, and stereotyped patterns of behavior, interests, and activities. (Criteria as for autism except that it is unnecessary to meet the criteria for number of areas of abnormality.)
C. The disorder meets criterion C for autism (F84.0).
D. The disorder does not fully meet criterion B for autism (F84.0).

F84.12 Atypicality in Both Age of Onset and Symptomatology

A. The disorder does not meet criterion A for autism (F84.0); that is, abnormal or impaired development is evident only at or after age 3 years.
B. There are qualitative abnormalities in reciprocal social interactions or in communication, or restricted, repetitive, and stereotyped patterns of behavior, interests, and activities. (Criteria as for autism except

that it is unnecessary to meet the criteria for number of areas of abnormality.)
C. The disorder meets criterion C for autism (F84.0).
D. The disorder does not fully meet criterion B for autism (F84.0).

F84.2 Rett Syndrome

A. Apparently normal prenatal and perinatal period and apparently normal psychomotor development through the first 6 months and normal head circumference at birth.
B. Deceleration of head growth between 5 months and 4 years and loss of acquired purposeful hand skills between 6 and 30 months of age that is associated with concurrent communication dysfunction and impaired social interactions and appearance of poorly coordinated/unstable gait and/or trunk movements.
C. Development of severely impaired expressive and receptive language, together with severe psychomotor retardation.
D. Stereotyped midline hand movements (such as hand wringing or washing) with an onset at or after the time that purposeful hand movements are lost.

F84.3 Other Childhood Disintegrative Disorder

A. An apparently normal development up to the age of at least 2 years. The presence of normal age-appropriate skills in communication, social relationships, play, and adaptive behavior at age 2 years or later is required for diagnosis.
B. A definite loss of previously acquired skills at about the time of onset of the disorder. The diagnosis requires a clinically significant loss of skills (and not just a failure to use them in certain situations) in at least two out of the following areas:
   1. expressive or receptive language;
   2. play;
   3. social skills or adaptive behavior;
   4. bowel or bladder control;
   5. motor skills.
C. Qualitatively abnormal social functioning, manifest in at least two of the following areas:
   1. qualitative abnormalities in reciprocal social interaction (of the type defined for autism);
   2. qualitative abnormalities in communication (of the type defined for autism);
   3. restricted, repetitive, and stereotyped patterns of behavior, interests, and activities including motor stereotypies and mannerisms;
   4. a general loss of interest in objects and in the environment.
D. The disorder is not attributable to the other varieties of pervasive developmental disorder; acquired aphasia with epilepsy (F80.6); elective mutism (F94.0); schizophrenia (F20–F29); Rett syndrome (F84.2).

F84.5 Asperger Syndrome

A. A lack of any clinically significant general delay in spoken or receptive language or cognitive development. Diagnosis requires that single words should have developed by 2 years of age or earlier and that communicative phrases be used by 3 years of age or earlier. Self-help skills, adaptive behavior, and curiosity about the environment during the first 3 years should be at a level consistent with normal intellectual development. However, motor milestones may be somewhat delayed and motor clumsiness is usual (although not a necessary diagnostic feature). Isolated special skills, often related to abnormal preoccupations, are common but are not required for diagnosis.

B. Qualitative abnormalities in reciprocal social interaction (criteria as for autism).

C. An unusually intense circumscribed interest or restricted, repetitive, and stereotyped patterns of behavior, interests, and activities (criteria as for autism; however, it would be less usual for these to include either motor mannerisms or preoccupations with part-objects or nonfunctional elements of play materials).

D. The disorder is not attributable to the other varieties of pervasive developmental disorder; schizotypal disorder (F21); simple schizophrenia (F20.6); reactive and disinhibited attachment disorder of childhood (f94.1 and .2); obsessional personality disorder (F60.5); obsessive-compulsive disorder (F42).

F84.8 Other Pervasive Developmental Disorders

F84.9 Pervasive Developmental Disorder, Unspecified

This is a residual diagnostic category that should be used for disorders that fit the general description for pervasive developmental disorders but in which a lack of adequate information, or contradictory findings, means that the criteria for any of the other F84 codes cannot be met.

DIAGNOSTIC ISSUES

Infantile autism (as it was then termed) was first clearly recognized 70 years ago (Kanner, 1943) but was not officially recognized as a diagnosis until 1980, when it was put in a new "class," of disorder the "pervasive developmental disorders (PDDs)." Earlier reports had noted children with similar clinical features but did not recognize the syndrome as such. Official recognition of autism after Kanner's report was delayed by early confusion, particularly about its relationship (or lack thereof) with schizophrenia, and the definition has evolved over time. The *Diagnostic and Statistical Manual of Mental Disorders Fourth Edition* (DSM-IV) approach included both autistic disorder and a number of other conditions including Asperger syndrome (social disability but with good verbal skills), childhood disintegrative disorder (a rare condition in which a condition like autism develops after a period of normal development), Rett disorder (a neurodegenerative disorder with a strong genetic basis), and pervasive developmental disorder not otherwise specified (PDD-NOS). The last is, somewhat paradoxically, the least well defined of the PDDs and least frequently studied, yet the most common type. The clinical features of the DSM-IV conditions are summarized in Table 43–1.

The DSM-5 approach abandons these distinctions in favor of a single autism spectrum disorder (ASD) and a new condition, social communication disorder, see Tables 43–2 and 43–3. There was general agreement that the use of the term autism spectrum was an advantage. However, two major conceptual decisions had a mixed effects—the decision to eliminate "subthreshold" categories throughout DSM and the decision to try to base definitions on data derived from research instruments. Although an impressive body of data from standard assessment instruments provides the foundation for the current definition (Huerta et al, 2012), the changes made have proven controversial. The controversy reflects concerns that in actual clinical use the definition is restrictive (see Smith et al, 2015, for a recent meta-analysis). These difficulties may reflect a decision to rely so strongly on assessment instruments. It appears that two groups are most strongly impacted—the very young and the more cognitively able. The background literature on the other "new" disorder proposed for DSM-5 (social communication disorder) is quite limited and clinical implications remain somewhat unclear.

▶ General Considerations

A. Epidemiology

Early studies on autism epidemiology reported a prevalence rate of 4.5 per 10,000. Subsequent studies have tended to report higher rates, on balance around 9 children per 10,000. Although there has been much interest in higher rates in recent years and whether the frequency of autism is "truly" increasing, several factors make it difficult to interpret the nature of the apparent increase. For example, diagnostic criteria have changed, and more recent approaches are designed to work well in children over the range of cognitive ability levels. Second, reported rates vary depending on other factors (e.g., sample size, with the highest rates reported in the smallest samples). There is also more general awareness of the condition (Lord C, Brugha TS, Charman T, et al. 2020). Given the importance of labels for service delivery (particularly in the United States), diagnostic substitution can be problematic, particularly for studies using reports from schools.

B. Demographic, Gender, Cultural, and Ethnic Issues

In Kanner's first paper (1943), many parents of autistic children were remarkably successful, leading to the impression of an association between social class and autism. Subsequent studies have failed to reveal such an association. Ethnic and

Table 43–1 Differential Diagnostic Features: Autism and Related Disorders

Feature	Autism	Asperger	Rett	CDD	PDD-NOS
Social disturbance	Severe	Moderate–severe	Variable	Severe	Variable
Language/communication impairment	Marked	Good verbal ability, poor communication	Very marked	Marked (previously normal)	Variable
Restricted interests	Marked, mannerisms, trouble with change, occasionally savant ability	Usually highly circumscribed interests (interfering with normal functioning)	Significant psychomotor retardation	Marked, as in autism	Variable—often troubled by change. Mannerisms may be less prominent
Motor issues	Often preserved early but poor later when imitation is required	Often clumsy, with fine and gross motor difficulties	Significant loss of motor abilities, hand-washing stereotypies	Often preserved but lose some self-care skills	Variable
Onset	Always before age 3 yr, often before age 1 yr. A minority regress after normal development	Problems often recognized in preschool. Motor delays may have been noted	Before age 5 yr (typically, onset with loss of skills)	By definition, child normal until age 2 yr; then major loss of skills and dramatic "autistic-like" picture	Variable

PDD-NOS, pervasive developmental disorder not otherwise specified; CDD, Childhood Disintegrative Disorder.

Table 43–2 DSM-5 Criteria for Autism Spectrum Disorder

Persistent deficits in social communication and social interaction	For example:
	Impairment in social-emotional responsiveness
	Problems with nonverbal communicative behaviors
	Difficulties in forming, sustaining, and comprehending relationships
Restricted, repetitive patterns of behavior, interests, or activities	For example:
	Repetitive or ritualistic physical actions, object manipulation, or verbal expressions
	Inflexible insistence on routines
	Restricted interests
	Heightened or reduced sensitivity to sensory stimuli, or an unusual fascination with sensory features of the environment
Severity	Severity based on social communication impairments and restricted, repetitive patterns of behavior
Other:	Symptoms must be present in the early developmental period
	Symptoms cause clinically significant impairment
	Disturbances not better explained by intellectual disability or global developmental delay
Specify if:	With or without accompanying intellectual impairment
	With or without accompanying language impairment Associated with a known medical or genetic condition or environmental
	Associated with another neurodevelopmental, mental, or behavioral disorder
	With catatonia

Table 43–3 DSM-5 criteria Social Communication Disorder

Criteria	Description
Criterion A: Persistent Difficulties in Social Use of Verbal and Nonverbal Communication	Deficits in using communication for social purposes, such as greeting and sharing information, in a manner appropriate for the social context. Impairment in adjusting communication to match context or the listener's needs (e.g., differentiating speech in different settings or to different individuals).
Criterion B: Deficits Interfere with Effective Communication	Challenges in adhering to conversation and storytelling rules (e.g., turn-taking, clarifying misunderstandings). Difficulty understanding implied or ambiguous language aspects (e.g., idioms, humor, metaphors).
Criterion C: Functional Impact	Resulting limitations in effective communication, social participation, relationships, academic achievement, or occupational performance. Manifestation in one or more of these areas due to communication deficits.
Criterion D: Onset and Development	Symptoms emerge early in development, although they may not fully manifest until demands exceed capacities for social communication. Onset during developmental period.
Criterion E: Exclusionary Criteria	Symptoms not attributable to medical or neurological conditions. Not explained by low abilities in word structure/grammar. Distinct from autism spectrum disorder, intellectual disability, global developmental delay, or other mental disorders.

DSM, *Diagnostic and Statistical Manual of Mental Disorders.*

cultural issues have been little studied in autism, but the condition may be underdiagnosed in minority groups. Gender differences have been consistently reported in autism, with boys being 3 to 4 times more likely than girls to be diagnosed with autism. However, this disparity is more marked at the upper end of the IQ distribution and, conversely, the ratio is less among children with more severe cognitive disability. This might reflect either a lower threshold for brain dysfunction in males and lower sensitivity for diagnostic assessments in girls, and/or factor(s) causing autism in females may be more severe (Fombonne, 2005; Zeidan, 2022).

C. Etiology

In the first decades after autism was identified, there was much speculation that experiential factors might be involved. However, as time went on, evidence (e.g., high rates of seizure disorder, persistence of primitive reflexes, and "soft" neurological signs) suggested brain involvement. When the confusion between autism and schizophrenia was clarified, the focus began to shift toward brain and genetic mechanisms.

The current understanding of ASD's etiology is a combination of genetic, neurobiologic, environmental, and possibly immunological factors that act during key developmental periods and alter a child's trajectory (Matelski L, Van de Water J. 2015). Environmental factors studied that may contribute to the development of autism have encompassed a wide range of factors including infections during pregnancy, environmental exposures, and immunologic factors (Hertz-Picciotti I, Lyall L, Schmidt R. 2014). These likely interact with underlying genetic risk impacting the expression and severity of ASD.

D. Genetics

The initial impression that there was no role for genetic factors in autism was discarded when the first twin samples were collected and the current evidence base supports a strong genetic contribution to ASD. Twin studies have revealed high levels of concordance for monozygotic twins compared to same-sex fraternal twins (although even in the latter the rate of autism was significantly increased over the population rate). Family studies reveal prevalence rates of between 2% and 10% in siblings. Even when siblings do not have autism, they have an increased risk for language, learning, and social development problems and there are higher rates of mood and anxiety problems in family members.

Although specific modes of inheritance are not yet well established, it is clear that autism is a strongly genetic disorder and the shared risk of autism in families has been shown to be best explained by shared genetics, not shared environmental factors. Of the likely multiple genes involved, very promising leads are now being followed up, with many genes mediating some aspect of neural development (State & Levitt, 2011). Increased genetic risk for older fathers having children with autism has also now been observed in several studies

(State & Levitt, 2011). Interest in developing polygenic risk scores (composite measures of common gene risk variants theoretically associated with a given disorder) in combination with other risk factors has grown regarding ability to inform both diagnosis and prognosis (Thapar & Rutter, 2021).

NEUROBIOLOGY

Many different brain systems have been studied regarding the neurobiology of autism (Parellada M, Penzol MJ, Pina L, et al. 2014). Given the diversity of symptoms and clinical features, it seems likely that multiple neural systems are involved (Veenstra-VanderWeele J, Blakely RD. 2012). On the other hand, it is clear that not all systems are involved, as often autism is seen in children with typical cognitive ability. Abnormalities in the limbic system and the temporal and frontal lobes have been suggested as have abnormalities in the microarchitecture and cortical "mini-columns." A recent finding has been the report of overall brain size increase in children with autism, but it remains unclear whether the increase is generalized or local and how these structural findings correlate to the clinical presentation. The focus of research recently has shifted to systems of connectivity and both the functional and structural brain connectivity differences in ASD when compared to healthy peers. Abnormal patterns of activation or connectivity have been seen in numerous studies in individuals with ASD compared to healthy controls. It remains unclear which brain networks and regions are most important in regard to connectivity differences seen in ASD.

▶ Clinical Findings

A. Signs & Symptoms

ASD is characterized by a wide range of symptoms and severity—over both age and developmental level. For example, less able children have significant behavioral problems and are typically nonverbal, whereas more able children are verbal and may only have unusual special interests. Difficulties with social interaction are the major commonality in ASD. As first noted by Kanner, social skills are a source of major difference and impairment from early in life. Early social deficits take the form of lack of interest in joint attention, abnormalities in eye contact, and flawed imitation. Social skills often do improve, but they remain a source of disability even for the most able individuals. Delays in language development are a core concern in ASD. When language develops, it is often associated with echolalia, pronoun reversal, and abnormal prosody and pragmatics. Many fail to develop symbolic–imaginative play.

In contrast to a relative lack of interest in the social environment, the nonsocial (inanimate) environment may seem highly relevant to the child with autism. Difficulties with change in routine, repetitive behavior and unusual attachments may be observed (e.g., the child may be fascinated with spinning objects).

ASD is a disorder of early onset. Increasingly, there has been a focus on early diagnosis, and autism is now often diagnosed in the first year of life. Other symptoms are not essential diagnostic features but are typically seen. These include problems with hyper- or hyposensitivity, problems with sleeping and eating, and difficulties with mood regulation.

B. Intellectual Functioning

Kanner's early impression of all individuals with autism having normal intellectual potential proved incorrect. It became apparent that, while children with autism often have strengths in nonverbal tasks (e.g., puzzles), they are often markedly deficient in verbal cognitive abilities. Most autistic children function, overall, in the normal intellectual capacity range, but scattered subtest scores are common (Rosello R, Martinez-Raga J, Mira A, et al. 2021). Approximately one-third of individuals with autism will also have a comorbid intellectual disability. It does appear that overall cognitive abilities improve with early detection and intervention. In autism, areas of weakness typically include verbal concept formation, abstract thinking, and social reasoning.

Islets of special ability ("savant skills") are sometimes observed. Highly developed skills in special areas such as drawing, musical performance, or calendar calculation are much greater than would be expected given overall IQ. Special ability is also reflected in the relatively frequent phenomenon of hyperlexia, a precocious interest in letters and numbers.

C. Laboratory Findings

At this point, no specific biological markers have been identified for the diagnosis of ASD. High peripheral levels of serotonin are observed but are not diagnostic. Genetic testing (chromosomal microarray and fragile X testing) is increasingly recommended in children diagnosed with ASD because of the significant genetic component of the disorder (Harris HK, Sideridis GD, Barbaresi WJ, Harstad E. 2020). However, this is often limited by the availability of genetic counseling and providers able to thoughtfully engage families with results of such testing. Electroencephalogram (EEG) abnormalities are observed, and epilepsy is fairly frequent—impacting 20–25% of children with more strictly diagnosed autistic disorder. Diverse types of seizures are noted with two peaks of onset: early childhood and adolescence.

D. Neuroimaging

Magnetic resonance imaging (MRI) studies have focused on both structure and function. For example, studies of the amygdala and hippocampus have not found differences in volume, but functional MRI (fMRI) studies have shown hypoactivity of the amygdala in tasks involving social and affective judgments. Probably the best replicated finding from fMRI has been the hypoactivation, relative to normal controls, of the fusiform gyrus during face perception tasks. This observation is consistent with an extensive literature on performance deficits in face processing tasks and facial expression recognition in autism and provides an important key to understanding the core social deficits in autism. Other research has focused on the regions of the prefrontal cortex presumed to be involved in social cognitive tasks (McPartland & Pelphrey, 2012).

These difficulties may, in part, account for some aspects of the social difficulty in autism.

Course of Illness

Although the outcome of autism is improving, autism is a lifelong disability. As many as 20% or more of autistic individuals now becoming adults may be able to function with independence and self-sufficiency. Gains can be made by individuals of all ages and levels of functioning, and more independent functioning has been seen with the increase in early intervention. Positive prognostic signs for autism include some communicative speech by the age of 5 or 6 years and average nonverbal cognitive skills. More able individuals, in particular with intact intellectual functioning and language, generally have the best outcome in terms of social outcomes and personal self-sufficiency (Howlin, 2014).

Differential Diagnosis (Including Comorbid Conditions)

ASD must be differentiated from other developmental disorders and sensory impairments. A detailed history and mental and physical examination are required. The early onset of problems in social interaction and communication is typical, and unusual behaviors often develop somewhat later (often around age 3 years). In intellectual disability, social skills are preserved and commensurate to cognitive level. In specific language disorders, language difficulties are seen in the context of good social skills. In obtaining historical information, aides to memory, such as baby books and videos, can be useful. A history of normal development followed by regression should prompt careful diagnostic investigation. Similarly, unusual features in the family history, child examination, and so forth may require specific investigation (Volkmar et al, 2005).

Treatment

A. Educational and Behavioral Interventions

Autism is a disorder of development. At the same time, development affects autism. The goal of treatment is to minimize the disruptive effects of autism on development and maximize normative developmental processes. Goals change with the child's age and level of functioning but always involve an explicit focus on social, language, and adaptive (self-help) skills. A structured, comprehensive program is needed with input from various professionals. The approaches used vary on several dimensions (e.g., how much they emphasize a child-centered or a developmental approach as contrasted to an adult-centered behavioral approach); however, all approaches share many features (Volkmar & Wiesner, 2009).

The focus of speech and language therapy is to expand the range of the child's communication skills. This should include teaching broader communication skills and, beyond, more vocabulary. Children who are not yet verbal can be helped by augmentative strategies (e.g., manual signing, picture exchange). For more advanced children, the focus is more on social language use. Behavioral interventions are used in the educational program. These techniques help with management of disruptive behavior and facilitate learning. Given the tendency of children with autism to learn things in isolation, the generalization of skills is important and is an essential aim.

B. Psychopharmacological Interventions

Medications do not affect the central social and communicative aspects of autism but may ameliorate the problem behavior that interferes with functioning. Neuroleptic medication, particularly the atypical neuroleptics, are effective in decreasing stereotypic behavior and agitation; however, side effects can be challenging. Two atypical antipsychotics, risperidone and aripiprazole, are FDA-approved for the treatment of irritability in ASD (risperidone in ages 5–16 and aripiprazole in ages 6–17). Multiple double-blind placebo-controlled studies have demonstrated the efficacy of risperidone (0.5 mg–3.5 mg/day) and aripiprazole (2.5–15 mg/day) in decreasing irritability, stabilizing mood, and decreasing aggression in youth with ASD. Weight gain and changes in metabolic parameters are the most common side effects when using risperidone or aripiprazole.

In addition, research continues on the SSRIs (selective serotonin reuptake inhibitors), given their potential for alleviating anxiety and behavioral rigidity. Results of controlled trials have been mixed regarding SSRIs and anxiety related to ASD (Doyle CA, McDougle CJ. 2012). However, because of the severity of anxiety individuals with ASD often experience, SSRIs are commonly prescribed clinically. It is recommended to start at low doses and slowly titrate to the maximally effective dose. Similarly, for the impulsivity and hyperactivity often associated with ASD, psychostimulants such as methylphenidate and dextroamphetamine remain the first-line treatments. Stimulant medication has also shown mixed results in controlled trials and, clinically, more side effects and lower response rates are seen in individuals with ASD when compared to neurotypical individuals treated with stimulants.

There remain no treatments approved for the core features of autism, but research continues into agents including glutamatergic agents (amantadine and memantine), cholinesterase inhibitors (donepezil, rivastigmine, and galantamine), oxytocin, and related compounds, but results remain mixed and there is no indication for these agents with the current level of evidence. Pharmacologic treatment remains a symptom-driven exercise, using medications to target the disruptive symptoms and individual with ASD experiences.

C. Psychotherapeutic Interventions

Early intervention is the mainstay of psychosocial interventions for children with ASD, but the type, intensity, and therapeutic modality vary. Modalities that focus on language, social reciprocity, and behavior supports have shown significant benefit in improving outcomes, in particular when initiated in early development. In addition, occupational therapy, in particular to meet the sensory needs of individuals with ASD, can have great benefit.

Many psychosocial interventions for autism are derived from the theoretical underpinnings of applied behavior analysis (ABA). A comprehensive review of ABA is outside the scope of this chapter but, in summary, is an intensive behavior therapy (several hours/session, several times/week) that focuses on increasing the frequency of desired behaviors, with a focus on social, communication, learning, and self-care skills. Lower intensity interventions are often parent-mediated interventions in which parents or caregivers are taught to increase awareness of child's communication signals and style and work to increase more joint engagement and social communication. As individuals with autism age into school age, adolescence, and adulthood, cognitive behavior therapy can be helpful in improving adaptive functioning, decreasing anxiety, and improving social interactions.

D. Alternative Treatments

Many different treatments have been proposed and most lack an empirical foundation. A majority of parents engage in such treatments, so practitioners should inquire about all forms of treatment a family is engaged in. Often, follow-up studies of nontraditional treatments demonstrated good outcome in a small number of cases without what, today, would be recognized as effective treatment—that is, some children do well anyway. Furthermore, there is a strong placebo (nonspecific treatment) effect. Occasionally alternative treatment is dangerous, either in terms of loss of access to effective programs or because of physical harm (Volkmar & Wiesner, 2009).

Websites
www.aspennj.org
www.autism.fm
https://www.autismspeaks.org/
www.quackwatch.com

Doyle CA, McDougle CJ. Pharmacologic treatments for the behavioral symptoms associated with autism spectrum disorders across the lifespan. *Dialogues Clin Neurosci.* 2012 Sep;14(3):263–279. doi: 10.31887/DCNS.2012.14.3/cdoyle. PMID: 23226952; PMCID: PMC3513681.

Fombonne E. Epidemiological studies of pervasive developmental disorders. In: Volkmar FR, Klin A, Paul R, et al, eds. *Handbook of Autism and Pervasive Developmental Disorders.* 3rd ed. Vol 1. Hoboken, NJ: Wiley; 2005:42–69.

Harris HK, Sideridis GD, Barbaresi WJ, Harstad E. Pathogenic yield of genetic testing in autism spectrum disorder. *Pediatrics.* 2020 Oct;146(4):e20193211. doi: 10.1542/peds.2019-3211. Epub 2020 Sep 16. PMID: 32938777; PMCID: PMC7786819.

Hertz-Picciotti I, Lyall L, Schmidt R. Environmental factors in ASD. In Volkmar F, Rogers S, Paul R, et al, eds. *Handbook of Autism and Pervasive Developmental Disorders.* 4th ed. Hoboken NJ: Wiley; 2014:424–456.

Howlin P. Outcome in autism spectrum disorders. In F. Volkmar F, S. Rogers S, Paul R, et al, eds. *Handbook of Autism and Pervasive Development Disorders.* 4th ed. Hoboken NJ: Wiley; 2014:97–116.

Huerta M, Bishop SL, Duncan A, et al. Application of DSM-5 criteria for autism spectrum disorder to three samples of children with DSM-IV diagnoses of pervasive developmental disorders. *Am J Psychiatry.* 2012;169(10):1056–1064.

Kanner L. Autistic disturbances of affective contact. *Nervous Child.* 1943;2:217–250.

Lord C, Brugha TS, Charman T, et al. Autism spectrum disorder. *Nat Rev Dis Primers.* 2020 Jan 16;6(1):5. doi: 10.1038/s41572-019-0138-4. PMID: 31949163; PMCID: PMC8900942.

Matelski L, Van de Water J. Risk factors in autism: thinking outside the brain. *J Autoimmun.* 2016 Feb;67:1–7. doi: 10.1016/j.jaut.2015.11.003. Epub 2015 Dec 22. PMID: 26725748; PMCID: PMC5467975.

McPartland JC, Pelphrey KA. The implications of social neuroscience for social disability. [Literature Review]. *J Autism Dev Disord.* 2012;42(6):1256–1262.

Parellada M, Penzol MJ, Pina L, et al. The neurobiology of autism spectrum disorders. *Eur Psychiatry.* 2014 Jan;29(1):11–19. doi: 10.1016/j.eurpsy.2013.02.005. Epub 2013 Nov 22. PMID: 24275633.

Rosello R, Martinez-Raga J, Mira A, et al. Developmental outcomes in adolescence of children with autism spectrum disorder without intellectual disability: a systematic review of prospective studies. *Neurosci Biobehav Rev.* 2021 Jul;126:590–603. doi: 10.1016/j.neubiorev.2021.04.010. Epub 2021 Apr 16. PMID: 33872683.

Smith IC, Reichow B, Volkmar FR. The effects of DSM-5 criteria on number of individuals diagnosed with autism spectrum disorder: a systematic review. *J Autism Dev Disord.* 2015;45(8):2541–2552.

State MW, Levitt P. The conundrums of understanding genetic risks for autism spectrum disorders. *Nat Neurosci.* 2011;14(12):1499–1506.

Thapar A, Rutter M. Genetic advances in autism. *J Autism Dev Disord.* 2021 Dec;51(12):4321–4332. doi: 10.1007/s10803-020-04685-z. PMID: 32940822; PMCID: PMC8531042.

Veenstra-VanderWeele J, Blakely RD. Networking in autism: leveraging genetic, biomarker and model system findings in the search for new treatments. *Neuropsychopharmacology.* 2012; 37(1):196–212.

Volkmar FR, Klin A, Paul R, et al, eds. *Handbook of Autism and Pervasive Developmental Disorders.* 3rd ed. Vol 1. Hoboken, NJ: Wiley; 2005.

Volkmar F, Wiesner L. *A Practical Guide to Autism.* Hoboken, NJ: Wiley; 2009.

Zeidan J, Fombonne E, Scorah J, et al. *Global prevalence of autism: a systematic review update. Autism Res.* 2022 May;15(5):778–790. doi: 10.1002/aur.2696. Epub 2022 Mar 3. PMID: 35238171; PMCID: PMC9310578.

Attention-Deficit Hyperactivity Disorder

44

Thomas J. Spencer, MD

International Statistical Classification of Diseases and Related Health Problems—10th Revision (ICD-10) Diagnostic Criteria for Attention-Deficit Hyperactivity Disorders (F90)

Attention-deficit hyperactivity disorders are behavioral disorders characterized by a marked pattern of inattention and/or hyperactivity–impulsivity that is inconsistent with developmental level and clearly interferes with functioning in at least two settings (e.g., at home and at school). At least some of the symptoms must be present before the age of 7 years. Although most individuals have symptoms of both inattention and hyperactivity–impulsivity, one or the other pattern may be predominant. Symptoms often attenuate during late adolescence although a minority experience the full complement of symptoms into mid-adulthood. The disorder is more frequent in males than females. The ICD-10 lists five separate subcategories (see below).

F90 Attention-deficit Hyperactivity Disorders

▶ F90.0 Attention-deficit hyperactivity disorder, predominantly inattentive type;

▶ F90.1 Attention-deficit hyperactivity disorder, predominantly hyperactive type;

▶ F90.2 Attention-deficit hyperactivity disorder, combined type;

▶ F90.8 Attention-deficit hyperactivity disorder, other type;

▶ F90.9 Attention-deficit hyperactivity disorder, unspecified type;

Reproduced with permission from ICD-10 Diagnostic Criteria for Attention-deficit hyperactivity disorders. Geneva, Switzerland; World Health Organization (WHO); 2003.

▶ General Considerations

A. Epidemiology

Attention-deficit hyperactivity disorder (ADHD) is the most common emotional, cognitive, and behavioral disorder treated in youth. It is a major clinical and public health problem because of its associated morbidity and disability in children, adolescents, and adults. Data from cross-sectional, retrospective, and follow-up studies indicate that youth with ADHD are at risk for developing other psychiatric difficulties in childhood, adolescence, and adulthood, including delinquency as well as mood, anxiety, and substance use disorders.

Early definitions, such as the Hyperkinetic Reaction of Childhood in Diagnostic and Statistical Manual of Mental Disorders Second Edition (DSM-II), placed the greatest emphasis on motoric hyperactivity and overt impulsivity as hallmarks of the disorder. The DSM-III represented a paradigm shift, as it began to emphasize inattention as a significant component of the disorder. DSM-IV defined three subtypes of ADHD: predominantly inattentive, predominantly hyperactive–impulsive, and a combined subtype. In DSM-5, the same 18 symptoms are used; however, there are six notable changes. First, descriptors are included to aid diagnosis at later ages; second, the cross-situational requirement has been increased to several symptoms in each setting; third, the age of onset criterion has been advanced to several symptoms before age 12; fourth, prior subtypes are now termed presentation specifiers; fifth, the existence of autism spectrum disorder does not preclude an ADHD diagnosis; and sixth, the minimum number of symptoms for adults has been reduced to five symptoms for either presentation specifier. The current ICD-10 criteria (see above) largely mirror the DSM-IV criteria.

A recent meta-analysis of 86 worldwide studies of children and adolescents determined an overall prevalence of 5.9–7.1%, depending on diagnostic procedure. There were no significant prevalence differences between countries after controlling for differences in diagnostic algorithms. Although ADHD was previously thought to remit largely in adolescence, a growing literature supports the persistence of the disorder and associated impairment into adulthood in a majority of cases.

Prevalence estimates of childhood ADHD in the United States are also estimated to be 5–8%. Estimates vary predictably depending on methodology. Definitions that require both symptom dimensions (hyperactivity/impulsivity and inattention) are more restrictive than those that require only one of these dimensions. Thus, estimates based on pre–DSM-III definitions or the ICD codes of hyperkinetic disorder produce lower estimates. In addition, the surveys that estimate based on symptoms alone and do not include impairment yield higher estimates. Other factors that affect apparent prevalence estimates include pervasiveness criteria, informants (teacher, parent, child), and use of rating scales versus clinical interviews as well as ascertainment issues. Community samples have higher rates than school samples.

Gender and age of the sample also affect estimates of prevalence. Girls more commonly have the inattentive presentation and also less commonly have accompanying oppositional defiant disorder/conduct disorder (ODD/CD), disruptive disorders, factors leading to lower rates of diagnosis. The original descriptions were derived from a child-focused perspective and do not reflect what are thought to be more salient aspects of adult ADHD: the executive function disorders of poor organization, poor time management, and memory disturbance associated with academic and occupational failure. The lack of appropriate description of adult symptoms may reduce the true prevalence of ADHD in adulthood.

B. Etiology

1. Biological adversity—Several biologic factors have been proposed as contributors to ADHD, including food additives/diet, lead contamination, cigarette and alcohol exposure, maternal smoking during pregnancy, and low birth weight. Although the Feingold diet for ADHD was popularized by the media and accepted by many parents, systematic studies showed that this diet was ineffective and that food additives have at best a very small effect on ADHD behaviors. Several investigators have shown that lead contamination can cause symptoms of ADHD. However, lead does not account for the majority of ADHD cases, and many children with high lead exposure do not develop ADHD. An emerging literature documents that maternal smoking and alcohol exposure during pregnancy, low birth weight, and psychosocial adversity are additional independent risk factors for ADHD.

Pregnancy and delivery complications (i.e., toxemia, eclampsia, poor maternal health, maternal age, fetal postmaturity, duration of labor, fetal distress, low birth weight, antepartum hemorrhage) appear to lead to a predisposition for ADHD. Several studies documented that maternal smoking during pregnancy is an independent risk factor for ADHD.

2. Psychosocial adversity—Findings of recent studies stress the importance of adverse family–environment variables as risk factors for ADHD. In particular, chronic family conflict, decreased family cohesion, and exposure to parental psychopathology (particularly maternal) are more common in ADHD families compared with control families. It is important to note that, although many studies provide powerful evidence for the importance of psychosocial adversity in ADHD, such factors tend to emerge as universal predictors of children's adaptive functioning and emotional health, rather than specific predictors of ADHD. As such, they can be conceptualized as nonspecific triggers of an underlying predisposition or as modifiers of the course of illness.

C. Genetics

Because ADHD is believed to be highly genetic, studies of twins have been used to establish its heritability or the degree to which this disorder is influenced by genetic factors. Based on numerous studies of twins, which varied considerably in methodology and definitions of ADHD, the mean heritability for ADHD was shown to be 77%. Five candidate genes continue to show statistically significant evidence of association with ADHD on the basis of the pooled odds ratio (1.18–1.46) across studies: DRD4, DRD5, DAT, HTR1B, and SNAP-25. However, the effect sizes are small and consistent with a model in which ADHD vulnerability is mediated by a number or genes. Investigators are currently examining gene–environment interactions as well as genome-wide association, copy number variation, and family-based studies of genetic susceptibility to ADHD.

▶ Clinical Findings

A. Signs & Symptoms

The diagnosis of ADHD is made by careful clinical history. A child with ADHD is characterized by a considerable degree of inattentiveness, distractibility, impulsivity, and often hyperactivity that is inappropriate for the developmental stage of the child. Other common symptoms include low frustration tolerance, shifting activities frequently, difficulty organizing, and daydreaming. These symptoms are usually pervasive; however, they may not all occur in all settings. Adults must have childhood-onset (by age 12), persistent, and current symptoms of ADHD to be diagnosed with the disorder. Adults with ADHD often present with marked inattention, distractibility, organization difficulties, and poor efficiency, which culminate in life histories of academic and occupational failure. In examining the stability of ADHD symptoms from childhood into adulthood, adult persistence was much greater for inattention than for hyperactivity/impulsivity. In addition, executive functioning symptoms are the most consistent and discriminating predictors of adult ADHD. Furthermore, there is renewed interest in deficient emotional self-regulation (DESR), as characterized by deficits in self-regulating the physiological arousal caused by strong emotions. Studies have shown that 40–60% of individuals with ADHD also have DESR. Individuals with the combined condition (ADHD + DESR) have been shown to have increased rates of emotional and psychosocial impairments and to be at higher risk for compromised outcomes.

B. Rating Scales

Rating scales are extremely helpful in documenting the individual profile of ADHD symptoms as well as assessing the response to treatments. It is important to emphasize that they should not be used for diagnosis without careful clinical confirmation and elicitation of the other criteria necessary for diagnosis. Although neuropsychological testing is not relied upon to diagnose ADHD, it may serve to identify particular weaknesses within ADHD or specific learning disabilities co-occurring with ADHD.

Rating scales are available for all age groups and can be useful in assessing and monitoring home, academic, and occupational performance. Increasingly, there has been a congruence of opinion in this area with a number of the most widely used scales consisting of Likert ratings of the existing DSM criteria, see Table 44–1. There are two types of scales in wide use, the so-called narrow scales that are specific for ADHD and "broad" scales that measure additional dimensions including comorbidity. The broad scales are useful for separating straightforward and complex cases, and the narrow scales are most useful for honing in on exclusively ADHD dimensions both for diagnosis and to monitor specific responses to treatment.

C. Psychological Testing

Psychological testing is not necessary for the routine diagnosis of ADHD and does not readily distinguish children with and without ADHD because of poor sensitivity. Nonetheless, psychometric testing can be valuable in narrowing

the differential diagnosis and identifying comorbid learning difficulties. Many children with ADHD have difficulties with abstract reasoning, mental flexibility, planning, and working memory, a collection of skills broadly categorized as executive functioning skills. They can also present with verbal and nonverbal performance skills and/or visual–spatial processing deficits. In such circumstances, neuropsychological assessments can be valuable and may help to clarify the diagnosis. Children with learning, language, visual–motor, or auditory processing problems usually perform poorly only in their particular problem area, whereas children with ADHD may perform poorly in several areas of evaluation.

▶ Laboratory Findings

Nonroutine laboratory studies are not indicated unless the history or physical examination is suggestive of seizures, neurodevelopmental regression, or localizing neurologic signs or if an acute or chronic medical disorder is suspected.

Neuroimaging

The neurobiology of ADHD is not completely understood, although imbalances in dopaminergic and noradrenergic systems have been implicated in the core symptoms that characterize this disorder. Many brain regions are candidates for impaired functioning in ADHD. Prefrontal hypotheses in ADHD have primarily involved the dorsolateral prefrontal cortex (DLPFC), associated with organizational, planning, working memory, and attentional dysfunctions, and orbital lesions associated with social disinhibition and impulse control disorders.

Structural imaging studies using computed tomography or magnetic resonance imaging (MRI) found evidence of structural brain abnormalities among ADHD patients, with the most common findings being smaller volumes in frontal cortex, cerebellum, and subcortical structures. Castellanos and colleagues found smaller total cerebral brain volumes from childhood through adolescence. This work suggested that genetic or early environmental influences on brain development in ADHD are fixed, nonprogressive, and unrelated to stimulant treatment. Numerous functional MRI (fMRI) studies have reported dorsal anterior cingulate cortex (dACC) hypofunction in ADHD on tasks of inhibitory control.

Brain imaging studies fit well with the concept that dysfunction in fronto-subcortical pathways occurs in ADHD. Three subcortical structures implicated by the imaging studies (i.e., caudate, putamen, and globus pallidus) are part of the neural circuitry underlying motor control, executive functions, inhibition of behavior, and the modulation of reward pathways. These frontal–striatal–pallidal–thalamic circuits provide feedback to the cortex for the regulation of behavior. The fronto-subcortical systems pathways associated with ADHD are rich in catecholamines, which are involved in the mechanism of action of stimulant medications used to treat

Table 44–1 Rating Scales Commonly Used in Assessing ADHD

Type of Scale	Name of Scale	Age Range
Broad	Child Behavior Checklist (CBCL)	6–18
	Conners Comprehensive Behavior Rating Scale	6–18
Narrow	National Institute for Children's Health Quality (NICHQ) Vanderbilt Assessment Scale	6–12
	Swanson, Nolan, and Pelham-IV (SNAP-IV) Questionnaire, which is for children aged 6–18 (also known as ADHD-RS-IV)	6–18

ADHD, attention-deficit hyperactivity disorder.

this disorder. A plausible model for the effects of medications in ADHD suggests that, through dopaminergic and/or noradrenergic pathways, these agents increase the inhibitory influences of frontal cortical activity on subcortical structures.

Imaging studies also implicate the cerebellum and corpus callosum in the pathophysiology of ADHD. The cerebellum contributes significantly to cognitive functioning, presumably through cerebellar–cortical pathways involving the pons and thalamus. The corpus callosum connects homotypic regions of the two cerebral hemispheres. Size variations in the callosum and volume differences in number of cortical neurons may degrade communication between the hemispheres, which may account for some of the cognitive and behavioral symptoms of ADHD.

Activation in brain regions exhibiting a strong positive temporal correlation is believed to be a component of intrinsic functional networks. One such network is the default mode network (DMN), which is composed of brain regions typically more activated during rest than during task performance (i.e., that are deactivated during task performance). Regions in the DMN often exhibit strong negative correlations (are anticorrelated) with other brain regions that are activated for working memory and executive function (task-positive networks), such as the DLPFC. Studies of ADHD in both adults and children report reduced correlations between midline regions of the DMN and also reductions in anticorrelations between DMN and task-positive networks.

There are now a sizeable number of studies that evaluated the impact of therapeutic oral doses of stimulants on the brains of ADHD subjects as measured with MRI-based neuroimaging (morphometric, functional, spectroscopy). Findings suggest that therapeutic oral doses of stimulants decrease alterations in brain structure and function in subjects with ADHD relative to unmedicated subjects and controls. These medication-associated brain effects parallel, and may underlie, the well-established clinical benefits.

Course of Illness

Samples ascertained before the publication of DSM-III relied on earlier definitions that highlighted hyperactivity as a hallmark of ADHD. Because it is hyperactivity that wanes earliest, it may be that older samples were enriched with subjects more likely to remit from ADHD than individuals identified today. There is evidence for this hypothesis in the data. In a recent analysis, the persistence rate was lowest in studies ascertained according to DSM-II ADD and highest in those studies ascertained according to DSM-III-R ADHD. The available data also suggest a continuation of childhood behavior problems and emerging antisocial behavior among many in this group of children. For example, researchers have noted the rate of CDs among children with ADHD to range between 25% and 50% at follow-up during adolescence. Reports also indicate that a majority of children with ADHD continue to exhibit deficits in attention and/or activity level in adulthood, with only

about 30% of children evidencing a remission of symptoms by adolescence and early adulthood. Recent work also suggests that ADHD youth disproportionately become involved with cigarettes, alcohol, and then drugs. Individuals with ADHD, independent of comorbidity, tend to maintain their addiction longer compared to their non-ADHD peers.

Differential Diagnosis (Including Comorbid Conditions)

A. Oppositional Defiant Disorder and Conduct Disorder

There are important nosologic distinctions between attention and hyperactivity per se and the associated symptoms common to the disruptive behavioral disorder category. ODD is characterized by a pattern of negativistic, hostile, and defiant behavior. ADHD and ODD/CD have been found to co-occur in 30–50% of cases in both epidemiologic and clinical samples. In contrast, CD is a more severe, and less common, disorder of habitual rule breaking defined by a pattern of aggression, destruction, lying, stealing, or truancy. Whereas CD is a strong predictor of substance abuse, ODD without CD is not.

B. Mood Disorders

Unipolar depression in a child may be apparent from a sad or irritable mood, or a persistent loss of interest or pleasure in the child's favorite activities. Other signs and symptoms include physiologic disturbances such as changes in appetite and weight, abnormal sleep patterns, psychomotor abnormalities, fatigue, and diminished ability to think, as well as feelings of worthlessness or guilt and suicidal preoccupation.

Classical mania in adults is characterized by euphoria, elation, grandiosity, and increased energy. However, in many adults and most children, mania is more commonly manifested by extreme irritability or explosive mood with associated poor psychosocial functioning that is often devastating to the patient and family. In milder conditions, additional symptoms include unmodulated high energy such as decreased sleep, excessive talkativeness, racing thoughts, or increased goal-directed activity (social, work, school, sexual) or an associated manifestation of markedly poor judgment such as thrill-seeking or reckless activities.

In epidemiologic studies and several controlled, prospective studies, higher rates of depression were found in ADHD. A baseline diagnosis of major depression predicted lower psychosocial functioning and a higher rate of hospitalization as well as impairments in interpersonal and family functioning. Similarly, higher rates of mania were detected in follow-up studies. ADHD children with comorbid mania at either baseline or follow-up assessment had other correlates expected in mania including additional psychopathology, psychiatric hospitalization, severely impaired psychosocial functioning as well as a greater family history of mood disorders.

C. Childhood Anxiety Disorders

Childhood anxiety disorders are often not suspected in an overactive child, just as ADHD is often not assessed in inhibited children. When present, both contribute to social, behavioral, and academic dysfunction. In addition, anxiety may be associated with intense intrapsychic suffering. Thus, having both ADHD and anxiety disorders may substantially worsen the outcome of children with both disorders. In the Massachusetts General Hospital follow-up study, ADHD children with comorbid anxiety disorder had increased psychiatric treatment and more impaired psychosocial functioning, as well as a stronger family history of anxiety disorders.

D. Cognitive Performance and Learning Disabilities

Children with ADHD perform more poorly than controls on standard measures of intelligence and achievement. In addition, children with ADHD perform more poorly in school than do controls, as evidenced by more grade repetitions, poorer grades in academic subjects, more placements in special classes, and more tutoring. The reported degree of overlap with comorbid learning disabilities varies by definition; the more restrictive definition has a rate of 20–25%.

E. ADHD Plus Tics

Children with ADHD have higher rates of tic disorders that may contribute additional dysfunction due to distractions and social impairments directly attributable to the movements or vocalizations themselves. A number of studies have noted that ADHD treatment is highly effective for ADHD behaviors, aggression, and social skill deficits in children with Tourette syndrome or chronic tics.

F. Substance Use Disorders

Combined data from retrospective accounts of adults and prospective observations of youth indicate that juveniles with ADHD are at increased risk for cigarette smoking and substance abuse during adolescence.

▶ Treatment

The ADHD adolescent and young adult are at risk for school failure, emotional difficulties, poor peer relationships, and trouble with the law. Factors identifiable in younger youth that predict the persistence of ADHD into adulthood include parental psychopathology, severe baseline symptoms, and psychiatric comorbidity—particularly aggression or delinquency problems. Although the literature provides compelling evidence that the diagnosis of ADHD in childhood predicts persistent ADHD and poor outcome in adolescence, these findings also suggest that such a compromised outcome is not shared by all ADHD children. The discussion thus far has not addressed a related clinical question: Can the functioning of ADHD children normalize in the context of persistent ADHD? We analyzed data from a 4-year longitudinal study of referred children and adolescents with ADHD to assess normalization of functioning and its predictors among boys with persistent ADHD.

Using indices of emotional, educational, and social adjustment, we found that 20% of children with persistent ADHD functioned poorly at follow-up in all three domains, 20% did well in all three domains, and 60% had intermediate outcomes. These findings suggested that the syndromatic persistence of ADHD is not associated with a uniform functional outcome but leads instead to a wide range of emotional, educational, and social adjustment outcomes that can be partially predicted by exposure to maternal psychopathology, larger family size, psychiatric comorbidity, and impulsive symptoms.

A. Psychopharmacologic Interventions

Medications remain a mainstay of treatment for children, adolescents, and adults with ADHD. In fact, multisite studies support that medication management of ADHD is a key ingredient in outcome for core ADHD symptoms in contrast to multimodal treatment. For example, in a large prospective and randomized long-term trial of ADHD youth, those receiving stimulants alone were observed to have similar improvement in core ADHD symptoms (inattention, hyperactivity, impulsivity) at 14 months follow-up compared to those randomized to receive stimulants plus psychotherapy.

The stimulants, alpha-adrenergic agonists, specific norepinephrine reuptake inhibitors (SNRIs), and certain antidepressants comprise the available agents for ADHD. Stimulants, SNRIs, and antidepressants have been demonstrated to have similar pharmacological responsivity across the life span, including school-aged children, adolescents, and adult groups with ADHD.

B. Stimulants

The stimulants are the most commonly prescribed agents for pediatric and adult groups with ADHD and the class of medication with the most evidence and largest effect sizes of about 1. The most commonly used compounds in this class include methylphenidate (Ritalin, Concerta, Metadate, Focalin, Quillivant, Cotempla, Aptensio, Jornay, generics, and others) and amphetamine (Dexedrine, Adderall, Vyvanse, Mydayis, Evekeo, Adzenys, generics, and others). Stimulants are sympathomimetic drugs, which increase intrasynaptic catecholamines (mainly dopamine) by inhibiting the presynaptic reuptake mechanism and releasing presynaptic catecholamines. Whereas methylphenidate specifically blocks the dopamine transporter protein, amphetamines also release dopamine stores and cytoplasmic dopamine directly into the synaptic cleft. Recent data suggest that acute tolerance to stimulants (tachyphylaxis) may develop rapidly necessitating an ascending—or pulsing—pharmacokinetic profile for ADHD efficacy.

Methylphenidate and D-amphetamine are both short-acting compounds, with an onset of action within 30–60 minutes and a peak clinical effect usually seen between 1 and 2 hours after administration lasting 2–5 hours. The amphetamine compounds (Adderall) and sustained-release preparations of methylphenidate and dextroamphetamine are intermediate-acting compounds with an onset of action within 60 minutes and duration of 6–8 hours.

Given the need to additionally treat ADHD outside of academic settings (i.e., social, homework) and to reduce the need for in-school dosing and likelihood for diversion, there has been great interest in extended-release preparations of the stimulants. Extended-release preparations greatly reduce untoward peak adverse effects of stimulants such as headaches and moodiness, as well as essentially eliminating afternoon wear-off and rebound.

A new generation of highly sophisticated, well-developed, safe, and effective long-acting preparations of stimulant drugs has reached the market and revolutionized the treatment of ADHD. These compounds employ novel delivery systems to overcome acute tolerance termed "tachyphylaxis." There are a number of long-acting methylphenidate and amphetamine formulations, whereas Concerta and Quillivant are 12-hour formulations, Focalin-XR is an 8- to 10-hour formulation, and Metadate-CD and Ritalin LA are 8-hour methylphenidate formulations. There is also a methylphenidate transdermal delivery system (patch) whose duration of activity varies by wear time. Vyvanse is a 13-hour amphetamine formulation, and Adderall XR is a 12-hour amphetamine formulation. Methylphenidate as a secondary amine gives rise to four optical isomers: D-threo, L-threo, D-erythro, and L-erythro. The active stereoisomer D-threomethylphenidate compound has been available in an immediate-release and long-acting form as Focalin and Focalin XR. There are generic versions of many but not all formulations.

Stimulants appear to work in all age groups of individuals with ADHD. Studies in preschoolers report improvement in ADHD symptoms and structured tasks as well as mother–child interactions; however, there may be a higher side effect burden and smaller effect size compared to other age groups. Similarly, in adolescents response has been reported as moderate to robust, with no abuse or tolerance noted. In addition, stimulant treatment has been found to be effective in adults with ADHD.

Predictable short-term adverse effects include reduced appetite, insomnia, edginess, and gastrointestinal upset. In adults, elevated vital signs may emerge, necessitating baseline and on-drug monitoring. There are a number of controversial issues related to chronic stimulant use. Although stimulants may produce anorexia and weight loss, their effect on ultimate height remains less certain. Although initial reports suggested that there was a persistent stimulant-associated decrease in growth in height in children, other reports have failed to substantiate this finding, and still others question the possibility that growth deficits may represent maturational

delays related to ADHD itself rather than to stimulant treatment. The FDA includes a warning about exacerbation of tics when taking stimulant medication. However, recent research does not support this association. A meta-analysis of 22 studies involving 2,385 children found there was no difference in the risk of new onset or worsening tics in those receiving stimulant treatment versus placebo. Type of stimulant, dose, age, or duration of treatment did not change the risk of tics (Cohen et al. 2015).There is a black box warning concerning the potential abuse of stimulants. Patients should be carefully assessed for past history and current substance use problems and risk of stimulant abuse at baseline and periodically during treatment. In addition, data suggest that diversion of stimulants to non-ADHD youth continues to be a concern. Families should closely monitor stimulant medication, and college students receiving stimulants should be advised to carefully store their medication. Despite the findings on efficacy of the stimulants, studies have also reported consistently that typically one third of ADHD individuals do not respond to or cannot tolerate this class of agents.

1. Specific norepinephrine reuptake inhibitors (atomoxetine)—Atomoxetine (Strattera) is one of a nonstimulant class of compounds known as SNRIs. Atomoxetine is the first nonstimulant that was FDA approved for ADHD. Atomoxetine may be particularly useful in stimulant failures or when abuse liability, anxiety, or tics co-occur within ADHD. After extensive testing, atomoxetine has been found to be generally safe and well tolerated, with a medium effect size of 0.64. However, there have been rare (2 out of 3 million patients) reports of potentially serious liver injury. Furthermore there is an uncommon risk of increased suicidality in children and young adults similar to that reported for antidepressants.

2. Antihypertensives—Long-acting versions of the alpha-adrenergic agonists clonidine (Kapvay) and guanfacine (Intuniv) have been approved both as monotherapies and as adjunctive therapies with stimulants for ADHD. Previously, alpha-adrenergic agonists have been used (off label) for the treatment of ADHD as well as associated tics, aggression, and sleep disturbances, particularly in younger children. Somnolence, sedation, and hypersomnia adverse events, although frequent, are typically mild to moderate and tend to diminish with continued treatment. Cardiovascular effects are consistent with their known antihypertensive effects and are generally modest in nature.

3. Antidepressants—A subgroup of antidepressants are second-line (non–FDA approved) drugs for ADHD. The tricyclic antidepressants (TCAs) as well as bupropion (Wellbutrin) block the reuptake of neurotransmitters including norepinephrine. In contrast, the serotonin reuptake inhibitors are not useful for ADHD. The TCAs are effective in controlling abnormal behaviors and improving cognitive impairments associated with ADHD but less so than the majority of stimulants. As minor increases in heart rate and electrocardiogram (ECG) intervals are predictable with TCAs, including potential increases in QTc intervals, ECG monitoring at baseline and at therapeutic dose is suggested.

4. Modafinil—Modafinil is an antinarcoleptic agent, which is structurally and pharmacologically different from other anti-ADHD agents. Although its use with ADHD is not FDA approved, testing in children has reported effectiveness in ADHD. Modafinil is generally safe and well tolerated; however, there have been concerns about uncommon occurrences of a severe exfoliating dermatitis possibly related to Stevens–Johnson syndrome.

C. Psychotherapeutic Interventions

The largest-scale study examining the relative and combined effectiveness of medical and nonmedical interventions for ADHD is the NIMH Multimodal Treatment Study for ADHD Study (MTA). In this 5-year, six-site project, 579 elementary-age children with ADHD were randomly assigned to one of four 14-month treatment conditions: behavioral treatment, medication management (mostly methylphenidate), combined behavioral treatment and medication management, and a community comparison group. Children in the behavioral treatment arm received a very intensive combination of treatments, including school consultation, a classroom aide, an 8-week summer treatment program, and 35 sessions of parent management training. Findings from the MTA study at 14 months indicate that medical intervention was significantly more effective than behavioral and community treatments, that behavioral treatment only modestly enhanced the effect of medication alone, and that behavioral treatment alone was no more effective than the treatment received by children in the community comparison group on core symptoms of ADHD (inattention, hyperactivity, impulsivity). However, intensive psychotherapy was increased in relative effectiveness for teacher rating social skills and equally as effective for ratings of parent–child arguing. Because of the heterogeneity of ADHD, it is important to match psychotherapeutic recommendations to the individual profile of the patient. Patients with primarily academic issues tend to need more organizational assistance, patients with behavioral problems need a greater focus on behavioral awareness and control, and patients with predominantly social problems may require interpersonal therapies.

▶ Complications/Adverse Outcomes of Treatment

If adult ADHD is a clinically significant disorder, then ADHD adults should show functional impairments in multiple domains. Several studies suggest this to be true. An increasing number of studies have documented that adults with ADHD had lower socioeconomic status, more work difficulties, and more frequent job changes. The adults with ADHD had fewer years of education and lower rates of professional employment. Similarly, others have shown that among patients with substance use disorders, ADHD predicts social maladjustment, immaturity, fewer social assets, lower occupational achievement, and high rates of separation and divorce.

▶ Prognosis

ADHD is a prevalent worldwide, heterogeneous disorder that often persists into adult years. The disorder is associated with significant impairment in occupational, academic, social, and intrapersonal domains necessitating treatment. Converging data strongly support a preponderant neurobiological and genetic basis for ADHD with catecholaminergic dysfunction as a central finding. Although psychosocial interventions such as educational remediation and cognitive–behavioral approaches should be considered in the management of ADHD, an extensive literature supports the effectiveness of pharmacotherapy not only for the core behavioral symptoms of ADHD but also for improvement in linked impairments including cognition, social skills, and family function.

American Psychiatric Association. *Diagnostic and Statistical Manual of Mental Disorders.* 5th ed. Washington, DC: American Psychiatric Association; 2013.

Biederman J, Mick E, Faraone S. Normalized functioning in youths with persistent ADHD. *J Pediatr.* 1998;133:544–551.

Biederman J, Petty CR, Woodworth KY, et al. Adult outcome of attention-deficit/hyperactivity disorder: a controlled 16-year follow-up study. *J Clin Psychiatry.* 2012;73:941–950.

Castellanos FX, Lee PP, Sharp W, et al. Developmental trajectories of brain volume abnormalities in children and adolescents with attention-deficit/hyperactivity disorder. *JAMA* 2002;288:1740–1748.

Cohen SC, Mulqueen JM, Ferracioli-Oda E, Stuckelman ZD, Coughlin CG, Leckman JF, Bloch MH. Meta-analysis: risk of tics associated with psychostimulant use in randomized, placebo-controlled trials. *J Am Acad Child Adolesc Psychiatry.* 2015 Sep;54(9):728–736. doi: 10.1016/j.jaac.2015.06.011. Epub 2015 Jul 2. PMID: 26299294.

Cortese S, Kelly C, Chabernaud C, et al. Toward systems neuroscience of ADHD: a meta-analysis of 55 fMRI studies. *Am J Psychiatry.* 2012;169:1038–1055.

Faraone SV, Mick E. Molecular genetics of attention deficit hyperactivity disorder. *Psychiatr Clin North Am.* 2010;33:159–180.

MTA Cooperative Group. A 14-month randomized clinical trial of treatment strategies for attention-deficit/hyperactivity disorder. The MTA Cooperative Group. Multimodal Treatment Study of Children with ADHD. *Arch Gen Psychiatry.* 1999;56:1073–1086.

Spencer TJ, Brown A, Seidman LJ, et al. Effect of psychostimulants on brain structure and function in ADHD: a qualitative literature review of magnetic resonance imaging-based neuroimaging studies. *J Clin Psychiatry.* 2013;74:902–917.

Willcutt EG. The prevalence of DSM-IV attention-deficit/hyperactivity disorder: a meta-analytic review. *Neurotherapeutics.* 2012;9:490–499.

Oppositional Defiant Disorder and Conduct Disorder

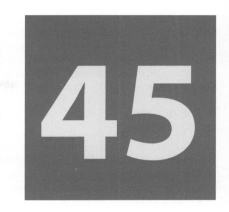

45

Mary M. LaLonde, MD, PhD
Jeffrey H. Newcorn, MD

Oppositional defiant disorder (ODD) and conduct disorder (CD)—together referred to as the disruptive behavior disorders (DBD) of childhood and adolescence—are frequently occurring and highly impairing disorders that share many core symptoms, associated features, and impairments. In the *Diagnostic and Statistical Manual of Mental Disorders*, Fifth Edition (DSM-5), ODD and CD have been placed with like-kind conditions that occur across the life span in the subgrouping "Disruptive, Impulse-Control, and Conduct Disorders." Each condition can present with disruptive behavior, academic underachievement, and poor social skills; impulsivity is also often present. ODD represents a risk factor for subsequent development of CD, and almost all youth with CD also have ODD. However, the two conditions also differ in important ways and are therefore best considered to be related, but distinct.

OPPOSITIONAL DEFIANT DISORDER

ESSENTIALS OF DIAGNOSIS

International Statistical Classification of Diseases and Related Health Problems—10th Revision (ICD-10) Diagnostic Criteria for Oppositional Defiant Disorder (ODD)

ODD (F91.3)

A conduct disorder (CD), usually occurring in younger children, is primarily characterized by markedly defiant, disobedient, disruptive behavior that does not include delinquent acts or the more extreme forms of aggressive or dissocial behavior. Caution should be employed before using this category, especially with older children, because clinically significant CD will usually be accompanied by dissocial or aggressive behavior that goes beyond mere defiance, disobedience, or disruptiveness. The key to distinguishing

ODD from other types of CDs is the absence of behaviors that violate the law and the basic rights of others.

Adapted with permission from International Statistical Classification of Diseases and Related Health Problems, 10th Revision (ICD-10). World Health Organization (WHO); 2010.

► General Considerations

As defined in DSM-5, ODD is categorized by a persistent pattern of age-inappropriate oppositional and defiant behavior toward adults (e.g., parents and teachers) and/or peers, and violation of minor rules and social conventions. Youth with ODD are often argumentative, defiant, annoying, irritable, resentful, and vindictive, and they tend to blame others for their own transgressions or omissions American Psychiatric Association. *Diagnostic and Statistical Manual of Mental Disorders*. 5th ed. Aggression, which is often but not always present, is predominantly verbal rather than physical. However, physical aggression can occur and does not necessarily signal the presence of CD. Aggression tends to be reactive (e.g., in response to imposition of unwanted rules by adults) rather than proactive or instrumental (e.g., bullying of peers for some perceived gain). It is more often overt (e.g., shouting) than covert (e.g., spreading malicious rumors), though there are important gender differences. Symptoms often begin early in life, though there are also later-onset cases. It is inconsistent if the behaviors persist into adolescence and adulthood in one form or another and, consequently, the diagnosis is relatively unstable. Clinical treatment and research are complicated by the high prevalence of comorbidity, which has an important role in moderating clinical presentation, response to treatment, and longitudinal course.

The definition of ODD as a categorical disorder is fraught with important and challenging questions. Specifically, it is unclear to what extent oppositional behavior is best considered to lie on a continuum between normal developmental limit-testing and pathologically disruptive behavior. While the

ICD-10 places ODD within the CD category and considers ODD to be a less pervasive and less severe developmental precursor to CD, DSM-5 treats ODD and CD as related but distinct entities. Moreover, oppositional and defiant behavior is seen in association with many childhood psychiatric conditions, which raises questions regarding divergent validity.

A. Epidemiology

ODD is highly prevalent, although there is considerable variability across studies—reflecting not only differences in populations but also variability in assessment methods and case definition. Worldwide prevalence estimates range from 1% to 11%, with an average of 3.3% (Canino et al, 2010). Male predominance (1.4:1) is found in pre-adolescent samples but not consistently in adolescent samples (Boylan et al, 2007). The National Comorbidity Survey—Replication (NCS-R) estimated the lifetime prevalence of ODD to be 10.2%, and somewhat higher for males (11.2%) than females (9.2%). ODD can begin as early as age 3, but is typically noted by age 8. The average age of onset is 6 years (Nock et al, 2007).

B. Etiology

Childhood oppositionality has heterogeneous origins. Because CD often evolves from earlier oppositional behavior, and because the two disorders have similar risk factors, ODD and CD are often discussed together.

1. Neurobiological factors—Although there is a paucity of research, recent studies examining mood dysregulation in the context of DBDs are relevant to ODD and represent the basis for the new DSM-5 diagnostic category, disruptive mood dysregulation disorder (DMDD). Specifically, children with severe, chronic irritability were found to have abnormally reduced activation in the left amygdala, bilateral striatum, parietal cortex, and posterior cingulate—areas implicated in emotion, attention, and reward processing (Deveney et al, 2013). Studies using quantitative electroencephalography (EEG) measures have found that the profile of low delta/high alpha activity is correlated with measures of emotion and behavior problems (McGough et al, 2013).

2. Psychological factors—Psychological and neuropsychological factors that have been linked to risk for ODD include difficult temperament, disturbed social cognition and reciprocity, negative and hostile attributions, and deficient inhibitory control and reward sensitivity. Many young children who exhibit oppositional defiant behavior had temperamental antecedents as infants, including early signs of emotional dysregulation such as irritability, inability to be soothed, and slow adaptation to new circumstances (Stringaris et al, 2010). Children with the combination of high novelty seeking, low harm avoidance, low reward dependence, and deficient inhibitory control are at greatest risk. These temperamental factors also likely interact with early life experiences and parent–child interactions; infants who exhibit disorganized attachment behavior are at risk for oppositional and disruptive behavior in middle childhood.

As children grow, they begin to develop stable patterns of social information processing and emotion regulation. These patterns are determined not only biologically but also through a complex interplay among temperament, psychological capacities, and experience in family, peer, and community environments. Three interrelated mental domains are found to be disrupted in aggressive children— punishment processing, reward processing, and cognitive control (Matthys et al, 2013). Aggressive children tend to have cognitive distortions in both the appraisal and problem-solving phases of social–cognitive processing. Thus, aggressive children have difficulties encoding incoming social information and accurately interpreting social events and others' intentions; importantly, they recall fewer nonhostile cues. Their deficits in problem solving are thought to be due to their desire for social domination and revenge. In addition, they often perceive aggressive behavior in a positive manner and expect that aggressive behavior will yield positive outcomes for them.

3. Environmental factors—Several studies have found that maternal use of alcohol, nicotine, cocaine, and other drugs of abuse during pregnancy substantially increases risk for behavior problems in offspring, possibly related to toxic effects on neurodevelopment of catecholamine systems and/or alterations in gene expression. However, determining causality is complicated by the fact that rates of conduct/antisocial disorders, ADHD, and substance abuse in offspring are likely increased in mothers with ADHD, behavior disorders, and substance use disorders (SUD) who use alcohol, nicotine, or other drugs during pregnancy. Thus, gene–environment interactions are likely important. A number of other environmental factors have been found to result in the co-occurrence of behavior problems with lower IQ and short attention span. For example, exposure to high or even moderate levels of lead increases risk for a variety of cognitive and behavioral problems. The magnitude of the relationship between lead exposure and conduct problems is similar to that for lead exposure and decreased IQ. Other studies suggest that exposure to environmental toxins, such as polychlorinated biphenyls (PCBs) and methylmercury, can increase the risk for attentional and conduct problems (Latimer et al, 2012; Carpenter & Nevin, 2010).

4. Social–familial factors—Numerous social–familial factors also have been shown to increase risk for ODD and CD (especially the latter) (Boden et al, 2010). Social adversity factors include large sibships, parental separation, single-parent households, early deprivation or neglect, parental conflict, adoption, and poverty. Compromised childrearing practices such as harsh physical discipline, low parental warmth, and poor supervision are associated with elevated risk for ODD and CD. In addition, parental depression, antisocial personality, and substance use increase risk for both disorders.

Recent data indicate that the experience of abuse, family violence, or other traumatic events in early childhood may be associated with increased risk for conduct and attention problems. The foregoing factors seem to operate in an additive fashion, with the probability of ODD/CD increasing linearly when there is aggregation of risk. Finally, a multitude of less serious but problematic parent–child interactions may influence the development and course of oppositional and disruptive behavior. The lack of positive reinforcement for acceptable behavior is often associated with negative attention gained through oppositional behavior. Often, there is inconsistent, unpredictable, and harsh punishment. Table 45–1 lists the characteristics of a coercive parent–child interaction and how these factors can be targeted for psychotherapeutic intervention (Templeman, n.d.).

C. Genetics

The genetics of ODD have not been studied apart from that of aggression and CD. Overall, genetic studies of aggressive behavior in children have demonstrated moderate heritability, with candidate genes involved in noradrenergic, dopaminergic, and serotonergic neurotransmission (Malmberg et al, 2008). (See the Conduct Disorder section for more detailed discussion.)

▶ Clinical Findings

A. Signs & Symptoms

The clinical assessment of ODD requires a thorough approach involving multiple methods and informants (Steiner et al, 2007). Generally, adults are considered to be the best informants of disruptive behavior in children, although older children and adolescents may be better able to provide information regarding mood and anxiety symptoms, cognitive difficulties, and infrequent or covert antisocial behaviors. Assessment requires information from caregivers and school professionals regarding the presence and severity of core and associated symptoms in school, home, and social settings; age of onset; duration of symptoms; presence of symptoms of frequently occurring comorbid conditions; and degree of impairment in age-appropriate functions.

The persistent, recurrent aggressive and defiant behavior associated with ODD may be restricted to one setting (e.g., home or school) or may be pervasive across settings. Symptoms are usually evident before 8 years of age but may emerge for the first time in adolescence. Oppositional, hostile, limit-testing behavior disrupts family relationships and can interfere with learning. At school, oppositional children or adolescents may be moody, irritable, and lacking in self-esteem. They often get into conflicts with teachers and other adults and often appear to have a "chip on their shoulder." In addition, they often annoy, argue with, or bully peers and, as a result, do not usually have satisfying and growth-enhancing peer relationships. Some oppositional adolescents may be solitary (e.g., those with callous and unemotional traits) or inclined to gravitate to the company of others who regard themselves as outlaws (e.g., those with predelinquent behavior). However, this is certainly not always the case. There is increased risk for early tobacco, alcohol, and other substance use—but this is more characteristic of youth with ODD who escalate to CD.

Table 45–1 Characteristics of the Parent-Child Coercive Cycle

Parent-Driven		Child-Driven	
The Cycle	**Breaking the Cycle**	**The Cycle**	**Breaking the Cycle**
Parent gives directive that is ignored by child (e.g., Do your homework. Get off the computer. Clean your room)	Parent gives directive that is ignored by child	Child makes demands that parent refuses (e.g., Give me back my phone! I want ice cream! I need to go to Riley's house!)	Child makes demands that parent refuses, and child acts out or argues
Parent (attacker) increases demands and child argues (counter-attack). Attack and counter-attack continue and escalate	Parent stops talking, removes a reinforcer (e.g. turns off TV), or removes child from reinforcement (e.g. moves away from toy aisle and time out)	Child acts out and parent gives up or backs off	Parent stops talking, removes reinforcers, or puts child in time out
Parent gives up or backs off, which reinforces arguing by child	Once child begins to comply, parent gives positive reinforcement (e.g., reacts positively, speaks positively, or provides other reinforcement)	Child quiets down. Cycle reinforces acting out by child	Once child calms, parent gives positive reinforcement. Parent makes counter-offer to child's request and stays engaged with child as long as child remains calm
Increases likelihood that same behavior will recur next time		Increases likelihood that same behavior will recur next time	

B. Clinical and Psychological Assessment

1. Rating scales—Broad-based rating scales survey a wide range of behaviors and are excellent for comprehensive assessment and screening of youth with ODD (Table 45–2). Commonly used broad-based scales are the Conners Parent and Teacher Rating Scales, the Achenbach Child Behavior Checklist and Teacher Report Form, and the Behavioral Assessment Scales for Children. Each of these instruments has one or more subscales for oppositional or aggressive behavior as well as several other domains of function. Rating scales, which more specifically evaluate DSM symptoms, include the Swanson, Nolan, and Pelham (SNAP) Parent and Teacher Rating Scales and the Vanderbilt ADHD Parent and Teacher Ratings Scales. Although these instruments are well known as scales for ADHD, the SNAP-IV and Vanderbilt include the DSM ODD items, and the Vanderbilt covers a variety of other mood, anxiety, and conduct problem behaviors. In addition, careful assessment of ADHD symptoms is essential, given the high degree of comorbidity (see later discussion).

Several instruments have been developed to specifically measure the spectrum of oppositional/aggressive behavior. The Inattention, Overactivity With Aggression (IOWA) Conners is made up of five items from the Conners for inattention/cognitive impairment and five items for aggression.

The New York Teacher Rating Scale includes the DSM items for both ODD and CD as well as a number of other disruptive and/or aggressive behaviors. The Overt Aggression Scale (OAS) is an observer-rated instrument designed to measure aggressive behavior in inpatient settings, whereas the Overt Aggression Scale—Modified (OAS-M) obtains this information via self/other report suitable for outpatient settings. The Buss–Perry Aggression scale is a self-report measure that has been used in adolescents as well as adults and provides information on four domains of aggressive behavior: physical aggression, verbal aggression, anger, and hostility. The Children's Aggression Scale (CAS) likewise measures the full range of physical aggression (verbal aggression, aggression against objects and animals, provoked physical aggression, unprovoked physical aggression, and use of weapons) but was specifically developed for children and adolescents.

Rating scales that measure key contextual factors related to parenting and/or family environment can also be helpful. The Alabama Parenting Questionnaire (APQ) measures several dimensions implicated in conduct problems: positive reinforcement, parental involvement, inconsistent discipline, poor monitoring and supervision, and harsh discipline. The Family Environment Scale (FES) is a 90-item inventory that contains subscales measuring family relationship, personal growth, and system maintenance and change. The

Table 45–2 Rating Scales for the Assessment of Oppositional/Aggressive Behavior

Scale	Description	References
Inattention, Overactivity With Aggression Conners'	Contains five items from the Conners for inattention/cognitive impairment and five items for aggression.	Loney and Milich 1982
New York Teacher Rating Scale (NYTRS)	Teacher report that includes DSM items for ODD and CD, as well as additional items for disruptive and/or aggressive behavior.	Miller et al. 1995
Overt Aggression Scale (OAS)—Modified	Modification of OAS for outpatient settings; rates behavior over a 1-week interval. Contains the same four domains of aggression. The addition of a 5-point response format allows assessment of both severity and frequency.	Sorgi et al. 1991
Buss–Perry Hostility Inventory	Modified version for youth with updated items, elimination of irrelevant items, and improved readability for youth with lower verbal abilities.	Buss and Perry 1992
Children's Aggression Scale (CAS) Parent and Teacher versions	Contains five factors: verbal aggression, aggression against objects and animals, provoked physical aggression, unprovoked physical aggression, and use of weapons. Distinguishes aggression (1) inside vs. outside the home and (2) against children vs. adults.	Halperin et al. 2002, 2003
Alabama Parenting Questionnaire (APQ)	Measures several dimensions implicated in conduct problems: positive reinforcement, parental involvement, inconsistent discipline, poor monitoring and supervision, and harsh discipline.	Frick 1991
Family Environment Scale (FES)	90-item inventory that contains subscales measuring family relationship, personal growth, and system maintenance and change.	Robertson and Hyde 1982
Parent–Child Conflict Tactics Scale (PCCTS)	Measures psychological and physical maltreatment and neglect of children by parents as well as nonviolent forms of discipline.	Straus et al. 1998
Parenting Stress Index (PSI) Child and Adolescent versions	Identifies stressful aspects of the parent and child relationship.	Loyd and Abidin 1985

Parent-Child Conflict Tactics Scale (PCCTS) primarily measures parental treatment of children, especially psychological and physical maltreatment and neglect. Finally, the child and adolescent versions of the Parenting Stress Index (PSI) identify stressful aspects of the parent–child relationship.

2. Diagnostic interviews—Several structured and semistructured clinical interviews have been designed for assessment of children and adolescents, including the Schedule for Affective Disorders and Schizophrenia for School Aged Children (K-SADS), Diagnostic Interview Schedule for Children (DISC-IV), Diagnostic Interview for Children and Adolescents (DICA), Child and Adolescent Psychiatric Assessment (CAPA), and Child Assessment Schedule (CAS).

3. Neuropsychological assessment—Neuropsychological testing is not required to diagnose ODD (or CD). However, neuropsychological and/or educational tests of cognitive, linguistic, perceptual, motor, and academic functioning can be used to augment clinical assessment by providing normed data required for the diagnosis of specific learning disabilities, which often co-occur, and to justify the need for supplemental services and school placement. Although neuropsychological assessment is often considered less important for assessment of ODD than ADHD, there is evidence that neuropsychological tests of executive function are impaired in individuals with ODD as well. Data obtained through neuropsychological evaluation can be helpful in the design of a comprehensive treatment plan.

C. Laboratory Findings

There are no physical findings or laboratory measures that reliably distinguish ODD and CD from each other, other disorders, or controls—although it is well established that reduced noradrenergic function is associated with behavioral overarousal and aggression.

D. Neuroimaging

There are no neuroimaging studies in youth with ODD apart from those conducted in youth with aggression, CD, or psychopathic traits. However, recent studies examining neural correlates of callous and unemotional traits in youth with aggression may be relevant to the spectrum of ODD behaviors. See the previous section on Neurobiological Factors in ODD.

E. Course of Illness

Onset of ODD can be as early as the preschool years and ODD symptoms are typically noted by age 8 (Steiner et al, 2007). Onset is rare after 16 years of age. There are several possible developmental trajectories. During the preschool years, transient oppositional behavior is very common. However, if oppositionality persists, there is heightened risk for escalation to more clinically significant disruptive behavior. In most oppositional children, who are usually not physically aggressive, oppositional behaviors peak in mid-childhood, around the age 8, and decline after that. In others, oppositional behavior increases and escalates to delinquent behavior. The early presentation of physical aggression is a key predictor of this latter trajectory, as physically aggressive children are more likely to progress from early oppositional behaviors to more severe and disabling conduct problems.

▶ Differential Diagnosis (Including Comorbid Conditions)

ODD should be differentiated from normal developmental limit-testing in toddlers and preschool children and from the challenging confrontations that occur between parents and typical adolescents who are seeking to be more independent. Developmental oppositional behavior is transitory, causes little impairment of note, and should not be diagnosed as ODD.

In the NCS-R, virtually all children with ODD (92.4%) also met criteria for at least one other lifetime DSM-IV-TR disorder, including mood (45.8%), anxiety (62.3%), impulse-control (68.2%), and substance-use (47.2%) disorders. Even after accounting for age and the presence of other disorders, the odds ratios for comorbid ADHD, depression, and anxiety were all significantly elevated in children with ODD (Nock et al, 2007). Given the high degree of comorbidity of ODD with other psychiatric disorders, assessment must thoroughly examine all symptom domains. One challenge in accomplishing this is that the conspicuous nature of disruptive behaviors can divert attention from less prominent or overt symptoms, despite their importance for treatment and prognosis.

1. Conduct disorder (CD)—Discrimination of ODD and CD is complicated by their frequent co-occurrence; however, there are important distinguishing features. Although both ODD and CD involve conduct problems that bring the child into conflict with parents and other adult authority figures, the behaviors of ODD are typically less severe than those of CD and do not necessarily include aggression toward people or animals, destruction of property, or a pattern of theft or deceit. Consequently, children with ODD generally demonstrate less impairment and are more socially competent than children with CD. Furthermore, ODD can also present with symptoms of emotional dysregulation that are less characteristic of CD. Finally, children with CD generally come from less advantaged families and have greater conflict with school and judicial systems than those with ODD only. Family adversity scores in children with ODD are usually intermediate between those of children with CD and typically developing children.

2. ADHD—Although there is very little overlap in the defining characteristics of ADHD and ODD, the frequent co-occurrence of inattention, hyperactivity, impulsivity, oppositionality, and aggression suggests that these symptoms are closely related. The core symptoms of ADHD and ODD are not identical, despite the very high rate of comorbidity. For example, ODD symptoms, such as "loses temper," "actively defies," and "swears," are not characteristic of children with ADHD only and can therefore be used to distinguish the two disorders. Children with ADHD who have high levels of hyperactive/impulsive symptoms are at greatest risk for also having ODD. Nonetheless, approximately 30% of children with ADHD and comorbid ODD have predominantly inattentive subtype.

3. Affective disorders—Distinguishing depressive and bipolar disorders from ODD and CD is often difficult, as it is not uncommon for children with depressive disorders to display poor frustration tolerance and irritability. However, these symptoms can be differentiated from the chronic mood problems seen in youth with ODD by their episodic nature. Several studies have suggested that a subgroup of children with severe impulsivity, hyperactivity, mood dysregulation, irritability, oppositionality, and conduct problems have underlying bipolar disorder, but results from other studies are inconsistent with this view. In youth with severe irritability and aggression, care must be taken to apply the diagnosis of bipolar disorder only in those children in whom manic or hypomanic symptom(s) represent a distinct episode of required duration and in whom irritability and mood dysregulation can be clearly distinguished from the individual's baseline. In children with disruptive behavior and persistent and severe irritability, the diagnosis of DMDD would be more appropriate. In DMDD, the severity, frequency, and chronicity of temper outbursts are greater than in children with ODD alone. Because of the obvious potential for overlap, when the disturbance in mood is severe enough to meet criteria for DMDD, a diagnosis of ODD is not given even if all criteria for ODD are met. See the CD Differential Diagnosis section on page 695 for further discussion of DMDD comorbidity.

4. Anxiety disorders—Generalized anxiety disorder (GAD) does not generally present with oppositional or defiant behavior; however, oppositional symptoms can occur in response to a perceived fear stimulus. When present, these behaviors do not reflect the individual's overall capacity for self-regulation, as in ODD. Children and adolescents with separation anxiety disorder may be oppositional in the context of being forced to separate from attachment figures, whereas children with social anxiety disorder may be defiant because of fear of negative evaluation by others.

5. Trauma and stress-related disorders—Posttraumatic stress disorder (PTSD) in children is most frequently comorbid with ODD and separation anxiety disorder, and the diagnosis of ODD may be cautiously made when defiance, oppositionality, irritability, and noncompliance occur in the context of chronic PTSD symptoms. As with affective and anxiety disorders, PTSD and adjustment disorder can present with alterations in conduct, but these conditions can be distinguished from ODD by obtaining a thorough longitudinal history of the behavioral problems and identifying a psychosocial stressor that preceded their onset.

6. Schizophrenia—It is not uncommon for the prodromal phase of schizophrenia to present with a variety of negative symptoms including academic underachievement, negativism, lack of motivation, and conduct problems—behaviors that are also present in many youth with ODD. Children with ODD will also frequently report perceptual disturbances such as auditory hallucinations telling them to do certain things to avoid blame and punishment. A careful history and description of the hallucinations should easily differentiate nonpsychotic from psychotic hallucinations.

7. Substance use disorders (SUD)—Because ODD is associated with early-onset substance use as well as heightened risk for SUD, it is crucial to evaluate for the presence of substance use and related behaviors, especially in adolescents. However, development of SUD is more often characteristic of youth with ODD who progress to CD.

8. Medical conditions—In addition to psychiatric comorbidity, a variety of medical conditions can co-occur with ODD (and CD), including epilepsy, sleep disorders, thyroid disease, postinfectious and/or posttraumatic encephalopathy, and sensory impairments. More often, it is important to rule out these conditions. Finally, many medications that are prescribed to children can produce behavioral dysfunction and mimic the symptoms of ODD. Examples include anticonvulsants (e.g., phenobarbital), antihistamines, decongestants, bronchodilators (e.g., theophylline), and systemic steroids, all of which are associated with disinhibition syndromes. Special attention to periodicity and the longitudinal course of symptoms is required for accurate diagnosis.

▶ Treatment

Given the wide-ranging deficits seen in youth with ODD, the high rates of comorbidity, and the presence of associated features such as academic underachievement, poor peer relations, and low self-esteem, a multimodal approach including both psychosocial and pharmacotherapeutic modalities is usually required (Steiner et al, 2007). In initiating psychosocial and/or medication therapy, it is important to identify specific target behaviors associated with impairment in one or more settings and to systematically assess change in the number and severity of these behaviors. In addition, it is important to assess comorbidity at baseline and over the course of treatment. As there are no specific medication treatments for ODD, it is important to identify specific symptom domains and/or comorbid disorders responsive to medication and use this information to guide treatment.

A. Psychopharmacological Interventions

The pharmacological treatment of ODD is less solidly evidence-based than that of comorbid disorders such as ADHD.

However, findings from recent studies suggest that ODD symptoms in youth with comorbid ADHD are reasonably well treated with off-label use of approved medications for ADHD (Steiner et al, 2007). Placebo-controlled trials have repeatedly demonstrated the efficacy of psychostimulants in treating aggressive and disruptive behaviors in youth with ADHD. Although there are limited studies examining the efficacy of stimulants in ODD independent of ADHD, the available data suggest this may also be the case (Pringsheim et al, 2015a). A major safety consideration regarding use of stimulants in youth with ODD (and especially CD) relates to the potential for misuse, abuse, and diversion of medication. It is therefore important to discuss issues related to abuse and diversion of medication with adolescents and to screen for signs and symptoms of substance abuse in monitoring treatment. It is also useful to consider using nonstimulants. There is mounting evidence for the utility of the alpha-2 adrenergic agonists clonidine and guanfacine and the selective norepinephrine (NE) reuptake inhibitor atomoxetine in treating oppositional symptoms in the context of ADHD (Garg et al, 2015; Pringsheim et al, 2015a). Serotonergic antidepressants can be potentially useful in the treatment of children and adolescents with aggressive and impulsive symptoms of ODD in the context of depression or anxiety. There are several open studies and case reports using fluoxetine in the treatment of children with DBD—both with and without comorbid mood disorder. One placebo-controlled study of depressed adolescents with high levels of oppositionality demonstrated that fluoxetine alone, cognitive–behavioral therapy (CBT) alone, and combination treatment were effective in reducing oppositional symptoms—although greater reductions in oppositional symptoms were seen in the fluoxetine arms (Jacobs et al, 2010). As of now, there is little evidence for the use of antipsychotic or mood-stabilizing medications in the treatment of ODD alone. However, recent data support the use of antipsychotic medication to augment response in youth with comorbid ADHD and aggression (Aman et al, 2014; Gadow et al, 2014). The systematic review by Gorman et al (2015) reported the most evidence for the antipsychotic medication risperidone for treating disruptive or aggressive behavior in patients who did poorly on stimulant or alpha agonist medications. However, risperidone only received a conditional recommendation, given its significant metabolic adverse effects.

B. Psychosocial Interventions

There are numerous evidence-based psychosocial interventions for youth with DBDs that have been found to be efficacious and cost-effective in improving child conduct problems, parental mental health, and parenting skills (Comer et al, 2013; Furlong et al, 2013). The broad array of interventions include parent training, family-centered therapy, behavioral modification, CBT, social skills training, and intensive summer treatment programs. Because family, peer, and school

Table 45–3 Components of Parent Management Training

Learn about developmentally appropriate behavior and how to analyze child's negative behaviors to see what maintains them.

Pay attention to the positives.

Ignore minor inappropriate behavior.

Communicate effectively by giving clear, brief commands, reducing task complexity, and eliminating competing influences (e.g., television).

Establish systems for natural or low-cost rewards to reinforce good behavior.

Use consequences such as time out and removing privileges for misbehavior.

Learn to stay calm and not react emotionally to child by learning how to handle negative emotions that arise when child is misbehaving.

Learn how to solve problems collaboratively with child.

interactions are important in the morbidity and maintenance of these disorders, it is important to target each of these areas with appropriate interventions.

For children under 12 years of age, treatment is provided primarily through parents (and sometimes teachers). Parents are educated concerning the origin and meaning of oppositional defiant behavior, taught about common impairments and how to anticipate them, and trained to restructure the environment and to replace coercive discipline with more effective childrearing techniques. Table 45–3 describes the essentials of effective parenting (Feldman & Kazdin, 1995).

1. Parent–child interaction therapy (PCIT)—PCIT is a form of behavioral parent training for children aged 2–7 with emotional and behavioral problems and their caregivers. Its emphasis is on improving the quality of the parent–child relationship and changing parent–child interaction patterns. PCIT is divided into two stages: relationship development, which is child-directed, and discipline training, which is parent-directed. The child-directed interaction portion aims to improve the parent–child relationship through play therapy. Parents are taught a list of "dos" and "don'ts" to use while interacting with their child during daily "special time." The parent-directed interaction portion aims to teach parents more effective ways of disciplining their child through a combination of play therapy and behavioral modification. PCIT has been shown to be effective in reducing oppositional/disruptive behaviors in DBDs as well as in other disorders, and the changes in behavior are maintained in long-term follow-up (Hood & Eyberg, 2003).

2. The Incredible Years—The Incredible Years is a multicomponent program that involves parents, children (3- to 8 years old), and teachers. It has been shown to be effective for reducing aggression, increasing positive social skills, and improving problem-solving and conflict-management skills. Although child treatment alone has been shown to be effective, co-delivery of the child and parent components is even more efficacious. Two thirds of children with an ODD/CD diagnosis no longer meet criteria for these diagnoses 5–6 years after completing the Incredible Years intervention (Drugli et al, 2010). The Incredible Years intervention was used to examine differential susceptibility (i.e., children with a certain trait function poorly under adverse conditions, whereas children with the trait function better than those without it under favorable conditions); children who exhibited the trait of emotionally dysregulated behavior had a greater decrease in conduct problems with improvement in parental care (Scott & O'Connor, 2012).

3. The positive parenting program (Triple P)—Triple P is a parenting and family support program that has been shown to decrease dysfunctional parenting behaviors, increase positive parenting behaviors, and decrease both internalizing and externalizing child behavior in the long term (Hahlweg et al, 2010). It can be delivered at five different levels that vary in breadth and depth. Each level of the Triple P system focuses on five main goals: promoting safe and engaging environments, creating positive learning environments, using effective discipline, creating clear and reasonable expectations, and encouraging parental self-care (Haggerty et al, 2013). Levels 1 and 2 provide information about parenting behavior and child development. Levels 3–5 are more intensive approaches that focus on children with mild to severe behavioral problems. Level 3, for example, is administered to parents of children with mild or moderate behavioral issues. The four-session counseling intervention consists of issue-specific psychoeducation and parent skills training. Level 4 is intended for caregivers whose children display moderate to serious behavioral problems. It provides more and longer sessions, and parents are taught key skills through modeling, rehearsal, and self-evaluation. Level 4 interventions have been found to reduce disruptive behaviors, a reduction that is maintained in long-term follow-up. If children in Level 4 continue to experience behavioral difficulties, they are referred to Level 5, where they receive additional family intervention.

4. CBT: The Coping Power Program—Several programs that use CBT techniques have been demonstrated to be effective in the treatment of DBDs, and most of these programs use similar core components of emotion awareness, perspective taking, anger management, social problem solving, and goal setting. Furthermore, most have a parent training component, as the combination of CBT and parent training is often more effective than either intervention alone.

The Coping Power Program is most appropriate for aggressive and disruptive children transitioning to middle school (grades 4–6). The child component consists of cognitive–behavioral group sessions with periodic individual sessions that are designed to help the child set short- and long-term goals; improve organization and study skills, anger management skills, social skills, and problem-solving skills; and learn how to resist peer pressure and enter into more positive peer groups. The parent component is also a series of group sessions interspersed with individual sessions aimed at helping the parent be more effective at providing positive attention, setting clear rules and expectations, promoting children's study skills, implementing appropriate discipline strategies, communicating, and problem solving. The Coping Power Program has been shown to reduce aggressive behavior, prevent substance use, reduce delinquent behavior, improve school functioning, and improve social competence and social information processing (Lochman et al, 2011).

5. The Family Check-Up—The Family Check-Up (FCU) program is grounded in coercion theory and aims to decrease family conflict while increasing parental monitoring. It is designed to support parents' accurate appraisals of their child's risk status and their own parenting practices. It then helps parents to identify appropriate family-centered interventions and implement change strategies. This is achieved through an initial interview, family assessment, and feedback session focused on parental motivation to improve parenting behaviors. Randomized trials have demonstrated the effectiveness of FCU to improve family management by parents, reduce coercive interactions between parent and adolescent, and improve adolescent behavior by decreasing deviant peer association, substance use, and antisocial behavior, while also improving school performance. The FCU has also been shown to decrease depressive symptoms in adolescents (Van Ryzin et al, 2012).

6. Problem-solving communication training (PSCT)—PSCT promotes more effective family communication and problem solving, helps the family generalize their new skills to the home environment, and reverses family structural and functional difficulties. Family communication and problem solving are addressed by eliciting the common causes of family disagreement and then ranking them in order of seriousness or difficulty. The family is directed to address one cause of dispute per session, starting with the least acrimonious, by first defining the problem, generating alternative solutions, taking turns evaluating each proposed solution, and then implementing the agreed-upon solution and evaluating its effectiveness. As the family addresses these problems, family communication difficulties can be remediated with the use of feedback, instruction, modeling, and behavioral rehearsal. In the course of treatment, the family's rigid, biased beliefs are revealed and targeted for cognitive restructuring. PSCT has been found to be effective in improving parent–adolescent conflict in adolescents with ADHD and ODD (Barkley et al, 2001).

▶ Prognosis

DSM-5 indicated a developmental link between ODD and CD, as virtually all youth with CD also have ODD, even though the majority of children with ODD do not develop CD. This developmental relationship was further supported by the findings of shared psychosocial, family, and individual risk factors including temperament, neurological deficits, and genetic liabilities. However, direct tests of this developmental relationship have yielded mixed results. Recent studies have demonstrated that different ODD symptom domains may have different outcomes (Rowe et al, 2010). Approximately one third of children with ODD will progress to CD, and one third of those with CD progress to antisocial personality disorder (ASPD) by age 25. Factors favoring the progression to CD include subthreshold CD symptoms, which are not independent of family and environmental factors, and persistent physical aggression. Family instability appears to be the most significant factor in this progression. There is some evidence that parental hostility and lower socioeconomic status may be associated with comorbid ODD/CD. Boys are at greater risk of developing CD, whereas no sex differences have been found in "pure" ODD. In the ODD to CD pathway, in which ODD precedes CD, the onset of CD is typically before the age 10 (childhood onset CD) and onset is uncommon at later ages (Rowe et al, 2010). Despite the uncommon occurrence of pure ODD progressing to pure CD, youth in either of these "pure" categories have higher levels of subthreshold symptoms of the other diagnosis compared to youth with neither diagnosis. In children with late-onset CD (i.e., after age 10), symptoms of ODD and ADHD are usually not present during early childhood. About 50% of youth continue to exhibit ODD in late childhood and adolescence, whereas 25% will cease to meet criteria for either ODD or CD. The presence of either active or remitted ODD significantly predicts subsequent onset of other disorders. Both early-onset ODD (before age 8) and ODD plus comorbidity predict a more chronic course, with less robust and less immediate improvement following treatment. Coexistent ADHD speeds the escalation to more severe conduct problems, resulting in elevated rates of ASPD and SUD in adulthood. Moreover, the ODD symptom clusters of negative affect (angry/irritable mood) appear to predict later depression and anxiety, whereas oppositional behaviors (argumentative/defiant) predict later CD.

CONDUCT DISORDER

 ESSENTIALS OF DIAGNOSIS

ICD-10 Diagnostic Criteria for Conduct Disorder (CD)

CDs (F91)

Disorders characterized by a repetitive and persistent pattern of dissocial, aggressive, or defiant conduct. Such behavior should amount to major violations of age-appropriate social expectations; it should therefore be more severe than ordinary childish mischief or adolescent rebelliousness.

Examples of the behaviors on which the diagnosis is based include excessive levels of fighting or bullying, cruelty to other people or animals, severe destructiveness to property, fire-setting, stealing, repeated lying, truancy from school and running away from home, unusually frequent and severe temper tantrums, and disobedience. Any one of these behaviors, if marked, is sufficient for the diagnosis, but isolated dissocial acts are not.

Duration of behavior should be 6 months or longer.

Exclusion criteria include serious underlying conditions such as schizophrenia, hyperkinetic disorder, or depression.

Specify if CD is confined to family context or peer relationships or whether individual is well integrated in peer network.

CD Confined to Family Context (F91.0)

Disorder involving dissocial or aggressive behavior, in which the abnormal behavior is entirely, or almost entirely, confined to the home and to interactions with members of the nuclear family or immediate household.

Unsocialized CD (F91.1)

Disorder characterized by the combination of persistent dissocial or aggressive behavior with significant pervasive abnormalities in the individual's relationships with other children.

Socialized CD (F91.2)

Disorder involving persistent dissocial or aggressive behavior occurring in individuals who are generally well integrated into their peer group.

Mixed Disorders of Conduct and Emotions (F92)

A group of disorders characterized by persistently aggressive, dissocial, or defiant behavior with overt and marked symptoms of depression, anxiety, or other emotional upsets. The criteria for both CDs and emotional disorders of childhood or an adult-type neurotic disorder or a mood disorder must be met.

Specify depressive CD when there are marked depressive symptoms (F92.0). For persistent and marked emotional symptoms such as anxiety, obsessions or compulsions, depersonalization or derealization, phobias, or hypochondriasis, other mixed disorders of conduct and emotions, unspecified (F92.8) can be used.

Adapted with permission from International Statistical Classification of Diseases and Related Health Problems, 10th Revision (ICD-10). World Health Organization (WHO); 2010.

▶ General Considerations

CD describes a repetitive and persistent pattern of dissocial, aggressive, or defiant conduct, in which major age-appropriate social expectations are violated. It is worth noting several significant differences in the classification of conduct problems between ICD-10 and DSM-5. ICD-10 allows for peer influence on conduct problems (socialized vs. unsocialized CD) and also allows for specification of conduct problems that present only within the family context. Unlike ICD-10, DSM-5 subtypes CD by age of symptom onset, with childhood onset diagnosed when one of the behaviors was present before age 10 and adolescent onset diagnosed when all symptoms began after age 10. DSM-5 also has a "limited prosocial emotions" specifier, which includes: (1) lack of remorse or guilt unless the individual is caught or faces punishment and lack of concern about negative consequences of his or her actions; (2) callous lack of empathy for the feelings of others even if the individual's actions result in substantial harm; (3) being unconcerned about performance at school, work, or other important activities as manifested by lack of effort and blaming of others for poor performance; and (4) shallow or deficient affect characterized by superficial and insincere-appearing affect or use of emotional expression for personal gain. The limited prosocial emotions specifier is used only if these behaviors represent a typical pattern of functioning. In DSM-5, CD is further specified as mild, moderate, or severe—based on the degree of harm to others and the number of symptoms present in excess of the three required for diagnosis American Psychiatric Association. *Diagnostic and Statistical Manual of Mental Disorders*. 5th ed.

A. Epidemiology

The prevalence of CD is considerably lower than that of ODD in childhood, with rates estimated to be as low as 1% in school-age children but increasing several fold in adolescence. However, the gender bias is greater, with recent estimates of the male–female ratio being approximately 2:1. Males predominate before adolescence, but prevalence rates among the genders are closer by age 15 years because of an increase in covert, nonaggressive delinquent behavior among girls. The prevalence of CD does not seem to vary by race/ethnicity, but the rate is higher in youth without a high school education, in urban populations, and in the western United States. Worldwide prevalence estimates of CD are fairly consistent across different countries (Canino et al, 2010). An epidemiological birth sample found that 10.5% of boys with conduct problems had childhood onset of CD symptoms and maintenance of CD symptoms through adolescence. Several other subgroups were identified: 19.6% developed conduct problems for the first time during adolescence, 24.3% had conduct problems in childhood but subsequently desisted, and 45.6% had persistent but low levels of conduct problems and did not meet criteria for CD. Longitudinal studies have found that childhood-onset (<12 years) CD in girls is predicted by paternal ASPD, whereas adolescent-onset CD (≥12 years) is associated with family conflict.

B. Etiology

1. Neurobiological factors

Neurochemical—Reduced noradrenergic function in children with CD is suggested by findings of low cerebrospinal fluid (CSF) concentration of the methoxyhydroxyphenylglycol (MHPG) metabolite of NE and reduced activity of the enzyme dopamine-β-hydroxylase (which converts dopamine [DA] to NE), perhaps reflecting the role of NE in behavioral arousal. Other research has examined central serotonergic function in aggression and antisocial behavior because antisocial adults have consistently been characterized as having a hypo-serotonergic state—as indicated by reduced CSF levels of 5-hydroxyindoleacetic acid, a serotonin metabolite. One study correlated defiance and aggression with low levels of whole-blood 5-hydroxytryptamine; another suggested a relationship between DBD and lower concentrations of CSF somatostatin. Research examining the relationship between testosterone and aggressive crime has yielded inconsistent results. Results of the foregoing studies must be interpreted with caution, given that many of the children who participated experienced severe maltreatment and other contextual problems that could have affected the neurochemical systems in question.

Neuroanatomy and neurocircuitry—Studies of children with ADHD with comorbid CD have demonstrated reduced right temporal lobe and right temporal gray matter volumes and possibly reduced prefrontal volumes. Youth with CD in the absence of ADHD have also been found to have decreased cortical thickness in the superior temporal cortex, decreased gyrification of the ventromedial frontal cortex, and decreased amygdala and striatum volumes (Wallace et al, 2014). Furthermore, right temporal cortical thickness was found to be inversely proportional to severity of callous-unemotional traits. Additional neuroimaging studies have demonstrated both structural and functional differences in brain areas associated with affect regulation and affect processing, such as reduced activation in both anterior cingulate cortex and amygdala, dysfunction of the "hot" ventromedial orbitofrontal-limbic system, and impaired functional connectivity in frontotemporal limbic white matter tracts in youth with callous-unemotional traits (Finger et al, 2012). In youth with ODD or CD with psychopathic traits, functional differences in reward and social information processing pathways have also been demonstrated, such as decreased orbitofrontal-caudate responsiveness to reinforcement and rewards (White et al, 2014; Finger et al, 2011) and reduced amygdala response to fearful expressions (White et al, 2012). It is important to consider that many of the ODD/CD neuroimaging studies have included DBD youth with psychopathic traits (i.e., callous-unemotional traits), and this ODD/CD subgroup may very well have unique structural and functional brain development.

Neurophysiology—Childhood-onset, aggressive CD is associated with low tonic physiologic arousal, low autonomic reactivity, and rapid habituation. These characteristics may be associated with an impairment of avoidance conditioning to social stimuli, a failure to respond to punishment, and deficient behavioral inhibition. An imbalance between central reward and inhibition systems has been postulated. It is unclear whether these physiologic phenomena are inherent, whether they are secondary to disruptive experiences in early childhood, or whether they are the result of a chaotic environment.

Numerous studies have demonstrated: (1) hyporeactivity of the sympathetic nervous system and orbitofrontal cortex to incentives and reward and altered DA functioning; (2) low basal heart rate and heart rate variability; (3) low punishment sensitivity, as indicated by reduced cortisol reactivity to stress, and hypoactivity of the amygdala to negative stimuli; (4) impairments in executive functions; (5) impaired functioning of the paralimbic system, encompassing the orbitofrontal and cingulate cortex, which suggest impaired cognitive control over emotional behavior; and (6) decreased hypothalamic–pituitary–adrenal (HPA)-axis activity.

2. Psychological factors

Neuropsychological—Cognitive testing in delinquent populations has consistently demonstrated that IQ is about 8 points below that of nondelinquent peers, a difference that persists when socioeconomic status is statistically controlled. This discrepancy is primarily the result of deficits in word knowledge, verbally coded information, verbal reasoning, verbally mediated response regulation, and metalinguistic skills. The most impulsive/aggressive subjects exhibit the widest discrepancy between verbal and performance IQs. These deficits probably antedate school entry and are associated with learning problems.

Temperamental—Research into temperamental factors that could potentially increase risk of conduct problems has yielded inconsistent results. However, several factors have emerged repeatedly, including impulsivity, sensation seeking, and external locus of control. See ODD section for additional details.

Social cognition—Youth with CD often have an interpersonal style characterized by hostile attribution (e.g., assuming negative intent when it is not there), distorted information processing (e.g., not including all information in decision making), and affording undue influence to like-minded peers. Aggressive children have been found to underutilize social cues, interpret neutral or ambiguous cues as hostile, generate few assertive solutions to social problems, and expect that aggressive behavior will be rewarded. Refer to ODD section for detailed discussion.

3. Social–familial factors

Adverse parenting practices—The following adverse parenting practices convey a risk for antisocial behavior: lack of parental warmth and involvement in childrearing, poor supervision, and harsh, punitive discipline. Characteristic parent–child interactions involve unclear communication; lax and inconsistent monitoring; lack of follow-through; unpredictable, explosive, coercive, harsh, and overly punitive verbal or physical discipline; and a failure to provide verbal reinforcement for desirable behavior. Thus parent–child interactions reinforce negative behavior, fail to model and reinforce desirable behavior, and contribute to the development of negative and hostile attributions toward authority figures. There is a bidirectionality between child temperament and behavior, which affects parenting practices parent–child interactions, and vice versa. Parenting practices are further influenced by complex interactions between multiple factors including the parent's experience of being parented and by the parent's underlying psychopathology.

Child maltreatment—Marital conflict, domestic violence, parental neglect, and child maltreatment are also associated with later-onset antisocial behavior. The effect of divorce on child behavior is likely mediated by exposure to marital discord before, during, and after parental separation. Physical abuse is related to later aggressive behavior and can be transmitted from generation to generation. The prevalence of sexual abuse among girls with CD is very high. According to a study of delinquent girls placed in therapeutic foster care, the girls first engaged in sexual activity at an average age of 6 years. The risk for child maltreatment is also increased by parental psychopathology and other parent factors, including parent criminality, parent substance use, and single or teenage parenthood.

School environment and peer interactions—Youth with externalizing behaviors (with frequently comorbid impairments in verbal reasoning) are often rejected by more prosocial peers and often have inaccurate perceptions of acceptance by peers. This leads them to associate with like-minded companions and more deviant peer groups, which increase the probability of antisocial behavior. Furthermore, parents of disruptive children are likely to have difficulty in preventing their children from associating with deviant peers who promote further delinquent behavior.

Family and community factors—Many of the same sociological risk factors for ODD have also been found to increase risk for the development of conduct problems. Family adversity, family transitions, and low socioeconomic status are particularly likely to be associated with childhood-onset, aggressive CD. However, the effect of low socioeconomic status is nullified when the effect of adverse parenting practices is statistically controlled. Adverse family circumstances therefore appear to affect the child via adverse parenting.

The main sociological theories concerning the development of conduct problems and delinquency include: (1) social segregation theory—in which disadvantaged social or ethnic groups become relegated to decaying neighborhoods which then become battlegrounds for competing ethnic groups and spawn criminogenic cultural organizations (Mesch et al, 2008); (2) social disorganization theory, which posits that individuals who live in disadvantaged neighborhoods are more likely to engage in antisocial behavior than those who live in advantaged neighborhoods, due to disruption of social ties (Lei et al, 2014); (3) culture conflict theory, which relates the antisocial behavior of the children of socially disadvantaged immigrants to the confusion and disempowerment of immigrant parents, leading to a conflict between traditional parental control and the influence of the new society (Einat & Herzog, 2011); (4) criminogenic social organization theory—which posits that the informal organization of street gangs is driven by focal concerns with masculinity, toughness, status, the capacity to outwit others, a hunger for excitement, and the belief that life is dictated by fate rather than planning (Stewart & Simons, 2010); and (5) blocked-opportunity theory, which emphasizes the function of the gang as an illegitimate means to acquire desirable amenities in a materialistic society that accords high status to affluence.

C. Genetics

Twin studies indicate moderate heritability of aggression/CD (Gelhorn et al, 2005). In 10 twin comparison studies, the concordance rates for adult criminality were approximately 50% for monozygotic twins and 20% for dizygotic twins. Candidate genes that have been studied as possible contributors to CD or aggression include those that affect serotonergic (5-HT) neurotransmission (e.g., 5-HT transporter and 5-HT receptor 1B and 2A genes), based on the well-accepted role of 5-HT neurotransmission in modulating impulsive/aggressive behavior (Fowler et al, 2009). Other studies have examined the potential role of genes regulating catecholaminergic function. For example, the catechol-O-methyltransferase (COMT) gene encodes an enzyme that degrades DA and NE. Studies have demonstrated that children with ADHD who express a less active version of the enzyme, which results in higher brain levels of DA in the prefrontal cortex, have a higher prevalence of comorbid DBD, conduct symptoms, and aggressive behavior (Caspi et al, 2008). Furthermore, in one study, the presence of the dopamine receptor D2 (DRD2) T allele conferred an increased risk of CD for subjects who did not have the dopamine receptor D4 (DRD4) 7R allele, whereas there was no risk associated with the DRD2 T allele in DRD4 7R carriers (Mota et al, 2013). Risk of CD is increased in families where a parent or sibling has CD and in families where a parent has severe alcohol use, depression or bipolar disorder, schizophrenia, or ADHD.

The potentially confounding effects of gender as well as a variety of family and environmental risk factors have complicated the study of genetic influences on CD and aggression. Three kinds of gene–environment interactions have been postulated in the development of adolescent chronic antisocial behavior: (1) parenting practices can dampen the impact of genes, (2) genes can alter the impact of traumatic environmental experiences, and (3) individuals and environments influence each other dynamically in developmental sequences (Dodge & McCourt, 2010). The developmental trajectories of the DBDs illustrate the principles of heterotypic continuity (the tendency of behavior patterns to evolve and change with development) and differential susceptibility (a certain trait leads to compromised functioning under adverse conditions, whereas the same trait can lead to improved functioning under favorable conditions). For example, heterotypic continuity can be seen when temperamental impulsiveness and oppositional defiant behavior in early childhood may evolve to antiauthoritarian behavior and stealing during middle childhood; to assault, risky sexual behavior, and substance abuse in adolescence; and to criminality in adulthood. Differential susceptibility is exemplified by a child with a certain genetic vulnerability developing conduct problems under harsh punitive parenting practices, while another child with that same genetic vulnerability is able to thrive with consistent and controlled parenting. Studies of gene–environment interactions have found that certain alleles of the serotonin transporter gene, the DA receptor gene, and the monoamine oxidase A gene interact with adverse environments to increase the risk of aggression and violence (Simons et al, 2012).

▶ Clinical Findings

A. Signs & Symptoms

CD represents a pattern of severe, persistent, and pervasive dysfunction that is intolerably disruptive or dangerous at home, in school, or in the community. Youth with CD violate the basic rights of others and/or major societal norms. These behaviors fall into four main categories: aggression toward people and/or animals, destruction of property, a pattern of deceitfulness or theft, and serious violations of rules. Onset of conduct symptoms may occur as early as the preschool years but usually begins during a period from middle childhood to middle adolescence. Onset after age 16 is rare. The course of CD after onset is highly variable, and symptoms vary with age and development. In addition to the age-of-onset specifier (childhood vs. adolescent), the CD diagnosis can be further described "with limited prosocial emotions." This specifier is used in individuals whose usual pattern of interpersonal and emotional functioning reflects a lack of remorse, callous lack of empathy, unconcern about performance, and/or a shallow or deficient affect. A minority of individuals with CD exhibit these characteristics.

Associated features of CD are often highly predictive of impairment (note that many of these are also characteristic of ODD). Key features include: (1) problems related to learning, academic underachievement or occupational attainment, (2) problems in affect regulation or anger management, (3) being unable to understand or appreciate social cues and/or social context, (4) problematic family and/or peer relationships, (5) aggression, (6) low self-esteem, and (7) substance abuse. The degree to which these features are present relates to the nature and severity of the presenting symptomatology but cannot always be anticipated from these alone.

For example, academic and vocational underachievement may be related to the presence of comorbid learning disorders (LD) but may be seen independent of LD. Persistent academic underachievement can lead to school failure and premature termination of educational pursuits. Social impairments are frequently present but need not reflect specific cognitive/skill deficits.

B. Clinical and Psychological Assessment

The clinical assessment of CD requires a multimodal, multisource approach similar to that described for ODD. Refer to the ODD section for a detailed discussion of assessment procedures.

C. Laboratory Findings

There are no physical findings or laboratory measures that reliably distinguish ODD and CD from each other, other disorders, or normal controls—although it is well established that reduced noradrenergic function is associated with behavioral overarousal and aggression. Lower resting heart rate, reduced autonomic fear conditioning, and low skin conductance are all documented findings in CD at the group level, but none are diagnostic.

D. Neuroimaging

Although neuroanatomical and neurophysiological studies of children with CD have demonstrated reduced volumes in the right temporal lobe and prefrontal cortex, reduced activation of the anterior cingulate cortex and amygdala, and dysfunction of the "hot" ventromedial orbitofrontal-limbic system (see earlier discussion), neuroimaging is not used in the clinical assessment and diagnosis of CD.

E. Course of Illness

Onset of CD can be as early as the preschool years; however, it is rare after 16 years of age. The developmental course of CD is highly gender dependent. In boys, symptoms of CD often begin in preschool years, with age of onset peaking in mid-childhood, and average age of onset at 10–12 years. In girls, CD symptoms are less often aggressive in nature and have their onset at a later age, with the average age of onset at 14–16 years. Earlier CD onset and a larger number of CD symptoms predict worse prognosis and increased risk for ASPD and SUD. Lifetime CD significantly predicts academic, psychiatric, and sexual behavior problems in girls with ADHD at follow-up.

Approximately one third of children with ODD will progress to CD, and one third of those with CD progress to ASPD by age 25. The early presentation of physical aggression is a key predictor of this ODD–CD–ASPD trajectory, as physically aggressive children are more likely to progress from early oppositional behaviors to more severe and disabling conduct problems. In cases where ODD precedes CD, the onset of CD

is typically before age 10 (childhood onset CD). In children with late-onset CD (i.e., after age 10), symptoms of ODD are usually not present during early childhood. Although it has been suggested that ODD and CD are not separate diagnostic entities but rather lie on a continuum, more recent work suggests that the two conditions are better understood as distinct entities (Rowe et al, 2010). Different models have been postulated to link childhood emotional–behavioral problems to ASPD in early adulthood (Diamantopoulou et al, 2010).

Other developmental trajectories have also been suggested. The exclusive substance abuse pathway involves progression from less serious to more dangerous illicit drugs, without aggressive or nonaggressive delinquency. The covert, nonaggressive pathway proceeds from minor theft to serious property violations. The aggressive, versatile path has an early onset, is associated with early hyperactivity and impulsivity, and involves increasingly violent behavior (e.g., from frequent fighting to assaultive behavior). A fourth pathway, authority conflict, is described as progressing from oppositionality to serious antiauthoritarianism. Many youths with CD cross over from one trajectory to another.

▶ Differential Diagnosis (Including Comorbid Conditions)

As with ODD, a lifetime diagnosis of CD was also strongly associated with DSM-IV-TR comorbidity in the NCS-R. The NCS-R found increased odds ratios of any mood disorder (2.7), any anxiety disorder (3.0), any impulse-control disorder (7.7), and any substance disorder (5.9) among those with a lifetime diagnosis of CD. In a nationally representative British sample, 39% of girls and 46% of boys with CD met criteria for at least one other DSM disorder. Even after accounting for age and the presence of other disorders, the odds ratios for comorbid ADHD, depression, and anxiety were all significantly elevated in children with ODD and CD. A large, clinically referred sample reported rates of comorbidity of ODD/CD to be as high as 80–90% for ADHD, 30–55% for major depression, 20–45% for bipolar disorder, 30–40% for anxiety disorders, 10% for Tourette disorder, and 20% for language disorders (Nock et al, 2007).

1. ODD—Although CD and ODD have related symptoms that bring youth into conflict with parents and other authority figures, ODD behaviors are much less severe in nature. ODD behaviors may or may not include aggression toward people, but in the case of ODD this is more often reactive in nature and not motivated. Aggression toward animals, property destruction, theft, and deceitfulness are characteristic of CD but not ODD. Furthermore, youth with ODD often have difficulties with emotion dysregulation that are less common in CD alone. When both ODD and CD criteria are met, both disorders can be diagnosed.

2. ADHD—CD is very often though not always comorbid with ADHD. Data from several studies indicate that among children with ODD and/or CD, 40–60% also have ADHD. However, the majority of this comorbidity is with ODD. The prevalence of comorbid ADHD/ODD/CD/aggression is thought to be higher in clinical than epidemiologic samples because the co-occurrence of these conditions is highly impairing and often leads to referral. Rates of comorbidity appear to vary across clinical settings, with an overrepresentation in psychiatric compared to pediatric settings. Although the hyperactive and impulsive symptoms of ADHD can be disruptive, youth with ADHD do not violate societal norms or the rights of others.

3. Affective disorders—Irritability, aggression, and conduct problems can be seen in youth with affective disorders. Depression in children is frequently accompanied by the acute onset of irritability and behavior problems, with 60% of youth with major depression meeting criteria for CD. In addition, anxiety and depression frequently are comorbid. The co-occurrence of ADHD with these other disorders is also not uncommon, meaning that three or more disorders are often present. Suicidal ideation, suicide attempts, and completed suicides occur at higher rates than expected in individuals with CD.

A somewhat controversial subject has been the co-occurrence of childhood bipolar disorder and CD. Prevalence rates of childhood bipolar disorder vary widely by sample, with some estimates as high as 15%. It is unknown what impact the new DSM-5 diagnosis DMDD will have on prevalence rates of other disorders characterized by temper outbursts, irritability, and externalizing behaviors, including bipolar disorders and ODD/CD. However, a recent study found that comorbidity with another disorder was present in most cases of DMDD; 57–70% had comorbid ODD and 18–23% had comorbid CD. Episodes of mania, however, were relatively rare in this study (see related section for ODD).

4. Intermittent explosive disorder (IED)—Both CD and IED have high levels of aggressive behavior. Whereas the aggressive behavior in IED is impulsive and not committed for personal gain, aggression in CD is more often premeditated and goal-driven. Furthermore, IED does not include the nonaggressive symptoms of CD as part of its criteria.

5. Trauma and stress-related disorders—As with ODD, parent–child relational problems are quite common in CD. Parental factors including parental psychopathology, harsh or inconsistent discipline, and abuse have consistently been identified as risk factors for CD. Aggressive punishment and coercive interactions have been associated specifically with childhood aggressive behaviors and low parental warmth with oppositional behaviors. Sexual or physical abuse, neglect, and other extremely harsh and traumatic parenting behaviors specifically increase the risk for CD and, ultimately, ASPD. Childhood trauma and abuse are risk factors for many types of psychopathology, but physical abuse may increase risk of aggressive conduct symptoms

more specifically. PTSD is also commonly comorbid with CD. While both disorders may follow from abuse or other traumatic events, it has been hypothesized that early onset conduct problems, whether genetically or environmentally influenced, could lead to a higher risk of exposure to traumatic experiences later in life.

6. Substance use disorders—CD is highly associated with early-onset substance use and rapid progression to serious substance abuse. Childhood-onset CD is more likely to be associated with comorbid substance use than is adolescent-onset CD.

7. Psychotic disorders—Careful history taking, mental status examination, neuropsychological testing, and EEG of violent juvenile offenders often reveal hallucinatory experiences, episodes of thought disorder, lapses of concentration, memory gaps, suspiciousness, explosive aggression, and nonspecific electroencephalographic abnormalities. These findings, along with the history of physical abuse often encountered among violent delinquents, have suggested that some antisocial youth may be experiencing covert psychosis or subclinical epilepsy caused by traumatic brain injury.

8. Medical conditions—As in ODD, a variety of other medical conditions can co-occur with CD, including sleep disorders, thyroid disease, postinfectious and/or posttraumatic encephalopathy, sensory impairments, and medication-induced disinhibition syndromes.

Treatment

As with ODD, CD requires a multimodal approach using individually tailored biological, psychosocial, and ecological interventions. The principles underlying the psychosocial interventions for youth with CD are the same as those discussed for ODD (Steiner et al, 2007). However, one important difference between treating youth with ODD and CD is that the occurrence of motivated aggression (more characteristic of CD) is not responsive to medication. Hence, there is a primacy for psychosocial intervention (with adjunctive medication if there is also impulsive or affective symptomatology) in youth with CD.

A. Psychosocial Interventions

1. Head Start REDI—Early intervention programs such as Head Start may have a preventative function as these programs not only help prepare preschoolers for kindergarten but also educate parents about child development and offer support in times of crisis. The Head Start REDI (Research-Based, Developmentally Informed) enrichment intervention was designed to complement and strengthen the impact of existing Head Start programs in the areas of preschool social–emotional competency as well as language and literacy skills (Nix et al, 2013). At the 1-year follow-up, children who received the REDI intervention were found to have improved learning engagement, improved social problem-solving skills, and reduced aggressive behavior (Bierman et al, 2014).

2. Positive Parenting Program (Triple P) and Fast Track—The Triple P and Fast Track provide intensive parent education to correct adverse parenting practices including difficulties with communication, consistency, effective discipline, and modeling/rewarding prosocial behaviors that frequently accompany CD. Both Triple P and Fast Track have demonstrated promising short- and long-term effects. Refer to the ODD section for a detailed discussion of the Triple P program.

Fast Track is a multicomponent intervention for children at high risk of developing conduct problems. The intervention takes place in both home and school settings. The intervention components target several risk factors for developing persistent conduct problems. The program was found to positively impact parenting and discipline practices, peer relations, and social cognitive skills such as emotion regulation and social problem solving. Although the intervention had a significant impact on development of CD in the highest risk groups, it did not prevent CD in the moderate risk group (Dodge & McCourt, 2010). The Fast Track intervention, unfortunately, has also not significantly improved long-term school outcomes.

3. Therapeutic foster homes—There is significant evidence that it is ineffective to treat adolescents who have CD in community or institutional groups, as the reinforcement of antisocial behavior generated by antisocial youth groups likely counteracts any benefit derived from group-oriented therapeutic programs. For that reason, therapeutic foster homes have been developed. Specially trained foster parents provide daily structure and support, institute an individualized point program, and ensure close supervision of peer associations, consistent nonphysical discipline, and social-skill-building activities supplemented by weekly individual psychotherapy. Although there are high levels of behavioral and mental health problems in youth placed into therapeutic foster treatment, these levels are lower than those seen in youth in residential treatment centers (Baker et al, 2007). Therapeutic foster care has been found to lead to a significant reduction in offending in the 12 months following discharge as compared to group care. The most significant treatment differences between therapeutic foster care and group care were in the ability of therapeutic foster care to prevent the adolescent from associating with deviant peers and in the quality of discipline provided. There is also evidence that therapeutic foster care prevents violence (Fisher et al, 2009; Hahn et al, 2005).

4. Multisystemic treatment (MST)—MST provides home-based community treatment for violent antisocial and substance-abusing youth. It aims to empower parents with parenting skills and to enable youth to cope with family, peer, school, and neighborhood problems. Multisystemic interventions target specific problems, particularly adverse sequences of behavior within and between ecological systems (e.g., between child, family, and school). Interventions are designed to promote the generalization and long-term maintenance of therapeutic change. Family therapy, parent training, CBT, and community consultation are combined as part of individualized treatment plans. Deviant peer contact is monitored, discouraged, and counteracted. Parent–teacher communication is promoted. Several controlled evaluation studies have demonstrated the efficacy of multisystemic therapy in decreasing criminality and violence in adolescents (Hahn et al, 2005).

5. Multidimensional treatment foster care (MTFC)—MTFC has been shown to prevent recidivism and decrease violent behavior, risky sexual behaviors, pregnancy rates, depressive symptoms, self-harm, and suicidal ideation among girls within the juvenile justice system (Rhoades et al, 2013; Fisher et al, 2009).

B. Psychopharmacologic Interventions

The treatment of CD is more complex than that of its frequently comorbid disorders ODD and ADHD, with many available medications used off-label, none of which can be recommended as fully evidence-based.

1. Psychostimulants—Placebo-controlled trials have repeatedly demonstrated the efficacy of stimulants in treating aggressive and disruptive behaviors in youth with ADHD. Methylphenidate has been shown to reduce oppositional and hostile behavior in youth with or without comorbid ADHD. Stimulant treatment is also associated with improvement in oppositionality, behavioral noncompliance, impulsive aggression, peer interactions, family dynamics, and ratings of self-esteem. Recent data indicate that the utility of stimulants for aggression is equivalent in children (note: adolescents were not studied) with and without callous and unemotional traits (Blader et al, 2013), possibly because of the co-occurrence of instrumental and reactive aggression in many children with DBDs. Because of the potential for misuse, abuse, and diversion of stimulant medication in this population, it is critical to directly discuss these issues with adolescents and young adults and to screen for signs and symptoms of substance abuse as part of treatment monitoring.

2. Alpha-2 adrenergic agonists—Several studies have demonstrated the effectiveness of the alpha-2 adrenergic agonists guanfacine and clonidine in addressing impulsivity, oppositional, and conduct symptoms (see ODD section).

3. Serotonin reuptake inhibitors—There is some evidence for the efficacy of fluoxetine and citalopram in treating aggressive and impulsive symptoms in children with comorbid CD and depression. The efficacy of selective serotonin reuptake inhibitors (SSRIs) implicates serotonergic mechanisms in aggression, which may in part explain the frequent comorbidity of CD in youth with depression. However, SSRIs cannot be recommended for the treatment of CD and aggression in the absence of depression.

4. Antipsychotic medications—Neuroleptic medications have been used for decades to treat children with severe behavioral problems characterized by aggression and combativeness. Several first-generation antipsychotics such as chlorpromazine, thioridazine, and haloperidol were FDA approved for this indication; however, these medications are rarely used now. More recent studies have focused on the atypical neuroleptics. Risperidone currently has the most extensive data, with several controlled trials documenting utility in treating aggressive symptoms and conduct problems in youth with DBDs (Gorman et al, 2015; Aman et al, 2014; Loy et al, 2012). Risperidone has FDA approval for the treatment of aggression in autistic spectrum disorders. Open studies and case reports are available for several of the other atypical antipsychotic medications—most notably quetiapine and aripiprazole—but currently there is not enough evidence to support their use in youth with DBDs. There are also no research data for children under 5 years of age.

5. Mood and behavior stabilizing medications— Mood-stabilizing medications have been utilized off-label in the treatment of aggression and episodic dyscontrol, although efficacy in the treatment of CD has not been established. Studies with lithium have yielded mixed results. Several antiepileptic medications have also been investigated, again with mixed results, although there continues to be substantial off-label use. The best data are for sodium valproate, which was shown to be effective in reducing overt aggression and improving global functioning in several controlled trials of adolescents with aggression, chronic temper outbursts, and mood lability. One study of divalproex added to methylphenidate increased the likelihood of remission of aggressive behavior in children with ADHD and chronic aggression that had been refractory to stimulants. Several other antiepileptic medications may also be relevant for youth with CD— including carbamazepine, topiramate, and lamotrigine—but there is a paucity of data (for a recent review, see Pringsheim et al, 2015b).

C. Combined Treatments

Combination treatment is almost always required for highly aggressive youth with CD. In the Multimodal Treatment Study of Children with ADHD (MTA), children with ODD/CD showed benefit from combined treatment over medication alone. In a follow-up to the MTA, Van der Oord and colleagues (2008) compared methylphenidate monotherapy to methylphenidate combined with multimodal behavioral therapy and also found significant improvement in ADHD, ODD, and CD symptoms in both arms. Another study examined stimulant use in combination with family behavioral therapy in ADHD, ODD, and CD and found

decreased aggression (Blader et al, 2013). A retrospective chart review, which examined the efficacy of combined risperidone and psychosocial treatment versus psychosocial treatment alone in adolescents with childhood-onset and persistent CD, found that the addition of risperidone yielded significant improvement on a composite measure of interpersonal behavior and rule compliance. Furthermore, in youth with ADHD, ODD/CD, and severe physical aggression, the addition of risperidone to optimized stimulant plus parent management training demonstrated moderate improvement in aggressive and other disruptive behaviors (Aman et al, 2014; Gadow et al, 2014).

▶ Prognosis

Developmental cascades in DBDs are the result of a complex interplay among biological, environmental, and ecological factors and reflect the aggregate effects of factors that act synergistically to influence levels of behavioral dysfunction. For these reasons, the prognosis for CD is highly variable.

Prognostically, it is important to differentiate early-onset persistent versus childhood-limited conduct problems (Barker & Maughan, 2009). Persistence of CD is more likely with childhood onset of conduct problems and those who qualify for the CD specifier "with limited prosocial emotions." There is also increased risk of persistence in individuals with comorbid ADHD, ODD, or substance abuse. ODD frequently precedes CD, and CD incorporates oppositionality; however, only about 25% of preschoolers with ODD progress to CD. The "headstrong" dimension of ODD significantly predicts later CD and substance use (Rowe et al, 2010). Approximately 40% of the comorbidity between ODD and CD can be accounted for by common risk factors (Boden et al, 2010). Similarly, whereas all adults with ASPD have manifested CD in adolescence, only 25–40% of adolescents with CD progress to ASPD.

Disruptive and aggressive behaviors are often refractory to medication monotherapy, combined medication treatments, and even multimodel therapies. This is most frequently true for patients with early age of onset, more severe symptoms, comorbidity, substantial psychosocial risk, and presence of callous-unemotional traits. Poor prognostic factors include age- and gender-atypical symptoms, comorbid mood disorders and/or substance use, low verbal ability, proactive non-impulsive aggression, and a lack of prosocial behaviors (Masi et al, 2013). For some patients with highly aggressive behaviors that have not been responsive to traditional multimodal treatments, psychiatric hospitalization or residential placement may be indicated.

Not only are childhood and adolescent DBDs frequently refractory to treatment, but unfortunately, their presence predicts young adult disorders and outcomes. Youth in all DBD groups (ODD, CD, and comorbid ODD/CD) are at increased risk for comorbid anxiety, depression, and SUD (Rowe et al, 2010). ODD predicts mood and anxiety disorders in young adulthood (Rowe et al, 2010; Copeland et al, 2009), whereas conduct problems predict both mood and disruptive disorders in adulthood (Reef et al, 2010). Youth with ODD only were not found to be at increased risk for ASPD in adulthood, but youth with childhood- or adolescent-onset CD were at significantly increased risk for ASPD.

Aman MG, Bukstein OG, Gadow KD, et al. What does risperidone add to parent training and stimulant for severe aggression in child attention-deficit/hyperactivity disorder? *J Am Acad Child Adolesc Psychiatry.* 2014;53(1):47–60.

American Psychiatric Association. *Diagnostic and Statistical Manual of Mental Disorders.* 5th ed. Washington, DC: American Psychiatric Association; 2013.

Baker AJ, Kurland D, Curtis P, et al. Mental health and behavioral problems of youth in the child welfare system: residential treatment centers compared to therapeutic foster care in the Odyssey Project population. *Child Welfare.* 2007;86(3):97–123.

Barker ED, Maughan B. Differentiating early-onset persistent versus childhood-limited conduct problem youth. *Am J Psychiatry.* 2009;166(8):900–908.

Barkley RA, Edwards G, Laneri M, et al. The efficacy of problem-solving communication training alone, behavior management training alone, and their combination for parent-adolescent conflict in teenagers with ADHD and ODD. *J Consult Clin Psychol.* 2001;69(6):926–941.

Bierman KL, Nix RL, Heinrichs BS, et al. Effects of Head Start REDI on children's outcomes 1 year later in different kindergarten contexts. *Child Dev.* 2014;85(1):140–159.

Blader JC, Pliszka SR, Kafantaris V, et al. Callous-unemotional traits, proactive aggression, and treatment outcomes of aggressive children with attention-deficit/hyperactivity disorder. *J Am Acad Child Adolesc Psychiatry.* 2013;52(12):1281–1293.

Boden JM, Fergusson DM, Horwood LJ. Risk factors for conduct disorder and oppositional/defiant disorder: evidence from a New Zealand birth cohort. *J Am Acad Child Adolesc Psychiatry.* 2010;49(11):1125–1133.

Boylan K, Vaillancourt T, Boyle M, Szatmari P. Comorbidity of internalizing disorders in children with oppositional defiant disorder. *Eur Child Adolesc Psychiatry.* 2007;16(8):484–494.

Buss AH, Perry M. The aggression questionnaire. *J Pers Soc Psychol.* 1992;63(3):452–459.

Canino G, Polanczyk G, Bauermeister JJ, et al. Does the prevalence of CD and ODD vary across cultures? *Soc Psychiatry Psychiatr Epidemiol.* 2010;45(7):695–704.

Carpenter DO, Nevin R. Environmental causes of violence. *Physiol Behav.* 2010;99:260–268.

Caspi A, Langley K, Milne B, et al. A replicated molecular genetic basis for subtyping antisocial behavior in children with attention-deficit/hyperactivity disorder. *Arch Gen Psychiatry.* 2008;65:203–210.

Comer JS, Chow C, Chan PT, et al. Psychosocial treatment efficacy for disruptive behavior problems in very young children: a meta-analytic examination. *J Am Acad Child Adolesc Psychiatry.* 2013;52(1):26–36.

Copeland WE, Shanahan L, Costello EJ, Angold A. Childhood and adolescent psychiatric disorders as predictors of young adult disorders. *Arch Gen Psychiatry.* 2009;66(7):764–772.

Deveney CM, Connelly ME, Haring CT, et al. Neural mechanisms of frustration in chronically irritable children. *Am J Psychiatry.* 2013;170(10):1186–1194.

Diamantopoulou S, Verhulst S, van der Ende J. Testing developmental pathways to antisocial personality problems. *J Abnorm Child Psychol.* 2010;38(1):91–103.

Dodge KA, McCourt SN. Translating models of antisocial behavioral development into efficacious intervention policy to prevent adolescent violence. *Dev Psychobiol.* 2010;52(3):277–285.

Drugli MB, Larsson B, Fossum S, Mørch WT. Five- to six-year outcome and its prediction for children with ODD/CD treated with parent training. *J Child Psychol Psychiatry.* 2010;51(5):559–566.

Einat T, Herzog S. A new perspective for delinquency: culture conflict measured by seriousness perceptions. *Int J Offender Ther Comp Criminol.* 2011;55(7):1072–1095.

Feldman J, Kazdin AE. Parent management training for oppositional and conduct problem children. *Clin Psychol.* 1995;48(4):3–5.

Finger EC, Marsh AA, Blair KS, et al. Disrupted reinforcement signaling in the orbitofrontal cortex and caudate in youths with conduct disorder or oppositional defiant disorder and a high level of psychopathic traits. *Am J Psychiatry.* 2011;168(2):152–162.

Finger EC, Marsh A, Blair KS, et al. Impaired functional but preserved structural connectivity in limbic white matter tracts in youth with conduct disorder or oppositional defiant disorder plus psychopathic traits. *Psychiatry Res.* 2012;202(3):239–244.

Fisher PA, Chamberlain P, Leve LD. Improving the lives of foster children through evidence-based interventions. *Vulnerable Child Youth Stud.* 2009;4(2):122–127.

Fowler TA, Langley K, Rice FJ, et al. Psychopathy trait scores in adolescents with childhood ADHD: the contribution of genotypes affecting MAOA, 5HTT and COMT activity. *Psychiatric Genetics.* 2009;19:312–319.

Frick PJ. *The Alabama Parenting Questionnaire.* Unpublished rating scale, University of Alabama; 1991.

Furlong M, McGilloway S, Bywater T, et al. Cochrane review: behavioural and cognitive-behavioural group-based parenting programmes for early-onset conduct problems in children aged 3 to 12 years (Review). *Evid Based Child Health.* 2013;8(2):318–692.

Gadow KD, Arnold LE, Molina BS, et al. Risperidone added to parent training and stimulant medication: effects on attention-deficit/hyperactivity disorder, oppositional defiant disorder, conduct disorder, and peer aggression. *J Am Acad Child Adolesc Psychiatry.* 2014;53(9):948–959.e1.

Garg J, Arun P, Chavan BS. Comparative efficacy of methylphenidate and atomoxetine in oppositional defiant disorder comorbid with attention deficit hyperactivity disorder. *Int J Appl Basic Med Res.* 2015;5(2):114–118.

Gelhorn HL, Stallings MC, Young SE, et al. Genetic and environmental influences on conduct disorder: symptom, domain and full-scale analyses. *J Child Psychol Psychiatry.* 2005;46:580–591.

Gorman DA, Gardner DM, Murphy AL, et al. Canadian guidelines on pharmacotherapy for disruptive and aggressive behaviour in children and adolescents with attention-deficit hyperactivity disorder, oppositional defiant disorder, or conduct disorder. *Can J Psychiatry.* 2015;60(2):62–76.

Haggerty KP, McGlynn-Wright A, Klima T. Promising parenting programs for reducing adolescent problem behaviors. *J Child Serv.* 2013;8(4):10.1108/JCS-04-2013-0016.

Hahlweg K, Heinrichs N, Kuschel A, et al. Long-term outcome of a randomized controlled universal prevention trial through a positive parenting program: is it worth the effort? *Child Adolesc Psychiatry Ment Health.* 2010;4:14.

Hahn RA, Bilukha O, Lowy J, et al; Task Force on Community Preventive Services. The effectiveness of therapeutic foster care for the prevention of violence: a systematic review. *Am J Prev Med.* 2005;28(2 Suppl 1):72–90.

Halperin JM, McKay KE, Grayson RH, Newcorn JH. Reliability, validity, and preliminary normative data for the Children's Aggression Scale—Teacher Version. *J Am Acad Child Adolesc Psychiatry.* 2003;42(8):965–971.

Halperin JM, McKay KE, Newcorn JH. Development, reliability, and validity of the children's aggression scale-parent version. *J Am Acad Child Adolesc Psychiatry.* 2002;41(3):245–252.

Hood KK, Eyberg SM. Outcomes of parent-child interaction therapy: mothers' reports of maintenance three to six years after treatment. *J Clin Child Adolesc Psychol.* 2003;32(3):419–429.

Jacobs RH, Becker-Weidman EG, Reinecke MA, et al. Treating depression and oppositional behavior in adolescents. *J Clin Child Adolesc Psychol.* 2010;39(4):559–567.

Latimer K, Wilson P, Kemp J, et al. Disruptive behavior disorders: a systematic review of environmental antenatal and early years risk factors. *Child Care Health Dev.* 2012;38(5):611–628.

Lei MK, Simons RL, Edmond MB, et al. The effect of neighborhood disadvantage, social ties, and genetic variation on the antisocial behavior of African American women: a multilevel analysis. *Dev Psychopathol.* 2014;8:1–16.

Lochman JE, Powell NP, Boxmeyer CL, Jimenez-Camargo L. Cognitive-behavioral therapy for externalizing disorders in children and adolescents. *Child Adolesc Psychiatr Clin North Am.* 2011;20(2):305–318.

Loney J, Milich R. Hyperactivity, inattention, and aggression in clinical practice. In: Wolraich M, Routh D, eds. *Advances in Developmental and Behavioral Pediatrics.* Vol 3. Greenwich, CT: JAI; 1982:113–147.

Loy JH, Merry SN, Hetrick SE, Stasiak K. Atypical antipsychotics for disruptive behaviour disorders in children and youths. *Cochrane Database Syst Rev.* 2012;9:CD008559.

Loyd BH, Abidin RR. Revision of the Parenting Stress Index. *J Pediatr Psychol.* 1985;10(2):169–177.

Malmberg K, Wargelius HL, Lichtenstein P, et al. ADHD and Disruptive Behavior scores—associations with MAO-A and 5-HTT genes and with platelet MAO-B activity in adolescents. *BMC Psychiatry.* 2008;23(8):28.

Masi G, Muratori P, Manfredi A, et al. Response to treatments in youth with disruptive behavior disorders. *Compr Psychiatry.* 2013;54(7):1009–1015,.

Matthys W, Vanderschuren LJ, Schutter DJ. The neurobiology of oppositional defiant disorder and conduct disorder: altered functioning in three mental domains. *Dev Psychopathol.* 2013;25(1):193–207.

McGough JJ, McCracken JT, Cho AL, et al. A potential electroencephalography and cognitive biosignature for the child behavior checklist-dysregulation profile. *J Am Acad Child Adolesc Psychiatry.* 2013;52(11):1173–1182.

Mesch GS, Turjeman H, Fishman G. Social identity and violence among immigrant adolescents. *New Dir Youth Dev.* 2008;Fall(119):129–150.

Miller LS, Klein RG, Piancentini J, et al. The New York Teacher Rating Scale for disruptive and antisocial behavior. *J Am Acad Child Adolesc Psychiatry.* 1995;34(3):359–370.

Mota NR, Bau CHD, Banaschewski T, et al. Association between DRD2/DRD4 interaction and conduct disorder: a potential developmental pathway to alcohol dependence. *Am J Med Genet.* 2013;162(6):546–549.

Nix RL, Bierman KL, Domitrovich CE, Gill S. Promoting children's social-emotional skills in preschool can enhance academic and behavioral functioning in kindergarten: findings from Head Start REDI. *Early Educ Dev.* 2013;24(7):10.

Nock MK, Kazdin AE, Hiripi E, Kessler RC. Lifetime prevalence, correlates, and persistence of oppositional defiant disorder: results from the National Comorbidity Survey Replication. *J Child Psychol Psychiatry.* 2007;48:703–713.

Pringsheim T, Hirsch L, Gardner D, et al. The pharmacological management of oppositional behaviour, conduct problems, and aggression in children and adolescents with attention-deficit hyperactivity disorder, oppositional defiant disorder, and conduct disorder: a systematic review and meta-analysis. Part 1: psychostimulants, alpha-2 agonists, and atomoxetine. *Can J Psychiatry.* 2015a;60(2):42–51.

Pringsheim T, Hirsch L, Gardner D, et al. The pharmacological management of oppositional behaviour, conduct problems, and aggression in children and adolescents with attention-deficit hyperactivity disorder, oppositional defiant disorder, and conduct disorder: a systematic review and meta-analysis. Part 2: antipsychotics and traditional mood stabilizers. *Can J Psychiatry.* 2015b; 60(2):52–61.

Reef J, van Meurs I, Verhulst FC, van der Ende J. Children's problems predict adults' DSM-IV disorders across 24 years. *J Am Acad Child Adolesc Psychiatry.* 2010;49(11):1117–1124.

Rhoades KA, Chamberlain P, Roberts R, Leve LD. MTFC for high risk adolescent girls: a comparison of outcomes in England and the United States. *J Child Adolesc Subst Abuse.* 2013;22(5):435–449.

Robertson DU, Hyde JS. The factorial validity of the Family Environment Scale. *Educ Psychol Meas.* 1982;42(4):1233–1241.

Rowe R, Costello EJ, Angold A, et al. Developmental pathways in oppositional defiant disorder and conduct disorder. *J Abnorm Psychol.* 2010;119(4):726–738.

Scott S, O'Connor TG. An experimental test of differential susceptibility to parenting among emotionally-dysregulated children in a randomized controlled trial for oppositional behavior. *J Child Psychol Psychiatry.* 2012;53(11):1184–1193.

Simons RL, Lei MK, Stewart EA, et al. Social adversity, genetic variation, street code, and aggression: a genetically informed model of violent behavior. *Youth Violence Juv Justice.* 2012; 10(1):3–24.

Sorgi P, Ratey J, Knoedler DW, et al. Rating aggression in the clinical setting. A retrospective adaptation of the Overt Aggression Scale: preliminary results. *J Neuropsychiatry Clin Neurosci.* 1991;3(2):S52–S56.

Steiner H, Remsing L. The Work Group on Quality Issues Practice. Parameter for the assessment and treatment of children and adolescents with oppositional defiant disorder. *J Am Acad Child Adolesc Psychiatry.* 2007;46(1):126–141.

Stewart EA, Simons RL. Race, code of the street, and violent delinquency: a multilevel investigation of neighborhood street culture and individual norms of violence. *Criminology*. 2010; 48(2):569–605.

Straus MA, Hamby SL, Finkelhor D, et al. Identification of child maltreatment with the Parent-Child Conflict Tactics Scales: development and psychometric data for a national sample of American parents. *Child Abuse Neglect*. 1998;22(4): 249–270.

Stringaris A, Maughan B, Goodman R. What's in a disruptive disorder? Temperamental antecedents of oppositional defiant disorder: findings from the Avon longitudinal study. *J Am Acad Child Adolesc Psychiatry*. 2010;49(5):474–483.

Templeman TL. *The Parent Child Coercive Cycle*. n.d. http://www.pendletonpsych.com/therapyhelpers/parent-child-coercive-cycle. Accessed on April 17, 2016.

Van der Oord S, Prins PJ, Oosterlaan J, Emmelkamp PM. Efficacy of methylphenidate, psychosocial treatments and their combination in school-aged children with ADHD: A meta-analysis. *Clin Psychol Rev*. 2008;28(5):783–800.

Van Ryzin MJ, Stormshak EA, Dishion TJ. Engaging parents in the family check-up in middle school: longitudinal effects on family conflict and problem behavior through the high school transition. *J Adolesc Health*. 2012;50(6):627–633.

Wallace GL, White SF, Robustelli B, et al. Cortical and subcortical abnormalities in youths with conduct disorder and elevated callous-unemotional traits. *J Am Acad Child Adolesc Psychiatry*. 2014;53(4):456–465.e1.

White SF, Fowler KA, Sinclair S, et al. Disrupted expected value signaling in youth with disruptive behavior disorders to environmental reinforcers. *J Am Acad Child Adolesc Psychiatry*. 2014;53(5):579–588.e9.

White SF, Marsh AA, Fowler KA, et al. Reduced amygdala response in youths with disruptive behavior disorders and psychopathic traits: decreased emotional response versus increased top-down attention to nonemotional features. *Am J Psychiatry*. 2012;169(7):750–758.

World Health Organization. *International Statistical Classification of Diseases and Related Health Problems, 10th Revision (ICD-10)*. Geneva: WHO; 1992. http://apps.who.int/classifications/icd10/browse/2010/en-/F90-F98. Accessed on April 10, 2016.

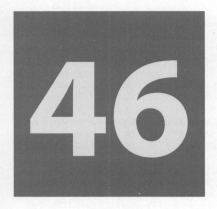

Substance-Related Disorders in Adolescents

Yifrah Kaminer, MD, MBA
Deborah R. Simkin, MD
Kara S. Bagot, MD

According to the biobehavioral developmental perspective and trajectories of adolescent substance use and substance use disorders (SUD), adolescents have not yet reached adulthood and therefore cannot be considered as simply "miniature adults." In addition, during adolescence and young adulthood, between the ages of 12 and 25 years, the nucleus accumbens, which drives reward-seeking behaviors, develops earlier than the prefrontal cortex, which is responsible for inhibitory and executive functioning. This leads adolescents to normatively seek out pleasurable activities, including high-risk sexual, driving, and substance-use experiences.

 ESSENTIALS OF DIAGNOSIS

ICD-10 Diagnostic Criteria

Mental and Behavioral Disorders due to Psychoactive Substance Use (F10–F19)

This characterization of disorders includes a greater spectrum of, and greater detail pertaining to, SUDs than the previous iteration of ICD coding. Substance Use Disorders are coded using the format F1x.xxx, where the third character of the code indicates substance used (i.e., alcohol) and the fourth plus characters indicate clinical state, including amount, extent of harm, or other related disorder (i.e., intoxication, dependence, medical comorbidity, psychosis). F10–F19 represents use of the following psychoactive substances, in numerical order: alcohol, opioids, cannabis, sedatives/hypnotics/anxiolytics, cocaine, stimulants, hallucinogens, nicotine, and other psychoactive substances or polysubstance use.

The fourth plus characters of the ICD-10 code represents the following designations:

.0 Acute Intoxication

A condition that follows the administration of a psychoactive substance resulting in disturbances in level of consciousness, cognition, perception, affect or behavior, or other psycho-physiological functions and responses. The disturbances are directly related to the acute pharmacological effects of the substance and resolve with time, with complete recovery, except where tissue damage or other complications have arisen. Complications may include trauma, inhalation of vomitus, delirium, coma, convulsions, and other medical complications. The nature of these complications depends on the pharmacological class of substance and mode of administration.

.1 Harmful Use

A pattern of psychoactive substance use that is causing damage to health. The damage may be physical (as in cases of hepatitis from the self-administration of injected psychoactive substances) or mental (e.g., episodes of depressive disorder secondary to heavy consumption of alcohol).

.2 Psychoactive substance abuse.

.3 Dependence

A cluster of behavioral, cognitive, and physiological phenomena that develop after repeated substance use and that typically include a strong desire to take the drug, difficulties in controlling its use, persisting in its use despite harmful consequences, a higher priority given to drug use than to other activities and obligations, increased tolerance, and sometimes a physical withdrawal state.

.4 Withdrawal Stat

A group of symptoms of variable clustering and severity occurring on absolute or relative withdrawal of a psychoactive substance after persistent use of that substance. The onset and course of the withdrawal state are time-limited and are related to the type of psychoactive substance and dose being used immediately before cessation or reduction of use. The withdrawal state may be complicated by convulsions.

.5 Withdrawal State with Delirium

A condition where the withdrawal state as defined in the common fourth character .3 is complicated by delirium as defined in F05-. Convulsions may also occur. When organic factors are also considered to play a role in the etiology, the condition should be classified to F05.8.

.6 Psychotic Disorder

A cluster of psychotic phenomena that occur during or following psychoactive substance use but that are not explained on the basis of acute intoxication alone and do not form part of a withdrawal state. The disorder is characterized by hallucinations (typically auditory, but often in more than one sensory modality), perceptual distortions, delusions (often of a paranoid or persecutory nature), psychomotor disturbances (excitement or stupor), and an abnormal affect, which may range from intense fear to ecstasy. The sensorium is usually clear but some degree of clouding of consciousness, though not severe confusion, may be present.

.7 Amnesic Syndrome

A syndrome associated with chronic prominent impairment of recent and remote memory. Immediate recall is usually preserved and recent memory is characteristically more disturbed than remote memory. Disturbances of time sense and ordering of events are usually evident, as are difficulties in learning new material. Confabulation may be marked but is not invariably present. Other cognitive functions are usually relatively well preserved and amnesic defects are out of proportion to other disturbances.

.8 Residual and Late-Onset Psychotic Disorder

A disorder in which alcohol- or psychoactive substance-induced changes of cognition, affect, personality, or behavior persist beyond the period during which a direct psychoactive substance-related effect might reasonably be assumed to be operating. Onset of the disorder should be directly related to the use of the psychoactive substance. Cases in which initial onset of the state occurs later than episode(s) of such substance use should be coded here only where clear and strong evidence is available to attribute the state to the residual effect of the psychoactive substance. Flashbacks may be distinguished from psychotic state partly by their episodic nature, frequently of very short duration, and by their duplication of previous alcohol- or other psychoactive substance-related experiences.

.9 Other Mental and Behavioral Disorder

.10 Unspecified Mental and Behavioral Disorder

Adapted with permission from International Statistical Classification of Diseases and Related Health Problems 10th Revision (ICD-10) Version for 2010. Geneva: World Health Organization; 2010.

ICD-10 criteria overlap considerably with Diagnostic and Statistical Manual of Mental Disorders, Fifth Edition (DSM-5) criteria in diagnosis of more severe SUDs, including the following features: inability or desire to decrease consumption, craving, failure to fulfill responsibilities, negative impact on social/academic/occupational functioning, and withdrawal. Mismatches between the two classification systems for mild-moderate SUDs may come from the inherent nature of each; ICD-10 criteria for SUDs is a categorical system, and DSM-5 is dimensional with a continuum of severity. 'Harmful use' ICD-10 criteria represent a narrower definition of mild substance use (must impair physical or mental health) as compared to DSM-5 criteria, which require 2–3 of 11 possible symptoms, resulting in fewer mild SUD diagnoses based on the ICD-10 classification system.

For both the ICD-10 and DSM-5 classification systems, diagnostic criteria for SUD for adolescents are the same as for adult populations. There has been some criticism regarding their appropriateness for youth. Compared with adults, adolescents are on an upward trajectory of use that plateaus by their mid-20s, when developmental brain changes in the prefrontal cortex are commonly completed. Due to age and environmental restrictions on substance use unique to youth (i.e., school attendance, residing with parents/guardians), adolescents are less likely to demonstrate an extended duration of use or "a pattern of substance use that is causing damage to health," with long-term physical consequences such as hepatitis. As such, adolescents demonstrating use consistent with mild SUD based on DSM-5 criteria may remain undiagnosed via the harmful use criteria of ICD-10. In regard to dependence, youth are less likely to manifest withdrawal and again may not experience great difficulty controlling use given inherent environmental restrictions. Further, "harmful consequences" of use may be related to developmentally related reward-seeking behaviors in adolescents. Lastly, adolescents are more likely to use in social contexts, decreasing the chance that they will meet the neglect of pleasurable activities/interests criterion.

However, the use of the term addiction and the requirement of only 2 of 11 symptoms to meet mild SUD criteria in the DSM-5 "Substance Use Disorders and Addictive Disorders" may be more stigmatizing and developmentally inappropriate for youth, as in many cases use may represent a behavior that is developmentally normative or sub-diagnostic, as compared to ICD-10 "Mental and Behavioral Disorders due to Psychoactive Substance Use" classification system.

American Psychiatric Association. *Diagnostic and Statistical Manual of Mental Disorders*, 5th ed. Washington, DC: American Psychiatric Association; 2013.

Chung T, Martin CS. Prevalence and clinical course of adolescent substance use and substance use disorders. In: Kaminer Y, Winters KC, eds. *Clinical Manual of Adolescent Substance Abuse Treatment*. Washington, DC: American Psychiatric Publishing; 2011:1–24.

Galvan A, Hare TA, Parra CE, et al. Earlier development of the accumbens relative to orbitofrontal cortex might underlie risk-taking behavior in adolescents. *J Neurosci.* 2006;26(25): 6885–6892.

Hoffmann NG, Kopek AM. How well do the DSM-5 alcohol use disorder designations map to the ICD-10 disorders? *Alcohol Clin Exp Res.* 2015;39(4):697–701.

Kaminer Y, Winters KC. Proposed DSM-5 substance use disorders for adolescents: If you build it, will they come? *Am J Addictions.* 2012;21(3):280–281.

Rutherford HJV, Mayes L, Potenza MM. Neurobiology of adolescent substance use disorders: Implications for prevention and treatment. *Child Adolesc Psych Clinics North Am.* 2010; 19(3):479–492.

Winters KC, Chung T, Martin CS. Substance use disorders in DSM-5 when applied to adolescents. *Addiction.* 2011;106:882–884.

▶ General Considerations

The use of alcohol and other drugs is associated with the three leading causes of mortality among adolescents: motor vehicle accidents, homicide, and suicide. Additional morbidity under the influence of substances has contributed to suicidal behavior, violence, sexual aggression, and unprotected sexual activity including unplanned pregnancy and sexually transmitted diseases.

A. Epidemiology

Lifetime prevalence of illicit substance and alcohol use among adolescents in grades 8–12 is 34.9% (illicit substances) and 46.4% (alcohol), respectively. Seven percent of youth aged 12–17 years need treatment for SUDs. Because of lack of motivation, limited resources, insufficient age-appropriate, quality programs, and lack of a broad consensus on preferred treatment strategies, only 10–15% of adolescents in need of treatment end up receiving services.

Although any nonmedical use of drugs (including tobacco and alcohol) by adolescents is illegal and can be regarded as a form of abuse, this viewpoint ignores some key epidemiological findings. Specifically, the high prevalence of alcohol and tobacco use underscores the fact that use of alcohol and tobacco is normative or at least not exceptionally deviant. By age 18 years, approximately 80% of youth in the United States have drunk alcohol, two thirds have smoked cigarettes, and 50% have used an illicit drug at least once. Among adolescents in grades 8–12, 1% report daily alcohol use, 3.3% daily marijuana use, and 3.6% daily cigarette smoking (1.4% smoke half a pack or more cigarettes per day). Substance use (marijuana in particular) among American youth rose alarmingly rates between 1992 and 1997. It then decreased significantly until 2007 and has since then decreased for alcohol, tobacco, and most drug classes including prescription opiates, heroin, MDMA (3,4-Methylenedioxymethamphetamine, commonly known as Ecstasy), and synthetic cannabinoids. The use of marijuana and nontraditional nicotine/tobacco products

(i.e., hookah, cigarillos, and e-cigarettes) and nonmedical use of stimulants have remained stable or increased. In 2012, marijuana use reached a 30-year high and has become more prevalent than tobacco use. Daily marijuana use (6%) eclipsed daily cigarette smoking (5.5%) among high school seniors for the first time in 2014. The annual Monitoring the Future (MTF) survey also showed that teens' perception of marijuana harmfulness is down, signaling a great challenge in curbing increases in use. This erroneous perception is contrary to accumulating data supporting harmfulness of marijuana use, including but not limited to decrease in attention and psychomotor skills, neurophysiology alterations leading to impaired planning and engagement in risky behaviors, increased risk of early-onset psychosis, and decrease in IQ among cannabis users with prolonged use trajectories (early initiators with persistent use through adulthood) or those with preexisting psychiatric or neurologic vulnerabilities. Furthermore, the growing trend of medicinalization, decriminalization, and legalization of marijuana use for adults is sending mixed messages to teens that may negatively impact prevention efforts. There is some evidence of higher prevalence of teen cannabis use and a lower perception of risks in states with medical marijuana laws compared with states without such laws, with potential increase in diversion of medicinal marijuana to teens in states with medical marijuana.

Most adolescents who engage in substance use do not develop SUD. It is thus imperative to understand adolescent substance use in the context of changing patterns of behavior and to distinguish normative behavior from a SUD.

Bagot KS, Milin R, Kaminer Y. Adolescent initiation of cannabis use and early-onset psychosis. *Subst Abus.* 2015;36(4):524–533.

Johnston LD, O'Malley PM, Miech RA, et al. *Monitoring the Future National Survey Results on Drug Use: 1975–2014: Overview, Key Findings on Adolescent Drug Use.* Ann Arbor: Institute for Social Research, The University of Michigan; 2015.

Substance Abuse and Mental Health Services Administration (SAMHSA), Office of Applied Studies. *Substance Use Treatment Need Among Adolescents (The NSDUH Report, 2010).* Rockville, MD: Author; 2011.

Wall MM, Poh E, Cerda M, et al. Adolescent marijuana use from 2002 to 2008: higher in states with medical marijuana laws. *Ann Epidemiol.* 2011;21:714–716.

B. Etiology

Substance use disorders are complex phenotypically and etiologically. Genetic and environmental components and interactions may predispose and predict adolescent expression of SUD over the course of development. The genetic contributions are likely to be complex traits involving multiple loci of small effect. Several individual genes that may contribute to the risk for dependence have been identified. In the case of alcohol, these include genes encoding alcohol and aldehyde dehydrogenases and gamma-aminobutyric acid (A) receptor subunits, and nicotine genes encoding orexin (hypocretin) have been implicated. Temperament has a pivotal role in the pathways leading from genetic risk and environmental exposure to the development of psychopathology. Temperament deviations have been shown to be associated with psychopathology and substance abuse. Children having a "difficult temperament" commonly manifest externalizing and internalizing behavior problems by middle childhood and in adolescence. High levels of behavioral activity have been noted in youth at high risk for substance abuse as well as in those with an SUD. High levels of behavioral activity also correlate with disorder severity, as do temperamental trait deviations including reduced attention span; high impulsivity, novelty and sensation seeking; negative affect states, such as irritability; and emotional reactivity. Temperament precursors such as impulsivity and sensation seeking tend to peak in late adolescence.

Kendler KS, Prescott CA, Myers J, et al. The structure of genetic and environmental risk factors for common psychiatric and substance use disorders in men and women. *Arch Gen Psychiatry*. 2003;60(9):929–937.

Meyers JL, Dick DM. Genetic and environmental risk factors for adolescent-onset substance use disorders. *Child Adolesc Psychiatr Clin N Am*. 2010;19(3):465–477.

Nishizawa D, Kasai S, Hasegawa J, et al. Associations between the orexin (hypocretin) receptor 2 gene polymorphism Val308Ile and nicotine dependence in genome-wide and subsequent association studies. *Mol Brain*. 2015;8:50.

Rutherford HJV, Mayes LC, Potenza MN. Neurobiology of adolescent substance use disorders: Implications for prevention and treatment. *Child Adolesc Psychiatr Clin N Am*. 2010;19(3): 479–492.

Tarter RE, Kirisci L, Mezzich A. Multivariate typology of adolescents with alcohol use disorder. *Am J Addict*. 1997;6:150–158.

▶ Clinical Findings

A. Assessment & Screening

Self-report of substance use by adolescents is generally valid and more sensitive than laboratory testing. Collateral reports of alcohol and drug abuse from parents or other adults have low to moderate sensitivity compared to self-report and urinalysis. It may be helpful, in interviewing an adolescent, to begin by asking whether illicit drugs are available at school, whether the patient has close friends who use drugs, and whether the patient has access to drugs. Examples of reliable and valid screening instruments include The Personal Experience Screening Questionnaire, the Substance Abuse Subtle Screening Inventory, the Drug Use Screening Inventory—Revised, the Problem Oriented Screening Instrument for Teenagers, and the easy-to-use CRAFFT. A score of 2 or higher on the CRAFFT is optimal for identifying any problem use. The **CRAFFT** questions are as follows: Have you ever ridden in a **C**ar driven by someone (including yourself) who was "high" or had been using alcohol or drugs? Do you ever use alcohol or drugs to **R**elax, feel better about yourself or to fit in? Do you ever use alcohol/drugs while you are by

yourself **A**lone? Do your **F**amily/friends ever tell you that you should cut down your drinking/drug use? Do you ever **F**orget things you did while using alcohol or drugs? Have you gotten into **T**rouble while you were using alcohol or drugs?

If the self-report is positive, then it is important to assess the severity of the problem using well-established semistructured interviews such as the Teen Addiction Severity Index, the Adolescent Drug Abuse Diagnosis, or the Personal Experience Inventory. Computerized assessment is possible; for example, the Teen Addiction Severity Index was modified into a self-report administered via a telephone or a website. Modern technology also allows the telephone interactive voice response which provides a daily record of risky situations and drug use.

Levy S, Winters KC, Knight JR. Screening and brief interventions for adolescent substance use in the general office setting. In: Kaminer Y, Winters KC (eds.). *Clinical Manual of Adolescent Substance Abuse Treatment*. Washington, DC: American Psychiatric Publishing; 2011.

Winters K, Kaminer Y. Screening and assessing adolescent substance use disorders in clinical population. *J Am Acad Child Adolesc Psychiatry*. 2008;47:740–744.

B. Signs & Symptoms

Signs and symptoms that could give a clue to substance use in adolescents include changes in social network and association with deviant peers, secretive behavior, isolative behaviors including withdrawing from family, excessive complaints about violation of privacy, and smell of alcohol or marijuana on clothing, the youth, or in the room. Inappropriate and atypical behaviors or signs may be present such as agitation or sedation, pupillary dilation or constriction, tachycardia, bloodshot eyes, diaphoresis, slurred speech, yawning, and unsteady gait. The presence of eye drops, prescription drugs, drug paraphernalia, or drugs aid in confirmation of use.

C. Laboratory Findings

Testing for drugs of abuse can be performed on urine, blood, breath, hair, saliva, and sweat. Urine testing is most widely used because it is noninvasive, simple to obtain, and yields a detectable concentration of most drugs of abuse. The best evidence for long-term drug use is the combination of a good history and a urine toxicology screen. Screening tests for single or multiple drugs of abuse are commercially available. These tests typically screen for many possible combinations of drugs including opioids, alcohol, cocaine, marijuana, and amphetamines. Validity and reliability of urine drug test results can be compromised by tampering with the sample. Requirements for notification or permission to obtain specimens vary by jurisdiction. Patients should be asked for permission to perform testing. Self-report is highly reliable as long as it is not associated with a legal contingency. Parental report tends to be deficient or unreliable, yet should be obtained for a complete picture and to improve parental participation in the diagnostic and treatment processes.

Arias JE, Arias AJ, Kaminer Y. Biomarker testing for substance use in adolescents. In: Kaminer Y, Winters KC, eds. *Clinical Manual of Adolescent Substance Abuse Treatment*. Washington, DC: American Psychiatric Publishing; 2011.

Buchan BJ, Dennis ML, Tims FM, Diamond GS. Marijuana use: consistency and validity of self-report, on-site urine testing and laboratory testing. *Addiction*. 2002;97(S1):98–108.

Burleson J, Kaminer Y. Adolescent alcohol and marijuana use: Concordance among objective-, self-, and collateral-reports. *J Child Adolesc Subst Abuse*. 2006;16:53–68.

D. Neuroimaging & Neuropsychology

It is difficult to make accurate generalizations or conclusive statements about the neuropsychological and neurobiological correlates of drug use, given variations in the nature or extent of deficits observed within or across different classes of agents. However, across substances, there is evidence of impairments in prefrontally mediated cognitive functions that underlie behavioral regulation, including decision making and inhibitory control. Marijuana, the illegal drug most commonly abused by youth, has been reported to affect decrease in attention, learning, recall, psychomotor skills, and changes in the brain areas involved in thinking.

Chambers RA, Taylor JR, Potenza MN. Developmental neurocircuitry of motivation in adolescence: a critical period of addiction vulnerability. *Am J Psychiatry*. 2003;160:1041–1052.

Kalivas P, Volkow ND. The neural basis of addiction: a pathology of motivation and choice. *Am J Psychiatry*. 2005;162(8):1403–1413.

Kumra S, Robinson P, Tambyraja R, et al. Parietal lobe volume deficits in adolescents with schizophrenia and adolescents with cannabis use disorders. *J Am Acad Child Adolesc Psychiatry*. 2012;51(2):171–180.

E. Course of Illness

According to the influential "gateway" theory, there are at least four distinct developmental stages of drug use: (1) beer or wine consumption, (2) cigarette smoking or hard liquor consumption, (3) marijuana use, and (4) other illicit drug use. Approximately 25% of adolescents who use marijuana progress to the next stage, compared with only 4% who have never done so. This theory has been challenged given increasing use of marijuana among youth with limited or no alcohol use and ongoing research will continue to be needed as the marijuana increases in availability. The best-supported hypothesis for the common comorbidity between alcohol and illicit drug dependence in adolescents is that comorbid disorders are alternative forms of a single underlying liability.

Long-term trajectories of SUD with and without treatment are important. Youth are at increased risk for onset or worsening of SUDs until their mid-20s. Findings of long-term follow-up of adolescents with SUDs indicate that indeed adolescents have heterogeneous trajectories. A characteristic paradigm is as follows: a small percentage demonstrating sustained recovery, one third with a pattern of intermittent recovery, less than one third with low rates of use throughout 2- to 8-year follow-up, and one third with sustained substance use problems.

Abrantes AM, McCarthy DM, Aarons GA, Brown SA. Trajectories of alcohol involvement following addiction treatment through 8-year follow-up in adolescents. *Alcohol Clin Exp Res*. 2003; 27:258–259.

Godley SH, Dennis ML, Godley MD, Funk RR. Thirty-month relapse trajectory cluster groups among adolescents discharged from out-patient treatment. *Addiction*. 2004;99(Supp 2):129–139.

Kandel DB. Epidemiological and psychosocial perspective on adolescent drug use. *J Am Acad Child Adolesc Psychiatry*. 1982; 20:328–347.

▶ Differential Diagnosis (Including Comorbid Conditions)

While all psychiatric disorders increase risk for SUD, the literature demonstrates a particularly strong link between disruptive, impulse control, and conduct disorders and SUDs. It has been suggested that internalizing (mood and anxiety disorders) and externalizing (disruptive, impulse control, and conduct disorders [e.g., conduct disorder, oppositional defiant disorder, and attention-deficit hyperactivity disorder]) disorders may influence substance use through differing mechanisms, externalizing through commonality of impulsivity as a risk factor for risk-taking behaviors and behavioral disinhibition and internalizing through reduction of anxiety or common genetic influence. Further, complicating these relationships, psychopathology can precede SUD, develop as a consequence of preexisting SUD, moderate the severity of substance use, or originate from a common vulnerability. However, psychiatric comorbidity is the rule rather than the exception in youth SUD. The prevalence of alcohol and substance abuse among youth with prior psychiatric diagnoses is approximately 10% (alcohol) and 15% (illicit drug), respectively. The risk of alcohol and substance abuse among this population is particularly high especially among those with anxiety (alcohol: 17% and drug use: 20%) or behavioral (alcohol: 16% and drug use: 24%) disorders. Rates of conduct disorder range from 50% to 80% in adolescent patients with SUD. ADHD is also frequently observed and is likely indirectly associated with SUD among youth through a high rate of comorbid behavioral and disruptive disorders that accompany ADHD. Mood disorders, especially depressive disorders, have been shown to precede SUD in adolescents. The prevalence of depressive disorders ranges from 24% to greater than 50% in adolescents with SUD.

Several studies have found a high rate of anxiety disorder among youth with SUD. In adolescent patients with SUD, the prevalence of anxiety disorder ranges from 7% to more than 40%. While social phobia has been shown to precede substance abuse, the evidence for nonphobic anxiety disorders such as panic and generalized anxiety disorder is inconclusive with some studies demonstrating SUDs preceding these anxiety disorders and others with anxiety preceding the SUD. Undetected learning disorders can increase the risk for developing later substance abuse. Finally, it was reported that pathological gambling in youth may be associated with substance abuse.

The self-medication theory has not been supported by studies describing treatment of youth with SUD and comorbid depression but has been shown for adolescents with SUD and comorbid anxiety disorders and some personality disorders. Antidepressants have not been found to be efficacious in reducing substance use or improving substance use-related outcomes among depressed adolescents. Also, it is noteworthy that concerns about drug–medication interactions in dually diagnosed youth have not been substantiated. Treatment of dually diagnosed conditions should be addressed simultaneously and not sequentially. Integrative psychosocial interventions or a combination of psychopharmacological and psychosocial interventions is the rule rather than the exception and should continue to be investigated.

Conway KP, Swendsen J, Husky MM, He JP, Merikangas KR. Association of lifetime mental disorders and subsequent alcohol and illicit drug use: results from the National Comorbidity Survey—Adolescent Supplement. *J Am Acad Child Adolesc Psychiatry*. 2016;55(4):280–288.

Hops HA, Davis B, Lewin LM. The development of alcohol and other substance use: a gender study of family and peer context. *J Stud Alcohol Suppl*. 1999;13:22–31.

Kaminer Y, (ed.) *Youth Substance Abuse and Co-Occurring Disorders*. American Psychiatric Publishing Association, Arlington, VA, 2015.

Kaminer Y, Goldberg P, Connor D. Psychotropic medications and substances of abuse interactions in youth. *Substance Abuse*. 2010;31(1):53–57.

King SM, Iacono WG, McGue M. Childhood externalizing and internalizing psychopathology in the prediction of early substance use. *Addiction*, 2014; 99:1548-1559.

McKernan LC, Nash MR, Gottdiener WH, et al. Further evidence of self-medication: personality factors influencing drug choice in substance use disorders. *Psychodyn Psychiatry*. 2015;43(2):243–275.

Simkin, D. Children and adolescents. Section 13, Chapters 99–108, in: Ries RK, Miller SC, Fielin DA, et al, eds. *Principles of Addiction Medicine*. 4th ed., Philadelphia: Lippincott Williams & Wilkins; 2009.

Zhou X, Qin B, Del Giovane C, et al. Efficacy and tolerability of antidepressants in the treatment of adolescents and young adults with depression and substance use disorders: a systematic review and meta-analysis. *Addiction*. 2015;110(1):38–48.

Prevention

Development of effective approaches to substance abuse prevention is a national priority; however, universal substance use prevention campaigns have historically demonstrated little efficacy among youth, due to lack of specificity for high risk, or at-risk youth. The most promising prevention strategies are public health and legal interventions, especially for alcohol and nicotine/tobacco use, and those that enhance social skills and drug refusal. A school curriculum, the Life Skills Training program, was initially developed as a universal prevention program involving the teaching of general life skills and of skills for resisting social influences designed to prevent adolescent tobacco, alcohol, marijuana use, and violence. This prevention program was led by older peers and classroom teachers. The investigators reported a lasting reduction in drug use 6 years later among the 12th-graders in the experimental condition compared to those in the control condition. The generalizability of Life Skills Training prevention to African-American and Hispanic youth has also been supported. To maximize outcome, an understanding of the heterogeneity of the adolescent population is required. Preventive efforts need to take into account the developmental staging of substance use behavior and address the needs of adolescents in different domains of life. Prevention programs sensitive to more broad ethnic differences must be designed. Finally, universal prevention programs may delay onset of drinking among low-risk baseline abstainers; however, there is little evidence of utility in high-risk adolescents. Evidence suggests that motivational interviewing (MI) in a harm-reduction framework is well suited for secondary prevention in high-risk adolescents.

Botvin GJ, Baker E, Dusenbury I, et al. Long-term follow-up results of a randomized drug abuse prevention trial in a white middle-class population. *JAMA*. 1995;273:1106–1112.

Catalano RF, Haggerty KP, Hawkins JD, et al. Prevention of substance use and substance use disorders: Role of risk and protective factors. In: Kaminer Y, Winters KC, eds. *Clinical Manual of Adolescent Substance Abuse Treatment*. Washington, DC: American Psychiatric Publishing; 2011.

Hornik R, Jacobsohn L, Orwin R, Piesse A, et al. Effects of the national youth anti-drug media campaign on youth. *Am J Public Health*. 2008;98(12):2229–2236.

Kumpfer KL. Identification of drug abuse prevention programs: a literature review. *Health Services Resource*, NIDA website: https://psycnet.apa.org/record/2004-21248-021.

Stockings E, Hall WD, Lynskey M, et al. Prevention, early intervention, harm reduction, and treatment of substance use in young people. *Lancet Psychiatry*. 2016;3(3):280–296.

Treatment

Significant progress has been made in conceptualizing, testing, and implementing treatment strategies and programs for adolescents with SUD. One of the challenges in the treatment of adolescent SUD has been the attempt to match the individual needs of the adolescent to appropriate treatment services and levels of care. As SUD is a chronic, relapsing, remitting disorder, a continuum of case management and case monitoring akin to that in chronic disease management is likely to have the greatest impact on treatment outcomes.

A. Systems of Care for Adolescents with SUD

Eighty percent of adolescents with SUD are treated in outpatient settings. Outpatient services usually deliver episodic care using group therapy without coordination or continuity of care. Although many adolescents with mild to moderate severity of use respond to some degree to brief interventions, many do not. Moreover, the higher the severity, the less likely response is seen. More characteristic is a relapsing/remitting course over a prolonged period of time across several episodes of care and levels of care, with different services and interventions. Because SUD is often associated with dysfunction in school, family, legal, and behavioral domains, the need for service coordination and multidisciplinary teamwork is clear. The American Society for Addiction Medicine Patient Placement Criteria are increasingly used for both youth and adults for assessment, diagnosis, and assignment of appropriate level of treatment based on objective criteria.

Fishman M. Treatment planning, matching, and placement for adolescent substance abuse. In: Kaminer Y, Winters KC, eds. *Clinical Manual of Adolescent Substance Abuse Treatment.* Washington, DC: American Psychiatric Publishing; 2011.

Libby AM, Riggs PD. Integrated services for substance abuse and mental health: challenges and opportunities. In: Kaminer Y, Bukstein OG, eds. *Adolescent Substance Abuse: Psychiatric Comorbidity & High Risk Behaviors.* New York: Routledge, Taylor & Francis Group; 2008.

B. Psychosocial Treatments

Psychosocial treatments that have shown promise for adolescent SUD include the following: multisystemic therapy (MST); multidimensional family therapy (MDFT); cognitive–behavioral therapy (CBT), conducted either in groups or individually; motivational enhancement therapy (MET); contingency management reinforcement; the Minnesota 12-step model; and other integrative models of treatment. There is little evidence to suggest that one therapy is more effective than another. Family therapy is the most researched treatment modality for adolescent substance abuse. MST is an intensive home-based family intervention that addresses schools, peer groups, parenting skills, family communication skills, and family relations. MST combines structural and strategic family therapy with CBT. Available evidence does not support the claim that MST is more effective than usual services or other interventions for youth with social, emotional, or behavioral problems. There is no evidence of harmful effects compared to alternative services. MST has several advantages in that it is comprehensive, based on current knowledge of youth and family problems, well documented, and empirical.

MDFT combines drug counseling with multiple systems assessment and intervention both inside and outside the family. The approach is developmentally and ecologically oriented, to the environmental and individual systems in which the adolescent resides. MDFT is manualized and delivered in 16–25 sessions over 4–6 months at home or in the office.

CBT views substance use and related problems as learned behaviors initiated and maintained by environmental factors. Most CBT approaches integrate classical conditioning, operant conditioning, and social learning theory. Recent studies involve rigorous designs, larger samples, random assignment, direct comparisons of two or more active treatments, improved measures, manualization, and longer-term outcome assessment. The focus in treatment has been on improved drug refusal skills and managing of high-risk situations. Improved self-efficacy is associated with better outcome. CBT can also be applied in group settings. Different adolescents are manageable in a group once a clearly communicated, behavioral contract for ground rules is established. Experienced therapists can address inappropriate behavior and employ troubleshooting techniques.

MI and MET are based on research on the process of change. MI pertains both to a style of relating and a set of techniques to facilitate that process. Five main strategies are used in applying this approach: (1) express empathy, (2) develop discrepancy, (3) avoid argumentation, (4) roll with resistance, and (5) support self-efficacy. For as long as treatment results for adolescent substance abuse have been reported, clinicians and researchers have noted the difficulty of keeping adolescents in treatment. To this end, brief motivational interventions have just begun to be investigated. A single session of MI, designed to reduce illicit drugs among young people between 16 and 20 years of age, produced significant decrease in cannabis use at 12-week follow-up compared with nonintervention. Several studies have successfully employed MI following a negative event (e.g., a motor vehicle accident with referral to the emergency room), an intervention exploiting a "teachable moment." MET may be suitable for adolescents because they do not have to admit to having a substance use problem in order to benefit from it. MI alone may not be sufficient for adolescents with severe alcohol use disorder or psychiatric comorbidity. However, it may be an effective preliminary approach.

The Cannabis Youth Treatment study is probably the most comprehensive study of psychosocial treatments for adolescent substance use to date. This randomized prospective field experiment compared five interventions, in various combinations, across the four U.S. implementation sites, for 600 adolescents. The study addressed the comparative efficacy of five treatments. Two group CBT interventions were offered. Both began with individual MET sessions, followed by either 3 or 10 sessions of group-administered CBT. A third intervention was MET/CBT plus a 6-week family psychoeducational intervention. A 12-session individual Adolescent Community Reinforcement Approach and a 12-week course of MDFT were also tested. The effectiveness of five treatment models was evaluated in a community-based program and an academic medical center. Although all five models were not implemented within each treatment site, the MET plus three sessions of group CBT was replicated across all four sites, making it possible to study site differences and conduct quasi-experimental comparisons of the interventions across the study arms. All five interventions produced a significant reduction in cannabis use and negative consequences of use, from pretreatment to the 3-month follow-up. These reductions were sustained through the 12-month follow-up. Changes in marijuana use were accompanied by amelioration of behavioral problems, family problems, school problems, school absences, argumentativeness, violence, and illegal activity. Despite considerable support for family intervention in the literature, the individual Adolescent Community Reinforcement Approach and individual MET plus three sessions of group CBT produced better outcomes than the family approach in terms of days of substance use at 3 months. However, these initial differences were not sustained at long-term follow-up. The best predictor of long-term outcome was initial level of change. In terms of cost effectiveness, MDFT was better than the other interventions. One of the important contributions of the Cannabis Youth Treatment to the knowledge base is the emphasis on community effectiveness and ecological validity compared to a demonstration of efficacy in specialized research setting.

Treatment of adolescents with substance-related problems often incorporates the 12-step philosophy advocated by Alcoholics Anonymous (AA) and Narcotics Anonymous (NA). A national survey of adolescent programs found that more than two thirds (67%) involved "12-step" concepts. Many of these programs encourage attendance at community AA and NA groups following treatment. A retrospective study found that youth who were more hopeless, had friends who did not use drugs, and who had less parental involvement during treatment were more likely to become involved in AA. Two studies found that more severely alcohol- and drug-involved youth, and those more motivated to achieve abstinence, were more likely to attend and become actively involved in AA/NA in the first 3 months posttreatment. An 8-year follow-up study found that, following inpatient treatment, more severe substance dependence, measured by the number of DSM-IV-TR dependence symptoms at the time of treatment, predicted AA/NA attendance throughout a 6-year follow-up period, but not at 8 years following treatment, after controlling for age, gender, and intake substance use indices.

An emerging area of treatment for youth is technology-based intervention. While few mobile health interventions have been developed for use in adolescent substance users, the adult literature describes technology-based interventions, including internet and mobile phone-based platforms, social media, SMS text, GPS location services, and mixed media, for three phases of treatment for SUDs, prevention, treatment, and recovery. The literature shows that technology-based secondary and tertiary prevention interventions in populations of nonillicit substance using college-aged youth may be efficacious (active treatment and briefly following treatment).

Technology-based treatment is a promising area of intervention as nearly 75% of adolescents own or have regular access to a smartphone, and 91% access the internet through a smartphone occasionally and 56% frequently. Technology-based intervention is appealing, in part, because it allows intervention in real time in response to environmental, physiological, and psychological cues and access to treatment during times of increased motivation to change and increased risk of relapse secondary to environmental triggers. Finally, this platform for delivery of intervention may facilitate easier access to continuity of care for substance use behaviors feasible. Due to the ubiquity of ownership and use of mobile technology among youth, the potential to reach rural communities with inadequate clinical services, those who desire anonymity in regard to health risk behaviors and receipt of treatment for these behaviors, and treatment dissemination to underrepresented populations who have reduced access to traditional treatment may result in significant public health impact. As such there is great potential for harnessing the acceptability, accessibility, and functionality of mobile technology for interventions for behavioral change.

As for treatment of substance-related problems in the context of co-occurring psychiatric disorders, the National Institute of Drug Abuse recommends integrated treatment of the psychiatric disorders as a core treatment principle. However, systemic and economic barriers impede the implementation of integrated care: insufficient numbers of treatment providers, difficulty accessing specialty care, and financing streams. Combined treatment of psychiatric disorder and SUD may produce a better outcome than mental health or SUD treatment alone. The optimal design of integrated treatment (e.g., simultaneous or sequential) and the treatment components and exposure have yet to be determined.

Burleson JA, Kaminer Y, Dennis M. Absence of iatrogenic or contagion effects in adolescent group therapy: findings from the cannabis youth treatment (CYT) study. *Am J Addict.* 2006;15(Suppl 1):4–15.

Dennis ML, Godley SH, Diamond G, et al. Main findings of the cannabis youth treatment randomized field experiment. *J Subst Abuse Treat.* 2004;27:197–213.

Kaminer Y, Godley M. Adolescent substance use disorders: from assessment reactivity to post treatment aftercare: are we there yet? *Child Adolesc Psychiatr Clin North Am.* 2010;19(3):577–590.

Pew Research Center: *Teens, Social Media and Technology Overview 2015.* http://www.pewinternet.org/2015/04/09/teens-social-media-technology-2015/. Retrieved April 2016.

Suffoletto B, Kristan J, Chung T, et al. An interactive text message intervention to reduce binge drinking in young adults: a randomized controlled trial with 9-month outcomes. *PLoS One.* 2015;10(11):e0142877.

Waldron HB, Turner CW. Evidence-based psychosocial treatments for adolescent substance abuse. *J Clin Child Adolesc Psychol.* 2008;37(1):238–261.

C. Psychopharmacological Interventions

In general, the same therapeutic principles and approaches valid for adults are recommended for youth including detoxification protocols and various treatments of drug dependence. However, lack of sufficient data, as well as concerns about safety, adverse effects, and necessary age-appropriate legal pathways, in particular for methadone maintenance, has limited the use of drug-specific pharmacotherapy in youth. The emerging consensus among treatment researchers is that a biopsychosocial, multidimensional, problem-oriented approach is necessary to meet the needs of adolescent SUD.

Balter RE, Cooper ZD, Haney M. Novel pharmacologic approaches to treating cannabis use disorder. *Curr Addict Rep.* 2014;1(2):137–143.

Kaminer Y, Marsch L. Psychopharmacology for adolescent substance use disorders. In: Kaminer Y, Winters KC, eds. *Clinical Manual of Adolescent Substance Abuse Treatment.* Washington, DC: American Psychiatric Publishing; 2011.

Marshall K, Gowing L, Ali R, Le Foll B. Pharmacotherapies for cannabis dependence. *Cochrane Database Syst Rev.* 2014;12: CD008940.

Simkin DR, Grenoble S. Pharmacotherapies for adolescent substance use disorders. *Child Adolesc Psychiatr Clin North Am.* 2010;19(3):591–608.

D. Aftercare

Relapse rates are over 60% 3–12 months after treatment. However, little has been done to link patients with aftercare likely due to lack of an evidence base providing guidance for aftercare programs, and scarcity of trained clinicians and coordinated continuing care. The lack of posttreatment support and monitoring leaves patients vulnerable to relapse. Finally, oftentimes it is unclear who is a candidate for aftercare, although most would probably benefit from continued monitoring and relapse prevention. Few programs describe the means of linking completers or noncompleters with aftercare. Adolescents referred from residential treatment to continuing care services are more likely to initiate and receive more continuing care services, to be abstinent from marijuana at 3 months postdischarge, and to reduce 3-month postdischarge days of alcohol use provided they are assigned to an assertive continuing-care protocol providing case management, home visits, and a community reinforcement approach. Additionally, aftercare has been found to reduce the likelihood of severe comorbid psychiatric symptomatology including suicidal ideation.

Many communities lack aftercare services, however, even in cases where youth are referred, many adolescents do not enter, or only participate minimally in, aftercare interventions. Godley and colleagues found that only 36% of adolescents discharged from residential treatment attended one or more aftercare sessions at community clinics. Aftercare is especially important for those adolescents who do not complete treatment as they are at the highest risk for poor substance use outcomes. At a minimum, providers should track linkage rates by type of discharge (i.e., treatment completers vs. nontreatment completers/discharged against medical advice) and determine whether the adolescent is referred to their own organization or another service provider to inform their linkage practice. Finally, new interventions and modalities such as technology-based or remote, tele-care, should be examined and offered if available. Recent reports have found that phone intervention is as efficacious as traditional aftercare therapy. Telepsychiatry should be used when distance from service providers and cost effectiveness are barriers for the provision of aftercare.

Godley SH, Garner BR, Passetti LL, et al. Adolescent outpatient treatment and continuing care: main findings from a randomized clinical trial. *J Drug Alcohol Depend.* 2010;110(1–2):44–54.

Kaminer Y, Burleson J, Burke R. Efficacy of outpatient aftercare for adolescents with alcohol use disorders: a randomized controlled study. *J Am Acad Child Adolesc Psychiatry.* 2008; 47(12):1405–1412.

▶ Complications

Substance use threatens the health and well-being of adolescents. Substance use contributes to many deaths from injuries, homicide, and suicide, the three leading causes of mortality in this age group. For example, adolescents who commit suicide are frequently under the influence of alcohol or other drugs at the time of death. Possible mechanisms underlying this relationship include the direct acute pharmacological and chronic neurological effects of psychoactive substances. Acute intoxication may be experienced as an intense dysphoric state, with behavioral disinhibition and impaired judgment. Substance use can also exacerbate preexisting psychopathology, especially impulse dysregulation, depression, and anxiety.

Other complications include impaired school performance, school failure, unintended pregnancies, and criminal behavior. Medical complications include the toxic effects of substances on the central nervous system or other organ systems, either as the result of chronic use or overdoses, or due to the simultaneous use of multiple agents. Intravenous drug abuse can cause infections including endocarditis, hepatitis, and human immunodeficiency virus (HIV). Up to 90% of illicit injection drug users will eventually become infected with hepatitis C virus. Prostitution to support drug habits frequently leads to sexually transmitted diseases including HIV infection.

Blum RW, Nelson-Mmari K. The health of young people in a global context. *J Adolesc Health.* 2004;35:402–418.

Goldston D. Conceptual issues in understanding the relationship between suicidal behavior and substance abuse during adolescence. *Drug Alcohol Depend.* 2004;76S:S79–S91.

▶ Prognosis

Early initiation of substance use is linked to increased risk of use of other substances and faster progression along the substance use trajectory. Early initiation is also associated with poorer neurobehavioral, psychiatric, and psychosocial outcomes. However, positive peer influences and social networks, and involvement of parents/guardians who demonstrate positive parenting behaviors are protective factors in substance use outcomes among adolescents.

Alcohol and substance use tends to increase until the early 20s, then plateaus as young adults moderate or even cease use. This decrease is accompanied by a change in cognitive structure. When substance use behavior at age 18 years is well controlled, there appears to be no significant relationship between the intensity and consequences of adolescent risk and adult substance use. The effect of child and adolescent risk factors on adult substance use is likely mediated by the intensity of substance use in late adolescence.

Programs aimed at reducing risk factors during adolescence may have a more beneficial effects if they limit drug use during the peak lifetime period, ages 18–21 years. Programs that focus on postadolescence should concentrate on concurrent risk factors that are not necessarily the same as those operating during adolescence. In early adolescence, prevention efforts should be directed at delaying onset and increase of drug use because drug use predicts future drug use, although not in an invariant fashion. Finally, although many adolescents manifest a chronic course into adulthood, others overcome their problem and transition into abstinence or normative drinking.

Bates ME, Labouvie EW. Adolescent risk factors and the prediction of persistent alcohol and drug use into adulthood. *Alcohol Clin Exp Res.* 1997;21:944–950.

Brooks-Russell A, Conway KP, Liu D, et al. Dynamic patterns of adolescent substance use: results from a nationally representative sample of high school students. *J Stud Alcohol Drugs.* 2015;76(6):962–970.

Luciana M, Feldstein Ewing SW. Introduction to the special issue: Substance use and the adolescent brain: developmental impacts, interventions, and longitudinal outcomes. *Dev Cogn Neurosci.* 2015;16:1–4.

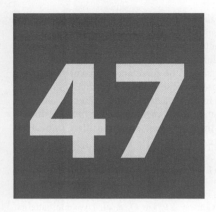

Depressive Disorders (in Childhood and Adolescence)

David A. Brent, MD
Fadi Maalouf, MD

In this chapter, we describe the characteristics and clinical features of unipolar depressive disorders in children and adolescents, etiologic risk factors for depression onset and recurrence, and assessment and differential diagnosis of depressive disorders. We review recommended psychosocial and pharmacological treatments, and in conclusion, suggest areas for future investigation.

▶ General Considerations

Child and adolescent depressive disorders are common, often recurrent, and generally continue into adulthood. These disorders are often familial and are associated with additional morbidity and mortality from comorbid substance abuse and from suicide and suicidal behavior. Patients also suffer educational and later occupational underachievement as well as relationship difficulties. Therefore, early identification and treatment of these conditions are important public health issues.

A. Epidemiology

The estimated prevalence of major depressive disorder (MDD) is 2% in children and 4–8% in adolescents (Avenevoli et al, 2015; Costello et al, 2003). After puberty, the risk for depression increases two- to fourfold, with a 20% incidence by the age of 18 years. The gender ratio in childhood is 1:1, and after puberty, the female/male ratio is 2:1. This may be related to higher rates of anxiety in females, changes in estradiol and testosterone at puberty, or socio-cultural issues related to female adolescent development (Angold et al, 1998).

It is important to differentiate childhood-onset from adolescent-onset depression. Depressive disorders in adolescence are much more likely to be recurrent into adulthood. In the context of significant family adversity, prepubertal depression is most often comorbid with behavioral problems (Harrington, 2000). A less common form of childhood

prepubertal depression is associated with strong familial loading for depression, high rates of anxiety, high risk for bipolar outcome, and recurrent mood disorder into adolescence and adulthood.

B. Etiology

Early-onset depression is multifactorial, including, but not limited to, familial factors, early life events, neuroendocrine changes, and genetics (Wilkinson & Goodyer, 2011). Twin studies show the importance of genetic and environmental factors, particularly in interaction. Familial risk factors for recurrent depressive disorders in youth include early-onset parental mood disorder. Nonfamilial depression has as risk factors parental substance-abuse disorder, parental criminality, family discord, and low family cohesion. Abuse may also be related to an earlier onset of depressive symptoms, as well as many other comorbid conditions. The contribution of early adverse life events is much greater in the setting of familial genetic risk factors (Wilkinson & Goodyer, 2011).

C. Genetics

The strongest single factor for developing MDD is familial loading for the disorder. The majority of studies including twin, adoption, and high-risk studies have shown a familial pattern with interaction of environmental and genetic factors. Family studies show a two- to fourfold increased risk for depression in offspring of depressed parents. Twin studies show a heritability for depression of 40–65% (Thapar & Rice, 2006). Evidence from twin studies shows greater genetic concordance in adolescent-onset depression than in childhood-onset depression, suggesting that very early onset depression is more related to environmental factors (Harrington, 2000; Thapar & Rice, 2006).

Twin studies show a strong cotransmission for depression and anxiety, with heritability of greater than 40% (Thapar & Rice, 2006). Genes imparting risk for anxiety may lead to youth depression by increasing sensitivity to adverse life events, another example of gene–environment interaction (Wilkinson & Goodyer, 2011). This model is further supported by the association of depression with the less functional genetic variant of the serotonin receptor in interaction with stressful life events.

 ## Clinical Findings

A. Signs and Symptoms

ESSENTIALS OF DIAGNOSIS

ICD-10 Diagnostic Criteria

Depressive Episode

In typical mild, moderate, or severe depressive episodes, the patient suffers from lowering of mood, reduction of energy, and decrease in activity. Capacity for enjoyment, interest, and concentration is reduced, and marked tiredness after even minimum effort is common. Sleep is usually disturbed and appetite diminished. Self-esteem and self-confidence are almost always reduced and, even in the mild form, some ideas of guilt or worthlessness are often present. The lowered mood varies little from day to day, is unresponsive to circumstances, and may be accompanied by so-called "somatic" symptoms, such as loss of interest and pleasurable feelings, waking in the morning several hours before the usual time, depression worst in the morning, marked psychomotor retardation, agitation, loss of appetite, weight loss, and loss of libido. Depending upon the number and severity of the symptoms, a depressive episode may be specified as mild, moderate, or severe.

F32.0 Mild Depressive Episode

Two or three of the above symptoms are usually present.

F32.1 Moderate Depressive Episode

Four or more of the above symptoms are usually present.

F32.2 Severe Depressive Episode Without Psychotic Symptoms

An episode of depression in which several of the above symptoms are marked and distressing, typically loss of self-esteem and ideas of worthlessness or guilt. Suicidal thoughts and acts are common and a number of "somatic" symptoms are usually present.

F32.3 Severe Depressive Episode with Psychotic Symptoms

An episode of depression as described in F32.2, but with the presence of hallucinations, delusions, psychomotor retardation, or stupor so severe that ordinary social activities are impossible; there may be danger to life from suicide, dehydration, or starvation. The hallucinations and delusions may or may not be mood-congruent.

F32.8 Other Depressive Episodes

Atypical depression
Single episodes of "masked" depression NOS

F32.9 Depressive Episode, Unspecified

F33.0–F33.9 Recurrent Depressive Disorder

A disorder characterized by repeated episodes of depression as described for depressive episode, without any history of independent episodes of mood elevation and increased energy (mania). There may, however, be brief episodes of mild mood elevation and overactivity (hypomania) immediately after a depressive episode, sometimes precipitated by antidepressant treatment. The first episode may occur at any age from childhood to old age, the onset may be either acute or insidious, and the duration varies from a few weeks to many months. Depending upon the number and severity of the current symptoms, a recurrent depressive episode may be specified as recurrent depressive disorder with current episode mild, moderate, or severe.

According to the *Diagnostic and Statistical Manual of Mental Disorders*, Fifth Edition (DSM-5), major depression involves depressed mood, irritable mood, or anhedonia, plus four other symptoms, and severity level is determined on the basis of impairment (American Psychiatric Association, 2013). Dysthymic disorder is pervasive and chronic, lasting at least 1 year, with fewer symptoms than MDD. Dysthymia may be complicated by major depressive episodes and is then often referred to as "double depression." Dysthymic disorder, or "minor depression," and subsyndromal depression can be disabling and may be precursors to MDD. Disruptive mood dysregulation disorder (DMDD) has been introduced in the DSM-5 as one of the depressive disorders and is characterized by persistent angry or irritable mood along with recurrent temper outbursts that are not consistent with developmental level. This chapter, however, primarily reviews MDD defined as having had at least one depressive episode, see the chapter on DMDD for more details regarding DMDD.

B. Psychological Testing

No psychological test is diagnostic of MDD. A comprehensive psychiatric diagnostic evaluation is the most useful tool to diagnose depressive disorders in children and adolescents. The Mood and Feelings Questionnaire (short-form) can be used to screen for depression and to monitor treatment (Myers & Winters, 2002). In adolescents, the Patient Health Questionnaire—2 (PHQ-2), a two-item screen, has been shown to be an efficient screen for adolescent depression in primary care (Richardson et al, 2010).

C. Laboratory Findings

No laboratory studies are diagnostic of major depressive episode; however, laboratory findings are abnormal in some patients with MDD symptoms. Alterations in sleep and provocative studies of noradrenergic, hypothalamic–pituitary–adrenal axis, and serotonergic systems have been found to be abnormal in depressed child and adolescent patients, but this is particularly true of patients exposed to trauma or severe life stressors (Birmaher et al, 2007; Rao et al, 2009).

Subclinical hypothyroidism, anemia, and nutritional deficiencies including vitamins B_6 and B_{12}, D, and folate are associated with depressive symptoms (Birmaher et al, 2007). Although these are more common in adults, screening laboratories including thyroid function testing, complete blood count, electrolytes, blood sugar, and B_6 and B_{12} and folate levels may be indicated, in cases of chronic or unresponsive depression. The rates of depression are higher than in the community in patients with central nervous system (e.g., epilepsy, migraine) or inflammatory disorders (e.g., asthma, inflammatory bowel disease) (Birmaher et al, 2007). There is growing evidence of the involvement of inflammatory processes, either as a contributor to or a consequence of depression in youth, and that cytokines may mediate part of the relationship between early adversity and depression (Mills et al, 2013).

D. Neuroimaging

Differences in morphometric and functional magnetic resonance imaging (fMRI) have contributed to our understanding of the neural circuitry underlying the development of depressive disorders. Cortical thinning of the lateral half of the right hemisphere and the medial aspect of the left hemisphere has been reported to be a familially transmitted intermediate phenotype for early-onset depression, occurring even in those at familial risk who are not affected (although youth with those features showed impaired attention and visual memory; Peterson & Weissman, 2011). Smaller hippocampal volume has been associated with risk for and onset of depression, especially in interaction with early life adversity (Rao, 2010). fMRI studies in depressed youth, as well as youth at risk for depression, demonstrate neurocircuitry related to biased information processing (greater attendance to negative emotional cues), greater limbic activation to emotional cues, and less ability to deploy prefrontal cortical resources to attenuate these exaggerated emotional responses (Hulvershorn et al, 2011). Depressed and at-risk youth also show attenuated striatal response to reward cues, correlating with an impaired ability to experience positive affect (Forbes & Dahl, 2012).

▶ Course of Illness

The average duration of major depressive episode in community samples is 3–6 months, with slightly longer duration in referred samples of 5–8 months (Birmaher et al, 2002). Approximately 1 in 5 adolescents will have resistant depression lasting more than 2 years (Lewinsohn et al, 1998). In contrast, depressive episodes may remit spontaneously without treatment. Comorbidity, especially with dysthymic disorder, increased severity, presence of suicidal ideation, parental depression, and absence of a supportive environment, contributes to longer duration and intractability of episodes (Birmaher et al, 2002).

Depression is a chronic and recurrent disorder. Estimates of the risk for recurrence from one study of primary childhood depression indicate a 40% rate of recurrence by year 2 and over 70% within 5 years, although childhood depression comorbid with externalizing disorders may be much less likely to recur (Harrington, 2000; Birmaher et al, 2002). Estimates of recurrence for adolescent depression are between 30% and 70% in 1–2 years of follow-up (Birmaher et al, 2002). Youth in whom there is incomplete symptom remission, presence of dysthymia, history of abuse, continued social impairment, or parental history of early-onset depression are more likely to experience recurrence. Children and adolescents with persistent depression are at risk for sequelae, including suicidal behavior, personality disorders, substance use disorders, psychosocial dysfunction, obesity, and underachievement (Birmaher et al, 2002, 2007). Manic episodes, with a consequent diagnosis of bipolar disorder, occur in 10–20% of clinically referred samples of child and adolescent depression and is most common in psychotically depressed patients and those with a strong family history of mania (Birmaher et al, 2002, 2007).

The majority of children and adolescents presenting for treatment of depression have a co-occurring disorder (Angold et al, 1999). Commonly, patients suffer from comorbid anxiety disorders, which can predate the onset of depressive symptoms. This should be differentiated from dysphoria, which resolves with removal of stress. Children with a history of childhood abuse are predisposed to development of depression (Brown et al, 1999). In these children, posttraumatic stress disorder and other disorders of extreme stress are prevalent. Substance use disorders can lead to depression and, conversely, distress from depression and anxiety can lead to substance abuse or dependence (Horwood et al, 2012). Attention-deficit hyperactivity disorder (ADHD) is often diagnosed in depressed youth and may be cotransmitted in some families (Faraone & Biederman, 1997). There is some evidence that depression can lead to conduct disorder and vice versa. Specifically, the irritability and emotion dysregulation that are often part of the picture of oppositional defiant disorder and ADHD may mediate the relationship between externalizing disorders and eventual development of depression (Stringaris et al, 2009; Hipwell et al, 2011).

One serious concern in children and adolescents with depression is their increased risk for suicide and suicidal behavior. All depressed patients should be assessed for the presence of suicidal ideation. Depressed youth with suicidal ideation require additional monitoring and treatment targeting improvement of suicidality. If suicidal ideation is present with intent, and the patient and family cannot adhere to a safety plan, then the patient requires a more intensive and restrictive setting, such as inpatient care (Birmaher et al, 2007).

▶ Differential Diagnosis

In light of the high degree of comorbidity in child and adolescent depression, differential diagnosis is both crucial to appropriate care and challenging. Identification and treatment of the disorder contributing to the greatest impairment should be prioritized. For example, treatment of a preexisting anxiety disorder may result in the resolution of depressive symptoms. Patients may not initially disclose anxiety symptoms, particularly in cases of ongoing trauma or obsessive–compulsive disorder. Such disorders require intervention beyond usual treatment for depression. Untreated ADHD may result in depressive symptoms because of functional impairment and interpersonal difficulty attributable to ADHD. In this disorder, treatment of symptoms of inattention and impulsivity may alleviate symptoms attributed to depression, as well as reasons contributing to low mood (e.g., peer rejection, school failure). Substance use disorders, particularly involving depressogenic substances, such as alcohol and opiates, may mimic or actually lead to a depressive disorder, but patients may be euthymic after detoxification and substance-abuse treatment. Substance abuse can also lead to an increased risk for depression (Lynskey et al, 2004). In the setting of psychotic disorders, affective flattening and the patient's unwillingness to share symptoms of psychosis can contribute to a misdiagnosis of depression. Finally, differential diagnosis should always include consideration of bipolar diathesis, as risk for this diagnosis in the setting of early-onset depression is as high as 10–20%. Children with a bipolar diathesis may present with decreased need for sleep, increased energy levels including marked change in behavior, flight of ideas, rapid speech, grandiosity, or psychosis (Birmaher et al, 2007). In the depressed phase, some studies suggest that depressive symptoms of hyperphagia, hypersomnia, and psychosis are predictive of bipolar outcome (Birmaher et al, 2007).

▶ Treatment

The treatment approach to and response of children and adolescents with depression may vary with severity, duration, and comorbidity of the presenting illness. Treatment should always include an acute and a continuation phase, with the availability of longer-term maintenance treatment for chronic or recurrent depression. Psychoeducation, support, and involvement of family and school are fundamental to any treatment plan and, in cases of very mild depression,

may be adequate. In cases of moderate to severe depression, the use of evidenced-based psychotherapies (described later), pharmacotherapy, or a combination is indicated (Birmaher et al, 2007).

A. Psychopharmacologic Interventions

A meta-analysis of all available clinical trials, both published and unpublished, revealed that selective serotonin reuptake inhibitors (SSRIs) are more efficacious than placebo, with response rates of 60% versus 49% on placebo and with greatest treatment gains early in treatment (Bridge et al, 2007; Varigonda et al, 2015). Fluoxetine is the only medication approved by the Food and Drug Administration (FDA) for the treatment of both child and adolescent depression, is the best studied, and has demonstrated the greatest difference between medication and placebo. Escitalopram is FDA-approved for the treatment of adolescent depression, and there are modestly positive placebo-controlled trials for sertraline, venlafaxine, and nefazodone (Bridge et al, 2007), but the last is not widely used because of a risk of hepatotoxicity.

In some studies there are significant effects for adolescents but not for children (Bridge et al, 2007). In addition, although tricyclic antidepressants show a positive response rate in adults, evidence does not support their use for the treatment of depression in children and adolescents (Hazell et al, 2002).

Dosing recommendations for children and adolescents are to start at half the usual adult starting dose for 1 week (i.e., the equivalent of 10 mg of fluoxetine) and to then increase the dose to 20 mg of fluoxetine or equivalent for another 3 weeks. Dosing increases should occur at no less than 4-week intervals to allow the medication to reach a steady state. Adequate concentration and adherence may both contribute to a successful outcome in treatment of depressed youth with SSRIs (Sakolsky et al, 2011; Woldu et al, 2011). Children and adolescents may require relatively higher doses of citalopram, sertraline, or fluvoxamine, based on pharmacokinetic studies (Findling et al, 2006). There is evidence that, in order to prevent relapse, treatment should be continued for at least 6 months after complete symptom remission, in the case of a first episode of MDD, and for at least 12 months after a recurrent episode (Emslie et al, 2008).

In view of its more extensive efficacy data, fluoxetine should be used as a first-line agent. For patients who have not responded to an adequate trial with an SSRI, studies show that a switch to another SSRI is as efficacious as a switch to venlafaxine, with fewer side effects; moreover, for resistant depression, a combination of medication and CBT is superior to medication monotherapy (Brent et al, 2008). In depression that has been refractory to monotherapy with adequate doses of at least two SSRIs, although empirical data are lacking, clinical experts recommend augmentation, or switching strategies can include bupropion, lithium, or lamotrigine (Maalouf et al, 2011). However, before embarking on additional medication trials, it is important to first establish adherence to the previous trial and that the dosage and duration were adequate, and that there were not untoward psychosocial stressors (e.g., parental depression, family discord, peer victimization) or an undiagnosed comorbid condition or misdiagnosis that might be contributing to treatment resistance (Maalouf et al, 2011). Psychotherapy, if not started previously, is also indicated. Other considerations in the pharmacotherapeutic treatment of depression include the management of contributing comorbidity. Milder cases may respond to psychoeducation alone or in combination with brief psychotherapy.

B. Psychotherapeutic Interventions

1. Cognitive–behavioral therapy—CBT has been shown to be an efficacious psychotherapy for the management of child and adolescent depression, with or without concomitant use of pharmacotherapy. CBT is based on the premise that depressed individuals have distorted information processing, thoughts, and core beliefs. Distortion manifests itself in a negative attributional style and beliefs that lead to, exacerbate, or perpetuate depression, particularly during times of stress. CBT uses cognitive techniques and skills building to attenuate cognitive distortions and maladaptive processing. The content of various CBT treatments varies widely, ranging from the highly structured CWD-A (Coping with Depression for Adolescents) to much less structured, principle-based treatments like those based on Beck CBT and to hybrids like those used in the Treatment of Adolescent Depression Study (TADS) or the Treatment of Resistant Depression in Adolescents (TORDIA) study (Brent et al, 1997, 2008; March et al, 2004).

Based on TADS, CBT alone may be best for less severe cases of depression, although in TADS, those treated with CBT monotherapy did not respond until 18 weeks from the initiation of treatment (March et al, 2004, 2007). On the other hand, combination of CBT and antidepressant medication produced the most rapid and complete response in most, but not all, clinical trials (March et al, 2004; Brent et al, 2008; Goodyer et al, 2007). Predictors of poorer response to CBT, from the TADS and TORDIA studies, include greater severity, history of abuse, history of nonsuicidal self-injury, parental depression, and anhedonia (Curry et al, 2006; McMakin et al, 2012; Asarnow et al, 2009). Conversely, CBT may be particularly favorable for those with high degrees of cognitive distortion and comorbidity (Curry et al, 2006; Asarnow et al, 2009).

In addition, a cognitive behavioral prevention program has been shown to decrease the incidence of depression in high-risk children of parents with a history of derision compared to squall care over a 6-year period (Brent et al, 2015), although effects are attenuated if one of the parents was depressed during the intervention.

2. Interpersonal therapy—Interpersonal therapy (IPT) is predicated on the exploration and recognition of precipitants of depression including interpersonal loss, role disputes and transitions, social isolation, and social skills deficits. IPT for adolescents (IPT-A) is an adaptation of IPT (Klomek & Mufson, 2006). It begins with an "interpersonal inventory" that includes the patient's interpersonal relationships. This inventory allows therapist and patient to make collaborative decisions about goals for treatment. IPT-A may be successful because it addresses role transitions, interpersonal difficulties with peers and family, and the development of social skills—all important developmental tasks of adolescence. IPT-A performs particularly well in youth with high levels of family and interpersonal discord and social dysfunction (Gunlicks-Stoessel et al, 2010). Comparisons of IPT and CBT for both prevention of depression and its treatment show that both are efficacious, and there is no clear evidence that either treatment is superior (Rossello & Bernal, 1999; Rossello et al, 2008; Horowitz et al, 2007).

3. Family therapy—Family therapy is often used as an adjunct to other treatments for depression. There have been both positive and negative studies regarding the use of family therapy. Interventions such as the management of parental depression, improvement of family communication, reduction of excess criticism, and enhancement of support are likely to be of benefit. More recently, family-based attachment therapy has been shown to reduce depressive symptomatology more than "usual" clinical management, and a family-based cognitive therapy has shown efficacy in the prevention of depression in at-risk youth (Diamond et al, 2010; Compas et al, 2011).

C. Other Interventions

Mentalization-based therapy (MBT), a year-long psychotherapy aimed at teaching youth and their families to be able to express the experience of emotions and situations, has been shown to reduce depressive symptoms in depressed, self-harming youth (Rossouw & Fonagy, 2012).

Light therapy has been shown to be beneficial for seasonal affective disorder (SAD) and as an adjunct for MDD with a seasonal component and may be as useful as a primary treatment for adolescents with mild depression or as an adjunctive treatment to accelerate antidepressant response (Swedo et al, 2007; Niederhofer & von Klitzing, 2011, 2012). Light therapy involves the daily use of full-spectrum light in the early morning; for SAD, light therapy is initiated in fall and winter months to counteract reduced daylight.

Although there is little controlled evidence about the use of electroconvulsive therapy (ECT) in adolescent depression, documented clinical experience supports a role for ECT in depression that is refractory to pharmacological and psychosocial management, as well as in severe psychotic depression, bipolar depression, and life-threatening depression (Walter & Rey, 2003).

Complications/Adverse Outcomes of Treatment

One of the primary concerns in the prescription of SSRI medications in children and adolescents has been the FDA "black-box warning" concerning risk of suicidal behavior with use of these medications (Bridge et al, 2007). These adverse events occurred relatively early in treatment and did not involve any actual suicides, and few suicide attempts. In the TADS study, adverse suicidal events were almost 4 times more likely to occur with fluoxetine than with placebo, although most studies have found around a twofold increase (Bridge et al, 2007; March et al, 2007). Data on whether the addition of CBT to SSRI antidepressant treatment protects against the occurrence of suicidal events are mixed: there is relatively little support in the treatment of primary depression, but some evidence of studies of depression comorbid with substance abuse is included (Dubicka et al, 2010; Cox et al, 2012). However, one meta-analysis found that the risk difference between antidepressant and placebo for suicidal events was only 0.9% and that the number of youth who responded to an antidepressant was 11 times the number who experienced a suicidal event (Bridge et al, 2007).

In addition to concern about suicide-related behavior, antidepressants can cause side effects such as agitation, akathisia, serotonin syndrome (particularly in combination with other agents), headache, dizziness, gastrointestinal symptoms, sleep cycle disturbance, sexual dysfunction, and platelet inhibition leading to bruising (Birmaher et al, 2007). In addition, in children at risk for bipolar disorder, it is important to consider that the risk of SSRI-induced mania has been reported as highest in children younger than 14 years of age (Martin et al, 2004). Because of platelet inhibition, SSRIs should be stopped prior to surgery. Medications such as fluoxetine interact with many medications via the cytochrome P-450 system, and this should be considered with each medication change or in cases of medical and psychiatric comorbidities requiring treatment.

Prognosis

Depression is a chronic and disabling illness that often starts in childhood or adolescence. It contributes to increased risk for suicide, substance use, and other psychiatric sequelae and interferes in the child or adolescent's personal development. Although some success has been experienced in the treatment of early-onset depression, up to 40% of youth do not remit at the end of clinical trials (March et al, 2007; Vitiello et al, 2011). Many children and adolescents do not experience complete recovery, and those who are symptomatic remain at risk for relapse (Birmaher et al, 2002; Emslie et al, 2008). Further information is needed about our current methods of treatment, the management of very early onset depression, the neurobiology of depression, identification of biomarkers for early response and suicidal events, and the interaction of biological, genetic, and environmental contributors to depression and to treatment response.

American Psychiatric Association. *Diagnostic and Statistical Manual of Mental Disorders.* 5th ed. Arlington, VA: American Psychiatric Publishing; 2013.

Angold A, Costello EJ, Erkanli A. Comorbidity. *J Child Psychol Psychiatry.* 1999;40:57.

Angold A, Costello EJ, Worthman CM. Puberty and depression: the roles of age, pubertal status and pubertal timing. *Psychol Med.* 1998;28:51.

Asarnow JR, Emslie G, Clarke G, et al. Treatment of selective serotonin reuptake inhibitor-resistant depression in adolescents: predictors and moderators of treatment response. *J Am Acad Child Adolesc Psychiatry.* 2009;48:330.

Avenevoli S, Swendsen J, He JP, et al. Major depression in the national comorbidity survey-adolescent supplement: prevalence, correlates, and treatment. *J Am Acad Child Adolesc Psychiatry.* 2015 Jan;54(1):37–44.

Birmaher B. Longitudinal course of pediatric bipolar disorder. *Am J Psychiatry.* 2007;164:537.

Birmaher B, Arbelaez C, Brent D. Course and outcome of child and adolescent major depressive disorder. *Child Adolesc Psychiatr Clin North Am.* 2002;11:619–637.

Birmaher B, Brent D, Bernet W, et al. Practice parameter for the assessment and treatment of children and adolescents with depressive disorders. *J Am Acad Child Adolesc Psychiatry.* 2007; 46:1503.

Brent DA, Brunwasser SM, Hollon SD, et al. Effect of a cognitive-behavioral prevention program on depression 6 years after implementation among at-risk adolescents: a randomized clinical trial. *JAMA Psychiatry.* 2015 Nov;72(11):1110–1118.

Brent D, Emslie G, Clarke G, et al. Switching to another SSRI or to venlafaxine with or without cognitive behavioral therapy for adolescents with SSRI-resistant depression: the TORDIA randomized controlled trial. *JAMA.* 2008;299:901.

Brent DA, Holder D, Kolko D, et al. A clinical psychotherapy trial for adolescent depression comparing cognitive, family, and supportive therapy. *Arch Gen Psychiatry.* 1997;54:877.

Bridge JA, Iyengar S, Salary CB, et al. Clinical response and risk for reported suicidal ideation and suicide attempts in pediatric antidepressant treatment: a meta-analysis of randomized controlled trials. *JAMA.* 2007;297:1683.

Brown J, Cohen P, Johnson JG, et al. Childhood abuse and neglect: specificity of effects on adolescent and young adult depression and suicidality. *J Am Acad Child Adolesc Psychiatry.* 1999;38:1490.

Compas BE, Forehand R, Thigpen JC, et al. Family group cognitive-behavioral preventive intervention for families of depressed parents: 18- and 24-month outcomes. *J Consult Clin Psychol.* 2011;79:488.

Costello EJ, Mustillo S, Erkanli A, et al. Prevalence and development of psychiatric disorders in childhood and adolescence. *Arch Gen Psychiatry.* 2003;60:837.

Cox GR, Callahan P, Churchill R, et al. Psychological therapies versus antidepressant medication, alone and in combination for depression in children and adolescents. *Cochrane Database Syst Rev.* 2012;11:CD008324.

Curry J, Rohde P, Simons A, et al. Predictors and moderators of acute outcome in the Treatment for Adolescents with Depression Study (TADS). *J Am Acad Child Adolesc Psychiatry*. 2006;45:1427.

Diamond GS, Wintersteen MB, Brown GK, et al. Attachment-based family therapy for adolescents with suicidal ideation: a randomized controlled trial. *J Am Acad Child Adolesc Psychiatry*. 2010;49:122.

Dubicka B, Elvins R, Roberts C, et al. Combined treatment with cognitive-behavioural therapy in adolescent depression: meta-analysis. *Br J Psychiatry*. 2010;197:433.

Emslie GJ, Kennard BD, Mayes TL, et al. Fluoxetine versus placebo in preventing relapse of major depression in children and adolescents. *Am J Psychiatry*. 2008;165:459.

Faraone SV, Biederman J. Do attention deficit hyperactivity disorder and major depression share familial risk factors? *J Nerv Ment Dis*. 1997;185:533.

Findling RL, McNamara NK, Stansbrey RJ, et al. The relevance of pharmacokinetic studies in designing efficacy trials in juvenile major depression. *J Child Adolesc Psychopharmacol*. 2006;16:131.

Forbes EE, Dahl RE. Research review: altered reward function in adolescent depression: what, when and how? *J Child Psychol Psychiatry*. 2012;53:3.

Goodyer I, Dubicka B, Wilkinson P, et al. Selective serotonin reuptake inhibitors (SSRIs) and routine specialist care with and without cognitive behaviour therapy in adolescents with major depression: randomised controlled trial. *BMJ*. 2007;335:142.

Gunlicks-Stoessel M, Mufson L, Jekal A, et al. The impact of perceived interpersonal functioning on treatment for adolescent depression: IPT-A versus treatment as usual in school-based health clinics. *J Consult Clin Psychol*. 2010;78:260.

Harrington R. Childhood depression: is it the same disorder? In: Rapoport J, ed. *Childhood Onset of "Adult" Psychopathology: Clinical and Research Advances*. Washington, DC: American Psychiatric Publishing; 2000:223.

Hazell P, O'Connell D, Heathcote D, et al. Tricyclic drugs for depression in children and adolescents. *Cochrane Database Syst Rev*. 2002;6:CD002317.

Hipwell AE, Stepp S, Feng X, et al. Impact of oppositional defiant disorder dimensions on the temporal ordering of conduct problems and depression across childhood and adolescence in girls. *J Child Psychol Psychiatry*. 2011;52:1099.

Horowitz JL, Garber J, Ciesla JA, et al. Prevention of depressive symptoms in adolescents: a randomized trial of cognitive-behavioral and interpersonal prevention programs. *J Consult Clin Psychol*. 2007;75:693.

Horwood LJ, Fergusson DM, Coffey C, et al. Cannabis and depression: an integrative data analysis of four Australasian cohorts. *Drug Alcohol Depend*. 2012;126:369.

Hulvershorn LA, Cullen K, Anand A. Toward dysfunctional connectivity: a review of neuroimaging findings in pediatric major depressive disorder. *Brain Imaging Behav*. 2011;5:307.

Klomek AB, Mufson L. Interpersonal psychotherapy for depressed adolescents. *Child Adolesc Psychiatr Clin North Am*. 2006;15:959, ix.

Lewinsohn PM, Rohde P, Seeley JR. Major depressive disorder in older adolescents: prevalence, risk factors, and clinical implications. *Clin Psychol Rev*. 1998 Nov;18(7):765–794.

Lynskey MT, Glowinski AL, Todorov AA, et al. Major depressive disorder, suicidal ideation, and suicide attempt in twins discordant for cannabis dependence and early-onset cannabis use. *Arch Gen Psychiatry*. 2004 Oct;61(10):1026–1032.

Maalouf FT, Atwi M, Brent DA. Treatment-resistant depression in adolescents: review and updates on clinical management. *Depress Anxiety*. 2011 Nov;28(11):946–954.

March J, Silva S, Petrycki S, et al. Fluoxetine, cognitive-behavioral therapy, and their combination for adolescents with depression: Treatment for Adolescents With Depression Study (TADS) randomized controlled trial. *JAMA*. 2004;292:807.

March JS, Silva S, Petrycki S, et al. The Treatment for Adolescents With Depression Study (TADS): long-term effectiveness and safety outcomes. *Arch Gen Psychiatry*. 2007;64:1132.

Martin A, Young C, Leckman JF, et al. Age effects on antidepressant-induced manic conversion. *Arch Pediatr Adolesc Med*. 2004;158:773.

McMakin DL, Olino TM, Porta G, et al. Anhedonia predicts poorer recovery among youth with selective serotonin reuptake inhibitor treatment-resistant depression. *J Am Acad Child Adolesc Psychiatry*. 2012;51:404.

Mills NT, Scott JG, Wray NR, et al. Research review: the role of cytokines in depression in adolescents: a systematic review. *J Child Psychol Psychiatry*. 2013;54:816.

Myers K, Winters NC. Ten-year review of rating scales. II: scales for internalizing disorders. *J Am Acad Child Adolesc Psychiatry*. 2002;41:634.

Niederhofer H, von Klitzing K. Bright light treatment as add-on therapy for depression in 28 adolescents: a randomized trial. *Prim Care Companion CNS Disord*. 2011;13.

Niederhofer H, von Klitzing K. Bright light treatment as monotherapy of non-seasonal depression for 28 adolescents. *Int J Psychiatry Clin Pract*. 2012;16:233.

Peterson BS, Weissman MM. A brain-based endophenotype for major depressive disorder. *Annu Rev Med*. 2011;62:461.

Rao U. Comorbidity between depressive and addictive disorders in adolescents: role of stress and HPA activity. *US Psyc*. 2010;3:39.

Rao U, Hammen CL, Poland RE. Risk markers for depression in adolescents: sleep and HPA measures. *Neuropsychopharmacology*. 2009;34:1936.

Richardson LP, Rockhill C, Russo JE, et al. Evaluation of the PHQ-2 as a brief screen for detecting major depression among adolescents. *Pediatrics*. 2010;125:e1097.

Rossello J, Bernal G. The efficacy of cognitive-behavioral and interpersonal treatments for depression in Puerto Rican adolescents. *J Consult Clin Psychol*. 1999;67:734.

Rossello J, Bernal G, Rivera-Medina C. Individual and group CBT and IPT for Puerto Rican adolescents with depressive symptoms. *Cultur Divers Ethnic Minor Psychol*. 2008;14:234.

Rossouw TI, Fonagy P. Mentalization-based treatment for self-harm in adolescents: a randomized controlled trial. *J Am Acad Child Adolesc Psychiatry*. 2012;51:1304e3.

Sakolsky DJ, Perel JM, Emslie GJ, et al. Antidepressant exposure as a predictor of clinical outcomes in the Treatment of Resistant Depression in Adolescents (TORDIA) study. *J Clin Psychopharmacol*. 2011;31:92.

Stringaris A, Cohen P, Pine DS, et al. Adult outcomes of youth irritability: a 20-year prospective community-based study. *Am J Psychiatry*. 2009;166:1048.

Swedo SE, Allen AJ, Glod CA, et al. A controlled trial of light therapy for the treatment of pediatric seasonal affective disorder. *J Am Acad Child Adolesc Psychiatry*. 2007;36:816.

Thapar A, Rice F. Twin studies in pediatric depression. *Child Adolesc Psychiatr Clin North Am*. 2006;5:869, viii.

Varigonda AL, Jakubovski E, Taylor MJ, et al. Systematic review and meta-analysis: early treatment responses of selective serotonin reuptake inhibitors in pediatric major depressive disorder. *J Am Acad Child Adolesc Psychiatry*. 2015 Jul;54(7):557–564.

Vitiello B, Emslie G, Clarke G, et al. Long-term outcome of adolescent depression initially resistant to selective serotonin reuptake inhibitor treatment: a follow-up study of the TORDIA sample. *J Clin Psychiatry*. 2011;72:388.

Walter G, Rey JM. Has the practice and outcome of ECT in adolescents changed? Findings from a whole-population study. *J ECT*. 2003;19:84.

Wilkinson PO, Goodyer IM. Childhood adversity and allostatic overload of the hypothalamic-pituitary-adrenal axis: a vulnerability model for depressive disorders. *Dev Psychopathol*. 2011;23:1017.

Woldu H, Porta G, Goldstein T, et al. Pharmacokinetically and clinician-determined adherence to an antidepressant regimen and clinical outcome in the TORDIA trial. *J Am Acad Child Adolesc Psychiatry*. 2011;50:490.

Wood A, Harrington R, Moore A. Controlled trial of a brief cognitive–behavioural intervention in adolescent patients with depressive disorders. *J Child Psychol Psychiatry*. 1996 Sep;37(6):737–746.

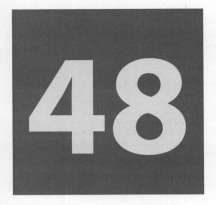

48

Pediatric Bipolar Disorder

Rasim Diler, MD
Benjamin I. Goldstein, MD, PhD, FRCPC
Boris Birmaher, MD

International Statistical Classification of Diseases and Related Health Problems 10th Revision (ICD-10) Diagnostic Criteria

In the ICD-10, bipolar disorder (BP) is included under mood (affective) disorders, conditions in which the fundamental disturbance is a change in affect or mood to depression (with or without associated anxiety) or to elation. The mood change is usually accompanied by a change in the overall level of activity; most of the other symptoms are either secondary to, or easily understood in the context of, the change in mood and activity. Most of these disorders tend to be recurrent and the onset of individual episodes can often be related to stressful events or situations.

F30 Manic Episode

All the subdivisions of this category should be used only for a single episode. Hypomanic or manic episodes in individuals who have had one or more previous affective episodes (depressive, hypomanic, manic, or mixed) should be coded as bipolar affective disorder (F31.).

F30.0 Hypomania

A disorder characterized by a persistent mild elevation of mood, increased energy and activity, and usually marked feelings of well-being and both physical and mental efficiency. Increased sociability, talkativeness, over-familiarity, increased sexual energy, and a decreased need for sleep are often present but not to the extent that they lead to severe disruption of work or result in social rejection. Irritability, conceit, and boorish behavior may take the place of the more usual euphoric sociability. The disturbances of mood and behavior are not accompanied by hallucinations or delusions.

F30.1 Mania Without Psychotic Symptoms

Mood is elevated out of keeping with the patient's circumstances and may vary from carefree joviality to almost uncontrollable excitement. Elation is accompanied by increased energy, resulting in overactivity, pressure of speech, and a decreased need for sleep. Attention cannot be sustained, and there is often marked distractibility. Self-esteem is often inflated with grandiose ideas and overconfidence. Loss of normal social inhibitions may result in behavior that is reckless, foolhardy, or inappropriate to the circumstances, and out of character.

F30.2 Mania with Psychotic Symptoms

In addition to the clinical picture described in F30.1, delusions (usually grandiose) or hallucinations (usually of voices speaking directly to the patient) are present, or the excitement, excessive motor activity, and flight of ideas are so extreme that the subject is incomprehensible or inaccessible to ordinary communication. Subtypes: 1) mood-congruent psychotic symptoms, 2) mood-incongruent psychotic symptoms, and 3) manic stupor.

F30.8 Other Manic Episodes

F30.9 Manic Episode, Unspecified (Mania NOS)

Bipolar Affective Disorder (F31)

A disorder characterized by two or more episodes in which the patient's mood and activity levels are significantly disturbed. One episode of these disturbances must be an elevation of mood and increased energy and activity (hypomania or mania) and the others are often (but not required to be) a lowering of mood and decreased energy and activity (depression). Repeated episodes of hypomania or mania only are classified as bipolar manic depression; manic-depressive (illness, psychosis, reaction): *Excl.*: bipolar disorder, single manic episode (F30), cyclothymia (F34.0).

F31.0 Bipolar Affective Disorder, Current Episode Hypomanic

The patient is currently hypomanic and has had at least one other affective episode (hypomanic, manic, depressive, or mixed) in the past.

F31.1 Bipolar Affective Disorder, Current Episode Manic Without Psychotic Symptoms

The patient is currently manic, without psychotic symptoms (as in F30.1), and has had at least one other affective episode (hypomanic, manic, depressive, or mixed) in the past.

F31.2 Bipolar Affective Disorder, Current Episode Manic with Psychotic Symptoms

The patient is currently manic, with psychotic symptoms (as in F30.2), and has had at least one other affective episode (hypomanic, manic, depressive, or mixed) in the past.

F31.3 Bipolar Affective Disorder, Current Episode Mild or Moderate Depression

The patient is currently depressed, as in a depressive episode of either mild or moderate severity (F32.0 or F32.1), and has had at least one authenticated hypomanic, manic, or mixed affective episode in the past.

F31.4 Bipolar Affective Disorder, Current Episode Severe Depression Without Psychotic Symptoms

The patient is currently depressed, as in severe depressive episode without psychotic symptoms (F32.2), and has had at least one authenticated hypomanic, manic, or mixed affective episode in the past.

F31.5 Bipolar Affective Disorder, Current Episode Severe Depression with Psychotic Symptoms

The patient is currently depressed, as in severe depressive episode with psychotic symptoms (F32.3), and has had at least one authenticated hypomanic, manic, or mixed affective episode in the past.

F31.6 Bipolar Affective Disorder, Current Episode Mixed

The patient has had at least one authenticated hypomanic, manic, depressive, or mixed affective episode in the past and currently exhibits either a mixture or a rapid alteration of manic and depressive symptoms.
Excl.: single mixed affective episode (F38.0).

F31.7 Bipolar Affective Disorder, Currently in Remission

The patient has had at least one authenticated hypomanic, manic, or mixed affective episode in the past, and at least one other affective episode (hypomanic, manic, depressive, or mixed) in addition, but is not currently suffering from any significant mood disturbance, and has not done so for several months. Periods of remission during prophylactic treatment should be coded here.

F31.8 Other Bipolar Affective Disorders

Bipolar II disorder, Recurrent manic episodes NOS

F31.9 Bipolar Affective Disorder, Unspecified

In contrast to the *Diagnostic and Statistical Manual of Mental Disorders, Fifth Edition* (DSM-5) nomenclature for BP and related disorders that require one manic episode to make the diagnosis, the ICD-10 criteria require at least two mood episodes, one of which should be manic or mixed (e.g., either a mixture or a rapid alteration of manic and depressive symptoms) episode and the other could be depressive, hypomanic, manic, or mixed episode, to make the BP affective disorder diagnosis. Duration for hypomanic and manic episodes has similar duration criteria (4 and 7 days, respectively) in both nomenclatures. However, BP-II disorder in DSM-5 (presence of hypomanic episode plus at least one major depressive episode) is categorized as "other bipolar affective disorders" in ICD-10. The ICD-10 criteria also do not mention 'impairment' but require that patient's mood and activity levels are significantly disturbed.

Several changes were made in DSM-5, in comparison to DSM-IV, for BP and related disorders such as:

▶ excluding mixed episodes,

▶ introducing the new specifier of "mixed features (presence of 3 or more depressive symptoms during the course of an manic episode),"

▶ introducing the new specifier of "anxiety features (presence of anxiety symptoms specifically during the course of an manic episode)," and

▶ the new requirement of "increased energy or goal-directed activity" as the main symptom criteria (in addition to "elated mood or irritability") for diagnosis of a manic episode.

▶ Essentials of Diagnosis

BP is a familial illness characterized by episodes of abnormally elevated mood that are above and beyond the child's developmental stage (Birmaher 2016; Birmaher et al, 2007; Diler & Birmaher, 2012). According to the *Diagnostic and Statistical Manual of Mental Disorders*, 5th ed. (DSM-5, American Psychiatric Association [APA], 2013), when accompanied by other symptoms of increased cognitive and physical activity and by major functional impairment, and lasting 7 days or longer (or requires inpatient treatment), these episodes are labeled "manic episodes." If the manic symptoms are milder and/or briefer (e.g., 4 days or longer with functional change), the episodes are labeled as "hypomanic episodes." In addition, to diagnose a youth with BP, the symptoms of mania or hypomania need to appear in clusters, be recurrent, and not be better accounted for by other psychiatric and medical conditions. Although not necessary for the diagnosis of BP-I, youth with this disorder often experience recurrent episodes of major depression (APA, 2013; Birmaher et al, 2009a).

BP is usually subdivided into several subtypes: BP type I (BP-I), BP type II (BP-II), cyclothymia, and unspecified/other-specified Bipolar and Related Disorder (in the past referred to as BP not otherwise specified, BP-NOS) (APA, 2004, 2013; Birmaher et al, 2009a; Goodwin et al, 2007). These subtypes are usually grouped under the label "BP Spectrum Disorders." BP-I can also be subdivided into manic, mixed (e.g., mixed features as in DSM-5), depressed, rapid cycling, and psychotic (Table 48–1). Each one of these subtypes is important because they have prognostic as well as treatment implications.

Our discussion includes the revisions in DSM-5, but it is important to note that all studies included in this chapter were carried out using the DSM-IV criteria for BP (APA, 2004, 2013).

General Considerations

Epidemiology

A meta-analysis of 12 epidemiological studies across the world and a recent epidemiological study in Canada and the United States of America reported a lifetime prevalence of 1–2% for BP-I/II and around 3–6% for subsyndromal manic symptomatology (Kozloff et al, 2010; Merikangas et al, 2012; Van Meter et al, 2011). There were no significant differences between the studies carried out within versus outside the USA for BP-I, but there were differences for BP-NOS indicating that subsyndromal BP is more prevalent in the USA than in other countries (Van Meter et al, 2011). These results may account, at least in part, for the relative increase in the diagnosis of unspecified BP observed in recent years in the USA and other countries (Holtmann et al, 2010; Moreno et al, 2007; Stringaris and Youngstrom, 2014).

The results, together with the fact that several studies in adults with BP carried out by different investigators across the world have consistently reported that up to 60% had the onset of their mood symptoms before the age of 25 years, give further validation to the observation that BP usually starts during adolescence (Chengappa et al, 2003; Goldstein and Levitt, 2006; Kozloff et al, 2010; Lish et al, 1994; Perlis et al, 2004; Van Meter et al, 2011). However, the foregoing figures need to be interpreted with caution because of the difficulties and controversies regarding the diagnosis of pediatric BP and the overlap of its symptoms with other psychiatric disorders.

In clinical populations the prevalence of BP has been reported to be between 0.6% and 20%, depending on the setting, the referral source, and the methodology used to ascertain and interpret the symptoms of BP (Pavuluri et al, 2005).

Etiology

1. Twin and adoption studies—Twin and adoption studies have demonstrated that BP in most part (~80%) is explained by genetic factors (Axelson et al, 2015; Birmaher et al, 2009b; Goodwin et al, 2007; Wozniak et al, 2012). However, identification of the genes associated with BP has been elusive because it seems that several genes and epigenetic factors are relevant to the manifestation of this illness. In addition, other factors, including variation in ascertainment, phenotype definition, control selection, and limited power, have led to inconsistent results.

2. High-risk family studies—Studies evaluating the risk for BP in offspring of parents with BP and in first-degree relatives of youth with BP have provided further evidence that BP specifically (i.e., to a meaningfully greater extent than non-BP disorders) runs in families (Birmaher et al, 2007; Birmaher et al, 2009b; Goodwin et al, 2007). In fact, offspring of parents with BP has up to 25-fold greater rates of BP when compared with offspring of control parents (Birmaher et al, 2009b; DelBello & Geller, 2001; Duffy, 2012; Mesman et al, 2013). Importantly, a large prospective high-risk BP study, the Pittsburgh Bipolar Offspring Study, suggested that offspring with mood lability, depression/anxiety, and particularly those with subsyndromal manic symptoms and whose parents had early-onset BP were at 50% risk to develop BP

Table 48–1 Subtypes of Bipolar (BP) Disorders

BP-Subtype	Clinical Characteristics
BP-Type I (BP-I) Mixed* episode (per DSM-IV) Rapid cycling Psychotic	Recurrent episodes of mania and often episodes of major depression. Concurrent symptoms of mania and depression* ≥4 episodes/year of mania, hypomania, mixed or major depression Presence of delusions and/or hallucinations
BP-Type II (BP-II)	Episodes of hypomania and at least one major depressive episode
Cyclothymia	For at least 2 years (*one year in children), the presence of numerous periods with hypomanic symptoms and numerous periods with depressive symptoms that do not meet criteria for a major depressive episode
BP Disorder Unspecified/ other-specified	• Episodes of mania and depression that meet symptom threshold criteria, but not minimal 7 days duration for mania, 4 days for hypomania, or 2 weeks major depression and cause functional impairment • Episodes of mania or hypomania that not have the meet symptom threshold criteria and cause functional impairment • Recurrent hypomanic episodes without depression

DSM, *Diagnostic and Statistical Manual of Mental Disorders.*

*In DSM-5, instead of mixed episode, "mixed" is used as a specifier for an episode of mania, hypomania, or major depression.

(Hafeman et al, 2016). However, it is important to note that children of parents with BP not only are at high risk to develop BP but also are at risk to develop depression, anxiety, attention-deficit/hyperactivity disorder (ADHD), and behavioral problems as well (Birmaher et al, 2009b).

In the same vein, there is a significant increased risk for BP and depression in first-degree relatives of children and adolescents with BP when compared with relatives of adolescents with other disorders (Biederman et al, 2013; Geller et al, 2006; Wozniak et al, 2010), further indicating that BP runs in families.

3. Psychosocial factors—Very few studies have evaluated the effects of psychosocial factors on the onset and maintenance of BP in youth. The few studies that have evaluated the effects of psychosocial factors on the onset and continuity of BP in youth have suggested that low socioeconomic status (SES), exposure to negative events, and high "expressed-emotion" (EE) in the family are associated with poor prognosis (Birmaher et al, 2009a; Bella et al, 2011; DelBello et al, 2007b; Geller et al, 2008; Miklowitz et al, 1988).

American Psychiatric Association (APA). *Diagnostic and Statistical Manual of Mental Disorders*. 5th ed. Washington, DC: American Psychiatric Association; 2013.

American Psychiatric Association (APA). *Diagnostic and Statistical Manual of Mental Disorders*. 4th ed. Washington, DC: American Psychiatric Association; 2004.

Axelson D, Goldstein B, Goldstein T, et al. Diagnostic precursors to bipolar disorder in offspring of parents with bipolar disorder: a longitudinal study. *Am J Psychiatry*. 2015;172(7):638–646.

Bella T, Goldstein T, Axelson D, et al. Psychosocial functioning in offspring of parents with bipolar disorder. *J Affect Disord*. 2011;133(1–2):204–211.

Biederman J, Faraone SV, Petty C, et al. Further evidence that pediatric-onset bipolar disorder comorbid with ADHD represents a distinct subtype: results from a large controlled family study. *J Psychiatr Res*. 2013;47(1):15–22.

Birmaher B. Pediatric bipolar disorder: epidemiology, pathogenesis, clinical manifestations and course. UpToDate. Accessed January 2016.

Birmaher B, Axelson D, Goldstein B, et al. Four-year longitudinal course of children and adolescents with bipolar spectrum disorders: the Course and Outcome of Bipolar Youth (COBY) study. *Am J Psychiatry*. 2009a;166(7):795–804.

Birmaher B, Axelson D, Monk K, et al. Lifetime psychiatric disorders in school-aged offspring of parents with bipolar disorder: the Pittsburgh Bipolar Offspring study. *Arch Gen Psychiatry*. 2009b;66(3):287–296.

Birmaher B, Axelson D, Pavuluri M. Bipolar disorder. In: Martin A, Volkmar FR, Lewis M, eds. *Lewis' Child and Adolescent Psychiatry: A Comprehensive Textbook*. 4th ed. London: Lippincott Williams & Wilkins; 2007.

Chengappa KN, Kupfer DJ, Frank E, et al. Relationship of birth cohort and early age at onset of illness in a bipolar disorder case registry. *Am J Psychiatry*. 2003;160(9):1636–1642.

DelBello MP, Geller B. Review of studies of child and adolescent offspring of bipolar parents. *Bipolar Disord*. 2001;3(6):325–334.

DelBello MP, Hanseman D, Adler CM, et al. Twelve-month outcome of adolescents with bipolar disorder following first hospitalization for a manic or mixed episode. *Am J Psychiatry*. 2007b;164(4):582–590.

Diler RS, Birmaher B. Bipolar disorder in children and adolescents. In: Rey JM, ed. *IACAPAP e-Textbook of Child and Adolescent Mental Health*. Geneva: International Association for Child and Adolescent Psychiatry and Allied Professions; 2012.

Duffy A. The nature of the association between childhood ADHD and the development of bipolar disorder: a review of prospective high-risk studies. *Am J Psychiatry*. 2012;169(12):1247–1255.

Geller B, Tillman R, Bolhofner K, Zimerman B. Child bipolar I disorder: prospective continuity with adult bipolar I disorder; characteristics of second and third episodes; predictors of 8-year outcome. *Arch Gen Psychiatry*. 2008;65(10):1125–1133.

Geller B, Tillman R, Bolhofner K, et al. Controlled, blindly rated, direct-interview family study of a prepubertal and early-adolescent bipolar I disorder phenotype: morbid risk, age at onset, and comorbidity. *Arch Gen Psychiatry*. 2006;63(10):1130–1138.

Goldstein B, Levitt AJ. Further evidence for a developmental subtype of bipolar disorder defined by age at onset: results from the national epidemiologic survey on alcohol and related conditions. *Am J Psychiatry*. 2006;163(9):1633–1636.

Goodwin FK, Jamison KR, Ghaemi SN. *Manic-Depressive Illness: Bipolar Disorders and Recurrent Depression*. New York: Oxford University Press; 2007.

Hafeman DM, Merranko J, Axelson D, et al. Toward the definition of a bipolar prodrome: dimensional predictors of bipolar spectrum disorders in at-risk youth. *Am J Psychiatry*. 2016;173(7):695–704.

Holtmann M, Duketis E, Poustka L, et al. Bipolar disorder in children and adolescents in Germany: national trends in the rates of inpatients, 2000–2007. *Bipolar Disord*. 2010;12(2):155–163.

Kozloff N, Cheung AH, Schaffer A, et al. Bipolar disorder among adolescents and young adults: results from an epidemiological sample. *J Affect Disord*. 2010;125(1–3):350–354.

Lish J, Dime-Meenan S, Whybrow P, et al. The National Depressive and Manic-depressive Association (DMDA) survey of bipolar members. *J Affect Disord*. 1994;31:281–294.

Merikangas KR, Cui L, Kattan G, et al. Mania with and without depression in a community sample of US adolescents. *Arch Gen Psychiatry*. 2012;69(9):943–951.

Mesman E, Nolen WA, Reichart CG, et al. The Dutch Bipolar Offspring Study: 12-year follow-up. *Am J Psychiatry*. 2013;170(5):542–549.

Miklowitz DJ, Goldstein MJ, Nuechterlein KH, et al. Family factors and the course of bipolar affective disorder. *Arch Gen Psychiatry*. 1988;45:225–231.

Moreno C, Laje G, Blanco C, et al. National trends in the outpatient diagnosis and treatment of bipolar disorder in youth. *Arch Gen Psychiatry*. 2007;64(9):1032–1039.

Pavuluri MN, Birmaher B, Naylor MW. Pediatric bipolar disorder: a review of the past 10 years. *J Am Acad Child Adolesc Psychiatry*. 2005;44(9):846–871.

Perlis RH, Miyahara S, Marangell LB, et al. Investigators S-B. Long-term implications of early onset in bipolar disorder: data from the first 1000 participants in the systematic treatment enhancement program for bipolar disorder (STEP-BD). *Biol Psychiatry*. 2004;55(9):875–881.

Stringaris A, Youngstrom E. Unpacking the differences in US/UK rates of clinical diagnoses of early-onset bipolar disorder. *J Am Acad Child Adolesc Psychiatry.* 2014;53(6):609–611.

Van Meter AR, Moreira AL, Youngstrom EA. Meta-analysis of epidemiologic studies of pediatric bipolar disorder. *J Clin Psychiatry.* 2011;72(9):1250–1256.

Wozniak J, Faraone SV, Martelon M, et al. Further evidence for robust familiality of pediatric bipolar I disorder: results from a very large controlled family study of pediatric bipolar I disorder and a meta-analysis. *J Clin Psychiatry.* 2012;73(10):1328–1334.

Wozniak J, Faraone SV, Mick E, et al. A controlled family study of children with DSM-IV bipolar-I disorder and psychiatric co-morbidity. *Psychol Med.* 2010;40(7):1079–1088.

▶ Clinical Findings

A. Signs & Symptoms

The literature has consistently shown that some children and adolescents meet the full DSM-5 criteria for BP (Axelson et al, 2006; Diler & Birmaher, 2012; Leibenluft & Rich, 2008). However, as discussed here, there was controversy regarding some of the symptoms by which mania manifests in youth, particularly the symptoms of elation, irritability, and grandiosity, and whether BP may be nonepisodic among youth. Also, it is important to note that there are developmental differences in the way that the symptoms of mania, hypomania, or depression manifest between children, adolescents, and adults (Birmaher et al, 2009c; Holtzman et al, 2015). Symptoms are often more difficult to ascertain and differentiate from symptoms of other psychiatric disorders (especially ADHD) or normal behaviors in children. Additionally, there are more rapid changes in polarity and more mixed states, further challenging accurate diagnosis. In contrast, both the manic/hypomanic and depressive symptoms among adolescents are more similar to those of adults (Birmaher et al, 2009c).

1. Mania—According to the DSM-IV, a manic episode is defined as a discrete period of abnormally and persistently elevated, expansive, or irritable mood, lasting at least 1 week (or any duration if the manic episode caused admission the hospital). Recently, the DSM-5 added to these symptoms **the criterion of "increased energy/activity as a core symptom" of mania**. During the period of excessive mood elevation or irritability as well as increased energy/activity, at least three or more of the manic symptoms (e.g., increased self-esteem, decreased need for sleep, more talkative/pressured speech, flight of ideas/racing thoughts, distractibility, increased goal-directed activity/psychomotor agitation, and excessive involvement in pleasurable activities) need to be present. These symptoms exist as a collection of concurrent symptoms and behaviors (i.e., "**cluster together**"), and most investigators agree that **the symptoms need to occur episodically** (Axelson et al, 2011a; Birmaher et al, 2007; Diler & Birmaher, 2012; Leibenluft & Rich, 2008). Also, some investigators have suggested that mania among youth is manifested more by irritability than elation (Wozniak, 2005). However, it appears that this finding was due to methodological issues with the ascertainment of manic symptoms and that, as in adults, most youth with BP have both elation and irritability, with a small proportion having irritability or elation only (Hunt et al, 2009, 2013). In these last cases, elation or irritability is not the only symptoms required to diagnose mania, but other symptoms such as grandiosity, increased energy/activity, or lack of need for sleep are required.

Also, to make the diagnosis, the manic episodes must impair the **youth's functioning**, and the symptoms must not be mainly accounted for by the use of medications, use of substances, or medical illness.

A recent meta-analysis of 20 published studies ($N = 2226$) evaluated the weighted rates of manic symptoms in youth (average age: 11.5 years, 64% male, mainly Caucasian) with BP-I and BP-NOS (Van Meter et al, 2016). The most common symptoms across BP subtypes included increased energy, irritability and mood lability, distractibility, and goal-directed activity (all approximately 75%), whereas hypersexuality, hallucinations, and delusions were the least frequent (all approximately 26%). Grandiosity and hypersexuality were the most specific symptoms, but they were less common (57% and 32%, respectively). As expected, youth with BP-I had more severe and greater number of symptoms than those with BP-NOS. The findings were similar to the meta-analysis published in 2005 (Kowatch et al, 2005b). However, because of methodological issues and probably also the way investigators conceptualize symptoms, there was significant variability in the prevalence of individual symptoms among the studies (Axelson et al, 2006; Diler, 2007; Kowatch et al, 2005; Van Meter et al, 2016). Some symptoms, such as not feeling tired or sleepy the day after having slept 3–4 hours during the night, or having inappropriate sexual behaviors not explained by exposure to sexual behaviors, should raise suspicion with regard to the diagnosis of BP. Perhaps due to the complexity of assessing psychosis in youth (particularly in children), the weighted rates of psychosis were unexpectedly high (31% hallucinations and 24% delusions) in the recent meta-analysis (Van Meter et al, 2016). Though it is not a symptom of mania per se and though schizophrenia is rare in children, the presence of psychosis (hallucinations and/or delusions) should also raise the question of whether the child has BP.

2. Hypomania—According to the DSM-5, hypomania refers to an episode of at least 4 days of less severe manic symptoms. Hypomania **usually causes functional changes**, but it is not associated with marked functional impairment or hospitalization. Moreover, sometimes hypomanic youth can improve their functioning, become more creative and "sharp," work many hours, and become more social and outgoing.

The identification of hypomania may be difficult not only because the youth can function better but also because the symptoms need to be differentiated from normal moods and behaviors usually observed in youth.

3. Major depression—To be diagnosed with DSM-5 major depression, a youth needs to have at least five depressive symptoms, and at least one of the symptoms must be either depressive/irritable mood or loss of interest (anhedonia) (APA, 2013). The symptoms should be present daily or for most of the day, or nearly daily for at least 2 weeks, and must be accompanied by impairment of functioning. Similar to the symptoms of mania or hypomania, they cannot be mainly caused by medications, drug abuse, or a medical condition (e.g., hypothyroidism) and should not be accounted for by other psychiatric disorders.

Depressive symptoms are noted to be prominent features in most phenomenological studies of pediatric BP, and BP adults frequently recall having significant depressive symptoms in childhood or adolescence (Chengappa et al, 2003; Diler, 2007; Duffy, 2012; Egeland et al, 2000; Goodwin et al, 2007; Uchida et al, 2015). Episodes of major depression usually precede the onset of mania/hypomania so that some youth who appear to have only symptoms of depression may actually have BP with depression as their initial presentation. Mild or transient manic symptomatology that does not meet the diagnostic threshold for mania or hypomania may also precede an episode of depression (Axelson et al, 2011b, 2015). All of these factors highlight the need to carefully probe for a history of manic symptoms in youth presenting with depression, particularly in the context of a family history of BP.

4. Subtypes of BP-I disorders

Mixed episodes—The majority of youth with BP have symptoms of depression interspersed in some manner with manic symptoms (Birmaher et al, 2007; Diler & Birmaher, 2012). However, only when there are enough symptoms of depression to fulfill the criteria for major depressive episode and at the same time the youth has symptoms of mania (e.g., agitation, expansiveness, and even euphoria) is the diagnosis of a "mixed episode" warranted as per DSM-IV. In DSM-5, "manic episode with mixed features" replaced mixed episodes and require co-occurring three or more depressive symptoms during the course of a manic episode. Youth with mixed presentations may be very irritable, confused, anxious, labile, agitated, depressed, suicidal, and sometimes psychotic. It appears that youth tend to have more mixed presentations than the adults (Birmaher et al, 2009a). This is important because the diagnosis and treatment of mixed BP are more complicated than for episodes of only mania or depression.

Rapid cycling—Rapid cycling is defined as four or more distinct mood episodes per year (APA, 2013). Similar to the mixed presentations, rapid cycling is associated with early onset and poor prognosis. Some studies have documented that BP youth have more frequent mood polarity changes than adults with BP (Birmaher et al, 2009a). However, it seems that these studies are not referring to the DSM definition of rapid cycling, but rather rapid mood changes within any given episode (Birmaher et al, 2007). For example, a single manic episode with mixed features could include numerous polarity changes or "cycles." Similar to the mixed presentations, the frequent variations in mood in youth make the diagnosis and treatment of BP more complex.

Subsyndromal mania/hypomania—A large proportion of youth do not fulfill the criteria for mania or hypomania because they do not have the time requirements of 7 days for mania or 4 days for hypomania noted in the DSM-IV and -5 (Axelson et al, 2011b). These youth usually are diagnosed with BP-NOS or currently labeled in the DSM-5 as unspecified/other specified bipolar and related disorders.

Youth with unspecified/other specified BP are younger and have more chronic course, irritability, mixed presentations with less euphoric mania than BP-I, but otherwise phenomenologically in continuum with BD-I (Axelson et al, 2011b; Birmaher et al, 2009; Hirneth et al, 2015). Moreover, youth with unspecified/other specified BP have similar psychosocial impairment, risk to develop substance abuse and suicidal behaviors, rates of comorbid disorders, and family history for mood disorders when compared with youth with BP-I (Axelson et al, 2011b; Birmaher et al, 2007). As described later, youth with unspecified/other specified BP are at high risk to convert into BP-I, especially if they have a family history of BP (Axelson et al, 2011b; Hafeman et al, 2016).

Psychosis—Sometimes during an episode of mania or depression, youth may experience delusions or hallucinations (Birmaher et al, 2009c; Kowatch et al, 2005a; Van Meter et al, 2016). For example, during an episode of mania, a child may have grandiose delusions and believe he/she has superpowers and act on these ideas. Also, a youth may be paranoid or, while depressed, have exaggerated guilty feelings. Hallucinations are usually of the auditory type, and youth may hear positive comments or derogatory and negative comments during mood episodes.

B. Assessments

The assessment of symptoms of mania, hypomania, and depression in youth requires careful probing and, in most cases, longitudinal assessments. In addition to the specific manic/hypomanic and depressive symptoms, it is important to ascertain the frequency, intensity, number, and duration (FIND) of the depressive and manic/hypomanic episodes (Diler & Birmaher, 2012; Kowatch et al, 2005a). Also, given that lack of insight can be associated with mania or hypomania, it is imperative to obtain information from caregivers or other significant adults who know the child well in order to accurately assess symptoms and potential change in functioning. Importantly, when assessing the levels of functional impairment or improvement, it is necessary to take into account the child's chronological age and intellectual capabilities and environmental factors.

The assessment of mood (and other psychiatric symptoms) can be facilitated by the use of psychiatric interviews and rating scales. These rating scales do not provide diagnoses but help to uncover symptoms that may alert clinicians to further asses for the presence of BP disorder.

1. Psychiatric interviews—There are several structured and semistructured interviews that can be used for the diagnosis of BP, including the Kiddie Schedule for Affective Disorders and Schizophrenia for school-age children—Present and Lifetime version (K-SADS-PL) (Kaufman et al, 1997). However, these interviews are lengthy and time-consuming and are mainly used for research purposes. Thus, symptom checklists based on the DSM criteria for BP as well as depressive disorders are also useful screens.

2. Clinician-based rating scales—Two clinician-based rating scales are currently used for the assessment of manic symptoms and their severity in youth, the Young Mania Rating Scale (YMRS) and the KSADS Mania Rating Scale that was derived from the KSADS-P mania module (KSADS-MRS) (Axelson et al, 2003; Youngstrom et al, 2005). However, further studies to evaluate the validity of these rating scales are necessary.

3. Youth, parent, and teacher rating scales—It appears that parental reports are more effective in identifying mania than youth or teacher reports (Youngstrom et al, 2005, 2015). The General Behavior Inventory (GBI), the parent version of the YMRS (P-YMRS), and more recently the Child Mania Rating Scale for Parents about their children (CMRS-P) (Youngstrom et al, 2005; Pavuluri et al, 2006) have been shown to have at least adequate psychometric properties and to be useful for the screening of BP symptoms in youth. However, further studies to evaluate the specificity of these instruments for BP are warranted.

The Children Behavior Checklist (CBCL), a parent-report instrument used to assess general psychopathology, has also been used to screen for BP in youth (Diler et al, 2008; Youngstrom et al, 2005). However, this instrument is not specific to assess mania (Diler et al, 2009).

4. Mood time lines or diaries—Mood time lines or diaries, using school years, birthdays, and holidays as anchors, are very helpful in the assessment of the onset and course of mood disorders. These instruments use a simple scale showing daily changes in mood. For example, they can include a scatter line in which 0 is being very sad, 10 exaggeratedly happy, and 5 is normal mood. Alternatively, depression can be measured from −1 to −10 and mania from +1 to +10 in a continuum scale along with the changes in energy levels from −10 to +10 (a.k.a. mood and energy thermometer) (Diler & Birmaher, 2012). The mood diary can include dosages of medications, sleep schedule, and stressors.

As noted before, it is important to evaluate for the presence of other psychiatric (e.g., anxiety, ADHD, and substance abuse) and medical conditions, suicidal and homicidal ideations, psychosocial functioning, presence of family psychopathology, and ongoing negative life events (e.g., family conflicts, abuse). Sometimes, if the child has learning problems, psychoeducational testing is necessary. It is worth noting, however, that cognitive dysfunction is commonly associated with BP, even in the absence of antecedent learning disorders.

Finally, the appropriate intensity and restrictiveness of care (e.g., hospitalization) need to be evaluated. The need for hospitalization will depend on the severity of mood symptoms, presence of suicidal and/or homicidal symptoms, psychosis, substance abuse, agitation, child's and parents' adherence to treatment, parental psychopathology, and family environment (Diler & Birmaher, 2012).

5. Psychological testing—None of the existing psychological tests help to diagnose BP. However, these tests may help to determine the IQ and the presence of comorbid learning and/or language problems that may worsen the prognosis of BP and need to be addressed.

Psychological testing may also provide some clues to the potential underlying cognitive deficits associated with BP. Several investigations have found several cognitive deficits, such as difficulties in attentional set-shifting, visuospatial memory, verbal memory, and executive function in BP youth (Joseph et al, 2008) that may persist during follow-up (Pavuluri et al, 2009). There is also widespread agreement that cognitive functioning independently and robustly predicts later functional outcomes in BP (Lee et al, 2013). However, a careful history-taking, ideally including school records, in order to help determine whether cognitive dysfunction predates BP, is secondary to BP, is secondary to comorbidities such as ADHD or anxiety, is secondary to the pharmacological treatments use to manage the symptoms of BP, or involves some combination of these factors.

6. Laboratory testing—To date, there are no laboratory, electroencephalography, or neuroimaging tests that can help with the diagnosis of BP (APA, 2013). These tests are requested, when indicated, to rule out medical or neurologic illness that may be accounting for the manic or hypomanic symptomatology.

Neuroimaging is also used as research tool to evaluate potential neural circuits associated with the etiopathogenesis of BP (Diler et al, 2013a). Current structural, functional, and connectivity brain imaging studies have suggested that several brain networks related to the cognitive (e.g., dorsolateral prefrontal cortex), emotional (e.g., amygdala, ventrolateral prefrontal cortex—vlPFC), and reward (e.g., striatum) functioning of the brain are affected in individuals with BP and at risk to develop BP (Phillips et al, 2008; Schneider et al, 2012). BP is conceptualized as parallel dysfunction in bilateral prefrontal cortical (especially vlPFC)–hippocampal–amygdala emotion processing and emotion regulation neural circuitries, together with an "overactive" left-sided ventral striatal–vlPFC–orbitofrontal cortex reward processing circuitry, which results in the characteristic behavioral abnormalities associated with BP: emotional dysregulation, heightened reward sensitivity, and predisposition to mania (Phillips & Swartz, 2014). However, further studies regarding specificity and predictive validity and whether the changes are trait or state characteristics are warranted.

American Psychiatric Association (APA). *Diagnostic and Statistical Manual of Mental Disorders.* 5th ed. Washington, DC: American Psychiatric Association; 2013.

Axelson DA, Birmaher B, Brent D, et al. A preliminary study of the Kiddie Schedule for Affective Disorders and Schizophrenia for School-Age Children Mania Rating Scale for Children and Adolescents. *J Child Adolesc Psychopharmacol.* 2003;13(4):463–470.

Axelson DA, Birmaher B, Findling RL, et al. Concerns regarding the inclusion of temper dysregulation disorder with dysphoria in the *Diagnostic and Statistical Manual of Mental Disorders,* Fifth Edition. *J Clin Psychiatry.* 2011a;72(9):1257–1262.

Axelson DA, Birmaher B, Strober M, et al. Phenomenology of children and adolescents with bipolar spectrum disorders. *Arch Gen Psychiatry.* 2006;63(10):1139–1148.

Axelson DA, Birmaher B, Strober MA, et al. Course of subthreshold bipolar disorder in youth: diagnostic progression from bipolar disorder not otherwise specified. *J Am Acad Child Adolesc Psychiatry.* 2011b;50(10):1001–1016 e3.

Axelson D, Goldstein B, Goldstein T, et al. Diagnostic precursors to bipolar disorder in offspring of parents with bipolar disorder: a longitudinal study. *Am J Psychiatry.* 2015;172 (7):638–646.

Birmaher B, Axelson D, Goldstein B, et al. Four-year longitudinal course of children and adolescents with bipolar spectrum disorders: the Course and Outcome of Bipolar Youth (COBY) study. *Am J Psychiatry.* 2009a;166(7):795–804.

Birmaher B, Axelson D, Pavuluri M. Bipolar disorder. In: Martin A, Volkmar FR, Lewis M, eds. *Lewis' Child and Adolescent Psychiatry: A Comprehensive Textbook.* 4th ed. London: Lippincott Williams & Wilkins; 2007.

Birmaher B, Axelson D, Strober M, et al. Comparison of manic and depressive symptoms between children and adolescents with bipolar spectrum disorders. *Bipolar Disord.* 2009c;11(1):52–62.

Chengappa KN, Kupfer DJ, Frank E, et al. Relationship of birth cohort and early age at onset of illness in a bipolar disorder case registry. *Am J Psychiatry.* 2003;160(9):1636–1642.

Diler, R.S. *Pediatric Bipolar Disorder: A Global Perspective.* New York: Nova Science Publishers; 2007a.

Diler RS, Birmaher B. Bipolar disorder in children and adolescents. In: Rey JM, ed. *IACAPAP e-Textbook of Child and Adolescent Mental Health.* Geneva: International Association for Child and Adolescent Psychiatry and Allied Professions; 2012.

Diler RS, Birmaher B, Axelson D, et al. The Child Behavior Checklist (CBCL) and the CBCL-bipolar phenotype are not useful in diagnosing pediatric bipolar disorder. *J Child Adolesc Psychopharmacol.* 2009;19(1):23–30.

Diler RS, de Almeida JR, Ladouceur C, et al. Neural activity to intense positive versus negative stimuli can help differentiate bipolar disorder from unipolar major depressive disorder in depressed adolescents: a pilot fMRI study. *Psychiatry Res.* 2013a;214(3):277–284.

Diler RS, Uguz S, Seydaoglu G, et al. Mania profile in a community sample of prepubertal children in Turkey. *Bipolar Disord.* 2008;10(4):546–553.

Duffy A. The nature of the association between childhood ADHD and the development of bipolar disorder: a review of prospective high-risk studies. *Am J Psychiatry.* 2012;169(12):1247–1255.

Egeland JA, Hostetter AM, Pauls DL, Sussex JN. Prodromal symptoms before onset of manic-depressive disorder suggested by first hospital admission histories. *J Am Acad Child Adolesc Psychiatry.* 2000;39(10):1245–1252.

Goodwin FK, Jamison KR, Ghaemi SN. *Manic-Depressive Illness: Bipolar Disorders and Recurrent Depression.* New York: Oxford University Press; 2007.

Hafeman DM, Merranko J, Axelson D, et al. Toward the definition of a bipolar prodrome: dimensional predictors of bipolar spectrum disorders in at-risk youth. *Am J Psychiatry.* 2016;173(7):695–704.

Hirneth SJ, Hazell PL, Hanstock TL, et al. Bipolar disorder subtypes in children and adolescents: demographic and clinical characteristics from an Australian sample. *J Affect Disord.* 2015;175:98–107.

Holtzman JN, Miller S, Hooshmand F, et al. Childhood-compared to adolescent-onset bipolar disorder has more statistically significant clinical correlates. *J Affect Disord.* 2015;79:114–120.

Hunt J, Birmaher B, Leonard H, et al. Irritability without elation in a large bipolar youth sample: frequency and clinical description. *J Am Acad Child Adolesc Psychiatry.* 2009;48(7):730–739.

Hunt JI, Case BG, Birmaher B, et al. Irritability and elation in a large bipolar youth sample: relative symptom severity and clinical outcomes over 4 years. *J Clin Psychiatry.* 2013;74(1):e110–e117.

Joseph MF, Frazier TW, Youngstrom EA, et al. A quantitative and qualitative review of neurocognitive performance in pediatric bipolar disorder. *J Child Adolesc Psychopharmacol.* 2008;18(6):595–605.

Kaufman J, Birmaher B, Brent D, et al. Schedule for Affective Disorders and Schizophrenia for School-Age Children-Present and Lifetime Version (K-SADS-PL): initial reliability and validity data. *J Am Acad Child Adolesc Psychiatry.* 1997;36:980–988.

Kowatch RA, Fristad M, Birmaher B, et al. Treatment guidelines for children and adolescents with bipolar disorder: child psychiatric workgroup on bipolar disorder. *J Am Acad Child Adolesc Psychiatry.* 2005a;44:213–255.

Kowatch RA, Youngstrom EA, Danielyan A, Findling RL. Review and meta-analysis of the phenomenology and clinical characteristics of mania in children and adolescents. *Bipolar Disord.* 2005b;7:483–496.

Lee J, Altshuler L, Glahn DC, et al. Social and nonsocial cognition in bipolar disorder and schizophrenia: relative levels of impairment. *Am J Psychiatry.* 2013;170(3):334–341.

Leibenluft E, Rich BA. Pediatric bipolar disorder. *Annu Rev Clin Psychol.* 2008;4:163–187.

Pavuluri MN, Henry DB, Devineni B, et al. Child mania rating scale: development, reliability, and validity. *J Am Acad Child Adolesc Psychiatry.* 2006;45(5):550–560.

Pavuluri MN, West A, Hill SK. Neurocognitive function in pediatric bipolar disorder: 3-year follow-up shows cognitive development lagging behind healthy youth. *J Am Acad Child Adolesc Psychiatry.* 2009;48(3):299–307.

Phillips ML, Ladouceur CD, Drevets WC. A neural model of voluntary and automatic emotion regulation: implications for understanding the pathophysiology and neurodevelopment of bipolar disorder. *Mol Psychiatry.* 2008;13(9):829.

Phillips ML, Swartz HA: A critical appraisal of neuroimaging studies of bipolar disorder: toward a new conceptualization of underlying neural circuitry and a road map for future research. *Am J Psychiatry.* 2014; 171(8):829–843.

Schneider MR, DelBello MP, McNamara RK, et al. Neuroprogression in bipolar disorder. *Bipolar Disord.* 2012;14(4):356–374.

Uchida M, Serra G, Zayas L, et al. Can unipolar and bipolar pediatric major depression be differentiated from each other? A systematic review of cross-sectional studies examining differences in unipolar and bipolar depression. *J Affect Disord.* 2015;176:1–7.

Van Meter AR, Burke C, Kowatch RA, et al. Ten-year update meta-analysis of the clinical characteristics of pediatric mania and hypomania. *Bipolar Disord.* 2016;18(1):19–32.

Wozniak J. Recognizing and managing bipolar disorder in children. *J Clin Psychiatry.* 2005;66(Suppl 1):18–23.

Youngstrom E, Meyers O, Demeter C, et al. Comparing diagnostic checklists for pediatric bipolar disorder in academic and community mental health settings. *Bipolar Disord.* 2005;7(6):507–517.

Youngstrom EA, Egerton GA, Van Meter AR. Multivariate meta-analysis of the discriminative validity of caregiver, youth and teacher rating scales for pediatric bipolar disorder: mother knows best about mania. *Arch Scien Psychology.* 2015;3:112–137.

▶ Course of Illness

Several prospective naturalistic studies have consistently shown that 70– 100% of children and adolescents with BP will recover (e.g., no significant symptoms for 2 months) from their index episode (Birmaher, 2007; Birmaher et al, 2009a, 2014; DelBello et al, 2007b; Geller et al, 2008). However, of those who recover, up to 80% will experience one or more recurrences in a period of 2–5 years. These studies have shown high rates of hospitalization and health service utilization, psychosis, suicide attempts and completion, switch from BP-NOS to BP-I or II and from BP-II to BP-I, substance abuse, unemployment, legal problems, and poor academic and psychosocial functioning (Birmaher et al, 2009a; Geller et al, 2008; Goldstein et al, 2009a, 2012, 2013). The persistent BP symptoms also have a negative impact on family, marital, and sibling relationships, as well as on family economics. The considerable impairment in psychosocial functioning reported in these studies is not only specific to the fact that most of the BP youth studies have been carried out in clinical samples, because similar findings have been reported in BP adolescents never referred for treatment (Lewinsohn et al, 2000).

Recent studies have shown that BP is not only manifested by recovery and recurrences but also by ongoing fluctuating syndromal and subsyndromal symptomatology (Birmaher et al, 2009a; DelBello et al, 2007b). In general, BP youth have syndromal and subsyndromal BP symptoms, particularly depressive and mixed symptoms, in about 60% of the follow-up time (Birmaher et al, 2009a). In addition, within each episode, youth manifest more fluctuations in mood than adults

with BP (Birmaher et al, 2009a). This may explain, at least in part, the difficulties encountered diagnosing and treating BP symptoms in youth. A recent study evaluated a more individualized course during a 9-year period using latent growth class analyses (Birmaher et al, 2014). Four longitudinal mood trajectories were found: "predominantly euthymic" course (24.0%), "moderately euthymic" course (34.6%), "ill with improving course" (19.1%), and "predominantly ill" course (22.3%). Within each group, youth were euthymic on average 84.4%, 47.3%, 42.8%, and 11.5% of the follow-up time, respectively. The fact that a substantial group of youth have good course gives youth and their families hope that BP disorder does not necessarily convey poor prognosis (Birmaher et al, 2014). Nonetheless, continued syndromal and subsyndromal mood symptoms in all four classes underscore the need to optimize treatment (Birmaher, 2016).

Overall, across the extant studies, early age of onset, long duration, low SES, mixed or rapid cycling episodes, psychosis, subsyndromal symptoms, comorbid disorders, exposure to negative life events, and family psychopathology are associated with worse course and outcome (Birmaher et al, 2009a, 2014; DelBello et al, 2007b; Geller et al, 2008).

When followed prospectively for approximately 5 years, about 50% of the youth diagnosed with BP-NOS convert into BP-I or -II (Axelson et al, 2011b). The main predictor of conversion is the presence of a family history of mania in first- or second-degree relatives. In a different study with offspring of BP parents, those with mood lability, depression/anxiety, and subsyndromal manic symptoms, and early-onset parental BP were at 50% risk to develop BP (Hafeman et al, 2016).

▶ Differential Diagnosis

A. Comorbid Disorders

The most common disorders found in youth with BP are ADHD, oppositional defiant disorder (ODD), conduct disorder (CD), and anxiety disorders (Axelson et al, 2006; Birmaher, 2016; Birmaher et al, 2007; Kowatch et al, 2005b; Miller et al, 2013). The prevalence of these disorders varies depending on the population studied and the methods used to ascertain them, but in general the rates fluctuate between 20% and 80%. Beginning in adolescence, the rate of comorbid substance abuse progressively increases (Goldstein et al, 2008, 2013; Wilens et al, 2004). The presence of these disorders affects the youth's response to treatment and prognosis, indicating the need to identify and treat them effectively.

In addition to the psychiatric comorbidity, the presence of medical illnesses is a major concern in BP. There are not many studies in youth, but cardiovascular disease in BP adults is both exceedingly prevalent and premature, leading to excessive cardiovascular mortality (Goldstein et al, 2009b). Although psychiatric medications are associated with metabolic disturbances, the association between BP and cardiovascular disease was observed before the advent of modern medications.

In youth, BP may also incur increased risk of medical comorbidities, with 28–36% suffering from multiple medical conditions, whereas this is true for only 8% of youth with other psychiatric disorders combined (Evans-Lacko et al, 2009; Jerrell et al, 2010). Obesity, hypertension, and diabetes are highly prevalent and often precede BP, and use of specialty cardiology services is doubled. Migraine, asthma, and neurological conditions such as epilepsy may also co-occur disproportionately with BP (Evans-Lacko et al, 2009; Jerrell et al, 2010). Clinicians should pay particular attention to these medical complications when assessing and following youth with BP spectrum disorders.

B. Difficulties Diagnosing Youth with BP

The following factors make the diagnosis of BP in youth challenging: (1) the inherent variability in the clinical presentation of BP—youth with BP can present clinically with different degrees of severity, various subtypes (e.g., BP-I or II), and phases of the illness (e.g., depression, manic, mixed); (2) the effects of development in symptom expression; (3) children's problems communicating their symptoms, in particular elation and grandiosity; (4) the presence of comorbid conditions, especially those whose symptoms overlap with the symptoms of mania (e.g., ADHD) manifested with symptoms of mania or hypomania; (5) the environmental context where BP is developing (e.g., family conflicts, parental symptomatology, parental viewpoints regarding symptoms); and (6) if the youth is on medications, their potential effects on the child's mood.

Regarding the effects of development (item 2), it is crucial to evaluate whether the mood symptoms are abnormal or clearly different from the child's usual mood and behavior given the context and developmental level. For instance, elevated mood, high activity level, and rapid speech would not be considered evidence of mania symptoms in a child who is very happy during his birthday party or in an amusement park. Also, it is common for young children to believe that they are the best players, dancers, and so forth. However, children usually do not perform extreme risky behaviors when they are acting out their fantasies (e.g., trying to fly from the third floor of a building because they think that they are Superman). Also, a school-age child is not likely to perform risky business ventures, drive recklessly, go on spending sprees, or have sexual relations with multiple partners. However, they can exhibit inappropriate sexual behavior (e.g., without having history of exposure to sex, they can touch others inappropriately, frequently masturbate, or draw sexually provocative pictures).

Concerning the presence of comorbid disorders (item 3), the main psychiatric conditions that can be difficult to differentiate from youth with BP are ADHD, disruptive disorders (ODD and CD), the new DSM-5 Disruptive Mood Dysregulation Disorder (DMDD) (most of these children also meet criteria for ODD and/or ADHD), unipolar depression, pervasive developmental disorders (PDD), schizophrenia, substance use disorders, and, although its use in youth below the age of 18 years is controversial, borderline personality disorder. Medical and neurological illnesses (e.g., head trauma, brain tumors, hyperthyroidism), and side effects of medications (e.g., corticosteroids, antidepressants, and stimulants) may be accompanied by mood fluctuations that may mimic BP. Also, normal mood variability sometimes may be misinterpreted as symptoms of hypomania.

Because the disruptive behavioral disorders and ADHD are the most frequent conditions that may be confused with BP, they deserve detailed assessment (Birmaher, 2004). There are some symptoms that mainly occur in BP youth and may help to differentiate between BP and these disorders, such as clinically relevant euphoria, grandiosity, decreased need for sleep, hypersexuality (without history of sexual abuse or exposure to sex), and hallucinations. The course of the symptoms over time is one of the more important factors helping differentiate BP from these disorders. Family history of BP may help, but offspring of parents with BP may suffer from other disorders such as ADHD and ODD. In general, chronic symptoms such as hyperactivity or distractibility generally should not be considered evidence of mania unless they clearly intensify with the onset of abnormal mood. Prolonged presentations of nonspecific manic-like symptoms that do not change in overall intensity should raise the possibility of an alternative psychiatric diagnosis.

Most depressed youth seen in psychiatric clinics are experiencing their first episode of depression (Birmaher et al, 2007, 2009a). The presence of psychosis, family history of BP, and pharmacologically induced mania/hypomania may indicate susceptibility to develop BP (Geller et al, 1994; Strober & Carlson, 1982; Uchida et al, 2014). However, the clinical picture of depression is not sufficiently specific to help differentiate between depressed youth with BP and those with unipolar depression. Thus, it is important to continue to follow these youth longitudinally and continue to evaluate for the presence of manic or hypomanic symptoms. Due to the controversy regarding irritability as a key symptom for the diagnosis of pediatric BP, the DSM-5 included a new disorder in the category of mood disorders entitled Disruptive Mood Dysregulation Disorder (DMDD). This disorder is characterized by frequent, severe, recurrent temper outbursts and chronically irritable and/or angry mood, both of which must be present for at least a year and cannot be accounted by other mood disorders (and cannot be diagnosed if the child meets criteria for BP diagnosis). Moreover, perhaps with the exception of severely irritable youth with positive family history of mania, longitudinal data indicate that youth with severe mood dysregulation (SMD), the condition from which DMDD was derived, are not at high risk to develop BD as they age (Towbin et al, 2013).

Schizophrenia is very rare in children. Thus, if a youth presents with symptoms of psychosis, mood disorders need to be ruled out. Youth with subsyndromal symptoms of autism spectrum disorders (a.k.a. PDD) including Asperger disorder (or mild autism) may have mood lability, aggression, and agitation and may be misdiagnosed as having BP. Substance abuse may also induce severe mood changes that may be difficult to differentiate from BP. Moreover, youth with mood disorders are at higher risk for using illicit drugs or alcohol for a number of reasons including self-medication, impulsivity, and reward seeking.

The use of medications such as the antidepressants may unmask or precipitate a manic or hypomanic episode in a susceptible individual (Martin et al, 2004). However, not every child who becomes agitated or giddy and excited with these or other medications has BP. Family history and the severity, length, and quality of manic symptomatology may help to differentiate between BP or agitation induced by these or other medications (Birmaher et al, 2007; Pavuluri et al, 2005). In the DSM-5, a new "medication/substance induced bipolar and related disorders" diagnosis is introduced for those who develop a manic episode during medication or substance use (APA, 2013).

Finally, although there is controversy about the validity of borderline personality disorder in youth, some BP teens, particularly those with BP-II, may be misdiagnosed as having this condition. Even in the absence of a full diagnosis, borderline personality-spectrum symptoms are common and associated with increased burden of psychiatric symptoms and impairment (Fonseka et al, 2015; Yen et al, 2015).

American Psychiatric Association (APA). *Diagnostic and Statistical Manual of Mental Disorders*. 5th ed. Washington, DC: American Psychiatric Association; 2013.

Axelson DA, Birmaher B, Strober M, et al. Phenomenology of children and adolescents with bipolar spectrum disorders. *Arch Gen Psychiatry*. 2006;63(10):1139–1148.

Axelson DA, Birmaher B, Strober MA, et al. Course of subthreshold bipolar disorder in youth: diagnostic progression from bipolar disorder not otherwise specified. *J Am Acad Child Adolesc Psychiatry*. 2011b;50(10):1001–1016 e3.

Birmaher B. *New Hope for Children and Teens with Bipolar Disorder*. New York: Three Rivers Press; 2004.

Birmaher B. Longitudinal course of pediatric bipolar disorder. *Am J Psychiatry*. 2007;164(4):537–539.

Birmaher B. Pediatric bipolar disorder: epidemiology, pathogenesis, clinical manifestations and course. UpToDate. Accessed January 2016.

Birmaher B, Axelson D, Goldstein B, et al. Four-year longitudinal course of children and adolescents with bipolar spectrum disorders: the Course and Outcome of Bipolar Youth (COBY) study. *Am J Psychiatry*. 2009a;166(7):795–804.

Birmaher B, Gill MK, Axelson D, et al. Longitudinal trajectories and associated baseline predictors in youth with bipolar spectrum disorders. *Am J Psychiatry*. 2014;171(9):990–999.

DelBello MP, Hanseman D, Adler CM, et al. Twelve-month outcome of adolescents with bipolar disorder following first hospitalization for a manic or mixed episode. *Am J Psychiatry*. 2007b;164(4):582–590.

Diler RS, Birmaher B. Bipolar disorder in children and adolescents. In: Rey JM, ed. *IACAPAP e-Textbook of Child and Adolescent Mental Health*. Geneva: International Association for Child and Adolescent Psychiatry and Allied Professions; 2012.

Evans-Lacko SE, Zeber JE, Gonzalez JM, Olvera RL. Medical comorbidity among youth diagnosed with bipolar disorder in the United States. *J Clin Psychiatry*. 2009;70(10):1461–1466.

Fonseka TM, Swampillai B, Timmins V, et al. Significance of borderline personality-spectrum symptoms among adolescents with bipolar disorder. *J Affect Disord*. 2015;170:39–45.

Geller B, Fox LW, Clark KA. Rate and predictors of prepubertal bipolarity during follow-up of 6- to 12-year-old depressed children. *J Am Acad Child Adolesc Psychiatry*. 1994;33(4):461–468.

Geller B, Tillman R, Bolhofner K, Zimerman B. Child bipolar I disorder: prospective continuity with adult bipolar disorder in adolescents; characteristics of second and third episodes; predictors of 8-year outcome. *Arch Gen Psychiatry*. 2008;65(10):1125–1133.

Goldstein BI, Fagiolini A, Houck P, Kupfer DJ. Cardiovascular disease and hypertension among adults with bipolar I disorder in the United States. *Bipolar Disord*. 2009b;11(6):657–662.

Goldstein BI, Strober M, Axelson D, et al. Predictors of first-onset substance use disorders during the prospective course of bipolar spectrum disorders in adolescents. *J Am Acad Child Adolesc Psychiatry*. 2013;52(10):1026–1037.

Goldstein BI, Strober MA, Birmaher B, et al. Substance use disorders among adolescents with bipolar spectrum disorders. *Bipolar Disord*. 2008;10(4):469–478.

Goldstein T, Ha W, Axelson DA, et al. Predictors of prospectively examined suicide attempts among youth with bipolar disorder. *Arch Gen Psychiatry*. 2012;69(11):1113–1122.

Goldstein TR, Birmaher B, Axelson D, et al. Psychosocial functioning among bipolar youth. *J Affect Disord*. 2009a;114(1–3):174–183.

Hafeman DM, Merranko J, Axelson D, et al. Toward the definition of a bipolar prodrome: dimensional predictors of bipolar spectrum disorders in at-risk youth. *Am J Psychiatry*. 2016;173(7):695–704.

Jerrell JM, McIntyre RS, Tripathi A. A cohort study of the prevalence and impact of comorbid medical conditions in pediatric bipolar disorder. *J Clin Psychiatry*. 2010;71(11):161–168.

Kowatch RA, Youngstrom EA, Danielyan A, Findling RL. Review and meta-analysis of the phenomenology and clinical characteristics of mania in children and adolescents. *Bipolar Disord*. 2005b;7:483–496.

Lewinsohn PM, Klein DN, Seeley JR. Bipolar disorder during adolescence and young adulthood in a community sample. *Bipolar Disord*. 2000;2:281–293.

Martin A, Young C, Leckman JF, et al. Age effects on antidepressant-induced manic conversion. *Arch Pediatr Adolesc Med*. 2004;158(8):773–780.

Miller S, Chang KD, Ketter TA. Bipolar disorder and attention-deficit/hyperactivity disorder comorbidity in children and adolescents: evidence based approach to diagnosis and treatment. *J Clin Psychiatry*. 2013;74(6):628–629.

Pavuluri MN, Birmaher B, Naylor MW. Pediatric bipolar disorder: a review of the past 10 years. *J Am Acad Child Adolesc Psychiatry*. 2005;44(9):846–871.

Strober M, Carlson G. Bipolar illness in adolescents with major depression: clinical, genetic, and psychopharmacologic predictors in a three- to four-year prospective follow-up investigation. *Arch Gen Psychiatry*. 1982;39(5):549–555.

Towbin K, Axelson D, Leibenluft E, et al. Differentiating bipolar disorder-not otherwise specified and severe mood dysregulation *J Am Acad Child Adolesc Psychiatry.* 2013;52(5):466–481.

Wilens TE, Biederman J, Kwon A, et al. Risk of substance use disorders in adolescents with bipolar disorder. *J Am Acad Child Adolesc Psychiatry.* 2004;43(11):1380–1386.

Yen S, Frazier E, Hower H, et al. Borderline personality disorder in transition age group in youth with bipolar disorder. *Acta Psychiatr Scand.* 2015;132(4):270–280.

▶ Treatment

A. General Considerations

The treatment of BP is subdivided into acute and maintenance phases. The main aim of the acute treatment is to stop the acute mood symptoms and related functional decline. The maintenance phase aims to prevent relapses and recurrences (new episodes).

In each one of these phases, the treatment may change according to the polarity of the episode (mania, hypomania, mixed, rapid cycling, psychosis, and depression). In addition, the type, dosage, and length of treatment depend of the age of the child, presence of comorbid psychiatric and medical illness, and tolerance to the side effects induced by these treatments.

All types of treatments require comprehensive education for the parents and the youth and other people such as teachers about the nature of the illness and consequences if it remains untreated. In addition, the education should encompass a review of the existent psychosocial and pharmacological treatments with their positive and potential negative consequences and need to adhere to the treatment to avoid relapses and further recurrences.

The vast majority of randomized controlled trials (RCT) for youth with BP pertain to the acute treatment of youth with BP-I with manic or mixed presentations (Liu et al, 2011). There are no controlled studies for youth with BP-II, and there are limited studies focusing on maintenance and prevention (recurrences). Thus, until further studies become available, the management of these conditions is strongly informed by the adult literature. However, it is important to note that not all the treatments that seem to work or are well tolerated in adults will be appropriate for the treatment of youth.

When medications are employed, the minimum clinically effective dose with the fewest side effects should be used. Unless there are significant side effects, in the presence of ongoing symptoms, the medications should be increased to the maximum tolerated dose found to be safe in youth to determine the full efficacy of the medication. This process of dose optimization should be undertaken before adding another medication. Ongoing evaluation of adherence and barriers to adherence, including side effects (which could reduce adherence), is warranted (Diler & Birmaher, 2012; Kowatch et al, 2005a).

It is important to assess the risk of overdose, whether accidental or purposeful. If necessary, regardless of the youth's age, a responsible adult should manage the medications. This is also true for cases where diversion of medication (stimulants and benzodiazepines in particular) might be an issue. Providing a limited supply of the medication or changing to another medication may be necessary in these cases.

B. Psychopharmacologic Interventions

1. Acute treatment phase

BP-I manic or mixed episodes—Monotherapy with traditional mood stabilizers (lithium, valproate, and carbamazepine) and second-generation antipsychotics (SGAs) (e.g., risperidone, olanzapine, aripiprazole, quetiapine, and asenapine) is indicated for the acute treatment of BP-I manic or mixed episode without psychosis (Correll et al, 2010; DelBello et al, 2005, 2007a, 2008; Findling et al, 2009, 2013, 2015a, 2015b; Geller et al, 2012; Haas et al, 2009; Liu et al, 2011; Pathak et al, 2013; Tohen et al, 2007; Wagner et al, 2006, 2009). Of these medications, most acute RCTs have shown that the SGAs (response: 50–68%) are more effective than the traditional mood stabilizers (response: 23–55%) and yield a quicker response (Correll et al, 2010; Findling et al, 2013, 2015a, 2015b; Fraguas et al, 2011; Kowatch et al, 2000; Meduri et al, 2016). However, as noted later, it is not yet well known whether the SGAs are also useful and safe for the prevention of further mood recurrences in youth with BP. Lithium was approved for youth 12 years and older with BP-I before any RCT in youth, and the recent RCT with lithium in youth aged from 7 to 17 years old with mixed or manic episodes suggested that 47% of youth responded to lithium (very much/much improved on Clinical Global Impression) compared to 21% of those to placebo (Findling et al, 2015b). Open treatment with carbamazepine indicates that this medication appears to be effective and safe for BP youth, but RCTs are needed to confirm this (Findling et al, 2014). An RCT for oxcarbazepine was negative (Wagner et al, 2006).

Further validation for the acute efficacy of the SGAs was given by a recent large controlled, randomized 8-week parallel comparison of risperidone, lithium carbonate, and valproate (Geller et al, 2012). Youth responded significantly better to risperidone (68.5%) than to lithium (35.6%) or valproate (24%) However, there were site differences, with some sites also showing good respond to lithium. As expected, risperidone was associated with more metabolic side effects.

The dosages for each of the foregoing medications are noted in Table 48–2. It is important to emphasize that the dosages of lithium, valproate, and carbamazepine depend on their respective blood levels (0.6–1.1 mEq/L, 70–150 mEq/L, and 8–12 mEq/L, respectively). However, minimal blood levels for each of these medications are mainly derived from the adult psychiatric literature and may not be completely applicable for children. It is not clear why lithium and valproate do not seem to work as well for BP youth as for their

Table 48–2 Major Randomized Controlled Studies of Secondary Generation of Antipsychotics and Mood Stabilizers in Acute Mania[*]

Medication	Citation	N	Age (Years)	Duration (Days)	Mean Dose (mg/day)	% Responders
Olanzapine	Tohen et al (2007)	161	13–17	21	10.4	49%[**] 22% (placebo)
Risperidone	Haas et al (2009)	169	10–17	21	0.5–2.5 (low) 3–6 (high)	59% (low)[**] 63% (high) 26% (placebo)
Aripiprazole	Findling et al (2009)	296	10–17	28	10 (low) 30 (high)	45% (low)[**] 64% (high) 26% (placebo)
Quetiapine	Pathak et al (2013)	284	10–17	21	400 (low) 600 (high)	64% (low)[**] 58% (high) 37% (placebo)
Ziprasidone	Findling et al (2013)	238	10–17	28	80–160	62%[**] 35% (placebo)
Asenapine	Findling et al (2015a)	403	10–17	21	2.5 mg bid, 5mg bid, or 10 mg bid	42–54%[**] (each dose was significant vs. placebo) 28% (placebo)
Lithium	Findling et al (2015b)	81	7–17	56	Blood level: 0.98 mEq/L	47%[†] 21% (placebo)
Valproate	Wagner et al (2009)	150		28	Mean blood levels: 79.9 µg/ml (end of the study)	24%[**] 27% (placebo)
Topiramate	DelBello et al (2005)	56	6–17	28	400	34.5%[†] 22.2% (placebo)
Oxcarbazepine	Wagner et al (2006)	116		28	1515	42%[**] 26% (placebo)
Risperidone Lithium Valproate	Geller et al (2012)	89 90 100	6–16	32	2.6 Blood level: 1.09 mEq/L Blood level: 113.6 µg/ml	68.5%[†] 35.6% 24.0%
Risperidone Valproate	Kowatch et al (2015)	46	3–7	42	0.5 mg Blood level: 81 mEq/L	88%[†] 50% 0% (placebo)

Data from Kowatch et al (2005b) and Correll (2010).

[*]Except for the study in preschool children (Kowatch et al, 2015), only randomized controlled trials with samples above 50 subjects were included.

[**]≥50% reduction in the Young Mania Rating Scale (YMRS) scores.

[†]Clinical Global Improvement Scale (CGI-I).

adult counterparts. Possible causes include the fact that in youth BP is usually manifested with more mixed and rapid-cycling presentations, and these subtypes tend not to respond well to lithium and sometimes to valproate, even in adults with BP. Also, it is possible that in comparison with adults with BP, youth may require higher dosages of lithium because it seems that in comparison to the adults, youth have lower ratios of brain-to-serum lithium concentration (Moore et al, 2002), that duration of the acute RCTs was too short, and that the studies included a significant proportion of youth who in reality did not have BP with distinct manic episodes but other disorders that usually do not respond to lithium or valproate, such as ADHD and/or ODD.

An analysis of the benefits of either an add-on or a switch of antimanic medications for an 8-week period in partial and nonresponders, respectively, showed better response to risperidone than lithium or valproate (Walkup et al, 2015). A small 6-week study comparing valproate versus risperidone versus placebo for preschool BP also showed that risperidone was efficacious but not valproate (Kowatch et al, 2015). These studies have also suggested that the combination of two mood stabilizers such as lithium and valproate or a mood stabilizer with an atypical antipsychotic appears to be superior to mood stabilizer monotherapy, with responses ranging from 60% to 90% (Delbello et al, 2002; Findling et al, 2003, 2005; Kafantaris et al, 2001; Pavuluri et al, 2004).

For youth with only moderate to minimal improvement with optimal dosages and appropriate duration of monotherapy treatment (e.g., at least 4–6 weeks), augmenting with either another mood stabilizer or an atypical antipsychotic is recommended. In fact, taking into account methodological limitations, some studies have suggested that the combination of two traditional mood stabilizers, such as lithium and valproate, or a traditional mood stabilizer and an atypical antipsychotic appears to be superior to mood stabilizer monotherapy for the acute treatment of manic or mixed episodes (DelBello et al, 2002, 2005; Walkup et al, 2015).

For youth having no response to initial monotherapy, or for youth having intolerable side effects, monotherapy with another agent is recommended. Importantly, before declaring a youth as having a condition "resistant" to treatment, several factors need to be considered. First, the clinician should explore if each current diagnosis is correct. If the diagnosis is accurate, the clinician should consider whether the pharmacological treatment for this diagnosis was the most appropriate, whether the medications were administered for a sufficient length of time, and whether the youth was adherent to the treatment. If adherence is a problem, exploring the reasons for poor adherence and working with the youth and the family to solve these issues could lead to resolution of the symptoms. If adherence to treatment was good, other factors such as the presence of another undiagnosed psychiatric or medical condition (e.g., substance abuse, eating disorder, epilepsy) or other factors (e.g., exposure to stressors fewer supports) could be accounting for the lack of response to treatment (Diler & Birmaher, 2012).

For youth with BP-I, manic, or mixed episodes with psychosis, a mood stabilizer combined with a SGA is recommended. Once the psychosis has subsided, the SGA can be tapered down. However, as noted earlier, SGA monotherapy may be considered as an alternative.

If polypharmacy is indicated, it is important to introduce only one medication at a time in order to effectively evaluate the response to each medication, except in emergencies.

Depression—Youth with BP usually have more recurrent and long periods of syndromal or subsyndromal depressive symptoms than manic presentations (Birmaher et al, 2007, 2009a), but evidence-based treatment remains limited. Recently, lurasidone received Food and Drug Administration (FDA) approval for the treatment of pediatric patients (aged 10–17) with BP-I experiencing an acute depressive episode. In a 6-week randomized, double-blind, placebo-controlled trial, lurasidone showed significant efficacy in the treatment of pediatric BP depression in patients aged 10–17 within the dose range of 20 mg/day–80 mg/day (Delbello et al. 2017). The FDA has also approved the combination olanzapine/

fluoxetine (OFC) medication for BP depression in youth aged 10–17. OFC showed superiority to placebo in an 8-week RCT; however, youth experienced significant weight gain and metabolic side effects (Detke et al, 2015). In addition, there is one small RCT with quetiapine in depressed youth with BP-I that reported a 71% response rate, which was not superior to placebo (DelBello et al, 2009). Two open-label studies in depressed BP youth reported response rates of 48% with lithium alone in BP-I (Patel et al, 2006) and 84% with lamotrigine (adjunct or monotherapy) in BP-I, BP-II, and BP-NOS (Chang et al, 2006). Few of the open-label studies in the treatment of mania assessed improvement in depression, and response rates for depressive symptoms ranged from 35% to 60% for SGAs (aripiprazole, olanzapine, risperidone, and ziprasidone), 43% for carbamazepine, and 40% with omega-3 fatty acids (Liu et al, 2011). A secondary analysis of the TEAM study showed that depressive symptoms, present in the acutely manic/mixed phase of BP, equally improved with risperidone, lithium, and valproate (Salpekar et al, 2015). However, risperidone yielded more rapid improvement than the other two medications. Sometimes, after the patient is stabilized with mood stabilizers or the SGAs, a serotonin reuptake inhibitor or bupropion may be used, but careful monitoring is needed because this can induce mania, a mixed episode, or rapid cycling (Diler & Birmaher, 2012).

An open-label study with omega-3 fatty acids showed minimum to modest improvement in depressive symptoms in BP depressed youth (Wozniak et al, 2007) with good tolerance. In a RCT with a small sample of prepubertal children with mild to moderate BP spectrum disorders, combined treatment of omega-3 fatty acids plus inositol reduced symptoms of depression (and manic symptoms) (Wozniak et al, 2015). A recent RCT with omega-3 supplementation in youth with subsyndromal BP disorder suggested a modest effect size (d = 0.48) for depressive symptoms (Fristad et al, 2015). For subjects with recurrent seasonal depression, light therapy may also be considered, although this too has the potential to precipitate mania. Transcranial magnetic stimulation (TMS) is suggested as a treatment option for unipolar depression, but it has not been well studied for youth (Diler & Birmaher, 2012; Wall et al, 2016).

2. Maintenance treatment phase—There are few data in youth regarding the maintenance treatment for BP disorder (Findling et al, 2005, 2012, 2015c), and most of the guidance for this phase of treatment is derived from adult studies (Fountoulakis et al, 2012; Podawiltz, 2012; Popovic et al, 2011; Post et al, 2013). Until further research is available, unless there are side effects, it is recommended to continue the same treatment that helped during the acute phase.

Lithium, lamotrigine (especially for depression), some SGAs, and, to a lesser extent, valproate are efficacious compared to placebo for the prevention of new episodes in adults with BP (Connolly & Thase, 2011; Fountoulakis et al, 2012; Post et al, 2013; Podawiltz, 2012; Popovic et al, 2011;

Stovall et al, 2013). The optimal duration of psychosocial treatment for pediatric BP has not been established; however, continuing psychosocial interventions for subthreshold symptoms may be helpful (Miklowitz et al, 2011). It is reasonable to provide ongoing psychosocial support, crisis management, and therapy booster sessions as appropriate.

Duration of treatment—There are no clear guidelines to help determine how long medications need to be maintained. The duration of treatment usually depends on the severity and length of the illness, the disorder(s) that underlie the severe mood swings, exposure to stress, availability of psychosocial interventions at home and school, parental psychopathology, social supports, and other family and social conditions.

BP is generally considered a lifelong illness, and as a consequence, the medications should not be discontinued. However, given that some BP youth have a predominantly euthymic course (Birmaher et al, 2009a), for youth with 1–2 years of euthymia, especially if the first episode was mild or short-lived or if the diagnosis of BP was questionable, it is recommended to slowly taper the medications after 12–24 months of euthymia. If the symptoms recur, the youth's situation should be reassessed, as the relapse may not be due to the lack of medication but to other causes. If needed, the medication may be increased once more to target particular symptoms. If the child is taking more than one medication, only one medication should be discontinued at a time, starting with any medications that could be causing any side effects and/or do not seem to be helping.

For cases in which the manic episode was severe or long and in cases in which the youth had two or more episodes of mania, long-term or even lifelong treatment may be warranted. In this case, as with other chronic illnesses such as epilepsy or diabetes, psychotherapeutic approaches may be beneficial in helping the youth and family gain acceptance of the concept of chronic disease management.

C. Psychotherapeutic Interventions

Supportive psychotherapy is indicated as part of the acute and maintenance treatment for youth with BP and their families. In addition, specific psychosocial treatments including have been developed including the Child and Family Focused Cognitive Behavior Therapy (CFF-CBT) (West et al, 2007, 2014), Multi-Family Psychoeducation Groups (MFPG) and Individual Family Psychoeducation (IFP) (Fristad, 2006; Fristad et al, 2015), Family Focused Therapy (FFT) (Miklowitz et al, 2011, 2014), Dialectical Behavior Therapy (DBT) (Goldstein et al, 2007, 2014), and Interpersonal and Social Rhythm Therapy (IPSRT) (Goldstein et al, 2013; Hlastala & Frank, 2006; Hlastala et al, 2010). RCTs for some of these therapies have shown their efficacy, particularly for depression (Miklowitz et al, 2011).

These psychotherapies are administered as adjunctive to the pharmacotherapy treatment. Their primary aims are to help the youth to control and cope with the acute mood symptoms and prevent relapses and recurrences. They improve the youth's coping and social skills, mood and sleep regulation, adherence to treatment, and family problem-solving and communication skills, and they help manage comorbid conditions. In addition, psychotherapy helps youth to manage stress and the psychological "scars" or side effects of the illness. It bolsters protective effects of the family, increases acceptance of the disorder, protects and maintains developmental trajectory, and enhances social, school, and family functioning. Usually parents are also engaged in their child's therapy and, if necessary, referred for treatment themselves.

RCTs have demonstrated the efficacy of several of the psychotherapy approaches for BP in adults (Oud et al, 2016). However, to date the only RCT using FFT has been carried out in adolescents with BP-I/II (Miklowitz et al, 2008). This study showed that compared with three sessions of psychoeducation, FFT was associated with faster recovery from depression, less time in depressive episodes, and lower depression severity scores over 2 years. Additionally, a RCT examined whether FFT-A could be a beneficial early intervention for mood-disordered adolescents (i.e., those with BP-NOS, cyclothymia, or depression) with a family history of BP (Miklowitz et al, 2011, 2013). This study showed more rapid recovery from mood symptoms, more weeks symptom-free, and fewer manic symptoms over 1 year among high-risk youth receiving FFT-A as compared with those receiving a single session family educational intervention; effects were more pronounced among high-EE families (Miklowitz et al, 2013).

D. Other Interventions

Case series exist on the effectiveness of electroconvulsive therapy in the treatment of acute mania and BP depression in adolescents, and practice parameters were introduced (Ghaziuddin et al, 2004). Also, the use of light therapy and the omega-3 fatty acids appears to be beneficial and well tolerated for some BP youth, but further research is necessary (Diler & Birmaher, 2012; Fristad et al, 2015; Wozniak et al, 2007, 2015).

▶ Complications of Treatment

1. General issues—All medications used for the treatment of BP may induce acute and long-term side effects. However, there is a lack of long-term safety data available in youth.

It is beyond the scope of this chapter to describe the side effects of each medication in detail. In general, most medications use to treat BP may induce tiredness, somnolence, increased weight, and gastrointestinal, skin, movement, and cognitive problems (Birmaher et al, 2007; Diler & Birmaher, 2012). Sometimes, slow titration and adjustment of dose timing can be helpful in reducing some of these effects. It is very important that patients and family members be aware of the initial symptoms of these side effects and to contact their physicians if they occur.

Given the nature of BP with multiple presentations (depression, mania, and mixed episodes) and the presence of comorbid disorders, polypharmacy is commonly employed for the management of BP. As a consequence, it is important to take into account potential drug-to-drug interactions. There are several websites (e.g., Medscape) and smartphone applications (e.g., Micromedex Drug Information by Thomson Reuters, Medscape, Epocrates) that may assist clinicians with this information.

Depending on which medication is used, height and weight (e.g., body mass index [BMI]), vital signs, and waist circumference should be recorded at each visit. A detailed clinical, physical assessment and, as appropriate, laboratory tests at baseline and during the follow-ups are indicated. Given the potential side effects of some of the medications used for the treatment of BP, pregnancy tests should be performed as needed (Correll et al, 2009, 2010).

2. Second generation of antipsychotics (SGA)—Most of the SGAs are associated with weight gain and metabolic problems (diabetes mellitus, hyperlipidemia, and elevation of liver function tests) (Bobo et al, 2013; Correll et al, 2009, 2010; Nielsen et al, 2014; Rummel-Kluge et al, 2012; Vitiello et al, 2009). Thus, it is crucial to monitor weight, BMI, fasting glucose, and lipid profile at baseline and subsequently at least every 6 months. Even though the SGAs have been associated with fewer extrapyramidal symptoms (EPS) and less tardive dyskinesia than the first-generation antipsychotics, it is important to evaluate for the presence of these potential side effects. They also may induce cognitive problems, sedation, tiredness, neuroleptic malignant syndrome, prolactin elevation, and cardiac conduction problems.

There are important differences among the SGAs. For example ziprasidone rarely increases weight, but clinical impression seems to indicate that dose-for-dose it seems to be less efficacious for controlling rages and mood swings when compared to other SGAs. At higher dosages, it may increase the heart-rate corrected QT interval and overly sedate the youth. Olanzapine tends to cause more weight gain and metabolic side effects than the other SGAs. Risperidone causes a larger increase in prolactin and has a higher risk for EPS. Aripiprazole has been associated with more dyskinesia and tremor, and in contrast to adults, it does not seem to be weight-neutral among treatment-naive youth (Correll, 2008). Some of the SGAs, like quetiapine, appear to have a short half-life that could necessitate dosing two or three times a day.

3. Mood stabilizers—The mood stabilizers may produce sedation, tiredness, weight gain, metabolic disturbances, tremors, dermatological problems (e.g., rashes and loss of hair), and cognitive difficulties (Birmaher et al, 2007; Diler & Birmaher, 2012). The anticonvulsants may induce hematological and dermatological problems and, although controversial, increase the risk for suicidality. Some specific side effects for each of the mood stabilizers are described next.

Lithium has a narrow therapeutic index, and blood levels above 1.5 mEq/L (and sometimes less) may cause severe metabolic, neurological, and kidney problems. Therefore, there is a need for careful monitoring through physical examinations and laboratory tests. Blood levels should be obtained as early as 5–6 days after each dose increase, immediately if clinical symptoms of toxicity occur and periodically during the maintenance phase (e.g., each 6 months). Lithium is associated with distal hand tremors, exacerbation of acne, hypothyroidism, polydipsia, polyuria, and changes in renal function. Laboratory tests to monitor kidney, thyroid, and parathyroid functioning are required at baseline and during follow-up. Youth and parents should be informed about clinical symptoms of lithium toxicity including dizziness, clumsiness, unsteady gait, sedation, confusion, blurred vision, slurred speech, coarse distal hand tremor, nausea and/or vomiting, and diarrhea. Lithium levels can increase by mistake, as consequence of an overdose, secondary to dehydration (e.g., excessive exercise, hot weather, gastrointestinal illness) or after taking certain medications such as the nonsteroidal anti-inflammatory drugs (e.g., ibuprofen).

Valproate has been associated with hair loss, polycystic ovarian syndrome, and rash, and baseline menstrual history and a gynecological consultation are required for any female who develops significant changes in her menstrual cycle and/or hirsutism while on this medication. Valproate carries a "black-box" warning about rare, but potentially life-threatening, pancreatitis.

Carbamazepine is not a first-line medication for youth with BP. If used, it is important to emphasize that it usually induces the metabolism of other medications (e.g., oral contraceptives) as well as its own through cytochrome P450 1A2 and 3A4 isoenzymes and may decrease the blood level and reduce its own and other medications' effectiveness. Also, it usually reduces the number of white cells and platelets, requiring frequent blood tests, and may induce significant dizziness, nausea, somnolence, diplopia, fatigue, and rash.

Lamotrigine is usually well tolerated with relatively lower risk for weight gain and sedation. However, particularly when a high starting dose is used, when the dose is increased rapidly, and/or when it is used in conjunction with valproate (or other medications that increase its blood levels), it may cause serious dermatological reactions such as Stevens–Johnson syndrome or toxic epidermal necrolysis. This risk is higher among youth than among adults. Unless a new rash is clearly attributable to another cause (e.g., contact dermatitis) other than lamotrigine, treatment should be suspended immediately. Also, lamotrigine should be reinitiated from the starting dose of 12.5 mg/day or 25 mg/day if it is held or stopped for many days. The rate of serious dermatological reactions may be reduced by current dosing recommendations (prescribing small doses with a gradual escalation, e.g., 25 mg/day in ≥12-year-olds with increases of 25 mg every 2 weeks given twice a day until 100 mg/day is reached). The dose of lamotrigine should be halved if combined with valproate. It may take 6–8 weeks to increase the dose of lamotrigine to a therapeutic level because of this slow titration schedule, making it difficult to use in acute treatment settings (e.g., inpatient care).

Oxcarbazepine and topiramate do not appear to be efficacious for adults, and one RCT trial comparing oxcarbazepine and placebo in youth was negative (Wagner et al, 2006). However, some clinicians still use it for the management of BP in youth. Oxcarbazepine has similar side effects like those of carbamazepine, but it does not induce hepatic enzymes, does not require blood level monitoring, and does not seem to have similar hematological side effects. Topiramate does not increase weight, but it shares other side effects like those of other anticonvulsants as well as significant cognitive difficulties.

4. Antidepressants—The selective serotonin reuptake inhibitors (SSRIs) may be helpful for the treatment of BP depression and anxiety symptoms (Birmaher et al, 2007; Diler & Birmaher, 2012; Stovall, 2016). However, particularly in people with BP-I and history of mixed presentations and rapid cycling, it can deregulate their mood and trigger mania, hypomania, mixed episodes, or rapid cycling (Birmaher et al, 2007; Diler & Birmaher, 2012; Goodwin et al, 2007). Thus, families and youth should be informed about risks versus benefits of using antidepressants (including increased risk for suicide with antidepressants). It is not clear whether concomitant use of a mood stabilizer or a SGA protects the person against these complications.

Management of Comorbid Conditions

BP in youth usually presents with comorbid conditions that may worsen the prognosis of BP (Birmaher et al, 2007; Kowatch et al, 2005b; Sala et al, 2014; Yen et al, 2016). Thus, it is crucial to recognize and treat them appropriately. In general, before treating the comorbid disorder(s), it is recommended to first stabilize the symptoms of BP, especially if the youth's apparent "comorbid symptoms" (e.g., ADHD, behavior problems) appear to be secondary to the mood disorder (mania, depression, or both). If the comorbid conditions cannot be attributed to BP or do not improve after the symptoms of mania/hypomania subside, treatment for both the BP and the comorbid conditions is indicated (Birmaher, 2016; Birmaher et al, 2007; Diler & Birmaher, 2012; Wozniak, 2005).

Because some of the medications used for treatment may worsen mood symptoms, if appropriate, psychosocial treatments should be tried first. If medications are indicated, they should be used systematically, introducing only one at a time and waiting until it exerts its effect and does not induce side effects before increasing the dose or changing to other medications. As a rule, unless there is a contraindication, the medications that have been demonstrated to be more efficacious for the management of the specific psychiatric disorders should be chosen.

Prognosis and Future Directions

BP severely affects the normal development and psychosocial functioning of the youth and increases the risk for suicide, psychosis, substance abuse, and behavioral, academic, social, and legal problems (Birmaher et al, 2009a; Diler & Birmaher, 2012; Pavuluri et al, 2005).

BP is often a chronic and disabling illness. Early-childhood BP has a lower rate of recovery, with a longer duration of mixed and rapid cycling episodes, more symptoms, and more frequent polarity changes than BP later in life (Birmaher et al, 2009a, 2009c). Compared with adults, adolescents with BP often have a prolonged early course and are less responsive to treatment. Youth with BP show high lifetime rates of psychosis, which is associated with poor prognosis. Adolescents with BP are at increased risk for suicide relative to children with other psychiatric disorders. Comorbid substance use disorders further increase the suicide risk. Nevertheless, open treatment studies and small randomized trials of both pharmacological and psychosocial intervention suggest reason for cautious optimism.

Future studies evaluating possible preventative strategies for youth at high risk for BP, especially offspring at very high risk to develop BP, are indicated (Hafeman et al, 2016). Genetic and other biological studies including pharmacogenetic, neuroimaging, and the presence of inflammatory markers and studies correlating the effects of treatment and biochemical changes on the brain are urgently needed (Diler et al, 2013a, 2013b; Goldstein et al, 2011, 2015). Furthermore, studies to prospectively assess the contributions of risk protective factors (e.g., cognitive development, social and coping skills, environmental factors) to outcome are warranted.

Birmaher B, Axelson D, Goldstein B, et al. Four-year longitudinal course of children and adolescents with bipolar spectrum disorders: the Course and Outcome of Bipolar Youth (COBY) study. *Am J Psychiatry*. 2009a;166(7):795–804.

Birmaher B, Axelson D, Pavaluri M. Bipolar disorder. In: Martin A, Volkmar FR, Lewis M, eds. *Lewis' Child and Adolescent Psychiatry: A Comprehensive Textbook*. 4th ed. London: Lippincott Williams & Wilkins; 2007.

Birmaher B, Axelson D, Strober M, et al. Comparison of manic and depressive symptoms between children and adolescents with bipolar spectrum disorders. *Bipolar Disord*. 2009c;11(1):52–62.

Bobo WV, Cooper WO, Stein CM, et al. Antipsychotics and the risk of type 2 diabetes mellitus in children and youth. *JAMA Psychiatry*. 2013;70(10):1067–1075.

Chang K, Saxena K, Howe M. An open-label study of lamotrigine adjunct or monotherapy for the treatment of adolescents with bipolar depression. *J Am Acad Child Adolesc Psychiatry*. 2006;45(3):298–304.

Connolly KR, Thase ME. The clinical management of bipolar disorder: a review of evidence-based guidelines. *Prim Care Companion CNS Disord*. 2011;13(4).

Correll C, Manu P, Olshanskiy V, et al. Cardiometabolic risk of second-generation antipsychotic medications during first-time use in children and adolescents. *JAMA*. 2009;302(16):1765–1773.

Correll CU, Sheridan EM, DelBello MP. Antipsychotic and mood stabilizer efficacy and tolerability in pediatric and adult patients with bipolar I mania: a comparative analysis of acute, randomized, placebo-controlled trials. *Bipolar Disord.* 2010; 12(2):116–141.

DelBello MP, Chang K, Welge JA, et al. A double-blind, placebo-controlled pilot study of quetiapine for depressed adolescents with bipolar disorder. *Bipolar Disord.* 2009;11(5): 483–493.

DelBello MP, Correll CU, Carlson GA, et al. Pharmacological management of bipolar disorder in a youth with diabetes. *J Am Acad Child Adolesc Psychiatry.* 2007a;46(10):1375–1379.

DelBello MP, Findling RL, Kushner S, et al. A pilot controlled trial of topiramate for mania in children and adolescents with bipolar disorder. *J Am Acad Child Adolesc Psychiatry.* 2005;44(6):539–547.

DelBello MP, Findling RL, Wang PP, et al. Safety and efficacy of ziprasidone in pediatric bipolar disorder. Presented at the 55th Annual Convention and Scientific Program of the Society of Biological Psychiatry; Washington, DC; 2008.

DelBello MP, Goldman R, Phillips D, Deng L, Cucchiaro J, Loebel A. Efficacy and safety of lurasidone in children and adolescents with bipolar I depression: a double-blind, placebo-controlled study. *J Am Acad Child Adolesc Psychiatry.* 2017 Dec;56(12):1015–1025. doi: 10.1016/j.jaac.2017.10.006. Epub 2017 Oct 13. PMID: 29173735.

DelBello MP, Hanseman D, Adler CM, et al. Twelve-month outcome of adolescents with bipolar disorder following first hospitalization for a manic or mixed episode. *Am J Psychiatry.* 2007b;164(4):582–590.

DelBello MP, Schwiers ML, Rosenberg HL, et al. A double-blind, randomized, placebo-controlled study of quetiapine as adjunctive treatment for adolescent mania. *J Am Acad Child Adolesc Psychiatry.* 2002;41:1216–1223.

Detke HC, DelBello MP, Landry J, Usher RW. Olanzapine/Fluoxetine combination in children and adolescents with bipolar I depression: a randomized, double-blind, placebo-controlled trial. *J Am Acad Child Adolesc Psychiatry.* 2015 Mar;54(3):217–224. doi: 10.1016/j.jaac.2014.12.012. Epub 2014 Dec 29. PMID: 25721187.

Diler RS, Birmaher B. Bipolar disorder in children and adolescents. In: Rey JM, ed. *IACAPAP e-Textbook of Child and Adolescent Mental Health.* Geneva: International Association for Child and Adolescent Psychiatry and Allied Professions; 2012.

Diler RS, Ladouceur CD, Segreti A, et al. Neural correlates of treatment response in depressed bipolar adolescents during emotion processing. *Brain Imaging Behav.* 2013b;7(2):227–235.

Diler RS, Segreti AM, Ladouceur CD, et al. Neural correlates of treatment in adolescents with bipolar depression during response inhibition. *J Child Adolesc Psychopharmacol.* 2013a; 23(3):214–221.

Findling RL, Cavus I, Pappadopulos E, et al. Efficacy, long-term safety, and tolerability of ziprasidone in children and adolescents with bipolar disorder. *J Child Adolesc Psychopharmacol.* 2013;23(8):545–557.

Findling RL, Chang K, Robb A, et al. Adjunctive maintenance lamotrigine for pediatric bipolar i disorder: a placebo-controlled, randomized withdrawal study. *J Am Acad Child Adolesc Psychiatry.* 2015c;54(12):1020–1031.

Findling RL, Ginsberg LD. The safety and effectiveness of open-label extended release carbamazepine in the treatment of children and adolescents with bipolar I disorder suffering from a manic or mixed episode. *Neuropsychiatr Dis Treat.* 2014;10:1589–1597.

Findling RL, Landbloom RL, Szegedi A, et al. Asenapine for the acute treatment of pediatric manic or mixed episode of bipolar I disorder. *J Am Acad Child Adolesc Psychiatry.* 2015a;54(12):1032–1041.

Findling RL, McNamara NK, Gracious BL, et al. Combination lithium and divalproex sodium in pediatric bipolarity. *J Am Acad Child Adolesc Psychiatry.* 2003;42:895–901.

Findling RL, McNamara NK, Youngstrom EA, et al. Double-blind 18 month trial of lithium versus divalproex maintenance treatment in pediatric bipolar disorder. *J Am Acad Child Adolesc Psychiatr.* 2005; 44:409–417.

Findling RL, Nyilas M, Forbes RA, et al. Acute treatment of pediatric bipolar I disorder, manic or mixed episode, with aripiprazole: a randomized, double-blind, placebo-controlled study. *J Clin Psychiatry.* 2009;70(10):1441–1451.

Findling RL, Robb A, McNamara NK, et al. Lithium in the acute treatment of bipolar I disorder: a double-blind, placebo-controlled study. *Pediatrics.* 2015b;136(5):885–894.

Findling RL, Youngstrom EA, McNamara NK, et al. Double-blind, randomized, placebo-controlled long-term maintenance study of aripiprazole in children with bipolar disorder. *J Clin Psychiatry.* 2012;73(1):57–63.

Fountoulakis KN, Kasper S, Andreassen O, et al. Efficacy of pharmacotherapy in bipolar disorder: a report by the WPA section on pharmacopsychiatry. *Eur Arch Psychiatry Clin Neurosci.* 2012;262(Suppl 1):1–48.

Fraguas D, Correll CU, Merchán-Naranjo J, et al. Efficacy and safety of second-generation antipsychotics in children and adolescents with psychotic and bipolar spectrum disorders: comprehensive review of prospective head-to-head and placebo-controlled comparisons. *Eur Neuropsychopharmacol.* 2011;21(8):621–645.

Fristad MA, Young AS, Vesco AT, et al. 2015. A randomized controlled trial of individual family psychoeducational psychotherapy and omega-3 fatty acids in youth with subsyndromal bipolar disorder. *J Child Adolesc Psychopharmacol.* 2015;25(10):764–774.

Geller B, Luby JL, Joshi P, et al. A randomized controlled trial of risperidone, lithium, or divalproex sodium for initial treatment of bipolar I disorder, manic or mixed phase, in children and adolescents. *Arch Gen Psychiatry.* 2012;69(5):515–528.

Ghaziuddin N, Kutcher SP, Knapp P and the Work Group on Quality Issues. Practice parameter for the use of ECT with adolescents. *J Am Acad Child Adolesc Psychiatr.* 2004; 43:1521–1539.

Goldstein BI, Collinger KA, Lotrich F, et al. Preliminary findings regarding proinflammatory markers and brain-derived neurotrophic factor among adolescents with bipolar spectrum disorders. *J Child Adolesc Psychopharmacol.* 2011;21(5):479–484.

Goldstein BI, Lotrich F, Axelson DA, et al. Inflammatory markers among adolescents and young adults with bipolar spectrum disorders. *J Clin Psychiatry.* 2015;76(11):1556–1563.

Goldstein TR, Axelson DA, Birmaher B, Brent DA. Dialectical behavior therapy for adolescents with bipolar disorder: a 1-year open trial. *J Am Acad Child Adolesc Psychiatry.* 2007; 46(7):820–830.

Goldstein TR, Fersch RK, Axelson DA, et al. Early intervention for adolescents at high risk for the development of bipolar disorder: pilot study of Interpersonal and Social Rhythm Therapy (IPSRT). *Psychotherapy*. 2013;51(1):180–189.

Goldstein TR, Fersch-Podrat RK, Rivera M, et al. Dialectical Behavior Therapy (DBT) for adolescents with bipolar disorder: results from a pilot randomized trial. *J Child Adolesc Psychopharmacol*. 2014;25(2):140–149.

Goodwin FK, Jamison KR, Ghaemi SN. *Manic-Depressive Illness: Bipolar Disorders and Recurrent Depression*. New York: Oxford University Press; 2007.

Haas M, Delbello MP, Pandina G, et al. Risperidone for the treatment of acute mania in children and adolescents with bipolar disorder: a randomized, double-blind, placebo-controlled study. *Bipolar Disord*. 2009;11(7):687–700.

Hafeman DM, Merranko J, Axelson D, et al. Toward the definition of a bipolar prodrome: dimensional predictors of bipolar spectrum disorders in at-risk youth. *Am J Psychiatry*. 2016;173(7):695–704.

Hlastala SA, Frank E. Adapting interpersonal and social rhythm therapy to the developmental needs of adolescents with bipolar disorder. *Dev Psychopathol*. 2006;18:1267–1288.

Hlastala SA, Kotler JS, McClellan JM, McCauley EA. Interpersonal and social rhythm therapy for adolescents with bipolar disorder: treatment development and results from an open trial. *Depress Anxiety*. 2010;27(5):457–464.

Kafantaris V, Coletti DJ, Dicker R, et al. Adjunctive antipsychotic treatment of adolescents with bipolar psychosis. *J Am Acad Child Adolesc Psychiatry*. 2001;40:1448–1456.

Kowatch RA, Fristad M, Birmaher B, et al. Treatment guidelines for children and adolescents with bipolar disorder: child psychiatric workgroup on bipolar disorder. *J Am Acad Child Adolesc Psychiatry*. 2005a;44:213–255.

Kowatch RA, Scheffer RE, Monroe E, et al. Placebo controlled trial of valproic acid versus risperidone in children 3–7 years of age with bipolar I disorder. *J Child Adolesc Psychopharmacol*. 2015;25(4):306–313.

Kowatch RA, Suppes T, Carmody TJ, et al. Effect size of lithium, divalproex sodium, and carbamazepine in children and adolescents with bipolar disorder. *J Am Acad Child Adolesc Psychiatry*. 2000; 713–720.

Kowatch RA, Youngstrom EA, Danielyan A, Findling RL. Review and meta-analysis of the phenomenology and clinical characteristics of mania in children and adolescents. *Bipolar Disord*. 2005b;7:483–496.

Liu HY, Potter MP, Woodworth KY, et al. Pharmacologic treatments for pediatric bipolar disorder: a review and meta-analysis. *J Am Acad Child Adolesc Psychiatry*. 2011;50(8):749–762 e39.

Meduri M, Gregoraci G, Baglivo V, et al. A meta-analysis of efficacy and safety of aripiprazole in adults and pediatric bipolar disorder in randomized controlled trials and observational studies. *J Affect Disord*. 2016;191:187–208.

Miklowitz DJ, Chang KD, Taylor DO, et al. Early psychosocial intervention for youth at risk for bipolar I or II disorder: a one-year treatment development trial. *Bipolar Disord*. 2011;13(1): 67–75.

Miklowitz DJ, Schneck C, George EA, et al. Pharmacotherapy and family-focused treatment for adolescents with bipolar I and II disorders: a 2-year randomized trial. *Am J Psychiatry*. 2014;171:658–667.

Miklowitz DJ, Schneck C, Singh M, et al. Early intervention for symptomatic youth at risk for bipolar disorder: a randomized trial of family-focused therapy. *J Am Acad Child Adolesc Psychiatry*. 2013;52(2):121–131.

Moore CM, Demopulos CM, Henry ME, et al. Brain-to-serum lithium ratio and age: an in vivo magnetic resonance spectroscopy study. *Am J Psychiatry*. 2002;159(7):1240–1242.

Nielsen RE, Laursen MF, Vernal DL, et al. Risk of diabetes in children and adolescents exposed to antipsychotics: a nationwide 12-year case control study. *J Am Acad Child Adolesc Psychiatry*. 2014;53(9):97–979.

Oud M, Mayo-Wilson E, Braidwood R, et al. Psychological interventions for adults with bipolar disorder: systematic review and meta-analysis. *Br J Psychiatry*. 2016;208(3):213–222.

Patel NC, DelBello MP, Bryan HS, et al. Open-label lithium for the treatment of adolescents with bipolar depression. *J Am Acad Child Adolesc Psychiatry*. 2006;45(3):289–297.

Pathak S, Findling RL, Earley WR, et al. Efficacy and safety of quetiapine in children and adolescents with mania associated with bipolar I disorder: a 3-week, double-blind, placebo-controlled trial. *J Clin Psychiatry*. 2013;74(1):e100–e109.

Pavuluri MN, Birmaher B, Naylor MW. Pediatric bipolar disorder: a review of the past 10 years. *J Am Acad Child Adolesc Psychiatry*. 2005;44(9):846–871.

Pavuluri MN, Henry D, Naylor M, et al. A prospective trial of combination therapy of risperidone with lithium or divalproex sodium in pediatric mania. *J Affect Disord*. 2004;82 (Suppl 1): 103–111.

Podawiltz A. A review of current bipolar disorder treatment guidelines. *J Clin Psychiatry*. 2012;73(3):e12.

Popovic D, Reinares M, Goikolea JM, et al. Polarity index of pharmacological agents used for maintenance treatment of bipolar disorder. *Eur Neuropsychopharmacol*. 2011;22(5):339–346.

Post RM, Keck P, Solomon D. Bipolar disorder in adults: maintenance treatment. UpToDate. Accessed March 15, 2013.

Rummel-Kluge C, Komossa K, Schwarz S, et al. Second-generation antipsychotic drugs and extrapyramidal side effects: a systematic review and meta-analysis of head-to-head comparisons. *Schizophrenia Bull*. 2012;38(1):167–177.

Sala R, Strober M, Axelson D, et al. Effects of comorbid anxiety disorders on the longitudinal course of pediatric bipolar illness. *J Am Acad Child Adolesc Psychiatry*. 2014;53(1):72–81.

Salpekar JA, Joshi PT, Axelson DA, et al. Depression and suicidality outcomes in the treatment of early age mania study. *J Am Acad Child Adolesc Psychiatry*. 2015;54(12):999–1007.

Stovall J. Bipolar disorder in adults: epidemiology and pathogenesis. UpToDate. Accessed January 2016.

Stovall J, Keck P, Solomon D. Bipolar disorder in adults: pharmacotherapy for acute mania, mixed states, and hypomania. UpToDate. Accessed March 15, 2013.

Tohen M, Kryzhanovskaya L, Carlson G, et al. Olanzapine versus placebo in the treatment of adolescents with bipolar mania. *Am J Psychiatry*. 2007;164(10):1547–1556.

Vitiello B, Correll C, van Zwieten-Boot B, et al. Antipsychotics in children and adolescents: increasing use, evidence for efficacy and safety concerns. *Eur Neuropsychopharmacol*. 2009;19(9):629–635.

Wagner KD, Kowatch RA, Emslie GJ, et al. A double-blind, randomized, placebo-controlled trial of oxcarbazepine in the treatment of bipolar disorder in children and adolescents. *Am J Psychiatry*. 2006;163(7):1179–1186.

Wagner KD, Redden L, Kowatch RA, et al. A double-blind, randomized, placebo-controlled trial of divalproex extended-release in the treatment of bipolar disorder in children and adolescents. *J Am Acad Child Adolesc Psychiatry.* 2009;48(5):519–532.

Walkup JT, Wagner KD, Miller L, et al. Treatment of early-age mania: outcomes for partial and nonresponders in initial treatment. *J Am Acad Child Adolesc Psychiatry.* 2015;54(12):1008–1019.

Wall CA, Croarkin PE, Maroney-Smith MJ, et al. Magnetic resonance imaging-guided, open-label, high-frequency repetitive transcranial magnetic stimulation for adolescents with major depressive disorder. *J Child Adolesc Psychopharmacol.* 2016;26(7):582–589.

West AE, Henry DB, Pavuluri MN. Maintenance model of integrated psychosocial treatment in pediatric bipolar disorder: a pilot feasibility study. *J Am Acad Child Adolesc Psychiatry.* 2007;46(2):205–212.

West AE, Weinstein SM, Peters AT, et al. Child and family-focused cognitive-behavioral therapy for pediatric bipolar disorder: a randomized clinical trial. *J Am Acad Child Adolesc Psychiatry.* 2014;53D11:1168–1178.

Wozniak J, Biederman J, Mick E, et al. Omega-3 fatty acid monotherapy for pediatric bipolar disorder: a prospective open-label trial. *Eur Neuropsychopharmacol.* 2007;17(6–7):440–447.

Wozniak J, Faraone SV, Chan J, et al. A randomized clinical trial of high eicosapentaenoic acid omega-3 fatty acids and inositol as monotherapy and in combination in the treatment of pediatric bipolar spectrum disorders: a pilot study. *J Clin Psychiatry.* 2015;76(11):1548–1555.

Yen S, Stout R, Hower H, et al. The influence of comorbid disorders on the episodicity of bipolar disorder in youth. *Acta Psychiatr Scand.* 2016;133(4):324–334.

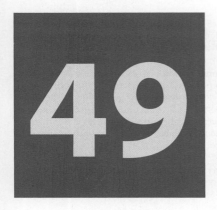

Suicidal Behavior in Children and Adolescents

49

Robert A. King, MD
Alan Apter, MD

ICD-10 Diagnostic Codes

R45.851 Suicidal Ideations

A condition characterized by suicidal thoughts or ideation.

T14.91 Suicide Attempt

A condition characterized by self-inflicted harm in an attempt to end one's own life; the unsuccessful attempt to kill oneself.

Z91.5 Personal History of Self-harm

A personal history of para-suicide, self-poisoning, or a suicide attempt. ICD-10 does not define para-suicide but lists as synonyms or specific examples of self-harm the following: attempted suicide, deliberate self-poisoning, and attempted self-mutilation or self-harm by physical trauma.

▶ General Considerations

Patients with strong or repetitive thoughts or urges to kill or hurt themselves, or who have acted deliberately to do so, pose a serious clinical challenge for assessment, treatment, and classification. Classification is challenging because although, at one extreme, there are those individuals who kill themselves with explicitly declared intent, in many more cases (as discussed in this chapter) the individual's intent and wish to die (or merely to self-injure) may be more ambiguous, ambivalent, and/or difficult to determine and variable over time. Similarly, the continuum from passing thought/urge, through persistent preoccupation, to tentative gesture, or on to action deliberately intended to harm or kill oneself is often difficult to demarcate clearly. As a result, working clinical and epidemiological definitions have varied.

The *Diagnostic and Statistical Manual of Mental Disorders, Fifth Edition* (DSM-5) (American Psychiatric Association, 2013) distinguishes two proposed conditions for further study: suicidal behavior disorder and nonsuicidal self-injury. As a feature of suicidal behavior disorder, suicide attempts are defined as a self-inflicted behavior done in the expectation that it will lead to death. In contrast, nonsuicidal self-injury consists of deliberate self-inflicted bodily damage with the expectation that the injury will not be lethal but will lead to only mild physical harm. The proposed criteria also suggest the self-injurious behavior is not motivated by a wish to die but rather to attain some positive feeling, relief from a negative state of mind, or to achieve some interpersonal end.

As discussed in this chapter, discerning intent in acts of self-harm is not always straight-forward, and there is much overlap in the risk factors for attempted suicide and nonsuicidal self-injury.

A. Epidemiology

1. Completed suicide—Completed suicide is rare in prepubertal children, with an annual rate in the United States on the order of 2.0 per 100,000 for female children aged 10–14 and 3.6 per 100,000 for male children aged 10–14 in 2020. This is rising in recent years, however, and was the second leading cause of death in this age group in 2020 and increased 100% in the years 2010–2019. Completed suicide in adolescents is also the second leading cause of mortality in the United States in this otherwise generally healthy age group, and in 2019 it accounted for the death of 10.5 teens, aged 15–19, per 100,000 (with the rates in that age group 15.8 per 100,000 for boys and 5.0 per 100,000 for girls). The most recent international data show a similar pattern of relatively low rates for youngsters aged 5–14 (ranging from 0 to 2.0 per 100,000), with higher rates for youth aged 15–24 (ranging from 1.6 to 25.8 per 100,000), making suicide the second leading cause of youth mortality worldwide. Although young male suicides substantially outnumber female suicides throughout much of the world, the pattern is reversed in rural parts of the developing world, such as India and China, perhaps because of ready access to lethal insecticides used in agriculture. Although variations in reporting practices make direct comparisons difficult, there are apparent wide international variations, with high rates of youth suicide associated with rapid political and economic changes, widespread gun availability, breakdown of traditional culture among indigenous peoples, and changes in the status of women.

Dramatic secular trends are also apparent internationally in the epidemiological data. According to the World Health Organization, youth suicide rates rose dramatically between the 1950s and mid-1980s in the United States, much of Europe, Mexico, and the Western Pacific; speculations as to the cause of this trend include rising divorce rates, increased adolescent substance use, demographic competition, erosion of religious/cultural taboos against suicide, and mass media coverage of celebrity and other suicides. The decades from 1990 to 2009 showed a decline in youth suicide rates in many but not all Western countries. The reasons for this decline are unclear, although greater awareness of adolescent depression and widespread availability of effective antidepressants have been speculated to play a role. Since 2010, however, adolescent suicide rates in the United States have again begun to climb and recent data show a significant increase in preadolescent suicide in particular.

2. Suicidal ideation and attempts—In contrast to completed suicide, suicidal ideation and attempts are far more common. The 2019 biennial national Youth Risk Behavior Survey found that, during the preceding 12 months, 17.2% of US high school students had seriously contemplated attempted suicide, 13.6% had made a plan to attempt suicide, 7.4% had actually attempted suicide 1 or more times, and 2.4% had made a suicide attempt involving an injury, poisoning, or overdose that had to be treated by a doctor or nurse.

Suicidal ideation or behavior is a common cause for pediatric emergency room (ER) visits. During the period 2006–2013, ER visits for attempted suicide or self-inflicted injury have increased, with the highest visit rate of 350.7 per 100,000 US population found among patients aged 15–19. (These data do not distinguish between suicide attempt and nonsuicidal self-injury; see later discussion.) Females had a significantly higher visit rate than their male counterparts. About 20% of such ER visits result in hospitalization. The annual hospitalization rate of youth with self-inflicted injuries is 44.9 per 100,000 5- to 20-year-olds. Among these hospitalized patients, the rate of cutting is 13.2%, hanging or suffocation 1.3%, and ingestion of acetaminophen 26.9%, antidepressants 14%, opiates 3.3%, and salicylates 10.2%.

3. Gender—Suicidal behavior varies markedly by gender. Attempted suicide is much more common in girls aged 15–19 years than in same-aged boys. Girls in this age group attempt suicide almost twice as often as boys, whereas boys complete suicide about 4 times more often than girls. Thus, for adolescent boys, the ratio of completed to attempted suicides is about 1:517, whereas it is 1:4000 for girls.

B. Etiology

1. Completed suicide

i. **Major psychiatric disorder**—The psychological autopsy is a procedure for reconstructing a decedent's life to understand the psychological antecedents and circumstances of the death. This process includes a review of available records and systematic interviews of knowledgeable informants regarding the decedent's lifestyle and expressed thoughts, feelings, and behaviors, especially those that might provide evidence of psychopathology. Such studies find that about 90% of adolescent suicide completers have at least one diagnosable major psychiatric disorder, especially depressive, substance abuse, and conduct disorders. In about half of adolescent suicides, one or more psychiatric disorders have been present for at least 3 years at the time of suicide.

From a screening and prediction perspective, although these diagnostic risk factors are sensitive (i.e., they are found in most cases of adolescent suicide), they are very nonspecific, because they are found in a very large number of adolescents who do *not* commit suicide. The small minority of adolescent suicides without a discernable major psychiatric diagnosis still show elevated rates, compared to community controls, of family psychiatric disorder, past suicidal ideation or behavior, legal or disciplinary problems in the prior year, and firearms in the home.

ii. **Psychopathological and psychosocial risk factors**—Additional psychosocial risk factors for completed suicide include isolative or impulsive character traits; recent life stressors, such as interpersonal loss or legal or disciplinary problems (especially in youngsters with substance abuse or disruptive disorders); and family history of suicide, depression, or substance abuse. Despite variations across ethnic and racial groups, completed suicide rates do not appear to be influenced by socioeconomic status per se. Troubled parent–child relationships and nonintact family of origin appear to be associated with youth suicide, although once parental or youth psychopathology is controlled for, the magnitude of this association is unclear.

iii. **Media and suicide "contagion"**—Clusters of apparently imitative suicide attempts and completions occur in adolescents and are estimated to account for 1–13% of youth suicides in the United States. Sensationalized media coverage of local, celebrity, or fictional suicides may provoke imitative suicidal behavior.

2. Suicidal ideation and attempts

i. **Psychopathology**—In community samples, adolescent suicidal ideation and attempts are associated with the presence of a psychiatric diagnosis such as substance abuse or mood, anxiety, and disruptive disorders; in adolescent girls, eating disorder also appears to be a potent risk factor for serious suicide attempts. In addition to these diagnostic risk factors, certain cognitive and personality traits, including impulsivity, aggression, hopelessness, poor emotional regulation, and impaired social and problem-solving skills, are important risk factors for adolescent suicidal ideation/behavior and provide targets for therapeutic or preventive intervention.

ii. Social and problem-solving skills deficits

a. Family factors—Family factors such as loss of a parent after death or divorce, residential instability, change in caretaking parent, living apart from parents (including foster care and running away from home), family conflict, and perceived low parental care and social support are all associated with adolescent suicide attempts. Sexual and physical abuse are potent risk factors for suicide attempts in youth, even after controlling for associated factors in the abusive parents such as mental disorder, impulsivity/aggression, suicidal behavior, substance abuse, parental discord, divorce, and step-parenting.

b. Problem behaviors—In light of these associations, it is not surprising that there is a high degree of overlap between adolescent suicidal ideation and attempts and the following: impulsive, sensation-seeking, or high-risk adolescent "problem behavior," such as substance use, fighting, and antisocial behavior (even at levels below threshold for the diagnosis of a substance abuse or disruptive disorder); the early onset of sexual intercourse; and weapon carrying.

c. Gender nonconformity—Transgender, bisexual, and homosexual youth, especially those who experience parental or peer rejection, stigmatization, or victimization (e.g., as part of a tumultuous "coming out" process), have an increased risk of attempted suicide, even after controlling for depression and other risk factors.

3. Precipitants—Children and adolescents usually manifest suicidal behavior as a desperate attempt to escape from unbearable affect, such as rage, intense isolation, or self-loathing. Feelings of inner deadness, intolerable anxiety, or fear of fragmentation (in the case of psychosis) less commonly play a role. These feelings are often intensified by different forms of interpersonal discord that activate suicidal ideation or behavior. Thus, although extraordinary acute stressors, such as physical assault or sexual abuse, may precipitate suicidal feelings or behavior, the commonest immediate triggers of adolescent suicide attempts are the commonplace travails of adolescence—disciplinary crises, teasing, arguments with a parent or romantic partner, or perceived failure, shame, or humiliation. Suicidal feelings and attempts can result when such upsets occur in a youngster with pessimism, hopelessness, and perceived helplessness due to depression or with poor affect regulation, impulsive decision making, impaired social and communication skills, and a propensity to aggression, especially if these risk factors have been exacerbated by substance use or sleep disturbance. In turn, the psychopathology associated with adolescent suicidality makes it more likely that the vulnerable adolescent will encounter or provoke interpersonal discord.

C. Genetic and Biological Factors

A family history of attempted or completed suicide is a significant risk factor for youthful suicidal behavior. Twin studies suggest that genetic factors predict 17–45% of the variance in suicidal behavior. The psychiatric disorders predisposing to suicidal behavior (especially mood disorders) have strong heritable components. Family studies suggest, however, that genetic factors contribute to the risk for suicidal behavior over and above the genetic contribution to the transmission of mood disorder. The familial transmission of suicidal behavior appears to be mediated by the transmission of a tendency to impulsive aggression; furthermore, sexual abuse in parent and child further increases the risk of suicidal behavior in the child, most likely by several mechanisms, such as shared genetic and environmental factors and gene–environment interaction.

These associations, together with the observation that greater family loading for suicidal behavior is associated with increased risk for, and earlier onset of, suicide attempts in, offspring, suggest opportunities for case finding and early intervention. Hence, prospective screening for children of parents with histories of mood disorder, suicide attempts, and childhood sexual abuse identifies at-risk children who would benefit from preventive intervention.

The specific genes that contribute to suicide risk are unknown. In adults, low cerebrospinal fluid levels of the serotonin metabolite 5-hydroxyindoleacetic acid are correlated with impulsive aggression and attempted and completed suicide. Data concerning the neurobiology of adolescent suicide attempters are considerably more sparse. Given the apparent centrality of impulsivity and aggression in attempted and completed adolescent suicide, genetic and neurobiological studies of adolescent suicide have focused on serotonergic regulatory genes and functioning. They have been largely inconclusive. Postmortem studies have found higher levels of 5-HT$_{2A}$ receptors and altered levels of second messenger–associated mRNA and regulatory kinases in the prefrontal cortex of adolescent suicides.

In addition to evidence of altered neurotransmitter regulation, some recent studies have found evidence linking depression or suicidal behavior to altered neuro-inflammatory processes, including microglial and cytokine abnormalities,

Convergent neuroimaging and postmortem studies point to structural and functional abnormalities in the frontolimbic and frontostriatal systems and their connections. Studies using empirically operationalized neuropsychological paradigms with adolescent suicide attempters have found deficits in affective decision making and risk assessment, findings that may provide clues concerning underlying neurobiological processes.

▶ Clinical Findings

The primary goals of clinical evaluation of the suicidal child are as follows: (1) determine the degree of acute suicidal risk;

(2) determine the immediate steps needed to ensure the child's safety; (3) assess the general psychiatric, psychological, family, and social context of the suicidal crisis; (4) identify what internal, interpersonal, and treatment resources are available; (5) design a treatment plan to address the immediate and persistent risk factors for suicide and enhance personal resources; and (6) maximize treatment compliance and follow-up.

A. Assessment of Suicide Risk

This involves systematic inquiry about the presence of suicidal ideation, whether the youngster had explicit plans for self-injury, and a detailed history of past incidents of actual self-harm (including their precipitants, context, and outcome). In the clinical setting, assessment is best done by means of a careful interview of the child and parents, separately and together. Careful inquiry can reveal suicidal ideation or behavior previously unsuspected by parents or other adults. A very large number of rating scales and structured instruments are available to help systematize such inquiry for research or screening purposes. Among the most commonly used are the widely translated Beck Scale for Suicidal Ideation and Suicide Intent Scale, which are useful for screening and assessing degree of intent in suicidal youngsters. The Suicidal Ideation Questionnaire and the broader and more elaborate Columbia Teen Screen have proven useful for school-based screenings. The Child Suicide Potential Index covers multiple risk domains associated with suicidal behavior and assesses risk for suicidal potential as well as suicidality per se. The Multi-Attitude Suicide Tendency Scale assesses conflictual attitudes toward life and death and can help discriminate suicidal youth from psychiatric and nonclinical youth. The Columbia–Suicide Severity Rating Scale (C-SSRS) was developed paralleling the Columbia Classification Algorithm for Suicide Assessment (C-CASA), which is a standardized system for classifying suicidal phenomena. The C-SSRS consists of a clinical interview that focuses on both ideation and behavior and can be administered during evaluation or risk assessment to identify the level and type of suicidality present. It can also be used during treatment to monitor clinical deterioration or improvement. Although this tool needs further assessment, it is an important step in the development of much-needed common terminology and assessment procedures.

B. Assessment of Intent, Motivation, and Lethality

Because the motivation of suicide attempts is usually ambivalent, it is important to assess the severity of intent, that is, the extent to which the youngster wished to die. Among the factors to be assessed are the following:

- *Did the patient truly wish to die?*
- *Did the patient believe the means (e.g., overdose hanging) was lethal?*
- *How intense and persistent was the patient's suicidal ideation preceding the attempt?*

- *Did the patient plan and take premeditated steps and over how long (e.g., hoarding pills, leaving a note)?*
- *Did the patient take measures to avoid or ensure discovery and rescue (e.g., finding an isolated location, seeking help, telling immediately, or not telling)?*
- *Did the suicidal ideation persist after the attempt?*

The severity of intent may range from a serious premeditated attempt of high lethality involving a clear wish to die and steps to avoid discovery, through impulsive overdoses of low lethality when someone else is either nearby or promptly sought and the wish to die is ambivalent or passing.

To understand the motive for the suicide attempt, it is important to comprehend the interpersonal and affective context of the attempt as well as the youngster's style of interpersonal relating and emotional regulation. Although about one half of adolescent suicide attempters endorse a wish to die (usually to obtain relief from an unbearable state of mind), one quarter to one half endorse interpersonal motives such as "to make people understand how desperate I was," "to show how much I loved someone," "to get help from someone," or "to find out whether someone really loved me." About a third of adolescents making serious suicide attempts are unable to describe any precipitant or motivation, stating, "I don't know why I did it; I was upset." Vagueness can reflect a difficulty articulating feelings, poor emotional regulation, and impaired social problem-solving skills.

The lethality of the attempt does not necessarily correspond to the intensity of a conscious intent to die. Youngsters with low suicidal intent may underestimate the toxicity of medication (e.g., a hepatotoxic acetaminophen overdose), whereas others with high suicidal intent can underestimate what is needed to kill themselves.

In assessing the degree of suicidal risk and the need for hospitalization, persistent suicidal ideation, high intent, high lethality of an attempt, or a history of multiple attempts are all associated with an increased risk of repetition and completion.

C. Laboratory and Imaging Studies

Although research studies of adolescent suicide have examined neuroimaging findings and neurobiological measures (e.g., neuroendocrine provocation paradigms and platelet or cerebrospinal fluid neurotransmitter parameters), these are not useful in ordinary clinical practice. Laboratory studies such as thyroid function tests may be indicated as part of the routine pediatric evaluation of persistent adolescent depression.

▶ Differential Diagnosis (Including Comorbid Conditions)

Having established the presence of significant suicidal ideation or behavior, the next task is to evaluate psychopathological, family, and social factors that underlie the youngster's suicidality.

A. Comorbid Psychiatric Disorder

Among the most potent risk factors for suicidality is the presence of mood disorder, chronic anxiety, disruptive behavior disorder (especially conduct disorder), and substance abuse. The risk of a suicide attempt increases with the number of comorbid disorders. The impact of these risk factors varies by gender, as illustrated by a landmark New York area case–control study of adolescent suicides. For boys, the risk of completed suicide was most increased by a history of a prior attempt (approximate odds ratio [OR] 22.5 compared to the general adolescent male population), followed by major depression (OR 8.6), substance abuse (OR 7.1), and previous antisocial behavior (OR 4.4). In contrast, for girls, major depression was the predominant risk factor (OR 49), followed by a history of a prior attempt (OR 8.6), and previous antisocial behavior (OR 3.2). Substance abuse did not contribute to suicidal risk in girls (OR 0.8). Although schizophrenia and bipolar disorder are major risk factors for suicide in adults, it is only in older adolescents that they play a significant role in youth suicide.

Substance abuse is an especially important risk factor, because, beyond its links to mood disorder and impaired social functioning, the depressogenic and disinhibiting effects of acute drug or alcohol intoxication facilitate the transition from suicidal ideation to impulsive action.

B. Psychopathological Traits

Over and above the presence of major psychiatric disorders, psychological characteristics such as hopelessness, poor impulse and affect regulation, impaired capacity to express emotion in words, and impaired problem-solving and social skills are important risk factors, the presence of which must be assessed and which may provide targets for clinical intervention.

▶ Treatment

A. Risk assessment and Determining the Level of Care

A crucial dispositional question in the initial evaluation of the suicidal youngster is whether immediate hospitalization is needed to ensure the child's safety or whether outpatient treatment is safe and feasible. For this complex question, there are no reliable, objective algorithms. High lethality, serious intent, persistent suicidal ideation, and/or a history of multiple attempts weigh in favor of hospitalization, as do serious depression, psychosis, or persistent, current, serious life stresses. Other factors to be considered are the youngster's and parents' attitudes toward the suicidal episode. Minimization by the youngster or punitiveness by the parents regarding the episode bode ill; the quality of parental support, supervision, and commitment to treatment are important determinants of the feasibility of effective outpatient treatment. For example, can the family guarantee that firearms, dangerous medicine,

and poisons in the house will be secured? Active substance abuse on a youngster's part is also problematic, because acute intoxication may cast to the winds any treatment alliance or "no harm" agreement (see later discussion). Family turmoil, with high expressed emotion, physical or sexual abuse, active parental substance abuse, or parental psychosis, makes outpatient treatment risky.

When these concerns lead to hospitalization, follow-up and long-term treatment compliance must be dealt with in the transition to less restricted care. Although hospitalization is often necessary to provide a safe environment for further assessment or stabilization, there are few systematic data on the impact of hospitalization on subsequent course.

B. Measures to Ensure Safety and Optimize Treatment Compliance and Follow-up

If the decision is made to send the youngster home with follow-up outpatient treatment, explicit steps are needed to help ensure the child's safety and increase the likelihood of aftercare.

1. Means restriction—The presence of a firearm in the house is a potent risk factor for adolescent suicide. Parents should be educated about the importance of preventing the youngster's access to guns at home. Similarly, steps should be taken to prevent access to lethal quantities of medication or poisons.

2. Safety plans—As part of establishing an initial treatment alliance with the youngster, the clinician should review the precipitant of the current suicidal episode and plan for the reasonable steps to be taken by the youngster and family if stresses recur. Coping measures may be devised, identifying the responsible adults who can be turned to for help, and clarifying how the clinician or other emergency mental health providers can be contacted. The culmination of the discussion should be a safety plan with an explicit agreement by the youngster to try to refrain from self-harm, to employ the alternatives agreed upon, and to contact the clinician if thoughts of suicide return. It is this process that is likely to be helpful, rather than resorting to a misleading pro forma agreement to which the youngster half-heartedly agrees to in order to avoid hospitalization.

C. Steps to Maximize Compliance

About half of adolescent suicide attempters receive little or no follow-up outpatient treatment. Different interventions have been developed to improve rates of treatment adherence. If possible, definite arrangements (specifying time and therapist) should be made before the child leaves the ER. More patients enter and complete treatment when the referring emergency clinician personally contacts the accepting agency rather than leaving it to the patient or family to do. The building of a preliminary alliance between family and mental health care system while the family is still in the ER is useful. Innovative ER-based interventions have been developed that successfully increase adolescent attempters' adherence to outpatient treatment. These include an ER-based problem-solving intervention and a program that helps families and youngsters in the ER reframe their understanding of the child's suicidal crisis by means of participation in an initial family therapy session.

D. The Focus of Treatment

When a major psychiatric disorder is diagnosed, the primary focus is the treatment of the underlying disorder. Furthermore, the family, social, school, and other stressors that precipitate, perpetuate, or exacerbate suicidal impulses must be explicitly addressed, as must hopelessness, emotional dysregulation, and impaired emotional and social problem solving. The sections that follow address treatment issues related to the presence of suicidal ideation or behavior. Because many drug and psychotherapy treatment studies of child and adolescent depression explicitly exclude suicidal subjects, the applicability of the extant treatment research is unclear. Nonetheless, despite the general correlation of depression and suicidality, the studies discussed here suggest that particular interventions can have divergent impacts on depression and suicidality.

E. Psychotherapeutic Interventions

There is a sizable research literature on psychosocial therapies for suicidal behavior in adults, including cognitive–behavioral therapy (CBT), dialectical behavior therapy (DBT), problem-solving therapy, and interpersonal psychotherapy (IPT). However, despite controlled trials demonstrating the efficacy of CBT and IPT for depression in children and adolescents, the impact of these interventions on suicidal ideation and behavior (which may be independent of their impact on depression) has not been well studied. Meta-analyses and systematic reviews suggest that certain psychosocial interventions are modestly effective in reducing recurrence of adolescent suicide attempts, namely DBT, CBT, and mentalization-based therapy. However, suicidal depressed adolescents may be particularly hard to engage and in some studies were more likely to drop out of treatment and improved less in depression than did depressed adolescents who were not suicidal. Hopelessness at intake is an important predictor of poor treatment response; hence, addressing motivation for treatment early on is important. Attention to bolstering protective factors such as family and peer support, as well encouraging sobriety, is also an important component. Suicidal adolescents assigned to nondirective therapy did especially poorly, suggesting that structured therapies may be preferable for suicidal depressed adolescents and that treatment should specifically target hopelessness early.

The Treatment of Adolescent Suicide Attempters (TASA) study showed that a combination of treatments seems to be the most effective. Comparing three treatment conditions in depressed adolescent suicide attempters—CBT combined with medication management, CBT alone, and medication management alone—the study found positive results for adolescents vigorously treated with a combination of medication and psychotherapy. Adolescents with depression who had recently attempted suicide showed rates of improvement and remission of depression comparable to those observed in nonsuicidal adolescents with depression.

F. Psychopharmacological Interventions

Although fluoxetine and other SSRIs appear more effective than placebo for the treatment of depression in children and adolescents, the balance of risk to benefit in this age group remains controversial. Most clinical trials of these agents have not been adequately designed or sufficiently powered to address their impact on suicidality. In the Treatment of Adolescent Depression Study, fluoxetine was markedly superior to CBT alone for the treatment of adolescent depression. However, although clinically significant suicidal ideation improved across all treatment groups (fluoxetine alone, CBT alone, CBT with fluoxetine, placebo), the groups that received CBT (either alone or with fluoxetine) showed the greatest improvement, suggesting specific beneficial effects of CBT on suicidal ideation.

Despite public and regulatory concern, the magnitude of suicidality potentially caused by antidepressant medication appears small. Meta-analytic studies of randomized clinical trials of the SSRIs for the treatment of adolescent depression find that the therapeutic benefits of the SSRIs outweigh their risks. The Treatment of Adolescent Depression Study found a statistically significant elevated risk for harm-related adverse effects in SSRI-treated patients in contrast to non-SSRI-treated patients and evidence for the protective effect of CBT.

▶ Prognosis

Compared to youngsters without a history of attempted suicide, youngsters with a history of attempted suicide have a markedly increased risk of completing suicide (a threefold increase in girls and a 30-fold increase in boys). Thus, about one quarter to one third of youth suicides have a prior history of a suicide attempt. Adolescent suicide attempters have high rates of subsequent repeat attempts and are also at elevated risk for motor vehicle and other accidental injuries and homicidal death. Adolescent male suicide attempters, especially those who are hospitalized, appear to have a worse prognosis than female adolescent attempters in terms of subsequent social functioning and risk of completed suicide.

Indeed, suicide attempts in youth are a predictor of ongoing psychosocial risk over subsequent decades. Longitudinal studies suggest that individuals with a suicide attempt in youth remain at long-term risk for persistent mental and physical health problems, violence, and social pathology, even after controlling for youth psychiatric diagnosis and social class.

▶ Prevention

The relative rarity of completed youth suicide poses formidable statistical challenges for screening, prediction, and prevention.

Prevention efforts are best directed against risk factors that appear to play a decisive role in a significant proportion of youth suicides and that are potentially modifiable at a reasonable cost.

In the case of adolescent suicide, the most important risk factors appear to be depression, substance abuse, conduct disorder, history of prior suicide attempt, family history of suicide, and ready access to lethal means.

Universal preventive interventions for adolescent depression and/or substance abuse focused on unselected populations have produced mixed results and appear less effective than targeted programs. Such untargeted, school-based approaches include curricula teaching the warning signs of depression and suicidality, but there is not good evidence supporting their efficacy. A newer generation of universal curriculum-based programs seeks to promote alternative responses to emotional distress, with a focus on improving coping and problem-solving skills. A large multinational randomized clinical trial examined one such manualized universal classroom intervention, which, in addition to increasing awareness about risk/protective factors for suicide, also included information about depression and anxiety and skill enhancement for dealing with stress and adverse life events; at 1-year follow-up, the intervention was effective in reducing both suicide attempts and severe suicide ideation.

Examples of targeted preventive interventions included those addressed to youngsters at high risk because of parental depression or identified as at risk because of self-reported depressive symptoms. Systematic school-based screening of adolescents, using self-reports and structured interviews such as the Columbia Teen Screen, has been studied as a means of facilitating case-finding as a prologue to referral and treatment. Such screening has been shown to identify students at risk with depression and/or suicidal ideation, most of whom were not previously known to school personnel as having significant problems. Furthermore, such screening does not appear to cause an iatrogenic increase in suicidal ideation. Although promising, institutional barriers remain to implementing such programs, and developing effective means of providing therapeutic intervention of teens identified as at risk remains an unsolved problem.

Additional approaches include educating "gatekeepers," such as school personnel and primary care physicians, to identify at-risk youngsters. Neither "gatekeeper" nor systematic screening approaches, by themselves, have been shown to be effective in reducing the incidence of adolescent suicide attempts, perhaps because to be effective they also require follow-up by parents or school and subsequent effective treatment.

Other community-based approaches include hotlines/crisis centers, means restriction (access to firearms or lethal quantities of medications or poisons), and minimizing contagion.

It is unclear whether hotlines reach the youngsters most in need of help or whether they affect outcome. There is some epidemiological evidence that stricter gun control and reduced availability of firearms decrease the youth suicide rate. On the clinical level, counseling parents of suicidal youngsters about preventing access to guns is an important intervention, although often ineffectually done. Restricting the amount of potentially lethal medications (such as acetaminophen) available per purchase or mandating the use of blister packaging (which makes it difficult to impulsively take a large number of loose pills) can successfully decrease rates of severe or fatal overdoses.

Because media publicity of suicides have been shown to increase attempted and completed suicides, school and media outlets need to implement available guidelines to avoid romanticizing or sensationalizing suicides, focusing instead on the causal connection to mental disorder.

Nonsuicidal Self-injury

Many research studies have failed to distinguish between suicidal behavior and acts of NSSI (i.e., purposefully hurting oneself without the conscious intent to die, such as self-cutting or burning). However, the majority of clinicians and researchers are now in agreement that there is a distinct type of nonsuicidal self-injurious behavior (NSSI) that some individuals engage in for reasons other than to end one's life. However, because a history of NSSI is an important predictor of suicidal behavior in individuals, there is a large amount of overlap in risk factors for suicide attempts and engagement in NSSI.

Estimates of the lifetime prevalence of NSSI range from 13.0% to 23.2%. The typical reported age of onset of NSSI falls between 12 and 14 years of age, peaking in mid-adolescence and decreasing into adulthood. Onset after early adulthood is very unusual. Reasons for engaging in NSSI include to regulate emotion and to elicit attention. Correlates of NSSI include a history of sexual abuse, depression, anxiety, alexithymia, hostility, smoking, dissociation, suicidal ideation, and suicidal behaviors.

By definition, the presence or absence of suicidal intent is used to distinguish between NSSI and suicide attempts. However, discerning suicidal intent clearly is sometimes difficult, as stated intent and circumstances may be ambiguous (or contradictory) and ambivalence toward death may be common in individuals engaging in self-injurious behavior. Furthermore, certain behaviors, such as overdoses and self-poisonings, are often reported in the literature as attempted suicides, regardless of self-reported intent to die. More definitive studies of the relationship of NSSI to suicidal ideation and behavior await a clearer classification system that permits sharper delineation between the various phenomena.

Brent DA, Brown CH. Effectiveness of school-based suicide prevention programmes. *Lancet*. 2015;385(9977):1489–1491.

Brent DA, McMakin DL, Kennard BD, et al. Protecting adolescents from self-harm: a critical review of intervention studies. *J Am Acad Child Adolesc Psychiatry*. 2013;52(12):1260–1271.

Bridge JA, Goldstein TR, Brent DA. Adolescent suicide and suicidal behavior. *J Child Psychol Psychiatry.* 2006;47(3–4):372–394.

Bridge JA, Iyengar S, Salary CB, et al. Clinical response and risk for reported suicidal ideation and suicide attempts in pediatric antidepressant treatment: a meta-analysis of randomized controlled trials. *JAMA.* 2007;297:1683–1696.

Brunstein Klomek A, Stanley B. Psychosocial treatment of depression and suicidality in adolescents. *CNS Spectr.* 2007; 12(2):135–144.

Canner JK, Giuliano K, Selvarajah S, Hammond ER, Schneider EB. Emergency department visits for attempted suicide and self harm in the USA: 2006-2013. *Epidemiol Psychiatr Sci.* 2018 Feb;27(1):94–102. doi: 10.1017/S2045796016000871. Epub 2016 Nov 17. PMID: 27852333; PMCID: PMC6999001.

Centers for Disease Control and Prevention. Youth risk behavior surveillance—United States, 2019. *MMWR Morb Mortal Wkly Rep.* 2016;65(6):1–175.

Centers for Disease Control and Prevention, WONDER Online Databases. http://wonder.cdc.gov/mcd-icd10.html. Accessed on July 1, 2016.

Clark TC, Lucassen MF, Bullen P, et al. The health and well-being of transgender high school students: results from the New Zealand adolescent health survey (Youth'12). *J Adolesc Health.* 2014 Jul; 55(1):93–99.

Cox Lippard ET, Johnston J, Blumberg HP. Neurobiological risk factors for suicide: insights from brain imaging. *Am J Prev Med.* 2014;47(suppl 2):S152–S162.

Finkelstein Y, Macdonald EM, Hollands S, et al. Long-term outcomes following self-poisoning in adolescents: a population-based cohort study. *Lancet Psychiatry.* 2015 Jun;2(6):532–539.

Gananç L, Oquendo MA, Tyrka AR, et al. The role of cytokines in the pathophysiology of suicidal behavior. *Psychoneuroendocrinology.* 2016 Jan;63:296–310.

Goldman-Mellor SJ, Caspi A, Harrington H, et al. Suicide attempt in young people: a signal for long-term health care and social needs. *JAMA.* 2014;71(2):119–127.

Gould MS. Suicide and the media. *Ann N Y Acad Sci.* 2001;932: 200–224.

Gould MS, Greenberg T, Velting DM, Shaffer D. Youth suicide risk and preventive interventions: a review of the past ten years. *J Am Acad Child Adolesc Psychiatry.* 2013;42(4):386–405.

Hawton K, Witt KG, Taylor Salisbury TL, et al. Interventions for self-harm in children and adolescents. *Cochrane Database Syst Rev.* 2015;12:CD012013.

Horowitz LM, Bridge JA, Pao M, Boudreaux ED. Screening youth for suicide risk in medical settings: time to ask questions. *Am J Prev Med.* 2014 Sep;47(3 Suppl 2):S170–S175.

Inagaki M, Kawashima Y, Kawanishi C, et al. Interventions to prevent repeat suicidal behavior in patients admitted to an emergency department for a suicide attempt: a meta-analysis. *J Affect Disord.* 2015;175:66–78.

Jacobson CM, Gould M. The epidemiology and phenomenology of non-suicidal self-injurious behavior among adolescents: a critical review of the literature. *Arch Suicide Res.* 2007;11(2):129-147.

King RA. Psychodynamic and family aspects of youth suicide. In: Wasserman D, ed. *The Oxford Textbook of Suicidology and Suicide Prevention: A Global Perspective.* Oxford: Oxford University Press; 2009;643–652.

Kõlves K, De Leo D. Adolescent suicide rates between 1990 and 2009: analysis of age group 15-19 years worldwide. *J Adolesc Health.* 2016 Jan;58(1):69–77.

Lewitzka U, Doucette S, Seemüller F, et al. Biological indicators of suicide risk in youth with mood disorders: what do we know so far? *Curr Psychiatry Rep.* 2012;14(6):705–712.

Mann JJ. The serotonergic system in mood disorders and suicidal behaviour. *Phil Trans R Soc Lond B Biol Sci.* 2013;368: (1615):20120537.

March J, Silva S, Petrycki S. Treatment for adolescents with depression study (TADS) team: fluoxetine, cognitive–behavioral therapy, and their combination for adolescents with depression: treatment for adolescents with depression study (TADS) randomized controlled trial. *JAMA.* 2004;292(7):807–820.

Mehlum L, Tørmoen AJ, Ramberg M, et al. Dialectical behavior therapy for adolescents with repeated suicidal and self-harming behavior: a randomized trial. *J Am Acad Child Adolesc Psychiatry.* 2014 Oct;53(10):1082–1091.

Mundt JC1, Greist JH, Jefferson JW, et al. Prediction of suicidal behavior in clinical research by lifetime suicidal ideation and behavior ascertained by the electronic Columbia-Suicide Severity Rating Scale. *J Clin Psychiatry.* 2013;74(9):887–893.

Nock MK. Future directions for the study of suicide and self-injury. *J Clin Child Adolesc Psychol.* 2012;41(2):255–229.

Nock MK, Green JG, Hwang I, et al. Prevalence, correlates, and treatment of lifetime suicidal behavior among adolescents: results from the National Comorbidity Survey Replication Adolescent Supplement. *JAMA* 2013;70(3):300–310.

Olfson M, Marcus SC, Bridge JA. Emergency department recognition of mental disorders and short-term outcome of deliberate self-harm. *Am J Psychiatry.* 2013;170(12):1442–1450.

Ougrin D, Tranah T, Stahl D, Moran P, Asarnow JR. Therapeutic interventions for suicide attempts and self-harm in adolescents: systematic review and meta-analysis. *J Am Acad Child Adolesc Psychiatry.* 2015 Feb;54(2):97–107.

Rossouw TI, Fonagy P. Mentalization-based treatment for self-harm in adolescents: a randomized controlled trial. *J Am Acad Child Adolesc Psychiatry.* 2012 Dec;51(12):1304–1313.

Ruch DA, Bridge JA. Epidemiology of suicide and suicidal behavior in youth. In: Ackerman JP, Horowitz LM, eds. *Youth Suicide Prevention and Intervention.* Cham: Springer; 2022. https://doi.org/10.1007/978-3-031-06127-1_1

Ting SA, Sullivan AF, Boudreaux ED, et al. Trends in US emergency department visits for attempted suicide and self-inflicted injury, 1993-2008. *Gen Hosp Psychiatry.* 2012;34(5):557–565.

Vitiello B, Brent DA, Greenhill LL, et al. Depressive symptoms and clinical status during the Treatment of Adolescent Suicide Attempters (TASA) Study. *J Am Acad Child Adolesc Psychiatry.* 2009;48(10):997–1004.

Wagner BM, Wong SA, Jobes DA. Mental health professionals' determinations of adolescent suicide attempts. *Suicide Life Threat Behav.* 2002;32(3):284–300.

Wasserman D, Hoven CW, Wasserman C, et al. School-based suicide prevention programmes: the SEYLE cluster—randomised, controlled trial. *Lancet.* 2015;385(9977):1536–1544.

World Health Organization. *Suicide prevention. Country reports and charts.* 2016. http://www.who.int/mental_health/suicide-prevention/en/. Accessed on July 1, 2016.

50

Anxiety Disorders for Children and Adolescents

Eli R. Lebowitz, PhD
Robert A. King, MD
Wendy K. Silverman, PhD

International Statistical Classification of Diseases and Related Health Problems, 10th Revision (ICD-10) Diagnostic Criteria

Anxiety Disorders

A group of disorders in which anxiety is evoked only, or predominantly, in certain well-defined situations that are not currently dangerous. As a result these situations are characteristically avoided or endured with dread. The patient's concern may be focused on individual symptoms like palpitations or feeling faint and is often associated with secondary fears of dying, losing control, or going mad. Contemplating entry to the phobic situation usually generates anticipatory anxiety. Phobic anxiety and depression often coexist. Whether two diagnoses, phobic anxiety and depressive episode, are needed, or only one, is determined by the time course of the two conditions and by therapeutic considerations at the time of consultation.

Separation Anxiety Disorder of Childhood F93.0 (209.21)

Should be diagnosed when fear of separation constitutes the focus of the anxiety and when such anxiety first arose during the early years of childhood. It is differentiated from normal separation anxiety when it is of a degree (severity) that is statistically unusual (including an abnormal persistence beyond the usual age period) and when it is associated with significant problems in social functioning.

*Note that while ICD-10 classifies separation anxiety disorder as an "emotional disorder with onset specific to childhood" (as was the case in *Diagnostic and Statistical Manual of Mental Disorders, Fourth Edition* [DSM-IV]), DSM-5 no longer groups separation anxiety in this category, rather grouping it along with the other anxiety disorders.

Social Phobia F40.1 (300.23)

Fear of scrutiny by other people leading to avoidance of social situations. More pervasive social phobias are usually associated with low self-esteem and fear of criticism. They may present as a complaint of blushing, hand tremor, nausea, or urgency of micturition, the patient sometimes being convinced that one of these secondary manifestations of their anxiety is the primary problem. Symptoms may progress to panic attacks.

Selective Mutism F94.0 (313.23)

Characterized by a marked, emotionally determined selectivity in speaking, such that the child demonstrates a language competence in some situations but fails to speak in other (definable) situations. The disorder is usually associated with marked personality features involving social anxiety, withdrawal, sensitivity, or resistance.

Specific (Isolated) Phobias F40.2 (300.2)

Phobias restricted to highly specific situations such as proximity to particular animals, heights, thunder, darkness, flying, closed spaces, urinating or defecating in public toilets, eating certain foods, dentistry, or the sight of blood or injury. Though the triggering situation is discrete, contact with it can evoke panic as in agoraphobia or social phobia.

Panic Disorder (Episodic Paroxysmal Anxiety) F41.0 (300.01)

The essential feature is recurrent attacks of severe anxiety (panic), which are not restricted to any particular situation or set of circumstances and are therefore unpredictable. As with other anxiety disorders, the dominant symptoms include sudden onset of palpitations, chest pain, choking sensations, dizziness, and feelings of unreality (depersonalization or derealization). There is often also a secondary fear of dying, losing control, or going mad. Panic disorder should not be given as the main diagnosis if the patient has a depressive disorder at the time the attacks start; in these circumstances the panic attacks are probably secondary to depression.

Agoraphobia F40.0 (300.22)

A fairly well-defined cluster of phobias embracing fears of leaving home, entering shops, crowds and public places, or traveling alone in trains, buses, or planes. Panic disorder is a frequent feature of both present and past episodes. Depressive and obsessional symptoms and social phobias are also commonly present as subsidiary features. Avoidance of the phobic situation is often prominent, and some agoraphobics experience little anxiety because they are able to avoid their phobic situations.

Generalized Anxiety Disorder F41.1 (300.02)

Anxiety that is generalized and persistent but not restricted to, or even strongly predominating in, any particular environmental circumstances (i.e., it is "free-floating"). The dominant symptoms are variable but include complaints of persistent nervousness, trembling, muscular tensions, sweating, lightheadedness, palpitations, dizziness, and epigastric discomfort. Fears that the patient or a relative will shortly become ill or have an accident are often expressed.

Reproduced with permission from International Statistical Classification of Diseases and Related Health Problems 10th Revision (ICD-10) Version for 2010. Geneva: World Health Organization; 2010.

SEPARATION ANXIETY DISORDER

General Considerations

A. Epidemiology

Separation anxiety disorder (SAD) is the most prevalent anxiety disorder among children younger than 12, and 90% of cases will have their onset before age 13. Onset can be as early as preschool age, and prevalence among children is approximately 3–4% (Kessler et al, 2005). Prevalence of SAD decreases over adolescence, and the disorder affects 1–2% of adolescents. SAD is among the most common causes of referral to child anxiety treatment. Some community samples have reported higher prevalence in girls than boys (Foley et al, 2004). SAD is highly comorbid with other anxiety disorders, particularly generalized anxiety disorder (GAD).

B. Etiology

Multiple factors, both biological and environmental, contribute to the development of abnormal anxiety in children including separation anxiety. SAD has been linked to parent anxiety and depression and to insecure attachment (Angelosante et al, 2013). Protective parenting and family accommodation of anxious symptoms by parents may contribute to the maintenance of SAD (Lebowitz et al, 2013). Life stressors such as death of a family member or serious illness often precede the appearance of SAD.

C. Genetics

SAD is heritable, and genetic influences account for at least some of the variance in developing SAD or symptoms of separation anxiety (Angelosante et al, 2013). Heritability for SAD may be greater in girls than in boys.

Clinical Findings

A. Signs & Symptoms

SAD is among the most common causes of referral to childhood mental health care with peak onset at around age 8. The core clinical feature of SAD is severe distress at actual or possible separation from primary attachment figures, most often the mother. Children may fear harm that could befall them during the separation (e.g., being kidnapped, becoming sick), or they may fear harm that could occur to the attachment figure (e.g., having a car accident). Children with SAD frequently resist sleeping alone, and either they sleep in the parents' bed or a parent sleeps in the child's bed. In some cases even brief separations such as a parent leaving a room can trigger significant distress and is avoided. Threat of separation can evoke marked arousal and physical symptoms including crying, yelling, vomiting, and trembling. School attendance is a common trigger for separation anxiety in children with SAD, and they may attempt to refuse to attend school or to separate from the parent, though school refusal can occur across other anxiety disorders as well. Children with SAD may repeatedly query parents about their plans or request reassurance that no separations are planned. Parents of children with SAD report significant family accommodation of the child's anxiety through participation in symptoms (e.g., sleeping next to the child) and modification of their or the family's routines (e.g., returning early from work). Very young children with SAD may not verbalize specific worries relating to the separation.

B. Psychological Testing

See end of chapter for integrated discussion of the anxiety disorders.

C. Laboratory Findings

There is no laboratory test for SAD and no testing is indicated. However, research indicates elevated hypothalamic–pituitary–adrenocortical (HPA) (Brand et al, 2011) function in children with SAD and greater sensitivity to CO_2-enriched air. Recent research has also linked separation anxiety to low levels of salivary oxytocin in children (Lebowitz et al, 2016).

Course of Illness

SAD is less persistent than other childhood anxiety disorders. Remission occurs in most cases, but there may be periods of exacerbation (Foley et al, 2004). Although SAD is frequently outgrown by adulthood, its presence in childhood predicts the onset of other, more persistent anxiety disorders (Aschenbrand et al, 2013). Chronic SAD that does not remit in childhood is more likely to be associated with other comorbid conditions or symptoms, particularly externalizing behaviors.

▶ Differential Diagnosis

See end of chapter for integrated discussion of the anxiety-disorders.

▶ Treatment

See end of chapter for integrated discussion of the anxiety disorders.

▶ Complications/Adverse Outcomes of Treatment

See end of chapter for integrated discussion of the anxiety disorders.

▶ Prognosis

See end of chapter for integrated discussion of the anxiety disorders.

Angelosante AG, Ostrowski MA, Chizkov, RR. Separation anxiety disorder. In: Vasa RA, Roy AK, eds. *Pediatric Anxiety Disorders*. New York: Springer Science; 2013:129–142.

Aschenbrand SG, Kendall PC, Webb A, et al. Is childhood separation anxiety disorder a predictor of adult panic disorder and agoraphobia? A seven-year longitudinal study. *J Am Acad Child Adolesc Psychiatry*. 2013;42(12):1478–1485.

Brand S, Wilhelm FH, Kossowsky J, et al. Children suffering from separation anxiety disorder (SAD) show increased HPA axis activity compared to healthy controls. *J Psychiatr Res*. 2011;45(4):452–459.

Foley DL, Pickles A, Maes HM, et al. Course and short-term outcomes of separation anxiety disorder in a community sample of twins. *J Am Acad Child Adolesc Psychiatry*. 2004;43(9):1107–1114.

Kessler RC, Berglund P, Demler O, et al. Lifetime prevalence and age-of-onset distributions of DSM-IV disorders in the National Comorbidity Survey Replication. *Arch Gen Psychiatry*. 2005;62(6):593–602.

Lebowitz ER, Leckman JF, Feldman R, et al. Salivary oxytocin in clinically anxious youth: Associations with separation anxiety and family accommodation. *Psychoneuroendocrinology*. 2016;65:35–43.

Lebowitz ER, Woolston J, Bar-Haim Y, et al. Family accommodation in pediatric anxiety disorders. *Depress Anxiety*. 2013;30(1):47–54.

SOCIAL PHOBIA

▶ General Considerations

A. Epidemiology

Social anxiety disorder (also termed social phobia and abbreviated here SoP to distinguish from SAD) is common and affects between 5% and 10% of children and adolescents. Most children with SoP report feeling anxious in a range of social situations and will not match the *performance only* specifier of the diagnostic criteria, which is assigned when the fear is restricted to speaking or performing in public (Burstein et al, 2011). Community samples of children and adolescents show significantly higher rates of SoP in females compared to males, but this difference has not been reported in clinical samples (Beesdo et al, 2009). Onset is earlier in females, with an average age of onset at 11 years compared to 14 for males. Selective mutism (SM) occurs in less than 1% of children and is more common in young children than adolescents. Most children with SM also have SoP.

B. Etiology

There is no single definitive etiology for SoP, SM, or any of the other anxiety disorders. Temperamental style in infancy has been linked to the likelihood of developing SoP in later life. In particular, behavioral inhibition, a pattern of exaggerated sympathetic arousal in response to aversive stimuli, avoidance of novelty, and hypervigilance, predicts vulnerability to SoP in childhood or adolescence (Lopes & Albano, 2013). Overprotective, rejecting, or controlling parenting as well as childhood maltreatment are risk factors for SoP (Taylor & Alden, 2006). Socially stressful events or situations such as being bullied in school or humiliated in front of others increase the likelihood of developing SoP. Parent accommodation of social avoidance (e.g., excusing a child from school, refraining from inviting guests to the home) may contribute to the maintenance of SoP. Social anxiety is the primary risk factor for SM, and factors that increase risk of SoP, such as behavioral inhibition and overly protective parenting, are additional risk factors for SM. Children with SM also tend to exhibit receptive language difficulties. Family accommodation of attempts to avoid speaking (e.g., speaking instead of the child) increase the likelihood of SM.

C. Genetics

SoP is heritable, and parents with SoP are more likely to have children with SoP than are parents without SoP (Lieb et al, 2000). Genetic heritability of underlying traits that predispose children toward SoP, such as behavioral inhibition, also contributes to the genetic heritability of SoP and SM.

▶ Clinical Findings

A. Signs & Symptoms

Children with SoP fear, and attempt to avoid, social situations involving peers. Adolescents are more likely than small children to verbalize their fear of being perceived negatively. For example, adolescents may say others will think they are weird, stupid, clumsy, or ugly. Avoidance may involve hiding in one's room when others arrive; not interacting with other children during recess in school; refusal to frequent public places such as malls, restaurants, or public restrooms (paruresis); and in severe cases, almost complete self-isolation in the child's room, often accompanied by a reversal of diurnal cycles. Children with SoP will generally prefer to play with one friend than in a group and will rarely initiate any social interaction with peers. Most children and adolescents with SoP will fear a variety of social situations, but in some cases the fear and avoidance are limited to explicitly performance-related activities such as making a presentation in front of a classroom (*performance only* type). Children with SoP will frequently adopt overly rigid body postures, have poor eye contact, and speak with abnormally high or low voices. Cultural expectations and norms (both family and broader sociocultural context) should be considered when considering a diagnosis of SoP.

Children with SM will avoid speaking in particular situations. These may include many situations (e.g., everywhere but inside their house) or specific situations (e.g., in class). The SM can lead to academic and social impairment, particularly as children mature. Many children with SM will rely on parents and/or friends to speak instead of them. Although children with SM usually have SoP, SM is not an "extreme" case of SoP and is not tightly associated with SoP severity.

B. Psychological Testing

See end of chapter for integrated discussion of the anxiety disorders. The Social Phobia and Anxiety Inventory for Children measures symptoms of SoP (Kuusikko et al, 2009).

C. Laboratory Findings

No laboratory tests are indicated.

▶ Course of Illness

Onset of SoP is usually between the ages of 8 and 15 but can occur in younger childhood as well. Onset of SoP will frequently follow a history of social or behavioral inhibition. The disorder tends to be chronic and persistent, rarely remitting spontaneously. SoP in children and adolescents does not show a waxing and waning pattern of severity but rather is generally stable or increasingly severe over time. Most children and adolescents with SoP do not seek treatment for the disorder, and response to treatment is poorer than in most anxiety disorders. The course of SM is variable. In many cases, SM may remit while comorbid SoP persists.

▶ Differential Diagnosis

See end of chapter for integrated discussion of the anxiety disorders.

▶ Treatment

See end of chapter for integrated discussion of the anxiety disorders.

▶ Complications/Adverse Outcomes of Treatment

See end of chapter for integrated discussion of the anxiety disorders.

▶ Prognosis

See end of chapter for integrated discussion of the anxiety disorders.

Beesdo K, Knappe S, Pine DS. Anxiety and anxiety disorders in children and adolescents: developmental issues and implications for DSM-V. *Psychiatr Clinic N Am.* 2009;32(3):483.

Burstein M, He JP, Kattan G, et al. Social phobia and subtypes in the national comorbidity survey-adolescent supplement: prevalence, correlates, and comorbidity. *J Am Acad Child Adolesc Psychiatry.* 2011;50(9):870–880.

Kuusikko S, Pollock-Wurman R, Ebeling H, et al. Psychometric evaluation of social phobia and anxiety inventory for children (SPAI-C) and social anxiety scale for children-revised (SASC-R). *Eur Child Adolesc Psychiatry.* 2009;18(2):116–124.

Lieb R, Wittchen HU, Hofler M, et al. Parental psychopathology, parenting styles, and the risk of social phobia in offspring: a prospective-longitudinal community study. *Arch Gen Psychiatry.* 2000;57(9):859–866.

Lopes VM, Albano AM. Pediatric social phobia. In: Vasa RE, Roy AK, eds. *Pediatric Anxiety Disorders.* New York: Springer Science; 2013:91–112.

Taylor CT, Alden LE. Parental overprotection and interpersonal behavior in generalized social phobia. *Behav Ther.* 2006;37(1):14–24.

SPECIFIC PHOBIA

▶ General Considerations

A. Epidemiology

Specific phobia (SP) is among the most common mental disorders of childhood, affecting approximately 5% of children and 15% of adolescents (Kessler et al, 2005). Median age of onset is between 7 and 11 years and average age of onset is around 10 years. The most common types of SP in children are *animal* and *natural environment. Situational* SP tends to have a later onset, in adolescence (Ollendick et al, 2013). Most children with SP fear more than one object or situation, frequently spanning multiple diagnostic types of SP (each of which is diagnosed separately). Prevalence rates for girls are higher than for boys, although rates of *blood–injection–injury* phobia are equivalent across genders.

B. Etiology

Multiple etiological pathways can lead to the development of SP in children and adolescents (Rachman & Costello, 1961). SP can appear following a stressful or traumatic event (e.g., being trapped in an elevator, witnessing a dog bite), but often no such event is reported. Some phobias, such as fear of situations that may result in choking, are much more likely to be preceded by a related stressful event than others. Some phobias are thought to be learned through vicarious conditioning, or the process of observing another person, particularly a parent, responding phobically to an object or situation. Verbal information provided by parents about potential threat may also contribute to elevated fear (Muris & Field, 2010). Overly protective or intrusive parenting has been associated with the development of childhood anxiety and may predispose a child to developing SP. Parent accommodation of child anxiety symptoms (e.g., sleeping next to a child who fears the dark) may contribute to the maintenance of the disorder.

C. Genetics

SP is heritable, and twin studies indicate a genetic component to the transmission of phobias. It is as yet unclear to what extent particular types of SP are heritable, as opposed to a general vulnerability to any SP type (Ollendick et al, 2013).

▶ Clinical Findings

A. Signs & Symptoms

SP must be differentiated both from typical fear responses toward stimuli generally perceived as aversive and from developmentally appropriate or transient fears often seen in children. A child with SP will exhibit a strong fear response nearly every time they are exposed to the phobic stimulus and may experience anxiety in anticipation of possible exposure. They will actively try to avoid confronting the phobic stimulus and may avoid a broad range of situations with the fear that they could lead to exposure (e.g., not watching movies because they may show dogs). Children with SP often rely on accommodations by parents and other family members to facilitate their avoidance (e.g., asking a sibling to enter a room before them to check for spiders). Children frequently express their fear through crying, tantrums, and clinging rather than verbalizing their fearful emotion or anxious thoughts.

B. Psychological Testing

See end of chapter for integrated discussion of the anxiety disorders.

C. Laboratory Findings

No laboratory tests are indicated. SP of the blood–injection–injury type is associated with vasovagal syncope (fainting) in the presence of blood or other phobic stimuli.

▶ Course of Illness

Average age of onset is around 10 years, and severity may wax and wane. SP can persist into adolescence and adulthood and is then unlikely to remit without treatment.

▶ Differential Diagnosis

See end of chapter for integrated discussion of the anxiety disorders.

▶ Treatment

See end of chapter for integrated discussion of the anxiety disorders.

▶ Complications/Adverse Outcomes of Treatment

See end of chapter for integrated discussion of the anxiety disorders.

▶ Prognosis

See end of chapter for integrated discussion of the anxiety disorders.

Kessler RC, Berglund P, Demler O, et al. Lifetime prevalence and age-of-onset distributions of DSM-IV disorders in the National Comorbidity Survey Replication. *Arch Gen Psychiatry*. 2005;62(6):593–602.

Muris P, Field AP. The role of verbal threat information in the development of childhood fear. "Beware the Jabberwock!". *Clin Child Fam Psychol Rev*. 2010;13(2):129–150.

Ollendick TH, Cowart MJW, Milliner, EL. Specific phobias. In: Vasa RE, Roy AK, eds. *Pediatric Anxiety Disorders*. New York: Springer Science; 2013:113–128.

Rachman S, Costello CG. The aetiology and treatment of children's phobias: a review. *Am J Psychiatry*. 1961;118:97–105.

PANIC DISORDER

▶ General Considerations

A. Epidemiology

Panic disorder (PD) is rare in children and increases in frequency through adolescence and young adulthood. Prevalence in adolescents is around 2–3%, with twice as many females affected as males. Patients with PD frequently have other comorbid anxiety and nonanxiety conditions, including substance abuse. Diagnosis of PD is also a risk factor for suicidal behavior.

B. Etiology

There is no single definitive etiology for PD or any of the other anxiety disorders. One model of panic links it to increased sensitivity to physiological arousal along with negative cognitive interpretations of these sensations (Barlow, 2002). Research has supported the link between anxiety sensitivity and PD. The suffocation model of PD describes panic attacks as oversensitivity to increases in CO_2 that trigger panic-like symptoms and fear. This model has been supported by the finding that patients with PD are more sensitive to breathing CO_2-enriched air. PD in adolescents is also associated with a history of SAD in childhood (Angelosante & Ostrowski, 2013).

C. Genetics

PD is heritable, and genetic influences account for significant proportions of variance in the disorder. Genetic influences may be more strongly associated with adolescent- compared to adult-onset PD. Genetic influences on underlying traits such as anxiety sensitivity, respiratory disturbance, or hypersensitivity to CO_2 contribute to the heritability of the disorder. Adolescents with PD are more likely to have parents and relatives with PD, but also with other anxiety disorders, depression, or respiratory illness.

▶ Clinical Findings

A. Signs & Symptoms

Children and adolescents with PD experience episodes of intense fear and anxious arousal and become preoccupied about experiencing another attack. Actual frequency of attacks varies widely. Many patients fear that the attacks are symptoms of a serious medical illness and may continue to experience them as life threatening even after diagnosis of PD. Adolescents are frequently anxious about social ramifications of having a panic attack in front of peers. To prevent having attacks or to limit where they occur, children and adolescents with PD may develop avoidant behaviors such as not leaving the home, missing school, or requiring parental accompaniment (see the section on agoraphobia). Parental accommodation of the avoidance may perpetuate the avoidance.

B. Psychological Testing

See end of chapter for integrated discussion of the anxiety disorders. Anxiety sensitivity (i.e., the fear of sensations relating to anxiety or the tendency to misinterpret them as harmful and dangerous) is linked to PD and can be assessed with the Childhood Anxiety Sensitivity Index (Silverman et al, 1991).

C. Laboratory Findings

No laboratory tests are indicated. However, adolescents with PD are more likely to respond with symptoms of panic to CO_2 and other agents with disparate mechanisms.

▶ Course of Illness

Although young children can and do report experiencing episodes of intense fear, PD is rare before adolescence. Adolescents and adults diagnosed with PD frequently report having panic-like symptoms in childhood. Severity of PD, in terms of both frequency of attacks and impairment, waxes and wanes after onset but is generally chronic. Patients who remit frequently relapse within 1–2 years. Stressful life events can trigger onset or exacerbate PD.

▶ Differential Diagnosis

See end of chapter for integrated discussion of the anxiety disorders. Full panic attacks and limited-symptom panic attacks (having fewer than four of the hallmark symptoms of panic) are common in the general population as well as in other anxiety disorders. When panic attacks occur in the context of another anxiety disorder, a specifier is included in the diagnosis (e.g., SAD with panic attacks).

▶ Treatment

See end of chapter for integrated discussion of the anxiety disorders. Treatments aimed at regulating CO_2 levels may have specific benefits for patients with PD.

▶ Complications/Adverse Outcomes of Treatment

See end of chapter for integrated discussion of the anxiety disorders.

▶ Prognosis

See end of chapter for integrated discussion of the anxiety disorders.

Angelosante AG, Ostrowski MA. Panic disorder. In: Vasa RE, Roy AK, eds. *Pediatric Anxiety Disorders*. New York: Springer Science; 2013:143–155.

Barlow DH. *Anxiety and Its Disorders: The Nature and Treatment of Anxiety and Panic*. 2nd ed. New York: Guilford Press; 2002.

Silverman WK, Fleisig W, Rabian B, Peterson RA. Childhood Anxiety Sensitivity Index. *J Clin Child Psychol*. 1991;20(2): 162–168.

AGORAPHOBIA

▶ General Considerations

A. Epidemiology

Agoraphobia is rare in childhood and affects between 1% and 2% of adolescents, with approximately twice as many girls affected as boys. Prevalence is greater in late, compared to early, adolescence. Agoraphobia was first included as an independent diagnosis in DSM-5, and relatively little research has looked at it outside of the context of PD.

B. Etiology

Approximately half of patients presenting with agoraphobia report having panic attacks before the onset of the disorder. However, most patients with PD also report having agoraphobic symptoms before onset of panic. Temperamental characteristics such as behavioral inhibition and anxiety sensitivity are associated with elevated risk of agoraphobia, as are stressful childhood events such as the death of a parent or being attacked. Parental overprotection and accommodation of anxiety symptoms are risk factors for anxiety, including agoraphobia.

C. Genetics

Agoraphobia is strongly heritable, with a majority of variance in agoraphobic symptoms attributable to genetic influences.

Clinical Findings

A. Signs & Symptoms

Agoraphobia can be very debilitating, frequently leading to severe functional impairment and complete limitation to the home. Children with agoraphobia may fear becoming lost if separated from parents outside of the home. Adolescents more frequently fear experiencing panic-like symptoms in agoraphobic situations. Agoraphobic adolescents frequently present as depressed or dysthymic. Children and adolescents may rely heavily on parents and other family members for accommodation of their symptoms and facilitation of the avoidance.

B. Psychological Testing

See end of chapter for integrated discussion of the anxiety disorders.

C. Laboratory Findings

No laboratory tests are indicated.

Course of Illness

Agoraphobia increases in prevalence through adolescence and into early adulthood. Once established, the disorder rarely remits without treatment. The severity of agoraphobia can wax and wane, and relapse is common in case of remission. Progressively generalized avoidance and reliance on others (e.g., parents) for symptom accommodation can lead to increasingly severe symptoms and impairment.

Differential Diagnosis

See end of chapter for integrated discussion of the anxiety disorders.

Treatment

See end of chapter for integrated discussion of the anxiety disorders.

Complications/Adverse Outcomes of Treatment

See end of chapter for integrated discussion of the anxiety disorders.

Prognosis

See end of chapter for integrated discussion of the anxiety disorders.

GENERALIZED ANXIETY DISORDER

General Considerations

A. Epidemiology

GAD affects about 1% of adolescents and is less frequent in young children, although a tendency toward worry and anxiety is often apparent before onset of the disorder. Prevalence is higher in girls than in boys.

B. Etiology

As with other anxiety disorders, multiple factors contribute to the etiology of GAD. Youth with GAD tend to exhibit attention bias toward threat and cognitive biases skewed toward negative outcomes and interpretations (Ginsburg & Affrunti, 2013). Parenting characteristics such as parents being overly controlling, protective, intrusive, or critical are associated with GAD in youth (Hale et al, 2006). However, there are indications of reciprocal influences between child anxiety and parental style in childhood anxiety disorders (Silverman et al, 2009). Temperamental risk factors include behavioral inhibition and negative affectivity, which are also risk factors for other anxiety disorders.

C. Genetics

Genetic factors contribute to the risk of GAD, and some of same genetic factors also elevate risk for depression and other anxiety disorders.

Clinical Findings

A. Signs & Symptoms

Children and adolescents with GAD are very often preoccupied with school performance and may exhibit maladaptive perfectionism. They tend to be highly critical of themselves and may avoid activities in which they are not confident they will excel. Youth with GAD often present with physical complaints such as headache or stomachache. Difficulty concentrating is common in GAD and may be attributable to the worry as well to the effects of sleep disturbance. Other common worries include health issues (for themselves or loved ones) and peer status (Pina et al, 2002; Weems et al, 2000). Family accommodation of child GAD symptoms is common and will often include answering repeated reassurance-seeking questions.

B. Psychological Testing

See end of chapter for integrated discussion of the anxiety disorders. The Penn State Worry Questionnaire for Children (Chorpita et al, 2007) is a self-report instrument that specifically assesses symptoms of worry in children and adolescents.

C. Laboratory Findings

No laboratory tests are indicated. Children presenting with chronic pain or similar somatic complaints should be evaluated for GAD.

▶ Course of Illness

Onset of GAD becomes more prevalent after puberty and is broadly distributed in the following years. It is frequently preceded by a history of anxiety and worry. Once established, GAD only rarely fully remits, and severity waxes and wanes over time. Earlier onset of GAD is associated with greater comorbidity, particularly depression.

▶ Differential Diagnosis

See end of chapter for integrated discussion of the anxiety disorders.

▶ Treatment

See end of chapter for integrated discussion of the anxiety disorders. Treatments that target cognitive or attention biases, such as attention bias modification training, may be helpful for GAD (Hakamata et al, 2010).

▶ Complications/Adverse Outcomes of Treatment

See end of chapter for integrated discussion of the anxiety disorders.

▶ Prognosis

See end of chapter for integrated discussion of the anxiety disorders.

Chorpita BF, Tracey SA, Brown TA, et al. Assessment of worry in children and adolescents: an adaptation of the Penn State Worry Questionnaire. *Behav Res Ther*. 1997;35(6):569–581.

Ginsburg GS, Affrunti NW. Generalized Anxiety Disorder in children and adolescents. In: Vasa RE, Roy AK, eds. *Pediatric Anxiety Disorders*. New York: Springer Science; 2013:71–90.

Hakamata Y, Lissek S, Bar-Haim Y, et al. Attention bias modification treatment: a meta-analysis toward the establishment of novel treatment for anxiety. *Biol Psychiatry*. 2010;68(11):982–990.

Hale WW 3rd, Engels R, Meeus W. Adolescent's perceptions of parenting behaviours and its relationship to adolescent Generalized Anxiety Disorder symptoms. *J Adolesc*. 2006;29(3): 407–417.

Pina AA, Silverman WK, Alfano CA, Saavedra LM. Diagnostic efficiency of symptoms in the diagnosis of DSM-IV: generalized anxiety disorder in youth. *J Child Psychol Psychiatry*. 2002;43(7): 959–967.

Silverman WK, Kurtines WM, Jaccard J, Pina AA. Directionality of change in youth anxiety treatment involving parents: an initial examination. *J Consult Clin Psychol*. 2009;77(3):474–485.

Weems CF, Silverman WK, La Greca AM. What do youth referred for anxiety problems worry about? Worry and its relation to anxiety and anxiety disorders in children and adolescents. *J Abnorm Child Psychol*. 2000;28(1):63–72.

INTEGRATED DISCUSSION

▶ Psychological Testing

Psychological testing for anxiety disorders relies primarily on structured or semistructured interviews and clinician, parent, or child rating scales. The Anxiety Disorders Interview Schedule for Child and Parent (Silverman et al, 2001) is a widely used semistructured interview that provides reliable diagnoses but requires training and significant time to administer. The Multidimensional Anxiety Scale for Children (March, 1997) and the Screen for Childhood Anxiety Related Emotional Disorders (Birmaher et al, 1999) are both self-report measures with parent and child versions. These measures provide indication of elevated anxiety in various domains but are not adequate for establishing diagnosis. The Pediatric Anxiety Rating Scale (RUPP Anxiety Study Group, 2002) is a clinician-rated scale that provides sound indication of anxiety diagnoses. General screening instruments for mental health such as the Child Behavior Checklist (Achenbach, 1994) can also provide indication of clinically significant elevated anxiety. Behavioral avoidance tests can be used to behaviorally assess phobic behavior.

Parent involvement in childhood anxiety symptoms should be assessed at evaluation. The Family Accommodation Scale—Anxiety (Lebowitz et al, 2013) provides an indication of parent accommodation, including participation in child anxiety symptoms and modification of family routines.

Differential Diagnosis

Anxiety disorders are highly comorbid with each other and have overlapping symptoms, so differentiating among the anxiety disorders can be difficult. Anxiety disorders are often difficult to differentiate from related disorders such as obsessive–compulsive disorder or posttraumatic stress disorder. Symptoms of GAD are easily confused with both physical illness and attention-deficit/hyperactivity disorder. Children with anxiety disorders may have physical complaints due to reluctance to attend school. SoP and SM should be differentiated from autism spectrum disorder and depression, and SM should not be mistaken for intellectual disability. Children and adolescents may manifest anxiety through irritability or temper tantrums. A child may be mistakenly diagnosed as oppositional, and some children use aggressive behavior to get to parents to accommodate to their anxiety symptoms.

Treatment

A. Psychopharmacological Treatment

Medication can be a generally safe and effective treatment for the core symptoms of childhood anxiety disorders and should be considered as one potential component in the comprehensive treatment planning for children with these disorders. Randomized clinical trials (RCTs) have generally found the selective serotonin reuptake inhibitors (SSRIs) (and, in a smaller number of cases, the mixed serotonin-norepinephrine reuptake inhibitor [SNRI] venlafaxine) to be more effective than placebo in reducing anxiety symptoms in child anxiety disorders; there is a low rate of discontinuation due to adverse effects, despite the medication being less well tolerated than placebo. Although these medications are widely used, many important clinical questions require further systematic study. Among these are the relative merits and optimum use of these agents alone or in combination with cognitive–behavioral therapy (CBT) over time; long-term safety and therapeutic benefit of these agents; optimum dosing strategies, treatment duration, and process for discontinuing treatment; differential efficacy across different subtypes of anxiety disorders and patterns of comorbidity; and differences in efficacy/tolerability between the various agents relative to individual patient characteristics. In addition to these empirical questions, practical considerations, such as the local availability of competent CBT therapists and patient and family compliance and attitudes toward medication/psychotherapy, often impinge on treatment planning and the choice to use medication or not.

Only a few methodologically rigorous RCTs have compared medication and CBT alone or in combination. The most ambitious of these, the CAMS (Child Adolescent Anxiety Multimodal Study) (Walkup et al, 2008), studied the efficacy of sertraline and CBT with a combination of the two or a pill placebo in 488 children with separation, social, or GAD. CBT and sertraline alone were comparably effective and superior to placebo, while the combination treatment was superior to either monotherapy or placebo on a variety of outcome measures.

Most clinicians and parents are predisposed to feel that if a child's symptoms are not overwhelming or seriously impairing, a carefully observed initial trial of CBT is preferable to assess the child's capacity for progress before any decision is made about medication. Early introduction of medication should be considered in cases where there is substantial impairment with the child's social or academic functioning, clinically significant comorbid depression, or reluctance or inability of the child to participate collaboratively in CBT. Often, a trial of medication may provide enough relief that a previously avoidant and reluctant child becomes willing and able to participate in CBT. However, although medication may provide at least transient relief from inhibiting anxiety, permitting a child to participate more actively in the world around her, medication alone does not teach coping or social skills. Hence, there remain important unanswered questions around the relative long durability/utility of medication versus CBT, alone or in combination, across various realms of development, over and above relieving the acuity of the core anxiety symptoms.

Among the childhood anxiety disorders, the largest body of RCT data concerns the treatment of OCD (covered in Chapter 40). There are fewer systematic studies concerning the pharmacotherapy of the childhood anxiety disorders. Most of these have examined the efficacy of the various SSRIs (for a summary see Ghalib et al, 2010 and Schwartz et al, 2019 and a relevant Cochrane review by Ipser et al, 2009). Of the SSRIs approved by the FDA for adult use—namely fluoxetine, fluvoxamine, sertraline, paroxetine, citalopram, and escitalopram—only a few have specific FDA indications for childhood anxiety. In general, the presence or absence of such an FDA indication is less a reflection of the drug's efficacy or safety profile than of an economic calculation on the part of the manufacturer as to whether there is sufficient economic incentive (in terms of patent life or perceived market) to warrant the regulatory costs and mandated clinical studies needed to obtain a specific pediatric indication for a given target population. Hence, much of the use of the SSRI/SNRIs is "off-label," drawing on the prescriber's experience, non-FDA studies, or safety and efficacy data regarding the given agent's use for other conditions. Among the childhood anxiety conditions for which the SSRIs have been found useful are GAD (sertraline, fluoxetine), SoP (paroxetine, fluoxetine, sertraline), and a mixed group of children with SAD, GAD, or SoP disorders. An older body of literature found imipramine, an older tricyclic antidepressant (TCA), useful for school refusal; however, since the advent of the SSRIs, the TCAs are rarely used as first-line agents for pediatric depression and/or anxiety, because of their comparatively higher level of adverse effects (primarily anticholinergic) and the need for periodic electrocardiograms and blood-level monitoring in children. The mixed noradrenergic–serotonin agent venlafaxine (extended-release form) has been shown to be superior to placebo for GAD and SoP. In addition, the noradrenergic–serotonin agent duloxetine has demonstrated benefit in pediatric GAD based on a 2015 randomized controlled trial in youth, aged 7–17. Open trials, case reports, and small individual multiple baseline studies also suggest the possible utility of the SSRIs for SM, PD, or SP in children, but robust RCT data are lacking.

Benzodiazepines, such as clonazepam, alprazolam, or lorazepam, may be useful for acute or time-limited situations (e.g., a plane trip in a phobic child), but they are potentially sedating, habituating, and disinhibiting and should be avoided in children except for very short-term use.

B. General Principles

The decision to try medication for a child with an anxiety disorder should be based on a comprehensive psychiatric assessment of the child, including the presence of comorbid psychiatric disorders and a full discussion of treatment options and their respective risks and benefits with the parents and, depending on age, with the child. There are not yet sufficient data from RCTs or pharmacogenetic studies regarding relative efficacy/adverse effects to provide clear guidance in choosing among the various SSRIs; instead, the choice is often made on the basis of pharmacokinetics, drug–drug interactions, and other affected family members' patterns of response.

▶ Psychotherapeutic Interventions

CBT in group or individual format is the psychotherapeutic intervention that has received the most empirical support for its efficacy in treating anxiety in youth (Silverman et al, 2008). CBT includes primarily systematic gradual desensitization to feared stimuli and situations and restructuring of maladaptive cognitions or beliefs. Exposure to previously avoided stimuli and situations is likely the most active and important element in treatment of childhood anxiety, and a course of treatment that does not integrate exposure and desensitization should generally not be considered a true trial of CBT. Exposure is usually done in a graded manner, such that a child becomes increasingly able to tolerate the feared situation. Cognitive restructuring entails identifying anxious thoughts as stemming from the anxiety disorder, challenging their veracity or accuracy so as to recognize biases and misperceptions, and formulating more rational or realistic alternatives. Parent involvement in treatment has not yet been shown to significantly enhance outcomes, but parent training aimed at reducing accommodation to anxiety symptoms could potentially enhance treatment effects or allow for treatment of children without capacity

or motivation for individual treatment (Lebowitz & Omer, 2013).

RCTs consistently show superior effects of CBT over wait-list or other nonactive treatment control conditions. The evidence for CBT's superiority over other more active treatment conditions such as educational support is less strong (James et al, 2013). Firm guidelines for optimal sequencing of psychotherapeutic and psychopharmacological interventions are still required, but it is generally advisable to start with CBT and augment or substitute with medication if necessary.

▶ Complications/Adverse Outcomes of Treatment

The main adverse side effects of the SSRIs are restlessness, agitation, insomnia, and gastrointestinal distress. The side effects of venlafaxine reflect its greater noradrenergic activity and include tachycardia, hypertension, and decreased appetite. In general, adverse effects can be minimized by beginning with a low dose, monitoring closely, and increasing dosage gradually as needed. Improvement may take as long as 4 weeks to be apparent, and maximum improvement may not be apparent until several weeks after full therapeutic dose is reached. If trial with one SSRI is not successful, switching to another SSRI may be.

In 2004, based on its review of all of the placebo-controlled RCTs of antidepressants in children, the FDA issued a "black box warning" that their use may increase the incidence of suicidal thoughts or behavior (4% in the medication group vs. 2% in the placebo group). Clinically, de novo suicidal ideation as an adverse drug reaction in children appears linked to intense restlessness or akathisia. A subsequent meta-analysis found that when used for treatment of anxiety disorders, the SSRIs/SNRIs were relatively more effective (number needed to treat [NNT] = 3) than when used to treat major depressive disorder (NNT = 10) and had a low risk of suicidal ideation/behavior (0.7%) (Bridge et al, 2007).

When the decision is made to stop an SSRI/SNRI that a child has been on for more than a brief period of time, it is important to gradually taper the dose down, rather than stopping abruptly, to minimize a potential withdrawal syndrome, consisting of headache, dizziness, or irritability. This is not an issue with fluoxetine, which has a very long half-life, but is more problematic with paroxetine, which has the shortest half-life of the group.

▶ Prognosis

SAD and SP have the best prognosis of the anxiety disorders. GAD and SoP are most likely to persist despite treatment. Without treatment, SAD and SM are most likely to remit, and other anxiety disorders will typically persist. Agoraphobia, GAD, PD, and SP tend to wax and wane in severity, whereas SoP will usually remain stable or increase in severity.

Achenbach TM. Child Behavior Checklist and related instruments. In: Maurish M, ed. *The Use of Psychological Testing for Treatment Planning and Outcome Assessment*. Hillsdale, NJ: Erlbaum; 1994:517–549.

Birmaher B, Brent DA, Chiappetta L, et al. Psychometric properties of the Screen for Child Anxiety Related Emotional Disorders (SCARED): a replication study. *J Am Acad Child Adolesc Psychiatry*. 1999;38(10):1230–1236.

Bridge JA, Iyengar S, Salary CB, et al. Clinical response and risk for reported suicidal ideation and suicide attempts in pediatric antidepressant treatment: a meta-analysis of randomized controlled trials. *JAMA*. 2007;297(15):1683–1696.

Ghalib KD, Vidair HB, Woodcome HA, et al. Assessment and treatment of child and adolescent anxiety disorders In: Martin A, Scahill L, Kratochvil C, eds. *Pediatric Psychopharmacology: Principles and Practice*. 2nd ed. New York: Oxford University Press; 2010:480–495.

Ipser JC, Stein DJ, Hawkridge S, Hoppe L. Pharmacotherapy for anxiety disorders in children and adolescents. *Cochrane Database Syst Rev* 2009;3:CD005170.

James AC, James G, Cowdrey FA, et al. Cognitive behavioural therapy for anxiety disorders in children and adolescents. *Cochrane Database Syst Rev* 2013;6:CD004690.pub3.

Lebowitz ER, Omer H. *Treating Childhood and Adolescent Anxiety: A Guide for Caregivers*. Hoboken, NJ: Wiley; 2013.

Lebowitz ER, Woolston J, Bar-Haim Y, et al. Family accommodation in pediatric anxiety disorders. *Depress Anxiety*. 2013;30(1):47–54.

March J. The Multidimensional Anxiety Scale for Children (MASC): factor structure, reliability, and validity. *J Am Acad Child Adolesc Psychiatry*. 1997;36(4):554–565.

RUPP Anxiety Study Group. The Pediatric Anxiety Rating Scale (PARS): development and psychometric properties. *J Am Acad Child Adolesc Psychiatry*. 2002;41(9):1061–1069.

Schwartz C, Barican JL, Yung D, Zheng Y, Waddell C. Six decades of preventing and treating childhood anxiety disorders: a systematic review and meta-analysis to inform policy and practice. *Evid Based Ment Health*. 2019 Aug;22(3):103–110. doi: 10.1136/ebmental-2019-300096. Epub 2019 Jul 17.

Silverman WK, Pina AA, Viswesvaran C. Evidence-based psychosocial treatments for phobic and anxiety disorders in children and adolescents. *J Clin Child Adolesc Psychol*. 2008;37(1):105–130.

Silverman WK, Saavedra LM, Pina AA. Test-retest reliability of anxiety symptoms and diagnoses with the Anxiety Disorders Interview Schedule for DSM-IV: child and parent versions. *J Am Acad Child Adolesc Psychiatry*. 2001;40(8):937–944.

Strawn JR, Prakash A, Zhang Q, et al. A randomized, placebo-controlled study of duloxetine for the treatment of children and adolescents with generalized anxiety disorder. *J Am Acad Child Adolesc Psychiatry*. 2015 Apr;54(4):283–293. doi: 10.1016/j.jaac.2015.01.008. Epub 2015 Jan 29.

Walkup JT, Albano AM, Piacentini J, et al. Cognitive behavioral therapy, sertraline, or a combination in childhood anxiety. *N Engl J Med*. 2008;359(26):2753–2766.

Wang Z, Whiteside SPH, Sim L, et al. Comparative effectiveness and safety of cognitive behavioral therapy and pharmacotherapy for childhood anxiety disorders: a systematic review and meta-analysis. *JAMA Pediatr*. 2017 Nov 1;171(11):1049–1056. doi: 10.1001/jamapediatrics.2017.3036. Erratum in: *JAMA Pediatr*. 2018 Oct 1;172(10):992.

Child Maltreatment

51

William Bernet, MD

CHILD MALTREATMENT

 ESSENTIALS OF DIAGNOSIS

ICD-10 Diagnostic Criteria

The legal definitions regarding child maltreatment vary from state to state. In general, **neglect** is the failure to provide adequate care and protection for children. It may involve failure to feed the child adequately, provide medical care, provide appropriate education, or protect the child from danger. **Physical abuse** is the infliction of nonaccidental injury by a caretaker. It may take the form of beating, punching, kicking, biting, or other methods. The abuse can result in injuries such as broken bones, internal hemorrhages, bruises, burns, and poisoning. Cultural factors should be considered in assessing whether the discipline of a child is abusive or normative (Giardino & Alexander, 2005; Helfer et al, 1999). **Sexual abuse** of children refers to sexual behavior between a child and an adult or between two children when one of them is significantly older or more dominant. The sexual behaviors include the following: touching breasts, buttocks, and genitals, whether the victim is dressed or undressed; exhibitionism; fellatio; cunnilingus; penetration of the vagina or anus with sexual organs or with objects; and pornographic photography. **Psychological abuse** occurs when a caretaker causes serious psychological injury by repeatedly terrorizing or berating a child. When serious, it is often accompanied by neglect, physical abuse, sexual abuse, and exposure to domestic violence (Hamarman & Bernet, 2000). Also, psychological abuse occurs when a person indoctrinates a child to fear or hate a parent without good cause, which is sometimes called parental alienation.

The psychiatric classification of abuse and neglect in the *International Classification of Diseases*, 10th Revision (ICD-10) appears in Chapter XIX, "Injury, Poisoning and Certain Other Consequences of External Causes," and in the section "Maltreatment Syndromes." The codes from ICD-10 related to child maltreatment are the following:

T74.0   Neglect or abandonment
T74.1   Physical abuse
T74.2   Sexual abuse
T74.3   Psychological abuse

Adapted with permission from the International Statistical Classification of Diseases and Related Health Problems 10th Revision, 5th edition, Geneva: World Health Organization; 2016.

Giardino AP, Alexander R. *Child Maltreatment: A Clinical Guide and Reference & A Comprehensive Photographic Reference Identifying Potential Child Abuse.* 3rd ed. St. Louis: GW Medical Publishing; 2005.

Hamarman S, Bernet W. Evaluating and reporting emotional abuse in children: parent-based, action-based focus aids in clinical decision making. *J Am Acad Child Adolesc Psychiatry.* 2000;39:928.

Helfer ME, Kempe RS, Krugman RD, eds. *The Battered Child.* 5th ed. revised. Chicago: University of Chicago Press; 1999.

▶ General Considerations

Practitioners in private practice, as well as those employed by courts or other agencies, see children who may have been emotionally, physically, or sexually abused. As a clinician, the practitioner may provide assessments and treatment for abused children and their families in both outpatient and inpatient settings. As a forensic investigator, the practitioner may work with an interdisciplinary team at a pediatric medical center and assist the court in determining what happened to the child.

A. Epidemiology

Each year about 3.9 million alleged incidents of child maltreatment (involving approximately 7.1 million children) are reported to protective services. Of those reports that were investigated in 2021, protective services determined that at least one child was found to be the victim of abuse and neglect in about 18% of the cases. Of those substantiated cases, about 76% involved neglect; about 16% involved physical abuse; and about 10% involved sexual abuse. About 1820 children die each year as a result of maltreatment (U.S. Department of Health and Human Services, 2021).

B. Etiology

Child maltreatment is a tragic and complex biopsychosocial phenomenon (Myers, 2010). There are various models to explain why child abuse occurs, but generally they consider the interaction of five levels of risk factors and protective factors: (1) The individual biological and psychological makeup of the child victim is important. For example, children who are premature, developmentally disabled, and physically handicapped are more likely to be abused. (2) The individual characteristics of the adult perpetrator. For example, child abuse occurs in all strata of society, but it is associated with lower parental education, parental mental illness, and parental substance abuse, especially alcoholism. (3) The family system refers to the family environment, parenting styles, and interactions among family members. Risk factors include single parenting and domestic violence. (4) The community in which the family lives may relate to both risk and protective factors. In general, child abuse is strongly associated with poverty, financial stress, poor housing, and social isolation. However, there may be protective factors in the community related to the parent's workplace, peer groups of family members, and formal and informal social supports. (5) Finally, the values and beliefs of the culture affect the occurrence of child maltreatment. During the twentieth century, for example, there were two major societal shifts that reduced the frequency of child abuse: the concept that child behavior should be socialized primarily through love, not harsh, physical discipline; and the realization that parental authority is not absolute, that is, parents are not entitled to unrestricted authority over their children.

Myers JEB, ed. *The APSAC Handbook on Child Maltreatment*. 3rd ed. Thousand Oaks, CA: Sage; 2010.

U.S. Department of Health and Human Services, Administration on Children, Youth and Families. *Child Maltreatment 2021*. Washington, DC: U.S. Government Printing Office; 2021. https://www.acf.hhs.gov/sites/default/files/documents/cb/cm2021.pdf

▶ Clinical Findings

A. Signs & Symptoms

Children who have been abused manifest pleomorphic symptoms in a variety of emotional, behavioral, and psychosomatic reactions. Abused children may have internalizing symptoms such as withdrawal, anxiety, depression, and sleep problems.

Abused children may exhibit externalizing symptoms, such as aggression. Children who have been sexually abused are likely to display inappropriate sexual behavior. Table 51–1 lists symptoms that are associated with child abuse: they are not specific or pathognomonic; the same symptoms may occur in the absence of a history of abuse.

The parents of physically abused children have certain characteristics. Typically, they have delayed seeking help for the child's injuries. The history given by the parents is implausible or incompatible with the physical findings. There may be evidence of repeated suspicious injuries. The parents may blame a sibling or claim the child injured himself or herself.

In cases of intrafamilial sexual abuse and other sexual abuse that occurs over a period of time, there is a typical sequence of events: (1) engagement, when the perpetrator induces the child into a special relationship; (2) sexual interaction, in which the sexual behavior progresses from less intimate to more intimate forms of abuse; (3) the secrecy phase; (4) disclosure, when the abuse is discovered; and (5) suppression, when the family pressures the child to retract his or her statements (Sgroi, 1988).

The child sexual abuse accommodation syndrome is sometimes seen when children are sexually abused over a period of time. This syndrome has five characteristics: (1) secrecy; (2) helplessness; (3) entrapment and

Table 51–1 Symptoms Associated with Child Maltreatment

Type of Abuse	Associated Symptoms
Any abuse	Psychological symptoms related to emotional distress, such as fear, anxiety, nightmares, phobias, depression, low self-esteem, anger, and hostility More serious psychological problems such as the following: suicidal behavior; posttraumatic stress disorder; and dissociative reactions, with periods of amnesia, trancelike states, and, in some cases, dissociative identity disorder
Sexual abuse	Sexual hyperarousal (open masturbation, excessive sexual curiosity, talking excessively about sexual acts, masturbating with an object, imitating intercourse, inserting objects into the vagina or anus) Sexually aggressive behavior (frequent exposure of the genitals, trying to undress other people, rubbing against other people, and sexual perpetration) Avoidance of sexual stimuli through phobias and inhibitions In adolescents: sexual acting out may occur with promiscuity and, possibly, homosexual contact Physical symptoms (such as somatic complaints, encopresis, and eating disorders) and somatoform symptoms (such as pseudoseizures)

accommodation; (4) delayed, conflicted, and unconvincing disclosure; and (5) retraction (Summit, 1983). The process of accommodation occurs as the child learns that he or she must be available without complaint to the parent's demands. The child often finds ways to accommodate by maintaining secrecy in order to keep the family together, by turning to imaginary companions, and by inducing in herself altered states of consciousness. Other children become aggressive, demanding, and hyperactive. The child sexual abuse accommodation syndrome is not intended for diagnosing sexual abuse, but it helps explain the counterintuitive behavior manifested by some abused children.

It is possible to distinguish the psychological sequelae of children who have experienced single-event and repeated-event trauma (Terr, 1991). The following four characteristics occur after both types of trauma: (1) visualized or repeatedly perceived intrusive memories of the event; (2) repetitive behavior; (3) fears specifically related to the trauma; and (4) changed attitudes about people, life, and the future. Children who sustain single-event traumas manifest full, detailed memories of the event; an interest in "omens," such as looking retrospectively for reasons why the event occurred; and misperceptions, including visual hallucinations and time distortion. In contrast, many children who have experienced severe, chronic trauma (e.g., repeated sexual abuse) manifest massive denial and psychic numbing, self-hypnosis, dissociation, and rage.

Sgroi SM. *Vulnerable Populations: Evaluation and Treatment of Sexually Abused Children and Adult Survivors*, Vol 1. New York: Free Press; 1988.

Summit RC. The child sexual abuse accommodation syndrome. *Child Abuse Negl.* 1983;7:177.

Terr LC. Childhood traumas: an outline and overview. *Am J Psychiatry.* 1991;148:12–20.

B. Clinical Evaluation

The professional who evaluates children who may have been abused has several important tasks: finding out what happened; evaluating the child for emotional disorder; considering other possible explanations for any disorder; being aware of developmental issues; avoiding biasing the outcome with his or her preconceptions; pursuing these objectives in a sensitive manner so as not to retraumatize the child; being supportive to family members; and keeping an accurate record, which may be subpoenaed for future court proceedings (American Academy of Child and Adolescent Psychiatry, 1997; Ludwig & Reece, 2001).

It is important to be familiar with the normative sexual behavior of children for two reasons. First, normal sexual play activities between children should not be taken to be sexual abuse. In assessing this issue, the evaluator should consider the age difference between the children; their developmental level; whether one child dominated or coerced the

other child; and whether the act itself was intrusive, forceful, or dangerous. Second, sexually abused children often manifest more sexual behavior than do typical children. Sometimes they have sexual knowledge beyond what would be expected for their age and developmental level. For example, behavior such as trying to undress other people, masturbating with an object, performing fellatio, and imitating sexual intercourse are red flags that suggest a child has been sexually abused.

1. Patient interview—The clinical interview may need modification when assessing a child who may have been abused. The following sections describe the components of an interview that is particularly suited for forensic evaluations (Poole & Lamb, 1998; Yuille et al, 1993). This outline is based on the National Institute of Child Health and Human Development Investigative Interview Protocol (Lamb et al, 2007).

i. **Build rapport and make informal observations**—Build rapport with the child and make informal observations of the child's behavior, social skills, and cognitive abilities.

ii. **Ask the child to describe two specific past events**—This is done in order to assess the child's memory and to model the form of the interview for the child by asking nonleading, open-ended questions, a pattern that will hold through the rest of the interview. For example, prior to interviewing the child, one can obtain specific information from the parent about a recent birthday party, trip to the zoo, etc.

iii. **Establish the need to tell the truth**—Reach an agreement that in this interview only the truth will be discussed, not "pretend" or imagination. For example, the interviewer can say, "If I said I'm wearing a purple hat today, would that be the truth or a lie?" Reach an agreement that it is fine to say, "I don't know." For example, the interviewer can say, "Do I have a dog named Charlie?" and the child should say, "I don't know."

iv. **Introduce the topic of concern**—Start with more general questions, such as, "Do you know why you are talking with me today?" Proceed, only if necessary, to more specific questions, such as, "Has anything happened to you?" or "Has anyone done something to you?" Drawings may be helpful in initiating disclosure. For example, either the child or the interviewer draws an outline of a person. Then the child is asked to add and name each body part and describe its function. If sexual abuse is suspected, the interviewer could ask, when the genitals are described, if the child has seen that part on another person and who has seen or touched that part on the child. If physical abuse is suspected, the interviewer could ask if particular parts have been hurt in some way.

v. **Elicit a free narrative**—Once the topic of abuse has been introduced, the interviewer encourages the child to describe each event from the beginning without leaving out any details. The child is allowed to proceed at his or her pace, without correction or interruption. If abuse has occurred over a period of time, the interviewer may ask for a description of the general pattern and then for an account of particular episodes.

vi. Pose general questions—The interviewer may ask general questions in order to elicit further details. These questions should not be leading and should be phrased in such a way that an inability to recall or lack of knowledge is acceptable.

vii. Pose specific questions, if necessary—It may be helpful to obtain clarification by asking specific questions. For example, the interviewer may follow up on inconsistencies in a gentle, nonthreatening manner. Avoid repetitive questions and the appearance of rewarding particular answers in any way.

viii. Use interview aids, if necessary—Anatomically correct dolls may be useful in developing exactly what sort of abusive activity occurred. The dolls are not used to diagnose child abuse, only to clarify what happened (Everson & Boat, 1994).

ix. Conclude the interview—Toward the end of the interview, the interviewer may ask a few leading questions about irrelevant issues (e.g., "You came here by taxi, didn't you?"). If the child demonstrates a susceptibility to suggestions, the interviewer would need to verify that the information obtained earlier did not come about through contamination. Finally, the interviewer thanks the child for participating, regardless of the outcome of the interview. The interviewer should not make promises that cannot be kept.

2. Parent interview—In order to evaluate a child who may have been abused, it is necessary to do more than simply interview the child and ask him or her what happened. It is also important to interview the parents and perhaps other caregivers. The parents should be able to provide information regarding the child's experiences with particular people; the duration and evolution of the child's symptoms; the child's developmental and medical history; and factors in the child's life, other than abuse, that might explain the symptoms. One or both parents may be able to explain the precise circumstances in which the allegations arose. It may also be important to assess the parents' motivations and psychological strengths and weaknesses. For instance, some parents (who perpetrated the abuse or allowed another individual to do so) may be motivated to deny or minimize the possibility that the child was abused. Other parents (who are vengeful or overly suspicious of another person) may be motivated to exaggerate the possibility that the child was abused or may even fabricate symptoms of abuse.

C. Psychological Testing

Although psychological testing cannot diagnose child abuse, it may be a useful part of the evaluation. For example, the Child Sexual Behavior Inventory (Friedrich et al, 2001) is a questionnaire to be completed by a parent, usually the child's mother. This questionnaire helps the clinician identify sexual behaviors that can be considered normative for the child's age and gender and sexual behaviors that can be viewed as relatively atypical for the child's age and gender, and which raise the suspicion of possible sexual abuse. Intellectual testing may be used to establish the child's developmental level. A general psychiatric evaluation may help with the differential diagnosis and clarify the child's treatment needs.

D. Record Review

In evaluating a child who may have been abused, it is frequently important to obtain information from outside sources such as medical, mental health, and educational records. It may be helpful to review the investigation conducted by child protective services, although those records may not be available.

American Academy of Child and Adolescent Psychiatry. Practice parameters for the forensic evaluation of children and adolescents who may have been physically or sexually abused. *J Am Acad Child Adolesc Psychiatry*. 1997;36:423.

Everson MD, Boat BW. Putting the anatomical doll controversy in perspective: an examination of the major uses and criticisms of the dolls in child sexual abuse evaluations. *Child Abuse Negl*. 1994;18:113.

Friedrich WN, Fisher JL, Dittner CA, et al. Child Sexual Behavior Inventory: normative, psychiatric, and sexual abuse comparisons. *Child Maltreat*. 2001;6:37.

Lamb ME, Orbach Y, Hershkowitz I, et al. A structured forensic interview protocol improves the quality and informativeness of investigative interviews with children: a review of research using the NICHD Investigative Interview Protocol. *Child Abuse Negl*. 2007;31:1201.

Ludwig S, Reece RM. *Child Abuse: Medical Diagnosis and Management*. 2nd ed. Philadelphia: Lippincott Williams & Wilkins; 2001.

Poole DA, Lamb ME. *Investigative Interviews of Children: A Guide for Helping Professionals*. Washington, DC: American Psychological Association; 1998.

Yuille JC, Hunter R, Joffe R, Zaparniuk J. Interviewing children in sexual abuse cases. In: Goodman GS, Bottoms BL, eds. *Child Victims, Child Witnesses: Understanding and Improving Testimony*. New York: Guilford; 1993.

▶ Differential Diagnosis

Children may make false statements in psychiatric evaluations. Sometimes they falsely deny abuse; sometimes they make false allegations. A number of mental processes, both conscious and unconscious, can result in false allegations. For example, a delusional mother, who believes that her ex-husband has been molesting their daughter, induces the girl to state that the father had rubbed against her in bed. By repeatedly asking leading or suggestive questions, inept interviewers have induced children to make false allegations of abuse. Some children manifest pathological lying in making false allegations. Young children may tell tall tales, making innocent statements that evolve or are molded into false allegations of abuse. Older children may lie about abuse for revenge or personal advantage. In the past, multiple allegations of abuse have been generated through group contagion or spread by parental panic and overzealous clinical investigation (Bernet, 1993, 2006).

Credibility refers to the child's truthfulness and accuracy, which sometimes is an issue in assessing children who allege abuse (Lamb et al, 1997). The following factors indicate that the child is credible: the child uses his or her own vocabulary rather than adult terms and tells the story from his or her own point of view; the child displays advanced sexual knowledge; the child reenacts the trauma in spontaneous play; sexual themes are excessively present in play and drawings; the child's affect is consonant with the accusations; the child's behavior is seductive, precocious, or regressive; the child has good recall of details, including sensory motor and idiosyncratic details; and the child has a history of telling the truth.

The following factors indicate the child is making unreliable or fictitious allegations: the child's account is vague and lacks details, due to lack of information, not resistance or defensiveness; the child's statements are dramatic or implausible, for example, involving the presence of multiple perpetrators or situations in which the perpetrator has not taken ordinary steps against discovery; the child's statements become increasingly inconsistent over time; and the child's accounts progress over time from relatively innocuous behavior to increasingly intrusive, abusive, and aggressive activities.

Bernet W. False statements and the differential diagnosis of abuse allegations. *J Am Acad Child Adolesc Psychiatry.* 1993;32:903.

Bernet W. Sexual abuse allegations in the context of child-custody disputes. In: Gardner R, Sauber S, Lorandos D, eds. *The International Handbook of Parental Alienation Syndrome: Conceptual, Clinical and Legal Considerations.* Springfield, IL: Charles C Thomas; 2006.

Lamb ME, Sternberg KJ, Esplin PW, et al. Assessing the credibility of children's allegations of sexual abuse: a survey of recent research. *Learn Individ Differ.* 1997;9:175.

Treatment

The first step in the management of child maltreatment is ensuring the child's safety and well-being. The child may need to be removed from an abusive or neglectful family. A clinician who suspects that a child has been abused should perform an assessment within the scope of the clinician's expertise—that is, the psychiatrist conducts a psychiatric evaluation, the pediatrician conducts a pediatric assessment. If the clinician continues to suspect child abuse after conducting his or her assessment, the local child protection agency must be notified (Kalichman, 1999).

Maltreated children who have significant psychological or behavioral symptoms should receive psychiatric treatment. Treatment should not be confused with forensic investigation. Although a specific treatment plan depends on the findings of a diagnostic evaluation, the psychotherapist would generally address issues such as self-esteem, worries, and fears; developing a therapeutic relationship built on trust, in which the child will not be exploited or betrayed; and gaining an understanding over time of the factors that contributed to the child's victimization (Pearce and Pezzot-Pearce, 2006; Runyon et al, 2004).

Abused children with posttraumatic stress disorder have been successfully treated with a trauma-focused cognitive behavioral treatment (Cohen et al, 2006, 2012) that has four components: psychoeducation, anxiety management, exposure, and cognitive therapy. **Psychoeducation** includes teaching the child and the caregivers about strategies to avoid future abuse. **Anxiety management** includes teaching children how to use relaxation and other coping strategies to reduce fearful responses to memories of abuse. **Exposure** refers to mastering traumatic anxiety through talking, drawing, or writing about the abuse experiences, either in ordinary conversation or through a variety of play, artistic, or other projective techniques. **Cognitive therapy** techniques help the child replace cognitive distortions about the event or negative feelings about himself or herself.

If an abused child has no symptoms related to the maltreatment, it is appropriate to provide brief psychoeducational counseling and suggestions for recognizing any problems that arise in the future. For a child whose abuse was a transitory unpleasant experience (e.g., a single, brief episode of fondling by a stranger), it may be adaptive for the child to forget the incident and move on.

Cohen JA, Mannarino AP, Deblinger E. *Treating Trauma and Traumatic Grief in Children and Adolescents.* New York: Guilford; 2006.

Cohen JA, Mannarino AP, Deblinger E. *Trauma-Focused CBT for Children and Adolescents: Treatment Applications.* New York: Guilford; 2012.

Kalichman SC. *Mandated Reporting of Suspected Child Abuse: Ethics, Law, and Policy.* 2nd ed. Washington, DC: American Psychological Association; 1999.

Pearce JW, Pezzot-Pearce TD. *Psychotherapy of Abused and Neglected Children.* 2nd ed. New York: Guilford; 2006.

Runyon MK, Deblinger E, Ryan EE, Thakkar-Kolar R. An overview of child physical abuse: developing an integrated parent-child cognitive-behavioral treatment approach. *Trauma Violence Abuse.* 2004;5:65.

Complications/Adverse Outcomes of Treatment

The most serious risk in evaluating and treating victims of child maltreatment is that the child will be retraumatized. This can happen if treatment requires the child to remember and relive the traumatic experiences to an unnecessary degree or if the child and family are too emotionally fragile to cope. Although many therapists believe it can be helpful for the child to recall and share painful experiences from the past, it is not therapeutic to dwell on these events repeatedly and endlessly. Retraumatization can also occur when the child, who has already lost important people in her life, develops an attachment to a therapist and that new relationship is interrupted in a premature or painful manner.

Another possible complication of therapy is the child's unwitting compulsion to reenact the aggressive or sexual aspects of the abusive relationship with new caregivers. That is, a seriously abused child may be placed with benevolent foster parents but behave in a way to provoke overly punitive behaviors by his new caregivers. Also, a seriously abused child may behave in a way to evoke rejection by an otherwise well-meaning therapist.

Treatment can have an adverse outcome if an overzealous therapist persists in looking for memories of past abuse when the abuse never happened in the first place. If a therapist repeatedly asks the patient—who can be a child or an adult—to remember abuse, the patient may "remember" it to please the therapist. To complicate the situation further, the patient may become convinced of the reality of these false memories.

▶ Prognosis

Sometimes child maltreatment causes no long-term psychological problems at all, but sometimes it causes severe psychological problems. Child maltreatment is more likely to cause subsequent emotional and behavioral disorders if the following factors are present: greater frequency and duration of abuse, greater force, physical injury, perpetration by a family member, the child already has poor coping skills, and lack of family support. Support from the nonabusive parent and validation of the child's statement are correlated with better prognosis.

The long-term psychological consequences of child maltreatment have been studied prospectively by following abused children for more than 30 years (Widom, 1999; Widom et al, 2012). The long-term psychological and physical effects of childhood maltreatment were also examined retrospectively in the Adverse Childhood Experiences Study (Dube et al, 2001; Anda et al, 2006). In general, individuals who experienced child maltreatment were more likely to have psychological problems—posttraumatic stress disorder,

dysthymia, suicidality, alcoholism, and antisocial personality disorder—than were individuals who had not been abused (Kendall-Tackett, 2003).

van der Kolk (2003) and D'Andrea et al (2012) have studied the long-term psychological and neurobiological effects of severe child maltreatment. Adults who were severely abused as children may develop a condition called complex posttraumatic stress disorder or a disorder of extreme stress not otherwise specified (DESNOS). The features of DESNOS are altered regulation of affect and impulses, altered attention and consciousness, altered self-perception, altered relationships, altered systems of meaning, and somatization.

The long-term consequences of child maltreatment may be affected by the victim's genetic makeup. Caspi et al (2003) found that children who had a variant allele of the serotonin transporter gene and also had been seriously abused as children were more likely to be depressed and suicidal as young adults. This research suggests a mechanism by which genetic makeup and life experience interact to influence psychosocial development and future attitudes and behaviors.

Anda RF, Felitti VJ, Bremner JD, et al. The enduring effects of abuse and related adverse experiences in childhood. *Eur Arch Psychiatry Clin Neurosci.* 2006;256:174.

Caspi A, Sugden K, Moffitt TE, et al. Influence of life stress on depression: moderation by a polymorphism in the 5-HTT gene. *Science.* 2003;301:386.

D'Andrea W, Ford J, Stolbach B, et al. Understanding interpersonal trauma in children: why we need a developmentally appropriate trauma diagnosis. *Am J Orthopsychiatry.* 2012;82:187.

Dube SR, Anda RF, Felitti VJ, et al. Childhood abuse, household dysfunction, and the risk of attempted suicide throughout the life span: findings from the adverse childhood experiences study. *JAMA.* 2001;286:3089.

Kendall-Tackett K. *Treating the Lifetime Health Effects of Childhood Victimization.* New York: Civic Research Institute; 2003.

van der Kolk BA. The neurobiology of childhood trauma and abuse. *Child Adolesc Psychiatr Clin N Am.* 2003;12(2):293.

Widom CS. Posttraumatic stress disorder in abused and neglected children grown up. *Am J Psychiatry.* 1999;156:1223.

Widom CS, Czaja SJ, Bentley T, Johnson MS. A prospective investigation of physical health outcomes in abused and neglected children: new findings from a 30-year follow-up. *Am J Public Health.* 2012;102:1135.

Posttraumatic Stress Disorder in Children and Adolescents Following a Single-Event Trauma

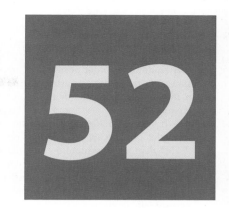

Brett McDermott, MD, FRANZCP

ESSENTIALS OF DIAGNOSIS

Children and adolescents frequently experience single-event traumas, for example, involvement in motor vehicle accidents, natural disasters, and other unexpected traumatic events such as being assaulted or raped. The experience of a single-event trauma is qualitatively different from the mental health sequelae of exposure to multiple traumatic experiences like the experience of protracted domestic violence, ongoing sexual assault, or experiences inherent in living in a war zone. Readers should consult the chapters on dissociative disorders and personality disorders and references to sexual abuse to further understand the sequelae of exposure to multiple-event trauma. The mental health outcomes following exposure to a single event trauma include posttraumatic stress disorder (PTSD), other anxiety disorders including specific phobias, and depressive presentations. The *Diagnostic and Statistical Manual* 5th edition (DSM-5) criteria for these conditions are detailed in Chapters xx, yy, and zz, respectively.

Diagnostic changes in DSM-5 are important in this area. PTSD is no longer a member of the anxiety group. Rather, it is in an overarching group of trauma- and stress-related disorders that includes dissociative disorders. The new PTSD criteria include four phenotypes: fear-based, anhedonic-dysphoric, externalizing, and dissociative. There have been changes in what events meet criteria: indirect exposure is now not included; rather, an individual must witness a traumatic event. Finally, and importantly for this chapter, there is a new preschool subtype with a greater focus on behavior rather than symptoms that relate to the individual's perception of their internal world. Further, adult constructs such as feelings of detachment have been changed to reflect the preschool experience. In this example the criteria are more about social withdrawal.

A valuable framework to help understand the effects of single-event trauma in children and adolescents is that of developmental psychopathology. Individuals function by integration of subsystems that interact vertically (e.g., gene to cell to organism) and horizontally (person to person, person to society). Infants, children, and adolescents also need to organize across time. Time course introduces new developmental constructs: novelty of cause and effect of inputs at different developmental stages (for example, negotiating the entry into elementary and high schools), differential rates of development across subsystems, critical periods, and negotiating developmental challenges such as the changing relationship between parent and child. A developmental psychopathology perspective subsumes other useful heuristics such as a bio-psycho-social and a systemic perspective. Inherent is the conceptualization of an individual's trajectory over the infant-child-youth developmental span, and abnormality is understood as deviance from a normal trajectory. The cumulative adversity inherent in experiencing repetitive traumatic events leads to a picture of continuity of developmental abnormality. That is, the child has been symptomatic and functionally impaired (developmentally the child is "under the normal trajectory") for some time. The mental health sequelae of a significant isolated, single event trauma is seen as a developmental discontinuity; a recent, obvious, subjective deviation from the developmental norm. For a more comprehensive account of the developmental approach see Costello and Angold (1996). The seminal paper of Lenore Terr advocated the useful nosology of Type I trauma describing the developmental discontinuity, and Type II the developmental continuity (Terr, 1994).

Costello EJ, Angold A. Developmental psychopathology. In: Cairns RB, Elder GH, Costello EJ, eds. *Developmental Science*. Cambridge, UK: Cambridge University Press; 1996:168–189.

Scheeringa MS, Myers L, Putnam FW, et al. Diagnosing PTSD in early childhood: an empirical assessment of four approaches. *J Trauma Stress*. 2012;25(4):359–367.

Terr L. Childhood traumas: an outline and overview. *Am J Psychiatry*. 1994;148:10–20.

▶ General Considerations

An adverse mental health outcome following a single-event trauma is not limited to PTSD. Clearly PTSD is of central importance; however, other postdisaster anxiety and depressive states are frequently reported. Current data are consistent in showing that individuals who experience greater disaster-related fear of death and event exposure are more likely to have a PTSD/anxiety outcome, whereas greater loss and grief predisposes to a depression outcome. However, PTSD-depression symptom concordance is great, and comorbid presentations are common. There are some recent data suggesting that posttrauma depressive symptoms are more persistent over time than PTSD symptoms.

The post–single-event trauma burden of mental illness is not restricted to new mental health presentations. Many individuals with preexisting mental illness will experience a postevent symptom relapse. Reasons may be pragmatic, such as difficulty obtaining medications or access to therapy in a postdisaster environment. Systemic issues such as an increased likelihood of parent distress and/or depression may be significant. Psychopathology may be related to event phase; immediately postevent individuals and service providers are appropriately focused on physical safety, water, food, and shelter needs. Mental health presentations and service provision generally begin in the weeks following the disaster. It is often the case that mental health issues come to dominate in the months and years postdisaster.

A. Major Etiological Theories

A potentially confusing range of causal theories have been advocated for PTSD presentations in childhood. Such theories are often extrapolated from adult research and include psychodynamic, behavioral, cognitive, and biological explanatory models. Given age-appropriate variations in a potential victim's integration of biological, emotional, and behavioral systems, it is not surprising that stressful events may affect individuals in different ways across the life span. Etiology has been influenced by research findings, often from epidemiological designs, that identify risk, vulnerability, and resilience factors. However, even seemingly simple associations such as gender and age and PTSD have proven difficult to clarify. It remains plausible that different traumatic events have differential gender impacts; a tragic example is the high rate of rape of girls during war, with boys more likely to experience the trauma of being forced to be a child soldier.

1. Risk factors—An overarching principle is whether the functioning of the individual with PTSD has diminished; it is below their pre-event trajectory. A second principle is whether the impaired functioning is due to a combination of event-related, proximal factors or distal factors intrinsic to the individual and present before the trauma. The event-related factor with the greatest empirical link to subsequent PTSD symptoms is traumatic event exposure. The event

exposure–PTSD association has been demonstrated in children more proximal to an earthquake's epicenter, those who experienced more hurricane damage, and those closer to gunfire or closer to actual wildfire flames. Note that high event exposure, although a useful summary variable, is itself a multifactorial construct that includes the perception of threat of death, concern about possible death of loved ones, witnessing serious physical injury of others, perceptual experiences such as smoke from fires, and witnessing the coping or lack of coping of parents, caregivers, and other adults. Relocation in the immediate aftermath of a disaster has been argued as both a positive factor, by decreasing disaster exposure, and a negative factor, given the lack of continuity with family and community; relocation also removes the opportunity to constructively engage in postdisaster recovery activities. Distal factors significantly associated with higher PTSD symptoms in children include high trait anxiety, a past history of emotional problems, children with a subjective sense of low self-efficacy and low social support, children employing poor coping strategies, and an internal causal attribution.

2. Cognitive factors—Information-processing theory postulates that there is the potential of being overwhelmed by the everyday volume of information requiring processing. To counter this, information is encoded and recalled in specific ways. Cognitive schemata are developed as a primary organizing heuristic. The interaction between incoming information and existing schemata influences subsequent memory encoding and retrieval. Information dissonance with existing schemata leads to conflict and the disruption of the usual memory encoding, comprehension, and memory retrieval sequence. The greater the dissonance, the greater is the likelihood of trauma symptoms and subsequent impairment.

One postulate is that there are specific schemata that, if violated, are more likely to precipitate trauma symptoms. Fundamental beliefs such as "good things happen to good people" may be radically undermined after a traumatic event such as the experience of being raped. Possible psychological responses to information dissonant to existing schemata include assimilation (altering information to fit preconceptions) and accommodation (changing existing schemata to account for and accept the new information). The latter may facilitate recovery. Unfortunately, accommodation may create a secondary impairment if, for instance, new schemata are punitive or self-deprecatory, undermine adaptive beliefs about safety or intimacy, and make the tasks of daily living more difficult. Child and adolescent trauma outcomes can be more complex given the added possibility of altered parent schemata about their child's safety. An example is the double jeopardy of the child who experienced a paroxysmal, single-event sexual assault that resulted in PTSD psychopathology. If, for a protracted period thereafter, altered parent–child safety schemata also lead to the child not being allowed to visit friends or go on school outings, "sleep-overs," and other events, the normal process of child–adolescent individuation-separation has been retarded generating a secondary impairment. As previously mentioned, psychological responses vary with the child's developmental stage. Accommodation in young children may manifest as self-blame for the event, heightened by a child's tendency to regress to a more egocentric worldview. Younger children may develop schemata that predict future disastrous events and ongoing extreme danger to themselves, friends, or family. Other common changed schemata include fears that the event will reoccur, that the event will become greater with a larger number of affected people, and that adults cannot protect children from future traumatic events.

3. Biological factors—Recent neuroimaging studies including young adult subjects with histories of child trauma have been informative. Results, some of which require replication, include reduced prefrontal cortical gray-matter volume in young adults exposed to harsh corporal punishment, reduced occipital cortex volume in women who have been sexually abused, and reduced hippocampal volume in physically abused individuals. The last suggests critical periods for different types of brain damage (see the work of Tomoda, Teicher, and colleagues). Neuroimaging is a burgeoning research area including new technologies to investigate potential white-matter changes. Other areas of research include neuroendocrine investigations focusing on dysregulation of the hypothalamus–pituitary–stress system following traumatic events. It is also anticipated that basic and animal research using system biology approaches (including epigenetics) will be applied to human populations and will be published over the coming years.

McDermott BM, Palmer LJ. Post-disaster emotional distress, depression and event-related variables: findings across child and adolescent developmental stages. *Aust N Z J Psychiatry.* 2002;36:754–761.

Meiser-Steadman R. Towards a cognitive-behavioural model of PTSD in children and adolescents. *Clin Child Fam Psychol Rev.* 2000;5(4):217–232.

Najarian LM, Goenjian AK, Pelcovitz D, et al. Relocation after a disaster: posttraumatic stress disorder in Armenia after the earthquake. *J Am Acad Child Adolesc Psychiatry.* 1996;35:374–383.

Ross MC, Heilicher M, Cisler JM. Functional imaging correlates of childhood trauma: a qualitative review of past research and emerging trends. *Pharmacol Biochem Behav.* 2021;211:173297. doi: 10.1016/j.pbb.2021.173297. Epub 2021 Nov 12. PMID: 34780877; PMCID: PMC8675038.

Song SH, Kim B, Choi NH, et al. A 30-month prospective follow-up study of psychological symptoms, psychiatric diagnoses, and their effects on quality of life in children witnessing a single incident of death at school. *J Clin Psychiatry.* 2012;73(5):e594–600.

Tomoda A, Polcari A, Anderson CM, et al. Reduced visual cortex grey matter volume and thickness in young adults who witnessed domestic violence during childhood. *PLoS One* 2012;7(12):e52528.

Weems CF, Russell JD, Neill EL, McCurdy BH. Annual research review: pediatric posttraumatic stress disorder from a neurodevelopmental network perspective. *J Child Psychol Psychiatry.* 2019;60(4):395–408. doi: 10.1111/jcpp.12996. Epub 2018 Oct 25. PMID: 30357832.

B. Epidemiology

Estimates of the prevalence of post–single-event PTSD vary greatly. Uniform PTSD rates would not be expected, given that every disaster or traumatic event is unique. PTSD estimate variability is also due to disparity in research design: the elapsed time of assessment since the event, developmental stage of participants, whether the child or parent was the primary informant, and the measure of psychopathology. Design considerations include bias due to selective mortality, recall and interview bias, and use of convenience samples. Significant "unpacking" of the event, both of event-related variables and the personal meaning of the event, is required for more meaningful between-event comparison.

Examples of prevalence variability include PTSD rates between 90% and 100% of children who were kidnapped and endured harrowing hours in captivity and children trapped in a school playground by sniper fire; intermediate rates of 40–60% in children who experienced major transport disasters; and lower rates of 5–15% of children screened after natural disasters. Occasionally studies report no children meeting diagnostic criteria for PTSD. Even in these low PTSD prevalence examples, limited-symptom PTSD and other anxiety disorder presentations are usually reported.

Single event-trauma research is often population-based initiatives following natural disasters. Significant research initiatives have followed the devastation of hurricanes, for example, Hugo (1989), Andrew (1992), Iniki (1992), and Katrina (2005). Female participants, younger age, high trait anxiety, and emotional reactivity during hurricanes independently predicted PTSD symptoms. Australian wildfire disasters have been subject to similar scrutiny, and both similar rates of child and adolescent PTSD have been reported, along with high rates of comorbid depression and similar proximal predictive values.

▶ Clinical Findings

A. Assessment & History Taking

No two single-event traumas are identical, and the notion that trauma exposure can be lumped into a nominal variable is simplistic. It is more typical that within the event setting, exposures vary widely. To help "unpack" a potentially traumatic event, a detailed, sometimes minute-by-minute chronological narrative is helpful. The clinician should consider potential traumatic stimuli in all sensory modalities—for example, what did the child see, hear, smell? What were the child's thoughts at different stages of the event? What is their understanding of what occurred and the meaning they gave to the event or the roles individuals played? What were the reactions of others, especially adults in the vicinity?

The type of traumatic event, for example, a motor vehicle accident, is usually identifiable in the PTSD symptom content as the subject matter of flashbacks, dreams and nightmares, and, if accessible, cognitions underlying avoidance behavior. Some individuals with intellectual impairment and the very young will not have a coherent verbal narrative of the event. In these cases, the clinician seeks to identify biobehavioral discontinuities, temporally related to event exposure, in various domains such as sleep, satiety, elimination, and regulation of mood, behavior, and impulsivity. Another useful exercise is to consider the event from a non–mental-health perspective. A societal and wider systems assessment is usually informative. Establish if there was environmental degradation, significant postevent economic hardship (short and long-term), disruption of services (electricity, water, sewer), and disruptions to institutions such as schools. Failure to provide services in the postevent setting may result in feelings of personal and collective powerlessness. Postevent concerns in these domains may be very significant in understanding overall impairment levels.

B. Signs & Symptoms Across Developmental Stages

The clinical presentation of child and adolescent PTSD is dependent upon the child's age; given age is a proxy for underlying developmental constructs such as cognitive, speech, and language development and sophistication of peer and societal relatedness.

1. Infants and preschool children—Recent research in preschool and infant school children has been informative (see Scheeringa) and influenced the creation of the new DSM-5 preschool (6 years or younger) subtype. The latter emphasizes that symptoms may be expressed during play (including flashbacks), that content of traumatic nightmares may not be obviously trauma related, and that emphasis is given to avoidance behavior, diminished interest, negative emotional states, and reduced positive emotions. Cluster D symptoms are largely unchanged, along with an acknowledgment of the possibility of posttrauma increased irritability and temper tantrums. Note that these empirically based changes are consistent with many previous qualitative findings such as posttraumatic play, in Terr's terminology "reenactments" given the absence of the fun element of play (Terr, 1994). Reenactments are compulsive, repetitive behavioral sequences that are unconsciously linked to the traumatic event. Importantly, these behaviors can place children in danger—for example, setting or playing with fire following a wildfire disaster. The clinician should also be vigilant for non-PTSD diagnoses such as depression, separation anxiety, and specific trauma-related fears.

2. Primary and high school children—With increasing age, symptomatology is more typical of adult PTSD. Age-related phenomena still exist, such as aggressive or withdrawn behavior; however, behavior becomes more sophisticated. Fear of death, separation anxiety, or fear of the event recurring are common. Magical thinking and ascribing omen status to events before the trauma is common in younger children; so, too, are phenomena such as nightmares and sleep disturbance. Flashbacks are reported; however, they often have more of a daydream quality than the sudden, intrusive adult phenomena. A fear generalization gradient has been described such that stimuli approaching the traumatic event evoked increasing distress. An example would be fear of seeing any car, but greater fear seeing the same color of car that was involved in a motor vehicle accident.

Denial and disavowal of the traumatic event is not often seen in childhood PTSD presentations that follow a single-event trauma. However, children can withhold the extent of their distressing experiences from their parents, either because of perceived difficulties talking to their parents following trauma or because children do not want to burden their parents with their feelings of distress. Another distinction from adult PTSD is that numbing and restriction of affect is not frequently reported by children, in part because of the difficulty younger children have in understanding and discussing these concepts.

C. Psychological Testing

Given research demonstrating low parent identification of their child's posttraumatic and other "internalizing" (e.g., depressive) symptoms, rating scales can play a valuable role in postevent screening and symptom identification. Some measures can be administered by a clinician as a semistructured interview or by child self-report. The developmental appropriateness of item wording is important; most children under 8 years of age will have difficulty with multiple response answer fields but can complete Yes/No formats. Questions to adolescents should include important comorbidities such as postevent substance abuse. See Chapter 36 for more details on specific measures.

D. Laboratory Findings & Imaging

There are currently no practice recommendations advising the routine use of specific laboratory tests or neuroimaging studies in children or adolescents who experienced single-event trauma.

▶ Differential Diagnosis

Early diagnostic closure on PTSD should be avoided. Care should be taken to also elicit symptoms of depression and other anxiety disorders, especially phobias, panic disorder with and without agoraphobia, and generalized anxiety disorder. For some children, the primary presenting complaint will be a sleep disorder or a restrictive eating pattern. Increased physical symptoms such as musculoskeletal complaints have been reported. In adolescents, postevent increased alcohol and substance use is an important consideration.

▶ Treatment

An important treatment consideration is that some single-event trauma, for example, natural disasters, potentially involves large numbers of individuals. In such circumstances a public health approach to service provision is justified. Such an approach may include screening for PTSD (consistent with the NICE guidelines), followed by universal and targeted responses to identified children, adolescents, and families. Recent studies such as the comparison of a stepped collaborative care model and a cognitive–behavioral therapy (CBT) intervention (see Zatzick and colleagues, 2009) provide information on how to increase service reach after large-scale disasters. As with assessment, the overarching treatment concern is the need to be developmentally appropriate, especially given the different communication style of children at different developmental stages.

A. Psychopharmacological Treatment

The Cochrane PTSD review of Stein and colleagues (2009) found no trials with pediatric subjects. Dedicated child and adolescent reviews concur with the absence of research in the pediatric domain. The UK NICE guidelines advise against prescribing for children and adolescents with PTSD, with the caveat that medication may have a role in acute postevent sleep disturbance. The recently published Australian Clinical Practice Guidelines recommend that pharmacotherapy should not be used as either a routine first-line treatment of PTSD in children and adolescents, or as a routine adjunct therapy to trauma-focused CBT. This does not exclude a role for serotonin reuptake inhibitor antidepressants for postevent presentations of depression.

Australian Guidelines for the Treatment of Acute Stress Disorder and Posttraumatic Stress Disorder. Melbourne: ACPMH; 2013.

Stein DJ, Ipser JC, Seedat S. Pharmacotherapy for posttraumatic stress disorder (PTSD). *The Cochrane Library.* 2009;Issue 1.

Taylor TL, Chemtob CM. Efficacy of treatment for child and adolescent traumatic stress. *Arch Pediatr Adolesc Med.* 2004;158(8):786–791.

Zatzick DF, Koepsell T, Rivara FP. Using target population specification, effect size, and reach to estimate and compare the population impact of two PTSD preventive interventions. *Psychiatry.* 2009;72:346–359.

B. Psychological Treatment

Current treatment guidelines emphasize that many individuals who experience a potentially traumatic event do not become symptomatic or have mild symptoms that spontaneously remit. There is currently no evidence that a single-session debriefing intervention will lead to better outcomes; indeed, some guidelines specifically advise against debriefing.

1. Psychological first aid (PFA)—PFA is an initiative of the National Child Traumatic Stress Network and the National Centre for PTSD, and its use is recommended. The *Field Operations Guide*, 2nd edition, is available from the NCTSN website. Along with PFA preparation and engagement issues, core intervention areas include safety, mental status stabilization, gathering essential information, practical assistance, facilitating social connectedness, psychoeducation about emotional trauma, and grief and service linkage. The NCTSN website also provides online PFA training and a free PFA Mobile app.

2. Trauma-focused cognitive–behavioral therapy (TF-CBT)—If PTSD symptoms persist for longer than 1 month or cause impairment, then treatment should be instigated. The treatment with the most evidence of effectiveness is TF-CBT. Although treatment of children will often include some element of play and creative expression, for effectiveness therapy must address the specific trauma memories and ameliorate the impact of such memories by CBT techniques such as exposure and habituation and/or cognitive restructuring. It is important to include parents and/or caregivers in a TF-CBT program, to educate and motivate parents to help their child attend sessions, to help and motivate their child to complete homework tasks, and to be aware there may be some initial worsening of symptoms as the child begins to talk about the traumatic experience. There is some emerging evidence favoring individual over group TF-CBT and TF-CBT programs delivered in school settings with greater treatment program retention. There is some evidence for the effectiveness of eye-movement desensitization and reprocessing in children; however, this literature is small compared to the TF-CBT literature. Comorbidities such as depressive symptoms may remit with PTSD therapy. If the severity of depressive or substance abuse symptoms prevents engagement in TF-CBT, these issues may need to be addressed first.

National Institute for Clinical Excellence (NICE). *Clinical Guideline 26. Post-traumatic Stress Disorder (PTSD): The Management of PTSD in Adults and Children in Primary and Secondary Care.*

The National Child Traumatic Stress Network. http://www.nctsnet.org

▶ Adverse Outcomes

Unnecessary treatment with medication or psychotherapy can occur following the good intentions of parents and clinicians to treat children who are exposed to a traumatic event. A competent assessment should prevent undue intervention. If a screening test is used, it is important to acknowledge that all screens have false-positive and -negative rates.

Negative screening results should not preclude subsequent referral for diagnostic clarification. In an ideal service provision scenario, an individual with a positive screening result on a self-report measure would then be offered an individual assessment to determine the need for an intervention.

▶ Prognosis and Course of Illness

For some individuals, time will diminish the emotional impact and symptoms of PTSD. Possible mechanisms include habituation to the reminders of a given event and a process of more normative forgetting. However, symptom reduction may be misleading. A perception of recovery from reexperiencing symptoms may in reality be greater emotional numbing and avoidance symptoms. Unfortunately, PTSD symptom chronicity is well described. One form of chronicity is anniversary reactions, which may increase over time, and often this occurrence is not immediately attributed to the traumatic event (Terr, 1994). Persistent symptoms of PTSD have been reported by children and adolescents 6 months after transport-related disasters, tsunamis, and wildfires; 18 months after earthquake disasters; and 2 years after bushfires. The few longer term outcome studies have also demonstrated symptom chronicity.

Cohen JA, Bukstein O, Walter H, et al; AACAP Work Group On Quality Issues. Practice parameter for the assessment and treatment of children and adolescents with posttraumatic stress disorder. *J Am Acad Child Adolesc Psychiatry*. 2010;49(4): 414–30. PMID: 20410735.

Korol MS, Kramer TL, Grace MC, Green BL. Dam break: long-term follow-up of children exposed to the Buffalo Creek disaster. In: LaGreca A, Silverman WK, Vernberg EM, Roberts MC, eds. *Helping Children Cope with Disasters: Integrating Research and Practice*. Washington, DC: American Psychological Association; 2002.

Tourette Syndrome, Tic Disorders, and Obsessive–Compulsive Disorder in Children and Adolescents

Michael H. Bloch, MD, MS
James F. Leckman, MD, PhD

TOURETTE SYNDROME AND TIC DISORDERS

ICD-10 Diagnostic Criteria

Tic Disorders

Syndromes in which the predominant manifestation is some form of tic. A tic is an involuntary, rapid, recurrent, non-rhythmic motor movement (usually involving circumscribed muscle groups) or vocal production that is of sudden onset and that serves no apparent purpose. Tics tend to be experienced as irresistible but usually they can be suppressed for varying periods of time, are exacerbated by stress, and disappear during sleep. Common simple motor tics include only eye-blinking, neck-jerking, shoulder-shrugging, and facial grimacing. Common simple vocal tics include throat-clearing, barking, sniffing, and hissing. Common complex tics include hitting oneself, jumping, and hopping. Common complex vocal tics include the repetition of particular words, and sometimes the use of socially unacceptable (often obscene) words (coprolalia), and the repetition of one's own sounds or words (palilalia).

Transient Tic Disorder F95.0 (307.21)

Meets the general criteria for a tic disorder but the tics do not persist longer than 12 months. The tics usually take the form of eye-blinking, facial grimacing, or head-jerking.

Chronic Motor or Vocal Tic Disorder F95.1 (307.22)

Meets the general criteria for a tic disorder, in which there are motor or vocal tics (but not both), that may be either single or multiple (but usually multiple), and last for more than a year.

Combined Vocal and Multiple Motor Tic Disorder [Gilles de la Tourette Disorder] F95.2 (307.23)

A form of tic disorder in which there are, or have been, multiple motor tics and one or more vocal tics, although these need not have occurred concurrently. The disorder usually worsens during adolescence and tends to persist into adult life. The vocal tics are often multiple with explosive repetitive vocalizations, throat-clearing, and grunting, and there may be the use of obscene words or phrases. Sometimes there is associated gestural echopraxia which may also be of an obscene nature (copropraxia).

F95.8 Other Tic Disorders

F95.9 Tic Disorder, Unspecified

Tic NOS

Adapted with permission from International Statistical Classification of Diseases and Related Health Problems 10th Revision (ICD-10) Version for 2010. Geneva: World Health Organization; 2010.

In contrast to the DSM-5 nomenclature for tic disorders, the ICD-10 criteria do not require explicitly that an individual must have a past history of both vocal and motor tics occurring for at least 1 year to qualify for a diagnosis of Tourette syndrome (TS). However, the 1-year threshold is in place for the ICD-10 criteria specific for a chronic motor or vocal tic disorder. Likewise, an individual who has had tics for less than a year qualifies for a diagnosis of a "transient tic disorder," termed "provisional tic disorder" in DSM-5. Individuals whose tics have an age of onset after 18 or are exclusively present during the use of substances known to induce tics such as amphetamines, stimulants, and crack/cocaine qualify for the diagnosis of Tic Disorder Otherwise Specified in DSM-5 and either Other Tic Disorder or Tic Disorder, Not Otherwise Specified (NOS) in ICD-10. In DSM-5, tic disorders, unlike most psychiatric disorders, do not possess an impairment criterion, so tics, even in the absence of any clinical, social, educational, or vocational impairment, are sufficient to make the diagnosis. The ICD-10 criteria also do not mention "impairment."

▶ General Considerations

A. Etiologic Theories

Our current understanding of TS provides a good working model to understand the pathogenesis of other childhood neuropsychiatric disorders: a genetically determined vulnerability; age-dependent expression of symptoms reflecting maturational factors; sexual dimorphism; stress-dependent fluctuation in symptom severity; and environmental influences on the phenotypic expression of tic severity. Recently, the role of the immune system has gained increasing attention as a potentially important etiological factor.

Strong evidence implicates basal ganglia and corticostriatal thalamocortical (CSTC) abnormalities as central to the pathogenesis of tics. Indirect evidence for the involvement of the basal ganglia comes from the association of other movement disorders such as Sydenham chorea, Huntington disease, hemiballismus, and Parkinson disease with basal ganglia pathology. Direct evidence supporting CSTC abnormalities in TS comes from neuroimaging, neuropathological, and neurosurgical studies.

CSTC loops are multiple, parallel, and partially overlapping neuroanatomical circuits, which relay information from most regions of the cortex to subcortical areas, particularly the striatum and thalamus, which in turn project to a subset of the original cortical areas. In CSTC loops, the basal ganglia can be viewed as a way station between intention and action (thought, affect, and movement). Tics and other repetitive and stereotyped movements are believed to arise from imbalances in basal ganglia circuits. For example, tics may arise through a failure of inhibition of a discrete population of striatal projection neurons. This disinhibition may activate specific cortical regions, which in turn trigger sensory urges and motor and vocal tics.

Altered dopaminergic functioning has been strongly implicated in the pathogenesis of TS. Evidence for abnormal dopamine neurotransmission in TS comes from two clinical observations. First, the blockade of dopamine receptors by neuroleptic drugs will suppress tics in most patients. In addition, dopamine-releasing drugs such as cocaine and amphetamines can precipitate or exacerbate tics. Indeed, it has been shown that TS patients release more dopamine at dopaminergic synapses in response to amphetamine compared to normal controls. Second, the importance of dopamine in TS is supported by brain imaging using dopamine ligands in single-photon-emission computed tomography and positron emission tomography (PET). In one twin study, tic severity was related to dopamine D_2 receptor binding in the head of the caudate nucleus. In addition to neuroanatomical factors, genetic, immune, and environmental factors have been implicated in TS.

B. Genetics

Although the majority of genetic factors responsible remain undiscovered, TS has a large heritable component. Early twin studies suggested that the concordance rate for TS among monozygotic twin pairs is greater than 50%, while the concordance of dizygotic twin pairs is about 10%. If co-twins with chronic motor tic disorder are included, these concordance figures increase to 77% for monozygotic and 30% for dizygotic twin pairs. Differences in the concordance of monozygotic and dizygotic twin pairs indicate that genetic factors play an important role in the etiology of TS and related conditions. However, the available data also suggest that nongenetic factors are involved in the nature and severity of the clinical syndrome.

The overall risk that an offspring of a parent with TS will develop TS is approximately 10–15%. The risk that their offspring will develop a tic disorder (20–29%) or obsessive–compulsive disorder (OCD) (12–32%) is slightly higher. Male offspring have a higher propensity to develop a tic disorder.

The analysis of a chromosomal anomaly in one TS patient led to the identification of other sequence variants in the *SLITRK1* gene in approximately 1% of TS cases. Specifically, among 174 unrelated probands with TS, one frame-shift mutation and two identical variants in the 3' untranscribed region of this gene were identified. None of these anomalies were demonstrated in over 3600 controls. *SLITRK1* mRNA is expressed in the human fetal brain at 20 weeks gestation in multiple neuroanatomical areas implicated in TS neuropathology including the cortical plate, striatum, globus pallidus, thalamus, and subthalamic nucleus.

A rare functional mutation in the *L-histidine Decarboxylase (HDC)* gene was discovered in two-generation family. *HDC* codes for the rate-limiting enzyme in histamine biosynthesis. This result suggests a potential link to the involvement of histaminergic neurotransmission in the pathophysiology TS. Although other genes of major effect are likely to be found, it is becoming clear that, in most cases, TS is a polygenetic disorder with complex gene–environment interactions yet to be fully elucidated.

C. Immune Factors

Emerging data implicate immune mechanisms in the pathophysiology of TS. A crucial role of microglia in the neural-immune crosstalk within TS and related disorders has been proposed by animal models and confirmed by a recent transcriptome analysis of postmortem brain tissue and by a PET study showing activated microglia in the caudate nucleus in children and adolescents with TS. These cross-sectional studies leave open the question of whether neuroinflammation plays a causal role. Prospective longitudinal studies of inflammatory cytokines, immunoglobulin levels, and the number of regulatory T cells in the peripheral circulation also point to the importance of the immune system. Indeed, immune mechanisms have been implicated in a number of neurodevelopmental disorders from autism to schizophrenia.

D. Environmental Factors

The existence of monozygotic twins discordant for tic severity emphasizes the importance of environmental factors in the phenotypic expression of TS. In monozygotic twins discordant for tic severity, the twin with more severe tics usually has lower birth weight and a greater number of dopamine receptor sites in the caudate nucleus. In observational and case control studies, low Apgar scores, stressful maternal life circumstances during pregnancy, and maternal first-trimester nausea have been found to be risk factors for TS.

Tic disorders have long been identified as "stress-sensitive" conditions. Typically, symptom exacerbation follows stressful life events. These events need not be adverse in character. Clinical experience suggests that, in some unfortunate instances, a vicious cycle can be initiated when tic symptoms are misunderstood by family and teachers, leading to active attempts to suppress the symptoms by punishment and humiliation. These efforts can lead to an exacerbation of symptoms and can increase the level of stress in the child's environment. Prospective longitudinal studies have begun to examine systematically the effect of intramorbid stress. It has been found that patients with TS experience more stress than matched healthy controls and that antecedent stress can play a role in subsequent tic exacerbation.

E. Epidemiology

Transient tics are common among school-age children, with estimates ranging between 4 and 24%. The number of children experiencing chronic motor tic disorders is roughly one-quarter this number. Once thought to be much rarer, the current lifetime prevalence estimate for TS ranges from 0.1 to 1%.

The prevalence of tic disorders peaks during the late first decade and early second decades due to the clinical course of the disorder. They are roughly one-third as prevalent in adulthood. Boys are twice as likely as girls to be affected by tic disorders.

Abelson JF, Kwan KY, O'Roak BJ, et al. Sequence variants in SLITRK1 are associated with TS. *Science.* 2005;310:317–320.

Ercan-Sencicek AG, Stillman AA, Ghosh AK et al. L-Histidine decarboxylase and Tourette's syndrome. *N Engl J Med.* 2010;362(20):1901–1908.

Findley DB, Leckman JF, Katsovich L et al. Development of the Yale Children's Global Stress Index and its application in children and adolescents with Tourette's syndrome and obsessive-compulsive disorder. *J Am Acad Child Adolesc Psychiatry.* 2003;42(4):450–457.

Hyde TM, Aaronson BA, Randolph C, et al. Relationship of birth weight to the phenotypic expression of Gilles de la TS in monozygotic twins. *Neurology.* 1992;42:652–658.

Kataoka Y, Kalanithi PS, Grantz H, et al. Decreased number of parvalbumin and cholinergic interneurons in the striatum of individuals with Tourette syndrome. *J Comp Neurol.* 2010;518(3):277–291.

Leckman JF, Vaccarino FM, Kalanithi PS, Rothenberger A. Tourette syndrome: a relentless drumbeat—driven by misguided brain oscillations. *J Child Psychol Psychiatry.* 2006;47(6):537–550.

Martino D, Zis P, Buttiglione M. The role of immune mechanisms in Tourette syndrome. *Brain Res.* 2015;1617:126–143.

Mataix-Cols D, Isomura K, Pérez-Vigil A, et al. Familial risks of Tourette syndrome and chronic tic disorders. A population-based cohort study. *JAMA Psychiatry.* 2015;72(8):787–793.

Peterson BS, Thomas P, Kane MJ, et al. Ganglia volumes in patients with Gilles de la Tourette syndrome. *Arch Gen Psychiatry.* 2003;60(4):415–424.

Scahill L, Sukhodolsky DG, Williams SK, Leckman JF. Public health significance of tic disorders in children and adolescents. *Adv Neurol.* 2005;96:240–248.

▶ Clinical Findings

A. Signs & Symptoms

Tics are sudden, repetitive movements, gestures, or phonic productions that typically mimic some aspect of normal behavior. Usually of brief duration, individual tics rarely last more than a second. Many tics occur in bouts with inter-tic intervals of less than 1 second. Individual tics can occur singly or together in an orchestrated pattern. They vary in intensity or forcefulness. Motor tics, which can be viewed as disinhibited fragments of normal movement, can vary from simple, abrupt movement such as eye blinking, nose twitching, head or arm jerks, or shoulder shrugs to more complex movements that appear to have purpose, such as facial or hand gestures or sustained looks. The two phenotypic extremes of motor tics are classified as simple and complex motor tics, respectively. Similarly, phonic tics can be classified as simple or complex. Simple vocal tics are sudden, meaningless sounds such as throat clearing, coughing, sniffing, spitting, or grunting. Complex phonic tics are more protracted, meaningful utterances, varying from prolonged throat clearing to syllables, words, or phrases and even to more complex behaviors such as palilalia, echolalia and, in rare cases, coprolalia.

The severity of tics in TS waxes and wanes through the course of the disorder. The tics of TS and other tic disorders are highly variable, from minute to minute, hour to hour, day to day, week to week, month to month, and even year to year. Tics occur in bouts, which also tend to cluster. Tic symptoms can be exacerbated by stress, fatigue, extremes of temperature, and external stimuli (i.e., hearing a word or phrase may lead to echolalia). In contrast, intentional movements can attenuate tic occurrence. Intense concentration on activities that require motor activity tends to dissipate tic symptoms.

Many individuals with tics, especially those advanced in age, are aware of premonitory urges (e.g., feelings of tightness, tension, or itching that are accompanied by a mounting sense of discomfort or anxiety) that can be relieved only by the performance of a tic. The premonitory urges are similar to the sensation preceding a sneeze or an itch. Premonitory urges cause many TS patients an endless cycle of rising tension and tic performance because the relief provided by tic performance is ephemeral. Thus, soon after the tic, the tension of the premonitory urge again rises to a crescendo. Most patients also report a fleeting sense of relief after a bout of tics has occurred, and most individuals can suppress their tics for short periods of time.

With increasing awareness of premonitory urges, TS patients begin to exhibit a variable degree of voluntary control over specific tics. In one study, 92% of TS subjects reported that their tics were partially or totally voluntary. However, this voluntary control should be likened to that governing eye blinking. Eye blinking and tics can both be inhibited voluntarily, but only for a limited period of time and only with mounting discomfort. Thus, some adult TS patients are able to demonstrate nearly complete control over the situation when their tics will occur. However, when complete or near-complete control of tics is present, resistance to the mounting tension of premonitory urges can produce mental and physical exhaustion even more impairing and distracting than the tics themselves.

The tics, which are the most prominent feature of TS, are often neither the first nor the most impairing psychological disturbance that TS patients endure. It has become apparent that children with TS have higher rates of OCD, attention-deficit/hyperactivity disorder (ADHD), and disinhibited speech and behavior, compared to individuals in the general population. In one study, 65% of TS patients in late adolescence regarded their behavioral problems (e.g., ADHD and OCD) and learning difficulties to have had an equal or greater impact on their life than the tics themselves. In the course of comorbid psychiatric illness in TS, ADHD symptoms, when they occur, typically precede the onset of tic symptoms by a year or two, whereas OC symptoms typically emerge after the onset of tics. Approximately half of all children with TS experience comorbid ADHD. Roughly one-half to one-third of TS patients experience clinically significant OCD during the course of their lifetime. Figure 53–1 depicts the clinical course of comorbid ADHD and OCD in children with tic disorder.

B. Instruments for Diagnosis and Measurement

Direct observation including video tic counting procedures is the most objective measure of tic severity. However, the frequency of tics varies dramatically according to setting and activity. Furthermore, many individuals with TS can suppress their symptoms for brief periods. Thus, clinical rating scales are the preferred method for assessing initial tic severity and measuring change in tic severity. The Yale Global Tic Severity Scale (YGTSS) is a clinician-rated, semistructured scale that begins with a systematic inventory of tic symptoms that the clinician rates as present or absent over the past week. Current motor and phonic tics are then rated separately according to number, frequency, intensity, complexity, and interference on 6-point ordinal scales (0 = absent; 1 through 5 for severity) yielding three scores: Total Motor, Total Phonic, and Total Tic Score. Self-report inventories such as the Yale Child

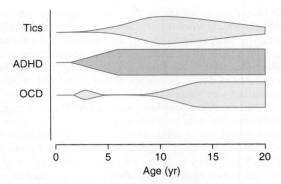

▲ **Figure 53–1** Clinical course of ADHD, OCD, and tic disorders. Age at which tics and coexisting disorders affect patients with TS. Width of bars shows schematically the amount the disorder affects a patient at a particular age. ADHD, attention-deficit/hyperactivity disorder; OCD, obsessive–compulsive disorder. (Reproduced with permission from Leckman JF. Tourette's syndrome. *Lancet.* 2002;360(9345):1577–1586.)

Study Center: TS Obsessive-Compulsive Disorder Symptom Questionnaire completed by the family prior to their initial consultation can be valuable ancillary tools to gain a long-term perspective of the child's developmental course and the natural history of the tic disorder. The YGTSS and Yale Child Study Center TS Obsessive-Compulsive Disorder Symptom Questionnaire are published and freely available for all interested in evaluating tic disorders.

C. Laboratory Findings and Imaging

At present, no laboratory testing or neuroimaging is useful in making a diagnosis of or guiding the management of tic disorders. Strong evidence from neuroimaging and from neuropathological and neurochemical studies implicates abnormalities in the basal ganglia and corticostriatal thalamacocortical circuits in the pathogenesis of TS. On volumetric magnetic resonance imaging (MRI), individuals with TS were found to have smaller caudate volumes than healthy controls. Reduced caudate volume in children with TS has also been associated with increased tic and OCD severity in adulthood. During tic suppression, functional neuroimaging has demonstrated increased activation of the frontal cortex and caudate during willful tic suppression. This increased activation of frontal cortex and caudate is in turn correlated with decreased activity of the globus pallidus, putamen, and thalamus. PET has demonstrated abnormalities of dopamine metabolism as well as evidence of neuroinflammation. Specific findings include increased striatal dopamine receptor and transporter densities and increased amphetamine-induced dopamine release in the putamen as well as activated microglia in the caudate nucleus bilaterally.

Bloch MH, Leckman JF, Zhu H, et al. Caudate volumes in childhood predict symptom severity in adults with TS. *Neurology*. 2005; 65:1253–1258.

Bloch MH, Peterson BS, Scahill L, et al. Adulthood outcome of tic and obsessive-compulsive symptom severity in children with TS. *Arch Pediatr Adolesc Med*. 2006;160:65–69.

Cohen SC, Leckman JF, Bloch MH. Clinical assessment of Tourette syndrome and tic disorders. *Neurosci Biobehav Rev*. 2013;37(6):997–1007.

Cheon KA, Ryu YH, Namkoong K, et al. Dopamine transporter density of the basal ganglia assessed with [^{123}I]IPT SPECT in drug-naive children with Tourette's disorder. *Psychiatry Res*. 2004;130:85–95.

Kumar A, Williams MT, Chugani HT. Evaluation of basal ganglia and thalamic inflammation in children with pediatric autoimmune neuropsychiatric disorders associated with streptococcal infection and Tourette syndrome: a positron emission tomographic (PET) study using ^{11}C-[R]-PK11195. *J Child Neurol*. 2015;30(6):749–756.

Leckman JF, Riddle MA, Hardin MT, et al. The Yale Global Tic Severity Scale: initial testing of a clinician-rated scale of tic severity. *J Am Acad Child Adolesc Psychiatry*. 1989;28:566–573.

Leckman JF, Walker DE, Cohen DJ. Premonitory urges in TS. *Am J Psychiatry*. 1993;150:98–102.

Leckman JF, Zhang H, Vitale A, et al. Course of tic severity in TS: the first two decades. *Pediatrics*. 1998;102:14–19.

Peterson BS, Skudlarski P, Anderson AW, et al. A functional magnetic resonance imaging study of tic suppression in TS. *Arch Gen Psychiatry*. 1998;55:326–333.

Peterson BS, Thomas P, Kane MJ, et al. Basal Ganglia volumes in patients with Gilles de la Tourette syndrome. *Arch Gen Psychiatry*. 2003;60(4):415–424.

Singer HS, Szymanski S, Giuliano J, et al. Elevated intrasynaptic dopamine release in Tourette's syndrome measured by PET. *Am J Psychiatry*. 2002;159:1329–1336.

Sukhodolsky DG, Scahill L, Zhang H, et al. Disruptive behavior in children with Tourette's syndrome: association with ADHD comorbidity, tic severity, and functional impairment. *J Am Acad Child Adolesc Psychiatry*. 2003;42(1):98–105.

▶ Differential Diagnosis

Tic disorders must be distinguished from movement disorders due to general medical conditions (e.g., Huntington disease, stroke, Lesch–Nyhan syndrome, Wilson disease, Sydenham chorea, multiple sclerosis, postviral encephalitis, head injury) or the direct effects of a substance (e.g., akathisia and tardive dyskinesias associated with neuroleptic medication). Table 53–1 defines the major types of movements that must be distinguished from tics. Usually medical and family history, movement morphology, rhythm, and modifying influences are sufficient to making the diagnosis. Onset of movements prior to age 18, waxing-and-waning course of symptoms, and the changing of the specific tic movements over time is characteristic of TS.

In children, tics often need to be distinguished from stereotyped movement disorder or pervasive developmental

Table 53–1 Differential Diagnosis of Tic Disorders

Movement	Description	Common Causes
Tics	Abrupt, stereotyped coordinated movements or vocalizations that often mimic aspects of regular behavior. Premonitory urges are common. Exacerbated by stress and relieved by distraction.	Tourette syndrome, Chronic Tic Disorder, Transient Tic Disorder
Stereotypies	Repetitive, purposeless, and apparently voluntary movements.	Autism, Pervasive Developmental Disorder, Mental Retardation, Stereotyped Movement Disorder
Chorea	Simple, random, irregular, and nonstereotyped movements. Have no premonitory component and increase when the person is distracted. Often flow from one body part to another.	Normal in children less than 8 months of age. Cerebral palsy, Sydenham chorea, hereditary choreas, kernicterus, Lesch–Nyhan syndrome, hypoxia, or stroke
Dyskinesia	Slow, protracted twisting movements interspersed with prolonged states of muscular tension.	Drug-induced, idiopathic torsion dystonia, anoxia or stroke, Wilson disease, Huntington disease, and Parkinson disease
Athetoid	Slow, irregular, writhing movements. Usually involving fingers and toes but occasionally the neck. A "slow chorea."	See Chorea
Myoclonia	Brief, simple, shocklike muscle contractions that may affect individualized muscles or muscle groups.	Physiologic—hiccups, anxiety, or exercise induced. Juvenile myoclonic epilepsy, metabolic encephalopathies, Creutzfeldt–Jakob disease, Wilson disease, and hypoxia
Synkinesis	Involuntary movement associated with a specific voluntary act, such as raising corner of mouth when closing one's eyes.	Physiologic

Table 53–2 Comparison of Tics and Stereotypies

	Tics	Stereotypies
Typical age of onset	4–8 years	2–3 years
Course of symptoms	Waxing and waning	Constant
Timing of movements	Brief and sudden	Continuous, rhythmic, and prolonged
Typical movements	Eye blinking, facial grimace, throat clearing	Arm flapping, rocking
Characteristics of movements	Typically unilateral	Often bilateral
Exacerbated by …	Stress, fatigue	Excitement
Premonitory urges	Present	Absent
Suppressibility	Often for short periods of time	Rare
Comorbid conditions	Obsessive–compulsive disorder, attention-deficit/hyperactivity disorder	Autism Spectrum Disorders
Treatment	Neuroleptics, alpha-2 agonists	No response to medication

disorders. Stereotypies typically have an earlier age of onset than tics, are bilateral rather than unilateral, and have a soothing quality. Table 53–2 contrasts tics and stereotypies. Complex tics often need to be distinguished from the compulsions of OCD. Making this particularly difficult is the high comorbidity between the two conditions. Compulsions are usually performed in response to an obsession and preceded by anxiety, worry, or concern, whereas tics are generally performed in response to a physical sensation or premonitory urges. Compulsions are typically more elaborate than tics and more likely to resemble "normal" behavior. Often, a diagnosis of OCD and a tic disorder is warranted in the same individual.

▶ Treatment

Given the usual waxing and waning course of tic disorders, it is probable that any intervention performed in response to symptom exacerbation will lead to clinical improvement. It is prudent to treat a patient's overall, long-term symptom severity rather than chasing the ebbs and flows of the natural course of the illness. Interventions should be started with the goal of reducing the severity of the tics (and the side effects of treatment) to a level that minimizes social and educational impairment rather than completely eliminating the tics (an aim that will be not be attained in the majority of cases). Many cases of TS can be successfully managed without medication.

When patients present with coexisting ADHD, OCD, depression, or bipolar illness, it is usually better to treat the "comorbid" condition first, as successful treatment of these disorders will often diminish tic severity.

Usual clinical practice focuses initially on educational, supportive, and cognitive–behavioral interventions. Pharmacological treatments are typically held in reserve. Psychoactive medication is best prescribed after educational and supportive interventions have been in place for a period of months and it is clear that the tic symptoms are persistently severe and a source of impairment of self-esteem, relationships with the family or peers, or the child's school performance.

A. Psychoeducation

Educational activities are among the most important interventions available to the clinician. They should be undertaken initially in all patients with tic disorders. Family psychoeducation focuses on the following points:

1. The tics are not voluntary or meant to be intentionally provocative. They typical occur in "bouts" when tics appear in rapid succession followed by tic-free intervals.

2. Premonitory urges are the physical sensations like an itch or before a sneeze that many patients experience prior to performing tics. TS is a sensorimotor disorder. There is also a momentary sense of relief following the tic.

3. Many patients are able to suppress their tics in the short term, but often this is at the expense of increasing discomfort and distraction. It is not uncommon for a child to have relatively minor tics at school and then return home to let loose a bout of tics.

4. Tics will wax and wane over time. Because of the natural ebb and flow of symptoms, any interventions started during an exacerbation of tic severity may appear successful as a result of a natural decline in symptom severity.

5. The illness tends not to be relentlessly progressive, and symptoms usually improve by adulthood. This information contradicts the impressions gained from lay literature that typically focuses on extreme cases—which typically do occur in adulthood.

6. Tics are exacerbated by fatigue, sleeplessness, stress, excitement, and possibly changes in temperature and infections. Tics are often alleviated when a child is deeply engaged in a motor activity such as sports, musical instruments, or dancing. The precise exacerbating and alleviating factors are highly individualized. Healthy habits such as good sleep hygiene and regular exercise can only improve tic symptoms.

7. Education on comorbid ADHD, OCD, learning disabilities, and disruptive or disinhibited behaviors is required. An improvement in these disorders often leads to an improvement in tics.

Resources to help educate parents about tic disorders are available at the Tourette Association of America (formerly called the Tourette Syndrome Association; http://tourette.org).

Perhaps equally important is educating a child's teachers about tic disorders. By educating the educator, clinicians can make significant progress toward securing a positive and supportive classroom environment. Teachers should respond to outbursts of tics with grace and understanding. Repeated scolding is counterproductive: the child may develop a negative attitude to authority figures and may become oppositional and/or reluctant to attend school, and classmates may feel more free to tease the child. A useful compendium of educational accommodations is available at http://www.tourettesyndrome.net/TouretteSyndrome_Plus/.

The education of peers is equally important. Many clinicians encourage patients, families, and teachers to educate peers and classmates about TS. It is remarkable what can be tolerated in the classroom and playground when teachers and peers know what the problem is and learn to disregard it.

B. Behavioral Intervention

Habit reversal training (HRT) is the first psychotherapeutic intervention that has shown promise in reducing tic severity in patients with TS. HRT has been shown to significantly reduce tic symptoms when compared to supportive therapy in randomized, blinded, clinical trials of both children and adults with TS.

HRT has two components: (1) awareness training; and (2) competing response practice. Awareness training has four activities designed to increase an individual's awareness of his own tics, including: (1) response description—in which an individual learns how to describe tic movements and re-enacts them into a mirror; (2) response detection—in which the therapist helps the patient detect the tic by pointing out each tic immediately after it occurs in the session; (3) the early warning procedure—in which an individual learns how to identify the earliest signs of tic occurrence; and (4) situational awareness training—in which an analysis is conducted to identify the high-risk situations where tics are most likely to occur. Competing response practice involves teaching individuals to produce an incompatible physical response (i.e., isometric contraction of tic-opposing muscles) contingent on the urge to perform a tic. At present, Comprehensive Behavioral Intervention for Tics is the frontline treatment for tics (http://tourette.org/Medical/CBIT.html). It includes HRT and psychoeducation aimed at making changes to the individual's day-to-day activities in ways that can be helpful in reducing tics.

C. Pharmacologic Intervention

Table 53–3 depicts the attributes of medication used to treat tic disorder. Neuroleptic medication, dopamine D_2 receptor antagonists, is the most effective tic-suppressant agents in the short term. Among the typical neuroleptics, haloperidol and pimozide are the most efficacious. Long-term experience, however, has been less favorable, and the "reflexive" use of these agents should be avoided. Common side effects include tardive dyskinesia, acute dystonic reactions, sedation, depression, school and social phobia, and weight gain. In many instances, by starting at a low dose and adjusting upward slowly, clinicians can minimize side effects. The goal should be to use as low a dose as possible to render the tics "tolerable." Efforts to stop the tics completely risk overmedication.

Because of the extrapyramidal side effects associated with typical neuroleptics, atypical neuroleptics such as risperidone, olanzapine, aripiprazole, and ziprasidone, are currently the most widely used medications for tic symptoms. These agents have potent $5\text{-}HT_2$ blocking effects as well as more modest blocking effects on dopamine D_2. Double-blind clinical trials have supported the efficacy of risperidone, olanzapine, and ziprasidone. Risperidone and olanzapine are often associated with weight gain and sedation. Ziprasidone use can be associated with QT prolongation in children; thus serial monitoring with electrocardiograms may be necessary.

There is emerging research regarding dopamine D1 receptor antagonists, including ecopipam. Two double-blind, randomized, placebo-controlled studies found ecopipam to be safe and effective for youth, age 7–17, in reducing tic severity and frequency notably without any weight gain (Gilbert et al, 2023, 2018).

Clonidine and guanfacine are potent α_2-receptor agonists that are thought to reduce central noradrenergic activity. Although less effective in relieving tics compared to neuroleptic medication, α_2-receptor agonists have the advantage of improving comorbid ADHD symptoms in patients with tics. The principal side effect associated with clonidine use is sedation. This occurs in 10–20% of subjects but usually abates with continued use. Other side effects are dry mouth, transient hypotension, and rare episodes of worsened behavior. Clonidine should be tapered and not withdrawn abruptly. Guanfacine is generally preferred to clonidine because it is less sedating and not associated with rebound hypertension following withdrawal. Randomized, placebo-controlled trials of the longer-acting formulations of α_2-receptor agonists are currently ongoing. There is no reason to expect better efficacy of patented longer-acting formulations compared to their cheaper, generic short-acting alternatives. In extreme cases, botulinum toxin injections can be used to weaken muscles associated with severe motor or vocal tics temporarily. The most common sites of injection are the neck, shoulders, and throat (for vocal tics).

When comorbid ADHD is the most impairing illness in a patient presenting with comorbid tics, methylphenidate, D-amphetamine, and Adderall are still first-line agents for the management of ADHD. Although there currently exists an FDA contraindication to the use of psychostimulants in children with tic disorders or a family history of TS, data from randomized controlled trials in children with ADHD

Table 53–3 Pharmacological Agents Used to Treat Tic Disorders

Medication	Starting Dose	Titration Schedule	Typical Dosage	Advantages	Side Effects
Neuroleptics					
Typical					
Haloperidol	0.25 mg per day	0.5 mg every 1–2 weeks	0.5–6.0 mg per day	Most effective medication for tics with longest record of use	Tardive dyskinesia, acute dystonic reactions, akathisia, sedation, depression, school and social phobias, and/or weight gain
Pimozide	1.0 mg per day	1.0 mg every 1–2 weeks	1–10 mg per day		
Atypical					
Risperidone	0.25–0.5 mg day	0.25–0.5 mg per week divided BID	1–6 mg per day	Most effective medications for tics, fewer side effects than typical neuroleptics, used to treat comorbid aggression and bipolar disorder	Weight gain, sedation, galactorrhea
Olanzapine	2.5–5 mg per day	2.5–5 mg every 1–2 weeks divided BID	5–20 mg day		Weight gain, sedation, galactorrhea
Ziprasidone	5 mg per day	5 mg every week with BID dosing	20–40 mg per day		Prolonged QT interval, rare heart arrhythmias
Aripiprazole	2 mg per day	2–5 mg every week	10–20 mg per day		Headache, weight gain, insomnia, nausea, akathisia
Alpha2-Agonists					
Guanfacine	0.5 mg QHS	0.5 mg weekly to TID dosing	2–4 mg divided TID	Helps treat comorbid ADHD	Sedation
Clonidine	0.025–0.05 mcg QD or BID	0.05 mcg added on weekly to TID or QID dosing	0.05–0.25 mcg/kg TID or QID		Sedation, hypotension, rebound hypertension on withdrawal

and comorbid tics suggest that these medications improve ADHD symptoms and do not worsen tics, on average. The combination of clonidine and methylphenidate is efficacious according to one large multisite, randomized controlled clinical trial. Atomoxetine, a nonstimulant medication used to treat ADHD, is beneficial to children with both conditions.

D. Neurosurgical Procedures

Neurosurgical intervention for TS is reserved to adults with intractable tics that severely affect social functioning. Originally, neurosurgical lesioning was used to treat the most severe, treatment-refractory cases. With the successful use of deep brain stimulation (DBS), a relatively reversible, stereotactic technique in the treatment of other movement disorders, DBS has been proposed as the preferred method of neurosurgical treatment for medically intractable tics. DBS has several advantages over previous neurosurgical lesioning procedures: it lacks many of the permanent complications associated with lesioning procedures (the electrodes can be removed); it allows access to otherwise inaccessible anatomical sites; and it enables bilateral stimulation. DBS thus holds great promise for adult patients with intractable tics. However, neither the appropriate site of electrode placement nor the parameters of electrode stimulation have been established in controlled clinical studies. In sum, DBS is not advisable for any but the most severely affected adults with TS. Children

with tics will probably get better with time. Those most severely affected with TS will probably benefit more from the procedure when the protocol has been refined over the coming years. Based on published case reports, the preferred sites of electrode placement are either the midline thalamic nuclei or the globus pallidus, pars internus (GPi). A patient who considers this intervention should be careful regarding the neurosurgical team. Every possible medical option should be exhausted first. The DBS team should consist of a neurosurgeon specialized in the stereotactic technique, a neurologist, a psychiatrist trained in movement disorders and their comorbidities, and a specially trained nursing staff. The utmost caution is warranted for everyone who applies this technique until the surgical method is improved and the method has undergone rigorous scientific testing.

Cohen SC, Mulqueen JM, Ferracioli-Oda E, et al. Meta-analysis: risk of tics associated with psychostimulant use in randomized, placebo-controlled trials. *J Am Acad Child Adolesc Psychiatry*. 2015;54(9):728–736.

Gilbert DL, Murphy TK, Jankovic J, et al. Ecopipam, a D1 receptor antagonist, for treatment of Tourette syndrome in children: a randomized, placebo-controlled crossover study. *Mov Disord*. 2018;33(8):1272–1280.

Gilbert DL, Dubow JS, Cunniff TM, Wanaski SP, Atkinson SD, Mahableshwarkar AR. Ecopipam for Tourette syndrome: a randomized trial. *Pediatrics*. 2023;151(2)

Piacentini J, Woods DW, Scahill L, et al. Behavior therapy for children with Tourette disorder: a randomized controlled trial. *JAMA*. 2010;303(19):1929–1937.

Scahill L, Chappell PB, Kim YS, et al. A placebo-controlled study of guanfacine in the treatment of children with tic disorders and attention deficit hyperactivity disorder. *Am J Psychiatry*. 2001;158: 1067–1074.

Shapiro ES, Shapiro AK, Fulop G, et al. Controlled study of haloperidol, pimozide, and placebo for the treatment of Gilles de la TS. *Arch Gen Psychiatry*. 1989;46:722–730.

Schrock LE, Mink JW, Woods DW, et al. Tourette syndrome deep brain stimulation: a review and updated recommendations. *Mov Disord*. 2015;30(4):448–471.

Tourette's Syndrome Study Group. Treatment of ADHD in children with tics: a randomized controlled trial. *Neurology*. 2002;58(4): 527–536.

Weisman H, Qureshi IA, Leckman JF, et al. Systematic review: pharmacological treatment of tic disorders—efficacy of antipsychotic and alpha-2 adrenergic agonist agents. *Neurosci Biobehav Rev*. 2013;37:1162–1171.

Wilhelm S, Peterson AL, Piacentini J, et al. Randomized trial of behavior therapy for adults with Tourette syndrome. *Arch Gen Psychiatry*. 2012;69:795–803.

Woods DW: Habit reversal treatment manual for tic disorders. In: Woods DW, Miltenberger RG, eds. *Tic Disorders, Trichotillomania, and Other Repetitive Behavior Disorders: Behavioral Approaches to Analysis and Treatment*. Boston: Kluwer Academic; 2001: 97–132.

Yoo HK, Joung YS, Lee JS, et al. A multicenter, randomized, double-blind, placebo-controlled study of aripiprazole in children and adolescents with Tourette's disorder. *J Clin Psychiatry*. 2013;74(8):e772–e780.

▶ Clinical Course and Prognosis

The onset of TS is usually characterized by the appearance of simple, transient motor tics that affect the face (typically eye blinking) around the age of 5–7 years. Over time, simple motor tics generally progress in a rostrocaudal direction, affecting other areas of the face, followed by the head, neck, arms, and, last and less frequently, the lower extremities. With time, vocal tics often appear, tics become increasingly complex, and premonitory urges appear. TS symptoms generally peak in severity between the ages of 10 and 12 years. Although the most severe TS cases are adults with relentless tics including self-injurious and dystonic tics, one-half to two-thirds of cases experience a marked reduction of symptoms by their late teens and early 20s, with one-third to one-half of these patients becoming virtually asymptotic in adulthood.

Given that tics in children are often ephemeral, producing social and educational impairment when the tics are at their worst but little afterward, the importance of minimizing the social consequences (peer teasing, poor self-esteem, social withdrawal) and educational consequences of tics cannot be overstated in determining long-term outcome. The proper management of and vigilance for psychiatric conditions comorbid with tic disorder, such as ADHD and OCD, is also crucial. Ensuring that adolescents and adults with a history of tic disorders refrain from using substances known to induce tics (such as amphetamines or crack/cocaine) likely improves their prognosis.

CHILDHOOD-ONSET OBSESSIVE COMPULSIVE DISORDER

ICD-10 Diagnostic Criteria

Obsessive-compulsive Disorder F42 (300.3)

The essential feature is recurrent obsessional thoughts or compulsive acts. Obsessional thoughts are ideas, images, or impulses that enter the patient's mind again and again in a stereotyped form. They are almost invariably distressing and the patient often tries, unsuccessfully, to resist them. They are, however, recognized as his or her own thoughts, even though they are involuntary and often repugnant. Compulsive acts or rituals are stereotyped behaviors that are repeated again and again. They are not inherently enjoyable, nor do they result in the completion of inherently useful tasks. Their function is to prevent some objectively unlikely event, often involving harm to or caused by the patient, which he or she fears might otherwise occur. Usually, this behavior is recognized by the patient as pointless or ineffectual and repeated attempts are made to resist. Anxiety is almost invariably present. If compulsive acts are resisted the anxiety gets worse.

Predominantly Obsessional Thoughts or Ruminations F42.0 (300.2)

These may take the form of ideas, mental images, or impulses to act, which are nearly always distressing to the subject. Sometimes the ideas are an indecisive, endless consideration of alternatives, associated with an inability to make trivial but necessary decisions in day-to-day living. The relationship between obsessional ruminations and depression is particularly close and a diagnosis of obsessive-compulsive disorder should be preferred only if ruminations arise or persist in the absence of a depressive episode.

Predominantly Compulsive Acts [Obsessional Rituals] F42.1 (300.2)

The majority of compulsive acts are concerned with cleaning (particularly hand washing), repeated checking to ensure that a potentially dangerous situation has not been allowed to develop, or orderliness and tidiness. Underlying the overt behavior is a fear, usually of danger either to or caused by the patient, and the ritual is an ineffectual or symbolic attempt to avert that danger.

Mixed Obsessional Thoughts and Acts F42.2

Other Obsessive-compulsive Disorders F42.8

Obsessive-compulsive Disorder, Unspecified F42.9 (300.3)

Reproduced with permission from International Statistical Classification of Diseases and Related Health Problems 10th Revision (ICD-10) Version for 2010. Geneva: World Health Organization; 2010.

A child must have either obsessions or compulsions, but not necessarily both, to qualify for a diagnosis of OCD. Obsessions are persistent ideas, thoughts, impulses, or images that are experienced as intrusive and inappropriate and that cause marked anxiety or distress. Compulsions are repetitive behaviors (e.g., hand washing, checking) or mental acts (e.g., counting, repeating words silently) the goal of which is to prevent or reduce anxiety or distress, not to provide pleasure or gratification. The current DSM-5 criteria, but not the ICD-10 criteria, require that the obsessions or compulsions be severe enough to cause significant distress or impairment or be time-consuming (taking up more than 1 hour a day). It is not uncommon for children, especially younger children with OCD, to have clinically significant compulsions without the insight or ability to articulate any obsessions. This condition is known in DSM-5 as OCD with poor insight. Tic-related OCD is also a "specifier" in DSM-5 indicating that the individual has a current or past history of a tic disorder.

▶ **General Considerations**

A. Major Etiologic Theories

Abnormalities in the serotonin system appear to be central to the pathogenesis of OCD. Evidence favoring the serotonin hypothesis for OCD comes from the fact that selective serotonin reuptake inhibitors (SSRIs) such as fluoxetine, fluvoxamine, sertraline, and paroxetine are the most effective medications for OCD. The relative effectiveness of clomipramine, a serotonin-selective tricyclic antidepressant for the treatment of OCD, compared to other tricyclic agents, lends strength to this hypothesis. Exacerbation of OCD symptoms with the administration of meta-chlorophenylpiperazine, a serotonin agonist, further supports the hypothesis. High platelet serotonin levels and a high cerebrospinal fluid concentration of 5-hydroxyindole acetic acid, a major metabolite of serotonin, are correlated with treatment response to clomipramine in children with OCD. Evidence for the presence of abnormalities in other neurotransmitter systems, especially dopamine, is evidenced by the successful augmentation of SSRI pharmacotherapy with neuroleptic

medication and the high comorbidity of childhood OCD with tic disorder.

Consistent with the serotonin hypothesis, basal ganglia—frontal lobe dysfunction has been implicated in the pathogenesis of OCD. Fluorodeoxyglucose-PET studies in children and adults with OCD have demonstrated hypermetabolism in the caudate, orbitofrontal cortex, and anterior cingulate, compared to normal controls, during resting conditions and during symptom provocation. These metabolic abnormalities were reversed with successful behavioral or pharmacological treatment. The high comorbidity of OCD with basal ganglia disorders such as TS and Sydenham chorea is consistent with this theory.

The frequent presence of obsessive–compulsive symptoms in Sydenham chorea suggests the importance of autoimmune processes in the pathogenesis of OCD. This observation led to the finding of a small subgroup of children with OCD or tic disorder who had pediatric autoimmune neuropsychiatric disorder associated with streptococcal infections (PANDAS). PANDAS cases characteristically have an abrupt, prepubertal onset of clinical symptoms (tic, OCD, or both) after an infection with group A β-hemolytic streptococcus (GAS). PANDAS cases typically have a dramatic, episodic course and usually have coexisting choreiform movements and a range of other neuropsychiatric symptoms. However, the diagnosis of PANDAS remains controversial and the proportion of true PANDAS cases among all children with OCD may be relatively small. Nonetheless, the observation of OCD symptoms in Sydenham chorea and the characterization of this unique PANDAS cohort of OCD and tic patients is consistent with the relevance of autoimmune and infectious factors to the pathogenesis of OCD.

The ongoing controversy about PANDAS has led to an effort to identify a more rigorously defined clinical phenotype (Pediatric Acute-onset Neuropsychiatric Syndrome [PANS]) while leaving open the potential etiological role of antecedent GAS infections or other postinfectious inflammatory processes. The cardinal feature of PANS is the sudden onset (within 24–48 hours) of OCD or of a restrictive eating disorder accompanied by two or more sudden-onset neuropsychiatric symptoms (anxiety, emotional lability, irritability, developmental regression, sudden deterioration in academic performance, motor abnormalities [tics, dysgraphia], and/or sleep disturbances, enuresis, or urinary frequency).

Leckman JF, King RA, Gilbert DL, et al. Streptococcal upper respiratory tract infections and exacerbations of tic and obsessive-compulsive symptoms: a prospective longitudinal study. *J Am Acad Child Adolesc Psychiatry.* 2011;50(2):108–118.

Murphy TK, Gerardi DM, Leckman JF. Pediatric acute-onset neuropsychiatric syndrome. *Psychiatr Clin North Am.* 2014; 37(3):353–374.

Rosso IM, Olson EA, Britton JC, S, et al., Brain white matter integrity and association with age at onset in pediatric obsessive-compulsive disorder. *Biol Mood Anxiety Disord.* 2014;4(1):13.

Saxena S, Rauch SL. Functional neuroimaging and the neuroanatomy of obsessive-compulsive disorder. *Psychiatr Clin North Am.* 2000;23(3):563–586.

Swedo SE, Leckman JF, Rose NR. From research subgroup to clinical syndrome: modifying the PANDAS criteria to describe PANS (Pediatric Acute-onset Neuropsychiatric Syndrome). *Pediatr Therapeut.* 2012;2:113. doi:10.4172/2161-0665.1000113

Swedo SE, Leonard HL, Mittleman BB, et al. Identification of children with pediatric autoimmune neuropsychiatric disorders associated with streptococcal infections by a marker associated with rheumatic fever. *Am J Psychiatry.* 1997;154(1):110–112.

B. Genetic, Immune, and Environmental Factors

Convincing evidence exists that OCD has a hereditable component. The strongest evidence of hereditability comes from family and twin studies. Four family studies, each examining between 300 and 500 first-degree relatives of OCD patients, have estimated the rate of OCD to be 5- to 10-fold greater in first-degree relatives of OCD patients compared to the relatives of psychiatrically healthy controls. Twin studies have suggested an 87% concordance rate among monozygotic twins with the disorder compared to 47% for dizygotic twins. Because monozygotic and dizygotic twins theoretically share similar environmental influences but different degrees of genetic relatedness, the higher rate of an illness among monozygotic twins is strong evidence of a hereditary component.

There is considerable evidence of a shared heritability of TS and OCD—that some of the same genes may contribute to the phenotypic expression of both conditions. The observation that relatives of OCD patients (without comorbid tics) have an elevated rate of tic disorder compared to controls, and that relatives of TS patients (irrespective of comorbid OCD) have significantly elevated rates of OCD compared to relatives of normal controls, supports this hypothesis. Early age of onset (<18 years) has also been found to be associated with increased familial risk.

Studies examining potential genetic mechanisms have yet to identify the genes involved in the phenotypic expression of OCD. Among the most promising candidate genes for OCD are the serotonin transporter (SLC6A4) on 17q11 and the high-affinity neuronal excitatory amino acid transporter (SLAC1A1/ECCA-1) located on 9p24.

Genetic studies of OCD have been hampered by the fact that OCD is a complex disorder with much heterogeneity in its clinical phenotypes, and the current ignorance of the molecular mechanisms underlying the disorder. It is hoped that the development of quantitative endophenotypes with clinical, neuropsychological, imaging, or electrophysiological measures will advance the field.

With the exception of the PANDAS hypothesis, systematic efforts to identify environmental factors associated with OCD have lagged behind genetic studies. In addition to antecedent GAS infections, current speculation focuses on perinatal adversity, parental child-rearing patterns, psychosocial stress (particularly the loss or threatened loss of close family members), traumatic brain injury, and exposure to drugs of abuse.

Browne HA, Gair SL, Scharf JM, Grice DE. Genetics of obsessive-compulsive disorder and related disorders. *Psychiatr Clin North Am.* 2014;37(3):319–335.

Hu XZ, Lipsky RH, Zhu G, et al. Serotonin transporter promoter gain-of-function genotypes are linked to obsessive-compulsive disorder. *Am J Hum Genet.* 2006;78(5):815–826.

Nestadt G, Samuels J, Riddle M, et al. A family study of obsessive-compulsive disorder. *Arch Gen Psychiatry.* 2000;57(4):358–363.

Pauls DL, Abramovitch A, Rauch SL, Geller DA. Obsessive-compulsive disorder: an integrative genetic and neurobiological perspective. *Nat Rev Neurosci.* 2014;15(6):410–424.

Pauls DL, Alsobrook JP, Goodman W, Rasmussen S, Leckman JF. A family study of obsessive-compulsive disorder. *Am J Psychiatry,* 1995;152(1):76–84.

Stewart SE, Yu D, Scharf JM, et al. Genome-wide association study of obsessive-compulsive disorder. *Mol Psychiatry.* 2013; 18(7):788–798.

Yu D, Mathews CA, Scharf JM, et al. Cross-disorder genome-wide analyses suggest a complex genetic relationship between Tourette's syndrome and OCD. *Am J Psychiatry.* 2015;172(1):82–93.

C. Epidemiology

Results from the Epidemiological Catchment Area study, which assessed more than 18,500 adults with structured diagnostic interviews, estimated the lifetime prevalence of OCD among adults between 1.9 and 3.3%. Epidemiological studies of adolescents provide similar estimates, in the range of 1.9–3.6%. The sex distribution of these epidemiologic studies suggests that OCD affects males and females equally after puberty. However, males have an earlier age of onset than females, their initial presentation typically occurring well before puberty.

Alvarenga PG, do Rosario MC, Cesar RC, et al. Obsessive-compulsive symptoms are associated with psychiatric comorbidities, behavioral and clinical problems: a population-based study of Brazilian school children. *Eur Child Adolesc Psychiatry.* 2016;25(2):175–182.

Flament MF, Whitaker A, Rapoport JL, et al. Obsessive compulsive disorder in adolescence: an epidemiological study. *J Am Acad Child Adolesc Psychiatry.* 1988;27(6):764–771.

Zohar AH, Ratzoni G, Pauls DL, et al. An epidemiological study of obsessive-compulsive disorder and related disorders in Israeli adolescents. *J Am Acad Child Adolesc Psychiatry.* 1992;31(6):1057–1061.

CHAPTER 53

▶ Clinical Findings

A. Signs & Symptoms

OCD is characterized by obsessions (unwanted, intrusive thoughts, images or impulses) and compulsions (repetitive behavioral or mental rituals) or both. Because obsessions and compulsions are usually recognized by the child as nonsensical, inappropriate, or unreasonable, they are often kept hidden from both parents and therapists. In these cases (especially in younger children), the parental observation of compulsive behaviors (i.e., repeated checking of locks, washing or cleaning objects, hoarding) or physical signs of compulsive behaviors (i.e., chapped hands or ulcerations from excessive washing) may be the only definite signs of the disorder. Because the vast majority of OCD patients have insight into their condition, a detailed clinical history of obsessive and compulsive behaviors from the child and his parents is sufficient to make a diagnosis of OCD. In order to qualify for the diagnosis of OCD, obsessions and compulsions must be time-consuming (longer than 1 hour a day), and cause both distress and impairment.

OCD has a bimodal distribution of age of onset. One peak of incidence occurs in the peripubertal years, and the other in early adulthood. There are several important differences between pediatric and adult-onset OCD. Pediatric-onset OCD has a male predominance (unlike adult-onset OCD cases where slightly more females are affected), has a stronger family history of OCD, and has higher rates of comorbid ADHD and tic disorders. The content of obsessions and compulsions in OCD also varies across the age range. Children with OCD have much higher rates of aggressive obsessions, such as fear of harm to self or others or a fear of a catastrophic event. They are also more likely to have limited insight, being unable to recognize that their obsessions and compulsions are excessive and unreasonable. Adolescents with OCD have a higher proportion of obsessions with sexual and religious themes, whereas cleaning- and contamination-related symptoms are prevalent at all ages. Those with OCD and comorbid tics have higher rates of intrusive violent or aggressive thoughts and images, concerns with symmetry and exactness, hoarding and counting rituals, and touching and tapping compulsions. Compulsions designed to eliminate a perceptually tinged mental feeling of unease, coined in the literature as "just right" perceptions, are characteristic of patients with OCD and comorbid tics.

There is also a very high degree of comorbid psychiatric illness in children with OCD. In clinical samples, around 80% of children with OCD had comorbid illness. Tic disorders, ADHD, and anxiety disorder, such as separation anxiety disorder, are particularly common among children with OCD, whereas depression and anxiety disorder are particularly common in adolescent patients. Each of these comorbidities affects one-fifth to one-third of OCD patients who reach

clinical attention. Proper screening for comorbid illnesses as well as the analysis of the particular content and character of each patient's OCD symptoms is crucial to designing a proper pharmacological and behavioral treatment strategy. The presence of comorbid tic disorder is a particularly important comorbidity to screen for, as evidenced in the new DSM-5 criteria. OCD patients with comorbid tics have been demonstrated to have a poorer response to SSRI pharmacotherapy and a greater likelihood of responding to antipsychotic augmentation.

Geller DA, Biederman J, Faraone S, et al. Developmental aspects of obsessive compulsive disorder: findings in children, adolescents, and adults. *J Nerv Ment Dis.* 2001;189(7):471–477.

Leckman JF, Grice DE, Bar LC, et al. Tic-related vs. non-tic-related obsessive compulsive disorder. *Anxiety.* 1994;1(5)208–215.

Leckman JF, Walker DE, Goodman WK, et al. "Just right" perceptions associated with compulsive behavior in Tourette's syndrome. *Am J Psychiatry.* 1994;151(5)675–680.

B. Instruments for Diagnosis and Measurement

The Yale–Brown Obsessive Compulsive Scale (Y-BOCS) is the standard clinical rating scale used to assess symptom severity in adults with OCD. The Y-BOCS is a 10-item ordinal scale (0–4) that rates the severity, separately, for both obsessions and compulsions according to the time occupied, the degree of interference, subjective distress, the level of internal resistance, and the subjective degree of control. The Children's Yale–Brown Obsessive Compulsive Scale (CY-BOCS) is a similarly designed scale for use in children with OCD. CY-BOCS and Y-BOCS scales differ only according to the accompanying symptom screening checklist, the CY-BOCS being more developmentally appropriate for children. Both scales have been validated for use in their representative patient populations, and both are sensitive to changes in symptom severity with treatment. Both scales rate OCD symptoms on a scale with range from 0 (no symptoms) to 40 (severe OCD). A score less than 8 is considered as subclinical, over 16 as clinically significant, and over 24 as moderate to severe. A reduction in the Y-BOCS score of 25 or 35% and a final Y-BOCS rating of less than 16, is considered the criterion for response to treatment. The Y-BOCS rating scale takes approximately 5 minutes to complete after the initial symptom checklist and serves as a good measure to assess symptom change.

As OCD is a heterogeneous condition with multiple genetic and environmental influences, researchers have stressed the importance of accurately characterizing the differences between types of OCD patients, so as to create more homogenous populations for genetic and neuroimaging studies. With this aim, the Dimensional Yale–Brown Obsessive Compulsive Scale (DY-BOCS) was created. The DY-BOCS uses a combination of self-report checklists and clinician ratings to assess the presence and severity of OCD symptoms in six thematically related dimensions of obsessions and compulsions. The six symptom dimensions are aggression/harm, cleaning/contamination, symmetry/ordering, religious/sexual, hoarding, and miscellaneous. The DY-BOCS rates symptom severity based on time occupied, subjective distress, and the interference living with obsessions and compulsions causes within these six domains.

Goodman WK, Price LH, Rasmussen SA, et al. The Yale–Brown Obsessive Compulsive Scale. I. Development, use, and reliability. *Arch Gen Psychiatry*. 1989;46(11):1006–1011.

Goodman WK, Price LH, Rasmussen SA, et al. The Yale–Brown Obsessive Compulsive Scale. II. Validity. *Arch Gen Psychiatry*. 1989;46(11):1012–1016.

Rosario-Campos MC, Miguel EC, Quatrano S, et al. The Dimensional Yale–Brown Obsessive-Compulsive Scale (DY-BOCS): an instrument for assessing obsessive-compulsive symptom dimensions. *Mol Psychiatry*. 2006;11(5):495–504.

Scahill L, Riddle MA, McSwiggin-Hardin M, et al. Children's Yale–Brown Obsessive Compulsive Scale: reliability and validity. *J Am Acad Child Adolesc Psychiatry*. 1997;36(6):844–852.

C. Laboratory Findings and Imaging

As yet, no laboratory or neuroimaging findings are useful in either diagnosing OCD or predicting treatment response or prognosis. Clinical findings are sufficient to make the diagnosis of OCD and to formulate a proper treatment strategy. Neuroimaging studies have supported the hypothesis that orbitofrontal-subcortical dysfunction is involved in the pathogenesis of the disorder. PET symptom provocation has demonstrated hypermetabolism in the anterior-lateral orbitofrontal cortex, caudate nucleus, and paralimbic areas when patients are exposed to situations that provoke OC symptoms compared to neutral stimulus periods. PET studies have implicated hypermetabolism in the orbitofrontal cortex and caudate nucleus in subjects with OCD compared to normal controls, during resting conditions. Hypermetabolism in these areas reverses with successful SSRI pharmacotherapy or CBT. Structural volumetric MRI studies of adults found increased left-sided gray orbitofrontal volumes and reduced overall orbitofrontal volumes compared to normal controls. MRI studies examining psychotropic-naive children with OCD found increased anterior cingulate gray matter and globus pallidus volumes, and reduced striatal volumes, compared to normal controls.

Brem S, Hauser TU, Iannaccone R, et al. Neuroimaging of cognitive brain function in paediatric obsessive compulsive disorder: a review of literature and preliminary meta-analysis. *J Neural Transm (Vienna)*. 2012;119(11):1425–1448.

Rosenberg DR, Keshavan MS, O'Hearn KM, et al. Frontostriatal measurement in treatment-naive children with obsessive-compulsive disorder. *Arch Gen Psychiatry*. 1997;54(9):824–830.

Saxena S, Rauch SL. Functional neuroimaging and the neuroanatomy of obsessive-compulsive disorder. *Psychiatr Clin North Am*. 2000;23(3):563–586.

Szeszko PR, MacMillan S, McMeniman M, et al. Brain structural abnormalities in psychotropic drug-naive pediatric patients with obsessive-compulsive disorder. *Am J Psychiatry*. 2004;161(6):1049–1056.

▶ Differential Diagnosis

Recurrent thoughts, images, and impulses similar to the obsessions present in OCD characterize many other mental disorders. For instance, in Major Depressive Disorder it is not uncommon for patients to have persistent thoughts about unpleasant circumstances, personal worthlessness, or possible alternative actions. The ruminative thoughts of depression can be distinguished from OCD by the fact that the ruminations are a mood-congruent aspect of depression, and ego-syntonic, compared to obsessions of OCD, which are ego-dystonic. There is a high comorbidity between depression and OCD; thus it is common for both ruminative thoughts of depression and OCD to be present in the same individual. The symptoms of other anxiety disorders can mimic the symptoms of OCD. Generalized Anxiety Disorder is characterized by excessive worry, but such worries can be distinguished from obsessions by the fact that the person experiences them as excessive concerns about real-life circumstances, whereas obsessions in OCD are generally experienced as excessive and unreasonable. Obsessions in OCD must also be distinguished from those mental disorders characterized by excessive worry about their appearance (body dysmorphic disorder, anorexia, and bulimia), a situation or circumstance (specific phobia), or a serious illness due to misinterpretation of normal bodily sensations (hypochondrias).

In children, the obsessions in OCD concerning the fear of harm coming to self or others must be distinguished from the concerns of harm to others typical of separation anxiety disorder. The two conditions can often be distinguished by the observation that obsessions in OCD are usually accompanied by specific compulsive rituals (i.e., checking or counting), whereas in separation anxiety disorder the compulsive actions are less stereotyped. Furthermore, the presence of other OCD symptoms besides fear of harm can aid in diagnostic clarification.

The repetitive stereotypies of children with autism spectrum disorders and intellectual impairment can resemble the compulsions of OCD. However, these stereotypies can usually be easily distinguished from OCD by the child's accompanying symptoms, as well as the fact that autistic stereotypies are usually soothing or pleasurable, whereas compulsions are ego-dystonic. Stereotypies can also be observed in children with normal social skills and cognitive ability. Complex tics in children with TS can also mimic the compulsions of OCD. Complex tics are usually preceded by a premonitory urge, whereas compulsions are preceded by anxiety or a specific obsession. The high comorbidity of tic disorders and OCD often makes this distinction difficult or arbitrary.

▶ Treatment

CBT and pharmacotherapy with serotonin reuptake inhibitors are effective therapies in the treatment of pediatric and adult OCD. CBT is a first-line treatment for OCD across all age ranges. However, the combination therapy of CBT and SSRIs is typically superior to either CBT or pharmacotherapy alone. Unless there is a strong clinical reason to do otherwise, all children with OCD at a minimum should be offered CBT.

A. Behavioral

CBT for children with OCD is based on exposure and response prevention (ERP). The therapist must first examine and take a detailed history of the nature of a child's specific OC symptoms. Symptom checklists such as those that accompany the CY-BOCS and Y-BOCS rating scales are useful. The therapist working with child and parent then develops a hierarchy of exposures, both direct and imaginary, which trigger the anxiety associated with obsessions of OCD (e.g., touching a toilet seat for a child with contamination concerns, or imagining a parent in a car accident for a child with fears of harm to others). The therapist enters into a contract with child and parent to work on completing these exposures over a set time frame, usually a couple of months. The therapist then engages in the specific exposures with the child (and sometimes the parent) over the next few treatment sessions, with the child agreeing not to engage in his compulsions in response to the anxiety produced. During exposures, the child reports on his level of anxiety, using subjective units of distress, a so-called anxiety thermometer. Child and parent are given similar exposure assignments to complete after each session. With increased duration of exposure and with subsequent exposures, the child's anxiety lessens (without performing the compulsions), helping him to overcome the OCD. ERP treatment manuals for children with OCD are freely available and also provide techniques for helping children deal with stress and anxiety, such as relaxation therapy, and exercises to illustrate other aspects of CBT, such as helping the child to recognize cognitive distortions common in OCD, such as overestimation of risk, all-or-nothing thinking, overcoming the need for certainty, and recognizing excessive feelings of responsibility or guilt. The most important piece during CBT is for parents to understand the concepts so that they can model and teach these behaviors to their children. If an ERP therapist is not available, there are multiple therapeutic manuals that present these treatments in a form that can be learned by a clinician in a time-efficient manner. Self-help

books are available to allow parents and children to engage in aspects of treatment themselves.

Another important behavior approach is with the parents to limit "family accommodation." Family accommodation describes changes that a parent makes in their own behavior to ostensibly help their child (e.g., repeatedly reassuring the child that they are "OK" when the child obsesses about harm coming to their parent). Family accommodation is associated with more severe psychopathology and poorer clinical outcomes. Indeed, family accommodation can lead to more severe OCD as it inadvertently reinforces the child's symptoms. It can also lead to coercive and aggressive behavior by the child that targets a caregiver (e.g., if the mother does not promptly comply with the child's request for reassurance, the child may get upset and act out). Supportive Parenting for Anxious Childhood Emotions is a therapeutic approach to family accommodation.

B. Pharmacologic

SSRIs and clomipramine are the first-line pharmacotherapy for children and adults with OCD. Clomipramine, fluoxetine, fluvoxamine, paroxetine, sertraline, and citalopram have demonstrated superior efficacy to placebo in randomized, double-blind, placebo-controlled clinical trials. Table 53–4 depicts the traditional starting and target doses for SSRIs across the age spectrum. The number-needed-to-treat (NNT) to produce a clinical treatment response (as defined by a 25–35% reduction in CY-BOCS scores) has ranged from 4 to 6 in double-blind, placebo-controlled studies. Based on cumulative studies, SSRI pharmacotherapy will lead to an average 6.5- to 9-point decline in CY-BOCS ratings and a 30–38% reduction in symptom severity. In a meta-analysis of pharmacotherapy trials for pediatric OCD, Geller et al (2003) reported that clomipramine was superior to the SSRIs for the treatment of pediatric OCD, and that the other SSRIs currently used to treat OCD were roughly equivalent. Clomipramine may be superior to other serotonergic agents because of its unique pharmacodynamic properties: it is metabolized into desmethylclomipramine, a secondary amine tricyclic antidepressant identical to desipramine with a chloride atom substitution. Desipramine has been reported to be effective in treating TS and ADHD. Clomipramine may thus be more effective in treating the comorbidities of OCD than traditional SSRIs are. However, the meta-regression results should be used with caution, considering that no studies have directly compared the efficacy of clomipramine to other SSRIs in children with OCD. Studies comparing these agents in adults have found no significant differences.

Despite modest evidence suggesting it might be more effective than SSRIs in children, clomipramine is rarely used as the initial pharmacological agent, because of its worse side-effect profile. Because of its potential arrhythmogenic properties, a baseline electrocardiogram and a detailed screening

Table 53–4 Pharmacotherapy for Obsessive–Compulsive Disorder (All Doses Listed Below Are mgs Per Day)

Medication	Starting Dose			Typical Dose Range	
	Child	Adolescent	Adult	Child	Adult
Clomipramine	12.5–25	25	25	50–200	100–250
Sertraline	12.5–25	25–50	50	100–200	150–250
Fluoxetine	5–10	10–20	20	20–80	20–80
Fluvoxamine	12.5–25	25–50	50	100–300	100–300
Paroxetine	5–10	10	10–20	20–60	40–60
Citalopram	5–10	10	20	20–40	40
Escitalopram	2.5–5	5	10	10–40	20–40

for a personal and family history for cardiac problems should be undertaken. Guidelines for unacceptable ECG indices for use of clomipramine have been issued by the FDA. They include: (1) PR interval >200 msec; (2) QRS interval >30% increased over baseline or >120 msec; (3) blood pressure >140/90; (4) heart rate >130 bpm, or (5) QTc >450 msec. Moreover, clomipramine also has a worse side-effect profile than SSRIs, with high rates of somnolence, gastrointestinal upset, reduced seizure threshold, and anticholinergic side effects. Despite these concerns, clomipramine is a valuable treatment for children who do not respond to pharmacotherapy with one or more SSRIs.

Thus, SSRIs are the initial pharmacologic treatment for children with OCD. There is no evidence in the currently available clinical trials literature that one SSRI is more effective than another. Starting and target doses for SSRIs in children are depicted in Table 53–4. Pharmacological treatment for patients with SSRIs should continue for 2–3 months at the maximal tolerated dose of medication before a child can be considered a nonresponder, as many OCD patients respond only after many weeks of SSRI monotherapy.

C. Augmentation Strategies

Approximately half of all children on SSRIs will fail to respond, despite adequate dosage. If CBT has not been tried, it should be done at this point. In adults with OCD, up to 25% of nonresponders respond if treated with another SSRI or clomipramine. Furthermore, augmentation with neuroleptic medications has been shown to be effective in the treatment of adults with OCD. The NNT to produce a clinically significant treatment response (35% reduction in Y-BOCS ratings) in adults with OCD was 4.5 (95% CI: 3.2–7.1). Neuroleptic augmentation is particularly effective in OCD patients suffering from comorbid tics (NNT = 2.3), a result not surprising because these medications are the mainstay of the treatment of tics. The dose of neuroleptic medication used to augment SSRIs is much lower than that used to treat psychosis or aggressive behavior.

Bloch MH, Landeros-Weisenberger A, Kelmendi B, et al. A systematic review: antipsychotic augmentation with treatment refractory obsessive-compulsive disorder. *Mol Psychiatry.* 2006;11(7):622–632.

Geller DA, Biederman J, Stewart SE, et al. Which SSRI? A meta-analysis of pharmacotherapy trials in pediatric obsessive-compulsive disorder. *Am J Psychiatry.* 2003;160(11):1919–1928.

Lebowitz ER, Scharfstein LA, Jones J. Comparing family accommodation in pediatric obsessive-compulsive disorder, anxiety disorders, and non-anxious children. *Depress Anxiety.* 2014;31(12):1018–1025.

Lebowitz ER, Omer H. *Treating Childhood and Adolescent Anxiety: A Guide for Caregivers.* Hoboken, NJ: John Wiley & Sons; 2013.

March JS, Mulle K. *OCD in Children and Adolescents: A Cognitive-Behavioral Treatment Manual.* New York: Guilford Press; 1998.

Pediatric OCD Treatment Study (POTS) Team. Cognitive-behavior therapy, sertraline, and their combination for children and adolescents with obsessive-compulsive disorder: the Pediatric OCD Treatment Study (POTS) randomized controlled trial. *JAMA.* 2004;292(16):1969–1976.

Pittenger C, Bloch MH. Pharmacological treatment of obsessive-compulsive disorder. *Psychiatr Clin North Am.* 2014;237(3):375–391.

Prognosis

Based on results from the Pediatric OCD Treatment Study and similarly designed randomized, double-blind clinical trials of pharmacological and behavioral treatments for OCD, one-third to one-half of children with OCD will experience a treatment response after 12 weeks of either behavioral or pharmacological treatment. The likelihood of a treatment response is higher when CBT and pharmacotherapy with an SSRI are combined. The durability of improvement with these two treatment modalities is less well studied.

A meta-analysis of long-term outcome in pediatric-onset OCD estimated that the persistence rate for full OCD was 41% and for full or subclinical OCD 60%, after 1–7 years of follow-up. Predictors of poor outcome are a poor initial treatment response, prominent hoarding symptoms (according to DSM-IV, not DSM-5, criteria), and comorbid psychiatric illness. The association of comorbid tic disorder in children with OCD has been associated with a good adulthood prognosis, suggesting that the trajectory of improvement in OC symptoms may follow that typically experienced by patients with a tic disorder.

Leonard HL, Swedo SE, Lenane MC, et al. A 2- to 7-year follow-up study of 54 obsessive-compulsive children and adolescents. *Arch Gen Psychiatry*. 1993;50(6):429–439.

Stewart SE, Geller DA, Jenike M, et al. Long-term outcome of pediatric obsessive-compulsive disorder: a meta-analysis and qualitative review of the literature. *Acta Psychiatr Scand*. 2004;110(1):4–13.

Developmental Disorders of Attachment, Feeding, Elimination, & Sleeping

Myo Thwin Myint, MD
Charles H. Zeanah, MD
Barry Nurcombe, MD[†]

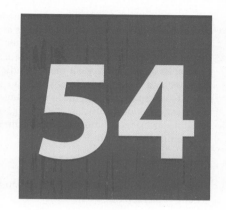

54

Human infants are born with the propensity to attach to their parents and to elicit care from them. Extremes of caregiving deficiencies—such as social and/or instrumental neglect, institutional rearing, or frequent changes in foster parents—increase the risk for a number of conditions such as reactive attachment disorder, disinhibited attachment disorder, rumination disorder of infancy, nonorganic failure to thrive, and psychosocial dwarfism. These conditions appear in infancy or early childhood and often are associated with cognitive, language, and social delays or deviancies and later functional impairment. Sleep problems usually appear in the first 2 years of life. Pica and elimination disorders are usually first diagnosed between 2 and 5 years of age.

REACTIVE ATTACHMENT DISORDER OF CHILDHOOD (F94.1)

ICD-10 Criteria

Starts in the first five years of life and is characterized by persistent abnormalities in the child's pattern of social relationships that are associated with emotional disturbance and are reactive to changes in environmental circumstances (e.g. fearfulness and hypervigilance, poor social interaction with peers, aggression toward self and others, misery, and growth failure in some cases). The syndrome probably occurs as a direct result of severe parental neglect, abuse, or serious mishandling.

Use additional code, if desired, to identify any associated failure to thrive or growth retardation.

Excl.:

Asperger syndrome (F84.5)
disinhibited attachment disorder of childhood (F94.2)
maltreatment syndromes (T74.-)

normal variation in pattern of selective attachment
sexual or physical abuse in childhood, resulting in psychosocial problems (Z61.4-Z61.6)

Reproduced with permission from International Statistical Classification of Diseases and Related Health Problems 10th Revision (ICD-10) Version for 2010. Geneva: World Health Organization; 2010.

▶ General Considerations

A. Epidemiology

Although this condition is believed to be rare, it has not been included in any population-based studies and its prevalence is unknown. Two studies of community samples of 2- to 5-year-old children recruited from pediatric clinics found no cases.

B. Etiology

Bowlby conceptualized attachment as the biologically based tendency for infants to seek comfort, support, nurturance, and protection from caregiving adults. The tendency for selective seeking of comfort is not apparent at birth, however. Following a period of interaction and comfort with adult caregivers during the first 6 months, two new infant behaviors become obvious: stranger wariness and separation protest, both at about 7–9 months of age. Stranger wariness describes an apparent discomfort with unfamiliar adults and selectively turning to those the child knows and trusts. Separation protest refers to the infant's tendency to protest separation from familiar caregivers. Although individual differences in the intensity and expression of these behaviors are clear, they may be considered universal. When these behaviors appear, the infant is said to be attached to one or more caregivers.

Infant behaviors that promote physical proximity to caregivers—such as crawling to, smiling at, clinging on—are known as attachment behaviors. Under species-typical rearing conditions, human infants gradually form attachments to a relatively small number of caregiving adults during the first year of life. Attachments form by 7–9 months of age and are

---

[†]Deceased

apparent when the infant begins to demonstrate stranger wariness and separation protest. Attachments are then described as "focused," "preferred," "discriminated," or "selected." When the infant is able to walk independently, usually by around 12 months of age, attachment motivates the child to use the caregiver as a secure base from which to explore and a safe haven to whom to return in the face of danger.

In extremes of insufficient caregiving, however, such as social neglect or institutional care, attachment may be seriously limited or even absent.

C. Genetics

The disorder is not heritable, and no studies demonstrate genetic vulnerabilities.

▶ Clinical Findings

A. Signs and Symptoms

Reactive attachment disorder (RAD) describes a constellation of aberrant attachment behaviors and other behavioral anomalies that are believed to result from social neglect and deprivation (Gleason et al, 2011; Rutter et al, 2009; Smyke et al, 2012; Zeanah et al, 2005). Essentially, RAD defines a condition in which the child fails to develop normal attachment to an attachment figure. As far as is known, the capacity for the affected child to form attachments is retained, and there is no age at which that capacity is lost. What is less clear is whether attachments that the child forms after being placed in a responsive caregiving environment are healthy and robust. In any case, the affected child demonstrates few if any efforts to seek or respond to comfort when distressed, reduced or absent social reciprocity, emotional constriction, and an apparent inability to derive pleasure from social contact or play.

B. Developmental Considerations

Because attachments do not form until the latter part of the first year of life, this disorder should not be diagnosed in children less than 10 months of age. Little is known about its later manifestations, so the diagnosis should be made with caution in children older than 5 years of age.

C. Course of Illness

Reactive attachment disorder is a serious condition that seems not to remit until the child is placed in a better caregiving environment (Gleason et al, 2011). Older studies reported significant mortality and severe psychosocial morbidity associated with this disorder. However, the adverse outcomes reported in these studies are compounded by the very poor quality of the institutions in which the studied children were housed. Some studies indicate that more than half of children raised in institutions have serious psychopathology. A number of investigations have compared the outcome of children raised in higher quality institutions with that of children adopted or placed in foster care. Children raised initially in institutions are at increased risk of becoming more restless, distractible, disobedient, oppositional, and irritable than children who were never institutionalized, and these problems often occur in conjunction with RAD. The signs of RAD remit after almost any family placement following severe deprivation.

▶ Differential Diagnosis (Including Comorbid Conditions)

RAD should be distinguished from autistic spectrum disorders, intellectual disabilities, and language disorders (Gleason et al, 2011). RAD shares some features with autistic spectrum disorders, including disturbances in emotion regulation, and impaired or absent social and emotional reciprocity. Children with either condition may have cognitive delay or exhibit stereotypies.

Autism spectrum disorder, on the other hand, is characterized by delays and deviance in the development of social relationships, cognition, and language. The impairment of social relationships in autism is profound and not reversible by effective parenting. Furthermore, a history of parental failure, maltreatment, or loss is not usually encountered. Importantly, there is no reason to expect children with RAD to display restricted or repetitive interests. In autism, language and pretend play are more delayed/impaired than one would predict from overall IQ.

Intellectual disability associated with parental neglect or maltreatment presents a difficult differential diagnosis. Young children with RAD should be distinguishable from children with intellectual disability because the latter group has social and emotional behavior consistent with developmental age, whereas children with RAD show clear evidence of deviance in their social responsiveness and regulation of emotion. Clearly, both conditions may occur in the context of neglect. Similarly, children with developmental language disorder do not demonstrate attachment pathology unless the language delay is associated with gross parental neglect.

Infants older than 6 months (the age at which the primary attachment figure is first recognized) react to separation from or loss of the attachment figure with the following sequence of behavior: (1) protest, (2) depression, and (3) detachment. Children in the stage of protest cry, demand that the parent return, and reject the attempts of others to comfort them. Depression and detachment are associated with sad face, anergia, insomnia, anorexia, loss of interest in surroundings, social withdrawal, "empty" clinging, and developmental arrest or regression. The child reacts to reminders of the primary attachment figure by ignoring or rejecting them or with a reactivation of protest. Once the child has become detached, they are likely to be indistinguishable from children with RAD in terms of the clinical picture. Only the history of loss of a caregiver can lead to a diagnosis of disrupted attachment.

Treatment

The first priority should be to provide a child with RAD an emotionally available attachment figure. Placing a child into a nonneglectful setting with a foster or adoptive parent will eliminate signs of the disorder within weeks to months (Smyke et al, 2012). Interventions such as Attachment and Biobehavioral Catch-up, Circle of Security, or Child Parent Psychotherapy assist parents to understand and respond more effectively to children who have experienced deprivation or other severe adversity. These interventions also may be useful in reconstructing attachment relationships between young, maltreated children and their parents.

Complications/Adverse Outcomes of Treatment

Dangerous treatments such as the coercive variations of "holding therapies" for reactive attachment disorder should be avoided. These treatments have proven fatal in several cases. Treatments that intentionally attempt to provoke anger are based on a flawed model, may re-traumatize already traumatized children, and may exacerbate the child's negative self-perceptions, further complicating the course of the disorder.

Prognosis

The prognosis for reactive attachment disorder is good if an affected child is placed in an adequate caregiving environment (Smyke et al, 2012). There seems to be no age at which RAD is irreversible. Less clear, however, is the degree to which recovery of interpersonal adaptation can be attained.

Gleason MM, Fox NA, Drury S, et al. The validity of evidence-derived criteria for reactive attachment disorder: indiscriminately social/disinhibited and emotionally withdrawn/inhibited types. *J Am Acad Child Adolesc Psychiatry*. 2011;50(3):216–231.

Rutter M, Kreppner J, Sonuga-Barke E. Emanuel Miller Lecture: attachment insecurity, disinhibited attachment, and attachment disorders: where do research findings leave the concepts? *J Child Psychol Psychiatry*. 2009;50(5):529–543.

Smyke AT, Zeanah CH, Gleason MM, et al. A randomized controlled trial of foster care vs. institutional care for children with signs of reactive attachment disorder. *Am J Psychiatry*. 2012;169(5):508–514.

Zeanah CH, Smyke AT, Koga S, Carlson E; BEIP Core Group. Attachment in institutionalized and community children in Romania. *Child Dev*. 2005;76(5):1015–1028.

DISINHIBITED ATTACHMENT DISORDER OF CHILDHOOD (F94.2)

ICD-10 Criteria

A particular pattern of abnormal social functioning that arises during the first five years of life and that tends to persist despite marked changes in environmental circumstances, e.g. diffuse, nonselectively focused attachment behaviour, attention-seeking and indiscriminately friendly behaviour, poorly modulated peer interactions; depending on circumstances there may also be associated emotional or behavioral disturbance.

> Affectionless psychopathy
> Institutional syndrome

Excl.:

Asperger syndrome (F84.5)
hospitalism in children (F43.2)
hyperkinetic disorders (F90.-)
reactive attachment disorder of childhood (F94.1)

Reproduced with permission for International Statistical Classification of Diseases and Related Health Problems 10th Revision (ICD-10) Version for 2010.WHO: 2010.

General Considerations

A. Epidemiology

Although this condition is thought to be rare, it has not been included in any population-based studies and its prevalence is unknown. Two studies of community samples of 2- to 5-year-old children recruited from pediatric clinics found no cases.

B. Etiology

Disinhibited attachment disorder (DAD) is caused by grossly insufficient caregiving, that is, severe social neglect or deprivation when caregiving adults fail to provide the child with basic emotional needs for comfort, stimulation, and affection (Gleason et al, 2011; Smyke et al, 2012; Rutter et al, 2009; Zeanah et al, 2005). Furthermore, repeated changes of primary caregivers that limit the opportunity for the child to form stable attachments (e.g., frequent changes in foster care) and rearing in settings that limit opportunities to form selective attachments (e.g., institutions with high child-to-caregiver ratios) have both been associated with DAD.

The clinical phenotype in DAD—indiscriminate behavior with strangers—also has been associated with Williams syndrome, a condition resulting from deletion of genes on the seventh chromosome. This means that only indiscriminate behavior occurring with a history of insufficient caregiving is sufficient to confirm the diagnosis.

C. Genetics

The disorder is not heritable. There is only one study to date implicating genetic vulnerability. That study showed that different polymorphic versions of the gene that codes for brain-derived neurotropic factor and the serotonin transporter gene confer environmental susceptibility, with odds for indiscriminate behavior higher in a more deprived environment and lower in a nondeprived environment. The other versions of alleles appear to cause intermediate levels of indiscriminate behavior whether they are in favorable or unfavorable caregiving environments.

Clinical Findings

A. Signs and Symptoms

DAD represents a failure of the infant to exhibit developmentally appropriate stranger wariness. The child fails to check back with the caregiver in unfamiliar settings, wanders away even in unfamiliar settings, and most importantly, willingly approaches, interacts with, and accompanies strangers. In addition, the child demonstrates a tendency to violate social boundaries by overly familiar physical closeness or later by verbal intrusiveness.

B. Developmental Considerations

Because attachments do not form until the latter part of the first year of life, the disorder should not be diagnosed in children less than 10 months of age. Less is known about the disorder and its manifestations after early childhood, though it has been described in school-aged children and adolescents. In older children, there seems to be a tendency for indiscriminate social behavior with peers.

C. Course of Illness

DAD is a persistent condition that does not always remit even when the child is placed in a more adequate caregiving environment (Rutter et al, 2009; Smyke et al, 2012). In fact, DAD has proven to be one of the most persistent social abnormalities following severe deprivation (Smyke et al, 2012). Among children living in deprived institutions, the disorder is even more persistent (Gleason et al, 2011; Zeanah et al, 2005).

Differential Diagnosis (Including Comorbid Conditions)

DAD has some features of attention-deficit/hyperactivity disorder (ADHD), especially impulsivity (Gleason et al, 2011). In DAD, the impulsivity is primarily social, whereas in ADHD, it is cognitive and behavioral. DAD and ADHD may co-occur, particularly in children who have experienced deprivation, but they do not always co-occur and may be distinguished clinically.

Treatment

The only treatment for DAD that has been studied is enhanced caregiving (Rutter et al, 2009; Smyke et al, 2012). This has been shown to be helpful for some but not all affected children. There is a clinical consensus that following adoption or placement in foster care, the child's contacts should be limited to a small number of caregivers (usually the immediate family) for several months before other social situations are introduced. The rationale is to allow the child to develop and consolidate attachments and reduce the likelihood of persistent indiscriminate behavior.

Complications/Adverse Outcomes of Treatment

As with RAD, coercive variations of holding therapy have been recommended for DAD, which is supposedly associated with psychopathic traits such as absence of guilt, shallow emotions, and manipulative behavior. These treatments have proven fatal in some cases and should be avoided. As noted, treatments designed to encourage expression of anger and rage are based on a flawed model, may re-traumatize already traumatized children, and can exacerbate the child's negative self-perceptions and further complicate the course of the disorder.

Prognosis

The evidence is mixed that the disorder resolves after placement in a more adequate caregiving environment (Rutter et al, 2009; Smyke et al, 2012). Work to date indicates that the sooner the child is removed from a deprived environment and receives adequate caregiving, the more likely it is that signs of the disorder will resolve, though some children continue to display indiscriminate behavior for years after they receive adequate caregiving.

Gleason MM, Fox NA, Drury S, et al. The validity of evidence-derived criteria for reactive attachment disorder: Indiscriminately social/disinhibited and emotionally withdrawn/inhibited types. *J Am Acad Child Adolesc Psychiatry*. 2011;50(3):216–231.

Rutter M, Kreppner J, Sonuga-Barke E. Emanuel Miller Lecture: attachment insecurity, disinhibited attachment, and attachment disorders: where do research findings leave the concepts? *J Child Psychol Psychiatry*. 2009;50(5):529–543.

Smyke AT, Zeanah CH, Gleason MM, et al. A randomized controlled trial of foster care vs. institutional care for children with signs of reactive attachment disorder. *Am J Psychiatry*. 2012;169(5):508–514.

Zeanah CH, Smyke AT, Koga S, Carlson E; BEIP Core Group. Attachment in institutionalized and community children in Romania. *Child Dev*. 2005;76(5):1015–1028.

FEEDING AND EATING DISORDERS OF INFANCY OR EARLY CHILDHOOD

FEEDING DISORDER OF INFANCY AND CHILDHOOD (F98.2)

ICD-10 Criteria

A feeding disorder of varying manifestations usually specific to infancy and early childhood. It generally involves food refusal and extreme faddiness in the presence of an adequate food supply, a reasonably competent caregiver, and the absence of organic disease. There may or may not be associated rumination (repeated regurgitation without nausea or gastrointestinal illness).

Rumination disorder of infancy

Excl.:

anorexia nervosa and other eating disorders (F50.-) feeding:

▶ difficulties and mismanagement (R63.3)

▶ problems of newborn (P92.-)

▶ pica of infancy or childhood (F98.3)

▶ General Considerations

A. Epidemiology

Nonorganic failure to thrive has been found to occur in 2–5% of admissions to pediatric hospitals. It appears to be equally common in both sexes. English studies that followed birth cohorts in a socially disadvantaged London health district identified 3.5–4.6% as having nonorganic failure to thrive by 12 months of age. Most of these children had never been referred for pediatric evaluation. About 20% of families living in a socially disadvantaged inner city area will have at least one child who fails to thrive. Late birth order in a large, closely spaced family is a risk factor.

B. Etiology

Organic and nonorganic failure to thrive are not sharply distinguished (Benoit, 2009). Aside from the 10% of cases of failure to thrive that are caused by clear-cut physical disease, subtle constitutional or temperamental factors in the infant often interact with a relative impairment of parenting capacity to cause this condition. However, all cases have the same final common pathway: insufficient food intake.

Among the subtle constitutional factors that interact with or trigger environmental failure are the following: hypotonic lips, poor sucking, tongue dysfunction, oral-motor impairment, poor coordination of sucking and swallowing, gastroesophageal reflux, minor forms of cerebral palsy, Sandifer syndrome (involving tension spasm and esophageal reflux), sleep apnea, and the aftermath of nasogastric, parenteral, or gastrostomy feeding. In some cases, feeding difficulties disrupt mother–infant interaction, engendering a vicious cycle.

Early studies implicated maltreatment and neglect as the cause of nonorganic failure to thrive. Better-controlled studies have cast doubt on the universality of this theory; however, follow-up studies of these children have demonstrated an increased risk of subsequent maltreatment.

Controlled studies of maternal characteristics have produced conflicting results. Some studies suggest an increased prevalence of depressive disorders, personality disorders, and substance use disorders. Controlled observations of the mother–infant interaction have demonstrated in these mothers less reciprocity, less sensitivity to the infant's cues, greater conflict over control issues, and more negative affect; in contrast, infants with nonorganic failure to thrive are relatively more inhibited, less cooperative, and more likely to avert their gaze from their mothers.

Although many case series have identified multiple risk and associated factors, they can be difficult to detect in controlled or population-based studies (Benoit, 2009).

C. Genetics

Organic failure to thrive occurs when there is an underlying medical cause. This may be genetically determined.

▶ Clinical Findings

Nonorganic failure to thrive is usually apparent in the first year of life. The infant is cachectic and prone to infection. Developmental delay is the rule, but the severity of the delay is variable. These children are listless and hypotonic, exhibiting abnormal postures and intense gaze. They prefer inanimate objects to people, and they are prone to self-stimulation. They look sad and are irritable, withdrawn, or hypervigilant.

Although in clinical studies the mothers of children with nonorganic failure to thrive have seemed to demonstrate psychopathology, controlled studies have yielded inconsistent findings. Higher rates of insecure and unresolved attachments have been noted in the mothers compared to mothers of infants hospitalized for conditions other than growth failure.

▶ Differential Diagnosis

Nonorganic failure to thrive and psychosocial dwarfism (discussed subsequently) must be distinguished from organic causes of failure to thrive and short stature, such as hereditary short stature, chromosomal abnormality (e.g., 46 X0, trisomy 23), dysmorphic short stature (e.g., Noonan syndrome, Russell–Silver syndrome), skeletal dysplasia (e.g., achondroplasia, hypochondroplasia), endocrinopathy (e.g., growth hormone deficiency, growth hormone resistance, hypothyroidism, hypercortisolism, congenital adrenal hyperplasia), other causes of malnutrition including food allergies and intolerances, or systemic disease (e.g., chronic pulmonary disease, congenital heart disease, gastrointestinal disease including malabsorption syndrome, renal disease, chronic anemia, and malignancies). Children with nonorganic failure to thrive or psychosocial dwarfism are within the normative range of birth weight but often at lower weight than their thriving counterparts. Differential diagnoses include other mental disorders such as reactive attachment disorder, autism spectrum disorder, anxiety disorders including specific phobia and social anxiety disorder, anorexia nervosa, obsessive–compulsive disorder, major depressive disorder, schizophrenia spectrum disorders, and factitious disorder.

Treatment

If the child's survival is in question, he or she should be removed from the home for hospitalization or placement into foster care. In extreme cases in which parents cannot provide the child with adequate nutrition for growth despite intensive intervention, parental rights may be terminated.

A variety of behavioral techniques have been used to counteract or remediate abnormal feeding behavior in infants. These techniques are used in tandem with individual psychotherapy aimed at enhancing maternal consistency and sense of competence and decreasing maternal stress. If the mother has a diagnosable psychiatric disorder (e.g., depressive or substance use disorder), it should be promptly treated. Casework can be provided in the home by a trained social worker or nurse, with attention given to financial, marital, or employment problems. Dyadic therapy involving both infant and mother is recommended when unresolved issues related to pathogenic maternal working models of attachment impede adequate childcare.

Complications/Adverse Outcomes of Treatment

Most children with nonorganic failure to thrive do not become psychosocial dwarfs. Failure to thrive is potentially reversible if the child is removed from the noxious home environment. However, if the child is returned to an adverse situation, developmental failure will recur. The later the onset, the better the prognosis for intellectual and language functioning.

Prognosis

Children with nonorganic failure to thrive who are not treated for an extended period of time may have difficulty "catching up" developmentally and socially. It has been reported that about half of children who experienced failure to thrive continued to have social and emotional problems or eating problems later in life. However, because of differences in definition and classification, it is difficult to predict prognosis (Kreipe & Palomaki, 2012).

Benoit D. Feeding disorders, failure to thrive, and obesity. In: Zeanah CH, ed. *Handbook of Infant Mental Health*. 3rd ed. New York: Guilford Press; 2009:377–391.

Kreipe RE, Palomaki A. Beyond picky eating: avoidant/restrictive food intake disorder. *Curr Psychiatry Rep*. 2012;14(4):421–431

PICA OF INFANCY AND CHILDHOOD (F98.3)

ICD-10 Criteria

Persistent eating of non-nutritive substances (such as soil, paint chippings, etc.). It may occur as one of many symptoms that are part of a more widespread psychiatric disorder (such as autism), or as a relatively isolated psychopathological behaviour; only the latter is classified here. The phenomenon is most common in mentally retarded children.

General Considerations

A. Epidemiology

The prevalence of pica varies widely. It is much more common among rural pregnant African American women and among institutionalized individuals with intellectual disability.

B. Etiology

The cause of pica is not known, but an association with iron deficiency has been reported. It is usually diagnosed only in those who are 2 years and older to avoid misdiagnosing developmentally typical behaviors. Specific craving for nonnutritive, nonfood substances can also occur during pregnancy.

C. Genetics

There are no known genetic factors specifically associated with pica.

Clinical Findings

Pica is defined as persistent craving and eating nonfood substances. Children or adults with pica eat dirt, stones, ice, paint, burned match heads, starch, feces, hair, and so on.

Differential Diagnosis (Including Comorbid Conditions)

The differential diagnosis of pica includes anorexia nervosa, factitious disorder, and self-injurious behaviors. Comorbid conditions include autism spectrum disorder and intellectual disability (Bryant-Waugh et al, 2010).

Treatment

The proper treatment of pica is unclear. Proper supervision of young children and behavioral techniques for older children are recommended.

Complications/Adverse Outcomes of Treatment

Laboratory studies are needed to rule out lead poisoning. In addition to lead poisoning, pica can lead to excessive weight gain, malnutrition, intestinal blockage, intestinal perforation, and malabsorption. Other complications such as poisoning, intestinal obstruction, intestinal perforation, and infections may occur from ingesting feces or dirt.

 Prognosis

The prognosis varies depending on the circumstances with regard to associated etiological conditions and the level of supervision.

Bryant-Waugh R, Markham L, Kreipe RE, Walsh BT. Feeding and eating disorders in childhood. *Int J Eat Disord*. 2010;43(2):98–111.

Rumination ICD-10 Criteria Rumination Disorder of Infancy (98.2)

A feeding disorder of varying manifestations usually specific to infancy and early childhood. It generally involves food refusal and extreme faddiness in the presence of an adequate food supply, a reasonably competent caregiver, and the absence of organic disease. There may or may not be associated rumination (repeated regurgitation without nausea or gastrointestinal illness).
  Rumination disorder of infancy

Excl.:
anorexia nervosa and other eating disorders (F50.-) feeding:

▶ difficulties and mismanagement (R63.3)

▶ problems of newborn (P92.-)

▶ pica of infancy or childhood (F98.3)

General Considerations

A. Epidemiology

The incidence of rumination in the general population of infants is unknown. Rumination among the intellectually disabled occurs more commonly in males, particularly among the profoundly disabled. The prevalence in institutional populations is 6–10%.

B. Etiology

In infants, rumination is thought to be associated with deprivation of maternal attention or neglect. In older individuals with intellectual disability, rumination has been ascribed to self-stimulation and is most often encountered in a setting of institutional deprivation. Gastroesophageal reflux, hiatus hernia, or esophageal spasm may be diagnosed, but the significance of these conditions is not clear, and it should not be assumed that, even if present, they cause rumination. Rumination has been interpreted as a complex, learned behavior reinforced by maternal attention or oral sensory gratification.

C. Genetics

Except when occurring in the context of various forms of intellectual disability, there are no known genetic factors specifically associated with rumination.

Clinical Findings

Ruminators stimulate their gag reflexes manually or adopt postures that facilitate regurgitation. The frequency can vary from several times per minute to once per hour. Regurgitated food fills the cheeks and may be stirred about by the tongue before being re-swallowed or spit out. Ruminators can sometimes be diverted from the practice temporarily, if they are offered interesting things to do after eating.

Differential Diagnosis

Rumination should be differentiated from other causes of vomiting and gastroesophageal reflux as well as from anorexia nervosa and bulimia nervosa.

Treatment

In infants, it may be sufficient to provide consistent, noncontingent, contact comfort, with holding, rocking, eye contact, and soothing vocalizations. In older children (e.g., in those with intellectual disability), or in infants for whom adequate nurturance has been insufficient to eliminate the condition, behavioral treatment will be required (Olden, 2001). The design of the specific treatment plan depends on a detailed behavioral analysis of the antecedents, the behavior, and its consequences. When the perpetuating reinforcer is intrinsic (e.g., self-stimulation in older patients) rather than extrinsic (e.g., operant vomiting reinforced by parental attention), treatment may need to be prolonged. The feeding of satiating quantities of high-caloric food is sometimes useful as a preliminary treatment in underweight patients. Habit-reversal training using diaphragmatic breathing as the competing response can also lead to substantial improvement. The provision of a substitute oral stimulant such as chewing gum after meals can also be helpful.

Complications/Adverse Outcomes of Treatment

Failure to diagnosis this condition and the extensive diagnostic testing in pediatric and adolescent patients prior to diagnosis can be a significant source of morbidity.

Prognosis

In general, rumination syndrome is a "benign" condition. However, there is a significant functional disability related to weight loss, school and work absenteeism, and hospitalization (Chial et al, 2003). In some cases, rumination has a serious prognosis. Unless treated successfully, it could lead to inanition and death.

Chial HJ, Camilleri M, Williams DE, et al. Rumination syndrome in children and adolescents: diagnosis, treatment, and prognosis. *Pediatrics*. 2003;111:158–162.

Olden KW. Rumination. *Curr Treat Option Gastroenterol*. 2001;4(4):351–358.

PSYCHOSOCIAL DWARFISM

ICD-10 Criteria Short Stature, not Elsewhere Classified (E 34.3)

Short stature:

▶ NOS

▶ constitutional

▶ Laron-type

▶ psychosocial

Excl.:

progeria (E34.8)
Russell–Silver syndrome (Q87.1)
short-limbed stature with immunodeficiency (D82.2)
short stature:

▶ achondroplastic (Q77.4)

▶ hypochondroplastic (Q77.4)

▶ in specific dysmorphic syndromes—code to syndrome—see Alphabetical Index

▶ nutritional (E45)

▶ pituitary (E23.0)

▶ renal (N25.0)

▶ General Considerations

A. Epidemiology

The incidence of psychosocial dwarfism in the general population of infants is unknown, although it is rare.

B. Etiology

Psychosocial dwarfism is caused by reversible hypopituitarism, with reduced growth hormone secretion (Munoz-Hoyos et al, 2011) leading to growth failure despite adequate caloric intake. The growth failure is eliminated when the child is provided with adequate caregiving—oftentimes even hospitalization leads to enhanced growth. The condition is usually associated with severe neglect, but it is not clear why only some children respond to a neglecting environment in this manner.

C. Genetics

Although mutations in the growth hormone receptor gene and related genes can lead to growth failure, psychosocial dwarfism is, by definition, a condition with an environmental etiology. There is no evidence of heritability.

▶ Clinical Findings

Psychosocial dwarfism is usually diagnosed between 18 months and 7 years of age. Severe growth retardation with cognitive and language delays is sometimes preceded by feeding problems in infancy. The child may exhibit polyphagia, food hoarding, pica, and insomnia, sometimes wandering at night apparently to look for food. Food fads, enuresis, encopresis, and self-induced vomiting are commonly associated with psychosocial dwarfism. Intellectual disability also may be present. The symptoms of psychosocial dwarfism have been associated with disorders of biological rhythms, self-regulation, mood, and social relationships. Sleep, appetite, and satiety are disturbed, and the children have a deficiency in the normally pulsed release of growth hormone into the bloodstream. The condition is reversible, at least in part, if the child is provided with adequate, nurturant surrogate care.

▶ Differential Diagnosis

Psychosocial dwarfism should be distinguished from short stature due to endocrine disorder, constitutional factors, or stress.

▶ Treatment

When children with psychosocial dwarfism are provided with adequate surrogate parental care, physical and mental growth occurs within a few weeks and the eccentric behavior characteristic of the condition recedes. However, the longer appropriate placement is delayed, the less likely it is that the child will catch up.

▶ Complications/Adverse Outcomes of Treatment

Parental psychopathology and compliance with treatment should be monitored. There is an increased risk of child maltreatment, including overt abuse and neglect.

▶ Prognosis

The prognosis is poor, unless adequate, surrogate parental care is provided. Short stature, delayed puberty, stunted intellectual development, and conduct problems are likely to result from untreated psychosocial dwarfism.

Munoz-Hoyos A, Molina-Carballo A, Augustin-Morales M, et al. Psychosocial dwarfism: psychopathological aspects and putative neuroendocrine markers. *Psychiatry Res*. 2011;188(1):96–101.

ELIMINATION DISORDERS

ENCOPRESIS

ICD-10 Criteria Non-Organic Encopresis (F98.1)

Repeated, voluntary or involuntary passage of faeces, usually of normal or near-normal consistency, in places not appropriate for that purpose in the individual's own sociocultural setting. The condition may represent an abnormal continuation of normal infantile incontinence, it may involve a loss of continence following the acquisition of bowel control, or it may involve the deliberate deposition of faeces in inappropriate places in spite of normal physiological bowel control. The condition may occur as a monosymptomatic disorder, or it may form part of a wider disorder, especially an emotional disorder or a conduct disorder.

Functional encopresis

Incontinence of faeces of nonorganic origin

Psychogenic encopresis

Use additional code, if desired, to identify the cause of any coexisting constipation.

Excl.:

encopresis NOS

Reproduced with permission for International Statistical Classification of Diseases and Related Health Problems 10th Revision (ICD-10) Version for 2010.WHO: 2010.

▶ General Considerations

A. Epidemiology

A Scandinavian population study revealed a prevalence of 1.5% among children aged 7–8 years. The sex ratio was 3.4:1 in favor of boys. A British study found a prevalence of about 1.5% among children aged 10–11 years, with a sex ratio of 4.3:1 in favor of boys.

B. Etiology

The etiology of encopresis is multifactorial. Normal continence and voiding requires the following sequence of neuromuscular events: (1) sensitivity to rectal fullness; (2) constriction of the external anal sphincter, puborectalis, and internal anal sphincter; (3) rectal contraction waves; (4) increase of intra-abdominal pressure following contraction of the diaphragm and abdominal muscles; and (5) relaxation of the sphincters.

Children with encopresis exhibit abnormal anorectal dynamics, such as a weak internal sphincter, or a failure of the external sphincter to relax in concert with rectal contraction waves and abdominal straining. There are two types of encopresis: (1) with constipation and overflow incontinence and (2) without constipation and incontinence. Toilet training involves the learning of the appropriate place and time for defecation; sensitivity to rectal fullness; and the sequential coordination of withholding, finding the right place, adopting the appropriate posture, relaxing the sphincters, and increasing intra-abdominal pressure. Most children are capable of learning the sequence by 18–24 months of age; however, learning may be interrupted by antecedent conditions or concurrent events. Particularly important are the parent's attunement to the infant's signals and the parent's capacity to introduce the child to the toilet calmly, offer praise and encouragement for a favorable result, and avoid discouragement, coercion, or punishment for failures.

A significant number of children who experience fecal retention were constipated in the first year of life. In other children, physiologic constipation has followed an attack of diarrhea. The preliminary constipation causes painful defecation, in some cases with anal fissure, which precipitates withholding. A pattern of withholding, fecal retention, and involuntary overflow may be created if withholding coincides with faulty toilet training (e.g., with coercion, harsh criticism, or physical punishment) or if the parent is emotionally unavailable or poorly attuned to the child (e.g., as a result of depression). Thus, an initially physiologic condition disrupts the mother–child relationship, and psychogenic retention culminates in abnormal anorectal dynamics, megacolon, rectal insensitivity, and leakage or involuntary voiding.

A small number of children with severe behavioral disturbance, often from neglectful or rejecting homes, exhibit no retention and constipation but deliberately defecate in closets or other inappropriate places. Two other nonretentive groups of encopretics are associated with (1) an apparent insensitivity to rectal fullness and the involuntary passage of feces or (2) the passage of (often liquid) feces when emotionally aroused by anxiety, fear, or laughter.

The degree to which encopresis is associated with psychopathology in the parent or child is unclear. Enuresis, oppositional-defiant behavior, tantrums, school refusal, fire setting, and developmental immaturities have been described as co-occurring, although it is uncertain to what degree these symptoms are primary or secondary to the encopresis.

C. Genetics

Although children with some genetically determined forms of intellectual disability, such as Fragile-X syndrome, are at greater risk for encopresis, this vulnerability related more to intellectual disability than a specific vulnerability.

▶ Clinical Findings

Some younger children who deliberately soil in inappropriate places do so at a time of stress or family change, for example, after the birth of a sibling. Others, as described earlier in this chapter, do so in reaction to severe neglect or rejection, as in psychosocial dwarfism. A second group appears to lose sphincter control when emotionally aroused. These are often anxious children exposed to emotional stress, for example, after a change of school.

The most serious cases are associated with constipation, retention, megarectum, megacolon, and the involuntary passage of small amounts of stool, together with liquefaction, fecal leakage, and virtually constant soiling, or the intermittent involuntary passage of large stools. Children with extreme megacolon can become disabled with abdominal distention, anorexia, and loss of weight.

Differential Diagnosis

The following causes of incontinence or constipation should be distinguished from encopresis: Hirschsprung disease, anal stenosis, and endocrine disorder. However, the combination of soiling; constipation; a ballooned, loaded rectum; and a loaded colon occurs only in encopresis. In females, urinary tract infection may be present. The clinician should evaluate the child for other developmental problems or psychiatric disorders (e.g., intellectual disability, learning problems, disruptive behavior disorder, and anxiety disorder).

Treatment

If the child has a full colon and rectum, it is likely that his or her rectum will be insensitive to distention. The colon should be washed out, and laxatives and stool softeners used (Navarro, 2008) until fecal masses can no longer be palpated and the child is passing regular stools of normal consistency. In severe cases, hospitalization is required.

Parents should be educated to administer a behavioral program. Coercion, punishment, and criticism should be avoided. It is ill advised, for example, to punish the child by making him or her clean soiled clothes. The child should be asked to sit briefly on the toilet at the same time twice per day: after breakfast and after school. All tension should be removed from the toileting experience. The child may be read to or may read to him or herself. The parent should make no comment if no bowel movement is passed; in contrast, the parent should praise and offer individualized reward to the child if toileting is successful. Star charts are useful both as a record and for reinforcement (see discussion on "Treatment" in section "Enuresis").

Depressed or compulsive parents often find it difficult to institute a consistent, gentle program of this type and may need treatment in their own right. Fathers should be involved in order to provide support and to cooperate in instituting the behavioral program. Marital problems may need attention.

The child may require individual and/or family psychotherapy for associated anxiety disorder, disruptive behavior disorder, or other psychopathology. Because the possibility of relapse is high, treatment is often needed for 1 or more years, with a combination of laxatives, stool softeners, a high-fiber diet, parental education, parental behavior management,

individual psychotherapy, and when necessary, psychiatric help for the parents. The results of this regimen are good, particularly in younger children. Success rates of 50–90% have been reported. Imipramine has been prescribed to treat encopresis, but no controlled studies of its effectiveness are available.

Complications/Adverse Outcomes of Treatment

Treatment complications are rare. Most children will improve with time and through the use of relatively innocuous interventions.

Prognosis

Most cases of encopresis resolve by adolescence, but 15% of children with functional nonretentive fecal incontinence remain symptomatic at the age of 18 years (Rajindrajith et al, 2013).

Navarro F. Management of constipation and encopresis in children. *J Pediatr Health Care*. 2008;22(3):199–204.

Rajindrajith S, Devanayana NM, Benninga MA. Review article: faecal incontinence in children: epidemiology, pathophysiology, clinical evaluation and management. *Aliment Pharmacol Ther*. 2013;37(1):37–48.

ENURESIS

ICD-10 Criteria Non-Organic Enuresis (F98.0)

A disorder characterized by involuntary voiding of urine, by day and by night, which is abnormal in relation to the individual's mental age, and which is not a consequence of a lack of bladder control due to any neurological disorder, to epileptic attacks, or to any structural abnormality of the urinary tract. The enuresis may have been present from birth or it may have arisen following a period of acquired bladder control. The enuresis may or may not be associated with a more widespread emotional or behavioural disorder.

Enuresis (primary)(secondary) of nonorganic origin
Functional enuresis
Psychogenic enuresis
Urinary incontinence of nonorganic origin

Excl.:

enuresis NOS (R32)

Reproduced with permission for International Statistical Classification of Diseases and Related Health Problems 10th Revision (ICD-10) Version for 2010.WHO: 2010.

General Considerations

A. Epidemiology

The sex ratio is equal until 5 years of age, after which males predominate (2:1 at 11 years of age). Boys are more likely to develop secondary enuresis. Scandinavian and New Zealand population studies have found the prevalence of enuresis at 7 and 8 years of age to be 9.8% and 7.4%, respectively. In the United States bedwetting is more common in African Americans and Asian immigrants than among other populations. Most enuretic children achieve continence by puberty. Approximately 3% of childhood enuretics are still incontinent at 20 years of age.

B. Etiology

The cause of enuresis is unknown. Enuresis correlates with other maturational delays, particularly in language, speech, motor skills, and social development. An association has been noted between the tendency to sleep for long periods each day, between 1 and 2 years of age, and later enuresis, but the significance of this finding is uncertain. Bedwetting occurs at any stage of sleep, and no abnormalities of sleep architecture have been identified.

Primary enuresis refers to enuresis without a period of continence. **Secondary enuresis** is enuresis after a period of normal bladder control. Two general population studies found that if toilet training is delayed until after 18 months, the prevalence of enuresis increases. Secondary enuresis, but not primary enuresis, is associated with psychosocial stressors. Secondary enuresis is more likely to be associated with behavioral disturbance. About 50% of enuretic children between 7 and 12 years of age have had a previous period of continence.

C. Genetics

A genetic contribution to enuresis is possible but as yet unidentified. Bedwetting runs in families (von Gontard et al, 2011) and is significantly more common in monozygotic than dizygotic twins.

▶ Clinical Findings

Daytime enuresis occurs after the child avoids urinating, whereas nocturnal enuresis occurs usually during rapid eye movement (REM) sleep, at times with a dream of urinating.

▶ Differential Diagnosis

Urinalysis, microurine, and urine culture should be ordered routinely. If daytime enuresis is present, if the patient has a history of urinary tract infection or other urinary symptoms (e.g., dysuria, urinary frequency, dribbling), or if the patient's urine grows bacteria, further urologic examinations are required in order to rule out urinary tract infection, bladder neck obstruction, neurogenic bladder, urethral valves, or other structural abnormalities. Epilepsy, diabetes mellitus, diabetes insipidus, and spina bifida should be excluded by history, physical examination, and urinalysis. Medication side effects also must be ruled out. Nocturnal enuresis can associate with sleep-disordered breathing (Jeyakumar et al, 2012).

▶ Treatment

A. Star Charts

The child is given a star to add to a calendar for each dry night. The star chart alone results in a cure for a minority of enuretic children. It also provides useful record of baseline and progress.

B. Surgical Treatment & Retention Control Training

The efficacy of radical surgical treatments such as urethral dilatation, bladder neck repair, cystoplasty, or division of the sacral nerves has not been demonstrated. Bladder training, which involves the retention of urine for longer and longer periods of time, is no longer used.

C. Psychopharmacologic Interventions

Heterocyclic antidepressants reduce the frequency of bedwetting in about 80% of patients and suppress it entirely in about 30%. However, most patients relapse within 3 months of withdrawal from the drug. The effective nighttime dosage is usually 1–2.5 mg/kg and occasionally as much as 3.5 mg/kg. This treatment essentially aims to suppress wetting while waiting for maturation in bladder control. The drug should be tapered and discontinued every 3 months and titrated back to a therapeutic level if enuresis recurs. The neuropharmacologic basis of the antienuretic effect is unknown.

The synthetic antidiuretic desmopressin acetate DDAVP (desamino-D-arginine vasopressin) is an antienuretic. It may be administered orally. Intranasal preparations are no longer indicated for enuresis because of risk of severe hyponatremia and seizure. Desamino-D-arginine vasopressin may operate by reducing urine volume below that which triggers bladder contraction. As with antidepressant therapy, relapse is common following withdrawal.

Sympathomimetic (e.g., ephedrine) and anticholinergic (e.g., belladonna) drugs are ineffective.

D. Psychotherapeutic Interventions

The alarm-and-pad technique (in which an alarm is triggered when the first drop of urine onto a pad closes an electrical circuit) has a 75–80% rate of cure and a 30% relapse rate. It is the most effective treatment available for both primary and secondary enuresis. Children with daytime enuresis, behavioral problems, and a lack of motivation may be resistant to behavioral treatment. Optimal improvement requires at least 6–8 weeks of treatment. For maximum benefit, the alarm-and-pad technique may be combined with antidepressant or antidiuretic medication and a star chart. If behavioral treatment is clearly the most effective method, why is it not the standard? Perhaps because it is cumbersome, lengthy, embarrassing, and requires good motivation, it is often resisted by parents and practitioners.

Complications/Adverse Outcomes of Treatment

Treatment complications are rare. Most children will improve with time.

Prognosis

Most cases of enuresis remit at one of two different ages, either between 5 and 7 years of age or 12 and 15 years of age. A minority of cases continue into adulthood.

Jeyakumar A, Rahman SI, Armbrecht ES, Mitchell R. The association between sleep-disordered breathing and enuresis in children. *Laryngoscope.* 2012;122(8):1873–1877.

von Gontard A, Heron J, Joinson C. Family history of nocturnal enuresis and urinary incontinence: results from a large epidemiological study. *J Urol.* 2011;185(6):2303–2306.

SLEEP DISORDERS

Sleep problems often occur before 2 years of age (see Chapter 40 for sleep disorders in older individuals).

INSOMNIA DISORDER

ICD-10 Disorders of Initiating and Maintaining Sleep (Insomnia) (G47.00)

General Considerations

Primary insomnia is most likely to be associated with psychosocial stress, maternal depression, inconsistent limits, and anxiety. It also occurs in association with sedative medication, Tourette syndrome, ADHD, intellectual disability, and autism spectrum disorder. Familial disposition has been observed (Zhang et al, 2009).

Parents have different tolerances for night waking. Thus, prevalence is a relative matter. Breastfed infants wake more often than those who are bottle fed. Waking is not associated with parity or sex; however, it is associated with perinatal adversity other than prematurity.

Clinical Findings

Night waking is sometimes associated with colic, a condition in which the child flexes the legs and cries paroxysmically as though in pain. The cause of colic is unknown. The condition seldom lasts beyond 4 months of age.

Differential Diagnosis

When considering diagnosis of insomnia disorder, normal sleep variation, situational/acute insomnia, circadian rhythm sleep–wake disorder, restless legs syndrome, breathing-related sleep disorders, narcolepsy, parasomnias, and substance/medication-induced sleep disorder should be considered.

Treatment

It is important to get a detailed history of the present illness, other concerning behavior, and family history. Treatment aims to help the child regulate his or her own sleep without disturbing the parents. Close, frequent follow-up is important, especially at the beginning of treatment. The treatment of marital problems, if any, should be reserved until a later date.

Complications/Adverse Outcomes of Treatment

Failures are most likely if the parents cannot establish daytime and nighttime routines, or if the father is not involved. Unfortunately, the practice of prescribing sedatives and hypnotics for pediatric insomnia is common among primary care providers, especially among patients with special needs. Empirical evidence supporting this practice is limited.

Prognosis

Chronic insomnia may increase the likelihood of later emotional and behavioral problems and may be a risk factor for later depression (Baglioni et al, 2011).

Baglioni C, Battagliese G, Feige B, et al. Insomnia as a predictor of depression: a meta-analytic evaluation of longitudinal epidemiological studies. *J Affect Disord.* 2011;135(1–3):10–19.

Zhang J, Li AM, Kong AP, et al. A community-based study of insomnia in Hong Kong Chinese children: prevalence, risk factors and familial aggregation. *Sleep Med.* 2009;10(9):1040–1046.

OBSTRUCTIVE SLEEP APNEA HYPOPNEA

ICD-10 Sleep Apnea (Obstructive) (G47.33)

General Considerations

Sleep apnea can be peripheral or central in origin. Obstructive apnea hypopnea is caused by oropharyngeal obstruction (e.g., by enlarged tonsilloadenoid tissue). The prevalence is 1–2% in children and increases with age. Obstructive apnea is strongly familial (Patel et al, 2008) and associated with obesity.

Clinical Findings

In obstructive sleep apnea hypopnea, the sleeping child's breathing stops intermittently and is then followed by snoring.

Differential Diagnosis

Obstructive sleep apnea or hypopnea should be distinguished from primary snoring and other sleep disorders, insomnia disorder, panic attacks, ADHD, and substance/medication-induced insomnia or hypersomnia. It may be associated with depression (Aloia et al, 2005).

Treatment

Prone sleeping and excessive bedding (e.g., blankets and comforters) should be avoided. Tonsillectomy and adenoidectomy may be necessary. Treatment with continuous positive airway pressure may be required.

Complications/Adverse Outcomes of Treatment

Children undergoing adenoidectomy (or other pharyngeal surgery) for treatment of upper airway obstruction have more frequent complications postoperatively and increased potential for serious respiratory compromise than those who undergo this procedure for other indications.

Prognosis

Chronic apnea can be associated with failure to thrive, attentional difficulty and other cognitive impairment, daytime drowsiness, and chronic headache.

Aloia MS, Arnedt JT, Smith L, et al. Examining the construct of depression in obstructive sleep apnea hypopnea. *Sleep Med.* 2005;6(2):115–121.

Patel SR, Larkin EK, Redline S. Shared genetic basis for obstructive sleep apnea and adiposity measures. *Int J Obes (Lond).* 2008; 32(5):795–800.

CENTRAL SLEEP APNEA

ICD-10 Sleep Apnea (Central) (G47.31)

General Considerations

Some sleep apnea is central as opposed to obstructive in origin. Central apnea occurs in the sudden infant death syndrome and may be associated with sleeping prone or excessive environmental temperature. Central sleep apnea includes idiopathic central sleep apnea, Cheyne–Stokes breathing, and central sleep apnea comorbid with opioid use (Yue & Guilleminault, 2010). The idiopathic type is thought to be a rare disorder with unknown prevalence, while Cheyne–Stokes breathing is commonly associated with low cardiac ejection fraction. Up to 30% of those who are on chronic opioid therapy have central sleep apnea cormorbid with opioid use (Wang et al, 2005). This is thought to be due to the effects of opioids on medullary anhypoxic/hypercapneic respiratory drive.

Clinical Findings

Central sleep apnea presents with sleepiness and insomnia. The characteristic breathing pattern can be observed using polysomnography.

Differential Diagnosis

Central sleep apnea should be differentiated from other breathing-related sleep disorders. It may coexist with obstructive sleep apnea hypopnea.

Treatment

Treatment should be targeted to associated conditions and comorbid disorders. Positive pressure therapy is recommended. Supplemental oxygen may be needed if hypoxemia is noted.

Complications/Adverse Outcomes of Treatment

Treatment complications are associated with the treatment of associated conditions.

Prognosis

The prognosis depends on the type and severity of disorder as well as other medical complications.

Wang D, Teichtahl H, Drummer O, et al. Central sleep apnea in stable methadone maintenance treatment patients. *Chest.* 2005;128(3):1348–1356.

Yue HJ, Guilleminault C. Opioid medication and sleep-disordered breathing. *Med Clin N Am.* 2010;94(3):435–446.

SLEEP-RELATED HYPOVENTILATION (G47.34-6)

General Considerations

Sleep-related hypoventilation includes idiopathic hypoventilation, congenital central alveolar hypoventilation, and most commonly, comorbid sleep-related hypoventilation. Congenital central alveolar hypoventilation is due to mutations of the *PHOX2B* gene (Weese-Mayer et al, 2010).

Clinical Findings

Sleep-related hypoventilation presents with daytime sleepiness, insomnia, and headache. During polysomnography, sleep-related hypoxemia and hypercapnia are noted.

Differential Diagnosis

Sleep-related hypoventilation should be distinguished from other medical conditions affecting ventilating and other breathing-related sleep disorders. It is associated with medication use (Yue & Guilleminault, 2010), hypothyroidism, pulmonary disorders, and neuromuscular disorders.

Treatment

Treatment should be targeted at associated conditions and comorbid disorders. Positive-pressure therapy is recommended. Sedatives should be used with caution.

Complications/Adverse Outcomes of Treatment

Treatment complications are associated with specific treatment of the associated conditions.

Prognosis

The prognosis depends on the type and severity of disorder as well as associated other medical complications.

Weese-Mayer DE, Berry-Kravis EM, Ceccherini I, et al. An official ATS clinical policy statement: congenital central hypoventilation syndrome: genetic basis, diagnosis, and management. *Am J Respir Crit Care Med.* 2010;181(6):626–644.

Yue HJ, Guilleminault C. Opioid medication and sleep-disordered breathing. *Med Clin N Am.* 2010;94(3):435–446.

NONRAPID EYE MOVEMENT SLEEP AROUSAL DISORDERS

ICD-10 Criteria Sleepwalking (Somnambulism)

A state of altered consciousness in which phenomena of sleep and wakefulness are combined. During a sleepwalking episode the individual arises from bed, usually during the first third of nocturnal sleep, and walks about, exhibiting low levels of awareness, reactivity, and motor skill. Upon awakening, there is usually no recall of the event.

ICD-10 Criteria Sleep Terrors (F51.4)

Nocturnal episodes of extreme terror and panic associated with intense vocalization, motility, and high levels of autonomic discharge. The individual sits up or gets up, usually during the first third of nocturnal sleep, with a panicky scream. Quite often he or she rushes to the door as if trying to escape, although very seldom leaves the room. Recall of the event, if any, is very limited (usually to one or two fragmentary mental images).

General Considerations

The disposition to sleepwalking and sleep terror is probably inherited. Sleepwalking and sleep terrors occurs in 1–5% of children. The prevalence of sleep terrors peaks at 18 months but decreases significantly with increasing age (Nguyen et al, 2008).

Clinical Findings

Sleep terrors, which occur during slow-wave sleep, are partial arousals in which motor functions are active though the brain is asleep. Sleep terrors must be distinguished from nightmares. In the latter, the child awakens and may recount a frightening dream but is consolable. In sleep terrors, the child appears terrified, usually sitting up, screaming, with wide eyes and autonomic arousal. Nevertheless, the child is not truly awake and is unresponsive to a parent's efforts to soothe. When the child calms, he or she resumes sleep and has no memory of the event on the following day. Unlike nightmares, the increase in heart rate is significant and occurs very quickly. Sleep terrors are most common in the first third of the night, when non-REM sleep is most evident, whereas nightmares most often occur in the latter third of the night when REM sleep is most evident.

In sleepwalking, the child walks about the house, unresponsive and blank-faced. As with sleep terrors, the child resumes sleep after the episode and has no memory of the episode.

Differential Diagnosis

Non-REM sleep arousal disorders must be distinguished from nocturnal complex seizures. Complex seizures are usually associated with violent thrashing about and stereotyped movements. Posttraumatic stress disorder should also be considered, as well as nightmare disorder, breathing-related sleep disorders, REM sleep behavior disorder, parasomnia overlap syndrome, sleep-related seizures, alcohol-induced blackouts, dissociative amnesia, malingering, panic disorder, medication-induced complex behaviors, and night eating syndrome. Non-REM sleep arousal disorders are associated with depression and anxiety disorders.

Treatment

The clinician should reassure the parents that the condition is probably a variant of normal development. The child should not be awakened during an episode but rather laid down or led back to bed. Anticipatory awaking has been used to treat. Extraneous sources of stress should be addressed. Safety intervention such as locking doors and windows and setting alarms should be instituted. Sleep deprivation should be avoided (Bloomfield & Shatkin, 2009). For those unresponsive to behavioral techniques, short-term treatment with low-dose benzodiazepine has been recommended.

Complications/Adverse Outcomes of Treatment

Treatment complications are rare. Most children will improve with time.

Prognosis

Sleep terrors typically resolve spontaneously in adolescence.

Bloomfield ER, Shatkin JP. Parasomnias and movement disorders in children and adolescents. *Child Adolesc Psychiatr Clin N Am.* 2009;18(4):947–965.

Nguyen BH, Pérusse D, Paquet J, et al. Sleep terrors in children: a prospective study of twins. *Pediatrics* 2008;122(6):e1164–e1167.

NIGHTMARE DISORDER

ICD-10 Criteria Nightmares (F51.5)

Dream experiences loaded with anxiety or fear. There is very detailed recall of the dream content. The dream experience is very vivid and usually includes themes involving threats to survival, security, or self-esteem. Quite often there is a recurrence of the same or similar frightening nightmare themes. During a typical episode there is a degree of autonomic discharge but no appreciable vocalization or body motility. Upon awakening the individual rapidly becomes alert and oriented.

General Considerations

Nightmares are more prevalent in association with anxiety, particularly posttraumatic stress disorder. Nightmares occur in 1–4% of preschool children (Simard et al, 2008). They often begin at 3–6 years of age, often after exposure to psychosocial stressors. A genetic predisposition to nightmares has been found in twin studies.

Clinical Findings

Following a nightmare, the child wakens and recounts a frightening, realistic dream but is consolable. Though rapid eye movements, mild shortness of breath, increased heart rate, and sweating may occur during nightmares, body movements and talking usually occur at the end of the nightmares since almost all nightmares develop during REM sleep with loss of muscle tone. They arise usually in the last third of the night (Simor et al, 2012).

Differential Diagnosis

Nightmares must be distinguished from sleep terrors (as above), as well as nocturnal complex seizures. Complex seizures are usually associated with violent thrashing about and stereotyped movements. Posttraumatic stress disorder should also be considered. Comorbid conditions include PTSD, insomnia disorder, anxiety disorders, adjustment disorders, and withdrawal from medications.

Treatment

Nightmares can be managed with behavioral techniques such as reassurance, rescripting, desensitization, hypnotherapy, and cognitive–behavioral therapy. If nightmares are associated with posttraumatic stress disorder, anxiety disorder, or environmental stress, the cause of the sleep disturbance should be treated or addressed.

Complications/Adverse Outcomes of Treatment

Treatment complications are rare. Most children will improve with time.

Prognosis

Most children who develop a nightmare problem outgrow it.

Simard V, Nielsen TA, Tremblay RE, et al. Longitudinal study of bad dreams in preschool children: prevalence, demographic correlates, risk and protective factors. *Sleep.* 2008;31(1):62–70.

Simor P, Horváth K, Gombos F, et al. Disturbed dreaming and sleep quality: altered sleep architecture in subjects with frequent nightmares. *Eur Arch Psychiatry Clin Neurosci.* 2012;262(8): 687–696.

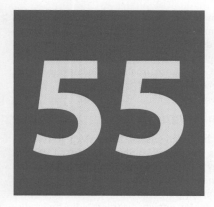

Gender Dysphoria in Children and Adolescents

Kenneth J. Zucker, PhD

▶ ## Essentials of Diagnosis

Different sets of criteria are used in the *Diagnostic and Statistical Manual of Mental Disorders, Fifth Edition* (DSM-5) to diagnose gender dysphoria (GD) in children versus adolescents (American Psychiatric Association, 2013). Both criteria sets emphasize incongruence between the experienced gender and the gender assigned at birth. The experienced gender can be either a traditional opposite-sex gender identity or some alternative, nontraditional gender identity that is inconsistent with the culturally specific gender roles associated with being a "man" or "woman." As with many diagnoses, an essential criterion is the presence of clinically significant distress or impairment of functioning in one or more important areas (e.g., social relationships, school). One should specify whether GD co-occurs with a disorder of sex development (DSD). For adolescents, one should also specify whether the patient has undergone a gender transition, including medical procedures to align the patient's physical appearance with his or her experienced gender identity.

In the ICD-11, several revisions have been proposed to the ICD-10 diagnoses of Transsexualism and Gender Identity Disorder of Childhood: (1) to rename these two diagnoses as Gender Incongruence of Adolescents and Adults and Gender Incongruence of Childhood; (2) for the child diagnosis, that it cannot be diagnosed before the age of 5 years and that the "incongruence" must be of at least 2 years in duration (unlike 6 months in the DSM-5); and (3) perhaps of most importance, to move these diagnoses out of the ICD section on Mental and Behavioural Disorders into a new section provisionally termed Conditions Related to Sexual Health (Drescher et al, 2012, 2016).

The proposal to create a new section of the ICD-11 to accommodate gender identity diagnoses has been influenced, in part, by some clinicians and transgender activists/organizations who want to "depathologize" and destigmatize gender dysphoria or gender incongruence (Drescher, 2015), yet at the same time to retain access to care, including mental health services, and insurance coverage for biomedical procedures, such as sex-reassignment (or "gender-affirming") surgery. The renaming of the diagnosis to Gender Incongruence (as opposed to GD as it is now called in the DSM-5) is because the proposed diagnosis does not require "distress" or impairment, as it does in the DSM-5. It is also of note that retaining any diagnosis at all for children is hotly contested. For example, a survey of members of the World Professional Association for Transgender Health found that about half were in favor of retention in the ICD and half were in favor of deletion (De Cuypere et al, 2016). Apart from these conceptual changes, one should note that the proposed rationale for a lower bound age of 5 years for the diagnosis in children has, as of yet, not been made clear. One could argue that this proposal is to alert clinicians to be cautious in offering any type of treatment recommendation for very young children; on the other hand, it could be argued that such a proposal will be a barrier to early treatment, and it is certainly the case that many children with this diagnosis are seen clinically prior to the age of 5 (see Cohen-Kettenis et al, 2003).

▶ ## General Considerations

A. Epidemiology

According to the DSM-5, data regarding the population prevalence of GD in children and adolescents are limited. The prevalence of adults seeking treatment for GD from specialty clinics has been used to provide estimates. The prevalence rates among natal adult males and females are 0.005–0.014% and 0.002–0.003%, respectively. These likely represent underestimates, however, because not all individuals who experience GD will present at specialty clinics for treatment and also because children or adolescents' GD symptoms may dissipate by adulthood. In any case, it is safe to conclude that GD in children and adolescents is relatively rare.

The sex ratio of natal males to females who are seen in specialty clinics for GD ranges from 2:1 to 4.5:1 among children (Wood et al, 2013). It is not clear whether this bias toward natal males reflects an actual childhood sex difference in the prevalence of GD. Instead, it may reflect differential reactions to cross-gender behavior in children, with feminine boys eliciting a stronger reaction than masculine girls. Among adolescents, the sex ratio of natal males to females who are seen in specialty clinics for GD is closer to parity, but more recently it appears that natal females have begun to outnumber natal males (Aitken et al, 2015).

B. Etiology

The etiology of GD appears to be multifactorial. Biological theories have focused on three areas: genetic factors, prenatal exposure to sex hormones, and maternal–fetal interactions. A twin study reported higher concordance for GD patients who were monozygotic (identical) versus those who were dizygotic (fraternal) twins, suggesting a role for genetic factors (Heylens et al, 2012). Individuals who were exposed to atypical prenatal sex hormone levels due to a DSD are more likely to experience cross-gender identification, suggesting a role for prenatal sex hormones in GD (e.g., girls exposed to elevated levels of androgens during gestation as in the case of congenital adrenal hyperplasia) (Pasterski et al, 2015). Regarding maternal–fetal interactions, some mothers might produce an immunological response toward male-specific proteins as a consequence of gestating successive male fetuses. This immunological response may limit masculinization and defeminization of the fetal male brain in later-born males. This immunological pathway is reflected in late birth order and excesses of older brothers among GD males—although this explanation appears to be limited to GD males who are also homosexual relative to their natal sex. GD females appear to have excesses of older sisters, but there are currently no hypotheses regarding the etiological significance of this finding (VanderLaan et al, 2014).

Psychosocial theories have often emphasized gender schema development or a complex family environment, but few psychosocial factors have been identified. Having rigid gender schemata or developmentally lagging in the formation of gender constancy may lead some children with stereotypically opposite-sex preferences (e.g., toy or activity preferences) to believe they are the opposite gender (Zucker et al, 1999). Psychodynamic perspectives have conceptualized cross-gender behavior and identification as an essential part of the child's attempt to cope with separation anxiety (Zucker et al, 2014). Parental factors also appear to be important. Persistence of GD is associated with lower parental socioeconomic status (Singh, 2012), although it is presently unclear why this association exists. Parental reactions to cross-gender behavior and identity also appear to be important. For example, GD is more likely to persist in children whose parents support a social gender transition (Steensma et al, 2013).

▶ Clinical Findings

A. Signs & Symptoms

Among children, the presence of GD is often inferred from the child's overt behavior. Many of the diagnostic criteria focus on concrete observations such as a marked preference for opposite-gender playmates, activities, and toys as well as avoidance of same-gender playmates, activities, and toys. Children with GD may also often make statements about being a member of the opposite gender or a strong desire to be of the other gender. In rare or extreme cases, children with GD may experience anatomic dysphoria and express the desire to alter their genitals (e.g., removing the penis) or behave as though they have the anatomy of the opposite sex (e.g., pretending to have breasts or to be pregnant in the case of boys or pretending to have a penis in the case of girls).

Adolescents with GD exhibit cross-gender identification or identify with some alternative gender category that is inconsistent with their gender assignment at birth. Anatomic dysphoria and the desire to undergo treatments to align their physical appearance via cross-sex hormone administration and/or surgical interventions (e.g., penectomy, hysterectomy) are common among adolescents with GD—although the degree of anatomic dysphoria and desire for such treatments can vary considerably between patients. Adolescents are often described as exhibiting either early- or late-onset GD. Early-onset GD pertains to those adolescents who recall experiencing cross-gender behavior and identification in childhood, whereas late-onset GD pertains to those adolescents whose GD was not evident in childhood. Asking adolescents (and their parents, if possible) whether the diagnostic criteria for GD in children applied to them as children can be useful for determining early versus late onset. The age of onset also appears to overlap with sexual orientation. The majority of early-onset adolescents are homosexual relative to their natal sex, whereas this is less true of late-onset adolescents. Late-onset natal males may also present with a history consistent with transvestic disorder.

As with many DSM diagnoses, a key criterion for a diagnosis of GD is the presence of clinically significant distress. This distress can be caused by the GD itself or can be a consequence of others' stigmatizing or discriminatory reactions to the gender-nonconforming behavior of the patient. Impairment in important areas of functioning (e.g., school performance) is considered to be a reliable indicator of underlying distress.

B. Psychological Testing

A number of measures have been developed for use in the clinical diagnosis of GD (Zucker, 2005; Zucker & Wood, 2011). These include parent- and self-report questionnaires, structured observations of play behavior, projective tests, and gender identity interview schedules. These measures show good discriminant validity (i.e., they distinguish between GD and control children) with low rates of false positives, and they also reliably distinguish those who satisfy the threshold for a DSM diagnosis of GD from those who are subthreshold for GD. Specialized measures for the diagnosis of GD should be complemented by more general measures such as the Child Behavior Checklist and the Youth Self-Report, as well as cognitive testing to provide a comprehensive assessment of other possible behavioral and/or psychiatric issues.

C. Neuroimaging

Data regarding brain differences between individuals who do and those who do not experience GD are largely limited to studies of adults (Altinay et al, 2020; Zucker et al, 2016). Before receiving any biomedical treatments for GD, GD individuals' brains are organized (at least in part) in an opposite-sex manner, but the extent to which this is true of particular neuroanatomical structures may differ for GD males and females. Natal GD males exhibit a shift toward female-typical white matter connectivity (Rametti et al, 2011) and cortical thickness in certain regions in the frontal, parietal, and temporal areas (Luders et al, 2012; Zubiaurre-Elorza et al, 2013). Natal GD males who are nonhomosexual in relation to their birth sex are more likely to exhibit male-typical brain structure (Savic & Arver, 2011), suggesting that GD brain anatomy varies by sexual orientation (similar data do not exist for nonhomosexual GD females). Natal GD females who are homosexual in relation to their birth sex show male-typical structure in the putamen (Zubiaurre-Elorza et al, 2013) as well as in the connectivity of brain white matter (Rametti et al, 2011), but appear to have female-typical cortical thickness (Zubiaurre-Elorza et al, 2013). Future research is needed to better characterize the neuroanatomical basis of GD.

Differential Diagnosis

In children and adolescents, GD is associated with an increased presence of internalizing, including suicidality, and externalizing problems (Aitken et al, 2016; Mason et al, 2023; Zucker et al, 2014). These problems may often be related to poor peer relations and experiences with bullying related to gender nonconformity (Shiffman et al, 2015). Separation anxiety is also often evident among boys clinically referred for GD (Zucker et al, 1996). There also appears to be a link between GD and autism spectrum disorders (ASD) (Van Der Miesen et al, 2016). Many GD children show elevations in repetitive behaviors and intense or obsessional interests, often revolving around a gender-related theme, and these behaviors and interests may be indicative of an overlap between GD and ASD (VanderLaan et al, 2015).

General risk factors should also be considered. Such factors include a family history of psychopathology. For example, parental psychopathology is positively associated with psychopathology among GD children (Zucker et al, 2014). Other factors that apply to youth more broadly, such as low cognitive functioning and socioeconomic background, should also be considered as potential influences on patient vulnerability.

GD and gender-nonconforming behavior more generally are elevated among individuals with certain DSDs (Berenbaum & Meyer-Bahlburg, 2015). The possible presence of a DSD should, therefore, be evaluated. Whether GD is concurrent with a DSD is one of the specifiers of the DSM-5 GD diagnosis.

Treatment

A. Psychotherapeutic Interventions

The focus of psychological therapy for children and adolescents with GD is informed by one's clinical formulation and etiological stance. If one views the distress associated with GD as a manifestation of the GD itself, then a primary goal might be to address the lack of congruence between the experienced gender identity and the one assigned at birth. Alternatively, if the cross-gender behavior is caused by some underlying anxiety (e.g., separation anxiety), therapeutic efforts might be most effective if they concentrated on assuaging the anxiety and/or helping the child use some coping strategy other than cross-gender behavior. In the event that the distress associated with GD is mainly owing to social ostracism, therapy might focus on coping skills and strengthening peer relations. If the GD is associated with a co-occurring ASD, then one might explore whether the GD is a consequence of an intense preoccupation with cross-gender objects and evaluate the likelihood that such a preoccupation gives rise to cross-gender identification and will continue to do so (de Vries et al, 2010).

There is no consensus regarding best practice when treating children with GD (Byne et al, 2012; Adelson & American Academy of Child and Adolescent Psychiatry (AACAP) Committee on Quality Issues (CQI), 2012). In younger children, gender identity is likely not yet fixed. It may, therefore, be possible to help a child feel comfortable with the gender identity that is consistent with his or her birth sex. However, one should be careful to not be critical. Instead, one may, for example, introduce same-sex peers who share similar interests, thereby helping the child feel comfortable as a member of his or her birth-assigned gender without challenging his or her preferences.

In treating adolescents, there is reasonable consensus that the best practice approach is to support a social gender transition and the initiation of biomedical treatments that permit an approximation of the phenotype of the desired gender (de Vries et al, 2014; Zucker et al, 2011). However, not all adolescents are immediate candidates for these treatments. For example, some adolescents express confusion about their gender identity or are exploring how their gender identity relates to their emerging sexual orientation. In such cases, the goal of therapy should be to help the adolescent work through these issues before making any decisions about a gender transition.

An important caveat is that therapeutic goals need to be clearly articulated and agreed upon with parents, especially when treating children. To begin with, parents' cultural and/or religious background may influence treatment recommendations. Parents may vary considerably in their goals for therapy. Some parents may request assistance with helping navigate a gender transition for their child (Olson et al, 2016). At the other extreme, parents might ask the therapist to avert a transgender or homosexual outcome. Most parents are somewhere in between these extremes and look to the therapist to guide them toward helping their child achieve the best psychosocial outcome possible. In general, it is recommended that therapists remain agnostic with respect to the particular gender identity or sexual orientation outcome that is ideal. That said, parents who wish for a homosexual outcome to be averted should be advised that there is no evidence that therapies directed toward altering sexual orientation are effective and are, in fact, harmful (Alempijevic et al, 2020). In sum, the therapist must gauge and consider parental goals in the context of tailoring therapy to maximize the patient's long-term functioning given his or her family environment.

B. Biomedical Interventions

Biomedical interventions designed to align an individual's physical appearance with his or her experienced gender identity can be used in the treatment of adolescents. For adolescents who have begun puberty (i.e., Tanner stage 2 or higher), it is common to prescribe gonadotropin-releasing hormonal therapy, which suppresses natural sex hormone production and the expression of sexually dimorphic characteristics (e.g., breast development and menses in females; facial hair and deepening of the voice in males). At approximately age 16, it is common to prescribe cross-sex hormone therapy, which promotes the development of sexually dimorphic characteristics associated with the opposite sex. Hormonal therapy appears to have a beneficial effect on behavioral and emotional problems (de Vries et al, 2014). Surgical interventions are not commonly employed below 18 years of age.

Complications/Adverse Outcomes of Treatment

Unfortunately, there are limited data from long-term follow-up studies examining potentially adverse outcomes of treatment, and which approach is optimal for treating GD in minors is controversial (Drescher & Byne, 2012). On the one hand, challenging the child's cross-gender identity may be experienced as invalidating and have negative long-term consequences. Alternatively, helping a child to be comfortable with his or her birth-assigned gender might help circumvent the long-term negative effects of social ostracism on behavioral and emotional problems. Ultimately, either of these could be true in any given case, and it is up to clinicians to use their best judgment in light of the current available information on long-term outcomes.

With respect to biomedical treatments, the goal should be to ensure that patients are unlikely to regret alterations to their body. It is thought that the effects of treatments to suppress puberty are mostly reversible, whereas those of cross-sex hormone administration are partially reversible (Kreukels & Cohen-Kettenis, 2011). Although this may be true for external anatomy, it is unclear what effects this therapy might have on the developing adolescent brain. In adults, cross-sex hormone administration can cause brain anatomy to be more similar to that of members of the opposite sex (Rametti et al, 2012; Zubiaurre-Elorza et al, 2014), but the effects during adolescence might be more profound given that adolescence is a much more dynamic period of brain development.

Prognosis

Long-term follow-up studies indicate that the majority of children will desist in their GD and exhibit a homosexual or bisexual sexual orientation as adults, whereas only a small percentage will persist in their GD (Drummond et al, 2008; Green, 1987; Steensma, 2013; Wallien & Cohen Kettenis, 2008). Low parental socioeconomic status, greater intensity of childhood GD, and early social gender transition appear to be associated with a higher likelihood of GD persistence, but the relative importance of these factors may differ for natal males and females (Singh, 2012; Steensma et al, 2013). Also, one study suggested that natal males who persist in their GD are also more likely to experience psychiatric problems, followed by those who desist and report a homosexual or bisexual sexual orientation, followed by those who desist and report a heterosexual sexual orientation (Singh, 2012). In adolescents, GD is likely to persist into adulthood, and many will seek biomedical treatments, including hormonal therapy and eventually sex reassignment surgery (Zucker et al, 2011).

Adelson SL; American Academy of Child and Adolescent Psychiatry (AACAP) Committee on Quality Issues (CQI). Practice parameter on gay, lesbian, or bisexual sexual orientation, gender nonconformity, and gender discordance in children and adolescence. *J Am Acad Child Adolesc Psychiatry*. 2012;51:957–974.

Aitken M, Steensma TD, Blanchard R, et al. Evidence for an altered sex ratio in clinic-referred adolescents with gender dysphoria. *J Sex Med*. 2015;12:756–763.

Aiken M, VanderLaan DP, Wasserman L, et al. Self-harm and suicidality in children referred for gender dysphoria. *J Am Acad Child Adolesc Psychiatry*. 2016;55(6):513–520 http://dx.doi.org/10.1016/j.jaac.2016.04.001.

Alempijevic D, Beriashvili R, Beynon J, et al. Independent Forensic Expert Group. Statement on conversion therapy. *J Forensic Leg Med*. 2020;72:101930. doi: 10.1016/j.jflm.2020.101930. Epub 2020 Feb 19. PMID: 32452446.

Altinay M, Anand A. Neuroimaging gender dysphoria: a novel psychobiological model. *Brain Imaging Behav*. 2020;14(4):1281–1297. doi: 10.1007/s11682-019-00121-8. PMID: 31134582.

American Psychiatric Association. *Diagnostic and Statistical Manual of Mental Disorders*. 5th ed. Arlington, VA: American Psychiatric Publishing; 2013.

Berenbaum SA, Meyer-Bahlburg HFL. Gender development and sexuality in disorders of sex development. *Horm Metab Res*. 2015;47:361–365.

Byne W, Bradley SJ, Coleman E, et al. Report of the American Psychiatric Association task force on treatment of Gender Identity Disorder. *Arch Sex Behav*. 2012;41:759–796.

Cohen-Kettenis PT, Owen A, Kaijser VG, et al. Demographic characteristics, social competence, and behavior problems in children with gender identity disorder: a cross-national, cross-clinic comparative analysis. *J Abnorm Child Psychol*. 2003;31:41–53.

De Cuypere G, Winter S, Green J, et al. The proposed ICD-11 gender incongruence of childhood diagnosis: a World Professional Association for Transgender Health membership survey. *Arch Sex Behav*. 2016;45(7):1605–1614.

de Vries ALC, McGuire JK, Steensma TD, et al. Young adult psychological outcome after puberty suppression and gender reassignment. *Pediatrics*. 2014;134:696–704.

de Vries ALC, Noens IL, Cohen-Kettenis PT, et al. Autism spectrum disorders in gender dysphoric children and adolescents. *J Autism Dev Disord*. 2010;40:930–936.

de Vries AL, Steensma TD, Doreleijers TA, et al. Puberty suppression in adolescents with gender identity disorder: a prospective follow-up study. *J Sex Med*. 2011;8:2276–2283.

Drescher J. Queer diagnoses revisited: the past and future of homosexuality and gender diagnoses in DSM and ICD. *Int Rev Psychiatry*. 2015;27:386–395.

Drescher J, Byne W. Gender dysphoric/gender variant (GD/GV) children and adolescents: summarizing what we know and what we have yet to learn. *J Homosex*. 2012;59:501–510.

Drescher J, Cohen-Kettenis PT, Reed GM. Gender incongruence of childhood in the ICD-11: controversies, proposal, and rationale. *Lancet Psychiatry*. 2016;3:297–304.

Drescher J, Cohen-Kettenis PT, Winter S. Minding the body: situating gender identity diagnoses in the ICD-11. *Int Rev Psychiatry*. 2012;24:568–577.

Drummond KD, Bradley SJ, Peterson-Badali M, et al. A follow-up study of girls with gender identity disorder. *Dev Psychol*. 2008;44:34–35.

Green R. *The "Sissy Boy Syndrome" and the Development of Homosexuality*. New Haven, CT: Yale University Press; 1987.

Heylens G, De Cuypere G, Zucker KJ, et al. Gender identity disorder in twins: a review of the case report literature. *J Sex Med*. 2012;9:751–757.

Kreukels BP, Cohen-Kettenis PT. Puberty suppression in gender identity disorder. *Nat Rev Endocrinol*. 2011;7:466–472.

Luders E, Sanchez FJ, Tosun D, et al. Increased cortical thickness in male-to-female transsexualism. *J Behav Brain Sci*. 2012;2:357–362.

Mason A, Crowe E, Haragan B, Smith S, Kyriakou A. Gender dysphoria in young people: a model of chronic stress. *Horm Res Paediatr*. 2023;96(1):54–65. doi: 10.1159/000520361. Epub 2021 Oct 21. PMID: 34673639

Olson KR, Durwood L, DeMeules M, et al. Mental health of transgender children who are supported in their identities. *Pediatrics*. 2016;137(3):e20153223.

Pasterski V, Zucker KJ, Hindmarsh PC, et al. Increased cross-gender identification independent of gender role behavior in girls with congenital adrenal hyperplasia: results from a standardized assessment of children 4- to 11-year-old children. *Arch Sex Behav*. 2015;43:1363–1375.

Rametti G, Carrillo B, Gómez-Gil E, et al. White matter microstructure in male to female transsexuals before cross-sex hormonal treatment. A diffusion tensor imaging study. *J Psychiatr Res*. 2011;45:949–954.

Rametti G, Carrillo B, Gómez-Gil E, et al. Effects of androgenization on the white matter microstructure of female-to-male transsexuals. A diffusion tensor imaging study. *Psychoneuroendocrinology*. 2012;37:1261–1269.

Savic I, Arver S. Sex dimorphism of the brain in male-to-female transsexuals. *Cereb Cortex*. 2011;21:2525–2533.

Shiffman M, VanderLaan DP, Wood H, et al. Behavioral and emotional problems as a function of peer relationships in adolescents with gender dysphoria: a comparison with clinical and nonclinical controls. *Psychol Sex Orientat Gend Divers*. 2015. doi: http://dx.doi.org/10.1037/sgd0000152.

Singh D. *A Follow-Up Study of Boys with Gender Identity Disorder*. Unpublished doctoral dissertation, University of Toronto; 2012.

Steensma TD. *From Gender Variance to Gender Dysphoria: Psychosexual Development of Gender Atypical Children and Adolescents*. Unpublished doctoral dissertation, Vrije Universiteit, Amsterdam; 2013.

Steensma TD, McGuire JK, Kreukels BP, et al. Factors associated with the desistence and persistence of childhood gender dysphoria: a quantitative follow-up study. *J Am Acad Child Adolesc Psychiatry*. 2013;52:582–590.

Van Der Miesen AIR, Hurley H, de Vries ALC. Gender dysphoria and autism spectrum disorder: a narrative review. *Int J Psychiatry*. 2016;28:70–80.

VanderLaan DP, Blanchard R, Wood H, et al. Birth order and sibling sex ratio of children and adolescents referred to a Gender Identity Service. *PLoS One*. 2014;9:e90257.

VanderLaan, DP, Postema L, Wood H, et al. Do children with gender dysphoria have intense/obsessional interests? *J Sex Res*. 2015;52(2):213–219

Wallien MS, Cohen-Kettenis PT. Psychosexual outcome of gender-dysphoric children. *J Am Acad Child Adolesc Psychiatry*. 2008;47:1413–1423.

Wood H, Sasaki S, Bradley SJ, et al. Patterns of referral to a Gender Identity Service for children and adolescents (1976–2011): age, sex ratio, and sexual orientation [Letter to the Editor]. *J Sex Marital Ther*. 2013;39:1–6.

Zubiaurre-Elorza L, Junque C, Gómez-Gil E, et al. Cortical thickness in untreated transsexuals. *Cereb Cortex*. 2013;23:2855–2862.

Zubiaurre-Elorza L, Junque C, Gómez-Gil E, Guillamon A. Effects of cross-sex hormone treatment on cortical thickness in transsexual individuals. *J Sex Med*. 2014;11:1248–1261.

Zucker KJ. Measurement of psychosexual differentiation. *Arch Sex Behav*. 2005;34:375–388.

Zucker KJ, Lawrence AA, Kreukels BPC. Gender dysphoria in adults. *Annu Rev Clin Psychol*. 2016;12, 217–247.

Zucker KJ, Wood H. Assessment of gender variance in children. *Child Adolesc Psychiatr Clin N Am*. 2011;20:665–680.

Zucker KJ, Bradley SJ, Kuksis M, et al. Gender constancy judgments in children with gender identity disorder: evidence for a developmental lag. *Arch Sex Behav*. 1999;28:475–502.

Zucker KJ, Bradley SJ, Lowry Sullivan CB. Traits of separation anxiety in boys with gender identity disorder. *J Am Acad Child Adolesc Psychiatry*. 1996;35:791–798.

Zucker KJ, Bradley SJ, Owen-Anderson A, et al. Puberty-blocking hormonal therapy for adolescents with gender identity disorder: a descriptive clinical study. *J Gay Lesbian Ment Hlth* 2011;15:58–82.

Zucker KJ, Wood H, VanderLaan DP. Models of psychopathology in children and adolescents with gender dysphoria. In: Kreukels BPC, Steensma TD, de Vries ALC, eds. *Gender Dysphoria and Disorders of Sex Development: Progress in Care and Knowledge*. New York: Springer; 2014:171–192.

Psychological Reactions to Acute and Chronic Systemic Illness in Pediatric Patients

Simona Bujoreanu, PhD
David R. DeMaso, MD

Acute and chronic physical illnesses are stressful for children and their families. The stresses of physical illness manifest as psychological reactions involving somatic symptoms (e.g., pain, dizziness, or fatigue), behavioral changes (e.g., acting out, nonadherence, or lifestyle alterations), emotional states (e.g., fear, sadness, or anxiety), and developmental challenges (e.g., incorporating medical information at different developmental stages). This chapter provides an overview of psychological reactions to physical illness, a differential diagnosis approach to these reactions, a review of selected childhood physical illnesses, and a summary of mental health interventions in children with physical illnesses.

Overview

Between 10 and 20 million U.S. children have a chronic physical illness or medical condition that significantly affects their functioning and life during at least 3 months of the year (American Psychiatric Association, 2000). Although children and their families are overall remarkably resilient in adapting to the challenges presented by a physical illness, at least 10% of children with physical illness have symptoms severe enough to have an impact on their daily living (Ingerski et al, 2010). With the advent of successful medical/surgical management for many childhood illnesses, pediatric psychosomatic medicine (including consultation–liaison psychiatry, pediatric psychology, and behavioral medicine) has developed as a specialty supporting children and their families with the emotional and behavioral impacts of acute and chronic systemic illness via psychological and pharmacological treatments (Bujoreanu et al, 2015; Snell & DeMaso, 2010).

Reactions to illness cover a spectrum of emotions and behaviors, from simple verbal expressions of discomfort, crying, or temporary withdrawal to disabling responses involving significant regression in social and emotional functioning (e.g., anxiety, depression, oppositional behaviors, or nonadherence). It is important to highlight that labeling a reaction as "normal" or "abnormal" is dependent not only

on a child's developmental stage but also on whose perspective is being considered. For example, parents and children are more focused on minimizing distress (hence withdrawal, unresponsiveness, or resistance), as compared to providers, who are often more interested in maximizing adherence to treatment (Rudolph et al, 1995). Furthermore, particularly for children with chronic physical conditions, past negative medical experiences are likely to increase a child's emotional distress during subsequent health care encounters (Siegel & Smith, 1989), and previous hospitalizations can lead to more troubling increases in separation anxiety, sleep difficulties, and pain perception, as well as changes in physiological indicators (Thompson, 1986).

Differential Diagnosis Approach to Psychological Reactions in Physical Illness

In the classic dichotomy, psychological reactions can be classified as internalizing or externalizing, depending on how the emotional tension is experienced by the child and the people around him/her. Depression, anxiety, and somatic complaints are markers of internalizing problems, whereas behavioral "acting out," aggression, or hyperactivity are typical symptoms of externalizing problems. For physically ill children, internalizing symptoms are the most frequently occurring presentation (Pinquart & Shen, 2011) and appear to be more frequent than in physically healthy children (Barlow & Ellard, 2006; Benton & DeMaso, 2010). The mechanism by which the internalizing struggles predominate in physically ill children has been hypothesized to be related to the loss of control over one's life, restrictions on positive activities, isolation from peers, and/or adverse medical experiences (Pinquart & Shen, 2011).

In the assessment and management of physically ill children presenting with significant psychological reactions, it is helpful to consider whether any of the following entities or combination of entities is responsible for the patient's presenting symptoms: (1) a primary mental disorder, (2) mental disorder due to a physical illness or its treatment, or (3) psychological factors affecting a physical illness. Although the presence of co-occurring mental disorder can certainly compound the diagnosis and management of the medical condition, both the direct effects (physiological effects and/or medications) and the indirect or reactive effects (e.g., hospitalizations or lifestyle changes) of the physical illness must be given consideration in the examination of the pediatric patient so as to fully understand a child's biopsychosocial functioning (DeMaso et al, 2009).

Presence of a Primary Mental Disorder

Associations between mental disorders and chronic health conditions have been estimated to be between 20 and 25% in the pediatric population (American Psychiatric Association, 2000; Wallander & Thompson, 1995), which is higher when compared with 8–20% rates of overall mental illness in community samples (Costello et al, 2004). In particular, children with central nervous system involvement (e.g., epilepsy) are three to six times more likely to develop psychopathology than the general population, particularly anxiety, depression, and disruptive disorders (Bujoreanu et al, 2011).

Neurovegetative symptoms of depression may mimic symptoms of a physical illness or its treatment. In children and adolescents, depression may present primarily with an irritable or cranky mood as well as troubling somatic symptoms (e.g., abdominal pain, headaches, whole-body pain). Symptoms of fatigue, lack of energy, changes in appetite associated with weight variations, and poor sleep may be misinterpreted as nonspecific symptoms of physical illness, when in fact they may reflect emotional struggles in younger patients. There are reports of increased rates of suicidal behaviors in physically ill children with comorbid mental disorders (e.g., depression) (Enujioke et al, 2020; Goldston et al, 1994). For some children, suicidal behavior may be manifested by the lack of action (passive suicidal behaviors) and nonadherence to medical treatment, which has equally dramatic effects on one's physical and emotional health. Anxiety symptoms and trauma stress reactions can be misinterpreted as asthma attacks, cardiac conditions, and/or gastrointestinal problems. Disabling somatic symptoms can place significant burden on the health care delivery system, as do misrecognized psychiatric illnesses, with heavy utilization of resources through repeated hospitalizations, consultations from different specialists, and investigations and treatments that are often ineffective and iatrogenic (Bujoreanu et al, 2014).

Mental Disorder Due to a Physical Illness and/or Its Treatment

Illness-related factors (e.g., metabolic imbalances, infections, neoplasms, or traumatic injury) or treatment-related factors (e.g., medications or surgery) can directly impact a child's mood and neurocognitive status (e.g., delirium or other neurocognitive disorders) with resultant changes in emotions and behaviors. The etiology for the psychological reactions in these situations is thought to be a direct physiological mechanism.

Psychological Factors Affecting a Physical Illness

In contrast, psychological factors can affect a physical illness and, consequently, impact the course of the medical condition. The etiology for these psychological reactions exists on a spectrum: at one end thought to be situational and developmental responses in reaction to the illness, and at the other end seen to reach intensity and severity levels significantly impacting a child's health and functioning (see Table 56–1 for diagnostic nomenclature). Many studies have shown significant resilience in patients and their families facing medical conditions (Hilliard et al, 2015; Hughes & Kleespies, 2001). For example, only a small percentage of patients undergoing medically traumatizing experiences appear to experience long-lasting psychiatric sequelae (Brosbe et al, 2013). Nevertheless, the impact of psychological factors on physical illnesses is underdiagnosed and underaddressed (LeBlanc et al, 2003).

Children's psychological reactions to their illness are generally attributed to a number of interrelated factors, including their coping style, temperament, family adjustment, and/or developmental stage. For example, an information-seeking coping style coupled with developmentally sensitive family

Table 56–1 Summary Comparison of ICD-10 versus DSM 5 Diagnostic Criteria for Psychological Reactions to Systemic Conditions

The ICD-10's diagnostic category entitled Psychological and Behavioral Factors Associated with Disorders or Diseases Classified Elsewhere (F54) is used to record the presence of psychological or behavioral influences thought to have played a major part in the etiology of physical disorders. The category includes psychological factors affecting physical conditions (e.g., asthma, dermatitis, gastric ulcer, irritable bowel syndrome, ulcerative colitis, and urticarial). Any resulting mental disturbances are usually mild, and often prolonged (such as worry, emotional conflict, or apprehension) and do not of themselves justify the use of any of the categories in this chapter.

This category is applicable to the DSM-5 category entitled Psychological Factors Affecting Physical Conditions (316), which recognizes the fact that psychological factors might contribute to the perpetuation and/or exacerbation of the symptoms, and might also impact treatment of the symptoms (e.g., via nonadherence). Unlike ICD-10, the DSM-5 allows for the recognition of various levels of severity regarding the impact of psychological factors affecting physical conditions.

Adapted with permission from *International Statistical Classification of Diseases and Related Health Problems* 10th Revision (ICD-10) Version for 2010. Geneva: World Health Organization; 2010.

education regarding the physical illness and its treatment is associated with better child psychological outcomes when confronting a medical stressor (Blount et al, 1991; Snell & DeMaso, 2010). In contrast, an anxious temperament along with symptoms of hyperactivity and distractibility has been found to be a risk factor in adjusting to a physical illness (Campo, 2007; Shaw & DeMaso, 2010).

Family responses to their child's acute or chronic medical needs have been proven to be a major contributor to their child's adjustment. Parents' reactions account for as much as 50% of the distress expressed by their child during an acute medical procedure (Mednick, 2010). Maternal depression and anxiety (Frank et al, 1995) and family conflict (Demaso & Bujoreanu, 2013; Manne & Miller, 1998) affect the long-term adjustment of the child with a chronic illness. The role of family coping and adjustment cannot be underestimated in a child's psychological reaction to acute or chronic illness. Awareness of parental distress, family cohesion, cognitive appraisal, problem-solving abilities, conflict, level of family disorganization, and level of support within the family and within the community widen the lens through which psychological reactions to acute and chronic pediatric illnesses are being understood, evaluated, and addressed (Bonner et al, 2010; Brosbe et al, 2013; Van Schoors et al, 2015).

A child's developmental stage influences the cognitive and emotional ability to process health-related information, to reason about causality and responsibility for the illness, and to adhere to medical regimens (Shaw & DeMaso, 2010; Thompson & Gustafson, 1996). Preschoolers are bound by magical thinking and concrete thought processes; separation from caregivers at this age is scary, and their expression of pain and fear is much more dramatic given the lack of emotional modulation and coping skills. School children may struggle with the lack of control experienced in managing illness and with the lifestyle changes; in addition, they maintain concrete thinking processes and might build faulty associations between the presence of physical illness and their perceived "wrongdoing." Adolescents' struggle with adherence to medical regimens despite having access to abstract thinking and better cognitive abilities to process complex medical information can be seen as part of their developmental striving for independence and identity definition and their use of denial as a primary coping strategy.

▶ Selected Physical Illnesses

Asthma

Asthma is the most frequent pediatric illness in the United States, with 9.4% of all children being affected (Bloom et al, 2011). Whereas asthma was seen as a "nervous disease" in the 1950s, it is now understood that allergic phenomena are central to this illness, with a behavioral component (conceptualized as stress) known to be linked with asthma (McQuaid & Abramson, 2009). Research has revealed a higher prevalence

of internalizing behaviors (16.3% have one or more diagnoses of anxiety and depressive disorders) compared to healthy peers (Katon et al, 2007). A direct relation has been found between asthma severity and the intensity of the behavioral problems (McQuaid & Abramson, 2009; Walker 2019), underscoring the undesirable connections among negative family emotional climate, child depression, reduced academic functioning, treatment nonadherence, emotional triggering of asthma episodes, and worse disease activity (Bender, 2006; Gutstadt et al, 1989; Miller et al, 2010). The physiological connection between the cholinergic and immune systems on one hand, and psychological stress and functioning in the child and the family on the other hand, has recently received scientific support highlighting not only the complexity of this illness and its management, but the intimate connection between physiological factors and the associated psychological correlates (Miller et al, 2010).

Cancer

Cancer remains one of the deadliest disorders for the pediatric population despite tremendous treatment advances resulting in significantly increased survival rates over the past decades (Jemal et al, 2009). Research on the psychological adjustment to pediatric cancer has revealed an interesting response pattern as the illness and treatment evolve over time. Initial high levels of distress at time of diagnosis and early treatment seem to normalize over the course of treatment (Vannatta et al, 2009), with a relatively high prevalence of depressive symptoms during treatment (32%), followed by only a 1.5-fold increased risk for developing depression post treatment (Germann et al, 2015; Schultz et al, 2007).

Although research supports the understanding that the majority of children with cancer do not exhibit significant psychopathology (Patenaude & Kupst, 2005), the late effects of cancer treatment may adversely affect neurological and neurocognitive functioning, leading to decline in IQ and struggles with executive functioning, attention, and memory. These struggles may further affect emotional functioning, leading to increased depression and anxiety as well as problematic social/peer relationships (Schultz et al, 2007).

Congenital Heart Disease (CHD)

CHD consists of a wide spectrum of heart disorders ranging from those that spontaneously resolve to those that are life threatening (DeMaso, 2004). CHDs are reported to be present in 5–8 of every 1000 live births (Botto et al, 2001). Innovative surgical techniques have allowed countless numbers of even the most seriously ill youngsters not only to survive but to resume healthy and active lives (DeMaso, 2004). Nevertheless, even with more advanced surgical repairs, those youth with complex cyanotic heart lesion (e.g., tetralogy of Fallot, transposition of the great arteries, or single ventricles) remain at significantly greater risk for attention, executive functioning, memory, and motor function problems

(Bellinger et al, 2011; Neal et al, 2015). Although emotional functioning of children and adolescents with CHD is generally not in the psychopathology range, there is evidence that youngsters with cyanotic heart defects are at more risk for attention-deficit/hyperactivity disorder and anxiety disorders (Bellinger et al, 2015; DeMaso et al, 2014).

Cystic Fibrosis

Approximately 1 in 3700 U.S. children are born with cystic fibrosis (CF) (Grosse et al, 2004). For children affected by CF, treatment adherence is a major challenge, as the regimen is time consuming, requiring 2–4 hours of the day invested in airway clearance and medication intake. Studies have shown that up to 50% of adolescents with CF do less than half of their prescribed therapies, 30% do none (DiGirolamo et al, 1997), and between 12 and 32% of parents report not understanding the physicians' prescriptions (Modi & Quittner, 2006). Evidence shows increased prevalence of psychiatric disorders in youth with CF as follows: anxiety disorder (37%), depressive disorder (22%), oppositional defiant disorder (23%), conduct disorder (12%), and enuresis (14%) (Smith et al, 2014; Thompson et al, 1990). Research within this illness population indicates that girls with CF report poorer quality of life than boys (Modi & Quittner, 2006).

Diabetes Mellitus Type 1 (DM1)

DM1 occurs in approximately 1 in every 400–600 children (Stanescu et al, 2012). Like CF, treatment for DM1 requires active involvement of the youth in managing a complex and multifaceted treatment, including daily insulin injections (or insulin pump oversight), blood glucose self-monitoring four to six times a day, regulation of carbohydrate intake, daily exercise, and the prevention or correction of blood glucose levels (Wysocki et al, 2009). Unlike in asthma, weak correlations were found between illness knowledge and either treatment adherence or glycemic control, highlighting yet another complex interplay between illness coordinates and personal, familial, cognitive, and environmental factors (Heidgerken et al, 2007; Rohan et al, 2015). DM1 is associated with increased prevalence for depressive, anxiety, and eating disorders as compared to healthy youth (Wysocki et al, 2009).

Psychological stress can also adversely impact DM1 management via nonadherence and/or maladaptive coping skills. High family conflict/dysfunction and overprotective parenting styles are risk factors for depression in youth with DM1. Struggles with adjustment at the time of diagnosis have predicted long-term difficulties in managing DM1 as well as psychiatric problems (Hanson et al, 1987).

The focus on eating and food intake inherent in DM1, both as treatment and via the side effects of weight gain, places adolescent females at risk for developing an eating disorder in which DM1 is used as a means to manipulate weight (e.g., bingeing and not using insulin). Warning signs of unexplainable fluctuations in blood sugar and delayed onset of puberty

have been suggested for monitoring and assessing for disordered eating in DM1 (Davidson, 2014; Jones et al, 2000).

Finally, a number of studies document that children with DM1 are at risk for learning disabilities subsequent to attention, processing speed, long-term memory, and executive dysfunction (McCarthy et al, 2003).

Epilepsy

By 20 years of age, 1% of the U.S. population can be expected to have developed epilepsy (Bujoreanu et al, 2011). Youth with epilepsy have approximately 2.5 times the risk for psychiatric disorders compared to children with other chronic physical illnesses that do not involve the central nervous system: Rates of psychiatric disorders were reported to be as high as 37% in children with epilepsy, in comparison to 11% in children with DM1 and 9% in healthy children (Davies et al, 2003). When compared with youth with asthma, DM1, or healthy siblings, the presence of epilepsy has been associated with higher scores on measures of internalizing, externalizing, attention, thought problems, and somatic complaints (Dunn et al, 2009). Similarly, reports of suicidal ideation have been found to be higher (20%) in children with epilepsy (Bell & Sander, 2009; Bujoreanu et al, 2011; Caplan et al, 2005).

Although the involvement of the central nervous system is associated with vulnerability for mental illness in youth with epilepsy, the iatrogenic side effects of antiepileptic medication may also play a part in the initiation, maintenance, or exacerbation of a patient's emotional and behavioral struggles (Bujoreanu et al, 2011).

Inflammatory Bowel Disease

Pediatric inflammatory bowel disease (IBD), which includes Crohn disease and ulcerative colitis, is a chronic physical illness that causes troubling symptoms such as abdominal pain, frequent and bloody diarrhea, weight loss, growth retardation, malabsorption, fatigue, and pubertal delay (Lakatos, 2006; Thompson et al, 2012).

Youths with IBD have been found to experience depression at much higher rates than physically healthy youths and those with other chronic physical conditions (Szigethy et al, 2014; Thompson et al, 2012). Similar to asthma, one explanation for these high depressive rates is a pathway involving inflammation. In addition, neural pathways exist between gastrointestinal sensory and motor functioning and emotions allowing for bidirectional communication (Campo & Gilchrist, 2010). An association between somatic symptoms of depression (e.g., fatigue, increased sleep, and physical complaints) and increased disease activity has been found in adolescents with IBD (Szigethy et al, 2014; Thompson et al, 2012).

Sickle Cell Disease (SCD)

SCD affects approximately 1 in every 500 African American children and 1 in every 1000–1400 Hispanic American children (Bonner et al, 2010). Similar to other chronic pediatric illnesses, over half of youth with SCD are at risk for internalizing symptoms (depression and anxiety) and poorer quality of life (Lemanek & Ranalli, 2009). In addition, social and peer difficulties (less liked, fewer friends) are frequent for this population, independent of the age group. For adolescents, studies have shown an increased risk for social anxiety, as mediated by delayed puberty and pain crises, which reduce social engagement. Gender research has shown differential results in psychosocial adjustment for this illness group; however, as opposed to the findings in the CF youth, females seem to have more active coping strategies and report better quality of life than males, who use more denial and have more internalizing and externalizing symptoms (Bonner et al, 2010; Lemanek & Ranalli, 2009).

As with DM1, youth with SCD have learning disabilities (e.g., deficits in attention, memory, verbal skills, and executive functioning). Interestingly, impairments in mental abilities and adaptive competencies for this population appear to increase with age independent of the presence of a cerebrovascular accident (Bonner et al, 2010; Casey et al, 2000).

▶ Mental Health Intervention Summary

The presence of co-occurring physical and psychiatric illnesses in childhood represents an added challenge to managing either illness alone. In general, youth with chronic physical illnesses suffer from a disproportionate burden of depression and anxiety. A survey of pediatricians and pediatric neurologists showed that the majority were not aware of the mental health needs of children with epilepsy and had limited knowledge of or access to mental health resources (Smith et al, 2007). In this context, an integrated behavioral health care approach that brings together pediatric and psychiatry clinicians is recommended. This approach, as exemplified in the pediatric medical home (Trivedi et al, 2011), offers the opportunity to reduce delayed recognition and/or misdiagnosis of psychiatric struggles while increasing access to effective treatment.

Psychotherapy

Individual psychotherapy should be considered for disabling emotional and behavioral problems in children with acute or chronic illnesses. This treatment modality can focus on building or strengthening existing coping mechanisms in order to promote continued psychological development and adaptation to illness (Szigethy & Noll, 2010). Various types of individual psychotherapies (e.g., cognitive–behavioral [CBT], interpersonal, narrative, and supportive therapies) have been found to be effective on target problems including depression, anxiety, and nonadherence. CBT has had the strongest empirical support among the types of psychotherapy with regard to the impact of illness on psychiatric functioning, with evidence coming from

interventions with IBD, CF, and cancer (Szigethy & Noll, 2010; Szigethy et al, 2015), as well as with patients with acute struggles with a medical condition (e.g., chemotherapy-induced nausea or maladaptive procedural behaviors) (Mednick, 2010). A comprehensive review of the use psychotherapy in children with physical illnesses can be found in Szigethy and Noll (2010).

Family Intervention

Families are a crucial factor in a child's psychological response to both acute and chronic physical illnesses. The working or treatment relationship between parents and pediatric medical providers is fundamental, in that working collaboratively and cooperatively can lead to optimal patient care (Demaso & Bujoreanu, 2013). Parents need to understand and implement the treatment at home for young children, or they need to coach or support older children and adolescents in gradually taking charge of their physical illness and treatment. The changes in the family system and dynamics imposed by a medical condition in the child are often an added stress on parents, who are already trying to deal with their own emotional reactions and fears about their child's health as well as daily life pressures (Sargent, 2010).

The national guidelines for the mental health assessment of the family proposed by the American Academy of Child and Adolescent Psychiatry (Birmaher et al, 2007) are relevant for youth with medical conditions. Several family interventions have been created to address the impact of a child's medical illness on family functioning and to increase the level of support for every family member. Families benefit from education (or factual information) given by their providers regarding their child's medical condition and its treatment (DeMaso & Bujoreanu, 2013). Formal family therapy has shown efficacy when addressing illness management skills, reducing concerns and fears, minimizing problem behaviors, decreasing associated stress and increasing psychological well-being, enhancing overall family functioning, improving problem-solving skills, and increasing family communication (Bujoreanu et al, 2011; Sargent, 2010). In response to the high demands on families' time and resources, family interventions can be delivered through a variety of modalities including family meetings, parent groups, phone interviews/conferences, or video conferencing.

Pharmacotherapy

Pharmacotherapy may play a role in treatment, especially when there is a lack of response to psychotherapy, there are barriers to accessing psychotherapy (severe psychopathology or illness, lack of available providers), and/or if there is family history of a first-degree relative who responded well to medications (Szigethy & Noll, 2010). Effective use of psychotropic medications in children with physical illness can be guided by identifying the presenting problem behaviors and targeting symptoms in the individual child: (1) anxiety—antidepressants, anxiolytics; (2) depression—antidepressants; (3) agitation/psychosis—atypical antipsychotics; (4) hyperactivity/inattention/impulsivity—stimulants, atomoxetine. A comprehensive review of the use of psychopharmacological interventions in children with physical illnesses can be found in Shaw et al (2010).

Conclusion

Children with physical illnesses are at increased risk for psychiatric comorbidities, either due to the copresence of primary psychiatric disorders, as consequence of the direct effects of the physical illness, and/or as reactions to the physical illness and associated personal and lifestyle demands. Despite this increased risk, adverse psychological reactions are often undetected or misdiagnosed. A developmentally informed biopsychosocial approach to the medical and psychiatric assessment of physically ill children will allow for a comprehensive understanding of their adaptation to and coping with their illnesses and will, in turn, provide opportunities for managing their illnesses by identifying not only points of intervention, but also areas of strength and resilience (DeMaso et al, 2009).

American Psychiatric Association. *Diagnostic and Statistical Manual of Mental Disorders.* 4th ed. *Text Revision.* Arlington, VA: American Psychiatric Association; 2000.

Barlow JH, Ellard DR. The psychosocial well-being of children with chronic disease, their parents and siblings: an overview of the research evidence base. *Child Care Health Dev.* 2006;32:19.

Bell GS, Sander JW. Suicide and epilepsy. *Curr Opin Neurol.* 2009;22:174.

Bellinger DC, Watson CG, Rivkin MJ, et al. Neuropsychological status and structural brain imaging in adolescents with single ventricle who underwent the Fontan procedure. *J Am Heart Assoc.* 2015;(12):e002302.

Bellinger DC, Wypij D, Rivkin MJ, et al. Adolescents with d-transposition of the great arteries corrected with the arterial switch procedure: neuropsychological assessment and structural brain imaging. *Circulation.* 2011;124:1361.

Bender BG. Risk taking, depression, adherence, and symptom control in adolescents and young adults with asthma. *Am J Respir Crit Care Med.* 2006;173:953.

Benton TD, DeMaso DR. Mood disorders. In: Shaw RJ, DeMaso DR, eds. *Textbook of Pediatric Psychosomatic Medicine.* Arlington, VA: American Psychiatric Publishing; 2010:77.

Birmaher B, Brent D, Bernet W, et al. Practice parameter for the assessment and treatment of children and adolescents with depressive disorders. *J Am Acad Child Adolesc Psychiatry.* 2007;46:1503.

Bloom B, Cohen RA, Freeman G. Summary health statistics for U.S. children: National Health Interview Survey, 2010. *Vital Health Stat 10.* 2011;250:1.

Blount RL, Davis N, Powers SW, Roberts MC. The influence of environmental factors and coping style on children's coping and distress. *Clin Psychol Rev.* 1991;11:93.

Bonner MJ, Puffer ES, Willard VW. Sickle cell disease. In: Shaw RJ, DeMaso DR, eds. *Textbook of Pediatric Psychosomatic Medicine.* Arlington, VA: American Psychiatric Publishing; 2010:259.

Botto LD, Correa A, Erickson JD. Racial and temporal variations in the prevalence of heart defects. *Pediatrics.* 2001;107:E32.

Brosbe MS, Faust J, Gold SN. Complex traumatic stress in the pediatric medical setting. *J Trauma Dissoc.* 2013;14:97.

Bujoreanu IS, Ibeziako P, DeMaso DR. Psychiatric concerns in pediatric epilepsy. *Pediatr Clin N Am.* 2011;58:973.

Bujoreanu S, Randall E, Thomson K, Ibeziako P. Characteristics of medically hospitalized pediatric patients with somatoform diagnoses. *Hosp Pediatr.* 2014;4(5):283–290

Bujoreanu S, White MT, Gerber B, Ibeziako, P. Effect of timing of psychiatry consultation on length of pediatric hospitalization and hospital charges. *Hosp Pediatr.* 2015;5(5):269–275.

Campo JV. Functional abdominal pain in childhood: lifetime and familial associations with irritable bowel syndrome and psychiatric disorders. *Prim Psychiatry.* 2007;14(4):54–68.

Campo JV, Gilchrist RH. Gastrointestinal disorders. In: Shaw RJ, DeMaso DR, eds. *Textbook of Pediatric Psychosomatic Medicine.* Arlington, VA: American Psychiatric Publishing; 2010:275.

Caplan R, Siddarth P, Gurbani S, et al. Depression and anxiety disorders in pediatric epilepsy. *Epilepsia.* 2005;46:720.

Casey R, Brown RT, Bakeman R. Predicting adjustment in children and adolescents with sickle cell disease: a test of the risk-resistance–adaptation model. *Rehabil Psychol.* 2000;45:155.

Costello EJ, Mustillo S, Keeler G, Angold A. Prevalence of psychiatric disorders in childhood and adolescence. In: Levin BL, Petrila J, Hennessy KD, eds. *Mental Health Services: A Public Health Perspective.* 2nd ed. Oxford, UK: Oxford University Press; 2004:111.

Davidson, J. (2014). Diabulimia: how eating disorders can affect adolescents with diabetes. *Nurs Stand.* 2014;29(2):44–49.

Davies S, Heyman I, Goodman R. A population survey of mental health problems in children with epilepsy. *Dev Med Child Neurol.* 2003;45:292.

DeMaso DR. Pediatric heart disease. In: Brown RT, ed. Handbook of Pediatric Psychology in School Settings. Mahwah, NJ: Erlbaum; 2004:283.

DeMaso DR, Bujoreanu IS. Enhancing working relationships between parents and surgeons. *Semin Pediatr Surg.* 2013;22:139.

DeMaso DR, Labella M, Taylor GA, et al. Psychiatric disorders and functioning in adolescent with d-transposition of the great arteries. *J Pediatr.* 2014;165:760–766.

DeMaso DR, Martini DR, Cahen LA, et al. Practice parameter for the psychiatric assessment and management of physically ill children and adolescents. *J Am Acad Child Adolesc Psychiatry.* 2009;48:213.

DiGirolamo AM, Quittner AL, Ackerman V, Stevens J. Identification and assessment of ongoing stressors in adolescents with a chronic illness: an application of the behavior-analytic model. *J Clin Child Psychol.* 1997;26:53.

Dunn DW, Austin JK, Perkins SM. Prevalence of psychopathology in childhood epilepsy: categorical and dimensional measures. *Dev Med Child Neurol.* 2009;51:364.

Enujioke SC, Ott MA. 50 years ago in The Journal of Pediatrics: suicide among adolescents with chronic illness: a path forward. *J Pediatr.* 2020;225:197. doi: 10.1016/j.jpeds.2020.04.016. PMID: 32977864.

Frank NC, Blount RL, Smith AJ, et al. Parent and staff behavior, previous child medical experience, and maternal anxiety as they relate to child procedural distress and coping. *J Pediatr Psychol.* 1995;20:277.

Germann JN, Leonard D, Stuenzi TJ, et al. Hoping is coping: a guiding theoretical framework for promoting coping and adjustment following pediatric cancer diagnosis. *J Pediatr Psychol.* 2015;40(9):846–855.

Goldston DB, Kovacs M, Ho VY, et al. Suicidal ideation and suicide attempts among youth with insulin-dependent diabetes mellitus. *J Am Acad Child Adolesc Psychiatry.* 1994;33:240.

Grosse SD, Boyle CA, Botkin JR, et al. Newborn screening for cystic fibrosis: evaluation of benefits and risks and recommendations for state newborn screening programs. *MMWR Morbid Mortal Wkly Rep.* 2004;53:1.

Gutstadt LB, Gillette JW, Mrazek DA, et al. Determinants of school performance in children with chronic asthma. *Am J Dis Child.* 1989;143:471.

Hanson CL, Henggeler SW, Burghen GA. Model of associations between psychosocial variables and health-outcome measures of adolescents with IDDM. *Diabetes Care.* 1987;10:752.

Heidgerken AD, Merlo L, Williams LB, et al. Diabetes Awareness and Reasoning Test: a preliminary analysis of development and psychometrics. *Child Health Care.* 2007;36:117–136.

Hilliard ME, McQuaid EL, Nabors L, Hood, KK. Resilience in youth and families living with pediatric health and developmental conditions: introduction to the Special Issue on Resilience. *J Pediatr Psychol.* 2015;40(9):835–839.

Hughes D, Kleespies P. Suicide in the medically ill. *Suicide Life Threat Behav.* 2001;31:48.

Ingerski LM, Modi AC, Hood KK, et al. Health-related quality of life across pediatric chronic conditions. *J Pediatr.* 2010;156:639.

Jemal A, Siegel R, Ward E, et al. Cancer statistics. *CA Cancer J Clin.* 2009;59:225.

Jones JM, Lawson ML, Daneman D, et al. Eating disorders in adolescent females with and without type 1 diabetes: cross sectional study. *BMJ (Clin Res Ed).* 2000;320:1563.

Katon W, Lozano P, Russo J, et al. The prevalence of DSM-IV anxiety and depressive disorders in youth with asthma compared with controls. *J Adolesc Health.* 2007;41:455.

Lakatos P-L. Recent trends in the epidemiology of inflammatory bowel diseases: up or down? *World J Gastroenterol.* 2006;12:6102.

LeBlanc LA, Goldsmith T, Patel DR. Behavioral aspects of chronic illness in children and adolescents. *Pediatr Clin N Am.* 2003;50:859.

Lemanek KL, Ranalli M. Sickle cell disease. In: Roberts MC, Steele RG, eds. *Handbook of Pediatric Psychology.* 4th ed. New York: Guilford Press; 2009:303.

Manne S, Miller D. Social support, social conflict, and adjustment among adolescents with cancer. *J Pediatr Psychol.* 1998;23:121.

McCarthy AM, Lindgren S, Mengeling MA, et al. Factors associated with academic achievement in children with type 1 diabetes. *Diabetes Care.* 2003;26:112.

McQuaid EL, Abramson NW. Pediatric asthma. In: Roberts MC, Steele RG, eds. *Handbook of Pediatric Psychology.* 4th ed. New York: Guilford Press; 2009:254.

Mednick L. Preparation for procedures. In: Shaw RJ, DeMaso DR, eds. *Textbook of Pediatric Psychosomatic Medicine.* Arlington, VA: American Psychiatric Publishing; 2010:475.

Miller BD, Wood BL, Smith BA. Respiratory illness. In: Shaw RJ, DeMaso DR, eds. *Textbook of Pediatric Psychosomatic Medicine.* Arlington, VA: American Psychiatric Publishing; 2010:303.

Modi AC, Quittner AL. Barriers to treatment adherence for children with cystic fibrosis and asthma: what gets in the way? *J Pediatr Psychol.* 2006;31:846.

Neal AE, Stopp C, Wypij D, et al. Predictors of health-related quality of life in adolescents with tetralogy of Fallot. *J Pediatr.* 2015;166(1):132–138.

Patenaude AF, Kupst MJ. Psychosocial functioning in pediatric cancer. *J Pediatr Psychol.* 2005;30:9.

Pinquart M, Shen Y. Behavior problems in children and adolescents with chronic physical illness: a meta-analysis. *J Pediatr Psychol.* 2011;36:1003.

Rohan JM, Huang B, Pendley JS, et al. Predicting health resilience in pediatric type 1 diabetes: a test of the Resilience Model Framework. *J Pediatr Psychol.* 2015;40(9):956–967.

Rudolph KD, Dennig MD, Weisz JR. Determinants and consequences of children's coping in the medical setting: conceptualization, review, and critique. *Psychol Bull.* 1995;118:328.

Sargent J. Family interventions. In: Shaw RJ, DeMaso DR, eds. *Textbook of Pediatric Psychosomatic Medicine.* Arlington, VA: American Psychiatric Publishing; 2010:439.

Schultz KAP, Ness KK, Whitton J, et al. Behavioral and social outcomes in adolescent survivors of childhood cancer: a report from the childhood cancer survivor study. *J Clin Oncol.* 2007;25:3649.

Shaw RJ, DeMaso DR, eds. *Textbook of Pediatric Psychosomatic Medicine.* Arlington, VA: American Psychiatric Publishing; 2010.

Shaw RJ, Spratt EG, Bernard RS, DeMaso DR. Somatoform disorders. In: Shaw RJ, DeMaso DR, eds. *Textbook of Pediatric Psychosomatic Medicine.* Arlington, VA: American Psychiatric Publishing; 2010:121–139.

Siegel LJ, Smith KE. Children's strategies for coping with pain. *Pediatrician.* 1989;16:110.

Smith BA, Cogswell A, Garcia G. Vitamin D and depressive symptoms in children with cystic fibrosis. *Psychosomatics.* 2014;55(1):76–81.

Smith K, Siddarth P, Zima B, et al. Unmet mental health needs in pediatric epilepsy: insights from providers. *Epilepsy Behav.* 2007;11:401.

Snell C, DeMaso, DR. Adaptation and coping in chronic childhood physical illness. In: Shaw RJ, DeMaso DR, eds. *Textbook of Pediatric Psychosomatic Medicine.* Arlington, VA: American Psychiatric Publishing; 2010:21.

Stanescu DE, Lord K, Lipman TH. The epidemiology of type 1 diabetes in children. *Endocrinol Metab Clin N Am.* 2012;41:679.

Szigethy E, Noll RB. Individual psychotherapy. In: Shaw RJ, DeMaso DR, eds. *Textbook of Pediatric Psychosomatic Medicine.* Arlington, VA: American Psychiatric Publishing; 2010:423.

Szigethy E, Youk AO, Benhayon D, et al. Depression subtypes in pediatric inflammatory bowel disease. *J Pediatr Gastroenterol Nutr.* 2014;58(5):574–581.

Szigethy E, Youk AO, Gonzalez-Heydrich J, et al. Effect of 2 psychotherapies on depression and disease activity in pediatric Crohn's disease. *Inflamm Bowel Dis.* 2015;21(6):1321–1328. doi: 10.1097/MIB.0000000000000358

Thompson RJ Jr, Gustafson KE. *Adaptation to Chronic Childhood Illness.* Washington, DC: American Psychological Association; 1996.

Thompson RJ Jr, Hodges K, Hamlett KW. A matched comparison of adjustment in children with cystic fibrosis and psychiatrically referred and nonreferred children. *J Pediatr Psychol*. 1990;15(6): 745–759.

Thompson RD, Craig AE, Mrakotsky C, et al. Using the Children's Depression Inventory in youth with inflammatory bowel disease: support for a physical illness-related factor. *Compr Psychiatry*. 2012;53:1194.

Thompson RH. Where we stand: twenty years of research on pediatric hospitalization and health care. *Child Health Care*. 1986;14:200.

Trivedi HK, Pattison NA, Neto LB. Pediatric medical home: foundations, challenges, and future directions. *Pediatr Clin North Am*. 2011;58(4):787–801, ix.

Vannatta K, Salley CG, Gerhardt CA. Pediatric oncology: progress and future challenges. In: Roberts MC, Steele RG, eds. *Handbook of Pediatric Psychology*. 4th ed. New York: Guilford Press; 2009:319.

Van Schoors M, Caes L, Verhofstadt LL, Goubert L, Alderfer MA. Systematic review: family resilience after pediatric cancer diagnosis. *J Pediatr Psychol*. 2015;40(9):856–868. doi: 10.1093/jpepsy/jsv055

Wallander JL, Thompson RJ Jr. Psychosocial adjustment of children with chronic physical conditions. In: Roberts MC, ed. *Handbook of Pediatric Psychology*. 2nd ed. New York: Guilford Press; 1995:124.

Walker VG. Exploration of the influence of factors identified in the literature on school-aged children's emotional responses to asthma. *J Pediatr Nurs*. 2017;33:54–62. doi: 10.1016/j.pedn.2016.11.008. Epub 2017 Jan 5. PMID: 28065421; PMCID: PMC5376515.

Wysocki T, Buckloh LM, Greco P: The psychological context of diabetes mellitus in youths. In: Roberts MC, Steele RG, eds. *Handbook of Pediatric Psychology*. 4th ed. New York: Guilford Press; 2009:287.

Disruptive Mood Dysregulation Disorder

57

Argyris Stringaris, MD, PhD, MRCPsych
Molly McVoy, MD
Pablo Vidal-Ribas Belil, MSc

▶ Essentials of Diagnosis

Disruptive mood dysregulation disorder (DMDD) was added in DSM-5 and is classified under the section of Depressive Disorders. This disorder is characterized by persistent irritable mood, and severe (i.e., out of proportion in intensity or duration) and frequent (i.e., three or more times per week) temper outbursts. These features should have been present for at least 1 year and began before age 10, although the diagnosis should not be made before age 6 or after age 18.

Research is beginning on DMDD itself since addition to DSM 5 (Benarous et al, 2017). Most of what we know about severe irritability as a category comes from the research done on severe mood dysregulation (SMD; see Table 57–1). This is a category of severe irritability created by Leibenluft et al (2003) as a means of empirically scrutinizing the notion that chronically irritable children may be suffering from bipolar disorder (BD). SMD and DMDD overlap considerably with two main differences. One is that in SMD, the requirement is for persistent negative mood (Criterion 2), which may be either irritability or sadness, whereas in DMDD only irritability or anger qualifies. The other difference is that DMDD does not include a hyperarousal criterion (Criterion 3 in SMD).

▶ Background

The main motivation of the American Psychiatric Association (APA) to create an irritability category can probably be traced back to the so-called pediatric bipolar debate (Leibenluft, 2011). Over the past two decades, the rates of BD diagnoses in children and adolescents in the United States have risen dramatically, in both inpatient units (Blader & Carlson, 2007) and outpatient services (Moreno et al, 2007). The increase in rates of BD diagnoses coincided with a rise in prescription rates of antipsychotic drugs (Olfson et al, 2006). Changes in diagnostic practice seem to be the most plausible explanation for the increased rates of BD diagnoses (Leibenluft, 2011;

Mikita & Stringaris, 2013), and irritability appears to have been central to this matter. The notion that mania may present differently in youths than in adults prompted researchers to suggest that *chronic, non-episodic irritability* may be a core characteristic of BD in children (Wozniak et al, 1995). It is crucial to note that this is not the episodic form of irritability that is a common presentation of mania. Indeed, the DSM-IV criteria for mania require a "distinct period of abnormally and persistently elevated, expansive or irritable mood." It is possible that not adhering to this requirement for an episodic mood change has resulted in many children with chronic irritability being misdiagnosed as suffering from BD. The APA attempted to tackle the dramatic increase of bipolar diagnoses in youth by introducing DMDD. The other motivation of the APA to create DMDD may have been to provide a diagnostic home for youth with severe irritability. These children are deemed to be severely impaired, but their irritability was not codeable under DSM-IV. Irritability, although a presenting problem for many young people (Stringaris, 2011), was either ignored or subsumed under conduct and oppositional disorders. Recognizing irritability as a mood and extreme irritability as a mood disorder is in keeping with a long tradition in psychopathology (Bleuler, 1983) that puts irritability alongside depression and elation as basic moods. It is also in line with psychological research (Stringaris, 2015; Stringaris & Taylor, 2015), where anger is one of the basic emotions.

▶ Epidemiology

Diagnostic instruments for DMDD are in their infancy (Boudjerida et al, 2022), and therefore studies so far have been conducted using items from existing instruments that were designed for assessing different disorders (McTate et al, 2017). The symptom of irritability is fairly common in the general population (Stringaris & Goodman, 2009a) with rates reaching up to 20% (Pickles et al, 2010). The category of SMD, which as explained earlier is closely related to DMDD, has been estimated to occur in about 3% of the population of

Table 57–1 Research Diagnostic Criteria for Severe Mood Dysregulation (SMD)

Inclusion criteria

1. Compared to his/her peers, the child exhibits markedly increased reactivity to negative emotional stimuli that is manifest verbally or behaviorally. For example, the child responds to frustration with extended temper tantrums (inappropriate for age and/or precipitating event), verbal rages, and/or aggression toward people or property. Such events occur, on average, at least three times a week.
2. Abnormal mood (specifically anger or sadness), present at least half of the day most days, and of sufficient severity to be noticeable by people in the child's environment (e.g., parents, teachers, peers).
3. Hyperarousal, as defined by at least three of the following symptoms: insomnia, agitation, distractibility, racing thoughts or flight of ideas, pressured speech, intrusiveness.
4. The symptoms in 1, 2, and 3 are currently present and have been present for at least 12 months without any symptom-free periods exceeding 2 months.
5. Aged 7–17, with the onset of symptoms before age 12.
6. The symptoms are severe in at least one setting (i.e., violent outbursts, assaultiveness at home, school, or with peers). In addition, there are at least mild symptoms (distractibility, intrusiveness) in a second setting.

Exclusion criteria

1. Exhibits any of these cardinal manic symptoms:
   • Elevated or expansive mood.
   • Grandiosity or inflated self-esteem.
   • Episodically decreased need for sleep.
2. The symptoms occur in distinct periods lasting more than 1 day.
3. Meets criteria for schizophrenia, schizoaffective disorder, pervasive development disorder, or posttraumatic stress disorder.
4. Meets criteria for substance abuse disorder in the past 3 months.
5. IQ <70.
6. The symptoms are due to the direct physiological effects of a drug of abuse, or to a general medical or neurological condition.

9- to 16-year-olds (Brotman et al, 2006). A study by Copeland et al (2013) using data from two different studies showed that prevalence estimates of DMDD varied between 0.8 and 1.1% for children between 9 and 17 years of age. More recently, Althoff et al (2016) found that the prevalence of DMDD in a large sample of adolescents ranged between 5.26 and 0.12%, depending on how conservative the diagnostic criteria applied were. In any case, these are relatively low prevalence rates compared to estimates for other disorders such as attention-deficit/hyperactivity disorder (ADHD) or oppositional defiant disorder (ODD) (see Chapters 44 and 45). It is also likely that these figures are an overestimate because, for example, the authors of the study by Copeland et al (2013) had included "sadness," rather than chronic irritability only, as a mood criterion for DMDD. However, the authors also showed that the prevalence would reach 3.3% if DMDD were diagnosable in preschoolers (Copeland et al, 2013), which

is in line with the higher rates—up to 8.2%—found more recently in a preschool sample (Dougherty et al, 2014). Prevalence of DMDD in clinical samples is around 30% (Axelson et al, 2012; Freeman et al, 2016). A consistent finding in the literature is that children with DMDD suffer from substantial psychosocial impairment and require high levels of service use (Althoff et al, 2016; Copeland et al, 2013; Dougherty et al, 2014). Importantly, DMDD co-occurs with other emotional and behavioral disorders (mainly depression, ADHD, and ODD) in between 65 and 90% of cases (Brown et al, 2009; Copeland et al, 2013; Dougherty et al, 2014).

▶ Etiology

Very few research findings are available on DMDD as such. However, it is useful to discuss DMDD etiology on the basis of the data available on SMD and dimensional constructs of irritability. Here we discuss three overall etiological questions. The first concerns the relationship of DMDD and irritability more generally with other psychiatric disorders; the second, the relationship of DMDD and irritability more generally with personality constructs. The third concerns genetic findings, mainly in the form of family and twin studies, about irritability.

1. DMDD and irritability: relationship with other psychiatric disorders

Overview—An important question is whether DMDD is a category that is separable from other disorders. As we have seen, up to 90% of children with DMDD also have another psychiatric disorder. Some of this overlap is due to item overlap and therefore artificial: DMDD has temper outbursts as its main criterion and anger is one of its characteristics; both these symptoms are also listed as criteria for ODD. Similarly, in the Copeland study (Copeland et al, 2013), sadness—a depression criterion—was also used to ascertain DMDD. It will be important to establish whether, after excluding such artificial overlap, DMDD shows more comorbidity than is characteristic of other established psychiatric disorders, for example, ADHD. A related question is whether the irritability that defines DMDD is a phenomenon that arises secondary to other disorders. For example, it could be that a child with ADHD manifests symptoms of DMDD because his or her hyperactivity/impulsivity colludes with the environment and causes frustration. It seems unlikely that irritability is only a secondary phenomenon. First, irritability is highly predictive of future impairment and future psychopathology even after controlling for other disorders (Stringaris & Goodman, 2009a). Adolescents scoring high on irritability have been found to be at increased risk of suffering from depression and generalized anxiety and to face socioeconomic adversity in a 20-year follow-up study (Stringaris et al, 2009). Importantly, these adverse outcomes persisted even after adjusting for psychiatric disorders at baseline (Stringaris et al, 2009). Indeed, a series of papers have demonstrated that irritability is a predictor of future depression or distress disorders more generally, independently of baseline depression (Brotman et al, 2006; Leibenluft et al, 2006; Stringaris & Goodman, 2009a; Stringaris et al, 2009; Whelan et al, 2013). These results are summarized in a recent systematic review and meta-analysis about the longitudinal correlates of irritability (Vidal-Ribas et al, 2016). In this review, the authors searched for articles in which dimensional or categorical (i.e., DMDD or SMD) irritability was a predictor of any future psychiatric outcome. Twenty-four of 163 reviewed articles met inclusion criteria. The results revealed that irritability was a significant predictor of depression and anxiety but not of BD, conduct disorder (CD), ADHD, or substance abuse. In the following, we discuss the overlap between DMDD and irritability for some of the main psychiatric diagnoses.

Relationship with bipolar disorder—As noted earlier, one of the important motivations for studying children with severe irritability was to find out whether they were suffering from an early form of BD, as had been previously suggested (Wozniak et al, 1995). The evidence suggests that severe irritability is not a precursor of BD. First, follow-up studies in community samples do not show a link between dimensional measures of irritability and later BD (Brotman et al, 2006; Leibenluft et al, 2006; Stringaris et al, 2009). Since BD is a relatively rare outcome in community samples, there is a possibility that these studies may have been underpowered to detect the link. However, the results are similar in referred samples. A follow-up study (median time 28.7 months) showed striking differences in the rate of manic symptoms between youth with SMD and those with classical BD. Only 1 of 84 SMD subjects (1.2%) experienced a (hypo-) manic episode during the study, whereas the frequency of such episodes was more than 50 times higher in those with narrowly defined BD (58/93, 62.4%) (Stringaris et al, 2010). Similarly, a study in a clinical sample of 706 children aged 6–12 years did not find an association between DMDD and future onset of BD (Axelson et al, 2010). More recently, in a study of 200 youth with SMD, only 1 participant developed BD at 4-year follow-up (Deveney et al, 2015).

In keeping with these findings, SMD and BD were found to differ in family history (Brotman et al, 2007). The parents of youth with classical (also called narrow phenotype) BD were significantly more likely to be diagnosed with BD (14/42, 33.3%) than parents of youth with SMD (1/37, 2.7%) (Brotman et al, 2006).

In addition to the clinical and family data, there has also been a surge of interest in the neurobiological differences and overlap between SMD and BD in youth. Compared to controls, children with either SMD or BD are significantly less accurate in labeling facial emotions (Guyer et al, 2007) and worse in recognizing facial expressions of emotions (Rich et al, 2008). Interestingly, SMD and BD differ in the brain mechanisms subserving these emotion deficits: a functional magnetic resonance imaging (fMRI) study showed that patients with SMD had reduced amygdala activity compared to those with BD during a face emotion-processing task (Brotman et al, 2010). The pattern of amygdala activation in SMD was similar to that of young people with depressive disorders (Beesdo et al, 2009). SMD and BD youth also differ in their response to frustration. Rich et al (2007) used a frustration task to show that although both SMD and BD youth displayed significantly more negative affect than healthy controls in response to negative feedback, patients with SMD differed from those with BD in their event-related potentials (Rich et al, 2007) and brain activation patterns (Rich et al, 2011). Similarly, children with SMD differ to those with BD in response reversal tasks, in which there are unexpected changes as to which stimulus is rewarded and which one is not (Dickstein et al, 2007). Youth with SMD but not those with BD showed reduced inferior frontal gyrus activation in response to errors on the task relative to healthy controls (Adleman et al, 2011). Of note, the same study found both SMD and BD youth to have reduced task-related caudate activation compared to healthy controls. More recently, a study using affective priming tasks with both masked and unmasked emotional faces found that youth with SMD showed lower activity in parietal, temporal, and frontal regions when processing neutral faces compared to youth with BD (Thomas et al, 2014). Aberrant response to emotional stimuli in the amygdala and frontal regions is consistent with recent findings in functional connectivity during resting state fMRI (Stoddard et al, 2015). In this study, youth with BD showed higher functional connectivity between the left basolateral amygdala and the medial superior gyrus and posterior cingulate than participants with SMD. There is also early evidence that irritability correlates of DMDD and BD differ in the processing of emotional faces (Wiggins et al, 2016). Taken together, these findings suggest that pathophysiological mechanisms differ between SMD and BD youth; however, they also show that there are shared pathways between the two conditions.

Relationship with oppositional and conduct problems—DMDD shows substantial overlap with ODD, not least because the irritability items of DMDD overlap with those of ODD (Mayes et al, 2015; Mayes et al, 2016). The DSM-5 introduced DMDD in order to give clinicians the opportunity to code the salient mood components, without having to use a label that implies antisocial behaviors. Stringaris and Goodman (2009c) proposed three distinct dimensions within oppositionality: an irritable dimension that predicts primarily depressive disorders and generalized anxiety disorder; a headstrong dimension related to ADHD and non-aggressive CD; and a hurtful dimension associated with aggressive conduct problems and callous/unemotional traits. These dimensions have been replicated in confirmatory factor analyses (Aebi et al, 2013; Burke et al, 2014; Herzhoff & Tacket, 2016), as well as in latent class analysis (Althoff et al, 2014), which aims to identify groups of people based on their response to a questionnaire and, therefore, is closer to the binary constructs of irritability such as DMDD or SMD. The differential associations of the three dimensions of ODD have been demonstrated in cross-sectional and longitudinal community-based samples (Aebi et al, 2010; Krieger et al, 2013; Rowe et al, 2010; Savage et al, 2015; Stringaris & Goodman, 2009b; Whelan et al, 2015). These findings are consistent with the recognition of irritability as a mood. Conduct problems and antisocial behavior can arise as a consequence of irritable mood, though the conditions under which this happens would need further study.

Relationship with depression and anxiety—Irritability shows substantial overlap with depressive disorders (major depressive disorder and dysthymia) and anxiety disorders. Moreover, irritability in children and adolescents appears to be a pathway leading to depression. It has previously been shown that ODD is one of the most robust predictors of future depression (Copeland et al, 2009). Results suggest that it is the irritable component of ODD that is specifically predictive of depression (Stringaris & Goodman, 2009b). As mentioned earlier, a recent systematic review and meta-analysis has shown that irritability, either continuous or categorically defined, is a predictor of future depression and anxiety rather than of other disorders (Vidal-Ribas et al, 2016). An important etiological question is why irritable children become depressed. A popular explanation has been that they follow a trajectory of failure—a variant of the so-called failure model (Capaldi, 1992), according to which irritable youth experience interpersonal difficulties that put them at risk for depression. Most findings so far argue against this failure model, however, and it appears that irritability and depression are tightly linked because of shared genetic risks (Savage et al, 2015; Stringaris et al, 2012a), as explained further in the genetics section.

2. DMDD and irritability: relationship with personality traits—Another question is whether severe irritability should be classed as a disorder at all or whether it would be more appropriate to consider it as a personality trait. Irritability has long been recognized as part of the temperamental dimension of negative affectivity (Caspi et al, 2005), so that severe irritability could simply be the extreme manifestation of a personality trait. The same could be said about a number of psychiatric disorders. For example, phobias and other anxiety disorders could be seen as extreme manifestations of negative emotionality; the same may be true of ADHD hyperactivity, which could be seen as the extreme of the personality trait of activity. Increasingly, psychiatric symptoms are seen as part of continuous traits that exist as dimensions within a population (Plomin et al, 2009). Although thinking dimensionally can be helpful for research and for certain clinical purposes, clinical decisions are typically binary (e.g., to treat or not to treat; Rutter, 2011). Therefore, even if irritability were indeed best conceptualized as a dimension, recognizing a threshold would still be important for clinical work.

Genetics

Irritability is a heritable trait. In a study using self-reported irritability, Stringaris et al (2012a) found that about 30% of the inter-individual variance of adolescent-reported irritability was due to genetic factors. This is in keeping with studies in adult samples (Coccaro et al, 1997). Also, genetic influences on irritability seem to increase slightly over time in males and decrease in females (Roberson-Nay et al, 2015).

Stringaris et al (2012a) also showed that the overlap between irritability and depression is due to shared genetic effects. That is, as with other psychiatric phenotypes (Eley, 1997), irritability and depression differ from each other as a result of specific environmental effects; by contrast, they overlap in one and the same individual because of shared genes. This genetic covariance seems to be peak in early adolescence (Savage et al, 2015). Moreover, the impact of irritability on future depression/anxiety seems to be greater than the impact of depression/anxiety on future irritability. The genetic overlap between depression and irritability is in line with studies showing that a family history of depression is associated with irritability in the offspring (Krieger et al, 2013; Wiggins et al, 2014).

Although we know that the overlap between irritability and depression is mainly explained by genetic effects, at present, neither the shared genes between irritability and depression nor the unique environmental effects are known.

▶ Clinical Findings

Many young people present with irritability as their main problem in child and adolescent psychiatry clinics. However, symptoms of irritability are often not documented in sufficient detail or quantified. An initial evaluation should include a screen for symptoms of irritability. At a busy or a primary care setting, this initial screen can be done using scales such as the Strengths and Difficulties Questionnaire (Goodman, 1997) or the Child Behavior Checklist (Achenbach, 1991), which inquire about psychopathology in general and include a few items on irritability. In more specialist settings, it can include using scales designed for assessing irritability (Narrow et al, 2013; Stringaris et al, 2012b). Such screening should inquire about (1) the *threshold* for an angry reaction (e.g., how easily a child become annoyed compared to others); (2) the *frequency* of angry feelings/behaviors (e.g., frequency of temper tantrums); and (3) the *duration* of such feelings/behaviors. It has been shown that asking such questions can differentiate between groups of children with SMD to those with other psychopathology, such as BD (Stringaris et al, 2012b). After detecting problems in these domains, the clinician can inquire in more detail about the two main components of the DMDD diagnosis.

The first component is temper outbursts. These are often quite prominent, and parents will often volunteer information on them (although they may use different names to describe them, such as "meltdowns," "wobbly," "explosions," "rages"). It is useful to ask the parents to describe the most recent such tantrum and the worst they can remember. This enables the clinician and the patient or parent to create a common language about the problem. It is also useful to do a functional analysis of the tantrum. Finding out about what goes on before the tantrum (*antecedents*) can give clues about differential diagnosis and help plan treatment. This should also contain information about the place where these tantrums occur (home or school) and the particular circumstances or time of day. Establishing the *behaviors* that accompany the tantrums (e.g., is he or she smashing things) helps assess risks, burden, and impairment from the tantrums. Asking about what happens during the tantrum will help establish whether it is out of proportion with what would generally be expected given the circumstances (Criterion B). Enquiring about the *consequences* (e.g., does the child regret the tantrum) is also important. Such an analysis also helps the clinician understand how the parent or others in the young person's environment respond to the temper outburst. The criteria stipulate that temper outbursts should occur 3 or more times per week. Noting the average number of tantrums per week (or per day) at first assessment is important to monitor and guide therapy. The DSM criteria also stipulate that the temper outbursts should be out of keeping with the child's developmental level. This is may be a difficult judgment to make based on parent report only, and talking to teachers who see other children at similar developmental levels can be very helpful. After the first consultation, it is useful to ask the parents to complete a diary about temper outbursts, noting the circumstances and consequences. Observing a child–parent interaction leading to tantrums can also be helpful but may not always be feasible. Parents and young people are often happy to take videos of outbursts; discussing them in clinic can be particularly helpful.

The second major component of the DMDD diagnosis is the prevailing irritable mood between tantrums. A persistently irritable mood as specified in the DMDD criteria is probably less common than even severe tantrums. It is arguably also more difficult to ascertain: outbursts tend to be more memorable than a persistently negative mood. In addition, parents or teachers will often find it difficult to differentiate between frequent temper outbursts that occur, say, 5 or 10 times a day and a negative mood. A useful approach is to do a mood timeline, which will also help establish the age at onset of the problem. Parents may remember a time before their child's mood became persistently irritable or may recall short periods of time (e.g., during a holiday), when their child's mood was positive. The main purpose of such a timeline is therefore to identify contrasts and changes in mood, which makes it easier to tackle what may otherwise be a diffuse negative feeling. Asking the child about his or her experience of the mood is paramount. This will help distinguish between feelings of irritability and those of sadness—the two often coexist. Finding out about ruminations (e.g., thoughts of anger directed against self or others) and diurnal variation will be particularly helpful for planning treatment (see later discussion).

Psychological Testing

There is no diagnostic psychological test for DMDD. However, as discussed earlier, children with severe irritability do seem to perform worse on a range of cognitive tasks. Establishing whether a child has cognitive deficits (e.g., specific reading or learning difficulties) that lead to frustration and compound or maintain irritability in certain settings can prove helpful.

Laboratory Findings

There are no clinically useful laboratory findings for DMDD. However, as with other psychiatric disorders, routine physical and laboratory examinations can help exclude medical causes of mood disorders.

Neuroimaging

There are as yet no clinically useful imaging findings for DMDD. So far, as mentioned earlier, most of this research has focused on differentiating SMD from BD and healthy volunteers (HV). Early evidence suggests that, compared to HV, youth with SMD present amygdala *hypo*activity during explicit processing of face emotions (Brotman et al, 2010) while amygdala *hyper*activity is evident during implicit processing (Brotman et al, 2010; Thomas et al, 2013). Two studies using affective priming tasks with both masked and unmasked emotional faces found that youth with SMD show higher activation during viewing of angry faces in the posterior cingulate and superior temporal gyrus compared to HV (Thomas et al, 2014; Tseng et al, 2016). Under frustrating conditions, youth with SMD display aberrant amygdala, striatal, parietal, and posterior cingulate activations compared with HV (Deveney et al, 2013; Perlman et al, 2015), suggesting difficulties in emotion regulation, reward processing, and attentional control.

Course of Illness

As discussed earlier, severe irritability is associated with a range of future adverse psychiatric and social outcomes (Vidal-Ribas et al, 2016). Irritability in youth has been associated with lower financial and educational attainment (Copeland et al, 2014; Stringaris et al, 2009) as well as worse health outcomes in adulthood (Copeland et al, 2014). The association between irritability and future functional impairment has also been found in young children (Dougherty et al, 2014, 2016; Ezpeleta et al, 2015). Finally, one study found that irritability in adolescence was associated with suicidal behaviors in adulthood independent of affective diagnoses (Pickles et al, 2010).

The stability of irritability differs according to whether irritability is measured continuously or categorically. Studies employing dimensional approaches show that irritability is moderately stable over time (Leadbeater & Homel, 2015; Roberson-Nay et al, 2015; Stringaris et al, 2013; Whelan et al, 2013). On the other hand, DSM-5 field trials have shown poor test–retest reliability for DMDD (Regier et al, 2013). In a clinical sample of children with DMDD aged 6–12 years, only 19% met criteria at 1- and 2-year follow-up (Axelson et al, 2012). Similarly, findings over four time points in a large cohort study showed that most youth with SMD (82.5%) met SMD criteria in one wave, but only 1.4% met criteria in all four waves of assessment (Brotman et al, 2006). However, youths with either persistent anger or temper outburst had a 75% likelihood of having either persistent anger or temper outburst 1 year later (Copeland et al, 2015). In a recent study evaluating the main symptoms of DMDD (i.e., irritable-angry mood and temper outburst) in a community sample of children followed over 8 years, the authors found that whereas rates of symptom remission were high (71%), the prevalence of new cases was also considerable (55%). Moreover, 29% of the participants with frequent DMDD symptoms at baseline also displayed these symptoms at follow-up. In any case, a high proportion of children who do not meet current DMDD criteria in longitudinal studies still present with impairing chronic irritability and functional impairment (Deveney et al, 2015).

Differential Diagnosis

Before diagnosing DMDD, one must have excluded conditions that may lead to tantrums and grumpiness. These may include medical conditions (particularly in hospital or other medical settings), as well as other psychiatric problems that may be treatable in their own right.

Other emotional problems, particularly anxiety disorders, are often associated with severe tantrums (Stoddard et al, 2014). For example, about a third of children with obsessive–compulsive disorder (OCD) experience severe tantrums when their rituals are interrupted (Krebs et al, 2013). It is not uncommon that irritability is the presenting complaint and that the underlying and often treatable anxiety problem is missed.

As we have seen, DMDD often co-occurs with depression, and the two may be hard to separate, especially because depressive disorders may be diagnosed in youth with irritability as the cardinal mood, even in the absence of sad mood. A recent study has shown that about a third of youth with depression also experience episodic irritability and that they are significantly more likely to also have comorbid ODD and CD compared to those with depression who do not have episodic irritability (Stringaris et al, 2013). Differentiating DMDD from this subset of people with depression may be particularly difficult; however, identifying co-occurring symptoms of depression in irritable children will be important for treatment (see later discussion).

In DSM-5, ODD may not be diagnosed in the presence of DMDD. Tantrums and grumpiness often co-occur with arguing, fighting, and other conduct problems that may require diagnosis and treatment in their own right.

Irritability is also common in children with ADHD. Tantrums and grumpiness may be manifestations of frustration due to hyperactive or inattentive behavior. Identifying these can have important therapeutic implications (Blader et al, 2009).

The differentiation between DMDD and BD-I or BD-II should be straightforward. Episodes are the single most reliable way to differentiate the two conditions. Patients with DMDD do not have a course of illness with episodes that last for several days or weeks; instead their symptoms are chronic (a year or longer). By contrast, patients with BD report more-or-less clearly defined periods of either mania or depression. Mania is typically characterized by euphoria, although irritability alone can be the predominant mood in about 10% of cases (Hunt et al, 2013). Such irritability is episodic—it comes as a change from the child's baseline mood and parents describe it as something that is out of character. Occasionally, very severe tantrums can last for several hours and a child may experience phases where such longer-lasting tantrums cluster. With experience, clinicians should become able to differentiate such phasic exacerbations of tantrums from BD.

Recent evidence (Simonoff et al, 2012; Mikita et al, 2015) suggests that mood dysregulation is prominent in children with autism spectrum disorders (ASD). The DSM-5 criteria for DMDD stipulate that the patient's presentation should not be better explained by the presence of other conditions, including ASD. However, it can often be difficult to make this judgment, and the lack of evidence in this area compounds this. Pragmatically, clinicians will want to document and treat the severe irritability of children with ASD, even if they decide not to diagnose DMDD formally.

Treatment

There is no licensed treatment for DMDD yet (Kircanski et al, 2018), and the evidence base for treating severe irritability is thin. Identifying conditions that may underlie severe irritability or contribute to it (as discussed earlier) is an important first step in the treatment of children with severe irritability.

As with most medical conditions, it is important that the clinicians provide adequate information about the condition, its likely causes, and its treatment. This is best done in the form of psychoeducation, where the clinician cooperates with the patient and the caregivers to achieve optimal communication and information sharing. Although psychoeducation has yet to be tested as an intervention in DMDD, it is part of effective treatments for other conditions (Miklowitz et al, 2008) and has also been shown to be effective in adult samples with other disorders (Colom et al, 2003). Its benefits are partly derived through better adherence to treatment.

An adequately powered study has demonstrated that lithium is not effective in children with SMD (Dickstein et al, 2009). There is one randomized controlled trial in the treatment of DMDD, studying a selective serotonin reuptake inhibitor, as an add-on medication to stimulant treatment for youth, age 7–17, with DMDD. Towbin et al (2020) describe results from the addition of citalopram (average dose 28 mg daily) versus placebo (PBO) to optimized open-label methylphenidate treatment. After treatment, 35% of those randomized to citalopram showed improvements in irritability compared to 6% of those randomized to placebo. However, there were no differences in functional impairment between groups at the end of the trial (Towbin et al, 2020). In addition, there were no differences found in types or rate of adverse events between the groups.

Irritability and mood fluctuations in some children with ADHD may respond to treatment with stimulants (Blader et al, 2009; Fernandez de la Cruz et al, 2015). There are several open-label studies of stimulant medications, one with long acting methylphenidate (MPH) (Winters et al, 2018) and one with both amphetamine and MPH (Baweja et al, 2016). Both showed improvement in externalizing symptoms and irritability with stimulant treatment but did not see the response rate seen in ADHD alone. Sodium valproate appears effective in youth with ADHD whose aggression has not responded to stimulant treatment (Blader et al, 2009), although its effectiveness in irritability has yet to be demonstrated. Antipsychotic medication, such as risperidone and aripiprazole, has been used successfully to treat irritability in people with ASD (McCracken et al, 2002) and learning difficulties; however, it is not clear how much the irritability construct in these studies overlaps with irritability in typically developing children (Mikita et al, 2015). An open-label trial using low doses (1.2 ± 0.5 mg) of risperidone in children and adolescents with SMD showed significant reductions in irritability scores (Krieger et al, 2011), yet any benefits of such treatment should be balanced against its downsides, such as sedation and metabolic complications. There is one open-label study using a combination of aripiprazole and methylphenidate that showed improvement in irritability, externalizing symptoms, depression, anxiety, attention, and social problems in youth, age 7–17, with DMDD (Pan et al, 2018).

Parenting interventions (e.g., based on Webster-Stratton techniques) have been shown to be effective in children with ODD (Pilling et al, 2013) and ASD (Bearss et al, 2015). It also seems that children who suffer from ODD and show predominantly irritability may benefit specifically from parenting interventions (Scott & O'Connor, 2012), although this needs to be tested further.

Treating anger with cognitive–behavioral therapy (CBT) seems moderately effective according to meta-analytic studies (Lochman et al, 2011). A study suggests that severe tantrums in children with OCD respond to standard treatment with CBT (Krebs et al, 2013). Also, group CBT has been shown to be effective in one trial of youth with ADHD plus SMD (Waxmonsky et al, 2016).

In the authors' experience, using a functional analysis of behavior to identify circumstances during which tantrums occur can be helpful; similarly, characterizing the cognitions (particularly ruminative thoughts) that accompany anger and persistent irritability appears helpful in reducing symptoms of anger (Leigh et al, 2012), although the effectiveness of these approaches has yet to be formally tested in children with DMDD.

Achenbach TM. *Manual for the Child Behavior Checklist 4-18, 1991 Profile.* Burlington: University of Vermont, Department of Psychiatry; 1991.

Adleman NE, Kayser R, Dickstein D, et al. Neural correlates of reversal learning in severe mood dysregulation and pediatric bipolar disorder. *J Am Acad Child Adolesc Psychiatry.* 2011;50(11):1173–1185.e1172.

Aebi M, Asherson P, Banaschewski T, et al. Predictability of oppositional defiant disorder and symptom dimensions in children and adolescents with ADHD combined type. *Psychol Med.* 2010;40:2089–2100.

Aebi M, Plattner B, Metzke CW, Bessler C, Steinhausen HC. Parent- and self-reported dimensions of oppositionality in youth: construct validity, concurrent validity, and the prediction of criminal outcomes in adulthood. *J Child Psychol Psychiatry.* 2013;54(9):941–949.

Althoff RR, Kuny-Slock AV, Verhulst FC, Hudziak JJ, van der Ende J. Classes of oppositional-defiant behavior: concurrent and predictive validity. *J Child Psychol Psychiatry.* 2014;55(10):1162–1171.

Althoff RR, Crehan ET, He JP, Burstein M, Hudziak JJ, Merikangas KR. Disruptive mood dysregulation disorder at ages 13–18: results from the National Comorbidity Survey-Adolescent Supplement. *J Child Adolesc Psychopharmacol.* 2016;26(2):107–113.

Axelson D, Findling RL, Fristad MA, et al. Examining the proposed disruptive mood dysregulation disorder diagnosis in children in the Longitudinal Assessment of Manic Symptoms study. *J Clin Psychiatry.* 2012;73(10):1342–1350.

Baweja R, Belin PJ, Humphrey HH, et al. The effectiveness and tolerability of central nervous system stimulants in school-age children with attention-deficit/hyperactivity disorder and disruptive mood dysregulation disorder across home and school. *J Child Adolesc Psychopharmacol.* 2016;26(2):154–163.

Bearss K, Johnson C, Smith T, et al. Effect of parent training vs parent education on behavioral problems in children with autism spectrum disorder: a randomized clinical trial. *JAMA.* 2015;313(15):1524–1533.

Beesdo K, Lau JY, Guyer AE, et al. Common and distinct amygdala-function perturbations in depressed vs anxious adolescents. *Arch Gen Psychiatry.* 2009;66(3):275–285.

Benarous X, Consoli A, Guilé JM, Garny de La Rivière S, Cohen D, Olliac B. Evidence-based treatments for youths with severely dysregulated mood: a qualitative systematic review of trials for SMD and DMDD. *Eur Child Adolesc Psychiatry.* 2017;26(1):5–23.

Blader JC, Carlson GA. Increased rates of bipolar disorder diagnoses among U.S. child, adolescent, and adult inpatients, 1996–2004. *Biol Psychiatry.* 2007;62(2):107.

Blader JC, Schooler NR, Jensen PS, et al. Adjunctive divalproex versus placebo for children with ADHD and aggression refractory to stimulant monotherapy. *Am J Psychiatry*. 2009; 166(12):1392–1401.

Bleuler E. *Lehrbuch der Psychiatrie*. Berlin: Springer; 1983.

Boudjerida A, Labelle R, Bergeron L, Berthiaume C, Guilé JM, Breton JJ. Development and initial validation of the disruptive Mood Dysregulation Disorder Questionnaire among adolescents from clinic settings. *Front Psychiatry*. 2022

Brotman MA, Schmajuk M, Rich BA, et al. Prevalence, clinical correlates, and longitudinal course of severe mood dysregulation in children. *Biol Psychiatry*. 2006;60(9):991.

Brotman MA, Kassem L, Reising MM, et al. Parental diagnoses in youth with narrow phenotype bipolar disorder or severe mood dysregulation. *Am J Psychiatry*. 2007;164(8):1238.

Brotman MA, Rich BA, Guyer AE, et al. Amygdala activation during emotion processing of neutral faces in children with severe mood dysregulation versus ADHD or bipolar disorder. *Am J Psychiatry*. 2010;167(1):61–69.

Brown RA, Kuzara J, Copeland WE, et al. Moving from ethnography to epidemiology: lessons learned in Appalachia. *Ann Hum Biol*. 2009;36(3):248–260.

Bruno A, Celebre L, Torre G, et al. Focus on disruptive mood dysregulation disorder: a review of the literature. *Psychiatry Res*. 2019;279:323–330. doi: 10.1016/j.psychres.2019.05.043. Epub 2019 Jun 1. PMID: 31164249.

Burke JD, Boylan K, Rowe R, et al. Identifying the irritability dimension of ODD: application of a modified bifactor model across five large community samples of children. *J Abnorm Psychol*. 2014;123(4):841–851.

Capaldi DM. Co-occurrence of conduct problems and depressive symptoms in early adolescent boys: II. A 2-year follow-up at Grade 8. *Dev Psychopathol*. 1992;4:125–144.

Caspi A, Roberts BW, Shiner RL. Personality development: stability and change. *Annu Rev Psychol*. 2005;56:453–484.

Coccaro EF, Bergeman CS, Kavoussi RJ, Seroczynski AD. Heritability of aggression and irritability: a twin study of the Buss-Durkee aggression scales in adult male subjects. *Biol Psychiatry*. 1997;41(3):273–284.

Colom F, Vieta E, Martinez-Aran A, et al. A randomized trial on the efficacy of group psychoeducation in the prophylaxis of recurrences in bipolar patients whose disease is in remission. *Arch Gen Psychiatry*. 2003;60(4):402–407.

Copeland WE, Shanahan L, Costello EJ, Angold A. Childhood and adolescent psychiatric disorders as predictors of young adult disorders. *Arch Gen Psychiatry*. 2009;66(7):764–772.

Copeland WE, Angold A, Costello EJ, Egger H. Prevalence, comorbidity, and correlates of DSM-5 proposed disruptive mood dysregulation disorder. *Am J Psychiatry*. 2013;170(2):173–179.

Copeland WE, Shanahan L, Egger H, Angold A, Costello EJ. Adult diagnostic and functional outcomes of DSM-5 disruptive mood dysregulation disorder. *Am J Psychiatry*. 2014;171(6):668–674.

Copeland WE, Brotman MA, Costello EJ. Normative irritability in youth: developmental findings from the Great Smoky Mountains Study. *J Am Acad Child Adolesc Psychiatry*. 2015; 54(8):635–642.

Deveney CM, Connolly ME, Haring CT, et al. Neural mechanisms of frustration in chronically irritable children. *Am J Psychiatry*. 2013;170(10):1186–1194.

Deveney CM, Hommer RE, Reeves E, et al. A prospective study of severe irritability in youths: 2- and 4-year follow-up. *Depress Anxiety*. 2015;32(5):364–372.

Dickstein DP, Nelson EE, McClure EB, et al. Cognitive flexibility in phenotypes of pediatric bipolar disorder. *J Am Acad Child Adolesc Psychiatry*. 2007;46(3):341–355.

Dickstein DP, Towbin KE, Van Der Veen JW, et al. Randomized double-blind placebo-controlled trial of lithium in youths with severe mood dysregulation. *J Child Adolesc Psychopharmacol*. 2009;19(1):61–73.

Dougherty LR, Smith VC, Bufferd SJ, et al. DSM-5 disruptive mood dysregulation disorder: correlates and predictors in young children. *Psychol Med*. 2014;44(11):2339–2350.

Dougherty LR, Smith VC, Bufferd SJ, et al. Disruptive mood dysregulation disorder at the age of 6 years and clinical and functional outcomes 3 years later. *Psychol Med*. 2016;46(5): 1103–1114.

Eley TC. General genes: a new theme in developmental psychopathology. *Curr Direct Psychol Sci*. 1997;6:90–95.

Ezpeleta L, Granero R, de la Osa N, Trepat E, Domenech JM. Trajectories of oppositional defiant disorder irritability symptoms in preschool children. *J Abnorm Child Psychol*. 2015;44(1): 115–128.

Fernandez de la Cruz L, Simonoff E, McGough JJ, et al. Treatment of children with attention-deficit/hyperactivity disorder (ADHD) and irritability: results from the multimodal treatment study of children with ADHD (MTA). *J Am Acad Child Adolesc Psychiatry*. 2015;54(1):62–70 e63.

Freeman AJ, Youngstrom EA, Youngstrom JK, Findling RL. Disruptive mood dysregulation disorder in a community mental health clinic: prevalence, comorbidity and correlates. *J Child Adolesc Psychopharmacol*. 2016;26(2):123–130.

Goodman R. The Strengths and Difficulties Questionnaire: a research note. *J Child Psychol Psychiatry*. 1997;38(5):581.

Guyer AE, McClure EB, Adler AD, et al. Specificity of facial expression labeling deficits in childhood psychopathology. *J Child Psychol Psychiatry*. 2007;48(9):863–871.

Hendrickson B, Girma M, Miller L. Review of the clinical approach to the treatment of disruptive mood dysregulation disorder. *Int Rev Psychiatry*. 2020;32(3):202–211. doi: 10.1080/ 09540261.2019.1688260. Epub 2019 Nov 28. PMID: 31775528.

Herzhoff K, Tackett JL. Subfactors of oppositional defiant disorder: converging evidence from structural and latent class analyses. *J Child Psychol Psychiatry*. 2016;57(1):18–29.

Hunt JI, Case BG, Birmaher B, et al. Irritability and elation in a large bipolar youth sample: Relative symptom severity and clinical outcomes over 4 years. *J Clin Psychiatry*. 2013;74(1):e110–e117.

Kircanski K, Clayton ME, Leibenluft E, Brotman MA. Psychosocial treatment of irritability in youth. *Curr Treat Options Psychiatry*. 2018;5(1):129–40. doi: 10.1007/s40501-018-0141-5. Epub 2018 Feb 9.

Krebs G, Bolhuis K, Heyman I, et al. Temper outbursts in paediatric obsessive-compulsive disorder and their association with depressed mood and treatment outcome. *J Child Psychol Psychiatry*. 2013;54(3):313–322.

Krieger FV, Pheula GF, Coelho R, et al. An open-label trial of risperidone in children and adolescents with severe mood dysregulation. *J Child Adolesc Psychopharmacol*. 2011;21(3):237–243.

Krieger FV, Polanczyk GV, Goodman R, et al. Dimensions of oppositionality in a Brazilian community sample: testing the DSM-5 proposal and etiological links. *J Am Acad Child Adolesc Psychiatry*. 2013;52(4):389–400.

Leadbeater BJ, Homel J. Irritable and defiant sub-dimensions of ODD: their stability and prediction of internalizing symptoms and conduct problems from adolescence to young adulthood. *J Abnorm Child Psychol*. 2015;43(3):407–421.

Leibenluft E. Severe mood dysregulation, irritability, and the diagnostic boundaries of bipolar disorder in youths. *Am J Psychiatry*. 2011;168(2):129–142.

Leibenluft E, Charney DS, Towbin KE, Bhangoo RK, Pine DS. Defining clinical phenotypes of juvenile mania. *Am J Psychiatry*. 2003;160(3):430–437.

Leibenluft E, Cohen P, Gorrindo T, et al. Chronic versus episodic irritability in youth: a community-based, longitudinal study of clinical and diagnostic associations. *J Child Adolesc Psychopharmacol*. 2006;16(4):456.

Leigh E, Smith P, Milavic G, Stringaris A. Mood regulation in youth: research findings and clinical approaches to irritability and short-lived episodes of mania-like symptoms. *Curr Opin Psychiatry*. 2012;25(4):271–276.

Lochman JE, Powell NP, Boxmeyer CL, Jimenez-Camargo L. Cognitive-behavioral therapy for externalizing disorders in children and adolescents. *Child Adolesc Psychiatr Clin N Am*. 2011;20(2):305–318.

Mayes SD, Mathiowetz C, Kokotovich C, et al. Stability of disruptive mood dysregulation disorder symptoms (irritable-angry mood and temper outbursts) throughout childhood and adolescence in a general population sample. *J Abnorm Child Psychol*. 2015;43(8):1543–1549.

Mayes SD, Waxmonsky JD, Calhoun SL, Bixler EO. Disruptive mood dysregulation disorder symptoms and association with oppositional defiant and other disorders in a general population child sample. *J Child Adolesc Psychopharmacol*. 2016;26(2):101–106.

McCracken JT, McGough J, Shah B, et al. Risperidone in children with autism and serious behavioral problems. *N Engl J Med*. 2002;347(5):314–321.

McTate EA, Leffler JM. Diagnosing disruptive mood dysregulation disorder: integrating semi-structured and unstructured interviews. *Clin Child Psychol Psychiatry*. 2017;22(2):187–203.

Mikita N, Stringaris A. Mood dysregulation. *Eur Child Adolesc Psychiatry*. 2013;22:S11–S16.

Mikita N, Hollocks MJ, Papadopoulos AS, et al. Irritability in boys with autism spectrum disorders: an investigation of physiological reactivity. *J Child Psychol Psychiatry*. 2015;56(10):1118–1126.

Miklowitz DJ, Axelson DA, Birmaher B, et al. Family-focused treatment for adolescents with bipolar disorder: results of a 2-year randomized trial. *Arch Gen Psychiatry*. 2008;65(9):1053–1061.

Moreno C, Laje G, Blanco C, et al. National trends in the outpatient diagnosis and treatment of bipolar disorder in youth. *Arch Gen Psychiatry*. 2007;64(9):1032–1039.

Narrow WE, Clarke DE, Kuramoto SJ, et al. DSM-5 field trials in the United States and Canada, Part III: development and reliability testing of a cross-cutting symptom assessment for DSM-5. *Am J Psychiatry*. 2013;170(1):71–82.

Olfson M, Blanco C, Liu L, et al. National trends in the outpatient treatment of children and adolescents with antipsychotic drugs. *Arch Gen Psychiatry*. 2006;63(6):679–685.

an PY, Fu AT, Yeh CB. Aripiprazole/methylphenidate combination in children and adolescents with disruptive mood dysregulation disorder and attention-deficit/hyperactivity disorder: an open-label study. *J Child Adolesc Psychopharmacol*. 2018 28(10):682–689.

Perlman SB, Jones BM, Wakschlag LS, Axelson D, Birmaher B, Phillips ML. Neural substrates of child irritability in typically developing and psychiatric populations. *Dev Cogn Neurosci*. 2015;14:71–80.

Pickles A, Aglan A, Collishaw S, et al. Predictors of suicidality across the life span: the Isle of Wight study. *Psychol Med*. 2010;40(9):453–1466.

Pilling S, Gould N, Whittington C, et al. Recognition, intervention, and management of antisocial behaviour and conduct disorders in children and young people: summary of NICE-SCIE guidance. *BMJ*. 2013;346:1298.

Plomin R, Haworth CM, Davis OS. Common disorders are quantitative traits. *Nat Rev Genet*. 2009;10(12):872–878.

Regier DA, Narrow WE, Clarke DE, et al. DSM-5 field trials in the United States and Canada, Part II: test-retest reliability of selected categorical diagnoses. *Am J Psychiatry*. 2013;170(1):59–70.

Rich BA, Schmajuk M, Perez-Edgar KE, et al. Different psychophysiological and behavioral responses elicited by frustration in pediatric bipolar disorder and severe mood dysregulation. *Am J Psychiatry*. 2007;164(2):309.

Rich BA, Grimley ME, Schmajuk M, et al. Face emotion labeling deficits in children with bipolar disorder and severe mood dysregulation. *Dev Psychopathol*. 2008;20(2):529–546.

Rich BA, Carver FW, Holroyd T, et al. Different neural pathways to negative affect in youth with pediatric bipolar disorder and severe mood dysregulation. *J Psychiatr Res*. 2011;45(10):1283–1294.

Roberson-Nay R, Leibenluft E, Brotman MA, et al. Longitudinal stability of genetic and environmental influences on irritability: from childhood to young adulthood. *Am J Psychiatry*. 2015;172(7):657–664.

Rowe R, Costello J, Angold A, et al. Developmental pathways in oppositional defiant disorder and conduct disorder. *J Abnorm Psychol*. 2010;119(4):726–738.

Rutter M. Research review: Child psychiatric diagnosis and classification: concepts, findings, challenges and potential. *J Child Psychol Psychiatry*. 2011;52(6):647–660.

Savage J, Verhulst B, Copeland W, Althoff RR, Lichtenstein P, Roberson-Nay R. A genetically informed study of the longitudinal relation between irritability and anxious/depressed symptoms. *J Am Acad Child Adolesc Psychiatry*. 2015;54(5):377–384.

Scott S, O'Connor TG. An experimental test of differential susceptibility to parenting among emotionally-dysregulated children in a randomized controlled trial for oppositional behavior. *J Child Psychol Psychiatry*. 2012;53(11):1184–1193.

Simonoff E, Jones CR, Pickles A, et al. Severe mood problems in adolescents with autism spectrum disorder. *J Child Psychol Psychiatry*. 2012;53(11):1157–1166.

Stoddard J, Stringaris A, Brotman M, et al. Irritability in child and adolescent anxiety disorders. *Depress Anxiety*. 2014;31(7):566–573.

Stoddard J, Hsu D, Reynolds RC, et al. Aberrant amygdala intrinsic functional connectivity distinguishes youths with bipolar disorder from those with severe mood dysregulation. *Psychiatry Res*. 2015;231(2):120–125.

Stringaris A. Irritability in children and adolescents: a challenge for DSM-5. *Eur Child Adolesc Psychiatry*. 2011;20(2):61–66.

Stringaris A. Emotion, emotion regulation and disorder: conceptual issues for clinicians and neuroscientists. In: Bishop D, Pine D, Scott S, et al, eds. *Rutter's Child and Adolescent Psychiatry*. 6th ed. London: Wiley Blackwell; 2015.

Stringaris A, Goodman R. Mood lability and psychopathology in youth. *Psychol Med*. 2009a;39(8):1237–1245.

Stringaris A, Goodman R. Longitudinal outcome of youth oppositionality: irritable, headstrong, and hurtful behaviors have distinctive predictions. *J Am Acad Child Adolesc Psychiatry*. 2009b;48(4):404–412.

Stringaris A, Goodman R. Three dimensions of oppositionality in youth. *J Child Psychol Psychiatry*. 2009c;50(3):216–223.

Stringaris A, Taylor E. *Dsiruptive Mood. Irritability in Children and Adolescents*. New York, NY: Oxford University Press; 2015.

Stringaris A, Cohen P, Pine DS, Leibenluft E. Adult outcomes of youth irritability: a 20-year prospective community-based study. *Am J Psychiatry*. 2009;166(9):1048–1054.

Stringaris A, Baroni A, Haimm C, et al. Pediatric bipolar disorder versus severe mood dysregulation: risk for manic episodes on follow-up. *J Am Acad Child Adolesc Psychiatry*. 2010;49(4):397–405.

Stringaris A, Zavos H, Leibenluft E, et al. Adolescent irritability: phenotypic associations and genetic links with depressed mood. *Am J Psychiatry*. 2012a;169(1):47–54.

Stringaris A, Goodman R, Ferdinando S, et al. The Affective Reactivity Index: a concise irritability scale for clinical and research settings. *J Child Psychol Psychiatry*. 2012b;53(11):1109–1117.

Stringaris A, Maughan B, Copeland WS, Costello EJ, Angold A. Irritable mood as a symptom of depression in youth: prevalence, developmental, and clinical correlates in the Great Smoky Mountains Study. *J Am Acad Child Adolesc Psychiatry*. 2013;52(8):831–840.

Thomas LA, Kim P, Bones BL, et al. Elevated amygdala responses to emotional faces in youths with chronic irritability or bipolar disorder. *Neuroimage Clin*. 2013;2:637–645.

Thomas LA, Brotman MA, Bones BL, et al. Neural circuitry of masked emotional face processing in youth with bipolar disorder, severe mood dysregulation, and healthy volunteers. *Dev Cogn Neurosci*. 2014;8:110–120.

Towbin K, Vidal-Ribas P, Brotman MA, et al. A double-blind randomized placebo-controlled trial of citalopram adjunctive to stimulant medication in youth with chronic severe irritability. *J Am Acad Child Adolesc Psychiatry*. 2020;59(3):350–361.

Tseng WL, Thomas LA, Harkins E, et al. Neural correlates of masked and unmasked face emotion processing in youth with severe mood dysregulation. *Soc Cogn Affect Neurosci*. 2016;11(1):78–88.

Vidal-Ribas P, Brotman MA, Valdivieso I, Leibenluft E, Stringaris A. The status of irritability in psychiatry: a conceptual and quantitative review. *J Am Acad Child Adolesc Psychiatry*. 2016;55(7):556–570.

Waxmonsky JG, Waschbusch DA, Belin P, et al. A randomized clinical trial of an integrative group therapy for children with severe mood dysregulation. *J Am Acad Child Adolesc Psychiatry*. 2016;55(3):196–207.

Whelan YM, Stringaris A, Maughan B, Barker ED. Developmental continuity of Oppositional Defiant Disorder subdimensions at ages 8, 10, and 13 years and their distinct psychiatric outcomes at age 16 years. *J Am Acad Child Adolesc Psychiatry*. 2013;52(9):961–969.

Whelan YM, Leibenluft E, Stringaris A, Barker ED. Pathways from maternal depressive symptoms to adolescent depressive symptoms: the unique contribution of irritability symptoms. *J Child Psychol Psychiatry*. 2015;56(10):1092–1100.

Wiggins JL, Brotman MA, Adleman NE, et al. Neural correlates of irritability in disruptive mood dysregulation and bipolar disorders. *Am J Psychiatry*. 2016;173(7):722–730.

Winters DE, Fukui S, Leibenluft E, Hulvershorn LA. Improvements in irritability with open-label methylphenidate treatment in youth with comorbid attention deficit/hyperactivity disorder and disruptive mood dysregulation disorder. *J Child Adolesc Psychopharmacol*. 2018;28(5):298–305.

Wozniak J, Biederman J, Kiely K, et al. Mania-like symptoms suggestive of childhood-onset bipolar disorder in clinically referred children. *J Am Acad Child Adolesc Psychiatry*. 1995;34(7):867–876.

Wiggins JL, Mitchell C, Stringaris A, Leibenluft E. Developmental trajectories of irritability and bidirectional associations with maternal depression. *J Am Acad Child Adolesc Psychiatry*. 2014;53(11):1191–1205, 1205e1191–1194.

Emergency Psychiatry

Daniel H. Ebert, MD, PhD
Matthew N. Goldenberg, MD, MSc

Emergency psychiatry encompasses the urgent evaluation and management of patients with active symptoms. The definition of emergency is determined by the ability of the patient or the patient's social environment to tolerate these symptoms. Although these emergency evaluations are most commonly performed in hospital settings, mobile crisis teams permit completion of emergency assessment in community settings.

▼ GOALS OF EMERGENCY PSYCHIATRY

The goals of emergency psychiatric care are similar to those of emergency medical–surgical care: (1) triage, (2) expeditious, pertinent assessment, (3) accurate differential diagnosis, (4) management of acute symptoms, and (5) appropriate disposition planning.

▶ Triage

The triage function determines the degree of urgency of the patient's presentation and the initial pathway for evaluation of the patient. In many settings, the person responsible for the triage function is not a mental health specialist. The triage clinician must first distinguish between situations that constitute a genuine emergency and those that, although perceived as such by the patient or others, can safely await later assessment.

Next, the triage clinician must correctly identify, among a variety of emergency situations, those that reflect a need for psychiatric evaluation as a first step. This is a critical decision as patients may have both medical and psychiatric complaints or exhibit behavioral problems that may originate from a medical, neurological, or substance-induced disorder. A medical evaluation, including a brief history of the presenting complaint, and physical assessment, including vital signs, are critical components of this triage function.

Last, the triage clinician must ensure the safety of patients until they can be evaluated by a psychiatrist or other mental

health professional. In emergency room (ER) settings, where priority is often given to patients presenting with severe injuries or acute medical signs and symptoms, the needs of a well-appearing patient arriving with no obvious disorder may be overlooked. However, this patient may have suicidal or homicidal ideation that can be as life threatening as any other medical emergency and requires immediate attention to ensure the safety of the patient and others.

Although initial triage is most commonly undertaken by nursing personnel, the psychiatrist must assume an active role in the training and supervision of those clinicians and in the formulation of standards and clinical criteria applied during the triage "sorting" function. This includes appropriate safe placement of the patient in the ER, including whether a sitter is needed for psychiatric safety and other suicide precautions, as per protocols at the particular hospital. Triage is only as effective as the quality of the standards and the rigor with which they are applied.

▶ Assessment

Assessment of psychiatric patients under emergency circumstances focuses on the need to quickly evaluate the pertinent aspect(s) of the patient's presentation, with special attention paid to potential life-threatening issues. Although the patient may have had an initial brief medical evaluation and triage to psychiatry, the clinician should continue to be alert to the possibility that the patient has a medical disorder or substance-induced disorder underlying his/her presentation.

The clinician should assemble as much data as possible before addressing the patient directly. For example, if information suggests that the patient may be dangerous to themselves or to others, appropriate security arrangements should be made. The patient may need to have a staff member be assigned to sit with them to ensure safety or may need to be searched for potential weapons. It is also important to establish how the patient came to psychiatric attention (e.g., did he/she self-present or was he/she brought in by police/ambulance?). A review of prior records, if available, can be a vital part of the emergency assessment.

During the initial moments of the direct encounter with the patient, the clinician should form an overall impression of the patient. This impression may include data from sources such as the patient's level of consciousness, orientation, appearance, willingness to engage with the clinician, apparent mood and affect, psychomotor retardation or agitation, and initial conversation. This initial period of direct observation can be helpful in determining whether the patient has been triaged correctly or whether additional medical evaluation or security arrangements are required. The clinician should always be mindful of their own and their staffs' safety with agitated patients, including always having easy egress from the interview and known routines to obtain the presence of security or additional staff quickly.

Despite the common pressure to proceed expeditiously, clinicians should attempt to be thorough in both their medical or psychiatric evaluations. This is critical to properly assess psychiatric and medical safety, including risk of imminent harm to self or others, risk of withdrawal from alcohol or drugs, or active medical issue that is presenting with behavioral or psychiatric symptoms. The emergency assessment should include history of present illness, past psychiatric history, past and current medical problems, current engagement in medical and psychiatric treatment, current medications and adherence to the medical regimen, history of past and current substance abuse, social history, family history, review of symptoms, mental status examination, and screening laboratory workup.

In the history of present illness, the clinician should screen for presence of mood episode, psychosis, anxiety disorder, delirium, and cognitive disorder. In addition, clinicians will need to manage alcohol and drug withdrawal, particularly for longer length of stays in the ER. The clinician should assess psychosocial stressors that may have precipitated the patient's presentation in the ER. These stressors may include disruptions in housing and work or disruptions in important relationships, including romantic relationships, family relationships, and the patient's relationship with a current outpatient clinician. Events such as an argument with a family member or friend, or the vacation of an outpatient clinician, can precipitate a patient's presentation for emergency treatment. A good question is to understand why the patient is presenting today.

The past psychiatric history can help inform the safety assessment, including history of past suicide attempts, history of self-harm behaviors, and history and response to past psychiatric treatment. This history can help inform the right level of care for patient at this time, whether inpatient psychiatric hospitalization, crisis stabilization unit, substance use disorders program, or outpatient care is most appropriate. A social history, including assessments of early development, education, employment, significant relationship, children, trauma history, living situation, and legal history, can be obtained efficiently and will provide critical components to an assessment of the patient from multiple perspectives. In addition, a family history will aid in making a thorough psychiatric assessment, including possibility of inherited major mental illness.

Assessment of past medical history, review of symptoms, and physical examination, including neurological screening examination, can help inform whether there are medical issues that need to be addressed. It is important for the mental health side of the ER to think independently and collaboratively with the medical side of the ER to obtain differential diagnosis that assesses for possible medical components to the presentation. This assessment will help determine what other appropriate laboratory, toxicology, or imaging studies should be ordered.

An emergency psychiatric evaluation should involve gathering collateral information to complete a safety assessment. Collateral can be obtained from family members, friends, outpatient providers, school officials, law enforcement officers, or others. This collateral information often provides important context to the patient's presentation and can prove invaluable, particularly in cases when patients are unable or unwilling to provide a reliable history. In addition, this collateral information can be essential to making an informed safety assessment of imminent harm to self or others or ability to care for oneself, as well as for assessment of whether psychiatric treatment is required at this time.

▶ Diagnosis

The pressures of the emergency setting often do not allow the detailed diagnostic assessment possible in other settings. However, a diagnostic assessment can be obtained efficiently. The clinician should construct a differential diagnosis which can be utilized to guide further emergency evaluation. The major clinical syndrome(s) (e.g., psychosis, mood, anxiety, and cognition) should be identified. In constructing this differential diagnosis, a high priority must be given to medical, neurological, and substance-induced etiologies of the presenting problem. Table 58–1 lists four sequential questions that should be considered in making a differential diagnosis.

Table 58–1 Differential Evaluation

1. Is the disordered affect, thought, or behavior the product of detectable pathophysiology, especially that associated with a medical problem or substance induced toxicity?
2. If not, is the disordered affect, thought, or behavior of psychotic quality, especially that associated with schizophrenia or manic states?
3. If not, is the disordered affect, thought, or behavior compatible with some other formal diagnostic entity, especially anxiety states, depression, or personality disorder?
4. If not, is the disordered affect, thought, or behavior contrived to obtain an advantage or to avoid an undesirable consequence (e.g., incarceration)?

▶ Initial Treatment

Treatment interventions, when appropriate as an emergency procedure, will usually follow the diagnostic assessment. However, sometimes the clinician must intervene before gathering all the diagnostic information. This is particularly true when the patient must be kept safe because of concern about being a danger to self or others. In most circumstances, emergency interventions will fall into one or more of four categories: environmental management, medication, crisis intervention, and education.

A. Environmental Management

As noted earlier, clinicians must be attentive to providing a safe environment for patients with psychiatric emergencies. These interventions often occur before a full evaluation is completed. Care environments should be designed to reduce risk for injury to self or others (e.g., no sharps, cords, projectiles, ligature points) and to prevent elopement or suicide (e.g., via sitter or locked unit). Patients may benefit from having diminished stimulation in their environment. Availability of a "quiet room" is often helpful in reducing psychomotor agitation. Some ERs have specialized psychiatric care areas (constructed for patient safety) and psychiatrically trained staff to care for patients in crisis.

B. Medication Interventions

Pharmacologic interventions in the emergency setting are often reserved for the treatment of severe acute symptoms such as agitation, aggression, or anxiety. Clinicians in the emergency setting use medications such as benzodiazepines and antipsychotics in order to manage symptoms of psychomotor agitation. When a patient is acutely agitated or threatening, medications can be given intramuscularly to quicken onset of action. In addition, clinicians will need to manage alcohol and drug withdrawal, particularly for longer length of stays in the ER.

Clinicians in ER settings should exercise caution about initiating more routine pharmacological interventions for several reasons. First, initial diagnostic impressions may prove inaccurate. Second, the full laboratory assessment of the patient may not be complete. Third, treatment with medications may produce sedation, which can mask other signs of medical illness. Last, the clinician in the ER will likely not be treating the patient in follow-up. Therefore, in general, pharmacological interventions should be limited to those needed to help manage the patient in the emergency setting.

Giving a patient medication to manage symptoms until the patient is seen in outpatient treatment requires careful consideration of several factors including the patient's adherence, issues of safety, and the amount of time before outpatient follow-up care will begin. The possibility that the patient is seeking benzodiazepines or pain medication because of an addiction should be strongly considered. In general, patients should not be given more than a few days' supply of medication at any one time.

C. Crisis Intervention

Psychological strategies based on a biopsychosocial understanding of the situation can often de-escalate a crisis. Such techniques include ventilation, identification of alternatives, clarification of interpersonal roles, interpretation of meaning, or simply empathic listening. Meeting with the patient and his/her family or significant other can help resolve difficulties that may have led to the patient seeking care in an emergency setting.

D. Education

An important but often overlooked component of treatment in the ER is the opportunity for preventive education. The patient, family members, significant others, and even other caregivers will sometimes benefit greatly from education about psychiatric illness, coping strategies, and/or treatment or other community resources. For example, a patient with new-onset panic disorder may be able to avoid returning to the ER if sufficiently educated about the nature of the disorder. Clarification of the situation in a way that can avoid unwarranted guilt or confusion will be helpful to all involved. The patient, and others important to the patient, may avoid a sense of alienation, shame, and hopelessness by better understanding the diagnosed illness, its treatment, and its prognosis.

▶ Disposition Planning

Determining the appropriate intervention and next level of care is a primary task of an emergency psychiatric evaluation. Disposition planning from a psychiatric emergency depends on the resources that are realistically available. In general, at least five issues must be considered: (1) initial level of care, (2) the patient's willingness to seek treatment, (3) timing of initial follow-up care, (4) interval provisions, and (5) communication with the patient and subsequent caregivers.

A. Initial Level of Care

The objective of an emergency evaluation is to identify and ensure a safe transition to the least restrictive level of care that meets the patient's clinical needs. As the most restrictive and expensive alternative, 24-hour inpatient care should be used only after careful consideration of several factors. Commonly accepted criteria for such care include mental illness associated with imminent danger to self or others, grave impairment of functioning to a degree that prohibits self-preservation in the most supportive environment available, and diagnostic uncertainty that could result in a lethal outcome. Patients who do not obviously require hospitalization but whose symptoms do not allow for immediate discharge (e.g., those requiring further evaluation/information, those with symptoms thought likely to stabilize within 24 hours) may be placed in observation status in either an emergency department or another specialized unit. Those patients who can be safely discharged from the emergency department may be referred to care at less restrictive alternatives, including crisis housing with less intensive staff observation, partial or day hospitalization, and intensive or routine outpatient follow-up care.

At times, modifying the home environment of a patient may avoid a hospitalization. Providing alternative short-term housing during a crisis, respite care for an elderly patient, or emergency placement of a child can decrease the patient's symptoms.

The patient's ability to pay for different services is a factor that unfortunately can determine what follow-up care is able to be provided. In some settings, indigent patients may have access to more services than low-income patients with more limited entitlements.

B. The Patient's Willingness to Seek Treatment

A patient presenting for psychiatric evaluation may not present to the ER voluntarily. Frequently, police or family members bring an individual to the ER for treatment. If a determination is made that the patient requires inpatient level of care, he/she should be offered the opportunity to agree voluntarily to a hospitalization. However, if the patient is unwilling to be admitted, the clinician may need to initiate an involuntary hospitalization process. Although the administrative processes vary in each state, licensed physicians are able to involuntarily admit patients who meet standards of acute dangerousness to self or others or inability to care for themselves due to their mental illness.

In general, patients with psychiatric disorders have the same right to accept or refuse treatment that patients with other medical conditions have. In most instances, if a patient in an ER does not meet legal requirements for involuntary hospitalization and/or is unwilling to seek outpatient care, the patient's decision must be respected. Patients who report not wanting outpatient treatment should be provided options for accessing care should they change their minds after discharge from the ER.

C. Timing of Initial Follow-up Care

For patients interested in outpatient treatment, the discharge planning should include determination of the clinically permissible time interval before a less restrictive level of care is available. For example, a situation that requires urgent outpatient follow-up care should not be scheduled 2 or 3 weeks later.

If significant time will elapse before initial follow-up care can be scheduled, the patient and relevant others should be informed of what to do in the event of an intervening crisis such as calling crisis hotlines, attending a walk-in clinic, or returning to the ER.

D. Communication with the Patient & Subsequent Caregivers

A breakdown in communication with clinicians providing outpatient care often frustrates the patient and can lead to nonadherence with the plan of care developed in the emergency setting. The precise discharge plan should be written out and given to the patient (and, when appropriate, to the family, significant others, and clinicians who will assume the patient's subsequent care). An opportunity to raise questions, seek clarification of details, and better understand the clinical rationale of the discharge plan should be a routine part of this process.

Equally important is the timely communication with other professional caregivers who are to provide subsequent treatment. This communication should provide enough detail for other clinicians to begin active treatment with the patient. A smooth transition in care gives the patient a reassuring sense of continuity from emergency onset to final initiation of outpatient treatment.

▼ SPECIAL CONSIDERATIONS IN EMERGENCY PSYCHIATRY

Four issues merit special consideration in the setting of emergent psychiatric evaluation: suicide, homicide and other violence, disaster psychiatry, and the medico-legal aspects of psychiatric evaluation and treatment in the emergency setting.

▶ Suicide

Suicide accounted for 48,000 deaths in 2021 in the United States. The number of attempted suicides is many times greater. Up to 80% of individuals who commit suicide have seen a physician or other health care personnel within 2 weeks before their deaths; most often this health care professional was not in the mental health care field. Therefore, it is extremely important that all health care professionals be alert to the signals of distress and risk factors for suicide. This is especially true in emergency psychiatric settings, where assessment of patients with suicidal ideation is a common occurrence.

Perhaps the single most important element in the assessment of suicidal risk is constant awareness of the possibility that it exists. The patient may make no direct reference to self-destruction unless asked. Asking about suicidal thoughts and behaviors is an essential component of any emergency psychiatric evaluation. Assessment of risk factors known to predispose to suicide is one method to quantify the risk that the patient will attempt suicide (Table 58–2). However, many patients with serious mental illness, especially those with dual diagnosis (mental illness and a substance abuse disorder), will have many of the risk factors known to predispose to suicide. Clinical judgment and the patient's ability to work with the clinician to develop a treatment plan that mitigates certain

Table 58–2 Suicide Risk Factors

Age (especially adolescents and older adults)
Marital status (suicide is more common among single, widowed, or divorced adults)
Sex (females attempt suicide more often than do males, but males succeed more often than do females)
Ethnicity (Whites are more likely to commit suicide than Hispanics, African-Americans, or Asians)
Economic status (unemployment or economic reverses increase risk)
History of prior attempt
Family history of suicide
Recent separation or loss
Presence of a plan and available means to accomplish it
Lethality of an attempt (more lethal attempts increase risk)
Diagnosis (especially major depression, schizophrenia, alcoholism or other substance dependence, and borderline personality disorder)
Specific symptoms (especially command hallucinations, delusional thinking, and profound depression with hopelessness)
Lack of social support

Table 58–3 Homicide and Other Violence: Clinical and Epidemiologic Factors

Age (violent individuals tend to be young)
Sex (males predominate)
Criminality (some individuals violate social rules without significant psychological impairment)
History (physical or sexual abuse as a child, fire setting, or cruelty to animals)
Proposed victim is a family member or close associate
Environmental influence (violent subcultures beget violence)
Diagnosis (especially manic states, schizophrenia, alcoholism or other substance dependence, conduct disorder, antisocial personality disorder, and intermittent explosive disorder)
Specific symptoms (especially command hallucinations, agitation, and hostile suspiciousness)

stressors and risk factors will help determine whether the patient is able to safely leave the emergency evaluation setting or requires inpatient treatment. Obtaining collateral information can be essential in making a suicide risk assessment. Clear documentation of the assessment, including risk factor assessment, is critical in the evaluations of the suicidal patient.

Homicidal Ideation and Violence

The relationship between violence and mental illness is complex. Although intense media coverage of violence perpetrated by patients with mental disorders can lead one to think that this is a common occurrence, patients with serious mental disorders are more often victims of violence than perpetrators of violence. However, patients with severe mental illness, perhaps especially those with psychotic paranoid symptoms, can act on their delusions that someone is going to hurt them or their hallucinations telling them to harm another person. As with the assessment of suicidal ideation, many clinical and epidemiologic factors need to be considered in the assessment of homicidal ideation or violence risk (Table 58–3). The clinician who is called upon to make an emergency assessment must be aware of the legal ramifications (see Chapter 60), and he or she is best advised to approach the task with the admonition that justice is served best by thorough, objective, accurate assessment, and documentation.

Disaster Psychiatry

Interest in the psychiatric aspects of response to mass traumatic events such as terrorist attacks and natural disasters has grown. It is reasonable to expect that psychiatrists will be called on by communities and governments to provide leadership in the wake of future disasters. Although this is a rapidly developing field, some valuable lessons have already been learned. Broadly, successful responses to these situations should be shaped by the type of disaster and the affected populations. Among the different types of disasters are ones without warning (terrorist attacks, earthquakes), ones with some warning (hurricanes, floods), and those with potentially longer-term notice (infectious disease outbreaks). The impact of these events can be influenced by such variables as intensity and duration of the event, number of people and particular subpopulations affected, degree to which those people are affected, and postdisaster response issues such as ongoing safety and available resources. Psychological resilience in the face of disaster is the most common response. Evidence suggests that psychological debriefing of disaster victims may in fact worsen psychological outcomes. Instead, the most appropriate public health interventions in the wake of mass trauma are guided by principles of psychological first aid, including ensuring access to safe housing and food and assisting people in reconnecting with family members and friends. Following a disaster, initial attention is frequently directed at "new" casualties—the population presumed to have suffered psychologically as a result of the disaster. Recent experience has also shown the need to address two other critical populations at these times. People with preexisting mental health needs, including the severely mentally ill population, are particularly vulnerable to stress and can present in a decompensated state with records that can be inaccessible or destroyed. Last, the mental health needs of disaster responders, both mental-health and non–mental-health providers, must be carefully monitored as they try to provide services to patients in dire need and under extremely trying circumstances.

Medico-legal Aspects of Psychiatric Care in Emergency Settings

Given the acuity of patient presentations and the frequent risk assessments being completed, attending to the medico-legal aspects of emergency psychiatry is of great importance. Clear documentation of the patient's history, risk factors, and the clinician's decision-making process (including consultation with other clinicians and with legal counsel) and treatment plan is imperative. Awareness of local statutes regarding compulsory evaluation/treatment and involuntary commitment is mandatory. Clinicians working in emergency psychiatric settings must have access to legal advice and should have a low threshold to consult with legal counsel.

A. Involuntary Patients

As suggested earlier, patients may be brought to the ER by the police or by the family because of suicidal ideation, homicidal ideation, or other aberrant thoughts and behaviors. Once in the emergency setting, patients may decide they do not want to consent to evaluation or treatment. In general, if there is suspicion that a patient may be at risk of hurting themselves or others, common law principles would allow holding the patient until a full evaluation can be completed. Many jurisdictions have specific statues allowing for detainment to complete an appropriate assessment.

As noted earlier, all states have methods providing for involuntary hospitalization of patients evaluated to be at significant risk of injury to themselves or others. Clinicians working in these settings should be knowledgeable about how to apply these laws and what right of appeal patients may have.

B. Confidentiality

Patients have the right to expect clinicians to respect the confidentiality of their communications. There are some circumstances in which common law and case law may support breaching patient confidentiality. One common circumstance involves a patient refusing to allow communication with potential sources of collateral information such as an outpatient clinician or a family member. For example, the clinician may suspect a drug overdose and need to know the medications that the patient was taking. In this clear emergency setting, allowance would generally be made under common law to proceed with contacting the outpatient clinician. Clinicians are generally permitted to receive information *from* a collateral source of information even if they should not provide information *to* that source about a patient's condition. In situations in which there is a less clearly life-threatening situation, the clinician may need to respect the patient's confidentiality and not contact the outpatient clinician.

C. Duty to Warn/Protect

If a clinician working in an emergency setting believes that a patient poses a significant risk of injury to another person, strong consideration should be given to hospitalizing that patient. If, however, the patient leaves the ER without being admitted to the hospital inpatient unit, the ER clinician may be required to warn the individual thought to be at risk and/or contact authorities such as the police who might be able to provide protection to that individual. This Duty to Warn stems from California case law, *Tarasoff v. Regents of the University of California* (1976). This precedent has not been endorsed in all states.

▼ MAJOR CLINICAL SYNDROMES

Patients with a variety of clinical syndromes may present in a health care setting for emergency psychiatric treatment (Table 58–4). The following sections discuss the disorders most commonly requiring emergency treatment.

DEPRESSION

▶ Assessment

A common presentation to the psychiatric ER is a patient reporting depressed mood, often accompanied by suicidal ideation or behavior (see Chapter 26 and the discussion on suicide earlier in this chapter). In addition to identifying current stressors and probing for a history of depression, the clinician must pay close attention to comorbid conditions such as medical illness, psychosis, substance abuse, anxiety, and personality disorders. A suicide risk assessment is one of the major tasks of a psychiatric evaluation of the depressed patient.

▶ Disposition Planning

As noted previously in this chapter, an inpatient treatment is frequently the most appropriate setting for patients with significant suicidal ideation or attempt. The availability of a vigorous, reliable support system may allow a less restrictive alternative to be considered. Referral for outpatient follow-up care of a depressed patient with suicidal ideation requires forethought about many factors such as safety, availability of supportive monitoring, time interval to next visit, access to help in the event of recurrent emergency, and advisability of medication use. In general, the patient should not be given antidepressant medication in an ER setting, as the prescribing clinician will not be able to provide follow-up and there is increasing evidence that some antidepressants may precipitate suicidal ideation in the short term, especially in adolescent patients.

PSYCHOSIS

▶ Assessment

A psychotic state may occur either as a completely new event or as the exacerbation or reactivation of chronic psychotic disorder (see Chapters 24 and 25). The distinction is important because new-onset psychosis frequently warrants

Table 58–4 Clinical Syndromes that May Present as Psychiatric Emergencies

Syndrome	Assessment	Dispositions
Geriatric syndromes	Review of systems Laboratory tests Look for delirium, delirium with dementia, depression, and psychosis	Inpatient care Collaboration with medical team High-potency neuroleptics (e.g., haloperidol, 0.5–1 mg orally or intramuscularly) for agitation
Substance abuse	Look for intoxication or withdrawal	Quiet environment Inpatient care for neuropsychiatric signs Lorazepam (1–2 mg intramuscularly or orally) or haloperidol (5 mg orally or 2 mg intramuscularly) for agitation
Psychosis	New onset versus exacerbation? Rule out substance abuse and medical illness Evaluate for compliance, dangerousness, and ADL	Inpatient care for new-onset psychosis, dangerousness, or severely impaired ADL Collaboration with outpatient team
Depression	Evaluate for suicidal risk, comorbidities, current stressors, and substance abuse	Inpatient care for suicidal risk, agitation, or substance abuse Collaborate with outpatient team
Mania	Evaluate for dangerousness and substance abuse	Inpatient care for psychosis, dangerousness, or substance abuse Lorazepam (1–2 mg intramuscularly) or haloperidol (1–5 mg intramuscularly) for agitation
Catatonia	Two subtypes: withdrawn and excited Look for schizophrenia, mood disorders, and medical disorders (e.g., using amobarbital, 500 mg, 50 mg/min intravenously)	Inpatient care Lorazepam (1–2 mg, intramuscularly or intravenously)
Acute anxiety states	Types include panic disorder, acute stress disorder, posttraumatic stress disorder, conversion states, dissociative states Evaluate for ADL	Inpatient care if ADL markedly impaired Lorazepam (1–2 mg orally or intramuscularly)
Personality disorders	Evaluate for substance abuse, legal history, relationships, "micropsychotic" episodes, mood changes, aggression, and comorbidities	Interdisciplinary treatment Focus on "here and now" issues
Neuroleptic malignant syndrome	Look for sudden onset, autonomic changes, neuromuscular changes, elevated CPK, and leukocytosis	Medical emergency Inpatient care: stop neuroleptic and provide supportive treatment (rehydration, antipyretic) Dantrolene (2–3 mg/kg) or bromocriptine (2.5–10 mg three times daily)

ADL, activities of daily living; CPK, creatine phosphokinase.

hospitalization, whereas the chronic condition often can be managed readily in cooperation with an outpatient team. New-onset psychosis warrants strong consideration of a medical etiology. Because of the psychosis-inducing effects of some drugs of abuse as well as the high frequency of substance abuse disorders among patients with psychotic disorders, clinicians should strongly suspect substance use as contributing to new onset or exacerbations of psychosis. Assessment should also consider the patient's medical condition; adherence with prior treatment recommendations including psychiatric medications; the severity of impairment in activities of daily living; the patient's risk of dangerousness to self and others; the presence of delusions, command auditory hallucinations, or thought disorder; and impairment of judgment about potentially dangerous situations.

Treatment and Disposition Planning

New-onset acute psychotic conditions generally require hospitalization. Command hallucinations with suicidal or homicidal intent or impaired judgment and evidence of dangerous behavior may warrant involuntary hospitalization. Severe psychomotor agitation or threatening behavior may require physical restraint or psychopharmacologic intervention.

Determination of the most appropriate and least restrictive level of care should include consideration of inpatient treatment, partial hospitalization, and outpatient care. When outpatient follow-up care will suffice, attention must be given to appropriate inclusion of the patient's outpatient clinicians, case managers, family members, and other caregivers in developing the outpatient care plan. Initiation or adjustment of antipsychotic medication may be indicated after collaboration with the outpatient clinician and necessary laboratory studies are completed.

ALCOHOL USE DISORDERS

▶ Assessment

Alcohol-related disorders are among the most common psychiatric emergencies. Presentations to emergency settings are most frequently associated with acute alcohol intoxication and withdrawal, including withdrawal delirium. Mood and anxiety symptoms including suicidal ideation as well as behavior disturbances such as agitation, ataxia, or sedation are frequently related to alcohol use. Determination of patient's current blood alcohol level (BAL) is essential, as is the patient's history of recent and longer-term alcohol use and withdrawal symptoms. Because coingestion with other drugs of abuse is common, a toxicology screen is important. A thorough medical evaluation is warranted to exclude physical conditions that resemble intoxication or withdrawal. Patients presenting with alcohol use disorders should have a physical examination including neurological examination to ensure that the patient has not sustained injuries as a result of a fall or other accident while intoxicated.

▶ Treatment and Disposition Planning

After medical evaluation, patients who present to the ER intoxicated will usually be monitored until sobriety is achieved. Patients who are experiencing alcohol withdrawal syndromes should be monitored closely, and their withdrawal symptoms should be treated appropriate with benzodiazepines. Those experiencing or at high risk for complicated withdrawal symptoms (seizures, delirium tremens) should frequently be admitted to medical services for treatment.

Acute behavioral and/or emotional symptoms present during intoxicated states frequently improve dramatically or resolve on sobriety. A common and complex question is determining when a patient with alcohol intoxication or withdrawal is able to be safely discharged from the ER. After the BAL is below the legal limit for intoxication, the clinician must evaluate whether the patient continues to have significant mental or physical problems related to intoxication. If the patient is no longer acutely intoxicated, screening for other symptoms of psychiatric disorder such as depression or psychosis and for the presence of suicidal or homicidal ideation should be completed. Because substance abuse raises the risk of suicidal and violent behavior, a patient who exhibits these symptoms need to be evaluated and managed carefully, including consideration for inpatient treatment.

Patients with alcohol abuse often present with denial of their illness and should be interviewed in emergency settings in a manner consistent with the tenets of motivation enhancement. Clinicians should be knowledgeable about the availability of detoxification and treatment facilities in order to provide access to treatment if the patient is motivated.

When possible, it is preferable to discharge a patient with alcohol abuse or dependence accompanied by family or friends. Appropriate referral may include an outpatient or inpatient detoxification or rehabilitation program, partial hospitalization, intensive or routine outpatient treatment, and Alcoholics Anonymous.

OTHER DRUGS OF ABUSE

▶ Assessment

Clinical history, specific physical examination findings, and a toxicology screen may offer evidence of other drugs of abuse (Table 58–5).

▶ Treatment and Disposition Planning

The management of intoxication or withdrawal depends on the specific type of drug (Chapter 17). Associated physical and psychiatric symptoms must be factored into the immediate treatment plan in a manner similar to that described with alcohol intoxication. Certain drugs of abuse induce characteristic psychotic, mood, and anxiety symptoms during both intoxicated and withdrawal states.

Chemical restraints, seclusion, or physical restraints may be needed to manage violent behavior associated with drug intoxication. It is rarely indicated to start opiate detoxification in the ER setting, as withdrawal from opiates is not life threatening, and starting these agents may reinforce the idea

Table 58–5 Evidence of Other Drugs of Abuse

Drug	Physical Findings	Psychiatric Findings
Amphetamines	Increased blood pressure, mydriasis	Euphoria, hypervigilance
Cannabis	Tachycardia	Anxiety, social withdrawal
Cocaine	Increased temperature, tachycardia, tremor	Euphoria, hypervigilance
Hallucinogens	Mydriasis, tachycardia, tremor	Anxiety, paranoia
Inhalants	Nystagmus, arrhythmia	Belligerence, apathy
Opioids	Miosis in intoxication, mydriasis in withdrawal	Agitation, dysphoria
Phencyclidine	Nystagmus, increased blood pressure, arrhythmia	Labile mood, amnesia
Sedative-hypnotics	Decreased respiration, tremor	Aggression, mood lability

that the emergency setting can be used at times when opiates are not otherwise available. The principles of outpatient referral are the same as for alcohol.

MANIA

▶ Assessment

Patients in acute manic states are frequently referred for emergency evaluation. The manic patient generally does not initiate help-seeking behavior but is instead more frequently referred for treatment by those around him/her (e.g., family, friends, police) who notice concerning behavior.

Assessment of the manic patient should include determining whether patient is experiencing psychotic symptoms, gathering a past history of mood episodes (both depression and mania), and family history of bipolar disorder, as well as consideration of substance misuse including stimulant ingestion (cocaine, amphetamines, phencyclidine, and other medications such as steroids). Patients with cluster B personality disorders may also have mood instability, which can be difficult at times to differentiate from mania due to bipolar disorder, but such a distinction can be important for appropriate treatment planning. Determining a patient's risk to self and others is very important when evaluating a manic patient. Such a determination should include not only screening for suicidal ideation and/or homicidal ideation but also evaluating a patient's risk due to limited judgment (e.g., hypersexuality), aggression (e.g., fighting), and poor safety awareness (e.g., speeding).

▶ Disposition Planning

In the ER, an agitated patient with mania warrants immediate intervention. As in the case of acute psychosis, pharmacotherapy with or without physical restraint may be required. Pharmacotherapy would include use of antipsychotic, mood stabilizer, or benzodiazepine. The primary goal is to contain the patient's agitation as quickly as possible so that the patient may be transferred safely to an inpatient setting.

A clear-cut manic episode, especially if associated with psychotic symptoms, usually warrants inpatient care. A dual-diagnosis program should be considered when mania is associated with chemical abuse or dependence. Because acute manic states are often accompanied by poor patient insight, involuntary hospitalization can be necessary.

ACUTE ANXIETY STATES

▶ Assessment

Panic attacks or other acute states of anxiety (including acute and posttraumatic stress disorders) as well as dissociative states may lead patients to seek treatment in the ER (see Chapters 27, 28, and 33 for common presenting symptoms for these anxiety disorders).

Clinicians assessing patients presenting with anxiety disorders in emergency settings should be mindful of the events preceding the patient's presentation. For example, a patient with acute anxiety may not reveal to the triage staff that the precipitant for their anxiety was a traumatic event such as an assault or a rape or the use of an illicit drug. Clinicians in psychiatry emergency settings should be aware of hospital protocols for counseling rape victims and managing evidence collection.

▶ Treatment and Disposition Planning

Many patients with anxiety symptoms respond positively to supportive crisis-oriented psychological interventions. Panic and other acute anxiety states respond favorably and quickly to a benzodiazepine.

Most anxiety disorders can be managed on an outpatient basis with a balanced combination of pharmacotherapy and psychosocial interventions. A marked restriction of activities of daily living or other severe functional impairment may necessitate inpatient care. High levels of anxiety are a risk factor for suicide, so a suicide risk assessment should always be performed. Reassurance that outpatient treatment is available can be efficacious, and psychoeducation about panic and anxiety disorder can usually help avoid inpatient hospitalization for these patients.

PERSONALITY DISORDERS

▶ Assessment

Patients with cluster B personality disorders frequently present in the ER after experiencing acute emotional distress and/or committing an impulsive act (e.g., self-injury such as cutting), often in the context of an interpersonal difficulty. The assessment of the patient with personality disorder can be made difficult by their mood lability, irritability, and use of defense mechanisms such as displacement, projection, and splitting.

▶ Treatment and Disposition Planning

Identifying and managing one's own inner reactions to these patients and helping staff maintain therapeutic boundaries are key components to the treatment of patients with cluster B personality disorders. A "here and now" approach, focused on resolution of the current stressor, is important in this clinical situation. The patient may frustrate clinicians using this approach by refusing to provide permission to contact others important to resolving the presenting complaint. Evaluation of suicidal ideation is difficult in these patients, because their mood instability and impulsivity means that a suicide attempt can be precipitated in response to an event that was difficult to predict. Comorbid substance abuse disorders are frequently present and may worsen a patient's impulsivity, making the assessment of suicidality even more difficult.

It is extremely important to be in contact with the patient's treating clinicians and other caregivers in order to enlist them in helping to devise a treatment plan for the patient. Inpatient treatment can be counterproductive for these patients by allowing/encouraging regression. However, at times, inpatient care is unavoidable because of the patient's clinical presentation. Clinicians in emergency settings should have ongoing collaborative relationships with clinical programs such as dialectical behavioral treatment programs or case management programs that care for patients with severe personality disorders; these collaborations can minimize the disruptions and staff splitting that can occur when these patients make frequent use of emergency settings.

GERIATRIC CONDITIONS

▶ Assessment

Elderly patients presenting with a psychiatric emergency require careful medical assessment, as coexisting medical disorders and medical treatments often precipitate psychiatric presentation. A thorough review of systems, a complete physical examination, and appropriate screening laboratory tests, including a urinalysis, are imperative in this age group. A medically oriented evaluative approach may be more effective than a traditional psychiatric one.

In addition to determining whether the patient may have any sensory deficits, the clinician should speak clearly and slowly to geriatric patients. When a cognitive disorder is suspected, the clinician should ask short and simple questions in a straightforward manner, should repeat them as necessary, and should strongly consider a collateral source to ensure the accuracy of the history.

Common geriatric emergencies include delirium, dementia, depression, and psychosis. Delirium and dementia may coexist with each other and with depression and psychosis (Chapters 15, 24, and 25).

▶ Delirium

Because delirium is characterized by an acute change in mental status, presentation for emergency evaluation is not uncommon. Delirium is characterized by acute changes in sensorium, orientation, concentration, and memory, which may be accompanied by perceptual changes such as hallucinations or delusions and by behavior changes like psychomotor retardation or agitation.

Delirium is a medical emergency that has a potentially fatal outcome; the possibility that the patient is delirious should be high on the differential list for all elderly patients presenting in the ER with an acute change in mental status or behavior. As soon as the clinician suspects delirium, a thorough medical evaluation should be initiated to determine the etiology. Urinary tract or other infections, onset or worsening of a medical or neurological condition, and adverse drug interactions, drug side effects (especially anticholinergic side effects), or drug intoxication secondary to an unintentional overdose related to cognitive impairment are all potential causes of delirium.

▶ Dementia

Elderly patients with dementia are often brought to the psychiatric emergency setting with acute psychomotor agitation, including combativeness. If the psychomotor agitation is of new onset, delirium or pain must be suspected and a medical workup initiated. If no medical etiology is found, the possibility that the patient is in pain from constipation, urinary retention, fall, or other source should be investigated. If no such source is identified, the patient may have had onset of a psychotic component to the dementia. If no psychotic component is present, the patient may have been upset by something or someone in the environment and have been unable to express their frustration except through agitation or combativeness. A careful review of the events precipitating the crisis may reveal the environmental issue needing to be changed.

▶ Depression

Depressed elderly patients may minimize mood symptoms but exhibit marked diminishment in interest in activities. Suicidal risk can be high in this population, so assessment of risk and development of a treatment plan must be especially carefully considered for this population.

▶ Psychosis

Presentation with new-onset psychosis in the elderly necessitates review for coexisting delirium or dementia. However, a primary psychotic disorder can have late-life onset of illness.

▶ Treatment and Disposition Planning

Because of the high likelihood of a coexisting medical illness, elderly patients presenting in the psychiatry emergency setting are best treated in collaboration with a medical team.

For patients with cognitive disorders, the highly stimulating environment of the ER is difficult to tolerate. If available, these patients benefit from provision of a quieter, less chaotic environment.

Demented patients who present with psychomotor agitation or combativeness due to a frustration with their environment may be calm on removal from their environment and transfer to the emergency setting. Clinicians in the ER should work with caregivers to determine what the precipitant might have been and how to mitigate that precipitant in the future. When possible, it is preferable for elderly demented patients to be returned to their home environment, as hospital admission itself can predispose the demented patient to worsening of their cognitive status. Knowledge of community resources such as respite programs, adult daycare, and visiting nurse agencies with psychiatric or dementia care expertise can aid in returning the patient to the community.

If an elderly patient remains agitated and or combative in the emergency setting, clinicians should make efforts to determine whether the individual can be managed with close staff attention, diverting the patient's attention to other topics by talking about family or reading a magazine together. Because of the high incidence of side effects in the elderly, medication management in the emergency setting should be avoided if possible. If medication is necessary to control physical aggression, clinicians should try to avoid deliriogenic medications, including benzodiazepines and anticholinergic medications.

OTHER EMERGENT CONDITIONS

CATATONIA

Assessment

Catatonia is a clinical syndrome characterized by cluster of behavioral symptoms, defined by the presence of a subset of catalepsy, waxy flexibility, stupor, agitation, mutism, negativism, posturing, mannerisms, stereotypies, grimacing, echolalia, and echopraxia. Catatonia can occur in the setting of psychiatric disorder, such as mood or psychotic disorders, neurologic disorders, or general medical conditions. Catatonia has been documented to be under-recognized and missed by clinicians. Catatonia is an emergency situation that requires immediate assessment to ensure that medical problems such as encephalitis or other causes of delirium are not present. In malignant catatonia, a life-threatening condition, there is fever, autonomic instability, and rigidity. There is overlap of malignant catatonia with neuroleptic malignant syndrome (NMS) (described next).

Treatment and Disposition Planning

A thorough medical workup must be pursued in order to ensure that significant medical problems are not involved in the presentation. Inpatient care is often warranted because dehydration and poor oral intake can be major complications. Benzodiazepines can lead to quick improvement. Antipsychotics can exacerbate catatonia. ECT may be required to treat catatonia.

NEUROLEPTIC MALIGNANT SYNDROME

Assessment

NMS is a serious and potentially lethal symptom complex. In NMS, three sets of symptoms appear very rapidly in response to antipsychotic (neuroleptic) treatment: (1) alteration in level of consciousness; (2) autonomic symptoms such as hyperthermia, tachycardia, labile hypertension, and tachypnea; and (3) neuromuscular symptoms such as "lead pipe" muscle rigidity. Elevated creatinine phosphokinase level and leukocytosis are common laboratory findings. Although the syndrome of altered mental status, muscle rigidity, elevated temperature, and hypertension should arouse the clinician's suspicion that NMS is present, the presence of even one of these elements can be cause for concern. NMS can appear at any time in a patient's treatment course, not just shortly after initiation of the antipsychotic. Clinicians should evaluate the patient for other disorders, especially infections, that might be present.

Treatment

Antipsychotic medication must be stopped at once, as NMS is frequently lethal. Supportive treatment such as fluids, cooling blankets, and medications to maintain blood pressure should be provided in a medical intensive care setting. The prescription of dantrolene or bromocriptine is indicated in situations where the patient is not responding to supportive interventions.

CONCLUSION

As in other fields of medicine, patients present with urgent psychiatric symptoms that may be life threatening and require emergency evaluation and treatment. The first duty of a well-prepared clinician is to recognize which of those situations is more critical than others, to identify the pertinent problem(s) correctly, and to intervene appropriately. Central considerations include whether the patient presents an imminent danger to self or others and whether the patient has grave psychological or behavioral impairment that prevents the patient from living safely in the community.

Common interventions include safety precautions, astute observation, sensitive inquiry, consideration of unsuspected medical conditions, crisis-oriented psychological treatment, judicious use of psychopharmacologic agents, and referral to the most appropriate and least restrictive level of follow-up care. Not to be overlooked is the admonition that psychiatric emergency care should always be provided in a respectful manner, no matter how disturbed or disruptive the patient may be.

Allen MH, ed. *Emergency Psychiatry*. Washington, DC: American Psychiatric Press Publishing; 2002.

Lukens TW, Wolf SJ, Edlow JA, et al: Clinical policy: critical issues in the diagnosis and management of the adult psychiatric patient in the emergency room. *Ann Emerg Med* 2006;47(1):79–99.

Slaby A, Dubin W, Baron D. Other psychiatric emergencies. In: Sadock B, Sadock V, eds. *Kaplan and Sadock's Comprehensive Textbook of Psychiatry*, Vol 2. New York: Lippincott Williams & Wilkins; 2005:2453–2471.

Consultation–Liaison Psychiatry

Catherine Chiles, MD
Thomas N. Wise, MD

INTRODUCTION

Consultation–Liaison Psychiatry is a centuries-old field of medical practice and research that bridges the biological, psychological, and social domains of psychiatric and medical illnesses. Since 2003, it has been recognized by the American Board of Medical Subspecialties as the psychiatric subspecialty *Psychosomatic Medicine*, based upon its historical nomenclature. In 2018, the Board changed the name of this added qualification to *Consultation–Liaison Psychiatry* to denote what the specialty entails. The term *psychosomatic medicine* has multiple meanings such as a theory of mind–body interactions, and research using biological and sociocultural variables as well as consultation-liaison psychiatry. The practice of *Consultation Psychiatry* usually occurs within general hospital settings. The standard consultation is performed at the request of the primary clinician and is a neutral collaboration with colleagues and patients in nonpsychiatric settings. Interview techniques in consultations may be open-ended for an individual patient's diagnostic evaluation or structured to screen for psychiatric disorders in a general population. Often a combination of both techniques is used. A central role of the consultation psychiatrist is to educate colleagues and patients about the psychiatric presentations or complications of medical illness and about illness behavior. *Liaison Psychiatry*, derived from the Latin "*to link*," expands the role of the psychiatrist to facilitate comprehensive treatment approaches within a system of care and to enhance communication among disciplines and across divisions in health care systems. The liaison psychiatrist is often a member of a multidisciplinary care team, performing psychiatric screenings, for example, in organ transplant surgery or oncology, when the risks of psychiatric comorbidity are increased due to the nature of the underlying disorders.

A. History of Psychosomatic Medicine

In the United States, the historical roots of psychiatry in the general hospital are found in the 1751 charter of the Pennsylvania Hospital, which provided for the care of "persons distempered in mind and deprived of rational faculties." At that time, outpatient psychiatric clinics both in the Philadelphia Hospital and New York's Bellevue Hospital were developed. Reports from these early centers contain themes emphasizing the significant rates of psychiatric disorders in medically ill patients and the need to integrate services.

In the modern era, the scientific approach to the relationship between psychiatric disorders and medical illness began with early studies in *psychosomatic medicine* that examined the relationship between psychological and medical disorders. Psychosomatic medicine as an area of research began with *psychoanalytic* studies of the mind–body relationship. Beginning in 1900, Sigmund Freud, as a young neurologist, described conversion hysteria as psychological symptoms imbued with deep psychic meaning, which manifested as or *converted* to somatic (physical) illness. In 1910, Sandor Ferenczi related conversion symptoms to the autonomic nervous system. In 1934, Franz Alexander proposed that "psychosomatic symptoms" were due to prolonged autonomic system arousal linked to repressed psychic conflict. Psychosomatic medicine advanced in the 1940s and 1950s with *psychophysiological* studies such as those by Hans Selye, who described the human stress response in relation to adrenocortical hormones. *Sociocultural* researchers Thomas Holmes and Richard Rahe in 1975 linked disease likelihood to the severity and number of stressful life events and further expanded the psychosomatic medicine framework. Zbigniew Lipowski in 1970 and George Engel in 1977 utilized *systems theory* to examine environmental influences on the mind–body–culture paradigm. All these works have shaped the *biopsychosocial perspective* of psychosomatic medicine extant today.

B. History of Consultation–Liaison Psychiatry

Concurrent with the development of psychosomatic medicine theories, psychiatrists returned to the general hospital they had left during the late nineteenth-century asylum movement. No longer isolated in psychiatric sanatoria or cloistered in consulting rooms, psychiatrists had begun to treat patients in general hospitals. In 1929, George Henry advocated the benefits of general hospital psychiatry that offered consultative services and was instrumental in the advancement of consultation practices. In addition to the emphasis that he placed on the diagnosis and treatment of psychiatric disorders seen in the medically ill, such as delirium, dementia, depression, and anxiety, he recognized that medical students and residents were more likely to utilize psychiatry for patients in medical settings than in isolated psychiatric facilities. Psychiatric consultation services developed further with support from the Rockefeller Foundation and grew with funding from the Psychiatry Education Branch of the National Institutes of Mental Health. By the end of the twentieth century, there was a significant cadre of trained consultation–liaison psychiatrists working within hospital settings and medical schools.

C. Psychosomatic Medicine as Subspecialty of Psychiatry

In May 2003, the American Board of Medical Subspecialties recognized the practice of consultation and liaison psychiatry in the general hospital as a discrete psychiatric subspecialty that requires advanced training and qualification by an examination conducted by the American Board of Psychiatry and Neurology. In recognition of its earliest scientific bases, the subspecialty was named Psychosomatic Medicine by the American Board of Medical Subspecialties to distinguish it from other consultative practices in medical subspecialties. Of note, this initial name was changed to *Consultation–Liaison Psychiatry* in 2018. In June 2005, the American Board of Psychiatry and Neurology administered the first examination to certify subspecialists in Psychosomatic Medicine. Psychiatric fellowship training programs in *Consultation–Liaison Psychiatry* (formerly *Psychosomatic Medicine*) qualify physicians in the *skills and techniques* of consultation–liaison psychiatry within the domain of psychiatric symptoms and disorders in medical settings, from both a clinical and research perspective.

▶ Is There a Need for Consultation–Liaison Psychiatry and Psychosomatic Medicine?

A. Evidence from Nonpsychiatric Settings

How does the work of a psychiatrist in a nonpsychiatric setting improve patient care? Numerous studies in the past decade have demonstrated that psychiatric consultation contributes to *reduced costs* in health care delivery and improves *access to mental health care*. Most importantly, psychiatric consultation improves the *detection* of psychiatric illnesses, many of which are life threatening. It is well known that, left undetected and untreated, psychiatric comorbidity increases hospital lengths of stay (and concomitant costs), even when demographics, medical diagnosis, and reasons for admission are taken into account.

Many studies have shown that patient outcome is markedly affected as a consequence of under-recognized or misdiagnosed psychiatric illness in nonpsychiatric settings. In primary care, where most patients with psychiatric illness present, the vast majority of patients do not receive treatment for psychiatric illness. Many factors collude in the limitation of care: psychiatric symptoms are difficult to distinguish from medical symptoms; patients fear stigma and minimize complaints; and time constraints, inadequate training, or the primary physicians' reluctance to stigmatize the patient may impede them from treating psychiatric symptoms.

Studies clearly demonstrate that psychiatric consultation in the hospital lowers morbidity, mortality, length of stay, and cost through the earlier recognition and treatment of psychiatric disorders, and it has an impact on quality-of-life measures of self-care. These findings mandate psychiatric education of colleagues, case-finding through psychiatric screening, and expansion of services by the consultation–liaison psychiatrist.

B. Evidence from Research in Psychosomatic Medicine

Psychosomatic medicine was first popularized when psychoanalytic theories of mind-body relationships suggested that psychotherapy could modify the course of medical disease. Although speculative, such theories posited that early life experiences (fostering unconscious conflicts) coupled with genetic (biological) vulnerability could cause disease states such as peptic ulcer or asthma. Although many of these ideas were erroneous, there are significant data in both animal and human research to demonstrate an effect of early life experiences on physiology and illness behavior.

Modern psychosomatic research has abandoned many of these early theories but continues to investigate the role of psychosocial variables in causing or maintaining disease states. It uses a variety of empirically based strategies; as an example, structured psychiatric interviews and reliable psychometric inventories are paired with biologic probes and immunologic measures to answer complex questions about the interrelationship between psychosocial and biologic variables.

An example of this research is the study of the biopsychosocial relationship between depression and cardiovascular disease. Landmark research in psychosomatic medicine beginning in the 1980s has revealed that individuals with major depressive disorders have significantly increased mortality risk following uncomplicated myocardial infarction (MI). The depressive episode often predates the acute coronary syndrome and is not a mere "reaction" to the cardiac event. Hostility and anger have been implicated in acute coronary syndromes. Biological factors that play a role in the genesis of coronary artery disease in depressed individuals include reduced heart rate variability, platelet dysfunction, and elevated cytokines. A shared genetic vulnerability for depressive disorders and cardiovascular disease underpins these truly psychosomatic relationships. Whether psychiatric treatment of the depressed patient following a cardiovascular event can prolong life continues to be a focus of research. The advent of sophisticated genetics and molecular biology holds the promise that such relationships will be further elucidated.

▶ **Chapter Overview**

This chapter considers the techniques, settings, and core concepts of *Consultation–Liaison Psychiatry* and *Psychosomatic Medicine*. At present, the general practice of the consultation–liaison psychiatrist includes the recognition and management of the following: (1) the impact of psychiatric disorders on medical illness, (2) comorbid psychiatric and medical disorders, (3) the etiologic role of medical illness in psychiatric disorders, (4) suicidal, homicidal, and violent behavior in medical-surgical settings, (5) legal and ethical principles in the psychiatric care of the medically ill, (6) pharmacological and therapeutic intervention in comorbid illnesses, (7) behavioral responses to medical illness, and (8) the physician–patient relationship.

The chapter condenses *Consultation–Liaison Psychiatry* and *Psychosomatic Medicine* into two sections: Clinical Consultations and Core Concepts in Psychosomatic Medicine. The first section on *Clinical Consultations* presents the standard skills and techniques used by practitioners in a general hospital, organized as follows: consultation–liaison psychiatry basics, diagnostic evaluation skills, screening techniques to identify psychiatric patients in general populations, consultation treatment, legal issues, emergency assessments, and finally, liaison psychiatry. The second section on *Core Concepts in Psychosomatic Medicine* presents the general conditions that the consultant is likely to encounter. These Core Concepts of diagnosis are based upon the framework proposed by Lipowski in 1967:

1. Psychiatric Disorders Caused by Medical Conditions
2. Psychiatric Disorders Affecting Medical Conditions
3. Psychological Reactions to Medical Illness
4. Somatic Presentations of Psychiatric Disorders

For detailed discussions of specific psychiatric diagnoses and treatments, the reader will be directed to relevant chapters in the book. A concluding section suggests future directions for clinical practice and research in the field of psychosomatic medicine.

CLINICAL CONSULTATIONS

▶ **Consultation–Liaison Psychiatry Basics**

The psychiatric consultant should serve as an ally to patient care provided by the physician (or primary team), the associated health care disciplines, and the system of care. In this alliance, *adaptability* and *diplomacy* enhance the care provided by the psychiatric consultant.

Adaptability is necessitated by the challenge of working in a general hospital. The modern hospital is a busy and crowded environment that usually limits privacy and is often unfamiliar to both patients and mental health professionals. Many hospital floors do not have interview rooms. Medical treatment rooms are often not conducive to psychiatric interviewing. Evaluations may have to be performed in hospital rooms occupied by other patients. Thus, the consultant must be both practical and flexible. Speaking in a soft voice to allow confidentiality is sometimes the only option. Patients may be critically ill and attached to devices such as intravenous lines, catheters, and respirators. If a patient cannot speak because of a tracheotomy or attachment to a ventilator, a signing board or pad and pen may be necessary. The interview may be interrupted by medical or nursing staff, or by transport personnel for ad hoc procedures. Patients may be obtunded or unable to give a comprehensive history; use of other sources of information is often necessary but raises concern about the right to privacy. Such issues challenge the consultant but also establish the psychiatrist as a physician with unique skills necessary in modern health care teams.

Diplomacy in consultation is rarely discussed but inherently useful in practice. It is based on the following qualities: awareness of the hierarchical and multidisciplinary nature of health care systems; respect for the roles and tasks a provider within a system assumes or is required to perform; regard for the boundaries or limitations of care, whether internal or external to the provider or system, affecting the patient's experience (e.g., economics determining hospital length of stay); and a collaborative or altruistic spirit that bolsters the care by the primary team through education and altered practice patterns. Examples of these qualities are the implementation of psychiatric care for organ transplantation patients and development of psychiatric screening in primary care settings. Consultation psychiatrists are ambassadors for the profession of psychiatry in large health care settings where communication between specialists can be limited.

▶ **Diagnostic Evaluation in the General Hospital**

Consultations requests may have many origins and serve varied needs for the patient, team, and system of care. Requests can be made by patients, primary providers, multidisciplinary teams, and family members. Requests can arise when a physician ponders the clinical status of the patient in regard to mood or affect (e.g., depressed after surgery), cognition (e.g., ability to make medical decisions), or behavior (e.g., agitated or threatening). Requests may seek assistance anywhere along the continuum of diagnosis, evaluation, treatment, and management. They may focus on a particular aspect of care, such as suicide risk assessment, or be more general in scope, such as the evaluation of a patient's reaction to medical illness.

Contacting the referring provider is important to understand the broader nature of the consultation request. The personal history of a psychiatric *disorder* may prompt a request for evaluation, although the consultant often is the first psychiatrist to evaluate the patient, even when the patient has a prior history of psychiatric *symptoms*. Some requests are urgent (e.g., "wants to leave against medical advice"), in which case contacting the referring clinician can provide important information to expedite the consultation. Often, a simple request such as asking for help in treating depression is really "the tip of the iceberg" heralding broader psychosocial difficulties within the patient and social system. Contacting the referring provider is the best way to elicit the "real story" behind the consultation request.

Collection of behavioral data from primary sources (nurses, medical students) is the next step. Prior to seeing the patient, consultants discuss the patient's status with nursing personnel who know the patient and are able to share observations regarding the patient's clinical status and interaction with family members. Nurses' notes are a trove of information about patient behavior (e.g., "lost returning from the bathroom") that can guide the review. Medical students also can offer keen observations of patient behavior.

Review of medical records can be approached in the manner of detective work. A discerning review of *medical notes* provides clues to the patient's behavior, cognitive status, and physical function. Admission summaries and off-service summaries are concise records from which to obtain a time line for the hospital course. Pertinent laboratory results and medication records reveal underlying medical conditions or areas that need further investigation. If the consultant is not clear about a medical illness, a review of the condition from available medical texts is done.

The review of medical records should search for *medication that acts on the central nervous system* (CNS), whether intended or as a side effect, and look for possible drug interactions (e.g., through cytochrome isoenzyme substrates and inducers). Substance-induced psychiatric disorders are common, not only for substances of abuse but also for prescribed medications (e.g., steroid-induced psychosis). In addition, a sedating (e.g., benzodiazepine) or activating (e.g., beta-agonist inhaler) medication administered prior to the evaluation can affect the assessment.

Review of pertinent *laboratory investigations* is informative. Metabolic derangements and end-organ disease can affect cognitive status. Awareness of the physiological status can focus the consultation examination and aid in the differential diagnosis. Radiological studies can hone the assessment.

Consent to interview the patient is obtained ideally by the primary team, prior to the consultant's interview, and this can be verified with the patient. The consultant should obtain permission from the patient to conduct the interview and to communicate findings with the treatment team. The consultant should adopt a neutral stance in order to increase patient participation. This way, the consultant is obtaining consent neither as a member of the medical team nor as a patient advocate. Patients with a prior psychiatric history may anticipate that individual psychiatric treatment is confidential; thus, they should be alerted to the consultant's role, particularly the need to confer with the primary team on the patient's behalf.

Diagnostic interviews aim to gather sufficient information to develop an answer to the consultation request. Following the preliminary actions described, the consultant introduces himself or herself as a psychiatric physician. First, ascertain whether the patient has been told that a psychiatric consultation has been requested. If the patient has not been informed, elicit his or her feelings about it and request permission to conduct the interview. Second, it is important that the patient be given privacy to speak openly to the psychiatrist. For this reason, it is better if a visitor or family member is excused from the interview. Even when assurances are offered by the patient to allow their involvement, privacy can be presented as a matter of policy for the initial interview. Patients are often in a vulnerable position and unable to ask openly for privacy; the psychiatrist should assume responsibility.

The approach to the interview must be guided by immediate safety concerns in emergent evaluations; this may require restricting the interview to a focus on acute intervention and behavioral management, as is discussed in more detail later in "Emergency Consultations" (also see Chapter 58). Often, a consultation is requested to assess the patient's level of anxiety or depression. The underlying task may be to assess how the patient is *adjusting to an illness*. A range of inquiries can provide an understanding of the patient's capacity to cope:

When and how was the disease diagnosed?

Were there delays in coming to treatment? Was there patient denial? Were there limitations to access?

How has the patient reacted to the treatment, medical or surgical, and to the primary team?

Have any medications been particularly difficult to take? Have any helped?

What knowledge does the patient have of others with similar disorders?

What has been the psychosocial and financial burden of the disease?

Has the illness forced changes in family roles and responsibilities? Is there a confidante?

Is there a support system? Is there neighborhood/religious/cultural/community support?

Does the patient have an accurate understanding of the prognosis? How does it affect the reaction to the illness?

Are there end-of-life issues that the patient is unable fully to address? Do supports know about the situation?

Some consultations focus on *cognitive capacity* and whether an individual has dementia or delirium. This mandates careful attention to the nursing notes and understanding the effects of the underlying disease process or medication on the CNS. A careful assessment of mental status is required for all patients, allowing for detection of psychopathological phenomena, affective symptoms, and cognitive integrity. Many patients fluctuate in their ability to attend; serial examinations can provide a more accurate assessment. Some patients are fearful that they will be judged "crazy" if they are experiencing hallucinations (e.g., due to medications such as opioids). Active inquiry about whether the patient has been confused or uncertain about their situation allows them to reveal their cognitive problems. Formal testing for cognitive status via the Folstein Mini-Mental State Examination (MMSE) provides a baseline cognitive assessment for the initial evaluation; the score is easily recognized by other specialists and can be followed serially.

General *review of symptoms* from the domains of mood, anxiety, psychosis, and substance use should be elicited. Even when they are not the focus of the consultation request, they may inform differential diagnosis and treatment plans. A detailed discussion of the principles of interviewing is provided elsewhere (see Chapter 4). Frequently, in medically ill patients, symptoms of prior concern to the patient are not reported to the primary team for a variety of reasons, whether omitted by the patient or missed by the team. The psychiatric consultant offers the patient a new opportunity to be heard and can also serve as a medical translator. If possible, the patient should give verbal consent during the interview to contact other sources of information.

Collateral information is important in situations in which the patient is unable to communicate accurately (e.g., altered consciousness, unreliable historian, cognitive impairments). The sources include spouse, family members, friends, case managers, or outpatient providers. The consultant must protect the patient's privacy; ideally patients can give consent to speak with others, but this is not always possible if the patient is impaired. In emergency situations, collateral information obtained from other sources can be vital, even if the consultant cannot provide information in return. Communication with family members can be essential. Reports from family members may differ from that of the patient and highlight problems. It is common to see elderly patients who believe that they can return to independent living arrangements while family members report numerous reasons to the contrary. Some patients deny substance abuse while family members contradict them. It is also useful to ascertain the patient's past adherence to treatment.

Consultation reports should summarize the data collected in a clear and legible manner; electronic charting is ideal for cogent communication. If consultations are dictated, put a brief note in the medical record immediately following the consultation with diagnostic or treatment suggestions that can be considered immediately. If time permits, a concise yet thorough summary of findings, expressed in an organized, standard format, is indicated (Figure 59–1). Differential diagnoses, diagnostic workup, symptomatic treatment, and, in most cases, cognitive capacity are documented. When the consultant seeks to narrow the differential diagnosis, it should be communicated to the treatment team that further investigations such as neuroimaging or specialized laboratory investigations are required (Figure 59–2).

Recommendations include further testing and medication advice. When psychopharmacologic recommendations are included, it is essential to outline side effects that may occur because the referring provider or treatment team may not be aware of them. The medically ill patient is particularly sensitive to drug side effects and may tolerate only a reduced dose. Oversedation may lead to aspiration while eating, and drug–drug interactions can cause toxic side effects. The consultant should warn about possible problems in the consultation report and in person with the consulting provider. Working with nurses and allied health professionals to ascertain the behavioral effects of medications is within the scope of consultation practice. Recommendations to assist with psychiatric disposition and capacity to live independently may rely on collaboration with social work services and liaison with outpatient mental health providers. Recommendations regarding cognitive status may include referral to or liaison with social workers or legal counsel, in accordance with hospital policies and local statutes. Consultation psychiatrists should be informed about the policies and laws that protect patient rights in every setting (see Chapter 60).

Discussions about end-of-life issues commonly arise in the medical setting, often when discussing the patient's coping strategies. Hospitalization itself can evoke fear in a seriously ill patient who is unprepared for death. Others may seek relief from suffering and express a passive wish to die interpreted by staff as suicidality, prompting a psychiatric consultation request. Family histories may reveal an early demise from a condition similar to that of the patient, causing the patient to be concerned about the current situation. This psychological connection may not be readily identified by the patient but expressed behaviorally, for example, by a refusal of procedures reminiscent of the deceased's medical course. A review of the patient's expectations for the future should be included in the initial diagnostic interview, although rapport should be developed sufficiently for the patient to explore his or her own mortality; premature introduction of a discussion of death may be unnecessarily alarming and better deferred to a follow-up session.

Follow-up of the patient is provided in collaboration with the treatment team and the frequency of contact determined by the patient's clinical status. For example, a patient experiencing delirium while the team conducts a search for the underlying causes may require daily mental status examinations by the psychiatric consultant to monitor progress. Alternatively, a patient unable to make decisions regarding a procedure may require little or no follow-up once a surrogate decision maker has been identified. Follow-up after the

	Demographic Data
	Reason for Consult
	History of Present Illness
	--- mood/anxiety/psychosis/cognition/substance (review of symptoms)
	--- acute stressors
	--- threats to safety
B	Past Medical History/Medications (drug interactions, side effects)
I	Family History (illnesses that recur in generations)
O	Substance Use History
P	Past Psychiatric History
S	--- challenges to medical adherence
Y	--- prior admissions
C	--- suicidal or violent acts
H	--- psychiatric disorders affecting (or caused by) medical illness
O	--- treatment history
S	Social History
O	--- childhood development, including early losses
C	--- level of education (validity of mental status examination)
I	--- military experience (exposure to trauma)
A	--- marital/family supports (community/religious/cultural)
L	--- socioeconomic stressors (finances/housing/access to care)
E	Physical Examination (targeted according to presentation)
X	Vital Signs (drug toxicity/withdrawal)
A	Laboratory Investigations (see Figure 59-2)
M	Mental Status Examination
I	
N	
A	
T	
I	
O	
N	
	Impression
	--- differential diagnosis
	--- diagnostic work-up
	--- symptomatic treatment
	--- safety and decision-making capacity assessments
	Recommendations

▲ **Figure 59–1** Standard format for consultation note.

initial consultation may allow the consulting psychiatrist to determine whether there should be changes in the initial recommendations. Each contact should be documented.

Screening Techniques to Identify Psychiatric Patients

In comprehensive medical and surgical care, often in outpatient settings, screening for comorbid psychiatric disorders can be time-efficient and cost-effective. Screening tests help nonpsychiatrists to uncover a symptom profile that heralds the need for evaluation by a psychiatrist. Screening tests are not a substitute for a psychiatric interview, but serve as a technique for *early detection.*

Endorsement of psychiatric symptoms may be elicited by self-administered patient questionnaires or by clinician-administered, structured interviews. Although myriad questionnaires are available, the self-administered questionnaire that is well standardized to detect depression, anxiety, and alcohol use in the primary care setting is the PRIME-MD Patient Health Questionnaire (PHQ). The PHQ-9 screens for depression and is available through its initial publication. The PHQ-2 is an abbreviated, standardized subset of the PHQ-9 that screens for depression in a general population, with high sensitivity (0.83) and specificity (0.92). The PHQ-2 is often added to a battery of health care questions completed in the outpatient waiting room. The Folstein MMSE, a structured, clinician-administered screen for dementia, is available through its initial publication. The MMSE is used in screening for cognitive disorders such as delirium but is standardized only for dementia. The Mini-Cog is an abbreviated, standardized test that uses

CBC/differential
Electrolytes
BUN/creatinine
Glucose
Calcium, Magnesium, Phosphate
Urinalysis/urine toxicology
Liver function tests
Thyroid function tests
Cyanocobalamin/Folate
Electrocardiogram
Chest X-ray
Oxygen saturation
RPR/VDRL
HIV
Lyme Titer
Electroencephalogram
Head CT/MRI

▲ **Figure 59–2** Common diagnostic laboratories/investigations.

the three-object recall item of the MMSE combined with the Clock Drawing Test; it has comparable sensitivity and specificity to the MMSE but taps additional regions in the brain. The CAGE questionnaire, a simple screen for detecting alcohol use, is utilized by psychiatric and nonpsychiatric clinicians and can prompt referral to substance treatment programs.

If the patient requires further evaluation after a positive screening questionnaire, referral to the psychiatric consultant is the next step. Patients reluctant to seek care in a psychiatric clinic may agree to evaluation by the consulting psychiatrist who, as a member of the primary care team, avoids the stigma of psychiatric referral. Consultation psychiatrists assist primary physicians who manage general psychiatric disorders directly and reserve referrals to psychiatric care for patients who are acutely ill or require a complicated medication regimen. There are good reasons for these strategies. Even though medical conditions, especially chronic conditions, increase the likelihood of a psychiatric condition, a minority of patients with a psychiatric disorder will be evaluated by mental health specialists. Moreover, half of all visits to physicians by patients with diagnosable psychiatric disorders occur in primary care clinics, and primary care physicians write most of the prescriptions for antidepressants and anxiolytics.

Psychiatric care provided in the medical setting in situ searches for untreated psychiatric patients. Psychiatric care within the setting of primary care closely resembles diagnostic evaluations in the general hospital in that it involves direct collaboration with the primary provider in the treatment of comorbid medical and psychiatric conditions. However, in response to early detection, whether through screening or by the astute primary provider, psychiatric consultation in primary care settings serves a greater number of psychiatric patients than in general psychiatric settings. The active consultation model has been developed to make hospital consultation more efficient by early detection. This model allows a psychiatric staff member (often a psychiatric nurse clinician or consultation psychiatrist) to embed with the medical unit's daily meeting that reviews new admissions. If an admission appears to be appropriate for a psychiatric consultation, the staff would be informed of that recommendation.

▶ Treatments in Consultation Psychiatry

A. Psychopharmacological Treatments

Special considerations are necessary in the treatment of medically ill patients with psychopharmacologic agents. The pharmacokinetic and pharmacodynamic properties of medications and the underlying clinical status of the patient are germane to the consultant's practice. A search for the cause of psychiatric symptoms is essential, but it also raises concern for the complex variables that affect the medicated, medically ill patient.

Pharmacokinetic changes in *absorption, distribution, metabolism,* and *excretion* often modify choice of agent and dosing regimens. *Absorption* of agents in patients who cannot take oral agents may be possible only via intramuscular, intravenous, or rectal routes. Novel routes of administration such as buccal wafer and topical patch offer options for the treatment of patients who cannot swallow. *Distribution* of drugs is altered in patients who are hypovolemic. Antacids, commonly prescribed for hospitalized patients, may slow the distribution and limit the onset of action of oral benzodiazepines. In patients who are chronically ill, there is often reduced protein binding available, which can create toxic levels of free agent. *Metabolism* by the liver transforms many psychotropic agents; thus, the presence of liver disease mandates reduced dosing. Drug–drug interactions can raise or lower drug level via inhibition or induction of metabolism by cytochrome P450 isoenzymes. Many psychiatric medications have narrow therapeutic indices in which the agent (substrate) has a narrow path for metabolism via a specific isoenzyme; altered function of the isoenzyme, through either its inhibition (immediate) or its induction (delayed), can markedly affect the blood level of the agent. Medical literature and online resources such as micromedex.com can provide this information.

Excretion via the kidneys is limited in acute and chronic renal failure; patients receiving medication dependent on renal function, such as lithium or bupropion, may require lower dosing. For patients on renal dialysis, lithium must be dosed very carefully. Only a single dose may be required following dialysis because it will not be excreted until the next dialysis.

Pharmacodynamic issues involve the alteration of a drug's intended pharmacologic effect by another drug or mechanism at the site of action. The serotonin syndrome exemplifies this phenomenon. Drugs such as meperidine or dextromethorphan interact with selective serotonin reuptake inhibitors (SSRIs) to provoke a potentially fatal syndrome characterized by confusion, ataxia, hyperreflexia, clonus, nausea, and hypertension. The putative effects of SSRIs in prolonging bleeding may have clinical consequences. The association of gastrointestinal bleeding in the elderly who are taking serotonin reuptake inhibitors should alert the clinician to minimize such agents in medical settings. Cumulative and excess anticholinergic effects from drugs can cause confusion and decrease bowel and bladder motility in vulnerable patients. Excess sedation in elderly patients can be due to the additive effects of sedatives such as benzodiazepines and hypnotics given together. Independent of sedation, benzodiazepines can increase the risk of falls in the elderly. The use of medication in the medically ill requires careful attention to all the medications a patient is currently taking, the contribution of underlying medical conditions, possible drug interactions, and possible dosage adjustments. Other variables include *nonadherence* to prescribed medication and *polypharmacy* in patients treated by several providers. Efforts to simplify medication regimens start with a polite inquiry into the indications for the prescribed agents, especially those suspected of CNS activity. Patients may be overwhelmed by the complexity of pill taking, which may prompt recommendations that the regimen be streamlined while the patient is hospitalized and thus directly observed. Some hospital units provide "self-medication" programs, allowing the patient to retain some autonomy in self-care. This can serve as an opportunity to further monitor illness behavior.

B. Psychotherapy in the Medically Ill

Psychotherapy for the hospitalized patient is usually brief and supportive. The type of intervention will depend upon the patient's cognitive status, disease state, and treatments. If a patient has had delirium, often there are gaps in memory that can foster fears of embarrassment and distortion of what happened. The psychiatric consultant should inquire about such issues and fill in the periods of time the patient does not recall, replacing misperceptions with accurate information. The patient who has had frightening hallucinations due to opiates or steroids requires reassurance that these were drug effects.

Even when cognitively intact, patients may be depressed and express feelings of helplessness and hopelessness. Patients who have witnessed the unsuccessful resuscitation of a roommate can benefit from gentle inquiry into the emotional sequelae of such an event. *Supportive psychotherapy* includes not only eliciting fears and emotions but also initiating helpful measures. For example, when patients are distressed by the conditions of hospitalization, they may respond to dietary supplementation from home if allowed or from room change when a noisy roommate disturbs sleep. Simple measures such as making a wall calendar available or locating eyeglasses can aid adaptation.

Common themes in *brief psychotherapy* are found in the exploration of the patient's ideas about the etiology of the illness, as well as the toll it has taken, and the exposure they have had to others with similar illnesses. Many patients fear discussing these issues with their primary physician. Distortions of causal factors, prognosis, and treatment effects should be corrected. This can alleviate anxiety if the patient is overly pessimistic. A contrasting situation occurs when the patient minimizes serious disease or the need for intervention. The diagnosis of denial requires that the patient be told the nature of both disease and treatment. Denial wards off the terror of diagnosis and must be managed slowly and carefully. If denial wards off the implications of disease such that refusal of care is at stake, it is essential to use available family supports to understand the factors that promote denial and decide how to intervene.

Long-term psychotherapy is usually conducted in ambulatory or rehabilitation settings. Limited data confirm that this treatment has efficacy for somatic syndromes such as irritable bowel disorder or chronic fatigue syndrome. Cognitive–behavioral therapy has been reported as effective for fibromyalgia. Graded exercise can help patients with chronic fatigue syndrome or fibromyalgia, whereas psychoeducation is important for patients undergoing treatment for a variety of disorders. Evidence is growing that psychotherapy and psychopharmacological treatment are synergistic in the treatment of depressive disorders, better than either treatment alone. In the context of genetic testing for some diseases such as breast cancer or Huntington disease, the patient needs full knowledge of the risks and benefits of such knowledge. This may generate a role for psychotherapeutic consultation.

C. Electroconvulsive Therapy

Electroconvulsive therapy (ECT) is a first-line treatment in medically ill patients with suicidal depression, psychotic depression, or depression during pregnancy, and in medical conditions that cause inanition or risk for cardiovascular collapse. Although generally reserved for refractory disorders and special circumstances, it is the most effective treatment for depressive disorders. The consulting psychiatrist may be in a position to initiate education of patient, family, *and* the patient's provider regarding the indications, potential side effects (retrograde amnesia and elevated blood pressure), and treatment outcomes of ECT. Many patients with a remote history of "shock treatment" require education about recent advances in ECT in order to inform them about the procedure.

▶ Legal Issues in Consultation Psychiatry

The legal issues that arise in consultation psychiatry are most commonly those of confidentiality, competency (decision-making capacity), and whether a patient has a right to die despite attempts to treat. Documentation of the patient's wishes in advance of the need to know often obviates many legal issues. Requests to leave against medical advice are a subset of competency assessments.

Confidentiality is mandated comprehensively by the Health Insurance Portability and Accountability Act. The consultation psychiatrist has a relative exemption from strict confidentiality when sharing information with the health providers who are treating the patient. The consultation note, as well, is exempt from the Health Insurance Portability and Accountability Act confidentiality. When obtaining corollary information from family members, the clinician should attempt to get verbal consent if the patient retains decision-making capacity. In some situations, information the patient divulges should remain confidential. Intimate details of a personal nature with no bearing on the issues that led to the consultation request are confidential and should not be revealed to other medical professionals or in the treatment record. Psychotherapy notes are considered private under the Health Insurance Portability and Accountability Act regulations and separate from the medical record. This does not mean that data from consultation follow-up visits that document diagnosis or response to treatment cannot be noted in the progress notes.

Competency is a broad concept that applies to a variety of acts and behavior. It is a legal issue, bestowed at birth. If the patient is impaired, a physician must provide evidence of erosion of competency to the legal system (in probate or "family" courts). Informed consent to a particular procedure or health care intervention, however, focuses upon the individual's ability to make a decision based on the capacity to understand the information, which *must be provided in a clear and understandable manner;* to recognize the options available (including the risks and benefits of each option); to use reason with regard to the information provided by the team; and finally, to make a rational decision that is sustained over time. Decisional incapacity, which is determined ultimately by a probate judge or other legal representative, does not automatically indicate incompetence in other activities of living.

Discharges *Against Medical Advice* (AMA) evoke legal fears and risk management concerns. In order to oppose the patient's free will to leave, the consulting psychiatrist must diagnose a condition that impairs judgment, such as delirium, dementia, or depression, of such severity that the patient's safety or the safety of others is threatened, either by direct threats to self or others, or by grave disability (inability to obtain food, shelter, or clothing). Issues of competency assessment described previously may apply. The challenge is to discriminate *subtly impaired* decisions (due to mental conditions, with or without physical conditions) from *bad* decisions (e.g., marginal capacity to provide for self, homelessness, refusing treatment). A rapid assessment of level of risk is required. Often efforts to address the pressing need for discharge reveal the origins of the AMA discharge request. Some patients require social worker assistance with responsibilities such as childcare, housing, or work mandates that are valid but impracticable in the face of serious illness. Finally, patients

who abuse substances sometimes request abrupt discharge. If no withdrawal state is observed, the consultant can enlist the help of family members to convince the patient to remain in the hospital; however, this is often impossible. In the circumstance where the patient demonstrates capacity to make a decision, albeit inconsistent with what is recommended, the patient retains the right to leave. Clinical status and attempts to contact support systems should be documented.

Right-to-die decisions require that the patient be judged competent and fully understand the nature of the disease state. Impairments in cognition or thought process (e.g., dementia or paranoia) may necessitate transferal of the decision to surrogates. Another complicated issue is of depression that causes a subtle erosion of decisional capacity. The seriously ill patient is often clinically depressed. If depression is aggressively treated, the wish to die may change. Family meetings in concert with the treatment team, and consultation with hospital ethics committees and legal counsel, maximize the opportunity for a fair appraisal of the request to withhold treatment.

Advance directives should be reviewed in the patient who has become cognitively compromised. Optimally, a surrogate decision maker has been identified for a future period of incapacity, and the consulting psychiatrist renders a second opinion to the team declaring that the time has come to utilize or *invoke* it. Advance preparation pays off for these patients, as they avoid the legal proceedings of competency. Social workers can assist with documentation of advance directives; these should be recommended for every patient found to retain the capacity to make such decisions.

▶ Emergency Consultations

A few situations need immediate attention, requiring a rapid assessment of a range of factors, including a scan of the physical situation (e.g., the patient might use medical equipment as a weapon) and the environment (e.g., multiple patient room or intensive care setting). Policies should be in place regarding clearing the room of sharp objects and having restraints available on medical and surgical floors. However, it may not be routine for staff in the usual medical setting to follow such policies, increasing the need for psychiatric consultant assistance.

Violent patients may be suffering from delirium or substance withdrawal. Such information can be obtained from a review of the medical record, focusing upon the disease status (e.g., presence of a mass lesion in the CNS) or prescribed medication fostering an encephalopathy. In such situations it is imperative that staff and other patients be protected. The concurrent presence of security guards allows safe assessment. The emergency use of psychotropic medication can diffuse these dramatic situations. Involving a family member can be helpful, but there may not be sufficient time to allow this.

Suicidal patients become emergencies if there is an attempt at self-harm or if drugs, knives, or weapons are detected that the patient is secretly storing to use for self-harm. Is the behavior a means of attention seeking, is it due to a mood or psychotic disorder, or is it an attempt to assume control when the situation has become so ominous that ending life is preferable to enduring a fantasized medical scenario? Following initial assessment, it is necessary to observe closely the patient who is acutely suicidal but too medically ill to be transferred to a psychiatric unit. Nursing personnel are trained in the monitoring of suicidal patients, but the psychiatric consultant may be sought for management advice. The care of high-risk individuals in such settings is eased by family supports, if available.

Liaison Psychiatry

The liaison psychiatrist is a regular member of a treatment team in transplant programs, cancer centers, or dialysis units. A subspecialized focus of liaison psychiatrists on diseases states (e.g., HIV psychiatry) or medical specialty (e.g., gynecology or pediatrics) has developed in recent years.

Transplantation psychiatry is important because of the psychological stress on patients and families who undergo lifesaving procedures or wait on a list for a limited number of available organs. The organ to be transplanted dictates the common psychiatric issues within each procedure. For related-donor kidney transplants, the psychiatric consultant may evaluate both overt and covert family pressures that the putative donor experiences and how the potential recipient feels in response. Treatment adherence is important, especially in patients with diabetes who have not followed diabetic regimens. The essential issue in liver-transplantation recipients who have been substance abusers is their history of abstinence. If potential recipients are still using alcohol or other substances of abuse, they need rehabilitation and abstinence before receiving a liver transplant, although candidacy is individualized and may vary according to the scarcity of the organ to be transplanted. Liaison psychiatrists may be called upon to assist with screening to identify latent psychiatric disorders and to assist with the psychological stressors as discussed. For heart transplantation patients, ongoing support is necessary during the waiting period before an available organ is found. Such patients commonly experience anxiety and depression and wrestle with mortality.

In *oncology* settings, central issues are depression in the terminally ill, delirious states due to diseases and treatments, and family reactions. In *nephrology* centers, patients who request termination of hemodialysis must be evaluated for delirium and dementia. The treatment of underlying depression may alter the request for cessation of hemodialysis. The role of the psychiatrist in nephrology also focuses on patients who resist dietary and fluid limitations, often in the context of depression and dementia. The psychiatrist will have many opportunities to teach health professionals to recognize and manage psychiatric disorders in chronic illness and end-of-life care.

CORE CONCEPTS IN PSYCHOSOMATIC MEDICINE

Psychiatric Disorders Caused by Medical Conditions

Psychiatric symptoms can occur as a direct consequence of an underlying medical condition. Many examples are catalogued in the *Diagnostic and Statistical Manual of Mental Disorders, Fifth Edition, Text Revision (DSM-5-TR)*. "Mental Disorder Due to Another Medical Condition" is diagnosed when there is evidence that the medical condition caused the psychiatric manifestation of the illness. The categories of psychiatric illness classified in the *DSM-5-TR* as caused by or "due to another medical condition" are as follows: Delirium, Major or Mild Neurocognitive Disorder, Catatonia, Personality Change, Psychotic Disorder, Bipolar and Related Disorders, Depressive Disorder, Anxiety Disorder, Obsessive Compulsive Disorder, and Narcolepsy. Each of these diagnoses is associated with the behavioral phenomena of a *psychiatric disorder;* however, when there is evidence of a causative *medical condition,* the *DSM-5-TR* does not regard these "due to" diagnoses as full-fledged *primary* psychiatric disorders. For example, Major Depression Disorder should not be diagnosed when there is a known medical etiology, but rather Depressive Disorder due to Another Medical Condition. Furthermore, the neurovegetative symptoms of Major Depressive Disorder (see Chapter 17) could also represent a medical symptom (e.g., decreased energy due to depression *or* anemia, *or* both). The confound of medical and psychiatric symptoms identical in their physical expression leaves consultation–liaison psychiatrists in a bit of a quandary. A recent example is the mounting evidence of neurological and psychiatric sequelae of coronavirus infection detected during the global pandemic that began in 2019. These conditions are manifesting acutely and over prolonged recovery periods and require further elucidation.

Most studies have led to the general consensus that all "potentially psychiatric" symptoms of the medical condition should be included in the diagnosis of the psychiatric disorder. In the case of depressive symptoms, for example, this strategy risks the psychiatric diagnosis of patients who do not meet full criteria of Major Depression (false positive) but avoids the failure to diagnose patients who do meet criteria (false negative).

Psychiatric symptoms caused by medical conditions have important implications, not only for diagnosis but also for evaluation, treatment, and management of both medical and psychiatric conditions. Detection and diagnosis of the medical cause often relies on the astuteness of the primary medical clinician; however, the patient with psychiatric symptoms might not present to medical care, but rather to a psychiatric setting, causing a possible delay in medical diagnosis. The patient with medically induced psychiatric symptoms who presents to medical settings may be dismissed as not medically ill. Treatment of the presenting psychiatric symptoms, without detection of the underlying medical condition, may actually exacerbate the medical condition. Clinical wisdom suggests that any nonresponder to psychiatric treatment de facto merits a review of the medical evaluation obtained at baseline and a repeat or expanded evaluation to search for undetected medical causes. Consultation–liaison psychiatrists identify those patients who elude diagnosis in primary care because of the prominence of the psychiatric presentation. They educate medical and psychiatric colleagues about the medical masquerade and may be a stalwart force toward completing the medical evaluation of a patient with psychiatric symptoms. The following section highlights this principle by clinical examples.

A. The Patient with Cerebrovascular Disease and Depression

Stroke, a rapidly occurring disturbance of brain function attributed to vascular disease, is the third leading cause of death in America after heart disease and cancer. The neuropsychiatric complications of stroke include cognitive deficit, and behavioral and emotional dysregulation. Depression following stroke is a frequent and adverse neuropsychiatric sequela of stroke, yet it is undiagnosed by most nonpsychiatric physicians. Depression has a negative impact on the patient's quality of life, not only from a psychosocial standpoint, but also by impeding the recovery of motor function. Depression in the aftermath of stroke (Post-stroke Depression and Post-stroke Pathological Affect) respond to aggressive treatment but escape detection when interpreted as an "understandable" response to the stroke. Post-stroke Pathological Affect is characterized by emotional dysregulation in which laughter or tears are expressed but are unrelated to mood and are exacerbated by minor cues. Post-stroke Pathological Affect can be severely disabling, causing patients to become isolative or agoraphobic. Post-stroke Depression and Post-stroke Pathological Affect are both responsive to antidepressant treatment.

B. The Patient with Postoperative Delirium

Delirium is an acute cognitive disorder with global impairment in brain function, and fluctuating consciousness and attention. Associated features include hyperactivity, hypoactivity, and reversal of the sleep–wake cycle. Delirium is a common presentation in hospitalized elderly patients, affecting up to 30% of elderly surgical patients. The most common predisposing surgical procedures are emergency hip fracture repair, gastrointestinal surgery, coronary artery bypass grafts, and lung transplants.

C. The Patient with Psychosis and Substance Use

Psychotic disorders due to medical illness or to substance use can originate from many conditions, such as brain diseases

---

PATIENT VIGNETTE 1

A 59-year-old divorced White man, right-handed graphic designer, with a history of hypertension, diabetes mellitus, and nicotine dependence, was brought to the hospital by his son after the sudden onset of slurred speech and inability to walk. Physical examination revealed aphasia and a dense right-sided paralysis; diagnostic investigations confirmed an ischemic stroke. Mr. S. was stabilized medically for 1 week and was then referred for physical rehabilitation. Despite aggressive efforts over the ensuing weeks by rehabilitation staff, the patient was increasingly unmotivated for physical therapy, socially isolative, and at times refused to eat. He mentioned in passing to a nursing aide that he would be "better off dead," prompting the team physician to request a psychiatric evaluation. Utilizing a communication board, Mr. S. expressed hopelessness about his career as a graphic designer and worries about his future financial situation. He also ruminated about past layoffs from work and financially compromising alimony payments. His speech was garbled and a source of immediate frustration. He was unable to write or draw designs with his paretic right hand. After a complete medical workup for additional underlying causes, the patient was started on a low dose of an SSRI. He had an early response to treatment, which was followed by improved participation in physical therapy.

(e.g., seizures, neoplasm, encephalitis, stroke), endocrine disorders (hyper- or hypothyroidism, Cushing syndrome), metabolic disorders (hypoglycemia, hyponatremia, uremia, thiamine deficiency/Korsakoff), and chemicals, including drugs of abuse, medications, or toxins. The most common substances that induce psychosis by intoxication are cocaine, amphetamines, and phencyclidine. The most common substances causing psychosis by withdrawal are sedative-hypnotics and alcohol. Psychosis due to general medical conditions or substance-related psychosis can be distinguished from a primary psychotic disorder by fluctuating level of consciousness, focal neurological signs, predominantly visual sensory involvement (e.g., visual hallucinations, illusions), perseverations in thought content, and abnormal vital signs (elevated blood pressure, heart rate).

▶ Psychiatric Disorders Affecting Medical Conditions

Psychiatric disorders may affect compliance with necessary medical treatment or even acceptance of the disease itself. Depression, hopelessness, and anhedonia can abet nonadherence to medication, dietary regulation, or ongoing surveillance for the recurrence of disease. Eating disorders are common in diabetic patients and can seriously compromise metabolic regulation. Even defensive mechanisms such as denial, not a psychiatric disorder in itself, can affect a

PATIENT VIGNETTE 2

A 45-year-old married man, construction worker, with a prior history of gastritis, pancreatitis, and anemia, was admitted for lumbar discectomy. Although he denied alcohol consumption during the preoperative visit, by the 4th postoperative day he displayed marked signs of alcohol withdrawal, delirium tremens, associated with autonomic instability and frank visual hallucinations. When he began to act in response to the hallucinations by seeking to climb out of bed and talk to an empty chair, psychiatric consultation was requested. Search for reversible causes of the mental status change was completed and did not alter the diagnosis of delirium tremens. Treatment with intravenous thiamine, multivitamins, and high doses of an intermediate-acting benzodiazepine led to amelioration of autonomic instability, but the psychotic symptoms persisted until an antipsychotic agent was added. After a protracted hospital course, the patient was referred for substance rehabilitation treatment and outpatient psychiatric care.

PATIENT VIGNETTE 3

A 24-year-old single man was evaluated for noncompliant behavior resulting in recurrent decubitus ulcers. Two years prior to the consultation, he had been involved in a motorcycle accident causing spinal cord injury and paraplegia. Confined to a wheelchair, the patient inconsistently attended rehabilitation. He spent many hours driving around in a van that had been equipped with hand controls. He did not use weight shifting or other approaches to minimize decubitus formation and consequently was hospitalized repeatedly. Upon evaluation, the patient was sullen and hostile and initially had nothing to say. Upon further questioning, he was clearly depressed and noted, "Who wouldn't be?" The patient complained that he had recurrent sleep problems. He ruminated about his accident. He began to talk about his loneliness and depression. Background evaluation revealed that the patient had a premorbid personality style involving impulsivity and activity. Social history revealed that he was raised in a single-parent family wherein his mother worked many hours to support his older sister and himself. He had dropped out of high school to work. Although his peers often used drugs he did not, but he did enjoy driving recklessly on a motorcycle he had purchased. Following his accident, his friends abandoned him.

After the evaluation, the psychiatric consultant held a few family meetings in which the evidence for depression was clear, as well as additional features of demoralization. The patient felt helpless and hopeless from his accident and saw no way to overcome his injury or life circumstances. Based on these meetings, the physical therapist introduced him to another patient who had successfully coped with a spinal cord injury. Although the intervention was initially hospital-based, it was many months before he was able to accept his injury better, pursue proper care, and complete his high school education in order to pursue a career in design.

medical condition because of poor compliance. Psychiatric medications with metabolic side effects can induce or interfere with the management of chronic medical conditions and warrant close monitoring in collaboration with primary providers.

A. Nonadherence to Treatment

Nonadherence is particularly common in certain medical illnesses. Psychiatric disorders such as depression or delirium can obstruct proper care. Whether hypertensive medication or more complicated treatments are involved, it is essential to understand the complexity of the regimen and the issues that prevent compliance, financial or psychological. A sense of hopelessness and lack of motivation can be fostered by premorbid characteristics, but also by depressive disorder. Multidisciplinary strategies to encourage compliance include collaboration with case managers, social work service, and primary clinicians who have long-standing relationships with patients. In patients with cognitive deficits, strategies to assist with medication compliance include dose-based pill boxes, simplification of dosing patterns, a switch to long-acting agents or an altered route of administration (e.g., topical patch), and parsimonious prescription patterns that reduce side effects. Written directions at the time of the visit, visiting nurse assistance, case management, and the enlisting of family support enhance adherence. Ensuring that underlying psychiatric conditions are adequately treated is important as well; inadequate dosing and inadequate duration are commonly associated with refractory depression in primary care settings, but nonadherence is equally important. In addition, psychotropic agents that interfere with other medications can cause the patient to choose among them.

B. Chronic Psychiatric Disorder Affecting Medical Condition

Patients with schizophrenia or bipolar disorder have increased rates of mortality. The shortened life span is due to the psychiatric disorder itself, as well as to treatment with medications such as antipsychotic agents, which can induce a metabolic syndrome leading to cardiovascular disease and diabetes. It is essential for the psychiatric consultant to work collaboratively with community mental health programs to develop treatment plans that promote health. If antipsychotic agents are used, clinicians should monitor the individual's weight and girth on a regular basis to avoid the development of serious metabolic consequences. Psychiatric patients are further at risk for obesity if they are isolated, avoid exercise, and follow sedentary lifestyles. The risks to general health from psychiatric disorders are compounded by the high rates of substance dependence such as cigarette smoking, which contributes to

A 47-year-old married woman, mother of two adult daughters, found a breast mass during routine self-examination. She quickly sought medical evaluation, which revealed she had a breast neoplasm. She was successfully treated with lumpectomy and chemotherapy. Lymph node dissection was negative. Despite these results, she dwelt on the possibility that her neoplasm might return. She experienced frequent crying spells, loss of concentration, sleep difficulties, and fatigue. She had no family history of either mood disorders or breast cancer. Psychiatric evaluation revealed a woman who was sad and cried during the interview. She reported she was having difficulty getting out of bed in the morning and that she could barely manage her work due to problems in concentration. She was not suicidal. She revealed that she believed she developed breast cancer due to promiscuity as a young adult prior to her marriage. In collaboration with her oncologist, the psychiatrist judged that none of her complaints were aspects of her neoplastic disease. The patient was treated with an antidepressant, which improved her sleep pattern and fatigue, and psychotherapy that allowed her to ventilate her guilty ruminations about her actions. As the treatment progressed, knowledge about her health dispelled beliefs that these were causal factors. Despite early side effects of nausea, she was encouraged to continue the medication. Over 6 weeks, she improved. After 12 weeks, she reported no symptoms of depression. She said she was very lucky to have "caught my cancer so early."

cardiovascular disease. Psychiatric consultation can have a role in prevention through education in primary care settings and collaboration with cessation programs.

C. Patient with Depression and Cardiac Disease

Depression is an independent risk factor for ischemic heart disease. It predicts higher morbidity and mortality after uncomplicated MI. For 6 months after the infarction, even up to 5 years, depression has an impact on cardiac mortality, eclipsing standard cardiac variables such as left ventricular ejection fraction. The possible mechanisms for these phenomena include a threefold increase in medication nonadherence, shared risk factors (smoking, diabetes, and obesity), lower heart rate variability, chronic inflammation (increased biomarkers such as C-reactive protein), platelet activation, and sympathoadrenal activation due to increased physiological stress. Studies to determine the role of psychiatric treatments aimed at lowering cardiac risk have indicated an improved quality of life but no clear reversal of increased mortality.

▶ Psychological Reactions to Medical Illness

Medical illness creates a crisis. The patient is faced with multiple emotional, physical, and financial challenges that can create serious psychological distress. The personal aspects of illness include pain, disability, and loss of function and autonomy due to the disease and/or its treatment. Loss of exercise tolerance in congestive heart failure, or pain and dietary limitations in short bowel syndrome, exemplify such challenges. The interpersonal aspects of illness create changes in roles and status such as the ability to be a fully active parent or employee and to be independent and supportive of others. Patients with HIV/AIDS face stigmatization. The patient with terminal cancer may be isolated when supports do not know how to interact with a dying individual. Finally, there is an intrapsychic challenge to disease due to fears of death, disfigurement, and pain.

People react differently to the challenges before them in accordance with their coping style, environmental circumstances, and the nature of the disease and its treatment. It is tempting to label a patient's reaction to a life-threatening illness as *understandable*. This rarely explains fully the diagnosis of depression or anxiety, and the patient's reaction does not always correlate with the level of functional disability or problems in activities of daily living. It is essential to evaluate the level of family support and the patient's ideas about the disease, knowledge about others with similar health problems, and the availability of community or national support groups.

A. The Hostile Patient

Premorbid personality style often shapes the reaction to a serious illness or hospitalization. The passive patient may tolerate a paternalistic approach, whereas the patient with obsessional and intellectual defenses will ask questions and seek more information. Patients with hysterical traits may be emotional and require compliments about the courage they display. Patients with borderline traits can split the medical team by idealization and devaluation of its hierarchical members; trainees may be particularly vulnerable to this behavior. Narcissistic patients have the sense that they are particularly important or deserving of preferential treatment. These broad-brushed descriptions are not pathological entities, but they describe coping mechanisms that emerge in stressful situations. Medical illness exaggerates such traits. The physician should not view these behaviors as challenges to professional competence or authority, but as demonstrations of fearfulness and regression during the crisis of illness.

B. The Demoralized Patient

Demoralization does not qualify for a primary psychiatric diagnosis. It is common in medical and surgical settings in the context of a reaction to acute or chronic stress, such as the onset of illness, its treatment (if particularly disabling or disfiguring), or illness that is terminal. The management of demoralization involves promotion of the primary physician's role in soothing the patient's fears about the illness through relevant information about treatment options. Treatment

PATIENT VIGNETTE 5

A 47-year-old married man, practicing attorney, sought emergency evaluation for chest pain. He reported tightness in his chest, which he interpreted as cardiac in origin. After a normal electrocardiogram and laboratory studies, he was reassured. The following day he began to worry that the tests could have been in error, causing increased anxiety. He openly admitted he was a "worrier" but felt that the tightness in his chest was a harbinger of a MI. Repeated medical evaluations found his physical status to be normal. He had no lipid abnormalities, and his blood pressure was normal. He requested that his physician refer him for cardiac catheterization to ensure that his coronary arteries were patent. He was referred for a psychiatric evaluation by his internist, after multiple negative medical evaluations for a variety of symptoms that the patient thought indicated cardiac disease. The patient reported that he exercised regularly and kept a careful diet but was preoccupied by the thought he would have a "heart attack." He had no family history of cardiac disease, but two of his legal associates had undergone bypass surgery in the previous 3 years. His wife reported that he tended to exaggerate minor viral illnesses or athletic injuries. His developmental history indicated that his mother always worried about his health. She prevented him from participating in normal sports activities when he was in school. Despite this, he became an outstanding tennis player. On full psychiatric evaluation, he was anxious and somewhat depressed. He recognized that his fears were not fully realistic but could not get the ideation of cardiac disease out of his head. Treatment involved pharmacological intervention for generalized anxiety with an SSRI and psychotherapy using cognitive–behavioral strategies. Over a period of 6 months, he limited calls to his internists to scheduled times and began to feel better. He still worried about cardiac disease when he heard about others with cardiac illness but was able to invoke cognitive strategies that he learned in therapy to reduce his anxiety and prevent maladaptive behavior such as emergency phone calls.

also involves reassurance by the consulting psychiatrist that the patient does not have a psychiatric disorder, but that low mood or anxiety symptoms are part of a natural response to stress and would be manifested by many patients in similar circumstances.

C. Distress in the Cancer Patient

Cancer is among the most feared diseases an individual can experience. Some level of anxiety or depression often occurs during the initial discovery of cancer but generally abates over time. Nevertheless, a significant number of patients experience sufficient anxiety or depression to merit treatment. These dysphoric states may not meet formal criteria for a psychiatric disorder but promote sufficient emotional pain that the concept of distress in the cancer patient has been developed. Distress in oncology patients is defined as "an unpleasant emotional experience that interferes with [the] ability to cope with a diagnosis of cancer or its treatments." This may include more than just noxious feeling states but behavioral and functional disruptions in work, social interactions, and adherence to treatments. Patients with previous psychiatric disorders, uncontrolled pain, and disfiguring lesions or surgery may be especially vulnerable to either distress or diagnosable psychiatric disorders. It is essential for the physician to inquire about what the patient is experiencing during the initial diagnosis and subsequent treatments. Therapy should be directed toward each of the identified problems. As in demoralization, use of both supportive psychotherapies and medications for depression and anxiety as well as effective pain control is essential to reduce suffering and pain, both emotional and physical.

▶ Somatic Presentations of Psychiatric Disorders

The common presentation of somatic concerns in primary care can be related to psychiatric disorder, most commonly anxiety or depression. Patients with major depression are more likely to present for care in primary care settings, and once there to complain of somatic illness. Chest pain is found in generalized anxiety and panic disorders. Fatigue, headache, and backache are common in major depressive disorders. These psychiatric illnesses are commonly underrecognized in busy outpatient settings. When the psychiatric disorder is identified and effectively treated, the somatic symptoms are alleviated.

Conversely, physical symptoms that are unexplained, not due to other psychiatric disorders such as depression and anxiety, and not intentionally produced may be due to a somatoform disorder. Somatoform disorders are grouped together because they require the exclusion of medical and substance-induced causes and are likely to present first to primary care or medical settings. Somatoform disorders include somatic symptom disorder, illness anxiety disorder, conversion disorder, psychological factors affecting other medical disorder, and factitious disorder (see Chapter 31). Psychiatrists consulting to these settings may be asked to assist in the diagnosis and management of these patients, who often exasperate caregivers. Strategies include maintaining the patient in primary care settings with one provider, when possible, and encouraging regular appointments that are scheduled at the end of each visit, not on an as-needed basis. In somatization disorder, the consultant may encourage the primary provider to "join in the patient's pessimism" by focusing on symptom management rather than cure.

The Patient with Illness Anxiety Disorder

When a patient has persistent fears about symptoms of an illness or beliefs about having an illness, and when no medical illness can be found, "worry" about illness becomes the disease itself: hypochondriasis. In this disorder, not only is worry about illness disabling, it becomes the focus of daily life. The course of illness tends to be chronic, but it has a better prognosis if the onset is acute and brief in duration, with no secondary gain.

FUTURE DIRECTIONS

Consultation psychiatry is the bridge between psychiatry and the rest of medicine. As medicine advances, there will be new psychological and emotional challenges for patients requiring the skills and techniques of consultation psychiatrists. Organ transplant technology will evolve into artificial organ transplant; the fear of recurrent pandemics such as that generated by SARS-CoV outbreaks in 2003 and 2019 will have an emotional toll for chronic neuropsychiatric sequelae and for the burdens placed on health care systems and providers. These are just a few examples that illustrate that there will be an increasing need for psychiatry at the interface with medicine. Consultation psychiatry is already dividing into subspecialized areas to accommodate the expansion of medicine. Consultation–liaison psychiatrists are focusing on HIV/AIDS, oncology, and nephrology as primary interests. Journals and books devoted to these topics complement the general consultation journals. Concurrently, the stresses of hospital life will continue, strained by the forces of economics, evolving demands, and health care policies.

The shift from hospital-based care to outpatient settings has expanded consultation services into outpatient clinics and specialized care facilities. The "stepped model" for care of depression in a medical population has been demonstrated to enhance both quality of life and effective treatments for a variety of disorders. By screening populations and using targeted case management, the psychiatric consultant can identify patients in need of increasing levels of treatment, at first from the primary care physician and advancing to the psychiatrist for those who continue to have significant psychiatric symptoms. As new psychiatric treatments emerge, the consult psychiatrist will provide them to patients underserved in nonpsychiatric settings.

Recognized over the past two decades as a discrete subspecialty, yet centuries old in practice, psychosomatic medicine has a new role in the ancient art of medicine. Graduate education programs with dedicated fellowship training in psychosomatic medicine will advance the mission to improve patient care. With increasing technologies and advances in biomedical knowledge, this subspecialty will provide the biopsychosocial elements of comprehensive patient care and clinical research to improve clinical outcome and enhance quality of life.

American Psychiatric Association. *Diagnostic and Statistical Manual of Mental Disorders*. 5th ed. *TR*. Washington, DC: American Psychiatric Publishing; 2022.

Boland R, Verduin, ML, Ruiz P. Somatic Symptom and Related Disorders In: *Kaplan and Sadock's Synopsis of Psychiatry*. 12th ed. Philadelphia: Lippincott Williams and Wilkins. 2022; 12:451-468.

Borson S, Scanlon J, Brush M, et al. The Mini-Cog as a screen for dementia: Validation in a population-based sample. *J Am Geriatr Soc*. 2003;51:1451-1454.

Chemerinski EC, Robinson RG. The neuropsychiatry of stroke. *Psychosomatics*. 2000;41:5-14.

Cozza KL, Scott CA, Jessica RO. *Concise Guide to Drug Interaction Principles for Medical Practice: Cytochrome P450s, UGTs and P-glycoproteins*. Arlington, VA: American Psychiatric Publishing. 2003;345-369.

Doyle F, Freedland KE, Carney RM, et al. Hybrid systematic review and network meta-analysis of randomized controlled trial of interventions for depressive symptoms in patients with coronary artery disease. *Psychosom Med*. 2021;83(5):423-431.

Evans D, Charney DS, Lewis L, et al. Mood disorders in the medically ill: Scientific review and recommendations. *Biol Psychiatry*. 2005;58:175-189.

Ewing JA. Detecting alcoholism: The CAGE questionnaire. *JAMA*. 1984;252:1905-1907.

Fava GA, Belaise C, Sonino N. Psychosomatic Medicine is a comprehensive field, not a synonym for consultation liaison psychiatry. *Curr Psychiatry Rep*. 2010 Jun;12(3):215-221.

Folstein, MF, Folstein SE, McHugh R. "Mini-mental state": a practical method for grading the cognitive status of patients for the clinician. *J Psychiatr Res*. 1975;12:189-198.

Frasure-Smith N, Lesperance F, Tlijic M. Depression following myocardial infarction: impact on 6 mo survival. *JAMA*. 1993; 270:1819-1825.

Groves JE. Taking care of the hateful patient. *N Engl J Med*. 1978; 298:883-887.

Holland JC, Bultz BD. National comprehensive cancer network (NCCN). The NCCN guideline for distress management: A case for making distress the sixth vital sign. *J Natl Compr Canc Netw*. 2007;5(1):3-7.

Katon W, Russo J, Lin EH, et al. Cost-effectiveness of a multicondition collaborative care intervention: a randomized controlled trial. *Arch Gen Psychiatry*. 2012;69(5):506-514.

Kroenke K, Spitzer RL, Williams JB. PHQ-15. *Psychosom Med*. 2002;64:258-266.

Levenson JL. Introduction. In: Levenson JL, ed. *Textbook of Psychosomatic Medicine*. Arlington, VA: American Psychiatric Publishing. 2005;19-21.

Lin EH, Von Korff M, Ciechanowski P, et al. Treatment adjustment and medication adherence for complex patients with diabetes, heart disease, and depression: A randomized controlled trial. *Ann Fam Med*. 2012;10(1):6-14.

Lipowski ZJ. Review of consultation–liaison psychiatry and psychosomatic medicine, II: Clinical aspects. *Psychosom Med*. 1967;29:201-224.

Lipowski ZJ. What does the word "psychosomatic" really mean? *Psychosom Med*. 1984;46(2):153-171.

Lipowski ZJ, Wise TN. History of consultation–liaison psychiatry. In: Wise MG, Rundell JR, eds. *Textbook of Consultation–Liaison Psychiatry: Psychiatry in the Medically Ill*. 2nd ed. Washington, DC: American Psychiatric Publishing. 2002;3-11.

Masand PS, Christopher EJ, Clary GL, et al. Mania, catatonia and psychosis. In: Levenson JL, ed. *Textbook of Psychosomatic Medicine*. Arlington, VA: American Psychiatric Publishing. 2005;242-250.

Powers PS, Santana CA. Surgery. In: Levenson JL, ed. *Textbook of Psychosomatic Medicine*. Arlington, VA: American Psychiatric Publishing. 2005;647-656.

Practice Guideline for the Psychiatric Evaluation of Adults, Third Edition. American Psychiatric Publishing. 2016.

Sharpe M, Toynbee M, Walker J. Proactive integrated consultation-liaison psychiatry: a new service model for the psychiatric care of general hospital patients. *Gen Hosp Psychiatry*. 2020;66(6): 9-15.

Slavney PR. Diagnosing demoralization in consultation psychiatry. *Psychosomatics*. 1999;40:325-329.

Smith FA, Querques J, Levenson JL, Stern TA. Psychiatric assessment and consultation. In: Levenson JL, ed. *Textbook of Psychosomatic Medicine*. Arlington, VA: American Psychiatric Publishing. 2005;3-4.

Spitzer RL, Kroenke K, Williams JB. Validation and utility of a self-report version of PRIME-MD: The PHQ primary care study. *JAMA*. 1999;282:1737-1744.

Stark D, Kiely M, Smith A, et al. Anxiety disorders in cancer patients: Their nature, associations, and relation to quality of life. *J Clin Oncol*. 2002;20(14):3137-3148.

Stern TA, Fricchione GL, Cassem NH, et al. *Handbook of General Hospital Psychiatry*. 5th ed. Philadelphia: Mosby. 2004.

Taquet M, Geddes JR, Husain, M. 6-Month neurological and psychiatric outcomes in 236,379 survivors of COVID-19: a retrospective cohort study using electronic health records. *Lancet Psychiatry*. 2021 May;8(5):416-427.

Wanji LCN, et al. Liver transplantation in alcohol-related liver disease and alcohol-related hepatitis. *J Clin Exp Hepatol*. 2023; 13(1):127-138.

Wise MG, Rundell JR. *Clinical Manual of Psychosomatic Medicine: A Guide to Consultation–Liaison Psychiatry*. Arlington, VA: American Psychiatric Publishing. 2005;1-7:68-69.

Forensic Psychiatry

Stephen Montgomery, MD
William Bernet, MD

PSYCHIATRY & THE LAW

Forensic psychiatry is the medical subspecialty, recognized by the American Psychiatric Association since 1991, in which psychiatric expertise is applied to legal issues. The American Board of Psychiatry and Neurology began in 1994 to examine individuals for "added qualifications in forensic psychiatry." There are about 50 1-year fellowship programs in forensic psychiatry accredited by the Accreditation Council for Graduate Medical Education, United States; eight fellowship programs are accredited by the Royal College of Physicians and Surgeons of Canada. A relevant professional organization is the American Academy of Psychiatry and the Law. Several major textbooks of forensic psychology and psychiatry are listed at the end of this section.

There are four divisions of forensic psychiatry. The first pertains to the legal aspects of general psychiatric practice, such as the civil commitment of involuntary patients, the doctrine of informed consent, the requirement to protect third parties from dangerous patients, and matters of privilege and confidentiality.

The second division of forensic psychiatry covers the assessment of mental disability. This includes the evaluation of individuals who have been injured on the job, the assessment of a plaintiff who claims that he or she was injured and is now seeking compensation from a defendant, and the assessment of the competency of individuals to perform specific acts such as making a will.

The third and most well-known aspect of forensic psychiatry deals with individuals who have been arrested. This division includes the evaluation of competency to stand trial, the evaluation of a person's competency to waive their *Miranda* rights, the assessment of criminal responsibility, evaluations that relate to sentencing, and the treatment of incarcerated individuals.

The fourth division of forensic psychiatry is forensic child psychiatry, which includes child custody evaluations, the evaluation of children who may have been abused, and consultation regarding minors who are involved with juvenile court.

Gold LH, Frierson, RL eds. *The American Psychiatric Textbook of Forensic Psychiatry.* 3rd ed. Washington, DC: American Psychiatric Publishing; 2018.

Gutheil TG, Appelbaum PS. *Clinical Handbook of Psychiatry and the Law.* 5th ed. Philadelphia: Lippincott Williams & Wilkins; 2019.

Lorandos D. *Litigator's Handbook on Forensic Medicine, Psychiatry and Psychology.* Egan, MN: West Group; 2023

Melton GB, Petrila J, Poythress NG, et al. *Psychological Evaluations for the Courts: A Handbook for Mental Health Professionals and Lawyers.* 4th ed. New York: Guilford Press; 2017.

Rosner R, Scott C eds. *Principles and Practice of Forensic Psychiatry.* 3rd ed. Boca Raton: CRC Press; 2017.

LEGAL ASPECTS OF PSYCHIATRIC PRACTICE

▶ Professional Liability

Psychiatrists are less likely than other physicians to be sued for professional negligence. However, most psychiatrists will be the subject of at least one professional liability claim during the course of their careers.

In a case of professional liability or malpractice, a patient (the plaintiff) sues the psychiatrist (the defendant). In order to prevail legally, the plaintiff must prove each of four elements: (1) the psychiatrist had a duty of care to the patient, (2) there was a breach of the duty to the patient, (3) the patient was injured, and (4) the negligent care was the proximate cause of the patient's injury. That is, if it were not for the negligent act, the injury would not have occurred. At a trial, the plaintiff will attempt to prove each of the four elements by a preponderance of the evidence. Both the plaintiff and the defendant may ask expert witnesses to testify.

Psychiatrists are at risk of being sued in many clinical situations. For example, a psychiatrist may be held responsible when a patient dies by suicide if: (1) the psychiatrist failed to perform a proper risk assessment, (2) the psychiatrist failed to take a proper history from the patient or other individuals, and/or (3) the psychiatrist failed to take appropriate precautions. A psychiatrist may be liable for negligent psychopharmacology if a patient sustains injury as a result of: (1) failure to obtain an adequate history, (2) use of a drug that is not efficacious or not indicated, (3) use of the wrong dosage of medication, or (4) failure to recognize or treat side effects. A particular concern is the occurrence of serious side effects of psychotropic medication, such as tardive dyskinesia (a movement disorder) and the metabolic syndrome (an increased risk for cardiovascular disease and diabetes), especially if the patient and family members were not warned of the risk and if the psychiatrist did not monitor the patient properly for side effects. A lawsuit may arise out of the use of electroconvulsive therapy if its use was inappropriate or if informed consent was not obtained. A lawsuit may arise out of the use of psychoanalysis if the patient did not give informed consent for this treatment—for example, if the patient was not advised of alternative treatments to consider.

Psychiatrists have been sued for engaging in sexual conduct with a patient or with the spouse of a patient. Because it has been clearly stated by professional organizations that sexual activity with patients is a breach of the psychiatric standard of care, the major issue in these cases is to prove that the sexual activity occurred. In some cases, patients have made false allegations of sexual conduct against psychiatrists. Even if the sexual activity never occurred, the psychiatrist may have mishandled the case through boundary violations that created the foundation for the false allegations (i.e., through negligent management of the transference) (American Psychiatric Association, 2013, 2024).

Informed Consent

Informed consent refers to the continuing process through which a patient understands and agrees to the evaluation and treatment proposed by the physician or mental health professional. Although informed consent is a concept that all psychiatrists claim to endorse, many practitioners do not understand what the concept means or give only lip service to its implementation (Grisso & Appelbaum, 1998).

There are three components to informed consent: mental competency, adequate information, and voluntariness. The assessment of competency is discussed later in this chapter.

Regarding the disclosure of adequate information, this generally means the patient should know the nature and purpose of the proposed treatment, the potential benefits and risks, and the alternative treatments that may be considered. The states have set different criteria for the amount of information that a physician should disclose. Some states have adopted the rule that a physician should disclose the amount of information that a **reasonable physician** would disclose in a similar situation. Most states have adopted a more progressive rule, that a physician should disclose the information that a **reasonable patient** would want to know about the proposed treatment. Regarding the requirement for giving consent voluntarily, this means the patient should not be coerced or offered inducements by the physician, other members of the treatment team, or family members.

Informed consent is more than just a signature on a form. As treatment progresses, there should be a continuing dialogue regarding the nature of the treatment and its possible side effects. In some circumstances, such as starting a psychotic patient on antipsychotic medication, the patient will be able to discuss these topics coherently only after treatment has begun. In some cases, informed consent should involve a discussion with close family members as well as the patient. When a chronically suicidal patient is being discharged from the hospital, for instance, it is useful for the immediate family to understand both the pros and cons of the discharge and for all parties (i.e., patient, family, and psychiatrist) to share and accept the inherent risks.

Civil Commitment

In some circumstances, psychiatric patients are hospitalized involuntarily. The legal bases for involuntary or civil commitment are the principle of *parens patriae* (i.e., the government may act as "father of the country" to protect individuals who are unable to take care of themselves) and the police power of the state (i.e., the government has the authority to protect society from dangerous individuals). Psychiatrists participate in this process by evaluating patients as to whether they meet criteria for civil commitment. Although the specific procedures vary from state to state, the criteria for involuntary commitment generally include all the following: (1) the patient has a serious psychiatric disorder, such as a psychosis or bipolar disorder, (2) there is significant risk that the patient will harm himself or others, and (3) hospitalization is the least restrictive alternative. In some jurisdictions, civil commitment is hard to justify (requiring an overt act rather than mere risk of danger) or less difficult to justify (allowing civil commitment if the patient is not likely to take care of basic personal needs).

The Rights of Patients

On many occasions, hospitalized psychiatric patients and institutionalized intellectually disabled persons have been railroaded, warehoused, and abused. As a result, state and federal courts and legislators have declared that patients have specific rights. For example, the right to treatment means that civilly committed mental patients have a right to individualized treatment. Likewise, patients also have the right to refuse treatment. That is, a patient who is civilly committed may still be competent to decide whether to agree to use psychotropic medication. If the psychiatrist proposes to use medication even though the patient refuses, the psychiatrist should follow the appropriate local procedures. Such procedures may include referring the question to a treatment review committee or asking the court to appoint a guardian for the patient.

In some jurisdictions, psychiatric patients have the following rights: to receive visitors; to send uncensored mail; to receive uncensored mail from attorneys and physicians, although other mail may be examined before being delivered; to confidentiality; to have medical records available to authorized individuals; and to a written statement outlining these rights. An important patient right is that seclusion and mechanical restraint will not be used unless required for the patient's medical or treatment needs. Seclusion and restraint may not be used for punishment or for the convenience of staff.

▶ Confidentiality

Psychiatric patients have a right to be assured that information they have related in therapy will not be revealed to other individuals. The American Medical Association (AMA) has promulgated ethical principles for many years, and these principles include the importance of confidentiality. The American Psychiatric Association has published both general principles and detailed guidelines regarding patient confidentiality. In some states, the medical licensing act or a separate statute defines the physician's obligation to maintain patient confidentiality.

In 1996, the United States Congress passed the Health Insurance Portability and Accountability Act (HIPAA) and, in 2000, the U.S. Department of Health and Human Services implemented "Standards for Privacy of Individually Identifiable Health Information" (the "Privacy Rule"), which created national standards to protect individuals' medical records and other personal health information (U.S. Department of Health and Human Services, 2000, periodically amended). The federal government took an important medical principle (Hippocrates said, "Whatsoever things I see or hear concerning the life of men, which ought not to be noised abroad, I will keep silence thereon, counting such things to be sacred secrets") and created a very detailed set of rules. Many providers responded by becoming unnecessarily legalistic and restrictive in the way they handle protected health care information.

The issue of confidentiality in clinical practice is complex. In some situations, confidentiality should be given great importance, but in other situations, it is therapeutically important to share information with other clinicians or people involved in the patient's daily life. For example, the treatment of chronically ill patients may require continuing collaboration with the individual's family members and close friends. The sharing of clinical information is almost always done with the patient's knowledge and consent. In treating a minor, the importance of confidentiality will depend on the patient's age and developmental level, their psychopathology,

their relationship with the parents, and the specific topic in question. For example, most therapists would maintain confidentiality regarding an adolescent's sexual activities and occasional drug usage that might be considered part of youthful experimentation. However, therapists would want parents to become aware of a teenager's sexual promiscuity, pregnancy, serious delinquent behavior, and serious substance abuse. The expectation of confidentiality is not absolute.

Table 60–1 lists some of the many exceptions to confidentiality in clinical and forensic practice, which are mentioned in the Privacy Rule that followed from the HIPAA. Clinicians have a strong impulse to discuss case material with colleagues, and these conversations sometimes occur in elevators, cafeterias, and other public places where they can be overheard by strangers. The urge to discuss cases occurs because clinical material is both extremely interesting (so the therapist wants to tell about it in order to show off in some way) and extremely anxiety provoking (so the therapist wants to find reassurance by sharing the case with a colleague). If a psychiatrist is concerned or puzzled about a clinical issue, he or she should confer in a formal setting with a consultant or a supervisor.

The clinician should be aware that any written record may later be read by the patient or by many other people. The wise psychiatrist will protect themselves from future chagrin by always keeping this in mind when they dictate an evaluation or write a progress note. Prospective patients should know the limits of confidentiality. One way that therapists can ensure patient understanding of such limits is to provide them with an office brochure that explains that the therapist values privacy very highly but that particular exceptions to confidentiality exist.

The right to confidentiality continues after a patient's death, but it must be balanced against the family's right to certain information. After a patient dies by suicide, for

---

Table 60–1 Exceptions to Confidentiality

The patient himself or herself.

Emergency circumstances to prevent a serious and imminent threat to the health or safety of a person or the public.

After a general consent is given, an individual's treatment providers can exchange health information for the purpose of carrying out treatment or health care operations.

Family members and close personal friends to the extent the information is directly relevant to that person's involvement with the individual's care.

Trainees can discuss their patients' psychotherapy with supervisors.

Information from an individual's psychotherapy can be disclosed to defend oneself in a legal action brought by the individual.

Reporting disease and injury to authorized public health authority.

Reporting victims of abuse, neglect, or domestic violence as required by law.

Reporting adverse events to the Food and Drug Administration.

instance, it may be appropriate for the patient's therapist to meet with family members and close friends and for all of them (i.e., including the therapist) to try to make sense of what happened. That meeting might involve the therapist's sharing certain kinds of information with the family (e.g., the diagnosis of bipolar disorder, the affection the deceased expressed toward a spouse), but it need not involve extensive or detailed revelations.

▶ Privilege

Confidentiality and privilege are related concepts because they both assert the privacy of information that one person has shared with another. "Confidentiality" is a broad concept that prohibits professionals from revealing information about a client to anyone. "Privilege"—a narrower concept—describes specific types of information that may not be disclosed in a legal setting. Privileged information is almost always confidential; not all confidential information is privileged.

A person has the right of testimonial privilege when they have the right to refuse to testify or to prevent another person from testifying about specific information. For instance, a woman may claim privilege and refuse to testify about conversations she had with her attorney because such discussions are considered private under the concept of attorney–client privilege. Likewise, a man may claim that his therapy is covered by physician–patient privilege and prevent the psychiatrist from testifying about him. On the other hand, the man may waive the right to physician–patient privilege and allow his psychiatrist to testify. It is up to the patient, not the psychiatrist, to make that decision. The psychiatrist should ordinarily go ahead and testify if the patient has waived his right to privilege.

▶ Protection of Third Parties

Occasionally, a patient may reveal that they have thoughts of harming a particular person. The psychiatrist should assess the seriousness of these thoughts. In addition, the psychiatrist should devise a treatment plan to protect the other person (i.e., the third party). Ideally, the psychiatrist and patient should cooperate in devising a safety plan. For example, a psychiatrist was treating a patient who had chronic schizophrenia and who expressed thoughts of hurting his parents. In response, the psychiatrist and the patient agreed to a joint telephone call to the parents to inform them of the danger, the patient's medication was adjusted, and the patient signed a written statement that he would not visit the parents until the crisis had been resolved.

If the psychiatrist and patient cannot agree on a safety plan or if it is clinically inappropriate to attempt such an agreement, the psychiatrist must take steps unilaterally to protect the third party. For example, an acutely paranoid man has told his psychiatrist that he intends to take revenge against his former boss. The psychiatrist protects both the patient and the boss by arranging for the patient's involuntary commitment to an inpatient facility.

Warning a potential victim is usually done with the patient's knowledge, if not with their permission. But this is not always possible. For example, an extremely angry and jealous man, who has been threatening his wife, has eloped from a supposedly secure inpatient program. It is no longer possible to discuss the issue therapeutically. The psychiatrist immediately notifies the wife and also the police.

State legislatures have adopted a variety of laws and local courts have held a variety of opinions, so psychiatrists should become familiar with the local standards. There could be contradictory practices as a professional moves from one state to another. Some states have laws that protect mental health professionals from liability if they disclose in good faith confidential information to the patient's intended victim.

In recent years there has been a growing concern that psychiatric patients may have an increased tendency toward violence with firearms and explosives. Some state legislatures have enacted additional laws that require mental health professionals to report potentially dangerous patients to law enforcement agencies; these are sometimes called "red flag laws."

American Psychiatric Association. *Opinions of the Ethics Committee on the Principles of Medical Ethics with Annotations Especially Applicable to Psychiatry*. Washington, DC: American Psychiatric Association; 2024.

American Psychiatric Association. *The Principles of Medical Ethics with Annotations Especially Applicable to Psychiatry*. Arlington, VA: American Psychiatric Association; 2013.

Grisso T, Appelbaum PS. *Assessing Competence to Consent to Treatment: A Guide for Physicians and Other Health Professionals*. New York: Oxford University Press; 1998.

Simon RI. *Preventing Patient Suicide: Clinical Assessment and Management*. Arlington, VA: American Psychiatric Press; 2011.

U.S. Department of Health and Human Services. *Standards for Privacy of Individually Identifiable Health Information*. 2000; 2013. https://www.hhs.gov/sites/default/files/hipaa-simplification-201303.pdf

ASSESSMENT OF MENTAL DISABILITY

There are several circumstances in which psychiatrists evaluate individuals to determine degree of disability, if any. These circumstances include claims under Workers' Compensation programs, personal injury lawsuits, and evaluations to determine mental competence to perform specific acts.

▶ Disability & Workers' Compensation

The Social Security Administration provides financial benefits for individuals who are not able to work at any occupation for at least 12 months because of a serious physical condition or psychiatric illness. Through the Department of Veterans Affairs, the federal government provides benefits to veterans who are partially or fully disabled because of a service-related condition. Individual states administer Workers' Compensation programs that provide defined and limited compensation to individuals who were injured during the course of their employment. Finally, some people have individual or group disability insurance policies and apply for benefits from an insurance company.

Individuals who are seeking disability benefits or Workers' Compensation should be evaluated in a thorough and systematic manner. The clinician should carefully read the referral information because the agency or company may be asking the evaluator to address very specific questions. In some cases, the cause or the date of onset of the illness may be very important. In other cases, the issue may be whether the person can currently engage in a particular occupation.

In addition to a thorough interview and mental status examination, a psychiatric disability evaluation may include the following: psychological testing, neuropsychological assessment, review of medical and psychiatric records, review of military and employment records, and interviews of family members and other informants. The evaluator should actively consider the possibility of malingering or exaggeration of either psychological (e.g., depression, anxiety, and fearfulness) or cognitive (e.g., problems with memory and concentration) symptoms (Rogers & Bender, 2020). The AMA has published guidelines for the assessment of physical and mental disability, which are updated annually (AMA, 2023).

▶ Personal Injury

Personal injury litigation is part of a large domain called tort law, the law of civil wrongs. A person who injures another can be arrested and tried (under criminal law) or sued (under tort law). A successful tort action requires proof of the four elements mentioned previously: (1) a duty was owed to the plaintiff by the defendant, (2) the duty was breached, (3) an injury occurred, and (4) the breach of duty directly caused the injury.

Courts allow plaintiffs to be compensated for both physical and psychological injuries. If a person was severely injured physically, it is easy to see how he or she may have sustained psychological damage as well. In some circumstances courts will allow compensation for psychological injury even when no physical injury occurred. This may happen when the plaintiff was so close to the incident (within the "zone of danger") that they could have been physically injured or when the plaintiff was not in the zone of danger but observed a close relative being injured.

Psychiatrists become involved in these cases by evaluating whether a plaintiff has been psychologically injured and whether the injury was the direct result of the negligent act by the defendant. The evaluator should interview the plaintiff carefully and collect information from other sources (e.g., prior medical and psychiatric treatment records, school

records, military records) in order to compare the person's psychological and social functioning before and after the alleged trauma. Several psychiatric conditions may follow a serious trauma: posttraumatic stress disorder, generalized anxiety disorder, phobias, panic disorder, adjustment disorder, and major depressive disorder. The evaluator should clarify whether the condition antedated the alleged trauma, whether other psychological stressors could have caused the symptoms, and whether there was a direct relationship between the alleged injury and the psychiatric disorder.

It is common for a psychiatrist to be asked to take on multiple roles with the same patient—for example, treating an individual and also describing the person's mental condition for some legal or administrative purpose. This is the problem of **dual agency** (Strasburger et al., 1997). For example, a psychiatrist may already have a treatment relationship with an individual who is injured on the job and subsequently requires an evaluation to support his claim for Workers' Compensation benefits. It is usually preferable for the psychiatrist to avoid taking on both roles, but recommend that the patient have a separate, independent medical evaluation for purposes of the claim for benefits. An independent medical evaluation is an examination by a physician who evaluates, but does not provide care for, the individual.

▶ Competence

In psychiatry, competence refers to a person's mental ability to perform or accomplish a particular task. Some writers make a distinction: "mental capacity" is assessed by a physician or a mental health professional, whereas "mental competency" is a legal finding determined by a court. Although the details of the competency evaluation will depend on the circumstances (Table 60–2) of the case, the general principles are the same. There are four functional abilities to consider in assessing competence (Grisso & Appelbaum, 1998).

Table 60–2 Circumstances in Which Competency Is an Issue

In criminal law
to waive Miranda rights
to stand trial
to testify
to be executed
In civil law
to write a will
to make a contract
to vote or hold office
to manage one's own funds
to care for a child
In medical practice
to consent to surgery or electroconvulsive therapy
to refuse surgery or electroconvulsive therapy

A. The Ability to Express a Choice

For example, an elderly woman who is making a will must be able to communicate her intentions verbally, in writing, or in some other manner. It may be important to interview the person on two or three occasions to make sure her choice remains consistent.

B. The Ability to Understand Relevant Information

For example, the elderly woman must understand that she is meeting with her attorney and they are preparing a legal document. She must know the extent of her property and who the potential heirs are.

C. The Ability to Appreciate the Significance of that Information for One's Own Situation

For example, the woman who is drafting her will must realize that her children will not receive anything if she puts her entire estate in a trust fund for her cats.

D. The Ability to Reason with Regard to That Information, Engaging in a Logical Weighing of Options

If the woman decides to leave her estate to her children—and not to the trust fund for her cats—the evaluator should assess whether her decision was made in a rational manner. A person who makes the "right decision" for the wrong reason, such as a delusion, would not be competent.

American Medical Association. *Guides to the Evaluation of Permanent Impairment.* 6th ed. Chicago: AMA Press; 2023.

Grisso T, Appelbaum PS. *Assessing Competence to Consent to Treatment: A Guide for Physicians and Other Health Professionals.* New York: Oxford University Press; 1998.

Rogers R, Bender, S. eds. *Clinical Assessment of Malingering and Deception.* 4th ed. New York: Guilford Press; 2020.

Strasburger LH, Gutheil TG, Brodsky A. On wearing two hats: role conflict in serving as both psychotherapist and expert witness. *Am J Psychiatry.* 1997;154:448.

INDIVIDUALS WHO HAVE BEEN ARRESTED

Forensic psychiatrists sometimes evaluate individuals who have been arrested and are awaiting trial. Usually, it is the defense attorney who is concerned about the defendant's mental competency to go to trial and their state of mind at the time of the alleged offense.

Competency to Stand Trial

In order to be competent to stand trial, the defendant must understand the charges that have been brought against them and the nature of the legal proceedings. For example, the defendant needs to understand the roles of the defense attorney, prosecuting attorney, judge, and jury. The defendant must be aware of the possible outcome of the legal proceedings (e.g., release to the community, imprisonment, capital punishment). Finally, the defendant must be able to cooperate with their attorney, disclose to the attorney the facts regarding the case, and testify relevantly.

If the defendant is found not competent to stand trial, the court will arrange for psychiatric treatment in the jail or at a state psychiatric facility. In some cases, a defendant becomes competent following psychotropic medication or psychoeducational intervention. A person who is permanently incompetent, such as someone with a severe intellectual disability, may never go to trial. They may simply be released or, if dangerous to self or others, civilly committed.

Competency to Waive *Miranda* Rights

Almost every U.S. citizen has heard the admonition: "You have the right to remain silent. Anything you say can and will be used against you in a court of law. You have the right to be speak to an attorney, and to have an attorney present during any questioning. If you cannot afford a lawyer, one will be provided for you at government expense." If the police have taken a person into custody, they must advise the person of their *Miranda* rights prior to interrogation. They must not continue to question a person who has asserted their right to remain silent or has requested an attorney. A person who has not been taken into custody may be questioned by police without any *Miranda* warning.

Forensic psychiatrists sometimes evaluate whether a criminal defendant was mentally competent to waive his *Miranda* rights after being arrested and prior to questioning by police. That is, whether the individual waived their *Miranda* rights in a knowing, intelligent, and voluntary manner. In general, **"knowing"** means the person is aware of what is happening and the possible consequences of making a statement to police, **"intelligent"** means the person has weighed the pros and cons in a logical manner, and **"voluntary"** means the lack of coercion. These criteria are comparable to the components of informed consent, in that "knowing" for the *Miranda* waiver is equivalent to "disclosure of adequate information" of informed consent and "intelligent" for the *Miranda* waiver approximates the ability to reason in a logical manner that is required for informed consent.

Some people are particularly vulnerable in the sense that they are overly willing to waive their *Miranda* rights. For example, individuals with intellectual disability may not understand the gravity of the situation and may be overly compliant in following the request of the police officer to answer questions. People with serious psychiatric disorders may be so mentally disorganized that they are incapable of exercising good judgment when they are arrested. Children and adolescents who have been arrested may simply assume that they should be obedient and do what the police officer wants them to do.

Criminal Responsibility

A person who has committed a crime is not held responsible for their behavior if they were legally insane at the time the crime was committed. In this sense, "insanity" is a legal term that implies a severe mental disorder or a significant degree of intellectual disability. The courts have applied several standards to define criminal insanity. The most common are the M'Naghten rule and the American Law Institute test (Perlin, 1994).

The **M'Naghten rule** provides for only a cognitive test for the insanity defense. That is, the person is held not responsible for a crime if "the party accused was labouring under such a defect of reason, from disease of the mind, as not to know the nature and quality of the act he was doing; or, if he did know it, that he did not know he was doing what was wrong."

The **American Law Institute test** provides for both a cognitive and a volitional test. That is, a defendant would not be responsible for criminal conduct "if at the time of such conduct as a result of mental disease or defect he lacks substantial capacity to appreciate the criminality of his conduct or to conform his conduct to the requirements of the law."

Insanity is determined by a person's mental functioning, not by a specific diagnosis. To be considered insane, however, the defendant must have a serious psychiatric condition such as bipolar disorder, schizophrenia, or another severe mental disorder. Some jurisdictions explicitly state in their insanity statute that "mental disease or defect" does not include any disorder that is manifested simply by antisocial conduct.

If a judge or jury finds a defendant not guilty by reason of insanity, the person does not go to prison. Nor does he or she go home. Usually the disposition is to a secure inpatient facility to determine if the person can be civilly committed to either hospital or outpatient treatment. Some states provide an alternative outcome, in that the defendant can be found guilty but mentally ill. That is, the defendant had a mental illness at the time of the alleged offense, but it was not severe enough to acquit them. The defendant found guilty but mentally ill goes to prison, where treatment is presumably available.

Diminished Capacity

Like insanity, the concept of diminished capacity also refers to the defendant's mental condition at the time of the alleged offense. In order to convict a defendant, the prosecution must prove that a criminal act occurred (referred to as the "actus reus") and that the perpetrator of the act had a particular mental state (referred to as the "mens rea"). For some crimes, it is simply required that the actor has the mental state of "knowing" what he or she is doing. For some crimes, it is required that the actor have the mental state of "intending" what they are doing, a higher level of mental activity than simply knowing. For some forms of first-degree murder, it is required that the actor has the mental state of "premeditation," a higher level of mental activity than either intending or knowing. States have various definitions for these terms.

Some states allow mental health professionals to testify regarding a person's capacity to form a particular mental state at the time of the alleged offense. For example, a forensic psychiatrist might be asked to evaluate whether a man who was very intoxicated by both alcohol and cocaine was mentally capable of premeditating a crime when he violently killed another person in a bar fight. If a judge or jury finds that the defendant was not capable of premeditation and therefore did not commit first-degree murder, the person is not usually acquitted and sent home. Usually, the person is found guilty of a lesser included offense such as second-degree murder or voluntary manslaughter. A successful insanity defense is exculpatory and the person is found not guilty of any crime; a successful diminished capacity defense usually means the person is found guilty of a crime with a shorter sentence.

Prison Psychiatry

American jails and prisons have much higher proportions of mentally ill and intellectually disabled individuals than are found in the general population. Forensic psychiatrists provide treatment to these individuals, who may have serious conditions manifested by chronic depression, violent and aggressive behavior, and overt psychosis (Scott, 2009).

AAPL Practice Guideline for Forensic Psychiatric Evaluation of Defendants Raising the Insanity Defense. *J. Am Acad Psychiatry Law.* 2014;42:4

Perlin ML. *The Jurisprudence of the Insanity Defense.* Durham, NC: Carolina Academic; 1994.

Scott CL, ed. *Handbook of Correctional Mental Health.* 2nd ed. Arlington, VA: American Psychiatric Publishing; 2009.

FORENSIC CHILD PSYCHIATRY

The interface between child and adolescent psychiatry and the law is a young discipline. The forensic child psychiatrist is likely to be consulted regarding child custody disputes, child maltreatment (such as physical, sexual, and psychological abuse), minors involved in the juvenile justice system, and personal injury (Benedek et al., 2010; Bernet et al., 2011).

Child Custody Evaluation

When parents divorce and disagree regarding the custody of the child, mental health professionals may evaluate the family and make recommendations to the court. Since the 1920s, lawmakers and courts have emphasized "the best interests of the child," which implies that the needs of the child override the rights of either parent. The American Academy of Child and Adolescent Psychiatry (1997) developed practice parameters for child custody evaluations. More recently, the Association of Family and Conciliation Courts (2022) and the American Psychological Association (2022) published guidelines for parenting plan evaluations in family law cases.

In conducting these evaluations, it is best to have access to all members of the family, including both parents. In some circumstances the psychiatrist may conduct a one-sided evaluation by interviewing only one parent and the child. In such a case the psychiatrist may make only limited observations and recommendations, such as commenting on the psychiatric condition of one parent and their relationship with the child. Usually, the psychiatrist would not be able to make any recommendations regarding custody because they had no way of evaluating the relative merits of the mother and father.

Typically, the psychiatrist has an initial conference with both parents together (if this is not too disruptive), meets with each parent individually in order to complete a psychiatric evaluation and to assess each person's parenting attitudes and skills, and meets twice with the child, so that each parent can bring the child for an appointment at least once. The psychiatrist may find it helpful to collect information from outside sources such as grandparents, babysitters, the pediatrician, and teachers. It is important to speak to previous and current psychotherapists of the child and of the parents.

Decisions regarding custody are guided by the best interests of the child, but there are no standard guidelines for the specific factors that should be taken into consideration and what weight should be given to each factor. The following factors are generally considered important: parental attitudes and parenting skills; which parent has been more involved with day-to-day childrearing; continuity of placement (it is usually presumed preferable to maintain the status quo unless there is good reason to change it); the physical health of the parents; the mental health of the parents (psychiatric diagnosis is less important than the person's parenting skills in the present and the future); each parent's willingness to encourage the child to have a good relationship with the other parent; substance abuse by the parents; the relative merits of the two households (e.g., whether the parent has remarried); allegations of physical or sexual abuse; the child's attachment to the parents; and the child's preference, if he or she articulates a definite preference for reasons that seem valid.

In a high-conflict divorce, the child may avoid visiting the noncustodial parent or refuse to have a relationship with one of the parents, which is called **contact refusal**. When that occurs, the custody evaluator should try to determine whether the contact refusal is a result of **estrangement** (i.e., the child refuses to spend time with a parent for a good reason, such as a history of child maltreatment or neglect) or **parental alienation** (i.e., the child refuses to spend time with a parent due to a false belief that the parent is evil, dangerous, or not worthy of affection) or some other family dynamic (Lorandos & Bernet, 2020, Bernet & Greenhill, 2022).

Child Maltreatment

Psychiatrists in private practice, as well as those employed by courts or other agencies, see children who are alleged to have been psychologically, physically, or sexually abused. The purpose of the evaluation may be to assist the court in determining what happened to the child, to make recommendations regarding placement or treatment, or to offer an opinion on the termination of parental rights. The evaluation of a child who is alleged to have been maltreated is described in Chapter 51.

Juvenile Justice

Forensic child psychiatrists may consult with the juvenile justice system to evaluate a juvenile's competency to go to trial and his or her state at the time of the alleged offense, if an insanity defense is being considered. Psychiatrists can also assist the court in determining if a juvenile who has been accused of committing an unusually serious offense should be tried as an adult ("waiver to adult court"); the evaluator takes into consideration the risk the child presents of violent or sexual offending, the reasons for the child's behavior, and the best disposition (Grisso, 2013).

American Academy of Child and Adolescent Psychiatry. Practice parameters for psychiatric custody evaluations. *J Am Acad Child Adolesc Psychiatr.* 1997;36 (Suppl 10):57S.

American Psychological Association. *Guidelines for Child Custody Evaluations in Family Law Proceedings.* Washington, DC: American Psychological Association; 2022.

Association of Family and Conciliation Courts. Guidelines for parenting plan evaluations in family law cases. Madison, WI: Association of Family and Conciliation Courts; 2022.

Benedek EP, Ash P, Scott CL. *Principles and Practice of Child and Adolescent Forensic Mental Health.* Arlington, VA: American Psychiatric Publishing; 2010.

Bernet W, Freeman BW, eds. Forensic psychiatry (special issue). *Child Adolesc Psychiatr Clin N Am.* 2011;20(3).

Bernet W, Greenhill L. The Five-Factor Model for the diagnosis of parental alienation. *J Am Acad Child Adolesc Psychiatr.* 2022;61:591.

Grisso T. *Forensic Evaluation of Juveniles.* 2nd ed. Sarasota, FL: Professional Resource Press; 2013.

Lorandos D, Bernet W, eds. *Parental Alienation—Science and Law.* Springfield, IL: Charles C Thomas; 2020.

THE PSYCHIATRIST IN COURT

The Written Report

The report should be carefully written. It will be read by several people, and the reader will tend to attach great significance to particular sentences or phrases. Probably the best approach is to make the report detailed enough for the reader to understand fully the procedure that was followed and the

Table 60–3 Outline for Typical Forensic Report

Identifying information: for example, names and birth dates.

Background information: a brief chronology of the situation and a statement about the circumstances of the referral and the specific purpose of the evaluation.

Procedure for this evaluation: an explanation of the various meetings that were held, the psychological testing utilized, and the outside information that was collected. It may be appropriate to state specifically that the evaluee gave informed consent for the evaluation.

Observations: a systematic presentation of the data that was collected during the evaluation.

Conclusions: a list of specific statements that the psychiatrist believes are supported by his or her data.

Recommendations: these should follow logically from the conclusions.

Appendixes: associated information, such as psychological testing.

Qualifications of the evaluator: may be a curriculum vitae.

basis for the conclusions and recommendations, but not to include every scintilla of data. Table 60–3 provides an outline of a typical forensic report.

Role Definition

There are many times when the psychiatrist must keep straight in their own mind, and for others, both who is the client and what precisely is the psychiatrist's role in the current situation. The client may be the person the psychiatrist is examining, or it may be somebody else. The psychiatrist may have the role of therapist, or simply that of an evaluator. In forensic work, any confusion regarding the psychiatrist's role will be magnified and highlighted by the legal process and will compromise their work, whether the psychiatrist is intending to be a therapist, an evaluator, a consultant, or an administrator.

The Problem of Bias

Psychiatrists and other mental health professionals may not realize how easily and how often they become biased in their work with patients and families. Despite all that is known about unconscious processes (such as countertransference) and conscious motivations (such as greed and the desire for popularity or fame), it is common for therapists to base their conclusions on a preconception rather than on the data that have been presented. Bias is more prevalent in forensic cases because the evaluator may be exposed to anger, threat, deceit, tragedy, innuendo, hypocrisy, flattery, or inducement. It is extremely important for the psychiatrist to be aware of their own motivations, as well as the agenda of the other professionals involved in the case.

Bias is a distorting glass through which the evaluator views the situation. For example, an evaluator who is a very strong believer in law and order may always interpret the facts to support criminal responsibility rather than a finding of not guilty by reason of insanity. The psychiatrist who enters a case with a particular bias is likely to change a situation despite a belief that they are studying it objectively. For example, an evaluator predisposed to find child abuse may interview children in such a suggestive manner that the children allege abusive acts that did not occur.

Several safeguards against bias are available. The psychiatrist should try to be aware of their own conscious and unconscious motivations. It may be helpful if the psychiatrist says something like this to themself: "My job is not to win this case. My task is to help the court by collecting accurate and pertinent data and organizing it in a way that is scientifically and medically valid." Another safeguard against bias is for the psychiatrist to carefully indicate in the written report the reasons for their conclusions, so that the court will truly understand the basis for the opinion.

Some forensic psychiatrists misuse their expertise by manipulating the court into believing something that may not be true. Sometimes, unscrupulous psychiatrists use obfuscating jargon in order to cloak shaky reasoning with a false air of certainty.

Degrees of Certainty

An important aspect of legal decisions is the standard of proof or the level of certainty that must be established in order for a particular decision or verdict to be reached. There are several levels of certainty.

The least exacting level of certainty to achieve is **probable cause**. In criminal law, probable cause is the set of circumstances sufficient to lead a reasonable man to suspect that the person arrested had committed a crime. In psychiatric practice, that may be a sufficient level of certainty to report a suspected instance of child abuse.

In civil cases, the side that prevails is the one that establishes a **fair preponderance of the evidence.** This can be expressed roughly as being at least 51% certain.

In some cases that involve psychiatric evidence; the level of certainty is **clear and convincing proof**, which is proof necessary to persuade by a substantial margin and more than a bare preponderance. In most states civil commitment, paternity suits, and legal insanity must be proven to a degree that is clear and convincing. In most circumstances, the proof that child abuse has occurred or that parental rights should be severed must be clear and convincing.

Criminal cases require proof that is **beyond a reasonable doubt**, which means that the jury is satisfied to a moral certainty that every element of a crime has been proven. The term means that no reasonable alternative could explain the evidence. To convict a specific person of child abuse would require proof beyond a reasonable doubt.

One of the most puzzling terms in forensic psychiatry is **reasonable degree of medical certainty.** When a physician testifies in court, they are frequently asked if their opinions are given with a reasonable degree of medical certainty. Unfortunately, there is no specific meaning for that term. At

Table 60–4 Important Cases in Forensic Psychiatry

Addington v. Texas, 441 U.S. 418 (1979). The U.S. Supreme Court found that the standard of proof for civil commitment is at least "clear and convincing evidence."

Ake v. Oklahoma, 470 U.S. 68 (1985). The U.S. Supreme Court said that an indigent defendant who raised the question of insanity has the right to a court-appointed psychiatrist to perform an evaluation and assist the defense in preparation of an insanity defense.

Canterbury v. Spence, 464 F.2d 772 (1972). The U.S. Court of Appeals for the District of Columbia stated that the proper criterion for informed consent is that the physician should warn the patient of all potential risks that a reasonable patient would want to know.

Daubert v. Merrell Dow, 61 U.S.L.S. 4805, 113 S. Ct. 2786 (1993). The U.S. Supreme Court held that judges in federal courts should consider factors such as the following when determining whether scientific evidence is relevant and reliable: whether the theory or technique can be and has been tested; whether it has been subjected to peer review and published; its error rate; and whether it has been generally accepted within the relevant scientific community.

Dillon v. Legg, 441 P.2d 912 (1968). The Supreme Court of California found that a person could be awarded damages for psychological injury that was caused by witnessing the physical injury of a close relative.

Dusky v. United States, 362 U.S. 402 (1960). The Supreme Court defined the test for competency to stand trial: whether the defendant "has sufficient present ability to consult with his lawyer with a reasonable degree of rational understanding—and whether he has a rational as well as a factual understanding of the proceedings against him."

In re Gault, 387 U.S.1 (1967). The U.S. Supreme Court defined the due process rights of a juvenile who has been arrested: written and timely notice of the charges; protection against self-incrimination; defense counsel; and right to cross-examination.

Miller v. Alabama, 132 S.Ct. 2455 (2012). Mandatory sentences of life without the possibility of parole may not be imposed on juveniles who are found guilty of homicide.

Landeros v. Flood, 551 P.2d 389 (1976). The Supreme Court of California established the standard of care for diagnosing the battered child syndrome, which was "whether a reasonably prudent physician examining this plaintiff. . . would have been led to suspect she was a victim of the battered child syndrome. . . and would have promptly reported his findings to appropriate authorities.. . ."

Miranda v. Arizona, 384 U.S. 436 (1966). The U.S. Supreme Court stated that the admissibility in evidence of any statement given during custodial interrogation of a suspect would depend on whether the police provided the suspect with four warnings: that a suspect "has the right to remain silent, that anything he says can be used against him in a court of law, that he has the right to the presence of an attorney, and that if he cannot afford an attorney one will be appointed for him prior to any questioning if he so desires."

Rennie v. Klein, 720 F.2d 266 (1983). The Third Circuit Court of Appeals found that civilly committed patients have a constitutional right to refuse treatment.

Tarasoff v. Regents of the University of California, 551 P.2d 334 (1976). The California Supreme Court found that the therapist of a dangerous patient "bears a duty to exercise reasonable care to protect the foreseeable victim of that danger."

Wyatt v. Aderholt, 503 F.2d 1305 (1974). The Fifth Circuit Court of Appeals said that civilly committed patients "unquestionably have a constitutional right to receive such individual treatment as will give each of them a realistic opportunity to be cured or to improve his or her mental condition."

one time or another, physicians have taken it to mean about the same as "beyond a reasonable doubt," the same as "clear and convincing," and even the same degree of certainty as "preponderance of the evidence." It has been proposed that reasonable medical certainty is a level of certainty equivalent to that which a physician uses when making a diagnosis and starting treatment (Rappeport, 1985). The implication is that the degree of certainty depends on the clinical situation. For example, the diagnosis of syphilis is accomplished with almost 100% certainty because there is a reliable laboratory test for that purpose. The determination that a patient has posttraumatic stress disorder as a result of a specific event can be made with considerably less certainty.

Testifying at Deposition and Trial

In many cases, the psychiatrist provides a written report, and the case proceeds without any further involvement of the psychiatric expert. At other times, however, the forensic evaluation culminates with the psychiatrist's testimony at a deposition and/or a trial. There are two kinds of depositions.

In a **discovery deposition**, the opposing attorney has an opportunity to question the expert about the details of her qualifications, her methodology in conducting the evaluation, and the bases for her conclusions; the principle is that the opposing attorney has a right to "discover" everything relevant about the expert and the evaluation process ahead of time, so there should be no surprises at the trial itself. In some cases, a **testimonial deposition** substitutes for testifying at the trial. For example, if the expert witness will be out of town at the time of the trial, the attorney who hired the expert may take a testimonial deposition and simply play back the video recording of the deposition when the trial occurs.

Testifying in court can be both a satisfying and harrowing experience. It is satisfying when the expert has an opportunity to educate the judge, the attorneys, and the jury members about some aspect of psychiatric practice that has an important bearing on the case before the court. In the best of circumstances, it feels like a dialogue between the expert witness and the other participants in the trial. For example, in some circumstances the judge may ask the expert questions in a manner that resembles a give-and-take conversation.

In some jurisdictions, jury members are allowed to submit questions for the expert, which are vetted by the judge and the attorneys before being asked.

Testifying as an expert can be difficult and nerve-wracking. During cross-examination, it is not uncommon for the opposing attorney to challenge the witness's expertise and even to ridicule the witness's conclusions and recommendations. It is important to think about such challenges and to plan ahead of time how to address them. There are several good books that give detailed advice and moral support to mental health experts who are anticipating testifying in court (Brodsky, 2022; Gutheil & Drogin, 2013). There are also books that give extensive guidance to attorneys on how to cross-examine mental health experts (Campbell & Lorandos, 2012).

Brodsky SL. *Testifying in Court: Guidelines and Maxims for the Expert Witness*. Washington, DC: American Psychological Association; 2022.

Campbell TW, Lorandos D. *Cross Examining Experts in the Behavioral Sciences*. Eagan, MN: Westlaw; 2001, 2021.

Gutheil TG, Drogin EY. *The Mental Health Expert in Court: A Survival Guide*. Arlington, VA: American Psychiatric Press; 2013.

Rappeport J. Reasonable medical certainty. *Bull Am Acad Psychiatry Law*. 1985;13:5.

CONCLUSION

Forensic psychiatry is an unusual medical specialty because of the diverse clinical situations and the broad scope of practice that it encompasses. For instance, a forensic evaluation might involve a very young child (regarding child maltreatment), a very old person (regarding competency to make a will), or anybody in between. The forensic practitioner must be familiar not only with the clinical literature but also with the applicable law and important legal precedents. Several important legal cases have influenced both the practice of law and the practice of psychiatry (Table 60–4).

In addition, it is challenging to apply psychiatric expertise to legal situations—both through written reports and oral testimony—in a manner that is evenhanded and unbiased. Finally, forensic psychiatrists experience a wealth of human relationships and a variety of roles. They may consult with clients and evaluees in the office, in the hospital, in jail, on death row, and in the corporate boardroom. After conducting an evaluation, they frequently take on the role of teacher or lecturer, as they explain their findings to family members, attorneys, and perhaps a judge and jury. The diversity of forensic psychiatry gives this medical specialty its own blend of suspense, accomplishment, and satisfaction.

Index

Page numbers followed by "f" denote figures and "t" denote tables.